2950

OCCUPATIONAL THERAPY

PRACTICE SKILLS FOR PHYSICAL DYSFUNCTION

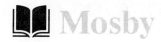

Editor Richard A. Weimer
Assistant Editor Rina Steinhauer
Project Manager Carol Sullivan Wiseman
Production Editing, Design, & Production, Inc.
Design Candace F. Conner
Cover Design Bradley C. Cowan

THIRD EDITION

The C.V. Mosby Company
11830 Westline Industrial Drive, St. Louis, Missouri 63146

Library of Congress Cataloging in Publication Data

Pedretti, Lorraine Williams, 1936–
    Occupational therapy : practice skills for physical dysfunction /
Lorraine Williams Pedretti, Barbara Zoltan. — 3rd ed.
      p.   cm.
    Includes bibliographies and index.
    ISBN (invalid) 0-301-63852-6
    1. Occupational therapy.   2. Physically handicapped-
-Rehabilitation. I. Zoltan, Barbara. II. Title.
    [DNLM: 1. Handicapped. 2. Occupational Therapy. WB 555 P371o]
RM735.P34   1990
615.8'515—dc20
DNLM/DLC
for Library of Congress
                                                        89-8360
                                                          CIP

GW/VH/VH 9 8 7 6

OCCUPATIONAL THERAPY

PRACTICE SKILLS FOR PHYSICAL DYSFUNCTION

LORRAINE WILLIAMS PEDRETTI, M.S., O.T.R.

Professor, Department of Occupational Therapy,
San Jose State University, San Jose, California

BARBARA ZOLTAN, M.A., O.T.R.

Consultant in Private Practice,
Saratoga, California

THIRD EDITION

with **371** *illustrations*

THE C. V. MOSBY COMPANY

ST. LOUIS • BALTIMORE • PHILADELPHIA • TORONTO   1990

Contributors

CAROLE ADLER, B.A., O.T.R.
Clinical Supervisor, Department of Occupational Therapy,
Santa Clara Valley Medical Center San Jose, California

ELIZABETH MARIA BIANCHI, B.S., M.S., O.T.R.
Senior Occupational Therapist, Stanford University
Hospital, Stanford, California;
Formerly Occupational Therapist, Cottage Hospital;
Consultant, Private Contractor, Hospital Home Health
and Community Clinics, Santa Barbara, California

HELEN BOBROVE, O.T.R.
Senior Occupational Therapist, Stanford University
Hospital, Stanford, California

SHIRLEY W. CHAN, O.T.R., C.V.E.
Supervisor, Hand Therapy Center, Davies Medical Center,
San Francisco, California;
Formerly Occupational Therapy Supervisor, Department of
Rehabilitation Therapy, St. Francis Memorial Hospital,
San Francisco, California

JAN ZARET DAVIS, O.T.R.
President, International Clinical Educators, Inc.;
Guest Faculty, Department of Occupational Therapy,
San Jose State University, San Jose, California;
Consultant/Lecturer, Los Gatos Rehabilitation Center,
Los Gatos, California

DENISE FODERARO, O.T.R.
Occupational Therapist, Private Practice, San Carlos,
California; Formerly Senior Occupational Therapist,
Cardiac Rehabilitation, Santa Clara Valley Medical Center,
San Jose, California

JOCELYN M. HITTLE, O.T.R.
Private practice, and Staff Occupational Therapist,
VNA Hand Rehabilitation Center, Watsonville, California;
Formerly Occupational Therapist, Arthritis and
Rheumatism Center, San Jose, California

MARY C. KASCH, O.T.R., C.V.E.
Director, Hand Rehabilitation Center of Sacramento,
Sacramento, California; Founding Active Member and Past
President, American Society of Hand Therapists

SHERI L. LIEBERMAN, O.T.R.
Clinical Coordinator of Occupational Therapy,
Department of Rehabilitation Services,
Stanford University Hospital, Stanford, California

GUY L. McCORMACK, M.S., O.T.R.
Associate Professor, Department of Occupational Therapy,
San Jose State University, San Jose, California

KAREN L. NELSON, O.T.R.
Director, Occupational Therapy, Meadowbrook
Neurologic Care Center, San Jose, California

JAN POLON NOVIC, O.T.R.
Occupational Therapist, Redwood City, California;
Formerly Clinical Coordinator of Neurological and
Intensive Care Units, Stanford University Hospital,
Stanford, California

STEPHANIE O'LEARY, M.S., O.T.R.
Occupational Therapist, Veterans Administration Spinal
Cord Injury Center, Palo Alto, California;
Formerly Occupational Therapist, Cardiac Rehabilitation,
Santa Clara Valley Medical Center, San Jose, California

SHARON PASQUINELLI, M.S., O.T.R.
Senior Occupational Therapist,
Fairmont Hospital, San Leandro, California

KAREN PITBLADDO, O.T.R.
Occupational Therapist, Fairport, New York;
Consultant, Strong Memorial Hospital and Eastpark
Rehabilitation Group, Rochester, New York;
Formerly Clinical Coordinator of Occupational Therapy
in Orthopedics, Stanford University Hospital,
Stanford, California

SARA A. POPE-DAVIS, M.O.T., O.T.R.
Manager of Occupational Therapy, Mills-Peninsula
Hospitals, San Mateo, California

SALLY A. ROOZEE, M.S., O.T.R.
Private Practice, Gerontology and Rehabilitation,
Danville, California

DIANE MEEDER RYCKMAN, M.A., O.T.R./L
Chief Occupational Therapist, Rehabilitation Medicine
Department, Kettering Medical Center, Kettering, Ohio

PATRICIA SMITH, M.S., O.T.R., C.V.E.
Owner and Director, Occupational Assessment and
Modification, Cupertino, California

GREGORY STONE, M.Ed., B.F.A., C.O.T.A.
(In Memoriam)
Formerly Assistant Professor, Department of Occupational
Therapy, San Jose State University, San Jose, California

Preface
to third edition

This book was designed for use by occupational therapy students in baccalaureate and entry-level master's degree programs and as a reference for clinicians. Its purpose is to support the preparation of the student for practice in occupational therapy for adults with acquired physical dysfunction. It is assumed that the readers of this text have knowledge of general psychology, anatomy and physiology, neuroanatomy and neurophysiology, kinesiology, orthopedic and neurological dysfunction, medical terminology, human growth and development, and theories of occupational therapy.

The content of the book is arranged according to the occupational therapy process. Part one is concerned with the foundations for treatment and includes a frame of reference for practice, psychosocial aspects of physical disabilities, treatment planning, and documentation of occupational therapy services. Part two covers evaluation and treatment procedures commonly used in occupational therapy for physical dysfunction.

Evaluation procedures include methods for assessing joint range of motion, muscle strength, muscle tone and coordination, reflexes and reactions, dysphagia, sensation, visual perception and perceptual motor skills, and cognition. Treatment methods most frequently used in physical disabilities practice are therapeutic activities (including principles of therapeutic exercise), activities of daily living, work hardening, four sensorimotor approaches to treatment and their neurophysiological basis, wheelchairs and wheelchair transfers, mobile arm supports and suspension slings, and hand splinting. Directions for many specific treatment procedures can be found in these chapters. The final part of the book, Part three, is concerned with the application of treatment principles, evaluation procedures, and treatment methods to specific dysfunctions. These include amputations, burns, arthritis, acute hand injuries, cardiac conditions, low back pain, hip fractures, lower motor neuron dysfunction, spinal cord injury, cerebral vascular accident, head injury, and degenerative diseases. These disabilities were selected because they are frequently encountered in practice and because principles that apply to them may be applied to other similar disabilities.

Each chapter concludes with review questions to assist the student to master content, achieve learning objectives, and prepare for evaluation of learning. Instructors may wish to use these questions for preparation of examinations or assignments.

Sample case studies and partial treatment plans are presented in each of the chapters in Part three. These are *not* intended to present the only approach to the treatment of the particular dysfunction or to imply that there is a stereotyped method of treating the dysfunction. Rather, they are intended to serve as models for the novice to complete the sample treatment plan and to construct diverse and alternate treatment plans for real or hypothetical patients encountered in their academic preparation. The terms *patient* and *client* have been used interchangeably in this book to designate the consumer of occupational therapy services.

The chapter contributors are gratefully acknowledged for their willingness to share their expertise in the production of the third edition of this text.

Our appreciation is extended to the artists Daryle Webb, Lydia Lopez, and Gregory Stone (in memoriam); to the photographers Amanda Hatherly, George Lamson, Romaldo Lopez and Steve Sloan; and typists Carolyn Beckum, Evelyn Messina, and Merrilee Cheetsos.

Gratitude is also extended to those who modeled for photographs: Deborah Van Buren, Michael Marsh, Morag Paterson, Diane M.T. Harsch and patients and former patients at the Santa Clara Valley Medical Center and Meadowbrook Neurologic Care Center.

Those who served as consultants and readers to whom we wish to express our appreciation are Lela Llorens, Ph.D., O.T.R., Carole Adler, O.T.R., Heidi McHugh Pendleton, M.A., O.T.R., Guy L. McCormack, M.S., O.T.R., Janet Jabri, O.T.R., Rosemary Shaw, O.T.R., Katie Schlageter, O.T.R., Karen L. Nelson, O.T.R., and Lawrence L. Mott of Otto Bock Orthopedic Industries, Inc. We gratefully acknowledge the following for their assistance in obtaining information and photographs: Dan Haney of Haney Labs, San Jose; Lawrence Williams of Williams Rents, San Jose; and Beth Gosnell of Everest and Jennings, Inc.

Special appreciation is extended to all of our professional colleagues who lent their support and assistance, and to our families for their patience and love.

Lorraine Williams Pedretti
Barbara Zoltan

Preface
to second edition

This book was designed for use by occupational therapy students in baccalaureate and entry-level master's degree programs. Its purpose is to support the preparation of the student for practice in occupational therapy for adults with acquired physical dysfunction. It is assumed that the readers of this text have knowledge of general psychology, anatomy and physiology, neuroanatomy and neurophysiology, kinesiology, orthopedic and neurological dysfunction, medical terminology, human growth and development, and theories of occupational therapy.

The content of the book is arranged according to the occupational therapy process. Part 1 is concerned with the foundations for treatment and includes a frame of reference for practice, psychosocial aspects of physical disabilities, and treatment planning. Part 2 covers evaluation procedures commonly used in occupational therapy for physical dysfunction and gives explicit instructions for their administration. Treatment methods most frequently used in physical disabilities practice are included in Part 3. This section covers therapeutic activities (including principles of therapeutic exercise), activities of daily living, four sensorimotor approaches to treatment and their neurophysiological basis, wheelchairs and wheelchair transfers, mobile arm supports and suspension slings, and hand splinting. Directions for many specific treatment procedures can be found in these chapters. The final part of the book, Part 4, is concerned with the application of treatment principles, evaluation procedures, and treatment methods to specific dysfunctions. These includes amputations, burns, arthritis, acute hand injuries, cardiac conditions, low back pain, hip fractures, lower motor neuron dysfunction, spinal cord injury, cerebral vascular accident, and head injury. These disabilities were selected because they are frequently encountered in practice and because principles that apply to them may be applied to other similar disabilities.

Each chapter concludes with review questions to assist the student to master content, achieve learning objectives, and prepare for evaluation of learning. Instructors may wish to use these questions for preparation of examinations or assignments.

Sample case studies and treatment plans are presented in each of the chapters in Part 4. These are *not* intended to present the only approach to the treatment of the particular dysfunction or to imply that there is a stereotyped method of treating the dysfunction. Rather, they are intended to serve as models for the novice from which to build diverse and alternate treatment plans for real or hypothetical clients encountered in their academic preparation. The terms *patient* and *client* have been used interchangeably in this book to designate the individual who is the consumer of occupational therapy services.

The chapter contributors are gratefully acknowledged for their willingness to share their expertise in the production of this text. My appreciation is extended to the artists, Karen Donaldson, Shirley W. Chan, Jan Zaret Davis, Gregory Stone, and Daryle Webb, and to the photographer Steven Sloan.

Appreciation is also extended to those who modeled for photographs: Joseph Brown, Janet Faubion, Roselle Fliesler, Guy L. McCormack, Morag Paterson, Julie Rasczewski, Deborah Stephany, Gregory Stone, Michael Swanson, and Norma Tanaka.

Those who served as consultants and to whom I wish to express my personal appreciation are Lela Llorens, Ph.D., O.T.R.; Amy Killingsworth, M.A., O.T.R.; Gregory Stone, M.Ed., B.F.A., C.O.T.A.; Vaunden Nelson, M.A.; and Peter I. Edgelow, R.P.T./O.T. All my colleagues in the Department of Occupational Therapy at San Jose State University are acknowledged with appreciation for their support and encouragement.

Finally, my husband Robert and my son Mark are lovingly appreciated for their unending patience, support, and assistance.

Lorraine Williams Pedretti

Preface
to first edition

This book was designed for use by students of occupational therapy at the baccalaureate level. Its purpose is to help prepare the student for entry-level practice in occupational therapy for adults with acquired physical disabilities.

The arrangement of content is based on the occupational therapy process. Methods of evaluation and treatment planning and descriptions of frequently used treatment methods are presented. This foundation is followed by chapters on the application of occupational therapy to several specific physical disabilities. These were selected because they are often encountered in practice, and each is considered representative of a major classification of physical dysfunction. A chapter that includes principles of hand splinting and a self-instruction program on splint construction is designed for independent study. Its purposes are to introduce students to the elements of hand splinting and to direct them in the construction of a basic splint. Each chapter concludes with review questions to assist the student to master content, achieve learning objectives, and prepare for evaluation of learning.

Congenital and acquired physical disabilities of childhood have not been included. The sample case studies and treatment plans presented are not intended to present the only approach to the treatment of the particular dysfunction. Rather, they are designed to provide students with guidelines to treatment from which to build diverse and more specific treatment plans for hypothetical or real clients encountered in their academic preparation.

For clarity and ease of reading in this book clients or patients will be referred to in the masculine gender and therapists in the feminine gender.

This book evolved out of a manual that was first printed in 1972 as a collection of teaching materials and lecture outlines for use in the occupational therapy curriculum at San Jose State University. The original manual underwent several revisions and in 1977 was printed and distributed under the title *Basic Practice Skills in Occupational Therapy for Physical Dysfunction*.

It is assumed that the readers of this text have prior knowledge of anatomy, physiology, kinesiology, neuroanatomy, neurophysiology, orthopedic and neurological dysfunctions, medical terminology, human growth and development, and basic occupational therapy theory.

It is the nature of human beings to be active. Mental and physical activity is essential to personal health and to the health and progress of the culture or society in which individuals exist. Conversely, inactivity can lead to mental or physical deterioration and can be a deterent to the progress of the culture or society in which human beings live.

At any age or stage in a person's life there is a desirable pattern and balance of optimum occupational performance for the maintenance of the health of the individual and the society. Disruptive forces, such as illness, injury, developmental disorders, and genetic defects, can alter the pattern and balance of occupational performance and place the organism in the state of disorder or imbalance so that it cannot achieve or maintain a desirable balance and pattern of occupational performance.

On these premises occupational therapy is viewed as an intervention agent whose roles are as follows:
1. Assess past and present patterns of occupational performance
2. Identify dysfunctions in occupational performance
3. Identify the dysfunctional performance components and their effect on occupational performance
4. Remedy or compensate for dysfunctions in occupational performance and performance components
5. Facilitate the structuring or restructuring of a pattern and balance in occupational performance that is suitable and optimal for the age, stage, and current life roles of the individual

Occupational therapy uses standardized testing procedures, clinical observations, and purposeful, goal-directed activity to achieve these objectives.

The chapter contributors, Mary C. Kasch, Jan Zaret Davis, Guy L. McCormack, Gregory Stone, Barbara

A. Baum, and Diane L. Meeder, are gratefully acknowledged for their willingness to share in the production of this text. My appreciation is extended to Linda Higgins for the cover design and illustrations and to Bart Favero for the photographs.

My gratitude is extended to those who modeled for photographs—my students Catherine Oberschmidt and Marianne Woodall, my niece Ramona Fournier, and my colleagues Morag Paterson and Gregory Stone, San Jose State University—and to Jana Hostetter, Rehabilitation Center of Los Gatos—Saratoga, for the loan of assistive devices to be photographed.

Manuscript reviewers and consultants to whom I wish to express my personal appreciation are Joyce Gorham, Santa Clara Valley Medical Center; Amy Killingsworth, Associate Professor, San Jose State University; Dr. William Lages, Santa Clara Valley Medical Center; and John G. Russell, Jr. Carol Feinour is gratefully acknowledged for typing the manuscript so expertly and for accommodating to my schedule and special needs.

All of my colleagues in the Department of Occupational Therapy at San Jose State University, especially Amy Killingsworth, Associate Professor, and Gregory Stone, Lecturer, are acknowledged with appreciation for their support and encouragement.

Last but not least, my husband Robert Leland Pedretti is lovingly appreciated for his unending patience, assistance, support, and encouragement. I thank my son Mark Samuel Pedretti, age 4, who frequently wondered when the "book" would be finished, for never touching my materials, and for waiting patiently for my attention.

Lorraine Williams Pedretti

Contents

PART ONE

FOUNDATIONS FOR TREATMENT OF PHYSICAL DYSFUNCTION

Chapter

1 A frame of reference for occupational therapy in physical dysfunction

LORRAINE WILLIAMS PEDRETTI
SHARON PASQUINELLI

A frame of reference is defined here as a conceptual structure around which a program, organization, or project is developed and organized.[1] It delineates a particular aspect of a profession and provides a central theme to which to refer for decisions regarding the appropriateness of the program design and content.[1,38] The frame of reference within which occupational therapy occurs influences the practitioner's choices and approach to treatment and thus gives unity, balance, and direction to the treatment program.[1,38]

The practice of occupational therapy in physical dysfunction should be guided by a unifying conceptual system. It is proposed that "occupational performance" is a frame of reference that can serve as this system and that treatment of physical disabilities can be carried out in its context.

OCCUPATIONAL PERFORMANCE

Occupational performance is

. . . the individual's ability to accomplish the tasks required by his or her role and related to his or her developmental stage. Roles include those of a "preschooler," student, homemaker, employee, and retired worker. Occupational performance includes self-care, work and play/leisure time performance.[2,43]

Performance Skills

Self-care, work, education, and play and leisure time activities are referred to as performance skills. Self-care includes feeding, hygiene, dressing, grooming, mobility, and object manipulation. Work activities include home and family management and employment. Education includes school and educational activities. Play and leisure include the play activities of childhood and the games, sports, hobbies, and social activities of adult life.[2,30]

Occupational performance requires learning and practice experiences with the role and developmental state-specific tasks and the utilization of all performance components. Deficits in task-learning experiences, performance components, and life space may result in limitations in occupational performance.[2,43]

Performance Components

Performance components are "the learned developmental patterns of behavior which are the substructure and foundation of the individual's occupational performance."[2,43] The performance components include (1) sensory-integrative functioning, (2) motor functioning, (3) social functioning, (4) psychological functioning, and (5) cognitive functioning.[1,2] These elements of human function affect an individual's ability to perform occupational tasks or performance skills.

The sensory-integrative component refers to the body scheme, posture, body integration, reflex and sensory functions, visual perception, and sensory-motor integration. The motor component refers to joint motion, muscle strength and tone, functional use of limbs and body, and gross and fine motor skills. The social component includes dyadic and group interaction skills. The psychological component includes emotional states, feelings, coping behaviors, defense mechanisms, self-identity, and self-concept. The cognitive component refers to written and verbal communication, concentration, problem solving, time management, conceptualization, and integration of learning.[1,2]

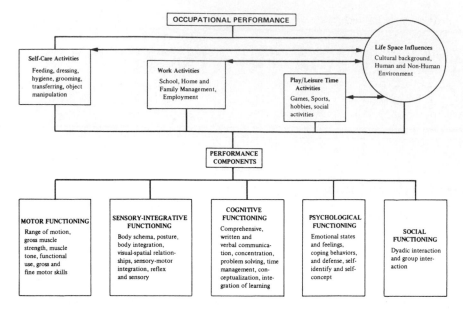

Fig. 1-1. The occupational performance frame of reference. From the American Occupational Therapy Association, Inc: A curriculum guide for occupational therapy educators, 1974.

Life Space

Life space refers to "the individual's cultural background and human and non-human environment"[1,2,43] (Fig. 1-1). Successful occupational performance occurs in the context of the individual's cultural requirements and is consistent with age and developmental stage.[30]

Origins of the Occupational Performance Frame of Reference

In 1973, the American Occupational Therapy Association published *The Roles and Functions of Occupational Therapy Personnel*.[2] In this publication, occupational performance, the performance skills, and the performance components were defined as outlined in the foregoing discussion.

The purpose was to describe the areas of expertise of the occupational therapist and the areas of concern within the profession.

The AOTA Task Force on Target Populations, in its publication in April 1974, stated that . . . "the generic foundation, or frame of reference [of ocupational therapy] is to be found in the concept of occupational performance." It was further stated that "the goal . . . of occupational therapy . . . is the improvement of occupational performance regardless of the target population."[3]

In 1974, the concept of the occupational performance frame of reference appeared in *A Curriculum Guide for Occupational Therapy Educators* published by the American Occupational Therapy Association.[1] In this publication, Figure 1-1 was shown as Dimension Two of a two-dimensional frame of reference, and its purpose was to diagram the content of occupational therapy practice and to identify the areas of concern of occupational therapy (Fig. 1-1). Dimension One (not shown here) diagrammed the processes in occupational therapy practice. The occupational performance frame of reference was presented again, with some modification, by Mosey in 1981.[38] She called it the "domain of concern for occupational therapy" and described it as "consisting of performance components within the context of age, occupational performance and an individual's environment." She defined "domain of concern" as "those areas of human experience in which practitioners of the profession offer assistance to others."[38]

Thus, the concept of the occupational performance frame of reference was developed from a series of task forces and committees of the AOTA. It was generated from professional conceptualizations of practice and described as a frame of reference for practice and a model for education.[32]

The Concerns of Occupational Therapy

In this frame of reference, the concerns of occupational therapy are the performance skills (self-care, work, education, and play and leisure activities) and the performance components which are the substructure of the performance skills.[1,30,38] Therefore, at any given time, the occupational therapy program may include treatment methods designed for the remediation of deficits or for the compensation for deficits in performance skills and performance components.[1] When working on a performance component (for example, motor skill development), it is essential that the methods be directed ultimately to the patient's ability to master performance skills. Functional independence is a core concept of occupational therapy theory and the goal of the occupational therapy process.[47]

Assumptions About this Frame of Reference

In an effort to interpret the occupational performance frame of reference, the following assumptions have been made.

1. Occupational roles of human beings can be categorized into the areas of self-care (including rest), play, leisure, education, and work (including family and home management).
2. Development, performance, and maintenance of occupational roles are influenced by elements from intrapersonal and extrapersonal space. Intrapersonal elements include genetic, physiological, developmental, and pathological factors. Extrapersonal elements include social, educational, cultural, familial, and environmental factors.
3. An appropriate balance of occupational roles is critical to the maintenance of health.
4. Appropriate balance changes with chronological/developmental age, life stage, and life circumstances.
5. Failure in development of occupational roles or loss, disruption, or change of occupational roles can be caused by intrapersonal and/or extrapersonal elements.
6. Adequate performance of occupational roles is dependent on the integrated functioning of the motor, sensory-integrative, social, psychological, and cognitive subsystems of the individual. These subsystems are called performance components in the occupational performance frame of reference.
7. Defect, disease, or injury affecting a performance component causes a failure of integration of the performance components subsystem and results in a failure or disruption in the performance skills and, thus, of occupational role performance.
8. The role of the occupational therapist is to facilitate both an appropriate balance and optimal performance of occupational roles.
9. The occupational therapist is concerned with remediaton of and compensation for defects in the performance components and performance skills.

10. Primary tools of the occupational therapist for the remediation of performance skills and performance components are purposeful and enabling activities.
11. The occupational therapist is also concerned with preparing the patient for performance of purposeful activity and may utilize adjunctive methods, such as exercise, facilitation and inhibition techniques, splints and sensory stimulation,[53] in the treatment continuum toward the development of ability to master the performance skills and to engage in functional activities appropriate to the patient's occupational roles.
12. Exclusive use of preparatory methods out of context of the patient's occupational performance are not considered occupational therapy.

Conceptualization of a Treatment Continuum Within the Occupational Performance Frame of Reference

As occupational therapy has evolved to be less dependent on medical direction, its role has expanded considerably. Occupational therapists have developed and demonstrated competence in many specific practice areas associated with physical dysfunction. The occupational therapist's concern, from the onset of the illness or injury, is for the patient to become as independent as possible in performance skills and to resume previously held occupational roles or to assume new and satisfying occupational roles. In many dysfunctions, occupational therapy intervention may begin at the time of surgery or in the early stages of acute care; thus, occupational therapy makes an important contribution at every stage in the treatment continuum.

Figure 1-2 is a model for the treatment continuum in physical disabilities practice. An occupational therapist may be responsible for only one or two stages on the continuum, but treatment is always within the context of occupational performance that guides the treatment process.

The stages in this treatment continuum overlap or can occur simultaneously in practice. The treatment continuum is not meant to demonstrate a strict step-by-step progression. It addresses the performance components and performance skills in the occupational performance frame of reference and takes the patient through a logical progression from dependence to resumption of life roles. The treatment continuum identifies the concerns of occupational therapy practice within the context of the occupational performance frame of reference.

STAGE ONE: ADJUNCTIVE METHODS. Procedures that prepare the patient for occupational perfor-

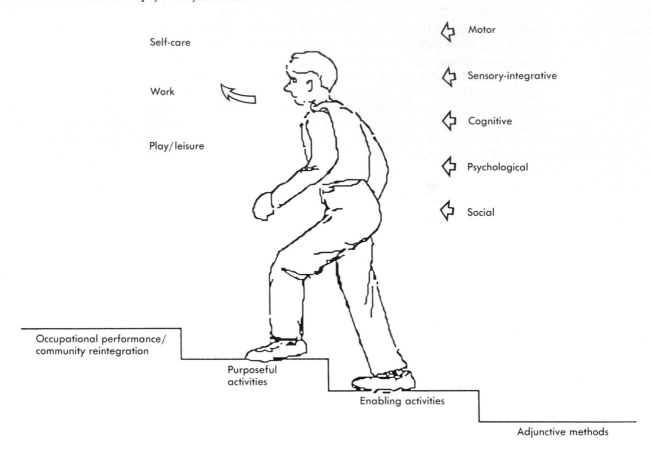

Self-care

Work

Play/leisure

Occupational performance/
community reintegration

Purposeful
activities

Enabling activities

Adjunctive methods

Motor

Sensory-integrative

Cognitive

Psychological

Social

Fig. 1-2. Treatment continuum within the occupational performance frame of reference. From a poster by Karin Boyce, OTS.

mance but that are preliminary to the use of the performance skills in treatment are necessarily the concerns of occupational therapy.[4] These procedures may include methods such as exercise, facilitation and inhibition techniques, positioning, splinting, sensory stimulation, and selected physical modalities.[53] These methods are often used in, but are not limited to, the acute stages of illness or injury. During this stage, the occupational therapist is likely to be most concerned with assessing and remediating performance components. It is important for occupational therapists to plan the progression of treatment so that maximum independence in performance skills is the ultimate outcome of the treatment program.

STAGE TWO: ENABLING ACTIVITIES. Purposeful activity has been defined as one that has an autonomous or inherent goal beyond the motor function required to perform the task.[4] Purposeful activity also requires the active participation of the patient and the coordination of physical, emotional, and cognitive systems.[23] Using these criteria, many methods used in occupational therapy cannot be considered purposeful but may constitute an integral step toward the

ultimate ability to perform purposeful activities. Such methods may be considered enabling methods.

Occupational therapists have created many such methods by simulating purposeful activities. Examples are sanding boards, stacking cones or blocks, practice boards for mastery of clothing fasteners and hardware, driving and work simulators, and tabletop activities such as pegboards for training perceptual-motor skills. Such activities are not likely to be as meaningful to the patient or to stimulate as much interest and motivation as purposeful activities. Yet, it may be necessary to use them as a preparatory or ancillary part of the treatment program.

In Stage Two, the therapist is still concerned with assessment and remediation of performance components and also begins to assess and teach performance skills.

STAGE THREE: PURPOSEFUL ACTIVITY. Purposeful activities include those activities that have an inherent or autonomous goal and are relevant and meaningful to the patient. Examples are feeding, hygiene, dressing, mobility, communication, arts, crafts, games, sports, and work activities. These are used to enhance performance skills and, ultimately, to resume occupational roles. They are carried out by the prescription or under the supervision of the occupational therapist in a health care facility or in the patient's home. At this stage, the occupational therapist is primarily concerned with assessing and remediating deficits in performance skills. Special equipment, such as wheelchairs, ambulatory aids, adaptive equipment, braces, splints, special clothing, communication devices, and environmental control systems, may be an integral part of the program to achieve maximum independence in the performance skills and assumption of occupational roles.

STAGE FOUR: OCCUPATIONAL PERFORMANCE AND COMMUNITY REINTEGRATION. In the final stage of the treatment continuum, the patient resumes or assumes occupational roles in his or her living environment and in the community. Appropriate tasks of self-care, work, education, and play and leisure are performed to the patient's maximum level of independence. Formal occupational therapy intervention is decreased and ultimately discontinued. At this stage, the individual is performing occupational roles following the remedial and compensatory measures of the early and intermediate rehabilitation programs. This performance is, of course, the ultimate goal and desired outcome of occupational therapy intervention.

For some patients, a Stage Four outcome will not be possible, and maximum functioning may be limited to partial independence in performance skills in a supervised living environment. The important goal of the occupational therapist is to facilitate the development of maximum functioning for each patient.

Relationship of the Occupational Performance Frame of Reference to Documents of the American Occupational Therapy Association

It is proposed that the occupational performance frame of reference is in concert with several important documents of the AOTA.

DEFINITION OF OCCUPATIONAL THERAPY

Occupational therapy is

. . . the art and science of directing man's participation in selected tasks to restore, reinforce and enhance performance, facilitate learning of those skills and functions essential for adaptation and productivity, diminish or correct pathology, and to promote and maintain health. Its fundamental concern is the development and maintenance of the capacity throughout the life span, to perform with satisfaction to self and others, those tasks and roles essential to productive living and to the mastery of self and environment.[39]

Relationship to Occupational Performance

In the definition just quoted *occupation* refers to the goal-directed use of time, energy, and interest.[39] The concept of occupation, then, includes all of the performance skills outlined in the occupational performance frame of reference: self-care, work, education, play and leisure. Another key phrase in the definition of occupational therapy is "participation in selected tasks." This implies that the patient's active involvement in his or her own treatment is essential to the effectiveness of the occupational therapy process and treatment outcomes. *Selected tasks* refers not only to those tasks that will best facilitate the achievement of the therapeutic objectives but also to those that will have meaning to the patient in terms of life roles and influences, which are also significant factors in the occupational performance frame of reference. The performance of tasks and roles essential to productive living throughout the lifetime is another central concept of the definition of occupational therapy. The occupational performance frame of reference has role performance as its unifying theme. The influence of the developmental process on occupational performance as a component of the frame of reference must always be considered when planning treatment programs. From these comparisons, it is concluded that occupational performance as a frame of reference is compatible with the definition of occupational therapy.

THE PHILOSOPHICAL BASE OF OCCUPATIONAL THERAPY

In 1979 the Representative Assembly of the American Occupational Therapy Association adopted a philosophical base for occupational therapy.[21] This philosophical base states:

Man is an active being whose development is influenced by the use of purposeful activity. Using their capacity for intrinsic motivation, human beings are able to influence their physical and mental health and their social and physical environment through purposeful activity. Human life includes a process of continuous adaptation. Adaptation is a change in function that promotes survival and self-actualization. Biological, psychological and environmental factors may interrupt the adaptation process at any time through the life cycle. Dysfunction may occur when adaptation is impaired. Purposeful activity facilitates the adaptive process.

Occupational therapy is based on the belief that purposeful activity (occupation) including its interpersonal and environmental components, may be used to prevent and mediate dysfunction, and to elicit maximum adaptation. Activity as used by the occupational therapist includes both intrinsic and therapeutic purpose.[21]

In addition to the adoption of this philosophical base, the Representative Assembly affirmed that

. . . there be universal acceptance and implementation of the common core of occupational therapy as the active participation of the patient/client in occupation for the purposes of improving performance [and that] the use of facilitating procedures is only acceptable as occupational therapy when used to prepare the patient/client for better performance and prevention of disability through self-participation in occupation.[21]

The philosophical base states that people can improve or influence their health through participation in purposeful activity (occupation). The term *purposeful activity* is a central theme of this philosophical base and was apparently used to mean *occupation,* as defined previously. It also implies that purposeful activity characterizes the tools of occupational therapy.

The affirmations accompanying the philosophical base emphasized that the active participation of the patient in purposeful activity is the core of occupational therapy and placed facilitating procedures in perspective as preparatory for purposeful activity. It is clearly stated that facilitating procedures are not acceptable as occupational therapy if they are used as ends unto themselves rather than as the means to the ultimate goal of occupational therapy, which is functional independence.

Position Paper on Purposeful Activities

When this philosophical base was presented, the AOTA had not yet adopted an official definition of *purposeful activity.* The term had been used and defined by many experts.[17,29,38] Each of their definitions described purposeful activity as possessing goals independent of therapeutic goals and as facilitating function, achievement, competence, and spontaneous action.[42]

In April 1983, the Representative Assembly of the AOTA adopted a position paper on purposeful activities. In this paper it is defined as

. . . tasks or experiences, in which the person actively participates. . . . Engagement in purposeful activity requires and elicits coordination between one's physical, emotional and cognitive systems. An individual who is involved in purposeful activity directs attention to the task itself, rather than to the internal processes required for achievement of the task. . . . Purposeful activities, influenced by the individual's life roles, have unique meaning to each person.[23]

The authors of the position paper on purposeful activities described the role of the occupational therapist as follows:

Occupational therapists evaluate clients to determine an individual's activity goals, the capacity to plan and perform purposeful activities, and the ability to meet the functional demands of the environment. Based on this evaluation, the occupational therapist designs activity experiences

that offer the client opportunities for effective action. These activities are purposeful in that they assist and build upon the individual's abilities and lead to achievement of personal goals.[23]

In both the philosophical base statement and the position paper on purposeful activities, a key theme is the active participation of the patient. This seems to be the essential factor that differentiates purposeful activity from other types of activity.

Brienes stated that all activities requiring both mental and physical involvement can be assumed to be purposeful activities.[8] Other important factors for consideration in determining whether a particular activity is purposeful are whether it is meaningful to the patient and whether it engages coordinated function of physical, emotional, and cognitive systems.

In describing the role of the occupational therapist, the emphasis is on the evaluation of role dysfunction and remediation through purposeful activities.

Relationship to Occupational Performance

The definition and discussion of purposeful activity and the role of the occupational therapist as set forth in these important documents are in concert with the occupational performance frame of reference. Because the performance skills, by their very nature, are purposeful and meaningful, they serve as appropriate treatment modalities in the domain of occupational therapy. Treatment modalities to remediate or compensate for deficits in performance components can also be adapted to be purposeful.

The philosophical base and the occupational performance frame of reference take into account the human developmental process. The philosophical base also speaks to the biological, psychological, and environmental influences that may disrupt the adaptive process. These parallel the life space influences element in the occupational performance frame of reference. Thus development, adaptation, internal and external factors influencing adaptation, purposeful activity, and active participation in the recovery of health are common elements of both the occupational therapy philosophical base and the occupational performance frame of reference.

TREATMENT APPROACHES AND THEIR RELATIONSHIP TO THE OCCUPATIONAL PERFORMANCE FRAME OF REFERENCE
Biomechanical Approach

The biomechanical approach to the treatment of physical dysfunction applies the mechanical principles of kinetics and kinematics to the movement of the human body.[44] These mechanical principles deal with forces acting on the body and the result of these forces on movement and equilibrium. Mechanics can be subdivided into (1) *statics*, which is concerned with the body in balance, and (2) *dynamics*, which is concerned with the body in motion. Dynamics is further subdivided into (1) *kinetics*, which deals with the forces that produce, arrest, or modify motion, and (2) *kinematics*, which is the geometry of motion. In biomechanics, equilibrium and motion are so closely interrelated that it is impractical to separate the static and dynamic aspects of human motion.[9] The biomechanical approach uses methods of treatment that employ principles of physics related to forces, levers, and torque.

The biomechanical approach is most appropriate for patients who have lower motor neuron or orthopedic disorders but whose central nervous system (CNS) is intact. Therefore, these patients possess control of isolated movement and specific movement patterns, although there is weakness, low endurance, or joint limitation. Examples of such disabilities are orthopedic dysfunctions, including rheumatoid arthritis, osteoarthritis, fractures, and amputations; hand trauma; burns; lower motor neuron disorders, such as peripheral nerve injuries, Guillain-Barré syndrome, and spinal cord injuries; and primary muscle diseases, such as muscular dystrophy.

The biomechanical approach includes those techniques of evaluation and treatment that use the application of forces to the body and employ principles of physics to select and direct those forces appropriatey. Some examples are joint measurement, muscle strength testing, therapeutic activity for kinetic purposes, therapeutic exercise, and orthotics. The purposes of the biomechanical approach are to (1) assess specific physical limitation in range, strength and endurance; (2) restore function of range strength, and endurance, and (3) reduce deformity.

RELATIONSHIP TO OCCUPATIONAL PERFORMANCE. Methods of evaluation and treatment that can be included in the biomechanical approach are primarily directed at restoration of motor functon. Therefore this approach addresses the motor performance component in the occupational performance frame of reference. Many of the techniques and modalities that can be considered adjunctive or enabling activities are biomechanical in nature. However, biomechanical principles can also be applied to purposeful activities and to performance skills. Biomechanical principles are used in activities, such as sawing wood, rolling out dough, and vacuuming a carpet. To place this approach appropriately within the frame of reference, it is important that the therapist use biomechanical methods to facilitate performance skills as a step in the progression of treatment toward functional independence. The exclusive use of biomechanical treatment methods for their physical restorative benefits would not be in concert with the occupational performance frame of reference.

Sensorimotor Approaches

Before the advent of the sensorimotor approaches to treatment, therapists tried to apply biomechanical principles to patients with a damaged CNS and met with many problems as a result. Because biomechanical treatment approaches demanded controlled voluntary movement, they were inappropriate for patients who lacked such control.

The sensorimotor approaches are used with patients who have CNS dysfunction. The normal CNS functions to produce controlled, well-modulated movement as a result of a balance between the inhibition and facilitation of motor responses.

In the damaged CNS, the inhibition and facilitation of motor responses are out of balance and are not working together to produce smooth, well-modulated, controlled movement. The result can be overfacilitation, producing hypertonic, hyperkinetic, or rigid states of muscle, or overinhibition, causing hypotonic or hypokinetic states of muscle.

In sensorimotor approaches to treatment, it is assumed that specific, controlled sensory input can influence motor responses and that abnormal motor responses can be inhibited and more normal motor responses can be learned by the CNS. All sensorimotor approaches to treatment use proprioceptive stimuli, such as stretching and resistance, to influence thresholds for inhibition and facilitation of movement.[55]

Cutaneous stimulation, which has been found to increase stretch receptor sensitivity, may be combined with proprioceptive stimulation to facilitate voluntary contraction of specific muscles. Exteroceptive stimuli, such as brushing to recruit touch receptors and icing to facilitate or inhibit muscle responses, are used. Reflex mechanisms may be used in some approaches. Some of these are the tonic neck and lumbar reflexes, righting and protective reactions, and associated reactions. The sequence in treatment may be based on the recapitulation of ontogenetic development, that is, the development of successive levels of CNS control—spinal, subcortical, and finally, cortical control of movement.[52]

Chapters 17 through 21 describe the sensorimotor approaches of Rood, Brunnstrom (movement therapy), Bobath (neurodevelopmental treatment), and Knott and Voss (proprioceptive neuromuscular facilitation). Treatment principles, some specific facilitation and inhibition techniques, and applications of the approach to purposeful activity are described.

RELATIONSHIP TO OCCUPATIONAL PERFORMANCE. All of the sensorimotor approaches use neurophysiological mechanisms to elicit a specific motor response. There are many similarities and differences among the approaches, but they are all directed to motor recovery and improvement of motor performance. None of these approaches considers motivation, arousal, attention, role dysfunction, or temporal adaptation and the influence of these factors on motor behavior.[13]

The sensorimotor approaches are primarily directed toward the remediation of the motor and sensory-integrative performance components in the occupational performance frame of reference. However, occupational therapists have expressed concern about the direct application of the techniques of these approaches. If they are to be considered part of the armamentarium of the occupational therapist using this frame of reference, it will be important to apply the principles of these approaches to purposeful activity and performance skills, as described in Chapters 20 and 21, for example. In so doing, it is possible to apply principles of sensorimotor approaches to performance skills. The direct application of the approach, not associated with activity, is often used "to prepare the client or patient for better performance and prevention of disability through self-participation in occupation."[21] Many occupational therapists have developed expertise in the application of these approaches. This is necessary if the approaches are to be scientifically applied during purposeful activity. The development of methods for their application to purposeful activity is limited at this time. These approaches need to be studied and their appropriate uses integrated into an occupational therapy framework. It is necessary to expand knowledge of the logical continuity beyond inhibition-facilitation techniques to activity and to the ways in which sensorimotor treatment principles can be applied during the performance of purposeful activity.[42] When used to precede and enable purposeful activity and as part of a purposeful activity, the sensorimotor approaches can be viable methods in the occupational performance frame of reference.

Rehabilitation Approach

The term *rehabilitation* means a return to ability, that is, the return to the fullest physical, mental, social, vocational, and economic usefulness that is possible for the individual. It means to be able to live and work with remaining capabilities.[24] Therefore, the focus in the treatment program is on abilities, rather than on disabilities.[44]

Rehabilitation is concerned with the intrinsic worth and dignity of the individual and with the restoration of a satisfying and purposeful life. In some sense, the rehabilitation approach uses measures that enable a person to live as independently as possible with some residual disability. Its goal is to help the patient learn to work around or compensate for physical limitations.[44]

The rehabilitation approach is a dynamic process and requires that the patient be a member of the rehabilitation team. It requires ongoing assessment and follow-up to maintain maximum function and, therefore, must keep pace with the scientific advances in methods and equipment (rehabilitation technology), social change and community resources to provide the best services and opportunities for each patient.[24]

RELATIONSHIP TO OCCUPATIONAL PERFORMANCE. In this approach, occupational therapy focuses on performance skills more than on performance components. The aim of the occupational therapy program is to effect role performance and to minimize the barriers of residual disability to role performance. The occupational therapist must assess the patient's capabilities and determine assets to facilitate overcoming the effects of the disability on function. The treatment methods of the rehabilitation approach include:

1. Self-care evaluation and training
2. Acquisition and training in assistive devices
3. Use of adaptive clothing
4. Homemaking and child care
5. Work simplification and energy conservation
6. Use of prevocational activities
7. Use of leisure activities
8. Prosthetic training
9. Wheelchair management
10. Home evaluation and adaptation
11. Transportation
12. Architectural adaptations
13. Acquisition and training in the use of communication aids and devices

INTEGRATION WITH OTHER APPROACHES. Frequently, the methods of the rehabilitation approach are used in combination with the biomechanical or sensorimotor approaches. First, biomechanical or sensorimotor principles can be applied during rehabilitation activities to enhance and reinforce the restoration of the motor or sensory-integrative components. Second, in reality, the treatment program often focuses on performance skills and performance components simultaneously. In this way, the restoration of motor, sensory-integrative, cognitive, and psychosocial functions are combined to improve performance skills and role function.

Cognitive, Psychologic, and Social Performance Components

In an examination of the aforementioned treatment approaches, the cognitive, psychological, and social performance components in the occupational performance frame of reference are not explicitly considered. The occupational performance frame of reference demands the consideration of life space influences, such as culture and human and nonhuman environments. These include genetic, biological, cultural, social, and environmental influences on the organisms. Di Joseph urges occupational therapists to consider not only motor control but motor behavior, that is, "a person acting purposefully within and upon his or her environment." She stated further that ignoring the emotive and cognitive aspects of motor behavior is a reductionistic approach that fails to consider all factors in the production of "purposeful action."[13] Treatment goals for patients must be based on a combination of mind, body, and environment; these goals should be reached through the use of activities that are compatible with the needs and values of the person and not necessarily with those of the therapist.[13] Interaction between the person and the environment is essential to the development of functional independence.[47] The person is mind and body, not just a motor system to be evaluated and "treated."

The occupational performance frame of reference is holistic in its application to the patient and, as such, demands consideration of the cognitive, social, and psychologic functions of the patient for its application. These components must be assessed and included in the treatment program. Therapeutic use of self, individual, and group approaches are ways of dealing with these components. These approaches can often be integrated with methods for improvement of motor and sensory-integrative functions, such as the use of a woodwork group or a dance and exercise program, for the improvement of motor function and the development of self-esteem and social skills.

CURRENT TRENDS

In the practice area of physical dysfunction, there is evidence that the use of purposeful activity as occupational therapy has declined and that the treatment methods used have changed significantly over the years.[6,12,16,35,49]

There has been a tendency toward reductionism in practice. The primary emphasis of reductionism is on a technique approach, and the focus of treatment is on one or more performance components and little integration with performance skills or vice versa. This continues to be a dominant influence in practice. Since the 1960s, there has been a growing awareness of the need to formulate a more adequate way to think about occupation and functional independence.[47]

Several authors contend the occupational therapy profession is currently in a state of crisis.[10,16,19,28] The crisis is considered a result of multidimensional internal and external factors, including the lack of a unified, systematic philosophy of occupational therapy practice. Gilfoyle suggests this crisis is partly a response to cultural, social, and political factors, including (1) the decline of patriarchal authority; (2) the decline of allegiance to a biomedical model; and (3) a shift in values, dimensions of practice, and education that form the reality of occupational therapy.[19]

To appreciate the current crisis in occupational therapy, it is necessary to review the historic development of the philosophy of occupational therapy.

Historical View

MORAL TREATMENT. Occupational therapy's philosophical roots extend to the period of moral treatment in early nineteenth-century America. The philosophy of moral treatment was derived from the cultural and political attitudes that predominated during that time and was based on the idea that mentally ill individuals need to be engaged in creative and recreational activity with their fellow citizens. According to Bockoven:

> The mentally deranged person best recovers his reason when accompanied by persons of sound mind and kindly nature who would help him by joining in the regimen of daily life. The regimen of daily life consisted of recreational and creative activity with others.[7]

The focus of moral treatment for the mentally ill consisted of providing activity programs, such as ward work, craft shops, gardening, and outdoor game areas. Adolf Meyer summed the philosophy of moral treatment by stating that the unique feature of people is their ability to organize time through activity.[34] Meyer believed that even under difficulty, people maintain a balance through actual doing or practice. Until the demise of moral treatment in 1900, activity was the fundamental medium of treatment for the neuropsychiatric patient.

1917 TO 1941. Occupational therapy formally began in 1917 as a result of the rebirth of moral treatment in psychiatry and of the number of chronically disabled soldiers returning from World War I. Occupational therapy services were extended to include the treatment of the physically disabled. According to Woodside, the role of "occupational therapy in rehabilitation was one of using crafts to reactivate the minds and motivation of the mentally ill and the limbs of the veterans, starting them on the way to vocational training."[56] Emphasis was placed heavily on craft and activity programs. The concept of activity was an effective philosophical base for the profession throughout the 1920s and 1930s. During that time, occupational therapy literature discussed activities as the fundamental treatment modality.[6] However, the depression years (1929 to 1941) had a substantial impact on the practice of occupational therapy. Budgets were cut and staff was limited. Therapists did not believe that occupational therapy could stand alone as a viable and independent profession. Occupational therapists sought alliance with the American Medical Association (AMA) to implement the Minimum Standards of Training to "establish standards for training institutions, and to accredit each new school . . . the powerful AMA came to the rescue."[46] The profession became a medical ancillary. Occupational therapy came under increasing pressure to think in reductionistic terms. The philosophy of activity was challenged by the medical community in both psychiatry and physiatrics.[28]

REHABILITATION MOVEMENT (1942 TO 1960). After World War II, occupational therapy joined the rehabilitation movement. As a result, the values, ideas, and activities related to the disabled were altered. According to Mosey:

> Once involved, occupational therapists were uncomfortable with their simple operating principles that it was good for disabled people to keep active and busy doing things they enjoyed. Rather the occupational therapist borrowed techniques from other disciplines.[36]

Emphasis was placed on acquiring techniques, such as progressive resistive exercises, neuromuscular facilitation, activities of daily living (ADL), prosthetic training, and making orthotic devices. The advantage of this trend was that physical disabilities therapists became proficient in the use of various treatment techniques. The disadvantage was that these techniques were practiced without integrating them into the concept of purposeful activity and without articulating a philosophical base. Emphasis was placed on technique acquisition rather than on development of a philosophical base.

1960 TO 1980. By the 1960s the profession recognized that occupational therapists had not only accepted reductionist thinking but that this mode of thinking had replaced the original emphasis on purposeful activity or occupation. Reductionism had led to a precise and extensive technology for the treatment of a wide range of physical disabilities. This technical orientation resulted in a gradual erosion of the philosophical base underlying the profession. There was a shift in practice from a broad philosophical base to a practice based on techniques.

Occupational therapy literature in the 1960s explored the need for change in the profession. There was and still is a growing concern over the inadequacies of the philosophical base supporting occupational therapy.[28]

1980 TO 1988. According to an article by Kielhofner, two different viewpoints regarding purposeful activity or occupation as the philosophical foundation of the profession currently exist.[26] The first viewpoint sees the development of the occupational therapy profession as being in a process of continuous adaptation. In adapting to meet the changing times and health care needs, the profession has disavowed "activity . . . as a generic philosophy."[26] Proponents of this first perspective consider purposeful activity or occupation to be an impractical philosophical premise.

In contrast, proponents of the second viewpoint argue that the profession's earlier philosophical premise regarding purposeful activity or occupation offered a unique and accurate theoretical base to occupational therapy. Current occupational therapy practice is viewed as seriously deviating from the early philosophical premises of the field.[27,49] This second viewpoint acknowledges that current beliefs must be reunited with the earlier philosophy of occupational therapy.

The term *occupation* or *occupational* is suggested as a concept that will enable the field to re-establish a continuity between current beliefs and the historical first beliefs of the profession.[19,25,26] Gilfoyle defines occupational as "a process of action in which the person is the action agent or 'doer.' "[19]

In an attempt to further clarify the term, Evans defines occupation as "the active or 'doing' process of a person engaged in goal-directed, intrinsically gratifying and culturally appropriate activity."[15] Inherent in this definition are the underlying concepts of biopsychosocial unity, hierarchy, developmental sequence, and adaptive capacities. Evans suggests that occupation is the core concept of occupational therapy, and as such, it determines the boundaries of the profession's domain.

Mosey states that the occupational therapy profession is too diverse to adhere to a monistic professional identity.[37] Instead, it is suggested that the profession consider a pluralistic approach. Monism is the belief that occupational therapy is defined by one basic principle, for example, a philosophical base, a legitimate tool, or a frame of reference. The one principle selected governs all other principles. Some of the monistic approaches that have been proposed for occupational therapy are purposeful activity, occupation, human growth and development, human occupation, occupational behavior, adaptive responses, and the systems model. On the other hand, a pluralistic approach to professional identity is the belief that many principles are needed to define a profession. There are several characteristics of a profession that support a pluralistic approach. Gilfoyle suggests that professional unity may not mean adhering to a single theory but, rather, to a set of theories.[19]

The Acceptance and Rejection of Activity

The use of purposeful activity or occupation has characterized the profession throughout its history. Since its conception, occupational therapy has been founded on the idea that being engaged in activity (1) restores health in individuals suffering from either mental or physical dysfunction and (2) maintains the well-being of the healthy individual.[12] Activity is not only viewed as the core of occupational therapy but also as the unique feature of the profession.

In physical disabilities practice there is evidence of a decline in the use of activities and a concomitant increase in the use of other treatment modalities.[6,16,49] Shannon called the profession's movement away from the traditional philosophy "the derailment of occupational therapy."[49] He stated that a new philosophy has developed that "views man as a mechanistic creature susceptible to manipulation and control via the application of techniques."[49] This "technique philosophy" contradicts the philosophy on which the profession was founded. According to Shannon, the profession is now faced with two alternatives. The first alternative is to ignore the crisis between the traditional and the contemporary "technique philosophy." The second alternative is to reinstate the traditional "values and beliefs on which the profession was founded and thereby arrest the process of derailment."[49]

A study by Bissell and Mailloux in 1981 explored the use of crafts in occupational therapy for the physically disabled.[6] This study employed a survey of 250 occupational therapists in the United States who chose physical disabilities as their specialty section. The results of this study showed that 72% of the respondents used crafts as a treatment modality. Of these, 51% used some crafts 20% or less of the treatment time. The greatest percentage of treatment time was devoted to self-care activities and therapeutic exercise. The authors concluded that "if therapeutic crafts are no longer considered a central concept of occupational therapy, there may be a need to revise the curricula pertaining to craft use."[6]

Fidler stated that occupational therapists have disclaimed activities and identified with the modalities of other professions to achieve credibility.[16] These modalities "eliminate the self as the doer-agent and place the causative agent outside the self."[16] According to

Fidler, "when occupational therapists are co[...] labeling a significant part of their practice as [...] ductive activity,' the fundamental principles o[...] pational therapy are denied."[16]

During the past two decades, newer sensorimotor and neurophysiologic approaches have developed. Clinical emphasis on these approaches has increased, whereas emphasis on activities has decreased. According to Cynkin, occupational therapists have incorporated these newer techniques into practice without looking at how they relate to an activity-oriented philosophical base for treatment.[12] In the process of acquiring these techniques, occupational therapists have disavowed the use of activities as the core of occupational therapy.[12]

Trend Reversal

In an attempt to reestablish activities as the core of occupational therapy, the Representative Assembly of the AOTA passed Resolution No. 531-79 in April 1979. The resolution stated that the Association shall adopt a single philosophical base of occupational therapy (cited previously).

Purposeful activity is the key concept in the philosophical base. Additionally, a survey of the professional literature from 1915 to 1977 revealed that purposeful activity was the second most frequently used term that consistently appeared in the literature.[20]

Despite the historical occurrence of the term, a definition of purposeful activity (cited previously) was not officially adopted by the profession until 1983.[23] Although open to interpretation, this definition of purposeful activity appears to be in concert with both the traditional philosophy of occupational therapy and the concept of human occupation.

In response to the attempt of the AOTA to promote the use of purposeful activity as the core of occupational therapy practice, several therapists expressed concern about the restrictions that purposeful activity would place on practice in the treatment of physical disabilities.[11,14,53] These restrictions include, but are not limited to, (1) jeopardizing reimbursement, (2) negating the skills and knowledge achieved by experienced clinicians, (3) jeopardizing referrals, and (4) excluding techniques, such as exercise, splinting, and inhibition-facilitation techniques.

These issues stem from an unclear or unacceptable definition of purposeful activity that excludes exercise.[53] These therapists believe that tying treatment methods to purposeful activity is not always appropriate or effective. Many patients receiving occupational therapy are not yet at an appropriate level of motor activity to participate in purposeful activity. In such circumstances, it is argued, the clinicians must use "adjunctive" treatment techniques to assist in the development of motor ability needed to participate in purposeful activity. Adjunctive techniques, as described by Trombly, include exercise, electrical stimulation, biofeedback, massage, whirlpool therapy, and thermal application. Therapists holding this viewpoint believe that the profession's history of purposeful activity should not be denied. However, they believe that the definition of purposeful activity needs to be expanded to incorporate contemporary treatment techniques. It is believed that, instead of attempting to redirect the focus of the profession, the profession needs to include current clinical practices that have proved effective on an empirical and a practical basis.[53]

Concern has been expressed that although purposeful activity may have been one of the unifying concepts of occupational therapy in the past this philosophical base no longer promotes cohesiveness in the profession.[33,42] Pedretti stated that purposeful activity "may have served to identify, define and articulate a disunity that has existed . . . for years."[42] Lyons reaffirmed this viewpoint in her statement that although purposeful activity "has been one of the unifying concepts of occupational therapy in the past, . . . today the use of this term seems more devisive than unifying."[33] She also stated that the phrase purposeful activity "has become an umbrella for a heterogeneous bag of human endeavors."[33] For some therapists, the term *purposeful activity* means crafts, games, or activities of daily living. Other therapists include exercise and physical modalities in their own personal definitions of purposeful activity. Lyons warned that, by allowing the term to "mean all things to all people," purposeful activity is loosing "its power to direct and influence" the profession.[33]

Trombly expressed the need for a clear definition of purposeful, goal-directed activity that takes into account theories of central motor control and motor acquisition. Such a definition would have to be a working one and tested by research.[53]

A definition of purposeful activity on a continuum that changes with the changing health status, values, and skills of the patient and that culminates in the performance of tasks essential to life roles could be developed to include both the enabling and "adjunctive" treatment modalities and modalities that have been traditionally considered purposeful activity.[42] Such a definition may satisfy both perspectives in the debate and would reflect the fact that occupational therapy has a service to offer at virtually every stage in the rehabilitation process. That service is one of the stimulation, integration, and continuous development of adaptive responses that enable and result in occupational performance.[42]

Rogers contends that, although the current debate tends to center around the use of arts and crafts in treatment, the real issue is whether a skills or subskills approach is best for dealing with the problems of the physically disabled in managing activities of daily living.[47] She proposes that the solution lies in the development of a philosophical base that will allow a synthesis of the skills and subskills approaches. The occupational performance frame of reference proposes such a synthesis with its emphasis on skills (self-care, work, education, and play and leisure) and subskills (motor, sensory-integrative, cognitive, social, and psychological components).

Yet the selection of appropriate treatment modalities (especially those that are directed to the remediation of the subskills) within this frame of reference continues to be debated. In addition, lawful use of modalities and competency to practice certain modalities are being questioned; they must be considered in the debate on treatment modalities appropriate for occupational therapy.[54]

An historical analysis conducted by Reed suggests that the following eight factors determine the treatment methods and media used by occupational therapists. "These factors are cultural, social, economic, technological, political, theoretical, historical, and research."[45] These factors operate singularly or in combination to influence the selection and elimination of the media and methods used in occupational therapy practice.

FUTURE DIRECTIONS
Frame of Reference/Philosophy

A view of the individual as an environment that requires balance for adaptation was proposed by Llorens.[31] If occupational therapists hold such a view, "the biological, psychological, and intrapersonal environment components of sensory, motor, psychological, sociological, and cognitive functions that permit interaction with the familial and cultural environment" must be considered.[31] The use of purposeful activity for self-care, work, play, leisure, and learning promotes such interactions.[31]

The occupational performance frame of reference makes the performance components, performance skills, and occupational theory operational in relation to the sociocultural and the biological-psychological environments. Occupational theory "refers to the inherent factors or properties of activity that elicit intrinsic reinforcement."[31] This theory is operative when occupational therapists prescribe and administer purposeful activity to bring about change in the individual's internal or external environment.[31]

The intrinsic goal of purposeful activity is generated from its inherent quality to arouse sensations, require processing of sensation, and elicit effective cognitive and motor responses that feed back into the individual system to effect balance.[31]

Purposeful activity is still a cornerstone of occupational therapy practice in the 1980s.[51] That purposeful activity facilitates change in the individual environment has been shown over time. It is generally accepted as a legitimate tool in the evaluation and treatment of physical and mental dysfunction. However, there is a need for controlled studies to measure the effectiveness and value of purposeful activity if its continued acceptance as the basic premise of occupational therapy is to be sustained.[31,51]

Llorens concluded that occupational therapy practice must be founded on a holistic philosophy that uses purposeful activity or occupation.[31] She claims that "the philosophy, theory, process in practice and frames of reference must be compatible" and that the techniques and modalities of occupational therapy must be congruent with its philosophical base, the science of occupation, occupational theory, and occupational behavior-performance frames of reference. The evaluation process and methods of the profession must allow the diagnosis of occupational dysfunction. Llorens made several recommendations to her colleagues. Among these were a commitment to (1) "unity of the profession"; (2) "the science of occupation"; and (3) "the ownership of the meaning of occupation and activity and the responsibility to explain the phenomenon."[31]

Rogers called for a study of human occupation. She stated that occupation is the medium of therapy and that, if it is to be used effectively, the occupational therapist needs a deep understanding of the health-enhancing nature of occupation.[48]

A definition of occupation cited by Rogers is that it is "volitional, goal-directed behavior aimed at the development of play, work, and life skills for optimal time management."[48] The study of human occupation is an important professional skill because applying knowledge of occupation to those whose occupational performance is at risk or is dysfunctional is the mission of occupational therapy. Three general areas of knowledge needed for effective application are "knowledge of normal occupational functions; knowledge of ineffective performance in occupational functions; and knowledge of the therapeutic properties of occupation."[48] A precise knowledge of occupation will allow occupational therapists to refine both the focus of their practice and the science of occupational therapy and to permit a more adequate definiton of the unique contribution of occupational therapy to health care.[48]

West summarized the positive and negative aspects of the current debate over a common philosophical base and appropriate treatment modalities.[54] Furthermore, she reviewed the origins, history, and possible causes of the loss of the scope of some of the traditional intervention strategies of occupational therapy and looked at the influence of social change and future social trends on occupational therapy practice. According to West, futuristic trends toward a more humanistic and holistic approach to disability and health is a significant reaffirmation of traditional philosophical and practice modes of occupational therapy.[54]

As a conclusion, several recommendations for the rerooting of occupational therapy in its philosophical traditions were offered. These included[54]

1. The consistent use and implementation of the concept and the term *occupation* as the common core of occupational therapy;
2. Speaking of the profession as serving the *occupational need of human beings* rather than as "treating the whole person," a claim that can be made by any of the health professions;
3. The definition and organization of occupational therapy around occupational performance dysfunction rather than in terms of disabilities;
4. The renewed commitment to the *mind-body-environment interrelationships* activated through occupation, one of the early tenets of occupational therapy.

There are many similarities in the recommendations of these experts. They are committed to the concept of occupation as the core of occupational therapy practice. The consideration of internal and external environmental interrelationships and the effect of occupation on the facilitation of these interrelationships are common themes of their writings. There is a strong recommendation for the focus of the profession to be on the occupational needs, roles, and role dysfunctions of the individual and on the foundation of occupational therapy on a holistic philosophy. The philosophy needs to be organized around occupational performance dysfunction rather than in terms of disabilities. Such a philosophy would expand the horizons of occupational therapy beyond the remediation of illness and disabilities to community and home settings. Perhaps those served by therapists in these settings have occupational performance dysfunctions because of environmental and sociocultural problems rather than only because of health problems.[31]

Modalities thought of as necessary for enabling the performance of purposeful activity have become commonplace in occupational therapy practice.[31] In some instances they are used exclusively and not tied to purposeful activity (occupation) in any way. Much debate has centered on the use of various modalities and their appropriateness in occupational therapy practice. Neither the occupational performance frame of reference nor the philosophical base of occupational therapy and the affirmations that accompanied it (adopted in 1979) negate the use of such preliminary activities.[1,21] Both, however, view such preliminary activities in the perspective of occupational role performance and recommend that they be used in that context. The selection of appropriate modalities, then, would provide a continuum of treatment from preparation, to sheltered trial, to satisfying occupational role performance, a process that is in progress in many treatment facilities. The selection of enabling treatment modalities must be guided by appropriate competency of the practitioner, lawful use, and their integration and relationship to *occupation* as the core concern of occupational therapy.

Practice

CHANGES IN HEALTH CARE. The health care system in the United States has undergone a "revolution" in the last 2 decades and change will continue.[5] The changes have created a significant challenge for health care delivery systems, health care administrators, and health care workers.[18] These changes may be viewed as problems, but at the same time, they present the profession of occupational therapy with significant challenges and opportunities for the future.[5,18] Changes in health care were generated by economic factors and the need for cost containment and gave rise to the industrialization of health care.[5,22] These factors resulted in a health care system that is more product-oriented than patient-oriented.[22]

The advent of Medicare (1965), Prospective Payment System (PPS) and Diagnostic Related Groups (DRG) (1983), health maintenance organizations (HMO), and the growth in home health care and the changing role of the occupational therapist in the public schools as a result of PL 94-142 are some of the major issues that have influenced health care and thus affected delivery of occupational therapy services.[5,22]

Until 1987, Medicare legislation excluded occupational therapy coverage under Medicare Part B (community practice). Reimbursement of occupational therapy was limited to acute hospital care and to the acute medical model.[22] After lengthy and extensive lobbying efforts of the AOTA, the Medicare amendment was passed in October 1986 and went into effect on July 1, 1987. The landmark legislation expanded the scope of occupational therapy services available to patients, and as a result, "occupational therapy has begun to come into its own as a fully respected health profession." The Medicare amendment expanded coverage of occupational therapy in skilled nursing

facilities, outpatient programs, and private practice. With this amendment, occupational therapy was permitted to charge Medicare directly, the only nonphysician provider service other than physical therapy able to do this.[41] This legislation ensures the role of occupational therapy as an integral member of the health care profession and its provision of needed occupational therapy services to patients who were formerly excluded.

The PPS forced external controls on the health care system and gave rise to making health care decisions based on cost.[5] The impact of the PPS and DRG on occupational therapy was studied by the AOTA in 1984. Hightower-Vandamm reported that the occupational therapists surveyed thought that patients were being discharged "sooner and sicker," that referrals to rehabilitation programs were often premature, and that referrals to outpatient occupational therapy increased significantly, as did "early referrals to occupational therapy, paper work, computerized record keeping, and quality assurance processes."[22]

HMOs have increased nationwide. The HMO is funded by monies from a percentage of each subscriber's dues. The physician and other health care professionals are paid out of this fund. At the end of the year, the money remaining in the pool is divided among the physicians in the HMO. This system is an incentive to cut costs by curtailing unnecessary referrals to specialists and other health care services. Under this system, physicians may be poorly motivated to refer patients for occupational therapy services.[22] HMOs traditionally offered limited rehabilitation services and often did not provide occupational therapy. Final Medicare regulations for HMOs published in the Federal Register (January 10, 1985) allowed Medicare beneficiaries to enroll in HMOs. Under these regulations, the HMO receives payment based on a predetermined monthly payment per enrollee—a PPS—rather than on a cost basis. The regulations require that the HMO provide the Medicare beneficiary services that meet Medicare regulations. Therefore occupational therapy must be available to the Medicare beneficiary enrolled in the plan on both an inpatient and outpatient basis. This program opened a new arena of health care delivery for occupational therapy.[40]

Home health care is currently the fastest growing health delivery system. Its continued growth is projected through 1990; however, this growth is not expected to continue. Federal and state governments are attempting to control the growth of home health care agencies by imposing standards, demanding certificates of need before new agencies can be established, imposing licensure, and freezing payments to home health care agencies as a way to curb increasing health care costs.[22] Such measures are likely to curtail home health care services, including occupational therapy.

Occupational therapists are employed in the public schools to fulfill the mandates of PL 94-142, the Education for All Handicapped Children Act. They are employed as teachers, are supervised by teachers, and their work is defined by teachers. Occupational therapists have worked as consultants to teachers and provided direct services to children. Occupational and physical therapists are developing "transdisciplinary treatment," which means that they provide treatment direction to the teacher, who then carries out the service. In so doing, occupational therapy can ultimately be deleted from the student's Individual Education Plan (IEP), as components of previously written treatment plans, described as the responsibility of teachers or teacher's aides, are included in the IEP. Thus teachers or aides may begin to provide "occupational therapy" services because they are anxious to maintain control of the education arena. Because of the shortage of occupational therapists, it has been difficult to meet the demands for occupational therapy in the public schools. Concomitantly, educators are seeking ways to fulfill the law, curtail budget, employ more teachers, and continue to provide necessary services. Thus they are setting standards that will decrease the need for occupational therapy. The public schools were developing as a strong practice arena, but this could be seriously eroded if the role of occupational therapy in the public school system is not protected.[22]

NEW ROLES FOR OCCUPATIONAL THERAPY.
Baum described five major types of health care delivery systems in which occupational therapy plays or can play an important role. These are (1) nonprofit, multihospital systems; (2) for-profit hospital systems; (3) health maintenance organizations; (4) industry; and (5) the public health care system. Baum conceptualized the role of occupational therapy in the hospital as developer of necessary plans for patients who are in acute care to receive rehabilitation services. The patient would progress from a hospital-based occupational therapy program to an outpatient occupational therapy program in appropriate agencies such

as home health, skill nursing, hospice, wellness, or designated rehabilitation beds in acute facilities; psychiatric facilities; or rehabilitation facilities.[5] Outpatient programs could focus on specific occupational therapy elements including life skills, work, industrial consultation, and driving, for example. Specialty clinical programs can be designed for specific diagnostic groups. Community-based programs, occupational therapy in the public schools, and occupational therapy in industry for the purposes of preventing work accidents, maintaining higher productivity, and promoting employee fitness are other practice areas that could be expanded.[5,22] An increase in the PPS will result in occupational therapy moving away from acute-care hospital settings to increased involvement in community-based health care and other arenas of practice.[22]

CONCLUSION

Fine stated that changes in the health care system can provoke unrest and anxiety for occupational therapists. However, these changes also present exciting challenges for the future of occupational therapy. Changes in health care delivery will necessitate changes in the role of occupational therapy.[18]

The potential to meet the challenge and demand for positive change is founded on valuable assets of the profession. The first is its "focus on function." The ability to function, as a treatment outcome, is a significant commodity and is of great benefit to the patient and society. The second asset is the growing need for occupational therapists; a demand for 8,000 more occupational therapists by 1995 has been projected. The third asset is the profession's belief "in interaction between biological, psychological, and social factors in human performance and adaptation."[18]

If occupational therapists are to emerge from the 1990s as principals in the rehabilitation of the disabled and in the promotion of health maintenance programs, Fine asserts that they must "anticipate needs, calculate economic advantages, influence public policy, and design, market, and deliver effective services to populations in need."[18]

REVIEW QUESTIONS

1. Define "frame of reference."
2. Why is a frame of reference necessary?
3. Briefly outline the elements in the occupational performance frame of reference.
4. What is the difference between a "performance skill" and a "performance component"? How are they related?
5. Define "enabling activities" as used in this chapter.
6. What is a key concept in the definition of occupational therapy? How is it related to the occupational performance frame of reference?
7. Define "purposeful activity."
8. Which treatment modalities can be thought of as primarily biomechanical in nature?
9. With which diagnoses is a biomechanical approach most likely to be used? Why?

10. How does the biomechanical approach fit into the occupational performance frame of reference?
11. For which diagnoses are the sensorimotor approaches most likely to be effective?
12. How can the sensorimotor approaches be integrated in an occupational performance framework?
13. Define what is meant by "rehabilitation approach."
14. List six treatment modalities that would be considered within the rehabilitation approach.
15. How is the rehabilitation approach integrated with the other approaches to treatment discussed in this chapter?
16. Discuss the current trends in occupational therapy practice in physical disabilities.
17. Identify the current controversy regarding philosophies and modalities and suggest possible solutions.
18. List and discuss five major factors that have influenced the role of occupational therapy in health care in recent years.
19. Discuss at least three possible new roles or directions for occupational therapy.

REFERENCES

1. American Occupational Therapy Association: A curriculum guide for occupational therapy educators, Rockville, MD, 1974, American Occupational Therapy Association.
2. American Occupational Therapy Association: The roles and functions of occupational therapy personnel, Rockville, MD, 1973, American Occupational Therapy Association.
3. American Occupational Therapy Association: Task force on target populations, Association report II, Am J Occup Ther 28:231, 1974.
4. Ayres AJ: Basic concepts of clinical practice in physical disabilities, Am J Occup Ther 12:300, 1958.
5. Baum CM: Growth, renewal, and challenge: an important era for occupational therapy, Am J Occup Ther 39:778, 1985.
6. Bissell JC and Mailloux Z: The use of crafts in occupational therapy for the physically disabled, Am J Occup Ther 35:369, 1981.
7. Bockoven JS: Legacy of moral treatment: 1800s to 1910, Am J Occup Ther 25:223, 1971.
8. Breines E: The issue is: an attempt to define purposeful activity, Am J Occup Ther 38:543, 1984.
9. Brunnstrom S: Clinical kinesiology, ed 3, Philadelphia, 1972, FA Davis Co.
10. Clark PN: Human development through occupation: theoretical frameworks in contemporary occupational therapy practice. Part 1, Am J Occup Ther 33:505, 1979.
11. Courtsunis DG et al: Purposeful activity restricts practice (Letters to the editor), Am J Occup Ther 36:468, 1982.
12. Cynkin, S: Occupational therapy: toward health through activities, Boston, 1979, Little, Brown & Co.
13. Di Joseph LM: Independence through activity: mind, body, and environment interaction in therapy, Am J Occup Ther 36:740, 1982.
14. English C et al: On the role of the occupational therapist in physical disabilities (The Issue) Am J Occup Ther 36:199, 1982.
15. Evans KA: Nationally speaking: definition of occupation as the core concept of occupational therapy, Am J Occup Ther 41:627, 1987.
16. Fidler GS: From crafts to competence, Am J Occup Ther 35:567, 1981.
17. Fidler GS and Fidler JW: Doing and becoming: purposeful action and self-actualization, Am J Occup Ther 32:305, 1978.
18. Fine SB: Nationally speaking: working the system; a perspective for managing change, Am J Occup Ther 42:417, 1988.
19. Gilfoyle EM: Transformation of a profession—1984 Eleanor Clark Slagle lecture, Am J Occup Ther 38:575, 1984.
20. Gillette N and Keilhofner G: The impact of specialization on the professionalization and survival of occupational therapy. Am J Occup Ther 33:20, 1979.
21. Highlights of actions taken by the Representative Assembly during its recent meeting, Occupational Therapy Newspaper, p. 1, Rockville, MD, June 1979. The American Occupational Therapy Association.
22. Hightower-Vandamm MD: Occupational therapy's journey: the implementation, challenge, and expectation, Am J Occup Ther 39:785, 1985.
23. Hinojosa J et al: Purposeful activities, Am J Occup Ther 37:805, 1983.
24. Hopkins HL, Smith HD, and Tiffany EG: Rehabilitation. In Hopkins HL and Smith HD, editors: Willard and Spackman's occupational therapy, ed 6, Philadelphia, 1983, JB Lippincott Co.
25. Kielhofner G: Health through occupation, theory and practice in occupational therapy. Philadelphia, 1983, FA Davis Co.
26. Kielhofner G: A heritage of activity: development of theory, Am J Occup Ther 36:723, 1982.
27. Kielhofner G and Burke JP: Occupational therapy after 60 years: an account of changing identity and knowledge, Am J Occup Ther 31:675, 1977.
28. Kielhofner G and Burke JP: A model of human occupation. I. Conceptual framework and content, Am J Occup Ther 34:572, 1980.
29. King LJ: Toward a science of adaptive responses, Am J Occup Ther 32:429, 1978.
30. Llorens LA: Application of a developmental theory for health and rehabilitation, Rockville, Md, 1976, American Occupational Therapy Association.
31. Llorens LA: Changing balance: environment and individual, Am J Occup Ther 38:29, 1984.
32. Llorens LA: Personal communication, July 6, 1988.

33. Lyons BG: The issue is: purposeful versus human activity, Am J Occup Ther 37:493, 1983.

34. Meyer A: The philosophy of occupational therapy, Am J Occup Ther 31:630, 1977.

35. Moore J: Changing methods in the treatment of physical dysfunction, Am J Occup Ther 21:18, 1967.

36. Mosey AC: Involvement in the rehabilitation movement: 1942-1960, Am J Occup Ther 25:234, 1971.

37. Mosey AC: A monistic or pluralistic approach to professional identity?—1985 Eleanor Clark Slagle lecture, Am J Occup Ther 39:504, 1985.

38. Mosey AC: Occupational therapy: configuration of a profession, New York, 1981, Raven Press.

39. Occupational therapy: its definition and functions, Am J Occup Ther 26:204, 1972.

40. Occupational Therapy News: New medicare regulations for HMOs open door for occupational therapy services, 39:4, April 1985, (p. 1), American Occupational Therapy Association, Rockville, MD.

41. Occupational Therapy News, The medicare amendment: accomplishment of a goal (pp. 1&7); Provisions of medicare amendment expand coverage for occupational therapy (p.4), 40:12, December 1986, American Occupational Therapy Association, Rockville, MD.

42. Pedretti LW: The compatibility of treatment methods in physical disabilities with the philosophical base of occupational therapy, Paper presented to the American Occupational Therapy Association National Conference, Philadelphia, May 1982.

43. Project to delineate the roles and functions of occupational therapy personnel, Rockville, MD, 1972, American Occupational Therapy Association. Cited in A curriculum guide for occupational therapy educators, Rockville, MD, 1974, American Occupational Therapy Association.

44. Reed KL: Models of practice in occupational therapy, Baltimore, 1984, Williams and Wilkins.

45. Reed K: Tools of practice: heritage or baggage?—1986 Eleanor Clark Slagle lecture, Am J Occup Ther 40:597, 1986.

46. Rerek MD: The depression years: 1929 to 1941, Am J Occup Ther 25:231, 1971.

47. Rogers JC: The spirit of independence: the evolution of a philosophy, Am J Occup Ther 36:709, 1982.

48. Rogers JC: The foundation: why study human occupation? Am J Occup Ther 38:47, 1984.

49. Shannon PD: The derailment of occupational therapy, Am J Occup Ther 31:229, 1977.

50. Shannon PD: Project to identify the philosophy of occupational therapy, Rockville, MD, 1983, American Occupational Therapy Association (unpublished). Cited in Rogers JC: The foundation: why study human occupation? Am J Occup Ther 38:47, 1984.

51. Steinbeck TM: Purposeful activity and performance, Am J Occup Ther 40:529, 1986.

52. Stockmeyer SA: An interpretation of the approach of Rood to the treatment of neuromuscular dysfunction, Am J Phys Med 46:900, 1967.

53. Trombly CA: Include exercise in purposeful activity (Letters to the editor), Am J Occup Ther 36:467, 1982.

54. West W: A reaffirmed philosophy and practice of occupational therapy for the 1980s, Am J Occup Ther 38:15, 1984.

55. Willard HL and Spackman CS, editors: Occupational therapy, ed 4, Philadelphia, 1971, JB Lippincott Co.

56. Woodside HH: The development of occupational therapy: 1910-1929, Am J Occup Ther 25:226, 1971.

Chapter

2 Psychosocial aspects of physical dysfunction

LORRAINE WILLIAMS PEDRETTI

PSYCHOSOCIAL CONSEQUENCES OF PHYSICAL DYSFUNCTION

The experience of loss of any physical part or function involves not only the painful distortion of body image and the image of oneself as a physical being but also the image of self as a social being whose family and social roles and vocational and leisure occupations may be unalterably changed. Independence, self-sufficiency, and autonomy may have to be given up partially or totally, temporarily or permanently.[13]

The onset of physical dysfunction necessitates a sudden change in daily life. The individual is likely to be thrown into the new world and lifestyle of a health care facility where there is enforced passivity and dependence. The newly disabled person must adapt to a new environment, new personnel, new food, and new time schedules. Privacy must be surrendered and virtual strangers must be allowed to probe the body. The person may be devastated by the drastic interruption of familial, vocational, and social roles.[22] Previous roles may be slightly changed, seriously impaired, or completely eliminated as a result of the disability. The damage to previously held roles may be due directly to the disability or may indirectly result from changed life circumstances brought about by the disability.[28]

The onset of physical disability affects the person who has the disability and all of those with whom he or she has contact. The individual's particular response and the responses of others to the disability will have a significant impact on rehabilitation personnel and on the rehabilitation process.[32] The disabled adult is first confronted with the task of survival, then with regaining essential physical skills, and finally, with the greater goals of resuming meaningful life roles. These are monumental and formidable tasks that require managing many overwhelming personal problems and overcoming external blockades to readjustment.[28]

Personal Reactions to Physical Dysfunction

As a result of the major life changes brought about by the onset of physical dysfunction, the individual's defense mechanisms are highly taxed as he or she attempts to deal with the changed social interactions and sexual patterns and the ability to direct his or her own life and to control the environment through physical action. Concomitantly the individual is dealing with fears, realistic and unrealistic, physical pain and suffering, and the symbolic meaning of the physical dysfunction. Changed attitudes of family and friends may provoke stress, fears, and expectations that others will react differently and reject him or her.[22,42]

Individual reactions to physical dysfunction depend on the previously held body image and compromise body image and the psychological meaning of the specific dysfunction in relation to the individual's personality.[42] For example, paraplegia may have a very different meaning to an athlete who defines self-worth in terms of physical performance and physique than to an office worker whose sense of self may be defined more in terms of use of head and hands.[25]

Although it is commonly believed that physical dysfunction generates only negative and disruptive psychological reactions, it has been found that opportunities and gratification may be generated as well.[38] The dysfunction may be regarded as a well-deserved punishment, especially if it is associated with a suicide attempt, asocial behavior, or the death of another. This attitude could gratify masochistic wishes and paradoxically lead to a greater sense of well-being.[22,42] The dysfunction may be seen as the final confirmation of a lack of self-worth and could precipitate a suicide or psychotic reaction.[42] The gratification of longed for dependency on a caring person leading to relative comfort may be satisfied by the dysfunction. Conversely, the reawakening of intolerable dependency longings and rage related to a lack of satisfaction of eary dependency needs can result in marked anxiety or a paranoid reaction.[22,42] Exhibitionistic wishes and the need to manipulate and control others may also be satisfied through the physical dysfunction. The dysfunction may be used as a means of expressing hostility or avoiding responsibilities by some individuals.[22] Conversely, the onset of dysfunction may lead to constructive, alternative life roles and offer social and career opportunities that were not previously contemplated by the individual.

Great emphasis and value are placed on productivity and physical attractiveness in the American culture. To not have achieved them or to be in the process of achieving them may evoke feelings of self-devaluation. Feelings of low worth tend to be all-or-none in quality. They may be evoked by consideration of only one characteristic of many by the disabled person, yet the person may conceive of self as all worthless. The feelings of low self-worth also tend to extend into the past and into the future so that the person can neither conceive of self as ever having been productive or attractive nor contemplate the possibility of future change.

The conclusions of worthlessness are in a sense true, because they are based on a self-definition in terms of degree of productivity and attractiveness. This is a distortion, since it bases the self-worth on deficits and overlooks the remaining assets and intrinsic worth. Although the concept of intrinsic worth, that is, the person is valued for self alone without external comparisons, is desirable and ideal, it is probably difficult or impossible to achieve for most people. In general, people in American society value themselves according to external standards of attractiveness, productivity, and achievements.

Disabled persons may conclude that they are worthless and of negative value and, therefore, feel that they are "awful" as well. They may expect and think that they deserve the rejection of others based on that notion. If they are not of any value to themselves, then others will not see them as valuable and, therefore, will reject them. This kind of thinking can persist for long periods of time and may account for withdrawal behavior or an intense search for approval and love. Some persons will draw this thinking process to what seems like a logical conclusion, which is that they are worth nothing to self or to others, therefore life is meaningless and empty, and they should not exist. This feeling may be especially strong in those who have intense guilt feelings.[14]

The meaning of the disability to the patient is the crucial factor in planning a sound approach in treatment and in aiding with the adjustment process. Therefore, treatment directed to aid psychosocial adjustment must be based on individual reactions to the circumstances rather than on reactions and characteristics assumed to be similar among patients with the same physical disability or the same degree of severity of disability.[38]

It has been assumed by many that a certain type of personality or adjustment pattern is associated with a specific physical disability or that the degree and type of dysfunction will cause psychological maladjustment. These premises have been refuted by research. It has been concluded that particular personality types or characteristics are not associated with specific dysfunctions, nor is there evidence to support the notion that the severity or type of disability is correlated with the degree of psychological adjustment.[38,39]

Psychological consequences of physical disability depend on many factors. The range of personal reactions varies widely from one individual to another. Some factors that may influence the patient's response to the dysfunction are (1) time of life in which the disability was acquired, (2) the extent and location of the defect, (3) whether or not it is obvious, (4) the social definition of the defect, (5) the attitudes of "significant others" toward the individual,[5] (6) the extent to which the disability interferes with functioning, and (7) the disruption of valued goals.

Societal Reactions to Physical Dysfunction

AVOIDANCE AND REJECTION. Attitudes of others toward physical disability affect attitudes toward oneself. In the newly disabled, devaluing attitudes toward the disabled, once an out-group, may now be directed to the self, with very serious consequences.[38] Physical dysfunction was once considered divine punishment or evidence of sinfulness. This is still the belief of some individuals. It is more likely to be viewed as ugly, loathsome, or, at the very least, discomforting. Few people are really comfortable with disabled or deformed individuals. Their presence constitutes a threat to the nondisabled about their own vulnerability. To avoid the threatening feeling, the nondisabled reject or avoid disabled or deformed persons.[42] The appearance of the injury or disability also engenders nonacceptance. If the disability is unsightly, this tends to be overestimated by the nondisabled and is a factor that prompts rejection or avoidance. The nondisabled may display unwarranted pity or excessive curiosity. The disabled person feels set apart from most "normal" people and is constantly striving to fight the negative implications of the physical dysfunction and to gain genuine social acceptance.[29]

NONACCEPTANCE. Nonacceptance exists in the nondisabled and stems from negative attitudes. It is a resistance or reluctance to enter into various degrees of social interchange with the disabled person and carries an aura of ostracism.

The disabled person may perceive an apparent, rather than a genuine, social acceptance by the nondisabled. The latter may be perceived as motivated by pity or duty and may offer empty gestures of acceptance devoid of meaning or real pleasure in the interchange. Apparent acceptance is not more desirable than nonacceptance. In each, the disabled see the underlying inability or unwillingness on the part of the nondisabled to know them as they really are.

Disabled individuals perceive a lack of patience on the part of the nondisabled toward performance ease and speed. Whether this attitude is maintained by the nondisabled or is projected by the disabled, it engenders the same feeling of nonacceptance in the disabled person.[29]

SPREAD FACTOR. Another tendency of the nondisabled is to judge the disabled not only in terms of the apparent physical limitation but also in terms of psychological factors assmed to be concomitant to the disability.[29] The nondisabled may treat the physically disabled as if they are limited mentally and emotionally as well.[11] The evaluation of the visible disability is "spread" to other characteristics that are not necessarily affected. The frequent assumption that a person who has cerebral palsy is also mentally retarded, and the practice of speaking loudly to a blind person as if he or she is also deaf are examples of this phenomenon. It is generally a devaluing process and the disabled person is thereby stigmatized and considered of lower social status and unworthy of acceptance.[29]

There is also a tendency for nondisabled persons to assess the limitations as more severe and restrictive than they actually are. Frequently when the nondisabled judge that the physical dysfunction precludes participation in a given activity or social situation, the disabled person knows that some level of participation is possible. The degree of difference between their assessments may make the difference between nonparticipation and nonacceptance. Because it is not possible for the nondisabled person to know the capabilities of the disabled person in a given situation, it is wise for the nondisabled to invite the participation of the disabled, thus allowing him or her to determine whether or not performance is feasible. Even if participation appears patently impossible to the nondisabled, the invitation still should be made to avoid rejection and to allow for the possibility of the disabled to participate in an alternative role from the roles most participants will be assuming. The disabled person may be willing to restructure the situation so that participation is possible. The changes devised to allow participation may be simple or complex but should be left to the discretion of the disabled person and not structured by the preconceived notions of the nondisabled. The role of the nondisabled is to provide opportunities for participation in social interchange for the disabled.[29]

LABELING. Words exist in the language of American culture that have a stigmatizing effect on the disabled. Expressions such as "retard," "crip," and "psycho" are examples. Within the language of the medical and allied health professions, these terms become formalized to "mentally retarded," "physically disabled," and "mentally ill." These terms have value for the classification of persons into diagnostic categories, but they stigmatize as well.[11] It follows that when rehabilitation workers refer to their patients as a diagnosis or disability (for example, "quad" or "hemi"), they are contributing to the stigmatization of those who they set out to help.

MINORITY GROUP STATUS. Stigma may be considered as negative perceptions or behaviors of normal people toward the physically disabled or toward all persons different from themselves. Physically disabled persons are regarded in much the same way as other minority groups in the population. They are subject to stereotyping and a reduced social status. Stigmatization is a basic fact of life for nearly all disabled persons. Interpersonal relationships between the nondisabled and the disabled tend to follow a superior-inferior pattern or to not exist at all. The nondisabled tend to demonstrate stereotyped, inhibited, and overcontrolled behavior in interactions with disabled persons. They tend to show less variable behavior, terminate interactions sooner, and express opinions less representative of their actual beliefs.[11]

SEGREGATION. There is substantial segregation of the physically disabled. Although some of this segregation is necessary (for example, institutionalization or special schools) and designed to assist disabled persons, it nevertheless sets them apart psychologically and evokes feelings of inferiority in relation to nondisabled peers. This kind of segregation should be minimized. The fact that restrictive legislation exists in reference to disabled persons testifies to the systematized stigmatization of the disabled within American society.[11]

UNFOUNDED POSITIVE IMAGES. In some instances, the disabled are also subjected to unfounded positive images. The belief that the other senses of the blind are sharpened to compensate for the loss of vision is such an example. This is the myth of "automatic compensation." The fact is that the blind and deaf learn to use their other senses more efficiently.[18]

Attitudes in the Health Care Facility

The health care facility can be considered a microcosm of society. There is a tendency for health care workers to believe that societal prejudices toward the disabled do not exist in the facility. The assumption is that rehabilitation personnel are immune from discriminatory attitudes and that patients are accepted as persons when they are accepted as patients.[15]

The attitudes of the professionals involved with the rehabilitation of the disabled are of great importance and, in fact, may be one of the most important determinants in the disabled person's response to rehabilitation. Negative attitudes held by health professionals will constrict the options of those in their care.[2]

Negative reactions will result in a negative response in the patient. Such reactions increase the patient's suffering and may result in negativistic behavior demonstrated by an apparent loss of motivation and uncooperative behavior.[22]

Benham cited several studies suggesting that there are more negative attitudes among health care professionals than may be expected. She compared the attitudes of occupational therapists toward the disabled with those of other health care professionals. The results of the study indicated that occupational therapists have a very positive attitude toward the disabled as compared with health care professionals described in other studies.[2]

Although the staff may hold the view that prejudice does not exist in the facility, in reality, the view of the staff is that the patient is one to be helped, a malleable individual who can be shaped and educated into a specific health status and behavior. Convictions of superiority are reinforced by the emergence of a teacher-student relationship, a superior-inferior pattern.[15] This pattern is further reinforced by the segregated dining areas, the uniforms of the staff, and the organizational hierarchy of the institution.

The patients view themselves as disabled and unable to perform and perceive themselves as applicants asking the knowledgeable, powerful, and authoritative others if they can regain the characteristics and skills of nondisabled persons. The patients confront a closed, self-sufficient subculture with an unfamiliar value system and are, in fact, outsiders in the facility seeking acceptance from omnipotent persons in authority. The patients occupy the lowest level in the status hierarchy of the institution and are manipulated by many forces over which they have no control. Individual life goals may be partly or completely determined by others and choices and decisions imposed under a facade of personal involvement and self-determination. There is segregation of staff and patients throughout the facility that parallels the exclusion of disabled persons by nondisabled persons in general society, and the physical impairment is the symbol of that exclusion.[15]

To change this, it is necessary for the rehabilitation worker to shed the role of teacher and authority and to assume the role of facilitator and guide. Segrega-

tion in the facility needs to be abandoned to the extent possible, for example, in the dining and recreation areas. The recognition and respect for different needs, goals, and value systems other than their own can change the attitudes of health care workers toward patients. Real involvement of the patient in the decision-making process for treatment and in patient government can also be helpful in reducing prejudice and equalizing the status of residents of the health care facility.

Roots of Societal Attitudes Toward the Disabled

Livneh outlined a classification system for sources of negative attitudes toward people with disabilities.[30] The major categories were:

1. Conditioning by sociocultural norms such as youth, health, attractiveness, athletic prowess, personal productivity and achievement. Also, socioeconomic level, society's delineation of the sick role, and the lower status attached to disability are factors in sociocultural conditioning.
2. The influence of childhood experiences on the child's beliefs and value system shapes attitudes toward the disabled. The reaction of parents and other caring adults, transmitted to the child through words, gestures, and tone of voice, perpetuate stereotypic beliefs and attitudes.
3. Psychodynamic mechanisms may evoke interaction strain with disabled persons. Such mechanisms as the "spread phenomenon," unresolved conflicts over scopophilia and exhibitionism, associating responsibility with etiology, fear of social ostracism, and guilt about being able-bodied tend to create unrealistic expectations and unresolved conflicts when interacting with the disabled.
4. Disability is seen as a punishment for personal or even ancestral sin. The disabled individual may be regarded as a dangerous person, that is, one who has committed a sin and, therefore, is evil, or one who was punished unjustly and may wish to get even. The nondisabled person, fearing imminent punishment, may tend to avoid the disabled person because of guilt for not being punished for past misdeeds or for fear of punishment by association.
5. Unstructured social, emotional, and intellectual situations have an inherent capacity to provoke confusion and anxiety. This applies to social interaction with the disabled, in which rules for proper social interchange are not well defined.
6. Aesthetic-sexual aversion, triggered by the sight of a visibly disabled person, evokes feelings of repulsion and discomfort in the nondisabled.
7. A threat to conscious and unconscious body im-

age is evoked by the presence of a disabled person. Such presence may reawaken castration anxiety, and evoke fear of losing one's physical integrity. Profound anxiety about the possibility of becoming disabled plays a critical part in the formation of prejudicial attitudes toward the physically disabled. Aversive attitudes may also develop from a fear of contamination or inheritance. Therefore social interaction with the disabled is avoided.

8. The disabled are in a marginal social group and are accorded minority group status in the society. Thus the same stereotypic reactions of devaluation and inferior social status that the nondisabled apply to other minority groups are applied to the disabled. Persons holding such attitudes may advocate isolation and segregation of the disabled.

9. The sight of a disabled person can evoke anxieties associated with dying in some individuals. The disability is a reminder of the death of a part or function that was an integral part of one's ego in the past. The disabled serve as a reminder of mortality and a denial of infantile omnipotence.

10. Certain behaviors of the disabled tend to provoke prejudice. Such behaviors as dependence, seeking secondary gains, acting fearful, insecure, or inferior can strengthen certain prejudices in the nondisabled.

11. Disability-related factors such as: functionality versus organicity (for example, alcoholism versus blindness); level of severity; degree of visibility; degree of cosmetic involvement; contagiousness versus noncontagiousness; body part affected; and degree of predictability (that is, whether curable) influence prejudicial attitudes toward the disabled.

12. Demographic and personality variables are also associated with attitudes toward the disabled. Factors such as age, sex, socioeconomic status, educational level, and certain personality traits are associated with negative and positive attitudes toward the disabled.[30]

Changing Negative Societal Attitudes

Several studies have suggested that society's attitudes and expectations toward the disabled may be critically important to the maintenance of their mental health. If this is so, it is important for health professionals to seek ways to influence attitudes positively.

Anthony cited several studies that involved contact, information, and contact plus information to effect change in attitudes toward the disabled.[1] Attitudes of the nondisabled toward the disabled can be positively influenced by providing them with an experience that involves both contact with disabled persons and information about the disability. Contact without information has only a limited positive effect and may actually reinforce negative attitudes. Information alone increases knowledge but has little effect on attitudes. Anthony recommended that health care professionals design contact plus information programs to facilitate attitude change in employers, school personnel, and students of various age groups.[1]

ORIGINS OF ATTITUDES TOWARD THE PHYSICALLY DISABLED

Aversion to the disabled is not natural or instinctive as it has been thought. Studies by animal psychologists and cultural anthropologists suggest that the existence of instinctive hostile attitudes toward the disabled is a myth.[9]

History

All societies probably have discriminated positively or negatively against the disabled. Examples of extreme forms of prejudice are the attribution of supernatural powers to the physically different on the positive end and the elimination of physically deformed infants on the negative end. More modern societies express their prejudice in more subtle ways such as excluding the disabled from employment opportunities and social interactions.[37]

The popularity of "freak" shows in circuses was testimony to paradoxic repulsion-attraction of the nondisabled toward the disabled and deformed. Negative attitudes toward the disabled are rooted in ancestral superstitions and mythologies and have evolved into the sophisticated bigotry of the present age.[18]

Because of the primacy of group survival, "primitive" societies did not tolerate those who were physically impaired. The physically weak were expendable and the law of survival of the fittest prevailed.[18]

Superstitions and folklore guided primitive peoples before the advent of organized religions. Evil spirits were thought to reside in the bodies of those who were sick or deformed. Therefore such individuals were to be avoided. Mental illnesses and physical afflictions were thought to be the work of evil spirits. If the spirits did not exit the afflicted body after considerable effort, it was believed that the individual was being punished and so such individuals were avoided or killed.[18]

In discussing the history and psychology of amputation, Friedmann noted that in ancient civilizations self-mutilation was practiced to appease the gods and, thus was a form of "religious rehabilitation." With few exceptions, the survival of deformed infants was not encouraged in any civilization. In some societies, transgressions of rules or crimes were punished by the amputation of a limb or part.[12] Thus the concepts that disability is a deserved punishment for misdeeds, that the disabled are not acceptable in society, and that disability as reparation for sin have ancient roots.

As societies became more civilized, methods of dealing with the disabled began to change. In a few societies, they were accepted and treated well. During the Middle Ages, the blind occupied a privileged position in France. In both Asia and the Mediterranean regions, progressive physicians called for humane treatment of the disabled. However, in most countries, inhumane treatment of the disabled persisted. Infants with disabilities were abandoned, drowned, or killed. Infanticide was practiced by nobility to maintain the purity of the bloodline. Children who escaped the fate of death roamed the country as beggars; some were subjected to slavery or forced into prostitution.[18]

During the Renaissance, more tolerant attitudes toward and improved treatment of the physically different developed. The Elizabethan English Poor Laws (1597-1601) were the legal foundation for the protection of the poor and disabled from degrading treatment and provided financial support for the unemployed, including those with disabilities. Gradually, the perception of the disabled began to shift from one of total worthlessness to one of their ability to be at least be marginally productive in society.[18]

In spite of this progress, it is evident that in early American history, there was little knowledge of and few resources available to the disabled. Medical care in the colonies precluded any rehabilitation. Medical knowledge and treatment began to improve in the nineteenth century. Medical personnel began to demand better facilities to treat the disabled. However, this attitude was not widespread and many physicians continued to demonstrate negative attitudes toward and inhumane treatment of the physically disabled. The myth that such afflictions were the result of evil spirits continued, and cures of "bleeding," potions, and ostracism continued.[18]

A few hospitals in New York and Philadelphia provided treatment to the physically disabled before the Civil War; the first sheltered workshop for the disabled was established in 1837. At the end of the nineteenth century, the Cleveland Rehabilitation Center was established and was the forerunner of present day rehabilitation centers. Among private organizations to help the disabled that began during this period were The Salvation Army (1880) and Goodwill Industries (1902).[18]

Ancient myths and stereotypes persist. Many people still associate disabilities with sin and the Devil or with evil. Disability becomes associated with *bad* and able-bodied with *good*. Metaphorical usage of these associations appear in the Bible. They also appear in both ancient and contemporary literature. This concept has been systematically instilled in children through books, television, and religious training.[18]

Literature and Media

Media images of the disabled are molded from early childhood through fairy tails and classical literature. The messages that different is ugly, that deformed is evil, and that the physically different deviate in other ways as well are conveyed.[9]

Traditional children's literature contributes to the stereotyping of the disabled. Physical deformity, illness, and, at the very least, unattractiveness often symbolize inner defects, evil natures, and villainous behavior in children's literature.[43] Some of the oldest and best known children's stories convey prejudices and stereotype the disabled. These stories can be a subtle form of teaching children scorn for the disabled. Examples of such characters are Cinderella's stepsisters, who were obese and unattractive, and Captain Hook of *Peter Pan*, who wore a prosthesis. The wicked witch of *Hansel and Gretel* was aged, arthritic, and had a kyphosis.[4] Gigantism affected the evil character in *Jack and the Beanstalk*.

An examination of these and other well-known stories reveals that physical attractiveness, health, and intactness of the body are usually features of the heroes and heroines, the noble, and the good, whereas the villains are often portrayed with some infirmity or unattractive features, such as large noses, wrinkles, and warts. The association of moral character and personality is thus made with the external appearance.[43]

Some stories show physical disability as a consequence of a misdeed. Pinocchio's nose grew as a result of his failure to tell the truth, whereas pirates lost eyes and limbs as a result of their violent behavior.[43]

There have been almost no average, ordinary physically abnormal individuals in children's stories in the past. More recently, several children's books that portray the disabled in a more favorable and matter-of-fact manner have been published.[3,8,35,36,43]

Although it is not possible to eliminate classical children's literature, it is possible for parents and others reading this literature to children to be aware of the biases that may be conveyed and to discuss and reflect on them with the children to minimize the unquestioned acceptance of these portrayals.[43] Fortunately, children today are much more matter-of-fact about disability, since they are likely to have disabled classmates, and there is open discussion of disability in the classroom.[4]

This same type of stereotyping occurs in television programs, movies, cartoons, comic strips, and adult fiction.

Currently, the disabled are being portrayed in more positive ways, performing ordinary life roles in movies, television programs, and television advertising.

Religion

The image of the physically disabled varies from society to society, and the dominant religion in a society may translate the disability into spiritual terms. The disability may be assigned a spiritual cause, such as possession, the consequences of sin, a special sign of God's grace, or a blessing.[9] Thurer believes that the stereotyping in literature reflects the subtle prejudice of the Judeo-Christian ethic that fosters the notion that God has smiled on those who are whole and successful, whereas those who are wrongdoers are punished with suffering and physical defects.[43]

Many people have grown up with the notion that God is all-wise, all-loving, and all-powerful. He is seen as a parent figure who rewards for obedience and who disciplines for disobedience. He protects those in His favor from harm and arranges for each person to get what he or she deserves in life.[27] If this premise is accepted, the question must be considered: "Why do bad things happen to good people?"[27] This question is raised when personal tragedy is experienced and when there are daily media confrontations with seemingly senseless tragedies that occur everywhere and to all types of people. It is troubling to know that suffering is distributed unfairly in the world. For many, this awareness raises questions about the goodness and even the existence of God. Kushner outlines various popular explanations of suffering based on this notion of God and discusses the faulty reasoning in each.[27]

Some of the most common notions of the causes of suffering that are based on scripture are that (1) suffering is punishment for sin (Isaiah 3:10-11 and Proverbs 3:7-8), (2) suffering is for personal growth or testing of spiritual strengths (Genesis 22), and (3) suffering is a cure for personality flaws (Proverbs 3:11-12).[6,27]

The New Testament introduces the concept of suffering as a share in the glory of Jesus Christ (Romans 8:17). Illness and disability are also sometimes shown as associated with the presence of demons (Matthew 8:16 and 8:28; Luke 9:37-43, 11:14, and 13:10-14). However, there are also many accounts of healings in which there is no association with sin or evil spirits (Matthew 8:8-13, Mark 8:22-26, and Luke 17:11-18[6]).

Someone who believes that suffering is punishment for sin will believe that the sufferers have gotten what they deserve. The difficulty arises when the individual cannot find a misdeed that deserves the punishment and may become angry at God or repress that anger to protect the perceived reputation of God as the fair and just parent.[27]

If the notion that suffering is for the enoblement of people to repair faulty aspects of the personality is accepted, it follows that suffering is for the individual's own good, that God teaches a lesson with suffering, and that everything happens for a purpose, although that purpose may be obscure and known only to God. Another explanation of suffering is that God tests only those whom he knows are strong of spirit.[27] This generates the idea that those with afflictions are privileged or chosen by God for a special role and may cause the believer to perceive the sufferer as elevated in God's sight. This idea does not explain all of those who break under the strain of their suffering and indeed those who do not appear strong enough to deal with it.[27]

If the presence of demons as a cause of illness and disability is accepted, it may follow that there is some spiritual illness or defect, and if the demons are driven out with prayers of healing, the sufferer will surely get well. Atlhough there are documented accounts of sudden and unexplained healings, it is not possible to say that there is a "formula" that works in every instance.

All of these responses or attempts at explaining tragedy assume that God is the cause of suffering. They attempt to explain why God would mete out suffering. Is it for the individual's own growth, is it divine punishment, or is it that God does not care what happens to human beings? Some approaches lead the believer to self-blame and foster the denial of reality and repression of true feelings. Kushner asks his readers to consider the possibility that God does not cause suffering and that maybe it occurs for reasons other than the result of the will of God.[27] Perhaps God does not cause bad things to happen, and the question is not "Why me?" but rather, "God see what is happening to me, can you help?" (Psalm 121:1-2).[6,27] There may be some things God does not control. Some of the misfortunes that happen to people may be the result of "bad luck," bad people, human weakness, random events, and the inflexible laws of nature.[27] Any health care worker or patient who is wrestling with this question is well advised to read Kushner's book, *When Bad Things Happen To Good People.*[27]

Spiritual counseling is a necessary aspect of the treatment program for many patients. Therapists should recognize this need and make the appropriate referrals.

ADJUSTMENT TO PHYSICAL DYSFUNCTION

Because there is no direct relationship between the type of physical dysfunction and personality structure, physical injury or illness resulting in disability should be regarded as one of several life stresses to which the individual brings a unique repertoire of coping mechanisms and response patterns.[41] There is usually little or no prolonged effect on personality resulting from physical dysfunction. Personality structure may be temporarily disordered by the crisis of physical change, but it appears to be capable of drawing on its resources and integrating the crisis experience into the self to become reestablished.[38]

The individual with physical dysfunction is faced with the problem of coping with fears and anxieties and maintaining a balance between conflicting needs and tendencies at a time when it is most difficult to cope and defenses are weakened. These anxieties may be managed through a variety of coping mechanisms.[22]

Coping Mechanisms and Their Implications for Rehabilitation

Emotions and behaviors that enable adjustment to problems are called coping mechanisms. Everyone uses coping mechanisms to maintain and restore emotional equilibrium. The struggle to maintain equilibrium occurs both consciously and subconsciously. The ability to keep anxiety at a manageable level is dependent on the appropriate regulation of feelings, beliefs, and actions.[18]

DEPRESSION. Depression is mourning the loss of function or loss of a part. It invariably occurs after the onset of physical dysfunction. The depression often occurs with the realization of the limitations imposed by the disability. The individual realizes that recovery will not be complete and that returning to "normal" is not possible. This confrontation with reality is likely to evoke a depression, and it may occur early or late in the course of the illness or injury. It may have occurred before the patient entered the rehabilitation phase of the treatment regime.

While the patient is depressed, progress in rehabilitation will be limited. During this time, it is important for rehabilitation personnel to maintain good communication with the patient. Areas for discussion are the patient's emotional pain, self-concept and self-esteem, goals and potential capabilities, and plans for the rehabilitation program. Such discussions need to be reinforced often and should focus on both the present and the future.[18]

DENIAL. The person with an acquired disability may deny its reality as a means of reducing its impact. Initially, the individual may believe that the situation will turn out to be just a bad dream. As the disability persists and is recognized as reality, there may be denial of the permanence of the disability.[9] Denial may be manifested by cheerfulness and an unrealistic lack of concern about the disabling condition.[22]

The failure to accept the reality of the circumstances results in unproductive behavior such as shopping for miracle cures or the "right" experts. Such patients may be difficult to work with in rehabilitation.[9,18] They do not accept the role of the disabled person and, consequently, do not want to work toward restorative and compensatory activities that would lead them to a productive life.[18]

Denial can also be helpful. It may help the patient to restore some emotional equilibrium and is usually followed by a more realistic attitude toward the disability.[18]

REPRESSION. Repression is the mechanism that removes painful memories from awareness. This mechanism may be necessary to the readjustment of some disabled persons. Selective forgetting of one's former attitudes toward the disabled may be necessary to self acceptance.[9] On the other hand, discussion of painful thoughts and memories may be necessary to achieving progress in restoring psychic equilibrium and in rehabilitation. Such discussion should be carried out only by well-trained persons, however.[18]

PROJECTION. Shifting responsibility for an act or a thought to another is the mechanism of projection. Its purpose is to avoid confronting failures or aggression.

The patient with an acquired disability may project previously held negative attitudes about the disabled onto others. They may attribute negative attitudes toward the disabled to rehabilitation personnel and family. Rehabilitation workers may expend much effort in getting patients to acknowledge their feelings and to accept responsibility for them so that they can gain control of their rehabilitation.[9,18]

DISPLACEMENT. In displacement, energy associated with one object or person is directed to a secondary target. For example, anger about the cause of the disability may be directed to the rehabilitation staff, which had nothing to do with its onset. The disabled person does not know who to blame and is asking the question, "Why did this happen to me?"

Negative energy associated with such inner conflict is often released on family, friends, and rehabilitation personnel. Sometimes the anger is internalized and leads to depression. Vacillation between anger and depression may occur.

Patients displaying displacement should be confronted about their behavior and made aware of its negative effect on loved ones and those engaged in their rehabilitation efforts. A disability does not give one the right to be rude or uncivil to others.[18]

SUBLIMATION. Sublimation is the process of channeling energy from prohibited goals to more socially acceptable ones. In rehabilitation, anger and aggression should be channeled into constructive activities. However, it is important not to replace interaction with others with activities. Resolution of interpersonal conflict is an important part of the rehabilitation process.[18]

AGGRESSION. Bravado and aggressiveness may be used to cover helplessness and dependency and to hide deep fears and anxieties.[22] Aggression can be directed inward to self or outward to others. As a coping style, it may take one of two forms—hostile aggression or aggressive behavior. Hostile aggression is not constructive in the rehabilitation process and is disruptive. Aggressive behavior, on the other hand, can be productive, as in aggressively pursuing rehabilitation goals. Aggressive behavior can be a way of asserting oneself. For some disabled persons, assertive behavior should be encouraged.[18]

DEPENDENCY. Dependency may be manifested by keeping family and personnel close by and having more attendant care than is realistically needed.[22]

The individual who uses dependency relies on others to perform activities of daily living (ADL). It is the behavioral symbol of a helpless attitude. All people are dependent to some extent; no one is capable of meeting all needs without some outside assistance. However, dependency tends to be regarded as a negative trait. Dependent persons may be thought of as lazy or lacking in initiative, but dependency really is a surrendering of independent problem-solving and the looking to others to find solutions to problems.[18]

Some patients will react against independence after some rehabilitation gains have been made. This is most likely to occur in late adolescents and young adults and those with long-standing, latent conflicts of dependency-versus-independence in the developmental phase of separation and individuation. It is important for the staff to understand the patient's developmental issues in order to plan appropriate intervention strategies.[25]

Patients whose premorbid personalities tended to be passive and dependent may have difficulty in rehabilitation and may resist efforts to end the sick role and associated dependency. For these patients, limits must be placed on regression, and the staff must be consistent in the use of clearly expressed expectations for cooperation and participation in the rehabilitation program.[25]

Some disabled persons present themselves as unable to do anything about their problems. Rehabilitation personnel must guard against allowing patients to become overly dependent on them. A balance between control and assistance must be maintained, since the ultimate goal of rehabilitation is to facilitate self-help.[18]

SELF-ABASEMENT. This is a passive coping mechanism characterized by humbling and denigrating oneself. It evokes the help of others. If the individual believes that the disability is the result of sin, self-abasement may be used as retribution. The belief of some disabled persons that they are inferior to others is another cause of self-abasement.

Those in helping roles should focus on positive attributes before directing attention to behavior that is in need of change. The success or failure of rehabilitation ultimately depends on the patient's ability to accept the self as a worthwhile human being.[18]

REGRESSION. Reverting to feelings, thoughts, and behaviors that worked well for coping in the past is sometimes used to relieve anxiety. Regression is a way of denying reality. Helpers may be seen as parents, lovers, or friends who met the patient's needs earlier in life. If the patient does not accept helpers for who they really are, the disability is not accepted, and the rehabilitation process is delayed. Rehabilitation workers must be careful not to get involved in the ego gratification that may be derived from thinking that they can replace others in the patient's life.[18] When some of the more significant problems are solved, the disabled person may regain enough confidence to resume more mature behavior.[9]

RATIONALIZATION. Justification of thoughts or behavior with reasons that are more acceptable to the ego than the actual reasons are is called rationalization. The process of rationalization is not often in the individual's consciousness. Rationalization may take four forms: (1) blaming incidental causes for problems, (2) devaluing unobtainable goals, (3) finding some advantage in an undesirable situation, and (4) mentally balancing negative and positive traits. An example of the first form occurs when disabled persons believe others do not like them because they are disabled. In the second instance, an example is the person who convinces himself or herself that it was all right to lose a job because the salary was too low.

An example of the third form can be found in the fable of the blind man who stated that being blind made him a better person because he no longer judged others by externals such as clothing or skin color. Beliefs such as "pretty women are dumb" or "disabled persons have more human understanding" are examples of the fourth form.[9]

COMPENSATION. Compensation is a way of making up for a deficit in one area by capitalizing on strengths in another. For example, a disabled person may excel in academics to compensate for the inability to excel in sports. Compensation is an unconscious decision. It may be necessary to bring it to consciousness so that the patient can make a self-assessment of strengths and weaknesses. Compensation may be helpful and wholesome if adjustment is personally and socially satisfying.[9,18]

FANTASY. Fantasy is the substitution of imaginary activities for actual activities.[18] It is a way to gain satisfactions not available in real life.[9] Continuous fantasy can be a sign of serious problems; however, the disabled person can use fantasy to cope until better solutions are found.[18] The use of fantasy can be channeled constructively in role-playing situations. The disabled person who is afraid to be seen in public or to participate in social situations can imagine doing so in role playing and become desensitized. It can be used to help the individual develop a repertoire of behaviors although he or she cannot be allowed to abandon the actual world for fantasy.[9,18]

PASSING. The denial of difference and attempts to conceal it is the process known as passing. This is a conscious behavior and not a true defense mechanism. Passing indicates shame and is a source of interaction strain. It requires constant vigilance, and denying the disability becomes a central focus of life. Acceptance, rather than denial, of the disability frees the person to utilize internal and external resources toward maximum rehabilitation.[18] Those whose disabilities are not apparent to others, such as persons with epilepsy or cardiac dysfunction, can use passing to some advantage. It allows the person to manage the initial stages of social interaction to permit essential personal traits to have primary influence on relationships.

When a disability is visible, passing is impossible. Such persons must manage tension in social encounters. The person who uses passing must manage tension as well as information about the disability. If the hidden disability is ultimately revealed, the person must deal with the discomfort when others learn the truth.[9]

Whether passing is a negative or positive behavior depends on the reasons for adopting this coping strategy. If it is not caused by a negative self-concept and serves a practical purpose, it can be a sign of adjustment and a concern for the discomfort of others. If it is used because the person is ashamed of the disability, it can be a sign of low self-esteem.[9]

The Compromise Body Image

According to Simon, the ultimate adjustment to the physical dysfunction is intimately related to the process of developing a new "compromise body image."[42] The body image consists of multiple perceptions about the body based on past experience, current sensations, and personal investment in the body. The development of the body image is influenced by the attitudes and values of the culture and the views, values, and fantasies of others in one's life. Parental attitudes about body parts and body functions are important factors in the development of the body image. All of the experiences and attitudes may result in an overvaluation of particular body parts and the perception of the body as good or bad, handsome or repugnant, lovable or unlovable. One may compare the body to the bodies of others and develop derogatory attitudes toward the body or its parts. One may also develop mechanisms of compensation to obscure perceived stigma.

The ego may feel anxiety, shame, or disgust in relation to the body image and may develop defenses to avoid the unpleasant effect of an unacceptable body image. By using such defenses as denial, sublimation, repression, and overcompensation, the person comes to accept the "compromise body image" that incorporates and modifies some of the unacceptable features. The compromise body image is an important factor in considering the emotional effects of physical dysfunction.

Most people who incur physical disability will initially experience worry and anxiety about the dysfunction. Old anxieties and fears about illness and disability will be evoked. The individual will experience realistic fears about the loss of security or loss of love from spouse, family, and friends. There is a loss of the fantasied future and a serious concern that the future may be dramatically altered.

Sadness and depression are to be expected for periods as long as 1 year. Depression is a mourning for the lost part or function. The lost part, function, and former body image are gradually surrendered, and there is resolution of anger. Psychic energy can then be freed for new activity, often for wholehearted involvement in rehabilitation efforts. The individual may compensate or even overcompensate for the loss in a healthy manner, and a new compromise body image emerges.[42]

Stages in Adjustment to Physical Dysfunction

Adjustment to physical dysfunction was described by Kerr and others as progressing through five stages. The adjustment process is analogous to the grief process described by Kübler-Ross.[20,24–26]

It is necessary to remember that the stages are points on a continuum and that all stages are not inevitable for all disabled persons. It is also important to understand the adjustment process, since there appears to be a relationship between the person's attitude toward the physical disability and the success of rehabilitation.

The stages as described by Kerr are as follows:[24]
1. Shock: "This isn't me."
2. Expectancy of recovery: "I'm sick but I'll get well."
3. Mourning: "All is lost."
4. Defensive A—healthy: "I'll go on in spite of it." Defensive B—pathological: Marked use of defenses to deny the effects of the disability.
5. Adjustment: "It's different but not bad."

SHOCK. Shock is an immediate reaction to trauma and occurs during the early diagnostic and treatment period.[25] It includes a sense of numbness and the inability to integrate or comprehend the magnitude of the event.[25]

The person lacks understanding that the body is ill or of the extent of the seriousness of the illness or injury. Because of these factors, there may be an apparent lack of anxiety that appears to be unrealistic. As the reality of the situation becomes more apparent to the person, the reacton is "This can't be me. It's a bad dream. I'll wake up, and this will all be gone." The disabled person is likely to blame the hospital and medical personnel for the lost ability to function. The feeling is "If I could only get out of here, I'd be all right." Psychologically, the person is still a normal, able-bodied person, pursuing the same goals and doing the same things as before the onset of the disabling condition.

There is an incompatibility between the person's real physical situation and the mental image. This incompatibility may account for the person's apparently inappropriate references to the disability, situation, recovery, and future performance. At this stage body image is more potent than perceptions. Perceptions incompatible with the self-image are rejected.

There is also an inevitable testing of reality that occurs after the onset of disability, and when the fact of changed function comes into focus, the psychological situation changes. A pathological "denial of illness" may occur and some persons previously considered psychologically healthy remain in this stage.[24]

EXPECTANCY OF RECOVERY OR DENIAL.[20,24,25] This stage lasts from a few days to 2 or 3 months. The patient may maintain that recovery will be quick and complete. It is a defense mechanism against the sudden, drastic change in functioning and the realization that his or her condition is generally permanent. Denial of the severity and irreversibility of the situation is maintained, and there is hope that the situation will be reversed in the future.[25] The patient may make frequent references to getting well or being whole again and may discuss future plans in which full recovery or a normally functioning body is essential.

The individual's only goal is to get well. This may lead to the search for a cure and "shopping" from one physician or health care agency to another. There is a preoccupation with the physical condition. Small improvements may be overestimated or misinterpreted. The person will do anything perceived as aiding recovery, since this is the primary goal. To the extent that it is believed that recovery will take place, motivation toward learning to function with a disability will be minimal.[24]

The person believes realistically that the disability is a barrier to everything in life that is important and worthwhile. A whole body is needed to attain important personal goals. Therefore full recovery must be achieved before anything else can be undertaken.[24]

Family, friends, and medical personnel may encourage denial by urging the individual not to think of his or her losses and may make false promises of recovery. The persistence of denial delays the healing process of grief.[20]

A change in this belief system or progress toward the next stage comes about when the person is moved toward a condition more similar to normal living than to the state of being temporarily ill. Being transferred from an acute care setting to the rehabilitation unit, being discharged in a wheelchair, having therapy terminated, having therapy redirected to learning to live with the disability, or being told that full recovery will not occur are some of the events that may precipitate mourning.[24]

MOURNING OR DEPRESSION. Mourning occurs when there is a shift from expectancy of recovery to the realization that the disability is permanent. This realization may be overwhelming and may require the intervention of specialists in psychiatry or psychology.[24]

Depression is a response to a sense of helplessness and a loss of self-esteem. Anxiety, sadness, and grief are natural and appropriate and are to be expected in the adjustment process. Self-esteem may be low and the individual may have a sense of helplessness and of being a burden to others. The initial depression involves difficulty in integrating the residual disability into a new self-concept.[25] All seems lost, and all former goals seem unattainable. Motivation to cope with the disability is gone. The person wants to give up and may contemplate suicide.[24,25]

Sadness is not easily expressed, and any overt expression may be associated with childishness. It is important for rehabilitation personnel to assure the patient that such sadness is normal and natural and to encourage its expression if the patient is to move beyond this stage. The mourning patient needs the opportunity to express and work out such feelings before progress in adjustment can be made.[20] If the individual is not allowed to express grief for the lost function or part because of the reprimands and attitudes of rehabilitation personnel and others, discussion of these feelings may be avoided and hostility toward those who forbid the expression of feelings may be demonstrated. The result is a "problem patient" who will not work and who spends much time complaining about the health care agency procedures and personnel.[24]

The patient may subsequently externalize hostility and blame for the loss to family, friends, physicians, and rehabilitation personnel. Hostility and anger must be channeled to productive activity to make rehabilitation gains.[25]

The person may become resigned to this fate, believing that he or she is worthless and inadequate, and may remain at this stage in the process. The person may adopt the role of the invalid and become a permanent resident of a health care institution.[28] He or she simply lives and remains dependent and, possibly, hostile.

The disability is now seen as an impenetrable barrier to important life goals, and unlike the hope for recovery that characterized the previous stage, the goal of recovery is now seen as unrealistic.

To effect progress to the next stage, the barrier imposed by the disability must be reduced. To the degree that this is possible, progress in adjustment and rehabilitation can be made. It may be possible to create situations in which previously held goals can be attained. However, because self-care activities were probably taken for granted, accomplishing them may not be seen as a positive goal by adults.[24]

The person in this stage may also begin to mourn the loss of some psychological characteristics. The patient may believe he or she has lost his "fight," "pride," or "faith," which can be more distressing than the physical loss. When this occurs, it may be important to expose the person to situations in which disabled persons can be observed demonstrating these qualities. The person can then begin to realize that the disability is irrelevant for the attainment of some more basic goals.[24]

DEFENSIVE A—HEALTHY. The defensive stage may be considered healthy if the person begins to deal with the disability and goes on in spite of it. Motivation to learn to function with the disability increases significantly. The person is pleased with his or her accomplishments and takes an active interest in being as normal as possible.

The disability barrier is being reduced and becomes less impenetrable. The person attains some goals that were held as a nondisabled person. Some treasured experiences, albeit small, are still possible. The barrier is still present, however, but there is the discovery of ways to circumvent it. The person learns to achieve previously held goals by other routes. Other goals may remain unattainable, and the person may remain distressed by the areas perceived to be unachievable.[24]

The movement toward adjustment comes through a changed need system. The need for a whole or normal body may be relinquished when important goals can be attained in spite of the disability. The goals are attainable, therefore the disability becomes less relevant. When physical impairment does in fact interfere with goal attainment, the person must relinquish the goals and discover equally satisfying ways of meeting important needs.[24]

DEFENSIVE B—PATHOLOGICAL. The defensive stage may be considered pathological if the person uses defense mechanisms to deny the continued existence of a partial barrier imposed by the disability. Diverse behavior may be displayed, depending on the defense mechanisms used. The person may try to conceal the disability; may rationalize and say he or she does not want the things that are unattainable; may project negative feelings to others, claiming that they cannot accept the disability although he or she has; and may try to convince others that he or she is well-adjusted. The existence of barriers imposed by the disability is denied.[24] A new compromise body image that can be accepted both consciously and unconsciously fails to develop. Psychotic reactions may result. Passive, dependent reactions may be manifested by a complete loss of motivation and a surrendering of all ambition. Psychological regression may become apparent, and pathological denial may be manifested by an inability to express negative feelings and by a repression of anger.[42]

Under some additional stress, the person may regress to an earlier stage and remain there permanently, or he or she may progress to adequate adjustment after a temporary regression.

ADAPTATION OR ADJUSTMENT. After grief, mourning, and hope of return are relinquished, new roles based on new functions can be achieved. An understanding of the patient's defense mechanisms and coping strategies will help facilitate the process of adaptation to functioning with a physical difference. The therapist can assess coping strategies by finding out how the patient customarily managed stresses. Coping strategies tend to be consistent, and stresses are handled by intensified use of previous strategies. If they can be identified, those strategies that can be used to enhance rehabilitation efforts can be maximized, whereas those that deter such efforts must be rechanneled.[25] If an adequate adjustment is attained, the person considers the disability as merely one of many personal characteristics. The disability is no longer considered a major barrier to be overcome. It is regarded as one of many assets or liabilities, and satisfying ways to meet personal needs and goals have been found.

It cannot be assumed that teaching the disabled person to do things will automatically lead to an adequate adjustment. Two other goals, held by many people, will need to be attained before adjustment is possible. The first goal lies in religion or personal philosophy. The person with religious beliefs must feel "right with God." All of the beliefs about the role of suffering in relation to God's influence on life must be resolved. The disability will be a barrier between the person and God as long as it is regarded as a punishment or if the person believes that God surely will heal those who love Him. Second is the goal of achieving a feeling of personal adequacy. Because of the tendency in our society to relegate the disabled to an inferior status, the disabled person must be helped to discriminate between adequate and inferior on the basis of characteristics rather than on physique and productivity.[24,44] The person must be helped to reach these more abstract goals before adjustment is attained.[24]

Sexual Adjustment

After pain, fear of death, and major discomforts of the disability have subsided, newly disabled persons begin to reassess life and relationships. Social concerns become more intense. Questions about attractiveness and the possibility of sexual relationships arise.[9] The sex-related limitations imposed by the disability and sexual taboos and prohibitions generate anxiety in the disabled person. Anxiety can be intensified by misunderstanding and misinformation in the patient, the professional staff, and the family. Anxiety increases if the patient's questions are not answered or concerns are not discussed. If such silence prevails, the patient receives the message that he or she is an asexual being and that sex should not be a concern.[19] Uncertainties about sexual matters will be influenced by the attitudes of helping professionals and the pre-

morbid beliefs of the disabled individual about the sexuality of the disabled.[9]

Professionals who are reluctant to address the patient's sexual concerns send the message to the patient that his or her fears are well-founded and that interest or efforts that do not focus directly on the disabling condition are of minor concern.[9,10] The predisability attitudes of disabled persons make them aware that others may regard them as asexual or incapable of any satisfying sexual activity.[9] Because sexual matters are regarded as very personal and private, patients are reluctant to discuss them. The patient may consider sexual concerns as separate from the disability and think that they are to be borne in silence and handled without assistance.[10]

Professional interest in the sexuality of disabled persons grew in the 1960s and 1970s. Initial interest and research was focused on persons with spinal cord injury and later extended to interest in other disabilities. Today, rehabilitation is incomplete if sexual rehabilitation is not addressed in the overall program.[9] Sexuality seems to play an important role for the patient coping with disability, and research has shown a relationship between sexuality and self-esteem.[34] Disability may have some effect on sexual functioning, but sex drives of the disabled are not different from those of the nondisabled. Problems encountered by the disabled person may be physiological, psychological, or social or any combination of these factors.[9]

Disabled persons are capable of participating in some form of sexual activity. They may engage in "normal" sexual behavior, alternative behaviors, or indulge only in casual expressions of tenderness. The focus of much of the available information has been on the mechanics of sex; however, sex is a complex behavior and must be considered from its perspectives as a biological drive, a learned behavior, and the expression of both drive and learned behavior in a relationship with another person. The disabled face their greatest problems in the area of sexual expression or sexuality.[9] Sexual problems and their management relative to specific disabilities have been outlined by several authors.[16,17,40]

Sexuality concerns and subsequent adjustment will be influenced by the age and developmental stage in which the onset of the disability occurred. The concerns of the adolescent with no previous sexual experience will be different from the concerns of the adult who has memories and experiences on which to draw.[10] Sexuality involves conversing, sharing interests, expressing feelings, and engaging in mutually satisfying sexual activities. Sexual fulfillment requires acceptance by another as a worthwhile, desirable companion and relating in other ways that are emotionally and physically satisfying.[9]

PSYCHOSOCIAL CONSIDERATIONS IN TREATMENT OF PHYSICAL DYSFUNCTION
Interpersonal Approaches in Treatment

ATTITUDES TOWARD THE PATIENT. In the treatment of physical dysfunction, the patient must be regarded as a whole person. The individual's capabilities, problems, interests, experiences, needs, fears, prejudices, beliefs, cultural influences, and reactions to the physical dysfunction are as important as the physical considerations in planning interaction strategies and the treatment program.[47]

To facilitate self-acceptance, the occupational therapist can demonstrate to the patient that he or she is accepted as a total person and that feelings of shame or guilt need not be associated with the disability. The therapist reacts to the patient as a person who happens to have a disability. Such an approach will reduce the fear and anxiety associated with being different. The therapist should demonstrate genuineness, empathy, and concern for the patient as a unique human being.[44]

The patient will reflect attitudes of personnel and family. The psychologic reactions and relationships between personnel and patient will affect the patient's reaction to the disability and, often, the degree of participation in the rehabilitation program.[22]

Becoming disabled alters a person's life situation not only in terms of functional performance but also in social interactions with others. The newly disabled person knows that there has not been a change in selfhood because of the disability, yet that person may be assigned an inferior status both by the nondisabled and by professional "helpers." Customary social behavior may stimulate responses very different from those that are usual or anticipated by the disabled individual. This may cause questioning of personal identity, appropriate roles, and expectations in performance ability. The early answers to such questions come from the rehabilitation personnel in everyday treatment situations. By their words and actions, personnel may communicate answers to critical and perhaps unspoken questions from the disabled person.[23]

Behavior of personnel that reflects respect for the rights, capabilities, and abilities of the disabled person to make judgments and be involved in the rehabilitation process communicates their belief in the disabled individual as a human being and a fully functioning adult. It is important for rehabilitation personnel to not automatically assign patients to an inferior status or to treat them as dependent children. The communication of a belief in the capacities of the disabled is essential. An attitude of helping the disabled person to explore and discover possibilities in performance skills and social interchange is much more helpful than preconceived notions and conclusions about their capacities by the "experts." Involvement of the patient on the rehabilitation team to the extent possible is a critical factor in communicating the belief that the disabled person can be a self-determining agent in the rehabilitation process.[23]

The focus of rehabilitation should be on helping the person to reformulate an approving self who wishes to continue with life despite important discontinuity with past identity. This requires the development of a new self-image based on a sense of worth rather than on deficiency and self-contempt.[41]

Adverse or negative reactions of rehabilitation workers toward patients may stem from a number of causes. Personality incompatibility or prejudicial reactions to a particular age, sex, ethnic group, or physical dysfunction are some of the factors that can evoke a negative reaction. Awareness and admission of adverse reactions are the first steps in coping with them constructively. Some signs of adverse reactions to patients are (1) failure to keep appointments; (2) offering less treatment time; (3) frequently arranging for the patient to be treated by an aide, student, or other therapist; (4) unnatural and excessive politeness and service to the patient; (5) a feeling of boredom when the patient is present; (6) a tendency to ignore the patient when others are present; (7) unrealistic optimism or pessimism about the patient's prognosis or potential achievements; and (8) giving the patient inadequate answers and instructions.[22]

To deal with adverse reactions to patients, rehabilitation personnel who become aware of these reactions may undergo a self-analysis or analysis with the aid of peers or a psychologic counselor to identify the underlying cause of the negative reaction, if it is not readily apparent. Discussion of such reactions with the patient who evokes them is sometimes appropriate. If the reaction is caused by an asocial or inappropriate behavior that is within the patient's capacity to change and if changed would aid in acceptance by others, discussion of the feeling with the patient may be helpful. Personnel may be able to change their reactions and reconstruct interaction with the patient more positively through ongoing counseling with peers or a professional counselor. If these measures fail and the negative reactions cannot be resolved, transferring the patient to the care of another is essential to progress.[22,42]

SELF-DEFINITION. Geis stresses self-definition and a sense of personal worth as critical factors in successful rehabilitation and suggests some methods for helping patients to value themselves positively.[14] If the disabled person is to achieve successful adjustment and adaptation, he or she cannot continue to value the self in terms of an unrealistic self-image.

The individual's definition of self is the crucial factor, determining the degree of sense of worth and self-satisfaction that can be achieved. Things outside of the patient do not satisfy him or her; rather, satisfaction is derived in terms of these things. The patient determines which things will bring satisfaction in terms of personal definition and concept of self. If this is the case, what kind of self-definition must be achieved for success, and how can rehabilitation personnel help the patient achieve a positive and worthwhile definition of self?

The goal of rehabilitation is to help the patient to change a self-defeating definition to one that is self-enhancing. When the patient's standards for attractiveness, productivity, or achievement are fixed, and he or she can only define self and measure individual value in terms of these standards, problems are encountered in the rehabilitation process and adjustment. Therapy involves helping the patient to experience the fact that a person does not have to achieve a certain standard of productivity to be worthwhile and that his or her need to do this is only a fixed belief. The patient needs to be directed to satisfactions that are attainable and helped to value goals and self preferentially rather than by some absolute standard.

In treatment, the traditional focus has been on helping the patient to develop better modes of "doing." An emphasis on doing only or becoming efficient at reaching performance goals may focus self-valuation on an extrinsic standard of productivity. What is needed is to add to treatment modalities techniques for helping the patient to simply "be" and to value things in themselves. Geis describes "being" as a spontaneous expressive activity that may be purposeless and nonstriving.[14] It exists during such pursuits as fiestas, ballet, dancing, and leisure activities and enjoying theatrical performances, comic events, and sports events, in which gratification is intrinsic and linked with the process rather than with the goal or end result of the activity. In contrast, "doing" activity has its satisfaction linked with the effect or ultimate achievement of the end-goal of the activity process. Before the onset of physical disability the patient's self-definition and sense of personal worth, in most cases, have been based largely on "doing" behavior. With the onset of physical dysfunction, there is a major loss of the self-satisfaction derived from "doing." This may evoke a reduced sense of self-worth, which can be improved by helping the patient derive gratification, and increase value to self as a result, from "being" experiences. Treatment methods that emphasize the patient's exploration, manipulation, personal interests and choices, enjoyment, delight, and play can facilitate self-satisfaction from "being."[14]

PREVENTING MALADJUSTMENT. Pathological reactions in adjustment may be prevented if personnel can recognize the stage of adjustment that the patient is experiencing and structure approaches and activities to accommodate the patient's particular emotional needs at that point in the adjustment process. Patients should be encouraged to express their fears, anxieties, worries, and sense of loss. This must be done with tact and understanding. Personnel must expect that strong emotions exist in the patient and must be prepared to invite the expression of these emotions and to cope with them. Personnel should not minimize the problems or enter into the patient's denial. Attitudes of acceptance of the individual with the physical dysfunction will help his self-acceptance. A cheerful and optimistic attitude is useful, but the appropriate expression of irritation and anger by personnel may help the patient realize that expressions of emotion are allowed and the acceptance of personnel will not be lost if such feelings are expressed.[22,42]

Early recognition of pathological reactions by personnel trained in personality development and the use of mental defense mechanisms is important.[22,31] Personnel should observe for deep depression, suicidal tendencies, undue guilt or preoccupation with symptoms, bizarre behavior, confusion, paranoid symptoms, or schizophrenic behavior.[22]

Personnel should share their observations for reality testing and for referral of problems to the appropriate specialists with other members of the rehabilitation team. There should be a concerted effort to deal with the normal adjustment process and minor problems. Assistance and special treatment by psychiatric or psychological specialists may be required to manage pathological reactions. Evaluation and treatment of the patient and counsel of personnel by these specialists may be helpful in dealing effectively with the patient, coping with feelings toward the patient, and helping the patient progress toward a healthy adjustment.[21]

ENHANCING ADJUSTMENT. The goal of rehabilitation then is to promote ego integrity and feelings of self-worth. Early rehabilitation efforts should be directed toward shaping basic life goals, and later efforts should shift to the emotional, physical, and technical resources necessary for their accomplishment.[41]

The job of rehabilitation workers is to help the disabled person feel that he or she, as a personality, still continues. Functional aid should be seen in the larger context of enhancing self-respect. Functional and physical progress can be ego builders and aid in the adjustment process. However, functional efforts in the early stages of rehabilitation should be strategies designed to help the patient see that performance is possible and should serve as a promise for the future. Emphasis on functional achievements as ends in themselves for specific skill development can serve as a means of avoiding the affective implications of physical dysfunction that must be manifested and resolved.

Therefore, the proper role of the rehabilitation worker is that of assistant to the patient. Unfortunately, most rehabilitation settings are founded on the medical model. The professionals assume the expert and authoritarian role, whereas the patients assume a passive, dependent, and compliant role. Passivity and authoritarian direction are inappropriate for persons with chronic, permanent conditions. Their role is the principal investment, and the roles of personnel are secondary.[41]

The patient's self-enhancement is supported when rehabilitation workers abandon their sense of omnipotence and see themselves as assistants to the patient as she or he goes about the job of restoring his or her life. The roles of the professional must shift from that of active authoritarian to a more passive mode of professional behavior. The role of the patient must shift from passive recipient of services to active doer. The rehabilitation approach is more suitable than the medical model approach when treating physically disabled persons. Except for the period of acute illness or injury and the subsequent maintenance of good health, issues are social, emotional, functional, and vocational performance problems to be solved, for which the medical model is not appropriate.[41]

The occupational therapist plays an important role in facilitating psychosocial adjustment to physical dysfunction. A primary and concrete role is that of teaching the patient to cope with activities of daily living (ADL). The frustrations of dealing with minor ADL can make the rehabilitation process unbearable. The occupational therapist teaches the patient to master ADL and to deal with the problems of everyday life. Through the process of the ADL program, the patient learns to solve problems and gains confidence that frustrations associated with the disability can be overcome.[44] The occupational therapist is in a unique position to observe the patient's psychological functioning when working closely with him or her and observing the performance of a variety of tasks. Psychological factors such as motivation, initiative, creativity, originality, and persistence can be assessed by performance observation.[31]

Watson described a psychiatric consultation-liaison program in an acute physical disabilities setting.[44] This is a method of delivering psychiatric services to the physically ill and addresses problems that interfere with the patient's treatment. The goal of the program was to facilitate adjustment to a lifestyle compatible with the patient's value system, disability, and prognosis. Depression was the most common reason for referral to the program. A team approach was used, and the members were the psychiatrist, the psychiatric nurse, and the occupational therapist.

The occupational therapist used functional activities to help the patient explore the meaning of the disability or illness. Participation in activity and the accompanying discussion ultimately had a positive outcome, although the patient sometimes directed negative behavior or attitudes toward the therapist as limitations were confronted. The occupational therapist used informal discussion to address fears, anxieties, feelings of helplessness, and vulnerability. The treatment program helped the patient redefine problems and assets.[46]

The goals of occupational therapy were to provide opportunities for mastery and control, reduce emotional distress, promote psychological competence, and help to maintain or establish an active support network. The occupational therapy evaluation assessed premorbid competencies and level of functioning; previously used coping methods; roles, responsibilities, values, and goals; past history and interests; available support network; and discharge plans. This information was attained through interviews and through observation during participation in activities. The occupational therapist encouraged the discussion and helped the patient to evaluate the situation.

The therapist's primary concern was to build rapport. This was accomplished by meeting the patient on his or her level, showing an understanding of the patient's emotional distress, and structuring the environment to promote psychological competence. Activities related to the patient's roles, interests, values, and responsibilities were important to promote psychological competence. Activities such as homemaking, cooking, crafts, games, and work simulations proved to be gratifying and motivating.

The focus in treatment was on ability rather than disability. The therapist structured treatment to ensure success. Making objects for others helped the patient resume the role of contributor. A treatment program focused on doing and giving, rather than on symptoms and complaints, helped to re-establish significant relationships and restore engagement in meaningful activities. The therapist gradually transferred responsibility for choice and control to the patient in the treatment situation. The therapist had to be continuously aware of the patient's emotional status and changing psychosocial needs. Easily accomplished, pleasant, and familiar activities were initially used to motivate and engage the patient. As emotional stresses decreased, more demanding physical rehabilitation activities were introduced.[46]

Group Approaches

Besides interpersonal interaction strategies to facilitate adjustment to physical dysfunction, several group approaches have been proposed, which can be applied in occupational therapy. Therapeutic communities, self-help groups, milieu therapy, group counseling, and sensitivity training may be helpful to facilitate the patient's adjustment and the development of a positive self-image.[11]

Kutner states that "in the diagnostic work-up and medical treatment plan of the recently disabled patient, it is rather rare to include a listing of 'role disorders' accompanying the illness or injury. . . . They require not the cursory attention typically accorded them but specific and purposeful therapy."[28] This statement has important implications for occupational therapy. The occupational therapist, concerned with the patient's occupational performance in self-maintenance, work, play, and leisure roles, is the expert in role definition, role analysis, and role change. Indeed a list of "role disorders" should appear in the medical record contained in the occupational therapy reports.

MILIEU THERAPY. Kutner suggests that milieu therapy may offer a solution for acquiring new roles, readapting old ones, and gaining the social and physical skills necessary to reach goals.[28]

Milieu therapy is particularly appropriate for use by occupational therapists, since it uses environmental or residential settings as a training ground for patients to practice social, interpersonal, and functional skills and to test their ability to deal with problems commonly encountered in the community. This approach to treatment has always been fundamental to occupational therapy practice.

The milieu therapy program engages the patient in a variety of social encounters, both group and individual, and exposes the patient to increasingly challenging problems. This same gradation can be applied to performance skills concomitantly. The experiences are structured to test social competence, judgment, problem-solving ability, and social responsibility.

The major therapeutic objective of milieu therapy is the maintenance of the achievements acquired in the rehabilitation program. It attempts to provide the patient with the necessary social, psychologic, and performance skills to overcome frustration, to deal effectively with new or risky social situations, to cope with rebuff or rejection, and to remain independent.

Most therapeutic efforts have been concentrated on physical restoration, with the assumption that personal and social readjustment follow automatically when physical integrity is restored. When adjustment difficulties occur, it has been customary to call on social, psychological, and psychiatric services to manage these special problems. In contrast, milieu therapy deals with the problems of adjustment to new or changed roles by structuring situations and environments to allow the patient to adopt and test roles as part of the treatment process.[28]

THE SELF-HELP GROUP. The self-help group model is another approach to managing psychosocial adjustment to physical dysfunction. Jaques and Patterson reviewed the growth and development of self-help groups in this country and described their effectiveness in the aid and rehabilitation of their members.[21] The self-help group is one that provides aid for each group member around specific problems or goals. Positive benefits to members of self-help groups include (1) gaining information and knowledge about the dysfunction or the problem, (2) learning coping skills from group members who are living successfully with the condition, (3) gaining motivation and support through communication with others who have similar experiences, (4) modeling the successful problem-solving behaviors of group members, (5) evaluating one's own progress, (6) belonging to and identifying with a group, and (7) finding self-help in a situation of mutual concern.

The mutual aid or self-help group is an excellent means of maintaining rehabilitation gain and preventing deterioration of function. It provides modeling by members who are coping with stigma and problems of functioning and reintegrating life roles.

Certain operational assumptions are characteristic of the self-help approach. Individuals with shared problems come together. All group members maintain peer status. Peers come together expecting to help themselves or one another. Behavior change is expected in each person at his own pace. Group members identify with the program, are committed to it, and practice its principles in daily life. There are regularly scheduled group meetings, but peers are available to one another as needed outside of group meetings. This allows for both individual and group modes of contact. The group process includes acknowledging, revealing, and relating problems; receiving and giving feedback; and sharing hopes, experiences, encouragement, and criticism. Members are responsible for themselves and their behavior. Leadership develops and changes within the group on the basis of giving and receiving help. Status comes from giving and receiving help effectively.

Many persons who were not helped in professional relationships and experiences turned to and received aid in self-help groups, which arose to meet needs that professionals could not meet. The professional process and self-help group models can share experiences with one another under certain conditions. The professional must meet the conditions of common problems, peer relationship, and mutual aid, and those professionals who cannot meet these conditions can act only as visitors or observers. A professional can act as a consultant or speaker to self-help groups if invited to do so by the group; however, professional therapeutic skills cannot be used as such inside the self-help group.[21]

The self-help group model, or some modification of it, has application in occupational therapy. It may have most potential for use in long-term rehabilitation programs, extended-care facilities, or community day care programs. Self-help groups could be initiated from the common needs of patients in the program. The focus on solving problems in functional performance can provide a safe area for sharing. Ultimately, as group relationships are cemented and mutual support is achieved, group members may move freely to emotional and social concerns and to problems of community reintegration. The occupational therapist and other concerned professionals could act as consultants, invited speakers, or group members, if the necessary conditions outlined previously are met.

GROUP COUNSELING. A group counseling approach to psychological rehabilitation for patients with spinal cord injuries was described by Mann, Godfrey, and Dowd.[31] The group was based on the proposition that self-concept is one of the factors determining psychological adjustment to physical disability. The goals of the group were to assist each patient in increasing self-concept to assist in total rehabilitation, to overcome depression, to provide a setting where problems with interpersonal relationships could be discussed and plans for their resolution could be made, and to modify perceptual distortions that patients may have about staff or other patients.

In the group, older patients assisted new patients in coming to terms with their disability and with planning a new life. Leadership was assumed by former patients. Patients were given feedback about their strengths and assets by leaders and other patients. This was done to correct negative self-evaluation. Group interaction focused on ways in which each patient could make maximum use of remaining function rather than on concentrating on lost abilities. Patients

were encouraged to share feelings with the group and reaped the benefit of knowing that others had similar feelings and experiences.

The group operated on an open basis, with members coming and going at will. Initially, patients were selected by the therapists, based on perceived need for psychological assistance, verbal ability, and ideas and resources that potential members could offer the group. Subsequently, members began to bring other patients with them, and they were allowed to join.

The sessions were informally structured and presented to the patients as an opportunity to discuss feelings and concerns. The sessions progressed from the discussion of things to the discussion of people, interpersonal relationships, and self exploration. The general focus of the sessions remained on the situational aspects of the disabilities rather than on psychodynamics. The leaders of the group were two occupational therapists and a psychologist.[31]

SEXUAL COUNSELING. Many patients make a satisfactory sexual adjustment without outside help, whereas others do not. Occupational therapists can provide support and information to facilitate adjustment.[40] Because occupational therapists are most concerned with the functional aspects of the patient's life, they are in an excellent position to provide information on sexual functioning.[33] Occupational therapy regards sexual functioning as an activity of daily living. As with other ADL, the occupational therapist's role is to facilitate the patient's achievement of an optimal level of independence.[34]

Therapists must be sensitive to the patient's concern about sexual readjustment. Accepting their sexuality may better enable the disabled person to accept the disability.[40] Changing social attitudes have made it easier for patients undergoing rehabilitation to seek assistance with sexuality and sexual functioning. Several different professionals may share in the responsibility for sexual counseling of the physically disabled. Psychological problems are likely to be handled by specialists in psychiatry, counseling, and social work. Physical problems with sexuality are most often managed by physicians, nurses, occupational therapists, and physical therapists within the domain of ADL.[7]

Rehabilitation personnel who are engaged in sexual counseling should be comfortable with their own sexuality, avoid projecting personal morals to the patient, be aware of their own limitations in providing counseling, and be willing to refer patients to other sources as necessary.[34]

Methods of counseling that are used include individual counseling, informal conversation, group sessions, and formal lectures. Some counselors prefer to have the patient's partner present, and counseling may be carried out in the ward, clinic, or the patient's home. Literature and films are media frequently used to disseminate information about sexuality counseling. Occupational therapists who do not feel qualified to do sexual counseling should obtain the necessary training, since it is an important part of the holistic approach to the patient.[34]

Neistadt and Baker described a program for sexual counseling of the physically disabled.[33] In preparation for the inception of the program, they reviewed the literature and attended relevant conferences. They attended the Sexual Attitude Reassessment Seminar (SARS) developed by Cole. Following this preparation, they organized the information into categories concerning the major functional problems encountered by the disabled and developed a list of suggested solutions for each problem. In-service meetings were provided to occupational therapy staff who could then engage in sexual counseling. In-service programs were conducted to inform other hospital personnel about the sexual counseling program.

Individual therapists decided when to initiate sexual counseling with their patients. Most found that a week or two before discharge from the facility was most suitable. They counseled patients about functional problems such as low endurance, contractures, sensory loss, incontinence, and communication problems. Different methods of counseling that were used included providing the patient with an informational booklet to be read privately, the booklet with discussion, and discussion without any written reference material. One counseling session was adequate for many patients, but therapists were available for additional sessions if needed. Serious psychological or medical problems were referred to the psychiatrist or physician.

Conine and others assessed the roles and attitudes of occupational therapists toward the sexual rehabilitation of the disabled.[7] They advised that evaluation of sexual dysfunction and sex education should be included in the patient's program with other ADL. These authors explored the specific tasks in sexual rehabilitation that were performed by the occupational therapist—whether therapists believed their performance of these tasks was important, whether they had adequate preparation to perform the tasks, and their attitude toward sexual rehabilitation in the context of occupational therapy and the rehabilitation process. The specific tasks identified were (1) sexual history taking as a part of the ADL evaluation; (2) training in personal care and hygiene related to sexual activity; (3) teaching management of indwelling catheters and diaphragms and other sexual devices; (4) providing information and intervention for the con-

trol of spasticity, pain, or phantom sensation; (5) advising on positioning; and (6) adapting the environment of prepartum and postpartum disabled women to their ADL needs and associated medical risks.

The results of this study indicated that occupational therapists are involved in a variety of tasks related to sexual rehabilitation. However, only about one third of the respondents were involved. Of the aforementioned tasks, occupational therapists were more likely to be involved in sexual history taking, providing sex education, advising on positioning, and remediating spasticity, pain, or phantom sensation. The lack of participation in other tasks may have resulted from role ambiguity and overlap of functions with other members of the rehabilitation team. These researchers concluded that there is a need for role delineation, content development, and education for sexual rehabilitation.[7]

Halstead presented a model for assessment and management of sexual problems.[17] Sexual history taking by the physician is the first part of the assessment. Sexual adjustment prior to the disability and present adjustment should be noted; potential outcomes of sexual counseling may be predicted on the basis of previous adjustment. Exploration of feelings of loss and setting realistic goals are important.

From the history, the physician or therapist can gain a general idea of the patient's knowledge of sexual function and activity, sexual satisfaction or dissatisfaction, and range of sexual behaviors. The physical examination by the physician focuses on strength, endurance, coordination, mobility, sensation, range of motion, and pain. Patients with longstanding, primary sexual dysfunction are referred to a specialist. Secondary dysfunction of recent onset, which may be related to the onset of the disability, can often be managed by rehabilitation practitioners.[17]

PLISSIT is an acronym for "Permission, Limited Information, Specific Suggestions, and Intensive Therapy." It is a model recommended by Halstead as an effective strategy for dealing with the sexual dysfunction of patients.[17] These elements are briefly described below:

1. *Permission.* The permission of an authority figure is often all that is needed for the patient to explore options and become sexually active.
2. *Limited information.* Providing information about anatomic and physiologic issues often gives adequate knowledge to make informed decisions and reduce fear and anxiety.
3. *Specific suggestions.* Guidelines for the particular problem or the specific disability must be provided.
4. *Intensive therapy.* Patients who do not respond to the first steps in the PLISSIT model should be

referred to a specialist for more intensive thera-peutic intervention.[17]

Hohmann offered nine precautions that should be considered in sexual counseling.[19] They are quoted here:

1. Do not put a person in conflict with his God.
2. Avoid extreme pressure on the patient to discuss sexuality.
3. Avoid forcing your morality and convictions on the patient.
4. Do not threaten the patient with your own sex-uality.
5. Do not make sex an all-or-none sort of experi-ence.
6. Do not assume that once the topic is discussed that you can leave it alone.
7. Do not conclude that there is only one way to convey information.
8. Be sure that the conjoint nature of sexual rela-tionship is held parallel.
9. Do convey the notion that all relationships, in-cluding the sexual one, are a matter of com-promise.

CONCLUSION

The occupational therapy program for patients with physical dysfunction must include objectives and methods designed to facilitate psychosocial adjust-ment. The treatment approaches include using ther-apeutic relationships, structuring a therapeutic envi-ronment, and using group and dyadic interpersonal experiences. Activities should aid the patient in ad-justing to the physical dysfunction and in restructur-ing his or her life style to achieve the maximum in-dependence possible.

Occupational therapy uses methods that demand the action and involvement of the patient in the re-habilitation process. In the initial stages of rehabili-tation when depression and denial are present and ego strength is poor, formal teaching or discussion groups fail because the patient cannot integrate verbal material that addresses psychological exploration. Therefore, social, recreational, special interest, and activity groups can be used to facilitate participation in rehabilitation tasks.

The group process may include discussion of needs and feelings, mutual support, and learning skills for working with the health care agency, its personnel, and the community. The therapist should plan and structure group experiences that enhance the devel-opment of social skills, allow opportunities to test in-teraction strategies, discover assets and new or mod-ified roles, and practice problem-solving behavior.

The occupational therapist can facilitate a collab-orative treatment program through the use of indi-vidual and group processes. The patient's involve-ment in treatment planning is critical because the pa-tient who uses individual skills in planning, sharing, playing, socializing, and making judgments is more likely to want to pursue daily living skills and other modalities for physical and functional improvements.

If the patient is involved in this kind of program-ming, it will not be necessary to point out that all skills have not been lost and that there are still assets and capabilities that can be used. There is usually a con-comitant and gradual increase in self-esteem and progress toward healthy adjustment and accommo-dation to the physical dysfunction.[45]

Professional health care workers must facilitate the achievement of self-acceptance and the development of coping strategies in their disabled patients. Public attitudes toward the disabled are a deterrant to suc-cessful psychosocial rehabilitation; they will be slow to change, but the occupational therapist can help a person apply physical and psychological resources to cope in a difficult world.[44]

REVIEW QUESTIONS

1. List some of the life changes that occur with the onset of physical dysfunction.
2. Describe the physical and psy-chologic suffering that may be caused by illness or injury.
3. What are some of the negative and positive secondary gains that may result from physical dys-function?
4. How do body image and self-val-uation affect the process of ad-justment to physical dys-function?
5. How does personality structure or adjustment pattern correlate with specific types of physical disabilities?
6. Describe two typical attitudes of the nondisabled toward the dis-abled.
7. Describe how rehabilitation workers may be demonstrating prejudice toward and suggesting reduced social status of their pa-tients.
8. Define "stigma."
9. Describe how the health care fa-cility is a microcosm of the soci-ety in which the disabled individ-ual will emerge? What can be done to minimize this phenome-non?
10. List and discuss two possible ori-gins of negative attitudes toward the disabled.
11. List and briefly describe the steps in the process of adjustment to physical dysfunction.
12. List the defense mechanisms that the disabled person may use to cope with physical dysfunction, and describe how they may be manifested.
13. What are the psychosocial factors that the therapist must consider in treatment planning?

14. How do the reactions of family, friends, and rehabilitation personnel affect treatment?
15. What is the role and helping pattern that rehabilitation workers should assume to facilitate the adjustment process?
16. List four signs of adverse reactions of personnel to patients.
17. Describe at least two ways adverse reactions of personnel to patients can be handled.
18. List signs of pathological adjustment to physical dysfunction.
19. What are some steps that should be taken if pathological reactions are recognized?
20. List three types of group approaches to treatment, and describe how each can aid in the psychosocial adjustment to physical dysfunction.
21. Describe the role of the occupational therapist in promoting sexual adjustment of the disabled.

EXERCISE

This is an empathy experience that is designed to help the student experience some of the personal and interpersonal reactions outlined in this chapter.
1. Select a wheelchair, walker, crutches, arm sling, or training arm prosthesis, and use the device as you would if you were so disabled.
2. Use the device for a minimum of 2 hours to tolerance.
3. Perform all of your usual daily living activities, and appear in public, perhaps to shop, eat in a restaurant, or look for an apartment during the experiential period.
4. During the experience, take notes and write a brief report describing your personal responses to people and objects, your affect and attitudes while performing daily living skills, reactions of others to you, your attitude toward dependency, if and how others offered assistance, and architectural barriers and how they foster dependency.

REFERENCES

1. Anthony WA: Societal rehabilitation: changing society's attitudes toward the physically and mentally disabled. In Marinelli RP and Dell Orto AE, editors: The psychological and social impact of physical disability, ed 2, New York, 1984, Springer Publishing Co, Inc.
2. Benham PK: Attitudes of occupational therapy personnel toward persons with disabilities, Am J Occup Ther 42:305, 1988.
3. Blume J: Deenie, Scarsdale, NY, 1973, Bradbury Press, Inc.
4. Burtoff B: Fairy tale stereotypes can harm, San Jose Mercury News, p 1C, January 26, 1980.
5. Castelnuevo-Tedesco P: Psychological consequences of physical defects and trauma. In Krueger DW, editor: Emotional rehabilitation of physical trauma and disability, New York, 1984, SP Medical and Scientific Books.
6. Catholic Biblical Association of America, The Bishops' Committee of the Confraternity of Christian Doctrine: The New American Bible, Nashville, Tenn, 1971, Thomas Nelson, Inc.
7. Conine TA et al: An assessment of occupational therapists' roles and attitudes toward sexual rehabilitation of the disabled, Am J Occup Ther 33:515, 1979.
8. Corcoran B: A dance to still music, New York, 1974, Atheneum Publishers.
9. De Loach C and Greer BJ: Adjustment to severe disability, New York, 1981, McGraw-Hill Book Company.
10. Diamond M: Sexuality and the handicapped. In Marinelli RP and Dell Orto AE, editors: The psychological and social impact of physical disability, ed 2, New York, 1984, Springer Publishing Co, Inc.
11. English RW: Correlates of stigma toward physically disabled persons. In Marinelli RP and Dell Orto AE, editors: The psychological and social impact of physical disability, New York, 1977, Springer Publishing Co, Inc.
12. Friedmann LW: The psychologi-

cal rehabilitation of the amputee, Springfield, IL, 1978, Charles C Thomas.
13. Garner HH: Somatopsychic concepts. In Marinelli RP and Dell Orto AE, editors: The psychological and social impact of physical disability, New York, 1977, Springer Publishing Co, Inc.
14. Geis HJ: The problem of personal worth in the physically disabled patient. In Marinelli RP and Dell Orto AE, editors: The psychological and social impact of physical disability, New York, 1977, Springer Publishing Co, Inc.
15. Gellman W: Roots of prejudice against the handicapped, excerpted from J Rehabil 25:4, 1959. In Stubbins J, editor: Social and psychological aspects of disability, Baltimore, 1977, University Park Press.
16. Griffith E, compiler: Sexual dysfunction associated with physical disabilities. In Marinelli RP and Dell Orto AE, editors: The psychological and social impact of physical disability, ed 2, New York, 1984, Springer Publishing Co, Inc.
17. Halstead LS: Sexuality and disability. In Krueger DW, editor: Emotional rehabilitation of physical trauma and disability, New York, 1984, SP Medical and Scientific Books.
18. Henderson G and Bryan WV: Psychological aspects of disability, Springfield, IL, 1984, Charles C Thomas.
19. Hohman GW: Reactions of the individual with a disability complicated by a sexual problem. In Marinelli RP and Dell Orto AE, editors: The psychological and social impact of physical disability, ed 2, New York, 1984, Springer Publishing Co, Inc.
20. Hughes F: Reaction to loss: coping with disability and death. In Marinelli RP and Dell Orto AE, editors: The psychological and social impact of physical disability, ed 2, New York, 1984, Springer Publishing Co, Inc.
21. Jaques ME and Patterson K: The self help group model: a review.

In Marinelli RP and Dell Orto AE, editors: The psychological and social impact of physical disability, New York, 1977, Springer Publishing Co, Inc.

22. Jeffress EJ: Psychological implications of physical disability, Videotape, San Jose State University, Instructional Resources Center.

23. Kerr N: Staff expectations for disabled persons: helpful or harmful. In Marinelli RP and Dell Orto AE, editors: The psychological and social impact of physical disability, New York, 1977, Springer Publishing Co, Inc.

24. Kerr N: Understanding the process of adjustment to disability. In Stubbins J, editor: Social and psychological aspects of disability, Baltimore, 1977, University Park Press.

25. Krueger DW: Emotional rehabilitation: an overview. In Krueger DW, editor: Emotional rehabilitation of physical trauma and disability, New York, 1984, SP Medical and Scientific Books.

26. Kübler-Ross E: On death and dying, New York, 1969, Macmillan Publishing Co, Inc.

27. Kushner HS: When bad things happen to good people, New York, 1981, Avon Books.

28. Kutner B: Milieu therapy. In Marinelli RP and Dell Orto AE, editors: The psychological and social impact of physical disability, ed 2, New York, 1984, Springer Publishing Co, Inc.

29. Ladieu-Leviton G, Adler DL, and Dembo T: Studies in adjustment to visible injuries: social acceptance of the injured. In Marinelli RP and Dell Orto AE, editors: The psychological and social impact of physical disability, New York, 1977, Springer Publishing Co, Inc.

30. Livneh H: On the origins of negative attitudes toward people with disabilities. In Marinelli RP and Dell Orto AE, editors: The psychological and social impact of physical disability, ed 2, New York, 1984, Springer Publishing Co, Inc.

31. Mann W, Godfrey ME, and Dowd ET: The use of group counseling procedures in the rehabilitation of spinal cord injured patients, Am J Occup Ther 27:73, 1973.

32. Marinelli RP and Dell Orto AE, editors: The psychological and social impact of physical disability, ed 2, New York, 1984, Springer Publishing Co, Inc.

33. Neistadt M and Baker MF: A program for sex counseling the physically disabled, Am J Occup Ther 32:646, 1978.

34. Novak PP and Mitchell MM: Professional involvement in sexuality counseling for patients with spinal cord injuries, Am J Occup Ther 42:105, 1988.

35. O'Dell S: Sing down the moon, Boston, 1970, Houghton Mifflin Co.

36. Robinson V: David in silence, Philadelphia, 1956, JB Lippincott Co.

37. Safilios-Rothschild C: Prejudice against the disabled and some means to combat it. In Stubbins J, editor: Social and psychological aspects of disability, Baltimore, 1977, University Park Press.

38. Shontz F: Physical disability and personality. In Marinelli RP and Dell Orto AE, editors: The psychological and social impact of physical disability, New York, 1977, Springer Publishing Co, Inc.

39. Shontz F: Six principles relating disability and psychological adjustment. In Marinelli RP and Dell Orto AE, editors: The psychological and social impact of physical disability, ed 2, New York, 1984, Springer Publishing Co, Inc.

40. Sidman JM: Sexual functioning and the physically disabled adult, Am J Occup Ther 31:81, 1977.

41. Siller J: Psychological situation of the disabled with spinal cord injuries. In Stubbins J, editor: Social and psychological aspects of disability, Baltimore, 1977, University Park Press.

42. Simon JI: Emotional aspects of physical disability, Am J Occup Ther 15:408, 1971.

43. Thurer S cited by Burtoff B: Fairy tale stereotypes can harm, San Jose Mercury News, January 26, 1980.

44. Vargo JW: Some psychological effects of physical disability, Am J Occup Ther 32:31, 1978.

45. Versluys H: Psychological adjustment to physical disability. In Trombly CA and Scott AD: Occupational therapy for physical dysfunction, Baltimore, 1977, Williams & Wilkins.

46. Watson LJ: Psychiatric consultation-liaison in the acute physical disabilities setting, Am J Occup Ther 40:338, 1986.

47. Willard HS and Spackman CS, editors: Occupational therapy, ed 4, Philadelphia, 1971, JB Lippincott Co.

Chapter

3 Occupational therapy evaluation of physical dysfunction

PRINCIPLES AND METHODS

LORRAINE WILLIAMS PEDRETTI

Evaluation of physical dysfunction is a process of gathering data and assessing occupational performance and performance components for the purpose of developing treatment objectives and treatment strategies based on the problems identified in the evaluation process. Evaluation takes place before treatment and periodically during the course of occupational therapy intervention.[8] Reevaluation is essential to assess the effectiveness of treatment and to modify it to suit current patient needs. This may involve eliminating unattainable goals, modifying goals that were partially or completely attained or achieved, and adding new goals as progress is made.

Evaluation provides the therapist with a specific and concrete method of determining his or her own effectiveness as a planner and administrator of treatment. It provides specific information that can be communicated to other members of the rehabilitation team. Furthermore, careful evaluation can enhance the development of occupational therapy. If evaluation data are collected systematically, they may be used for the development of more standardized evaluation instruments and may contribute to a better understanding of which evaluation and treatment techniques are suitable and effective in occupational therapy practice.

To be an effective evaluator, the therapist must be knowledgeable about the dysfunction, its causes, course, and prognosis; be familiar with a variety of evaluation methods, their uses, and proper administration; and be able to select evaluation methods that are suitable to the patient and the dysfunction. This means that an understanding of the possible dysfunctional performance, performance components, and applicable treatment principles is essential. In addition, the therapist must approach the patient with openness and without preconceived ideas about his or her limitations or personality. The therapist must have good observation skills and be able to enlist the trust of the patient in a short period of time.[11]

THE EVALUATION PROCESS

The evaluation process (Fig. 3-1) is initiated with *screening*, which refers to reviewing the potential patient's record, to determine the need for further evaluation and occupational therapy intervention.[14] Following the screening, an *initial evaluation* is conducted to determine whether occupational therapy services are needed and the kinds of services required.[8] The occupational therapist may interview the patient and administer selected tests and observations. The estimated time of treatment and the need to coordinate treatment with other services may also be determined at this time.[14]

The evaluation process continues with further *administration of specific tests* and clinical observations and with structured interviews. Standardized tests, performance checklists, and activities and tasks are used to evaluate specific performance abilities. Data necessary to plan treatment are obtained and interpreted.[14] The process concludes with an *analysis of the results* of the evaluation, interview, tests, and tasks.

An assessment of the individual's occupational roles and role dysfunction and a list of problems and assets to be used in planning occupational therapy intervention strategies is made.[8] Treatment objectives and methods are then selected on the basis of the data analysis. It is important that the patient be involved, to the extent possible, throughout the evaluation and treatment planning processes.

During the evaluation process, the occupational therapist must rely on clinical reasoning to guide decisions about the collection, classification, and analysis of data and, ultimately, to determine appropriate goals and methods of treatment. In a pilot study of clinical reasoning of a selected group of occupational therapists practicing in physical disabilities, Rogers and Masagatani outlined six stages of clinical reasoning used during the initial assessment.[9] During the first stage, the therapists obtained available information from the medical record, referral statement, and reports before meeting the patient to determine

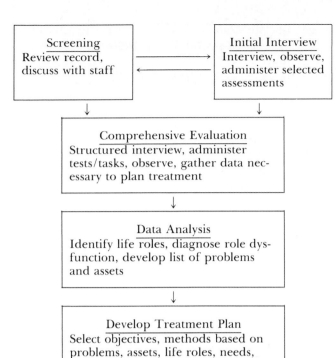

Fig. 3-1. Schematic of the evaluation process.

the diagnosis, prognosis, and severity of the condition. Next, the therapists selected assessments based on medical diagnosis, prognosis, and the patient's ability to cooperate and participate in the evaluation. In the third phase of the process, the therapists implemented the assessment plan by interacting with the patient and carrying out selected evaluations and tests. Patient problems were defined and possible causes were determined. In the fifth phase of clinical reasoning, treatment objectives based on the problem list were defined in conjunction with the patient. The selection of some treatment tasks and plans to carry out additional assessment also took place at this stage. Finally, the therapists evaluated the effectiveness of the assessment plan and the reliability of evaluation results.[9]

Rogers and Masagatani found that therapists used the medical diagnosis to select assessments, to recall standard problem lists for the diagnoses, and to select objectives and methods of treatment. This reflects a "recipe" approach to assessment and treatment planning and bypasses important considerations about the patient as a person that may be critical to effective treatment planning and treatment outcomes. The medical diagnosis is only one of several characteristics of the patient that must be considered in planning assessment and treatment. In physical disabilities practice, there may be a tendency to focus exclusively

on motor and sensory integrative performance components and self-care performance skills, with little attention given to the psychosocial component and work and play and leisure performance skills. This is an imbalance in the occupational therapy perspective that views humans as biopsychosocial beings.[9]

CONTENT OF THE EVALUATION

The initial occupational therapy evaluation should include an evaluation of the patient's goals, functional abilities and deficits in occupational performance, activities of daily living (ADL), including self-care skills, home, work, and school skills, and play and leisure skills.[12,13] Performance components should also be evaluated with particular attention to the motor and sensory-integrative components. Psychologic, social, and cognitive components are also evaluated or observed during the initial visits with the patient. The occupational therapist may need to plan remediation for these latter components and for the more obvious motor and sensory-integrative component, or refer the patient to the appropriate service for remediation.[12] The occupational therapist should obtain information about the patient's medical history, education, work history, family, and cultural background.[12] This information will provide a perspective of the patient from his or her own environmental and sociocultural context and should guide the therapist in selecting appropriate and meaningful treatment objectives and methods. Structuring treatment on the basis of the patient's needs, values, and sociocultural milieu is critical to eliciting his or her full participation in the treatment process.

METHODS OF EVALUATION
Medical Records

Data gathered from the medical record are an important part of the evaluation process. The medical record can provide information on the diagnosis, prognosis, current treatment regime, social data, psychologic data, and other rehabilitation therapies. Daily notes from nurses and physicians can give information about current medications and the patient's reactions and responses to the hospital, treatment regime, and persons in the treatment facility.

Ideally, the occupational therapist should have had the opportunity to study the medical record before seeing the patient to begin specific evaluation. This is not always possible, however, and the therapist may have to begin the evaluation without benefit of the information available in the medical record.

The information serves as a good basis for selecting methods of evaluation of and even of approach to the patient. It indicates problem areas and helps the therapist focus attention on the relevant factors of the case.[11]

Interview

The initial interview is a valuable step in the evaluation process. It is a time when the occupational therapist gathers information on how the patient perceives his or her roles, dysfunction, needs, and goals and a time when the patient can learn about the role of the occupational therapist and occupational therapy in the rehabilitation program.[11] An important outcome of the initial interview is the development of rapport and trust between therapist and patient.

The initial interview should take place in an environment that is quiet and ensures privacy. A specified period of time, known to interviewer and patient prior to the interview, should be set aside. The first few minutes of the interview may be devoted to getting acquainted and orienting the patient to the occupational therapy area and to the role and goals of occupational therapy in the treatment facility.

The therapist should plan the interview in advance to know what information must be acquired and to have some specific questions prepared. As the interview progresses, there should be an opportunity for the patient to ask questions as well. The therapist must have good listening and observation skills to gather maximum information from the interview.

It probably will be necessary to take notes or record the initial interview. The patient should be advised of this in advance, understand the reasons why, know the uses to which the material will be put, and be allowed to view or listen to the record if he or she desires.[11]

During the initial phase of the interview, the therapist should explain the role of the therapist, the purpose of the interview, and how the information is to be used. As the interview progresses, the therapist may seek the desired information by asking appropriate questions and guiding the responses and ensuing discussion so that relevant topics are addressed. The occupational therapist may wish to seek information about the patient's family and friends, community and work roles, educational and work histories, leisure and social interests and activities, and the living situation to which the patient will return. Information about how the patient spends and manages time is important. This can be determined by using a tool such as the daily schedule described in the following section or the activity configuration described by Watanabe and Cynkin.[4,15]

THE DAILY SCHEDULE. The therapist should interview the patient to get a detailed account of his or her activities for a typical day (or week) before the onset of physical dysfunction. Information that should be elicited is outlined as follows:

Rising hour
Morning activities with hours
  Hygiene
  Dressing
  Breakfast
  Work/leisure/home management
  Child care
  Luncheon
Afternoon activities with hours
  Work/leisure/home management
  Child care
  Rest
  Social activities
  Dinner
Evening activities with hours
  Leisure and social activities
  Preparation for retiring
Bedtime

The amount of time spent on each activity should be recorded carefully. During the interview, the therapist should be careful not to allow the patient to gloss over or omit any of the daily activities by cuing the patient with appropriate questions.

The therapist might ask "What time did you get up?" "What was the first thing that you did?" "When did you eat lunch?" "Who fixed it for you?" The review of the former daily schedule may evoke many recollections of family, friends, social, community, vocational, and leisure activities about which the patient may share information freely. At times, this digression from the schedule itself is desirable to elicit a well-rounded picture of the patient's roles and relationships and some ideas of his or her needs, values, and personal goals. In other instances, tangential conversation should be limited or discouraged to focus the patient's attention on the specific daily schedule.

If memory or communication disorders make the construction of the daily schedule impossible in the manner described, friends or family members may be consulted to get an approximation of the patient's activities pattern that may be helpful for setting goals and selecting activities.

A second daily schedule of present activities pattern in the treatment facility (or at home if the patient is an outpatient) is then constructed. It is important during this interview to ask the patient who helps him or her with each activity and how much assistance is needed and received. A discussion and comparative analysis of these two schedules between therapist and patient should yield valuable information about the patient's needs, values, satisfaction-dissatisfaction with the activities pattern, primary and secondary goals for change, interests, motivation, interpersonal relationships, and fears. On the basis of this information and the activity analysis, it becomes possible to set priorities for treatment objectives according to the patient's needs and values rather than to the therapist's priorities. Activities that will be meaningful to the patient as an individual and in his or her particular social group, which also may be appropriate for use in the intervention plan, begin to emerge. Their potential for facilitation of change may be presented, and selection of therapeutic modalities to meet objectives that have been agreed on can be made.

Throughout the interview, the therapist should sense the patient's attitude toward the dysfunction. The patient should have an opportunity to express what he or she sees as the primary problems and goals for rehabilitation. These may differ substantially from the therapist's judgment and must be given careful consideration when therapist and patient reach the point of setting treatment objectives together.

The two essential elements for a successful interview are a solid knowledge base and active listening skills. These abilities require study, practice, and preparation. The therapist's knowledge will influence the selection of questions or topics to be covered in the interview. The interview should reflect the therapist's knowledge and cover the areas that are relevant both to occupational therapy and to the construction of a meaningful treatment plan. The interviewer who actively listens demonstrates that he or she respects and is vitally interested in the patient.[1] In active listening, the receiver (therapist) tries to understand what the sender (patient) is feeling or the meaning of the message. The therapist then puts that understanding into his or her own words and feeds it back to the patient for verification, for example, by "This is what I believe you mean. Have I understood you correctly?" The therapist does not send a new message, such as an opinion, judgment, advice, or analysis. Rather, the therapist sends back only what he or she thinks the patient meant.[5]

The interview can be concluded with a summary of the major points covered, information gained, estimate of problems and assets, and plans for further occupational therapy evaluation.

This interview can reveal a good concept of the patient's life roles for the occupational therapist. Thus it enables the therapist to view the patient as a functioning human being rather than merely a diagnosis or disability. Treatment can then be based on the individual needs of the patient rather than on standard evaluation and treatment regimes established for a given disability. Knowing the patient's roles, interests, and activities is most helpful for diagnosing role dys-

function. It is valuable for determining the patient's values and establishing realistic possibilities for resumption of former roles or for structuring new ones.[10]

Observation

Some aspects of the evaluation of the patient will be based on the occupational therapist's observation of the patient during the interview and the evaluation procedures that follow. As treatment begins, the occupational therapist will be basing some of the reevaluation of the patient on observations during treatment. The occupational therapist can gain much information by observing the patient as he or she approaches or is approached. What is the posture, mode of ambulation, and gait pattern? How is he or she dressed? Is there obvious motor dysfunction? Are there apparent musculoskeletal deformities? What is the facial expression, tone of voice, and manner of speech? How are the hands held and used?

In addition to these observations, which can be made during the first few minutes of the initial contact with the patient, occupational therapists use observation to evaluate performance of self-care, home management, mobility, and transferring. Evaluation of these skills is usually carried out by observing the patient perform them in real or simulated environments. The therapist can determine the patient's level of independence, speed, skill, need for special equipment, and the feasibility for further training.

The rapport and trust that develops between the patient and the therapist will be based on the communication between them. The communication that occurs in the interview and observation phases of the evaluation will be critical to all subsequent interactions and thus to the effectiveness of treatment. The patient needs to have a sense that he or she has been heard and understood by someone who is empathetic and who has the necessary knowledge and skills to facilitate rehabilitation. The therapist needs to project self-confidence and confidence in the profession. This will set the tone for all future interaction with the patient. It will enhance the development of the patient's trust in the therapist and in the potential effectiveness of occupational therapy.[11]

Formal Evaluation Procedure

The evaluation of human performance is a major responsibility in occupational therapy. Along with the review of records, interview, and observations, the evaluation is carried out through the use of tests and assessments in occupational therapy. Relevant and accurate assessment is critical to decision-making for planning treatment, determining school and community living placement, considering admission and discharge to clinical programs, and other dispositions that may be based on test results. Thus in reporting evaluation data, it is essential that the information be supported by relevant and accurate assessment procedures.[2]

TYPES OF EVALUATIONS. Occupational therapists use both standardized and nonstandardized evaluations. A standardized evaluation includes stated instructions for administration and scoring and has statistical evidence of validity and reliability. It also has established norms, which allow the person being evaluated to be compared with a nondisabled population.[2] In contrast, a nonstandardized evaluation is subjective and has no criteria for scoring, nor does it provide information on interpreting results of the evaluation.[8] The results and interpretation of nonstandardized tests depend on the clinical skill, experience, judgment, and bias of the evaluator.[2] Many evaluation procedures in occupational therapy are neither standardized (objective) nor nonstandardized (subjective). These are procedures that provide some broad criteria for scoring and interpretation but still require the use of considerable subjective professional judgment.[8] The abilities required to administer the manual muscle test described in Chapter 7 is an example of the skill the therapist must have in using tests in occupational therapy.

It is assumed that standardized tests are superior to nonstandardized tests and that most clinicians would prefer to use standardized tests.[2] Yet there are few standardized evaluation procedures in occupational therapy.[8] Most assessments in current use have unknown reliability and validity. Many are informal instruments developed by occupational therapists to suit the needs of their own practice settings. Still others are adaptations of existing evaluation instruments and are used with patients other than those for whom they were designed. Standardized instruments designed by other professionals for their own disciplines are also used by occupational therapists.[3,17] The development of occupational therapy evaluation instruments that have reliability and validity and that are grounded in theory would increase confidence in occupational therapy practice. There is a need to broaden the repertoire of standardized tests used in occupational therapy evaluation and assessment.[2,3,17]

Watson encourages occupational therapists to use standardized measures to record information obtained from patients.[16] She maintains that using standardized tests improves the ability to formalize occupational therapy evaluations based on quantitative assessment. Results of the initial evaluation and follow-up evaluations can then be reported in a consistent, objective, and reliable manner. This will require

that the occupational therapist increase his or her knowledge and skill in testing and thus enhance professional credibility.[16]

Many standardized tests were designed by professionals other than occupational therapists for use in their own disciplines. Occupational therapists are using such tests in the areas of measuring achievement, development, intelligence, manual dexterity, motor skills, personality, sensorimotor function, and vocational skills.[3] The Buros Mental Measurements Yearbook is an excellent source of information about available standardized tests.[7] Current health care journals and psychological abstracts are other sources of information about standardized evaluations that may be relevant to occupational therapy.[2] Although it is desirable to have standardized and objective evaluations in occupational therapy, professional judgment and interpretation are always an important part of the evaluation procedure.[8]

COMPETENCIES FOR USE OF STANDARDIZED TESTS. To use standardized tests, the occupational therapist must possess certain skills; these are specified in a document of the American Occupational Therapy Association.[6] The occupational therapist using standardized tests must be able to (1) identify available tests in his or her area of practice; (2) identify the behavioral dimension measured by the tests; (3) interpret information on validity, reliability, and norms; (4) indicate a clinical or theoretic reason for the selection and use of the tests; (5) identify areas of occupational therapy practice in which test development is needed; (6) administer and interpret standardized and other tests that evaluate the patient's occupational performance and performance components; (7) identify the need for further evaluation of function; (8) integrate data from tests and evaluations to develop a treatment plan based on theory; (9) recognize the need for reassessment of the patient's performance; and (10) supervise evaluations performed by Certified Occupational Therapy Assistants (COTA).[6]

SUMMARY

The occupational therapy evaluation of the patient with physical dysfunction includes an examination of medical records, interview, observation, and the administration of specific formal and informal evaluation procedures. The treatment program is based on an analysis of the data gathered from all of these methods, which results in the identification of problems and assets in the patient's life. The evaluation process can help to determine if occupational therapy intervention is indeed appropriate.

Occupational therapists have developed many informal evaluation procedures that are useful to them in their particular treatment facilities. These include tests, checklists, and rating scales. These are useful tools and many of them can be or have been developed into standardized tests. In recent years, the need for reliable standardized tests has become more evident, and occupational therapists have recognized that they need to identify and employ tools that are commonly used to help establish the legitimacy of the profession.

The selection of the appropriate evaluation procedures will depend on the patient's diagnosis, medical history, lifestyle, interests, living situation, needs, and values. The information gathered throughout the evaluation process will determine the selection of objectives, methods, and treatment progression in the construction of the treatment plan.[11]

REVIEW QUESTIONS

1. Define "evaluation."
2. List four purposes of occupational therapy evaluation.
3. Which specific skills must the occupational therapist possess to be an effective evaluator?
4. List and describe the steps in the evaluation process.
5. List six stages of clinical reasoning during the evaluation process that were described by Rogers and Masagatani.[9]
6. Which specific occupational performance skills and performance components should be evaluated by the occupational therapist when treating patients with physical dysfunction?
7. Describe four categories of methods that the occupational therapist may use in the evaluation process.
8. Along with diagnosis and medical data, which other important factors about the patient should be considered by the occupational therapist during the assessment and later in treatment planning?
9. Compare the use of standardized and nonstandardized tests in occupational therapy evaluation. What are some advantages and disadvantages of each?
10. In order to use standardized tests, the occupational therapist must possess certain competencies. List at least five that were identified in the chapter.

REFERENCES

1. Allen C: The performance status examination, Paper presented at the American Occupational Therapy Association Annual Conference, San Francisco, October 1976. Cited in Smith HD and Tiffany EG: Assessment and evaluation: an overview. In Hopkins HL, and Smith HD: Willard and Spackman's occupational therapy, ed 6, Philadelphia, 1983, JB Lippincott Co.
2. Atchison B: Selecting appropriate assessments, Physical Disabilities Special Interest Section Newsletter, American Occupational Therapy Association, Inc, 10:2, June 1987.
3. Bowker A: Standardized tests utilized by therapists in the field of physical disabilities, Physical Disabilities Special Interest Section Newsletter, American Occupational Therapy Association, Inc, 6:4, 1983.
4. Cynkin S: Occupational therapy: toward health through activities, Boston, 1979, Little, Brown & Co.
5. Gordon T: PET: Parent effectiveness training, New York, 1970, The New American Library, Inc.
6. Maurer P, et al: Hierarchy of competencies relating to the use of standardized instruments and evaluation techniques by occupational therapists, Am J Occup Ther 38:803, 1984.
7. Mitchell JV, editors: Mental measurements yearbook, ed 9, Lincoln, NE, 1985, University of Nebraska. Cited by Atchison B: Selecting appropriate assessments, Physical Disabilities Special Interest Section Newsletter, American Occupational Therapy Association, Inc, 10:2, June 1987.
8. Mosey AC: Occupational therapy, configuration of a profession, New York, 1981, Raven Press.
9. Rogers JC and Masagatani G: Clinical reasoning of occupational therapists during the initial assessment of physically disabled patients, Occup Ther J Res 4:195, 1982.
10. Schwartz KB: Personal communication, October 13, 1987.
11. Smith HD, and Tiffany EG: Assessment and evaluation: an overview. In Hopkins HL, and Smith HD: Willard and Spackman's occupational therapy, ed 6, Philadelphia, 1983, JB Lippincott Co.
12. Standards of practice for occupational therapy services for clients with physical disabilities, Reference Manual of the Official Documents of The American Occupational Therapy Association, Inc, Rockville, MD, 1986, American Occupational Therapy Association.
13. Uniform occupational therapy evaluation checklist, Reference Manual of the Official Documents of the American Occupational Therapy Association, Inc, Rockville, MD, 1986, American Occupational Therapy Association.
14. Uniform terminology system for reporting occupational therapy services, Reference Manual of the Official Documents of The American Occupational Therapy Association, Inc, Rockville, MD, 1986, American Occupational Therapy Association.
15. Watanabe S: Regional institute on the evaluation process, Final Rep. RSA-123-T-68, New York, 1968, American Occupational Therapy Association.
16. Watson M: Analysis: Standardized testing objective, Physical Disabilities Special Interest Section Newsletter, American Occupational Therapy Association, Inc, 6:4, 1983.
17. Watts JH et al: The assessment of occupational functioning: a screening tool for use in long-term care, Am J Occup Ther 40:231, 1986.

Chapter
4 Treatment planning

LORRAINE WILLIAMS PEDRETTI

A treatment plan is the design or proposal for a therapeutic program. Pelland described it as "the core of occupational therapy practice."[5] A treatment plan should be based on one or more of the occupational therapy frames of reference. This determines which assessments, objectives, and methods will be most appropriate for the patient.[5,6] A treatment plan includes specific treatment objectives and methods for reaching those objectives and indicates how the program should progress.

The importance of writing a treatment plan cannot be overstated. It is necessary to have specific objectives outlined in an orderly and sequential manner. These, then, will be clear to the therapist, patient, and other concerned personnel. The treatment plan helps the therapist know how to proceed efficiently and provides a standard for measuring the progress of the patient and thus the effectiveness of the plan.

Therapists who do not write treatment plans may be working in a trial and error manner, wasting precious time and money. They may be poorly prepared to defend their course of action to themselves, the patient, or the rehabilitation team. They may tend to lack confidence in their reports about the patients assigned to them. The failure to have a well-written treatment plan available will also present many problems to other staff members who may have to apply treatment in the absence of the assigned therapist.

Perhaps one of the most important purposes for writing a treatment plan is that it allows the therapist to plan and analyze the proposed course of action. In so doing, the therapist should ask many questions. Some of these are (1) What is the most appropriate frame of reference or treatment approach on which to base the treatment plan? (2) What are the patient's capabilities and assets? (3) What are the patient's limitations and deficits? (4) What does occupational therapy have to offer this patient? (5) What are specific short-range objectives? (6) What are some long-range objectives? (7) Are the treatment objectives consistent with the patient's needs and personal objectives? (8) If objectives are not compatible, how do they need to be modified? (9) Which treatment methods are available to meet these objectives? (10) When should the patient have met the objectives? (11) What standards shall be used to determine when the patient has reached an objective? (12) How will the effectiveness of the treatment plan be evaluated?

The treatment plan affirms the therapist's competence and the professionalism of occupational therapy. It can provide a systematic method for gathering research data and documents the purposes and effectiveness of occupational therapy services. The treatment plan can enhance the quality of service and its effectiveness.

THE TREATMENT PLANNING PROCESS
Data Gathering

After the patient is referred for occupational therapy services, the therapist must gather data to develop an appropriate treatment plan. Sources for these data are the referral form; the medical record; social, educational, vocational, and play histories; interview of the patient or family and friends; and the results of evaluation procedures completed by occupational therapy and other services.

Data Analysis and Problem Identification

After data have been gathered, they are analyzed to identify functions and dysfunctions, and it is determined if occupational therapy can be employed to alleviate the problems.[6] From a careful analysis of all of the data gathered, a list of problems and assets should be developed, which forms the basis of the treatment plan. Those physical, psychosocial, cognitive, and performance skills deficits that may be amenable to occupational therapy intervention should be noted. Limitations that require intervention by other professional services should be communicated through the appropriate referral process. How the patient's assets can be used to enhance progress toward independence should be determined.

Selecting and Writing Treatment Objectives

The next step in the treatment planning process is to set objectives. Following the data gathering process, the selection of a frame of reference and one or more treatment approaches, some general kinds of treatment methods that would facilitate the patient's rehabilitation may be conceptualized. For example, following evaluation it may be apparent that the patient could benefit from training in activities of daily living (ADL) or from one of the sensorimotor approaches to treatment to influence muscle tone and movement patterns. Having ideas for such methods can facilitate the selection and writing of specific treatment objectives. The writing of objectives and selection of treatment methods actually are concurrent and mutually dependent processes.

Objectives should reflect the patient's needs and should be consistent with the more general objectives stated on the referral, although they need not be limited to these, if the referral agent approves. The occupational therapy objectives should complement objectives of ancillary services. Whenever possible, the therapist should select objectives and plan the treatment program in conjunction with the patient.

A treatment objective is a statement of intent describing a proposed change in a patient. The statement conveys clearly the physical function, performance skill, or behavior pattern the patient will demonstrate when the treatment procedure or program has been successfully completed.

The therapist must select objectives that the patient is to reach by the end of a treatment program so that treatment procedures relevant to those objectives may also be selected. Progress and evaluation will be based on the objectives selected.

When no clearly defined objectives have been stated, there is no sound basis for selecting appropriate treatment methods, and it is impossible to evaluate the effectiveness of the treatment program. It is important to state objectives to be able to evaluate the degree to which the patient is able to perform in the desired manner.

The method for writing treatment objectives, described below, is designed on models for writing-competency–based educational objectives described by Mager and Kemp.[3,4]

A meaningful objective conveys an idea of what the patient will be like when the objective has been achieved. The idea conveyed is identical to the one the therapist has in mind. Thus it succeeds in communicating the therapist's intent and describes the terminal behavior of the patient well enough to preclude misinterpretation. A comprehensive treatment objective has the following three elements.

1. *Statement of terminal behavior.* The physical changes, kind of behavior, or performance skill that the patient is expected to display.[4]

2. *Conditions.* The circumstances under which evaluation of performance will take place, for example, environment, special devices, and assistance required for the patient to perform the desired terminal behavior.[3,4]

3. *Criterion.* The performance standard or degree of competence the patient is expected to achieve, stated in measurable or observable terms.[3,4]

The following is an example of comprehensive treatment objectives and its analysis:

Given assistive devices, the patient will feed himself independently in 30 minutes.

CONDITIONS: Given assistive devices.
TERMINAL BEHAVIOR: The patient will feed himself.
CRITERIA: Independently in thirty minutes.

There are many variables and unknown factors in the growth and development or recovery of patients with physical dysfunction. Therefore the degree to which they can benefit from or participate or succeed in rehabilitation programs cannot be predicted with certainty. This often makes it difficult for therapists to write comprehensive treatment objectives. However, the therapist should attempt to write such objectives, using past experience with similar patients and knowledge gained from gathering pertinent data to describe desired terminal behavior, conditions, and criteria for each treatment objective. If this is not possible, it is recommended that a specific statement of terminal behavior be used until applicable conditions and criteria become apparent. The stated terminal behaviors can then be modified to become comprehensive objectives as treatment progresses.

The following are examples of specific statements of terminal behavior:

1. The joint range of motion (ROM) of the left elbow will increase.
2. The patient will operate the control systems of the left above-elbow prosthesis.
3. The patient will dress him/herself.
4. The patient will feed him/herself.

The conditions and, at times, the criteria are optional parts of the treatment objective. The criteria answer questions such as "how much," "how often," "how well," "how accurately," "how completely," and "how quickly."[3] If it is possible to estimate the patient's potential level of competence, it is important to include a criterion or performance standard in the objective. This is the only way the therapist can determine the achievement of the stated objective with certainty. The conditions describe any circumstances under which the performance will take place, and answer questions such as "Is special equipment needed?", "Is supervision or assistance necessary?", and "Are special cues necessary?"[3]

Adding one or more of these optional parts to the previous examples would make these objectives both more measurable and specific. For example:

1. The joint ROM of the left elbow will increase from 0-120 to 0-135 degrees. (Specifying the amount of increase in ROM adds a measurable criterion to the terminal behavior.)
2. The patient will be able to operate the control systems of the left above-elbow prosthesis without hesitation. (Specifying "without hesitation" adds an observable behavior as a criterion that could be indicative of automaticity of performance.)
3. Given assistive devices, the patient will be able to dress him/herself in less than 20 minutes. (The availability of assistive devices is a necessary condition to this patient being able to perform this task. The criterion or performance standard is set in terms of speed.)
4. Given equipment set-up and assistive devices, the patient will use mobile arm supports to feed him/herself independently. (The equipment set-up and the availability of assistive devices constitute the conditions for this objective, and the criterion for performance under these circumstances is "independently.")

Selecting Treatment Methods

When objectives have been selected, the treatment methods to help the patient achieve them are chosen. This is probably one of the most difficult steps in the treatment planning process. A treatment principle or assumption that is applied to the cause of an identified problem should underlie the selection of an appropriate treatment method.[1] For example, after peripheral nerve injury and repair and nerve regeneration is progressing, a principle would be that use of reinnervated muscles will maintain or increase their tone and strength. Therefore, graded therapeutic activity or exercise may be the method of choice to effect the desired goals. Many other factors will influence the selection of treatment methods. Some of the factors that should be considered in the selection of treatment methods are (1) What is the goal for the patient? (2) What are the precautions or contraindications that affect the occupational therapy program? (3) What is the prognosis for recovery? (4) What were the results of evaluations in occupational therapy and other services? (5) What other treatment is the patient receiving? (6) What are the goals of other treatment programs, and are the occupational therapy goals compatible with these? (7) How much energy does the patient expend in other therapies? (8) What is the

state of the patient's general health? (9) What are the patient's interests, vocational skills, and psychologic needs? (10) What roles will the patient assume in the community? (11) What kinds of activities or exercises will be most useful and meaningful to the patient?[2] (12) How can treatment be graded to meet the patient's changing needs as progression or regression occurs? (13) What special equipment or adaptations of therapeutic equipment are needed for the patient to perform maximally?

When treatment methods are selected, it should be clear to others reading the treatment plan exactly how the methods will be used to reach specific objectives. Sometimes several methods may be needed to achieve one objective, or the same methods may be used to reach several objectives.

Implementing the Treatment Plan

When at least one objective and one or more treatment methods have been selected, the treatment plan is implemented. The patient engages in the procedures that have been designed to ameliorate problems and capitalize on assets. A comprehensive treatment plan may evolve over a period of time. While a lengthy evaluation is in progress, for example, ADL assessment, the patient may have commenced a program of therapeutic activity to strengthen specific muscle groups. Thus as a comprehensive evaluation is being completed, an increasing number of problems may be identified, and additional objectives and methods may be added to the treatment plan.

Reevaluating the Patient and the Initial Treatment Plan

Once the treatment plan is implemented, its effectiveness is evaluated on an ongoing basis through continuous observation and assessment. The therapist must be an alert observer and ask: (1) Are the objectives suitable to the patient's needs and capabilities? (2) Are the methods most appropriate for fulfilling the treatment objectives? (3) Does the patient relate to the treatment methods and see them as worthwhile and meaningful? (4) Are the treatment objectives realistic, and are they consistent with the patient's personal objectives?

Scrutinizing the treatment plan in this way will enable the therapist to modify the plan as the need arises. The criterion for determining the effectiveness of the plan is the progress of the patient toward the stated objectives. Therefore periodic reevaluation of the patient, using the same tests and observations to determine baseline function, can provide objective evidence of maintenance or progress that validates the treatment plan.

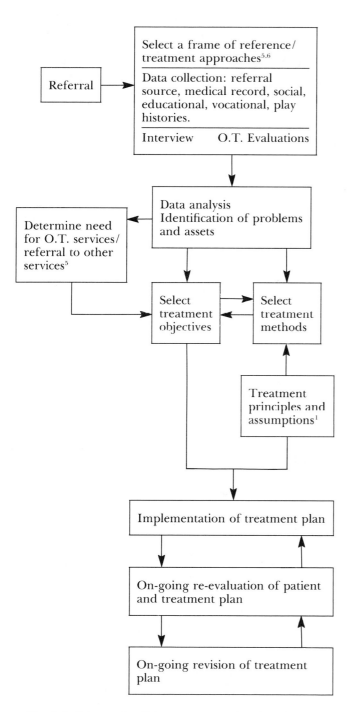

Fig. 4-1. Schematic of the treatment planning process.

Revising the Treatment Plan

The information gained from observations and reevaluation of the patient, as outlined above, may necessitate some revision or modification of the initial treatment plan. The patient's progress may be significant enough to increase such factors as duration, complexity, or resistance of the activity. In degenerative diseases, in which maintenance of optimal function is often a primary objective, resistance, duration, and complexity of activity may need to be decreased to accommodate the gradual inevitable decline of physical resources. The patient's motivation or inability to see the therapeutic program as helpful or meaningful may necessitate change in treatment approaches and methods.

Thus the initial plan is continually revised according to the patient's needs and progress. This process of reevaluation, revision, and reimplementation of the treatment plan goes on throughout the course of the therapeutic program (Fig. 4-1).[5,6]

A TREATMENT PLAN MODEL

The treatment plan model is useful for teaching treatment planning during academic preparation, and it may be modified for clinical use (Fig. 4-2).

The student is presented with a hypothetical case study or an actual patient and is directed to complete the treatment plan, using the Treatment Planning Guide. If given a hypothetical patient, the student is directed to complete the Evaluation Summary section of the treatment plan according to his or her knowledge of the particular diagnosis and its resultant disability.

Case study

Mr. P. is a 35-year-old electronics assembler. He completed the 10th grade in school. He is right-handed, married, and the father of two children under 8 years old. He suffered an injury of the right radial nerve at elbow level with minor involvement of the median nerve. The injury occurred 2 months ago, and partial to full recovery is expected to occur within 10 months.

Mr. P. is now supporting his family with insurance compensation payments but fears that these will terminate before recovery has occurred, and he is back on the job. He is worried and depressed about this.

The client is an outpatient and has been referred to occupational therapy for physical and functional restoration.

Muscle grades
Extensor carpi radialis brevis: F(3)
Extensor carpi ulnaris: P+(2+)
Extensor digitorum communis: F(3)
Supinator: P+(2+)
Extensor pollicis longus and brevis: P−(2−)
Abductor pollicis longus and brevis: P(2)
Extensor indicis proprius: P−(2−)

Case _____

Personal Data

   Name

   Age

   Diagnosis

   Disability

   Treatment aims stated in the referral

Other Services

Frame of Reference/Treatment Approach

O.T. Evaluation

   Performance components

     1. motor functioning

     2. sensory integrative functioning

     3. cognitive functioning

     4. psychological functioning

     5. social functioning

Performance skills

   1. self care

   2. work

   3. play/leisure

Evaluation Summary

Assets

Problem list

Outline treatment plan

   1. Problem

   2. Objective

   3. Methods

   4. Gradation of treatment

Fig. 4-2. Treatment plan model.

Treatment planning guide

The Treatment Planning Guide is a reference for filling out a treatment plan for either an actual or a hypothetical patient.

PERSONAL DATA. Fill in the requested information from the medical record or case study.

   Name
   Age
   Diagnosis
   Disability
   Treatment aims stated in the referral

OTHER SERVICES. List and give a brief statement of the roles of other services that the patient is undergoing.

   Physician
   Nursing
   Respiratory therapy
   Social service
   Speech pathology
   Physical therapy
   Vocational counseling
   Psychology/Psychiatry
   Educational services
   Spiritual Counseling
   Community social groups/Day care
   Home health care services
   Sheltered employment

FRAME OF REFERENCE/TREATMENT APPROACH. State the frame of reference and treatment approach on which the treatment plan is based. More than one may be necessary.

OT EVALUATION. From the list below, select the performance components and performance skills that should be evaluated. Indicate whether assessment would be determined by testing or by observation.

Performance components

Motor functioning
   Muscle strength
   ROM
   Physical endurance
   Standing tolerance
   Walking tolerance
   Sitting balance
   Involuntary movement
   Movement speed
   Level of motor development
   Equilibrium/Protective responses
   Coordination/Muscle control
   Spasms
   Spasticity
   Stage of motor recovery (stroke patients only)
   Postural reflex mechanism
   Functional movement patterns
   Hand function
   Swallowing/Cranial nerve functions

Sensory-integrative functioning
   Sensation—touch, pain, temperature, proprioception, taste, smell
   Body schema
   Stereognosis
   Visual perception
     Visual fields
     Spatial relations
     Position in space
     Figure-background
     Perceptual constancy
     Visual-motor coordination
     Depth perception

Continued.

Treatment planning guide—cont'd

Perception of vertical/horizontal elements
Eye movements
Motor planning
Functional auditory perception
Cognitive functioning
  Memory
  Judgment
  Safety awareness
  Problem-solving ability
  Motivation
  Sequencing
  Rigidity
  Abstract thinking
  Functional language skills
    Comprehension of speech/writing
    Ability to express ideas
    Reading
    Writing
  Functional mathematical skills
    Mental calculations
    Written calculations
Psychological functioning
  Self-identity
  Self-concept
  Coping skills
  Maturity (developmental level)
  Adjustment to disability
  Reality functioning
Social functioning
  Interpersonal skills—dyadic and group interactions

Performance skills
  Self-Care
  Feeding
  Dressing
  Hygiene
  Transferring
  Work/Work-Related Skills
  Work habits and attitudes
  Potential work skills
  Work tolerance
  Community mobility
  Home management
  Child care
  Play/Leisure
  Past and present leisure interests/play activities
  Modes of relaxation

EVALUATION SUMMARY. Summarize findings from tests and observations.

ASSETS. List the assets of the patient and his or her situation that can be used to enhance progress toward maximum independence.

PROBLEM LIST. Identify and list the problems that require occupational therapy intervention.

OBJECTIVES. Write specific treatment objectives in the comprehensive form described on p. 46. Each should be related to a specific problem in the problem list and identified by the corresponding number.

METHODS OF TREATMENT. Describe the treatment methods in detail that would be appropriate for the patient.

GRADATION OF TREATMENT. Briefly state how treatment methods will be graded to enhance the patient's progress.

Sample treatment plan

The following treatment plan is not a comprehensive plan for the hypothetical patient. Rather, it presents a sampling of parts of a proposed treatment program. The plan deals with four of the problems on the Problem List. The reader is encouraged to add objectives and methods to address additional problems and make the plan a more comprehensive one.

CASE STUDY

Mrs. R. is 49 years old. She has two sons. One is age 26 and married, and the other is age 17. Mrs. R. is divorced. She and her younger son live with her married son, his wife, and their 4-year-old boy. Before the onset of her illness, Mrs. R. lived in an apartment with her younger son.

Mrs. R. had Guillain-Barré syndrome. She has been left with residual weakness of all four extremities. Mrs. R. uses a standard wheelchair for mobility.

Mrs. R. appears thin and frail. She speaks in a weak voice and appears to be passive and discouraged. She feels she cannot accomplish anything. The home situation is poor. Mrs. R. does not communicate with her daughter-in-law, and there are conflicts between the couple and Mrs. R. concerning the management of the teenage son. Mrs. R. feels unable to assert her authority as his mother or to express her needs and feelings. The disability has brought about the loss of her independence and has changed her role in relation to her younger son.

Her daughter-in-law reported that Mrs. R. is dependent for self-care, never attempts to help with homemaking, and isolates herself in her room much of the time. She believes that her mother-in-law is capable of more activity "if only she would try." She says she is willing to allow Mrs. R. to do some of the household work.

Mrs. R. was referred for occupational therapy services as an outpatient for restoration or maintenance of motor functioning and increased independence in ADL.

TREATMENT PLAN

Personal data

Name: Mrs. R.

Age: 49

Diagnosis: Guillain-Barré syndrome

Disability: Residual weakness, upper and lower extremities

Treatment aims stated in referral: Restoration or maintenance of motor functioning; increased independence in ADL.

OTHER SERVICES

Physician: prescription of medication; maintenance of general health; supervision of rehabilitation program.

Physical therapy: muscle strengthening; ambulation and transferring training.

Social service: individual and family counseling.

Community social group: socialization

Continued.

FRAME OF REFERENCE
Occupational performance

TREATMENT APPROACHES
Biomechanical and rehabilitative

OT EVALUATION
Performance components
Motor functioning
  Muscle strength: test
  Passive ROM: test
  Physical endurance: observe, interview
  Walking tolerance: observe, interview
  Movement speed: observe
  Coordination: test, observe
  Functional movement: test, observe
Sensory-integrative functioning
  Sensation (touch, pain, thermal, proprioception): test
Cognitive functioning
  Judgment: observe
  Safety awareness: observe
  Motivation: observe, interview
Psychological functioning
  Coping skills: observe
  Adjustment to disability: observe, interview
  Social skills
  Interpersonal relationships: observe
Performance skills
Self care: observe, interview
Home management: observe, interview

EVALUATION SUMMARY
Muscle testing revealed that all muscles are the same grades bilaterally: scapula and shoulder muscles are F+ to G (3+ to 4); elbow and forearm muscles are F+ to G (3+ to 4); wrist and hand musculature is graded F+ (3+). Trunk muscles are G (4); all muscles of the hip are G (4), except adductors and external rotators, which are F+ (3+). Knee flexors and extensors are G (4). Ankle plantar flexors and dorsiflexors are F (3), and all foot muscles are F− (3−) to P (2).

All joint motions within normal to functional range. Physical endurance limited to 1 hour of light activity of upper extremities, with some ambulation, before rest Mrs. R. uses a wheelchair for energy conservation and propels it using both arms and legs. Slight incoordination, evident on fine hand function, caused by muscle weakness.

Sensory modalities of touch, pain, temperature, and proprioception are intact. No cognitive deficits were observed. Mrs. R. is passive and discouraged about her disability. She feels she cannot accomplish anything and tends to stay in her room alone.

Before onset of illness, Mrs. R. lived independently with her 17-year-old son. Since her illness, she and her son have moved in with her 26-year-old son, his wife, and their 4-year-old son. This arrangement has proved less than ideal. There is little communication between Mrs. R. and her daughter-in-law. There are conflicts between the couple and Mrs. R. about the management of her teenage son.

The disability has brought about the loss of Mrs. R.'s independence and has changed her roles as homemaker and mother. She feels unable to assert her authority as mother of her 17-year-old or to express her needs and feelings.

Mrs. R. manages some personal care such as face-washing and hair and teeth care. She needs some assistance with dressing and has difficulty with buttons and zippers. She requires an adaptive toothbrush and needs assistance in toilet transferring and showering. Mrs. R. does not perform any home management tasks but is potentially capable of light activities such as table setting, dusting, and folding clothes. Mrs. R.'s daughter-in-law is willing to allow her mother-in-law some household activities if understanding about their respective roles can be established.

ASSETS
Some functional muscle strength
Good joint mobility
Potential good living situation
Presence of able-bodied adults who can assist
Potential for some further recovery
Good sensation

PROBLEM LIST
1. Muscle weakness
2. Low physical endurance
3. Limited walking tolerance
4. Mild incoordination
5. Self-care dependence
6. Homemaking dependence
7. Dependent transferring
8. Isolation, apparent depression
9. Reduced social interaction
10. Lack of assertiveness

PROBLEM 1 Muscle weakness
Objective
Muscle strength of shoulder flexors will increase from F+ (3+) to G (4).
Method
Light progressive resistive exercise to shoulder flexion: patient is seated in a regular chair, wearing a weighted cuff one half the weight of her maximum resistance above each elbow. Lifts arms alternately through 10 repetitions and then rests. Repeated using three quarters' maximum resistance, then full resistance. Activities: reaching for glasses in overhead cupboard and placing them on the table, replacing glasses in cupboard when dry; rolling out pastry dough on a slightly inclined pastry board; wiping table, counter, and cupboard doors, using a forward push-pull motion; turkish knotting project with weaving frame set vertically in front of her and tufts of yarn on right and left sides, at hip level.
Gradation
Increase resistance, number of repetitions, and length of time as strength improves.

PROBLEM 1 Muscle weakness
Objective
Strength of wrist flexors and extensors and finger flexors will increase from F+ (3+) to G (4).
Method
Light progressive resistive exercises for wrist flexors and extensors: patient is seated, side to table, with pronated forearm resting on the table and hand extended over edge of table; a hand cuff, with small weights equal to one half of her maximum resistance attached to the palmar surface, is worn on the hand; patient extends the wrist through full range of motion against gravity for 10 repetitions, then rests. Exercise is repeated, using three quarters' maximum resistance and then full resistance. The same procedure is used to exercise wrist flexors, except that the forearm is supinated on the table, and the weights are suspended from the dorsal side of the

Continued.

Sample treatment plan—cont'd

hand cuff. Activities to improve finger flexors: tearing lettuce to make a salad; handwashing panties and hosiery. Progress to kneading soft clay or bread dough.

Gradation

Increase resistance, repetitions, and time.

PROBLEM 5 Self-care dependence

Objective

Given assistive devices, Mrs. R. will be able to dress herself independently within 20 minutes.

Method

Putting on bra: using a back opening stretch bra, pass bra around waist so that opening is in front and straps are facing up; fasten bra in front at waist level; slide fastened bra around at waist level so that cups are in front; slip arms through straps and work straps up over shoulders; adjust cups and straps. Putting on shirt: place loose fitting blouse on lap with back facing up and neck toward knees; place arms under back of blouse and into arm holes; push sleeves up onto arms past elbows; gather back material up from neck to hem with hands and duck head forward and pass garment over head; work blouse down by shrugging shoulders and pulling into place with hands; use button hook to fasten front opening. Putting on underpants and slacks: sitting on bed or in wheelchair, cross legs, reach down, and place one opening over foot; cross opposite leg, place other opening over foot; uncross legs, work pants up over feet and up under thighs; a dressing stick may be used to pull pants up if leaning forward is difficult; shift hips from side to side and work pants up as far as possible over buttocks; stand, if possible, and pull pants to waist level, then sit and pull zipper up with prefastened zipper pull; use Velcro at waist closure on slacks. Putting on socks: using stretch socks and seated, cross one leg, place sock over toes and work sock up onto foot and over heel; cross other leg and repeat. Putting on shoes: using slip on shoe with Velcro fasteners, use procedure for socks.

Gradation

Progress to more difficult dressing tasks such as pantyhose, tie-shoes, dresses, pullover garments.

PROBLEM 6 Homemaking dependence

Objective

Given assistive devices, Mrs. R. will perform homemaking activities in the home.

Methods

Using a dust mitt, patient dusts furniture surfaces easily reached from wheelchair such as lamp tables and coffee table; sits at sink to wash dishes; practices folding small items of clothing such as panties, nylons, children's underwear, while sitting at kitchen table; have Mrs. R.'s daughter-in-law observe activities at treatment facility; work out an acceptable list of activities and a schedule with both women. Discuss how Mrs. R. could make some contributions to home management routines; ask Mrs. R. to keep activity diary, noting of any performance difficulties and successes for review at next visit.

Gradation

Increase number of household responsibilities. Increase time spent on household activities.

PROBLEM 8 Isolation, depression

Objective

Mrs. R. will reduce time spent alone from 6 waking hours to 3 waking hours.

Method

Establish acceptable graded activity schedule between Mrs. R. and son and daughter-in-law; include homemaking tasks and socialization with family through playing games, watching TV, preparing and eating meals, and conversing; family members encourage Mrs. R. to be with them but to be accepting if she refuses; have Mrs. R. keep activities diary for review; determine how time is being spent and discuss how it could be more productive and enjoyable. Initiate avocational activity, such as needlework or tile mosaics, to complete at home; set goals for where and how much activity will be performed.

Gradation

Increase time spent out of own room; include friends, neighbors, family, in household social activities; plan a community outing for shopping or lunch.

REVIEW QUESTIONS

1. Define "treatment plan."
2. Why write a treatment plan?
3. Why base the treatment plan on a specific frame of reference?
4. List the steps for developing a treatment plan.
5. List, define, and give examples of the three elements of a comprehensive treatment objective.
6. If a comprehensive objective cannot be written, which one element would be *most* important to identify first?
7. List six factors to consider when selecting treatment methods.
8. Is it necessary to develop a complete comprehensive treatment plan before treatment can begin?
9. Is it ever necessary to change the initial treatment plan?
10. How is a plan evaluated?
11. How does therapist know when to modify or change plan?

EXERCISES

1. Analyze objectives and ask which characteristics of comprehensive objective each contains. Rewrite to include as many elements of a comprehensive objective as possible.
   a. Joint ROM at left elbow will increase.
   b. Patient will be more assertive among peers.
   c. Patient will be proficient in control and use of left below-elbow prosthesis.
2. Write treatment plan for patient described in case study.

REFERENCES

1. Day D: A systems diagram for teaching treatment planning, Am J Occup Ther 27:239, 1973.
2. Hopkins HL, et al.: Therapeutic application of activity. In Willard and Spackman's occupational therapy, ed 6, Philadelphia, 1983, JB Lippincott Co.
3. Kemp JE: The instructional design process, New York, 1985, Harper & Row.
4. Mager RF: Preparing instructional objectives, ed 2 (rev.), Belmont, CA, 1984, David S. Lake.
5. Pelland MJ: A conceptual model for the instruction and supervision of treatment planning, Am J Occup Ther 41:351, 1987.
6. Smith HD and Tiffany EG: Assessment and evaluation: an overview. In Willard and Spackman's occupational therapy, ed 6, Philadelphia, 1983, JB Lippincott.

Chapter

5 Documentation of occupational therapy services

LORRAINE WILLIAMS PEDRETTI

Documentation of occupational therapy services refers to the written record of all information relevant to the patient from occupational therapy admission to discharge. Documentation of occupational therapy services includes the referral form, evaluation forms or checklists, initial evaluation summary, treatment plan, progress notes, periodic progress reports, and discharge summary. There is no standard or single method for documenting occupational therapy services within the profession. The types of records and reports to be written may be determined by the individual treatment facility and by the funding agencies.[3,5]

Gleave defined a record as a written statement to preserve memory and to present accurate evidence of facts and events.[2] An example is the running progress note. A report is defined as a written summary of facts or occurrences to communicate the information. Examples are the progress report and discharge summary.[2]

Documentation should be clear, concise, objective, accurate, and complete. Omissions or errors in the record may present doubts about the accuracy of the entire record.[2] The record should contain pertinent information about the patient's status, progress, and performance. The occupational therapist is responsible for keeping accurate records and writing appropriate reports to document the treatment program and the patient's progress.

Purposes for Documentation

Many occupational therapists find documentation a time-consuming requirement and would like to reduce the amount of time spent doing it. However, current sources of funding for health care have required increased documentation. Therefore the occupational therapist is required to develop writing skills that reflect objectivity, clinical accuracy, conciseness, completeness, and a system of record keeping that is efficient. Documentation is a very important part of occupational therapy practice.

Documenting occupational therapy services (1) provides administrative control; (2) complies with the law and aids in litigation; (3) provides clear, objective data about the patient on which future treatment can be based; (4) communicates progress to the physician and other health care professionals; (5) provides justification for the cost of treatment; (6) interprets the treatment program to the patient, family, and other interested individuals or agencies; (7) facilitates continuity of treatment when staff changes occur; (8) facilitates in-service training and student education programs; (9) evaluates the effectiveness of occupational therapy intervention; and (10) provides data for research and the advancement of the professionalism of occupational therapy.[2,3,5]

RECORDS AND REPORTS
The Occupational Therapy Record

In some facilities the occupational therapy service will maintain separate records that do not necessarily become part of the patient's permanent medical record. The types of records that are included are detailed results of tests and observations such as the activities of daily living (ADL) checklist or muscle test form, treatment plans, and running daily progress notes. These records form the basis of the reports that do become part of the permanent record.[5]

Permanent Records

The information contained in the initial evaluation, progress reports, and discharge report usually become part of the patient's permanent record. In these reports the occupational therapist summarizes the content of the occupational therapy records. The detailed and lengthy results of a comprehensive evaluation, for example, are summarized into the initial evaluation summary or report. A series of daily progress notes are integrated to become a report of progress over a specific time period such as a week or a month. Progress reports are summarized in the discharge report and reflect a brief history of the initiation and progress of treatment and outcomes.[2]

CONTENT OF RECORDS AND REPORTS
(Fig. 5-1)
Records

The record should contain identification information, that is, the data base. This includes the patient's name, address, family roles, and educational and work histories. A description of the patient's physical and mental status at the time of admission to occupational therapy should be included. This information is gathered from the medical record, the occupational therapy evaluation, and the therapist's observations of the patient's performance and behavior during the evaluation process.[2]

EVALUATION DATA. The record should contain the detailed results of all evaluations that were carried out. These include the ADL and home management checklists; muscle testing, joint measurement, sensory evaluation, and perceptual/cognitive evaluation forms; and the record of any other tests or evaluation procedures that were performed.

TREATMENT PLAN. A brief or detailed treatment plan should be kept as part of the occupational therapy record. This includes identified problems and their corresponding goals and treatment methods, listed side by side or consecutively.

RUNNING PROGRESS NOTES. Many treatment agencies require daily or weekly running progress notes, which are later summarized to become a progress report for the permanent record. In some treat-

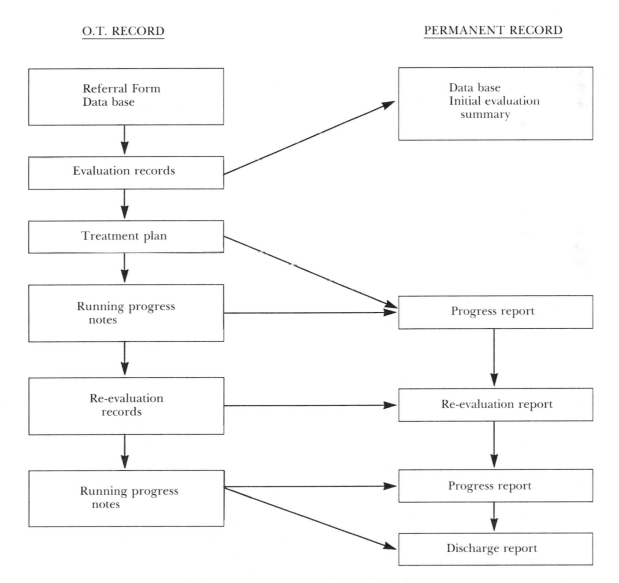

Fig. 5-1. Content and process of occupational therapy documentation.

ment facilities these notes are part of the permanent medical record. Progress notes should contain brief notations of the patient's problems, goals of treatment, specific treatment modalities, and the patient's response to treatment, that is, any gains or changes in performance.[2] Various styles or formats are used to ensure the consistency of the content of these notes in each facility. SOAP notes are frequently used in occupational therapy records. This acronym stands for Subjective (the patient's view of the problem), Objective (the clinical findings about the problem), Assessment (important data from the evaluation), and Plan (goals of treatment and modalities).[5] This method of recording information was based on the system designed by Weed in the Problem Oriented Medical Record.[4,6] Another format for a short daily note states the problem, progress, description of the treatment program, and future plans. Still another possibility is to record the length of attendance, goal, method, patient's response or progress, and future plan.

Sample of short running progress notes

11/4—Patient seen once since 11/2 for dressing training. Almost independent except for buttoning shirt, tying shoe laces, and buckling belt. Requires minimum assistance to stand and transfer to regular chair. Highly motivated for independence and cooperative. Continue dressing training.

11/6—Patient seen for dressing training. Button hook issued and patient trained in its use. Can button shirt independently now. Elastic shoe laces placed in shoes. Patient will try these and report at next visit. Patient expressing some feelings of discouragement today. Continue program to complete dressing training and to introduce light meal preparation.

Reports

INITIAL EVALUATION. The occupational therapy evaluation should be summarized in the initial evaluation report that becomes part of the patient's permanent record. It may include data such as the diagnosis and disability, date of admission to the service, the number of visits to date, any pertinent background information, tests used in evaluation, any special circumstances under which the tests were administered, results of the evaluation (with interpretation), analysis and identification of problems for occupational therapy intervention, and a statement about the planned treatment program.

Sample of initial evaluation report

10/24—The patient is 62 years old with onset of a left CVA on 9/1, resulting in right hemiplegia and mild expressive aphasia. He was first seen in the occupational therapy outpatient department on 10/10. He is scheduled for 1 hour of treatment three times a week and has kept all scheduled appointments, for a total of six visits to date.

The patient was working in a mill tending a mechanical loom at the time of his CVA. He lives in a small house with his wife and he liked gardening, cooking, and refinishing antique furniture in his spare time.

The patient ambulates slowly using a cane. He is able to maintain standing balance for up to 15 minutes but requires the support of the cane or nearby furniture. He tends to use his cane for support when rising from a chair. A safer method has been demonstrated and is being practiced by the patient.

The patient demonstrated ability to perform strong flexion and extension patterns of movement of the right upper extremity, in addition to some isolated movement on command. He has good grasp, finger extension, and opposition. Passive ROM at all upper extremity joints is within normal limits, except for slight limitation at the left shoulder and elbow resulting from previous injuries. However, impairment of touch and pain sensitivity, stereognosis, and proprioception prevents spontaneous functional use of available motor function. The patient complains of impairments of smell, taste, and hearing as a result of the CVA. These are scheduled for evaluation.

He reported that he was able to dress himself independently during hospitalization, but that his wife now assists him. He is capable of most dressing activities except that he requires moderate assistance for buttoning shirts, tying shoes, and managing belt buckles. Since his illness he has not prepared meals or independently performed any household activities for which he was responsible prior to his illness. He stated that he would like to resume performing some of them to increase his sense of usefulness.

Problems: (1) dependence in ADL, (2) sensory impairment, (3) limited functional use of right upper extremity, (4) poor standing balance, (5) loss of work role, and (6) loss of leisure role.

Goals: (1) achieve independence in ADL, (2) improve sensory functions, (3) increase functional use of right upper extremity, (4) increase standing balance and standing tolerance, (5) evaluate feasibility to return to work, and (6) increase performance of leisure activities at home.

Plan: ADL training, sensory retraining, sensorimotor training/bilateral functional activities, balance training and activities for standing tolerance, simulated work, and leisure activities.

PROGRESS REPORTS. The progress report should summarize the treatment program and progress of the patient over a specific period of time. This may include data such as the number of visits since the last report, problems, previous goals, specific treatment techniques, progress made toward stated goals, and the plan for future program.

Sample weekly progress report

11/15—The patient has attended three treatment sessions of 1 hour each since 11/7. He has demonstrated some improvement in ambulation, standing balance, and standing tolerance. He is able to walk for short periods while working. Sensorimotor training has resulted in some improvement in right upper-extremity movement. He is conscious of using his arm in bilateral activities and makes efforts to do so without cues from the therapist. Although some additional isolated movement is possible since the report of 10/31, this arm continues to function with gross movement patterns, and sensory impairment persists, limiting function. He is performing self-care activities independently with the aid of a button hook and elastic shoe laces. A Velcro fastener has been added to trousers to eliminate the need for a belt.

Goals and Plan: Continue sensorimotor training and activities to increase use of right upper extremity, continue training to increase standing balance and tolerance, introduce simulated work and leisure activities to explore feasibility of actual activities.

REEVALUATION REPORT. During the treatment program it is necessary to reevaluate the patient periodically. The results of reevaluations, if brief, may be included in the progress report. However, if a comprehensive reevaluation is carried out, a separate report may be required and should address all areas included in the initial evaluation and any new areas that were assessed.

DISCHARGE REPORT. The discharge report is a summary of the treatment program and its outcomes. It should clearly indicate the patient's performance at the time treatment was terminated. The report should contain data about the total number of visits, the treatment goals, a summary of the patient's progress, the reason for discontinuation of services, remaining problems, and recommendations for follow-up or referral to other services.

Sample discharge report

1/25—The patient is 62 years old and had a left CVA on 9/1, resulting in right hemiplegia and mild expressive aphasia. He was admitted to the occupational therapy outpatient clinic on 10/10 and was scheduled for 1 hour of treatment, three times weekly. He has attended regularly since admission. The purposes of the program were to (1) achieve independence in ADL, (2) improve sensory functions, (3) increase functional use of the right upper extremity, (4) increase standing balance and tolerance, (5) evaluate feasibility of returning to work, and (6) increase leisure activities at home.

Initially the patient ambulated slowly with the aid of a cane. He was unable to maintain standing balance without support for more than a few minutes. Gross flexion and extension patterns of movement were present in the right upper extremity, and some isolated movement was possible on command. Touch and pain sensation, proprioception, and stereognosis were impaired. These sensorimotor impairments resulted in minimum functional use of the right arm. The patient was partially dependent in dressing and dependent in performance of household tasks but expressed sincere motivation for greater independence.

As the treatment program progressed the patient's ambulation, standing tolerance, and standing balance improved to the degree that he walked more rapidly and for short distances around the clinic without his cane. Senses of touch and proprioception improved moderately, and purposeful use of the right upper extremity increased. Some sensory impairment persisted and limited his ability to use the available functional movement to fullest advantage. He is able to use the right upper extremity as a good

assist in nonhazardous activities. He achieved independence in dressing, light meal preparation, and light household tasks such as dusting and table setting.

The patient expressed feelings of worthlessness and a lack of inner drive. He related an interest in resuming household tasks, cooking, and furniture refinishing. Such activities were added to the program. He enjoyed these and gained pleasure, satisfaction, and improved self-esteem from the performance and end products. There was a remarkable improvement in level of interest, affect, and confidence in skills. Patient socialized more freely, showed an increased sense of humor, and an acceptance of the disability.

A home visit confirmed that the patient could manage safely in his own kitchen and bathroom. A basement workshop for furniture refinishing and repair was not suitable because of the number of steps to maneuver. Space in the garage was subsequently arranged for this purpose.

Work evaluation resulted in the determination that it would not be feasible for the patient to return to work at the mill because it required long periods of standing, rapid bilateral movement, fine coordination, and acute fingertip sensation to stop, adjust, and rethread the looms. He was able to retire with a pension.

The intensive phase of the occupational therapy program was discontinued on 1/15, with a status of "maximally improved" and a recommendation for check-up visits every 2 months.

In actual reports or records of the samples above, many of the words may have been abbreviated. For example, "moderate assistance" is often written "mod. a."; "right upper extremity" is "RUE"; an upward arrow represents the word "increase"; a downward arrow represents the word "decrease"; and PROM means "passive range of motion." Such abbreviations save time and space and are useful as long as all of the health care workers understand the given system used at the facility. The therapist may also write the record or report using short statements rather than complete sentences. This is another way to save time and space.

QUALITY OF DOCUMENTATION

It is necessary for occupational therapists to be able to convey their contributions to the treatment program of a patient verbally and in writing to all other health care providers. The development of good medical records demands continual, systematic reevaluation. Documentation of occupational therapy services is the medium through which, when well done, the profession commands respect.[2] As the public has demanded more accountability in health care, occupational therapy documentation has become more important.[5] Documentation is essential for quality control and maintainance of high standards of practice.

Documentation should be well organized, contain only pertinent information, and be accurate and objective. Brevity is important because space for records and reports is limited, as is the therapist's time. Many abbreviations are used as time- and space-saving device in documenting occupational therapy services. Some of these are universally used medical abbreviations, whereas many others are limited to use in a particular treatment facility. The therapist must learn and use them accurately and appropriately. A standardized system or outline for writing specific records or reports is very helpful for consistency in the occupational therapy program or facility and to ensure that the same data are included in all records and reports.

When writing records and reports, the occupational therapist should consider who will read them.[1] This influences how they are written, that is, whether abbreviations and medical terminology are appropriate or whether more detail in lay terms is necessary. Because funding for treatment, insurance payments, and sometimes legal claims will depend on documentation in the medical record, the manner in which it is done can be critical to the occupational therapy service and to the patient.

When writing records or reports, the occupational therapist should ask who will read them and what does the reader know about the patient, diagnosis, and occupational therapy services; how an accurate, complete picture of the problems, program, and progress can be best conveyed so that it is well understood by the reader and that the patient receives the fairest consideration and advantage as a result; and if the reader is a medical professional or an outside agent with no medical background.

The destination of the record and report is a key factor in the method of writing. The occupational therapist must be able to convert a brief report full of abbreviations, short statements, and jargon intended for other health care workers in the facility into a comprehensive detailed report to be read by an insurance agent, funding source official, or other concerned professional.

LEGAL IMPLICATIONS OF DOCUMENTATION

In the current health care system, there is close scrutiny of health care services, records, and costs. Laws have been enacted to ensure quality care and cost containment for the target population. The advent of the prospective payment system (PPS) in 1983 has had a significant impact on health care delivery. In this system payment of services is made according to a set fee determined before the delivery of the services. One of its primary purposes is to keep health care costs down.[1] The law requires that health care providers keep accurate, current records. The record must contain enough information to justify the treatment plan, treatment, and cost. It should reflect who administered the treatment, the treatment methods, and when the treatment was given. Progress, results, and a discharge summary should be included. The record must contain factual information and include no value judgments that may be prejudicial to the patient.[5,7]

Health care records may be used in litigation to settle insurance claims and may be examined by third party payers, fiscal intermediaries, Professional Standards Review Organization (PSRO), and other utilization review boards.[5,7] Therefore it is important that the record be accurate, objective, and reflect actual events and progress pertinent to the patient.

The review of health care records is governed by principles of ethical practice in relation to confidentiality and are under strict control of the physician or health care agency. No privileged information, verbal or written, can be released without written consent of the patient.[2] The patient has the right to know what is in the record and can ask for the information. The information must be given by the physician in a manner in which he or she sees fit.

REPORTING SYSTEMS
The Problem Oriented Medical Record[4,6]

The Problem Oriented Medical Record (POMR) was devised by Dr. Lawrence L. Weed at Case Western Reserve University.[6] It is based on a computer-compatible model and follows a systematic progression from evaluation to progress reporting. It is a problem-solving model that is easily accepted by occupational therapists and can be implemented in any setting. It offers a method by which evaluation and treatment standards can be documented and enforced.[4]

The POMR encourages all health care services to integrate information on one progress note sheet. The data base is composed of physical, social, and demographic information and is contained in one report. From this data base a problem list is formulated and kept at the front of the record. It serves as an index to all problems and may include anticipated problems. Each problem is numbered and named, and these designations remain the same for each hospitalization of the patient. All of the treatment plans must be titled and numbered according to the problem list, dated, and signed. For example, by reading all of the notes that refer to problem number 3, the health care worker can learn what each service is contributing to the patient's total rehabilitation at any given time.[4]

All progress notes are dated, numbered, and titled according to the problem to which they refer. All progress notes are recorded together. They are written according to the aforementioned SOAP outline. Progress notes are written whenever a staff member has relevant information to record. Frequency of entries to the record may reflect policies of the treatment facility, acuteness of the patient's condition, or need for continued evaluation.[4] The record concludes with a problem-oriented discharge summary.[6]

The POMR facilitates communications between health disciplines because all progress notes are intermixed and all personnel are bound by the same criteria for recording. All services are up to date on progress in other areas, and treatment can be adjusted accordingly. The patient can be educated to his condition and progress. The POMR allows for adequate documentation required for quality assurance and medical insurance purposes.

The accurate documentation of services is an outcome of the treatment process. The POMR offers a recording system that can improve the standards of documentation.[4] The reader is referred to the original source for further details about implementation of this system.[6]

The Occupational Therapy Sequential Client Care Record

The Occupational Therapy Sequential Client Care Record (OTSCCR) created by Llorens is unique to occupational therapy.[3] Rather than being based on medical or psychological reporting systems, it is organized according to a theoretical framework consistent with the characteristics, objectives, and goals of occupational therapy. As occupational therapy has progressed toward professional status, there has been an increased effort to measure the quality of care, achieve autonomy in decision making, be accountable to patients and funding agencies, and assume professional responsibility for services. Llorens described the client care record as the "key document for determining quality and effectiveness of care."[3]

The OTSCCR system combines the theoretical framework of Llorens's Occupational Therapy Developmental Analysis, Evaluation and Intervention Schedule, and the scientific method of the POMR for documenting care in occupational therapy. The OTSCCR includes a data base, information about the evaluation process, problem identification, occupa-

tional therapy plan, progress notes, and discharge summary. It is based on developmental and occupational performance frames of reference, and data are recorded and analyzed according to the performance skills and performance components of the occupational performance frame of reference.

The OTSCCR documents factual information about the client based on actual behavior. It is designed to span the total time the client is served by occupational therapy from admission to discharge. It is retained by the occupational therapy department for use in preparing reports and communicating with the client and other interested persons or agencies.[3] The reader is referred to the original source for details about the use of this system for documenting occupational therapy services.[3]

SUMMARY

Documentation of occupational therapy services consists of written records and reports that contain pertinent information about the patient's status, progress, and performance. The occupational therapist is responsible for keeping accurate records to document the treatment program and the patient's progress.

Documentation is necessary for administrative, educational, legal, and communications purposes. It is essential to justify the necessity and cost of treatment. It contributes to advancing the professionalism of occupational therapy. Occupational therapy documentation includes the referral form, evaluation data, initial evaluation summary, treatment plan, progress notes and reports, reevaluation reports, and discharge summary.

Records and reports should reflect clear, concise, accurate, and objective information about the patient, progress, and performance. The reader of the documents must be considered when records or reports are being written to avoid misunderstanding. Documentation should be well organized and developed according to an agreed-on system for internal consistency of the record. The POMR and the OTSCCR system are two methods for documenting occupational therapy services.[3,6]

REFERENCES

1. Baum CM and Luebben AJ: Prospective payment systems, Thorofare, NJ, 1986, Slack Inc.
2. Gleave GJ: Medical records and reports. In Willard HS and Spackman CS, editors: Occupational therapy, ed 4, Philadelphia, 1971, JB Lippincott Co.
3. Llorens LA: Occupational therapy sequential client care record manual, Laurel MD, 1982, Ramsco Publishing Co.
4. Potts LR: The problem oriented record: implications for occupational therapy, Am J Occup Ther 26:6(288), 1972.
5. Tiffany EG: Psychiatry and mental health. In Hopkins HL and Smith HD, editors: Willard and Spackman's occupational therapy, ed 6, Philadelphia, 1983, JB Lippincott Co.
6. Weed LL: Medical records, medical education and patient care, Chicago, 1971, Year Book Medical Publishers.
7. Welles C: The implications of liability: guidelines for professional practice, Am J Occup Ther 23:1(18), 1969.

METHODS OF EVALUATION AND TREATMENT FOR PATIENTS WITH PHYSICAL DYSFUNCTION

Chapter

Evaluation of joint range of motion

LORRAINE WILLIAMS PEDRETTI

Joint measurement is a primary evaluation procedure for those physical dysfunctions that could cause limitation of joint motion, for example, arthritis, fractures, burns, and hand trauma. Range of motion (ROM) is the arc of motion through which a joint passes. Passive ROM is the arc of motion through which the joint passes when moved by an outside force. Active ROM is the arc of motion through which the joint passes when moved by the muscles acting on the joint. Normally passive ROM is slightly greater than active ROM.[7] The instrument used for measuring ROM is the goniometer.

The purposes for measuring ROM are to (1) determine limitations that interfere with function or may produce deformity; (2) determine additional range needed to increase functional capacity or reduce deformity; (3) keep a record of progression or regression; (4) measure progress objectively; (5) determine appropriate treatment goals; (6) select appropriate treatment modalities, positioning techniques, and other strategies to reduce limitations; and (7) determine the need for splints and assistive devices.

PRINCIPLES OF JOINT MEASUREMENT

The evaluator should know the average normal ROM, how the joint moves, and how to position self, patient, and joints for measurement.[3] Before measuring, the evaluator should ask the patient to move the part through the available ROM, if muscle strength is a grade of Fair (3) or better, and observe the movement.[3] The evaluator should move the part passively through the ROM to see and feel how the joint moves and to estimate ROM.

Formal joint measurement is *not* necessary with every patient. When joint limitation is not a primary symptom, or the disability is of recent onset, with proper positioning and daily ROM exercises, limited ROM would not be anticipated. In such cases, however, ROM should be visually observed by using active ROM or by putting all joints through passive ROM. Normal ROM varies from one person to another. Establish norms for each individual by measuring the uninvolved part if possible.[3] If this is not possible, average ranges listed in the literature are used. The therapist should check records and interview the patient for the presence of fused joints and other limitations caused by old injuries. Joints should not be forced when resistance is met on passive ROM. Pain may limit ROM and crepitation may be heard on movement in some conditions.

METHODS OF JOINT MEASUREMENT
The 180° System

Using the 180° system of joint measurement, 0° is the starting position for all joint motions. For most motions the anatomic position is the starting position, and the 180° is superimposed as a semicircle on the body in the plane in which the motion will occur. The axis of the joint is the axis of the semicircle or arc of motion. All joint motions begin at 0° and increase toward 180°.[4,7] The 180° system is used later in this chapter to describe procedures for joint measurement.

The 360° System

Using the 360° system of joint measurement, movements occurring in the coronal and sagittal planes are related to a full circle. When the body is in the anatomic position, the circle is superimposed on it in the same plane in which the motion will occur with the joint axis as the pivotal point. "The 0° (360°) position will be overhead and the 180° position will be toward the feet."[4] Thus, for example, shoulder flexion and abduction are movements that proceed toward 0°, and shoulder adduction and extension proceed toward 360°.[4] The average normal ROM for shoulder flexion is 170°. Therefore using the 360° system, the movement would start at 180° and progress toward 0° to 10°. The ROM recorded would be 10°. On the other hand, shoulder extension that has a normal ROM of 60° would begin at 180° and progress toward 360° to 240°, and 240° would be the ROM recorded.[4] The total ROM of extension to flexion would be 240° minus 10°, that is, 230°.[4,5]

Some motions cannot be related to the full circle. In these instances a 0° starting position is designated, and the movements are measured as increases from 0°. These motions occur in a horizontal plane around a vertical axis. They are (1) forearm pronation and supination, (2) hip internal and external rotation, (3) wrist radial and ulnar deviation, and (4) thumb palmar and radial abduction (carpometacarpal flexion and extension).[4]

GONIOMETERS

Goniometers are used to measure the range of joint motion. They are made of metal or plastic, come in several sizes, and are available from medical and rehabilitation equipment companies.[4,7] The word *goniometer* is derived from the Greek, *gonia*, which means angle and *metron*, which means measure.[7,9] Thus goniometer literally means to measure angles.

The goniometer consists of a stationary (proximal) bar and a movable (distal) bar.[7] The body of the stationary bar is a small protractor (half circle) or a full circle printed with a scale of degrees from 0° to 180° for the half circle and 0° to 360° for the full circle goniometer.[3] The movable bar is attached at the center or axis of the protractor and acts as a dial. As the movable bar rotates around the protractor, the dial points to the number of degrees on the scale.

Two scales of figures are printed on the half circle. Each starts at 0° and progresses toward 180°, but in opposite directions. Since the starting position in the 180° system is always 0° and increases toward 180°, the outer row of figures is read if the bony segments being measured are end to end, as in elbow flexion. Similarly the inner row of figures is read if the bony segments are being measured are alongside one another, as in shoulder flexion.

Fig. 6-1 shows five styles of goniometers. The first (Fig. 6-1, *A*) is a full circle goniometer that can be used for both the 360° and the 180° systems, since it has calibrations for both printed on its face. This goniometer has longer arms and is convenient for use on the large joints of the body. Fig. 6-1, *B*, is a half circle instrument used for the 180° system. This par-

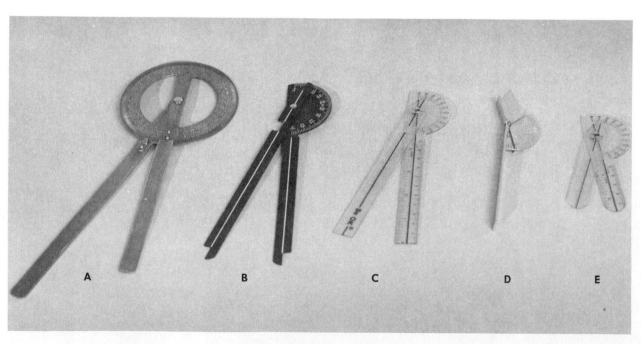

Fig. 6-1. Types of goniometers.

ticular goniometer is radiopaque and could be used during x-ray examinations if necessary. Its dial is notched at two places so that an accurate reading of motion can be taken regardless of whether the convexity of the half circle is directed toward or away from the direction of motion. The advantage of this is that the examiner does not have to reverse the goniometer, obscuring the figures on the scale from view. A special finger goniometer is shown in Fig. 6-1, *D*. Its arms are short and flattened. It is designed to be used over the finger joint surfaces rather than on their lateral aspects, as is done in most of the larger joint motions. Small plastic goniometers are shown in Fig. 6-1, *C* and *E*. These are inexpensive and easy to carry. The longer one can be used with both large and small joints. The dials of goniometers that are transparent are also marked or notched in two places like the goniometer in Fig. 6-1, *B*. The smaller of these two goniometers is simply a larger one that has been cut to be adapted as a finger goniometer.

One important feature of the goniometer is the axis or fulcrum. The nut or rivet that acts as the fulcrum must move freely, yet it must be tight enough to remain where it was set when the goniometer is removed from the body segment following the joint measurement.[3] Some goniometers have a locking nut for the fulcrum. This nut is tightened just before removing the goniometer so that the reading can be easily and accurately made.[4]

There are other types of goniometers. Some use fluids with a free-floating bubble that provides the reading after the motion is completed.[4] Others can be attached to a body segment and have dials that register rotary motions, such as pronation and supination.

RECORDING RESULTS OF MEASUREMENTS

When using the 180° system, the evaluator should record the number of degrees at the starting position and the number of degrees at the final position after the joint has passed through the maximal possible arc of motion.[7] Normal ROM always starts at 0° and increases toward 180°. A limitation is indicated if the starting position is not 0°. For example:
1. Elbow.
   Normal: 0° to 140°
   Extension limitation: 15° to 140°
   Flexion limitation: 0° to 110°
2. Abnormal hyperextension of the elbow may be recorded by indicating the number of degrees of hyperextension *before* the 0° starting position. The amount of motion before the 0° position is recorded with a minus sign.[7]
   Normal: 0° to 140°

Abnormal hyperextension: −20° to 0° to 140°
3. There are alternate methods of recording ROM. The evaluator is advised to learn and adopt the particular method required by the health care facility.

A sample of a form for recording ROM measurements is shown in Fig. 6-2.

Average normal ROM is listed on the form and in Table 6-1. It should be noted that movements of the shoulder (glenohumeral) joint are accompanied by scapula movement as outlined. Glenohumeral joint motion is highly dependent on scapula mobility, which gives the shoulder its flexibility and wide ranges of motion. Although it is not possible to measure scapula movement with the goniometer, the evaluator should assess scapula mobility before proceeding with shoulder joint measurements. If the scapula musculature is in a state of spasticity or contracture and the shoulder joint is moved into ROMs that require scapula mobility (for example, above 90° of flexion or abduction), joint damage can result.

When joint measurements may be performed in more than one position, for example, as in shoulder internal and external rotation, the evaluator should note on the record in which position the measurement was taken. The examiner should also note any pain or discomfort experienced by the subject, the appearance of protective muscle spasm, whether active or passive ROM was measured, and any deviations from recommended testing procedures or positions that were used.[7]

RESULTS OF EVALUATION AS A BASIS FOR TREATMENT PLANNING

Common causes of joint limitation include skin contracture caused by adhesions or scar tissue, muscle weakness, spasticity, displacement of fibrocartilage or presence of other foreign bodies in the joint, bony obstruction or destruction, and soft tissue contractures, such as tendon, muscle, or ligament shortening.[6] Following joint measurement, the therapist should analyze the results in relationship to the patient's life role requirements. The therapist's first concern should be to correct ROMs that fall below functional limits. Many ordinary activities of daily living (ADL) do not require full ROM.

Functional ROM refers to the amount of joint range necessary to perform essential ADL without the use of special equipment.[6] The first concern of treatment, then, would be to try to increase ROMs that are limiting performance of self and home maintenance tasks to "functional range of motion."[6] For example, a significant limitation of elbow flexion would affect ability to eat and perform oral hygiene. Therefore it would

JOINT RANGE MEASUREMENTS

Patient's name _____ Chart no. _____

Date of birth _____ Age _____ Sex _____

Diagnosis _____ Date of onset _____

Disability _____

LEFT				RIGHT		
3	2	1	SPINE	1	2	3
			Cervical spine			
			Flexion 0-45			
			Extension 0-45			
			Lateral flexion 0-45			
			Rotation 0-60			
			Thoracic and lumbar spine			
			Flexion 0-80			
			Extension 0-30			
			Lateral flexion 0-40			
			Rotation 0-45			
			SHOULDER			
			Flexion 0 to 170			
			Extension 0 to 60			
			Abduction 0 to 170			
			Horizontal abduction 0-40			
			Horizontal adduction 0-130			
			Internal rotation 0 to 70			
			External rotation 0 to 90			
			ELBOW AND FOREARM			
			Flexion 0 to 135-150			
			Supination 0 to 80-90			
			Pronation 0 to 80-90			
			WRIST			
			Flexion 0 to 80			
			Extension 0 to 70			
			Ulnar deviation 0 to 30			
			Radial deviation 0 to 20			
			THUMB			
			MP flexion 0 to 50			
			IP flexion 0 to 80-90			
			Abduction 0 to 50			
			FINGERS			
			MP flexion 0 to 90			
			MP hyperextension 0 to 15-45			
			PIP flexion 0 to 110			
			DIP flexion 0 to 80			
			Abduction 0 to 25			
			HIP			
			Flexion 0 to 120			
			Extension 0 to 30			
			Abduction 0 to 40			
			Adduction 0 to 35			
			Internal rotation 0 to 45			
			External rotation 0 to 45			
			KNEE			
			Flexion 0 to 135			
			ANKLE AND FOOT			
			Plantar flexion 0 to 50			
			Dorsiflexion 0 to 15			
			Inversion 0 to 35			
			Eversion 0 to 20			

Fig. 6-2. Form for recording joint ROM measurement.

Table 6-1 Average Normal ROM (180° Method)

Joint	ROM	Associated girdle motion	Joint	ROM
Cervical spine			**Wrist**	
Flexion	0° to 45°		Flexion	0° to 80°
Extension	0° to 45°		Extension	0° to 70°
Lateral flexion	0° to 45°		Ulnar deviation (adduction)	0° to 30°
Rotation	0° to 60°		Radial deviation (abduction)	0° to 20°
Thoracic and lumbar spine			**Thumb***	
Flexion	0° to 80°		DIP flexion	0° to 80°-90°
Extension	0° to 30°		MP flexion	0° to 50°
Lateral flexion	0° to 40°		Adduction, radial and palmar	0°
Rotation	0° to 45°		Palmar abduction	0° to 50°
Shoulder			Radial abduction	0° to 50°
Flexion	0° to 170°	Abduction, lateral tilt, slight elevation, slight upward rotation	Opposition	
			Fingers*	
Extension	0° to 60°	Depression, adduction, upward tilt	MP flexion	0° to 90°
			MP hyperextension	0° to 15°-45°
Abduction	0° to 170°	Upward rotation, elevation	PIP flexion	0° to 110°
Adduction	0°	Depression, adduction, downward rotation	DIP flexion	0° to 80°
			Abduction	0° to 25°
Horizontal abduction	0° to 40°	Adduction, reduction of lateral tilt	**Hip**	
Horizontal adduction	0° to 130°	Abduction, lateral tilt	Flexion	0° to 120° (bent knee)
Internal rotation		Abduction, lateral tilt	Extension	0° to 30°
Arm in abduction	0° to 70°		Abduction	0° to 40°
Arm in adduction	0° to 60°		Adduction	0° to 35°
External rotation		Adduction, reduction of lateral tilt	Internal rotation	0° to 45°
			External rotation	0° to 45°
Arm in abduction	0° to 90°		**Knee**	
Arm in adduction	0° to 80°		Flexion	0° to 135°
Elbow			**Ankle and foot**	
Flexion	0° to 135°-150°		Plantar flexion	0° to 50°
Extension	0°		Dorsiflexion	0° to 15°
Forearm			Inversion	0° to 35°
Pronation	0° to 80°-90°		Eversion	0° to 20°
Supination	0° to 80°-90°			

Data Adapted from American Academy of Orthopaedic Surgeons: Joint motion: method of measuring and recording, Chicago, 1965, American Academy of Orthopaedic Surgeons, and Esch D and Lepley M: Evaluation of joint motion: methods of measurement and recording, Minneapolis, 1974, University of Minnesota Press.
*DIP, Distal interphalangeal; MP, metacarpophalangeal; PIP, proximal interphalangeal.

be important to increase elbow flexion to nearly full ROM for function. Likewise, a severe limitation of forearm pronation would affect the performance of tasks, such as eating, washing the body, telephoning, child care, and dressing. To sit comfortably hip ROM must be at least 0° to 90°, so that if hip flexion is limited, a first goal might be to increase it to 90°. Of course, if additional ROM can be gained, the therapist should plan the progression of treatment to increase the ROM to the normal range.

In some instances the ROM limitations may be permanent, and it will not be possible to increase ROM. In such cases the role of the therapist is to work out

methods to compensate for the loss of ROM. These may include assistive devices, such as a comb, brush, or shoe horn with long handles, device to apply stockings, or adapted methods of performing a particular skill. See Chapter 15 for further suggestions of ADL techniques for those with limited ROM.

In many diagnoses, as with burns and arthritis, loss of ROM can be anticipated; the goal of treatment would be to prevent joint limitation with splints, positioning, exercise, activity, and application of the principles of joint protection, before it occurs.

Limitations of ROM, their causes, and the prognosis for increasing ROM will suggest treatment approaches. Some of the specific methods used to increase ROM are discussed elsewhere in this text. These include passive or active stretching exercise, resistive exercise, strengthening of antagonistic muscle groups, activities that require active motion of the affected joints through the full available ROM, splints, and positioning. To increase ROM the physician may perform surgery or may manipulate the part while the patient is under anesthesia. The physical therapist may employ manual stretching with heat and massage.[6]

PROCEDURE FOR JOINT MEASUREMENT

Average normal ROM for each joint motion is listed in Table 6-1, in Fig. 6-2, and before each of the following procedures for measurement. The reader should keep in mind that these are averages and that there may be considerable variation in ROM from one individual to another.

Normal ROM is affected by age, sex, and other factors such as lifestyle and occupation.[7] Therefore the subject in the illustrations may not always demonstrate the average ROM listed for the particular motion.

The goniometer in the illustrations is shown so that the reader can most easily see its correct positioning. However, the examiner may not always be in the best position for the particular measurement. For the purposes of clear illustration, the examiner is necessarily shown off to one side and may have only one hand on the instrument. Many of the motions require that the examiner be squarely in front of the subject or that the examiner's hands obscure the goniometer. The manner in which the examiner holds the goniometer and supports the part being measured is determined by factors such as degree of muscle weakness, presence or absence of joint pain, and whether active or passive ROM is being measured. The examiner and subject should be positioned for the greatest comfort, correct placement of the instrument, and adequate stabilization of the part being tested to effect the desired motion in the correct plane.

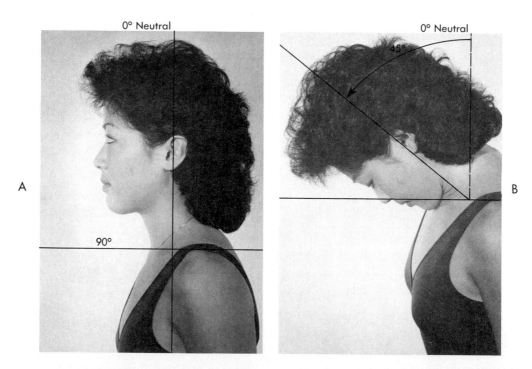

Fig. 6-3. Cervical flexion. **A,** Starting position. **B,** Final position.

Cervical flexion —0° to 45° (Fig. 6-3)[1]

POSITION OF THE SUBJECT: Sitting or standing erect.

MEASUREMENT OF MOTION: The subject is asked to flex the neck so that the chin moves toward the chest. The number of degrees of motion may be estimated, or the examiner may measure the number of inches or centimeters from chin to the sternal notch.[1,7] If a goniometer is used, the axis is placed over the angle of the jaw. The examiner grasps the corner of the protractor, which is positioned with the arc upward, and steadies her arm by resting it against the subject's shoulder. The arms of the goniometer are aligned with a tongue depressor, which the subject is holding between the teeth. As the subject performs neck flexion, the movable bar of the goniometer is adjusted downward to align with the new position of the tongue depressor.[3,7]

General procedure—180° method of measurement

1. Have subject comfortable and relaxed in appropriate position.
2. Explain and demonstrate to subject what you are going to do, why, and how you expect him or her to cooperate.
3. Uncover joint to be measured.
4. Establish bony landmarks for the measurement.
5. Stabilize joints proximal to joint being measured.
6. Move part passively through ROM to estimate available ROM and get the feel of joint mobility.[7]
7. Return part to the starting position.[7]
8. At starting position place axis of goniometer over axis of joint. Place stationary bar on proximal or stationary bone and movable bar on distal or moving bone. Avoid goniometer dial going off semicircle by always facing curved side away from direction of motion, unless the goniometer can be read when it moves in either direction.
9. Record number of degrees at starting position and remove goniometer. Do not attempt to hold goniometer in place while moving joint through ROM.
10. Evaluator should hold part securely above and below joint being measured and *gently* move joint through available ROM to determine full *passive ROM. Do not force joints.* Watch for signs of pain and discomfort.

Unless otherwise indicated, passive ROM should be measured.
11. Reposition goniometer and record number of degrees at final position.
12. Remove goniometer and gently place part in resting position.
13. Record reading at final position and any notations on the evaluation form.

DIRECTIONS FOR JOINT MEASUREMENT— 180° SYSTEM

The spine[1,3,7,8]

CERVICAL SPINE. Measurement of motions of the neck are the least accurate, since there are few bony landmarks and much soft tissue overlying bony segments.[3] X-ray is the best means to make an accurate measurement of the specific joints.[8] Approximate estimates of cervical flexion, extension, rotation, and lateral flexion may be made by using the goniometer or by estimating the number of degrees of motion, using a fixed axis and estimating the arc of motion from that point (Figs. 6-3 to 6-10.)[1,3]

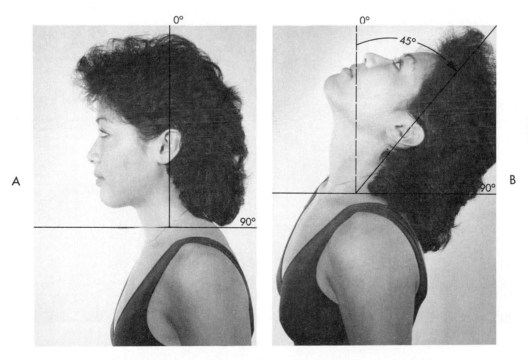

Fig. 6-4. Cervical extension. **A,** Starting position. **B,** Final position.

Cervical extension —0° to 45° (Fig. 6-4)[1]

POSITION OF THE SUBJECT: Sitting or standing erect.

MEASUREMENT OF MOTION: The subject is asked to extend the neck as if to look at the ceiling, so that the back of the head approaches the thoracic spine. The number of degrees of motion can be estimated. If a goniometer is used, the axis is again placed over the angle of the jaw. The examiner grasps the corner of the protractor, which is now positioned with the arc downward, and again steadies her arm against the subject's shoulder. The movable bar of the goniometer is moved upward to align with the tongue depressor as the subject extends the neck.[3,7]

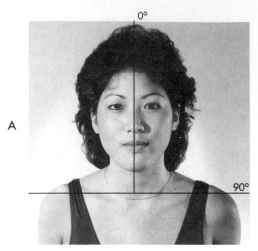

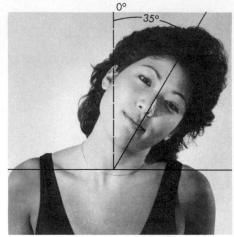

Fig. 6-5. Cervical Lateral flexion. **A,** Starting position. **B,** Final position.

Lateral flexion —0° to 45° (Fig. 6-5)[1]

POSITION OF THE SUBJECT: Sitting or standing erect.

MEASUREMENT OF MOTION: The subject is asked to flex the neck laterally, moving the ear toward the shoulder. The number of degrees of motion may be estimated, or the examiner may measure the number of inches or centimeters between the ear and shoulder.[1] If a goniometer is used, the axis is placed over the spinous process of the seventh cervical vertebra. The stationary bar may be over the shoulder and parallel to the floor so that the motion begins at 90°, or it may be aligned with the thoracic vertebra for a starting position of 0°. The movable bar is aligned with the external occipital protuberance.[1,7]

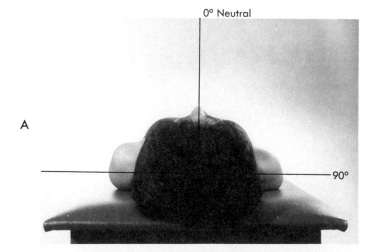

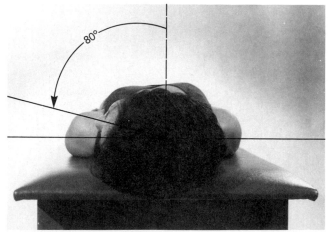

Fig. 6-6. Cervical rotation. **A,** Starting position. **B,** Final position.

Cervical rotation —0° to 60° (Fig. 6-6)[1]

POSITION OF THE SUBJECT: Lying supine.

MEASUREMENT OF MOTION: The subject is asked to rotate the head to right or left without rotating the trunk. The amount of rotation may be estimated in degrees from the neutral position.[1] If a goniometer is used, it is set at 90°, and the axis is placed over the vertex of the head. The stationary bar is held steady, parallel to the floor or to the acromion process on the side being tested. The movable bar is aligned with the tip of the nose.[3,7]

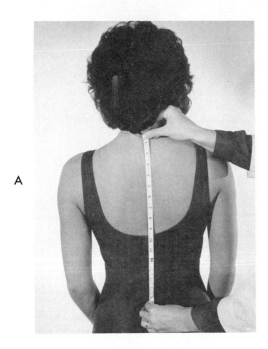

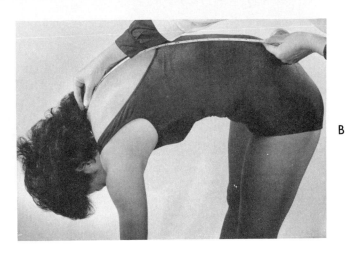

Fig. 6-7. Spine flexion. **A,** Starting position. **B,** Final position.

Thoracic and Lumbar Spine

Flexion —0° to 80° and +4 inches (Fig. 6-7)[1]

POSITION OF THE SUBJECT: Standing erect.

MEASUREMENT OF MOTION: Four methods of estimating the range of spinal flexion are (1) measuring the number of degrees of forward flexion of the trunk in relation to the longitudinal axis of the body. The examiner must hold the pelvis stable with the hands and any change in the subject's

normal lordosis should be observed; (2) indicating the level of the fingertips along the front of the subject's leg; (3) measuring the number of inches or centimeters between the subject's fingertips and the floor; and (4) measuring the length of the spine from the seventh cervical vertebra to the first sacral vertebra when the subject is erect and again after the subject has flexed the spine (Fig. 6-7).[7] This is probably the most accurate of these clinical methods.[1] In a normal adult there is an average increase of 4 inches in length in forward flexion of the spine. If the subject bends forward at the hips with a straight back, there will be no difference in length.

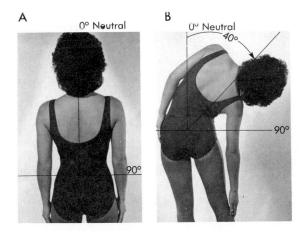

Fig. 6-8. Spine lateral flexion. **A,** Starting position. **B,** Final position.

Lateral flexion —0° to 40° (Fig. 6-8)[1]

POSITION OF THE SUBJECT: Standing erect.

METHOD OF MEASUREMENT: Several methods may be used to estimate the range of lateral flexion of the trunk. The steel tape measure may be held in place during the motion and used to estimate the number of degrees of lateral inclination of the trunk when compared with the vertical po-

sition. Other methods include (1) estimating the position of the spinous process of C7 in relation to the pelvis (Fig. 6-8); (2) measuring the distance of the fingertips from the knee joint in lateral flexion; and (3) using a long arm goniometer, placing the axis on S1, the stationary bar perpendicular to the floor, and the movable bar aligned with C7.[1,7]

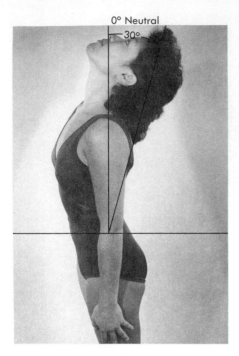

Fig. 6-9. Spine extension.

Extension —0° to 30° (Fig. 6-9)[1]

POSITION OF THE SUBJECT: Standing erect or lying prone.

METHOD OF MEASUREMENT: The subject is asked to bend backward while maintaining stability of the pelvis. The examiner may assist with this from the anterior when the measurement is taken in the standing position, if necessary. The range of extension is estimated in degrees from the vertical, using the superior iliac crest as the pivotal point in relation to the spinous process of C7.

Rotation —0° to 45° (Fig. 6-10)[1]

POSITION OF THE SUBJECT: Lying supine or standing.

METHOD OF MEASUREMENT: The subject is asked to rotate the upper trunk while maintaining neutral position of the pelvis. The examiner may fix the pelvis firmly to maintain the neutral position. This is especially important if the subject is in the standing position. This motion is recorded in degrees, using the center of the crown of the head as a pivotal point and the arc of motion made by the shoulder as it moves upward or forward.

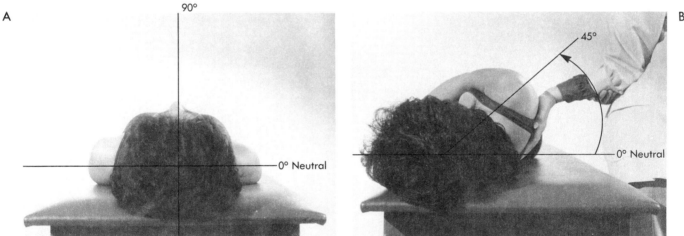

Fig. 6-10. Spine rotation. **A,** Starting position. **B,** Final position.

Upper extremity[1,2,4,7,8]

Shoulder

Flexion—0° to 170° (Fig. 6-11)

POSITION OF THE SUBJECT: Seated or supine with humerus in neutral rotation.

POSITION OF GONIOMETER: Axis is in the center of humeral head just distal to the acromion process on the lateral aspect of humerus. Stationary bar is parallel to trunk, and movable bar is parallel to humerus. Note that when the shoulder is flexed, the axis point moves upward and backward to the posterior surface of the shoulder. Thus when replacing the goniometer to take the measurement of the final position, it should be replaced on the lateral surface of the shoulder aligned with the end of the crease, which is formed over the deltoid mass.

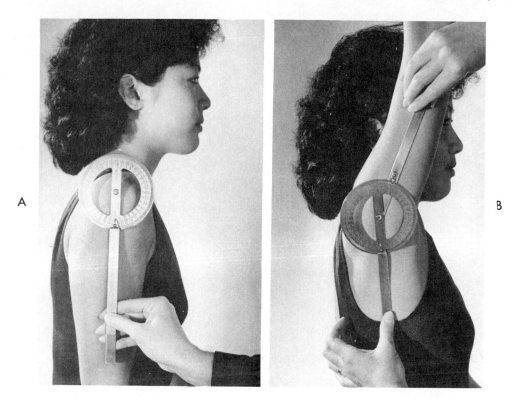

Fig. 6-11. Shoulder flexion. **A,** Starting position. **B,** Final position.

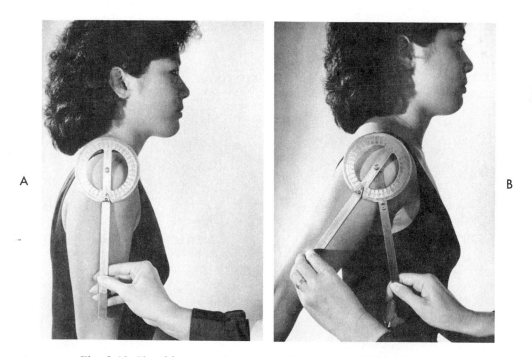

Fig. 6-12. Shoulder extension. **A,** Starting position. **B,** Final position.

Extension —0° to 60° (Fig. 6-12)

POSITION OF THE SUBJECT: Seated or prone, with no obstruction behind humerus and humerus in neutral rotation.

POSITION OF GONIOMETER: Same as for flexion, but the axis point remains the same for starting the final positions. Movement should be accompanied by slight upward tilt of the scapula. Excessive scapula motion should be avoided.

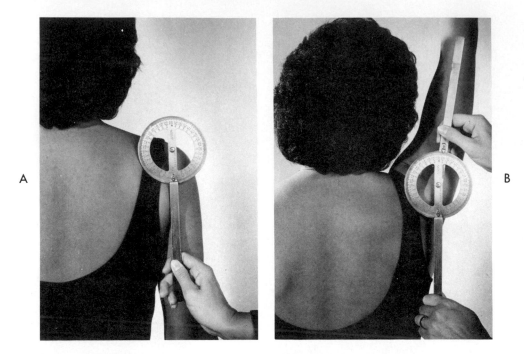

Fig. 6-13. Shoulder abduction. **A,** Starting position. **B,** Final position.

Abduction —0° to 170° (Fig 6-13)

POSITION OF THE SUBJECT: Seated or prone with humerus in external rotation. Measure on posterior surface.

POSITION OF GONIOMETER: Axis is on acromion process on posterior surface of shoulder. Stationary bar is parallel to trunk, and movable bar is parallel to humerus.

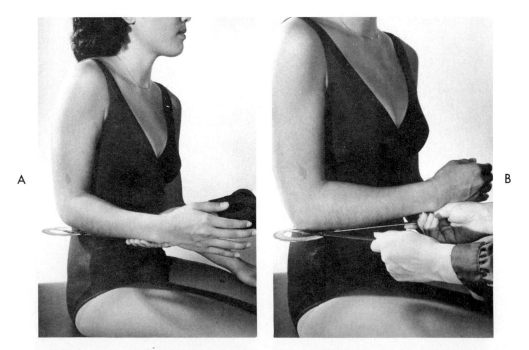

Fig. 6-14. Shoulder internal rotation, shoulder adducted. **A,** Starting position. **B,** Final position.

Internal rotation —0° to 60° (Fig. 6-14)

POSITION OF THE SUBJECT: Seated with humerus adducted against trunk, elbow at 90°, and forearm at midposition and perpendicular to body.

POSITION OF GONIOMETER: Axis on olecranon process of elbow and stationary bar and movable bar parallel to forearm.

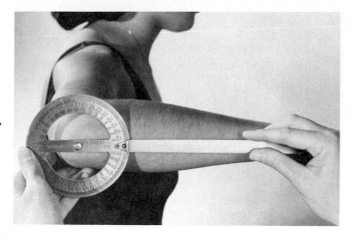
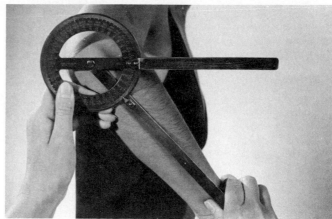

Fig. 6-15. Shoulder internal rotation, shoulder abducted; alternate position. **A,** Starting position. **B,** Final position.

Alternate position: Internal Rotation —0° to 70° (Fig. 6-15)

POSITION OF THE SUBJECT: Seated or supine with humerous abducted to 90°, elbow flexed to 90°.

POSITION OF GONIOMETER: Axis on olecranon process of elbow and stationary bar and movable bar parallel to forearm.

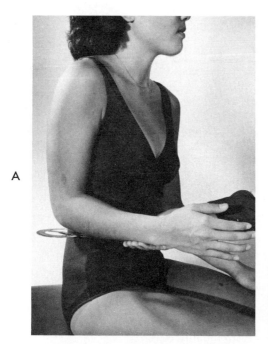
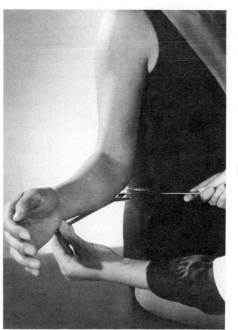

Fig. 6-16. External rotation, shoulder adducted. **A,** Starting position. **B,** Final position.

External rotation —0° to 80° (Fig. 6-16)

POSITION OF THE SUBJECT: Humerus adducted, elbow at 90°, and forearm in midposition, perpendicular to the body.

POSITION OF GONIOMETER: Axis on olecranon of elbow. Stationary bar and movable bar parallel to forearm.

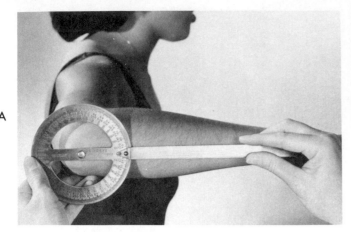
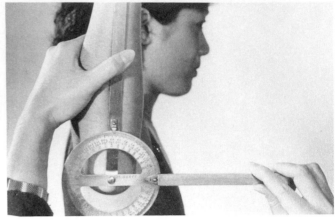

Fig. 6-17. Shoulder external rotation, shoulder abducted; alternate position. **A,** Starting position. **B,** Final position.

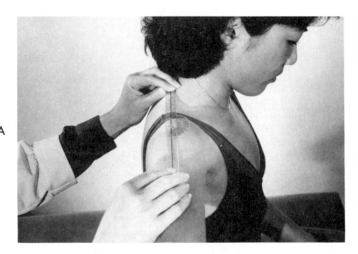
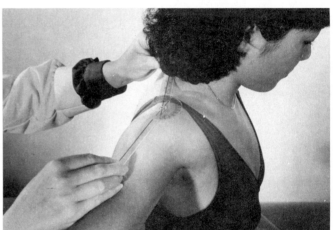

Fig. 6-18. Shoulder horizontal abduction. **A,** Starting position. **B,** Final position.

ALTERNATE POSITION: *External rotation* —0° to 90° (Fig. 6-17)

POSITION OF THE SUBJECT: Seated or supine with humerus abducted to 90°, elbow flexed to 90°, and forearm pronated.

POSITION OF GONIOMETER: Axis on olecranon process of elbow and stationary bar and movable bar parallel to forearm.

Horizontal abduction —0° to 40° (Fig. 6-18)

POSITION OF THE SUBJECT: Seated erect with the shoulder to be tested abducted to 90°, elbow extended, and palm facing down.

POSITION OF GONIOMETER: The axis is centered over the acromion process. The stationary bar is parallel over the shoulder toward the neck, and the movable bar is parallel with the humerus.

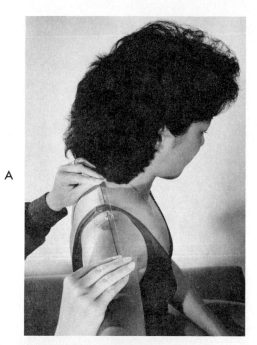

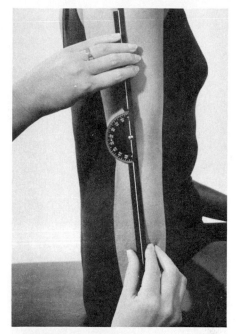

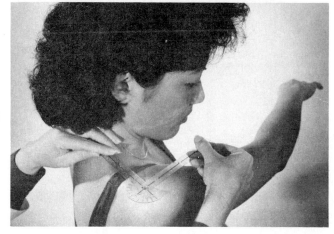

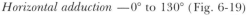

Fig. 6-19. Shoulder horizontal adduction. **A,** Starting position. **B,** Final position.

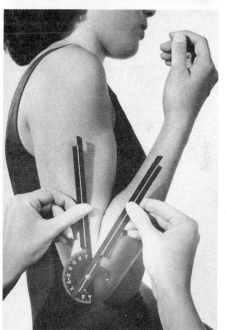

Fig. 6-20. Elbow flexion. **A,** Starting position. **B,** Final position.

Horizontal adduction —0° to 130° (Fig. 6-19)
POSITION OF SUBJECT AND GONIOMETER: Same as for horizontal abduction.
Elbow

Extension to flexion —0° to 135°-150° (Fig. 6-20)
POSITION OF THE SUBJECT: Standing, sitting, or supine with humerus adducted and externally rotated and forearm supinated.
POSITION OF GONIOMETER: Axis is placed over the lateral epicondyle of humerus at end of elbow crease. Stationary bar is parallel to midline of humerus, and movable bar is

parallel to radius. After the movement has been completed, the position of the elbow crease changes in relation to the lateral epicondyle because of the rise of the muscle bulk during the motion. The axis of the goniometer should be repositioned so that it is over, although will not be directly on, the lateral epicondyle.

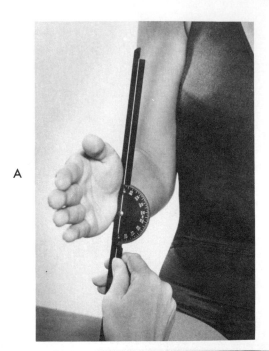

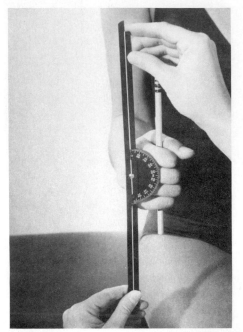

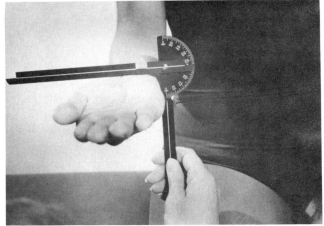

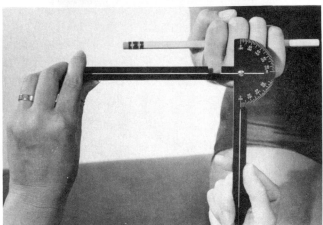

Fig. 6-21. Supination. **A,** Starting position. **B,** Final position.

Fig. 6-22. Forearm supination, alternate method. **A,** Starting position. **B,** Final position.

Forearm

Supination —0° to 80° or 90° (Fig. 6-21)

POSITION OF THE SUBJECT: Seated or standing with humerus adducted, elbow at 90°, and forearm in midposition.

POSITION OF GONIOMETER: Axis is at ulnar border of volar aspect of wrist, just proximal to the ulna styloid. Movable bar is resting against the volar aspect of the wrist, and the stationary bar is perpendicular to the floor. Note: After the forearm is supinated, the goniometer should be repositioned so that the movable bar rests squarely across the center of the distal forearm.

ALTERNATE METHOD: Supination (Fig. 6-22)

POSITION OF THE SUBJECT: Seated or standing with humerus adducted, elbow at 90°, and forearm in midposition. Place pencil in hand so it is held by subject perpendicular to floor.

POSITION OF GONIOMETER: Axis is over the head of third metacarpal, and stationary bar is perpendicular to floor. Movable bar is parallel to pencil.

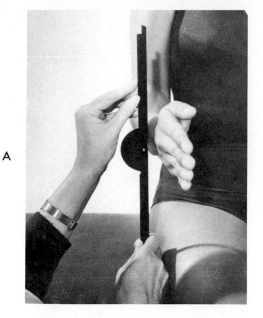

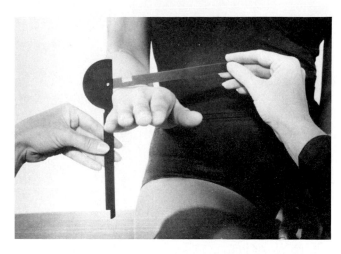

Fig. 6-23. Pronation. **A,** Starting position. **B,** Final position.

Pronation —0° to 80° or 90° (Fig. 6-23)

POSITION OF THE SUBJECT: Seated or standing with humerus adducted, elbow at 90°, and forearm in midposition.

POSITION OF GONIOMETER: Axis is at the ulnar border of the dorsal aspect of the wrist, just proximal to the ulna styloid. The movable bar is resting against the dorsal aspect of the wrist and the stationary bar is perpendicular to the floor. Note: After the forearm is pronated, reposition the goniometer so that the movable bar rests squarely across the center of the dorsum of the distal forearm.

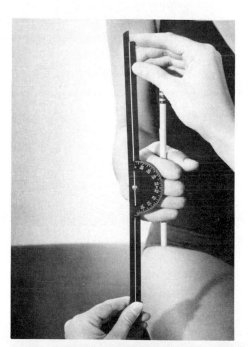

ALTERNATE METHOD: Pronation (Fig. 6-24)

POSITION OF THE SUBJECT: Seated or standing with humerus adducted, elbow at 90°, and forearm in midposition. A pencil is placed in the hand so that it is held perpendicular to the floor.

POSITION OF GONIOMETER: Axis is over the head of the third metacarpal, and stationary bar is perpendicular to the floor, and movable bar is parallel to pencil.

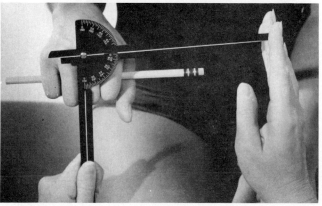

Fig. 6-24. Pronation; alternate method. **A,** Starting position. **B,** Final position.

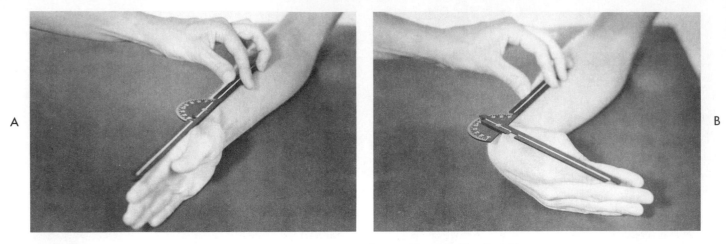

Fig. 6-25. Wrist flexion. **A,** Starting position. **B,** Final position.

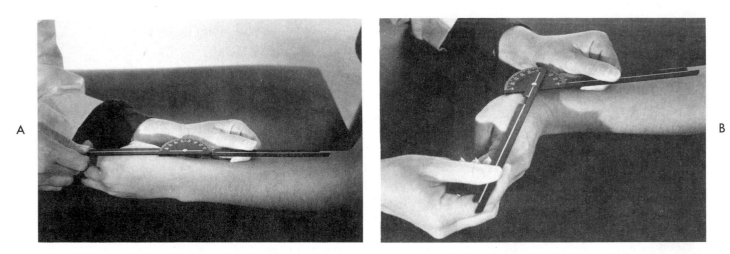

Fig. 6-26. Wrist extension. **A,** Starting position. **B,** Final position.

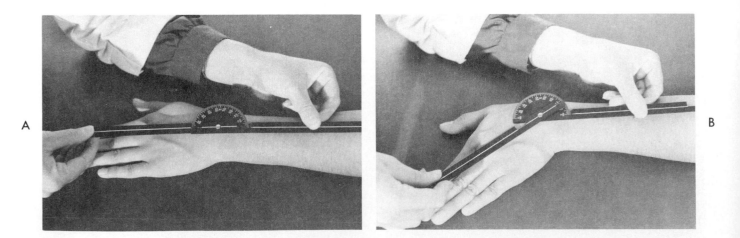

Fig. 6-27. Wrist ulnar deviation. **A,** Starting position. **B,** Final position.

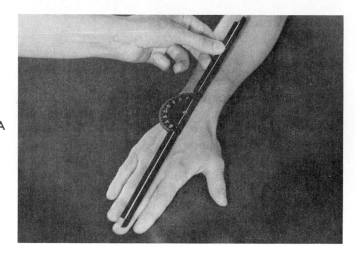

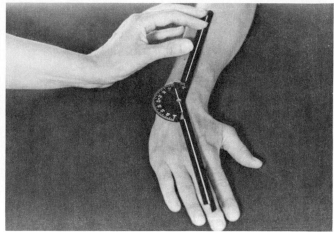

Fig. 6-28. Wrist radial deviation. **A,** Starting position. **B,** Final position.

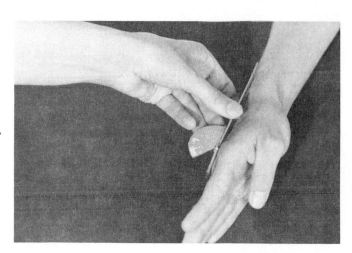

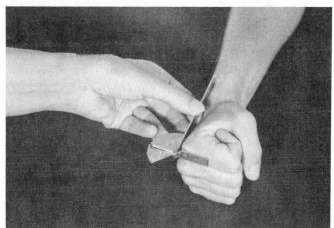

Fig. 6-29. MP flexion. **A,** Starting position. **B,** Final position.

Wrist

Flexion —0° to 80° (Fig. 6-25)

POSITION OF SUBJECT: Seated with forearm in midposition and hand and forearm resting on table on ulnar border.

POSITION OF GONIOMETER: Axis is on lateral aspect of wrist just distal to radial styloid in anatomical snuff box. Stationary bar is parallel to radius, and movable bar is parallel to metacarpal of index finger.

Extension —0° to 70° (Fig. 6-26)

POSITION OF SUBJECT AND GONIOMETER: Same as for wrist flexion.

Ulnar deviation —0° to 30° (Fig. 6-27)

POSITION OF THE SUBJECT: Seated with forearm pronated and palm of hand resting flat on table surface.

POSITION OF GONIOMETER: Axis is on dorsum of wrist at base of third metacarpal. Stationary bar is parallel to third metacarpal.

Radial deviation —0° to 20° (Fig. 6-28)

POSITION OF SUBJECT AND GONIOMETER: Same as for ulnar deviation.

Fingers

Metacarpophalangeal (MP) flexion —0° to 90° (Fig. 6-29)

POSITION OF THE SUBJECT: Seated with forearm in midposition, wrist at 0° neutral, and forearm and hand supported on firm surface on ulnar border.

POSITION OF GONIOMETER: Axis is centered on top of middle of MP joint. Stationary bar is on top of metacarpal, and movable bar is on top of proximal phalanx.

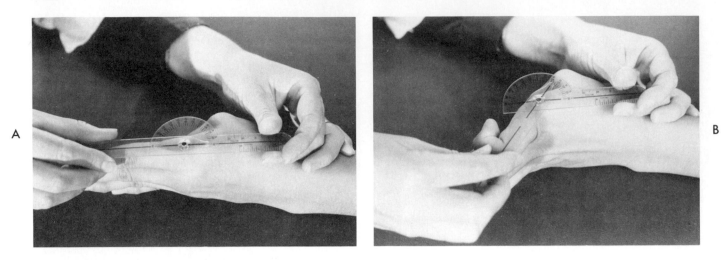

Fig. 6-30. MP hyperextension. **A,** Starting position. **B,** Final position.

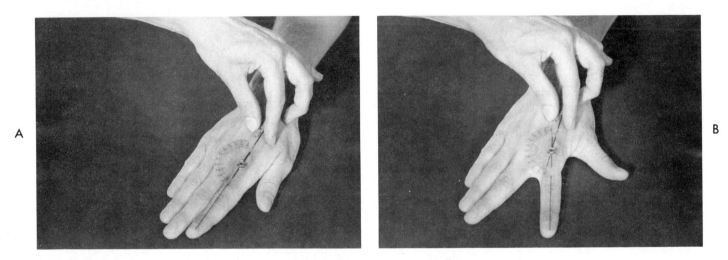

Fig. 6-31. MP abduction. **A,** Starting position. **B,** Final position.

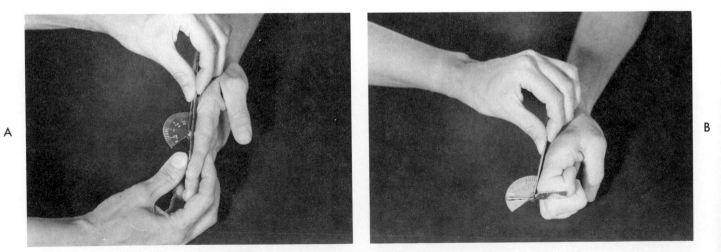

Fig. 6-32. PIP flexion. **A,** Starting position. **B,** Final position.

MP hyperextension —0° to 15°-45° (Fig. 6-30)

POSITION OF THE SUBJECT: Seated with forearm in mid-position, wrist at 0° neutral, and forearm and hand supported on a firm surface on ulnar border.

POSITION OF GONIOMETER: Axis is over lateral aspect of MP joint of index finger. Stationary bar is parallel to metacarpal, and movable bar is parallel to proximal phalanx. Fifth finger MP joint may be measured similarly. ROM of third and fourth fingers can be estimated by comparison.

MP abduction —0° to 25° (Fig. 6-31)

POSITION OF THE SUBJECT: Seated with forearm pronated and hand palm down, resting on firm surface. Fingers straight.

POSITION OF GONIOMETER: Axis is centered over MP joint being measured. Stationary bar is over corresponding metacarpal, and movable bar is over corresponding proximal phalanx.

Proximal interphalangeal (PIP) flexion —0° to 110° (Fig. 6-32)

POSITION OF THE SUBJECT: Seated with forearm in mid-position, wrist at 0° neutral, and forearm and hand supported on a firm surface on ulnar border.

POSITION OF GONIOMETER: Axis is centered on dorsal surface of PIP joint being measured. Stationary bar is placed over the proximal phalanx, and movable bar is over distal phalanx.

Distal interphalangeal (DIP) flexion —0° to 80° (Fig. 6-33)

POSITION OF THE SUBJECT: Seated with forearm in mid-position, wrist at 0° neutral, and forearm and hand supported on the ulnar border on a firm surface.

POSITION OF GONIOMETER: Axis is on dorsal surface of DIP joint. Stationary bar is over middle phalanx, and movable bar is over distal phalanx.

Thumb

MP flexion —0° to 50° (Fig. 6-34)

POSITION OF THE SUBJECT: Seated with the forearm in 45° of supination, wrist at 0° neutral, and forearm and hand supported on a firm surface.

POSITION OF GONIOMETER: Axis is on dorsal surface of MP joint. Stationary bar is over thumb metacarpal, and movable bar is over proximal phalanx.

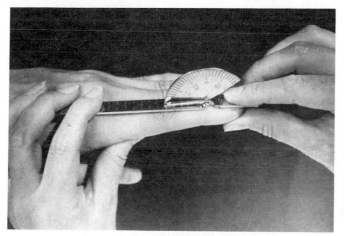
A

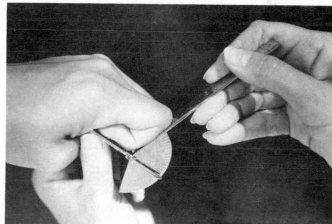
B

Fig. 6-33. DIP flexion. **A,** Starting position. **B,** Final position.

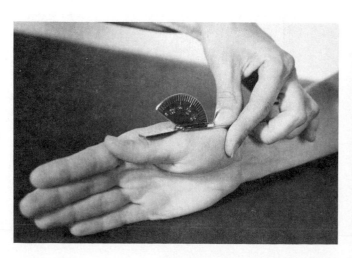
A

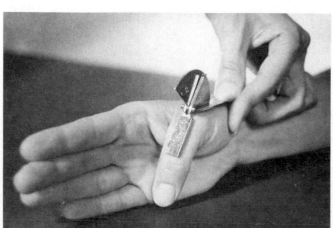
B

Fig. 6-34. Thumb MP flexion. **A,** Starting position. **B,** Final position.

Interphalangeal (IP) flexion —0° to 80°-90° (Fig. 6-35)

POSITION OF THE SUBJECT: Same as described for PIP and DIP finger flexion.

POSITION OF GONIOMETER: Axis is on dorsal surface of IP joint. Stationary bar is over proximal phalanx, and movable bar is over distal phalanx.

Radial abduction (carpometacarpal [CMC] extension) —0° to 50° (Fig. 6-36)

POSITION OF THE SUBJECT: Seated with forearm pronated and hand palm down, resting flat on firm surface.

POSITION OF GONIOMETER: Axis is over CMC joint at base of thumb metacarpal. Stationary bar is parallel to radius, and movable bar is parallel to thumb metacarpal.

ALTERNATE METHOD: Radial abduction (Fig. 6-37). Subject is positioned same as described in first method. Axis is over the CMC joint at the base of the thumb metacarpal. The stationary and movable bars are together and parallel to the thumb and the first metacarpals. Neither will be directly over these bones.

Palmar abduction (CMC Flexion)—0° to 50° (Fig. 6-38)

POSITION OF THE SUBJECT: Seated with forearm at 0° midposition, wrist at 0°, and forearm and hand resting on ulnar border. The thumb is rotated so that it is at right angles to the palm of the hand.

POSITION OF GONIOMETER: Axis is over CMC joint at base of thumb metacarpal. Stationary bar is over radius, and moveable bar is over thumb metacarpal.

ALTERNATE METHOD: (Fig. 6-39). Subject is positioned same as described in first method. Axis is over the CMC joint at the base of the thumb metacarpal. The stationary and movable bars are lined up together parallel to the thumb and the first metacarpals.

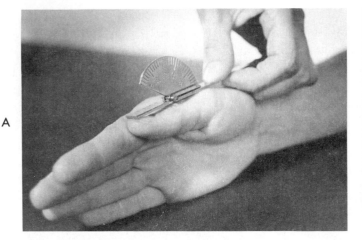
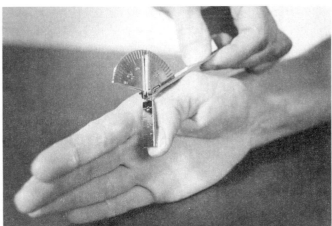

Fig. 6-35. Thumb IP flexion. **A,** Starting position. **B,** Final position.

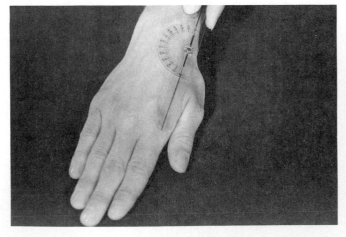
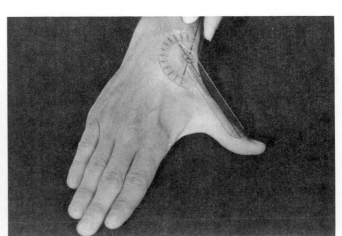

Fig. 6-36. Radial abduction. **A,** Starting position. **B,** Final position.

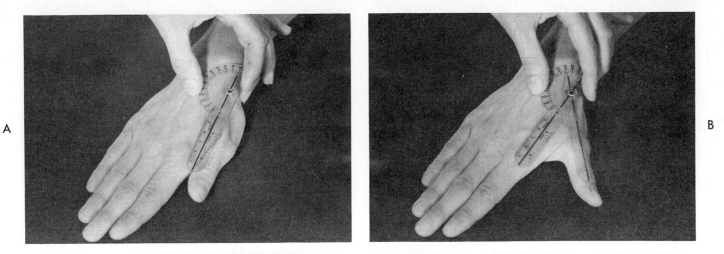

Fig. 6-37. Radial abduction; alternate method. **A,** Starting position. **B,** Final position.

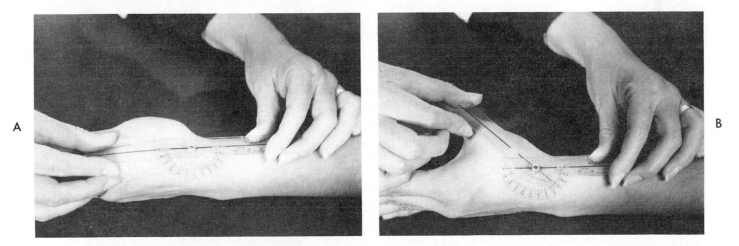

Fig. 6-38. Palmar abduction. **A,** Starting position. **B,** Final position.

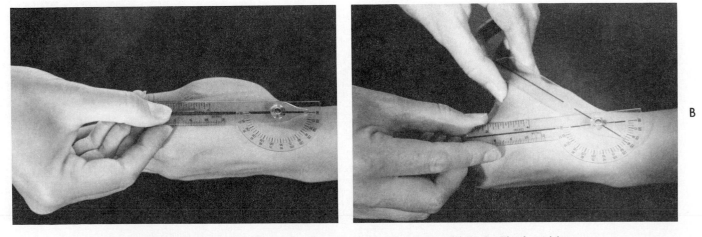

Fig. 6-39. Palmar abduction; alternate method. **A,** Starting position. **B,** Final position.

Opposition —(Fig. 6-40) Deficits in opposition may be recorded by measuring distance between pad of the thumb and pad of fifth finger with a centimeter ruler.

Lower extremity[4,5,7]

Hip

Flexion —0° to 120° (Fig. 6-41)

POSITION OF THE SUBJECT: Supine lying with hip and knee in extension.

POSITION OF GONIOMETER: Axis is on lateral aspect of hip over greater trochanter of femur. Stationary bar is centered over the lateral aspect of the pelvis, and movable bar is parallel to long axis of femur on lateral aspect of thigh. Knee is bent during the motion.

Extension (hyperextension) —0° to 30° (Fig. 6-42)

POSITION OF THE SUBJECT: Prone lying with hip and knee at 0° neutral extension.

POSITION OF GONIOMETER: Same as for hip flexion.

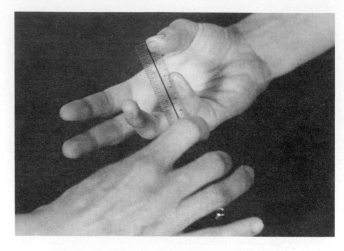

Fig. 6-40. Thumb opposition to fifth finger.

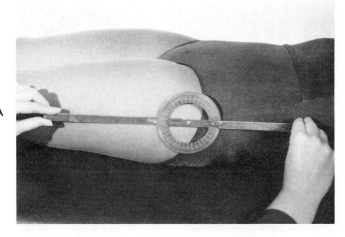

A

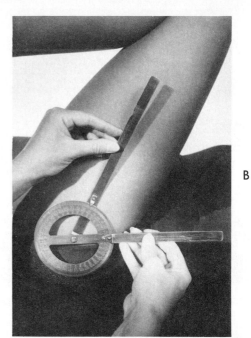

B

Fig. 6-41. Hip flexion. **A,** Starting position. **B,** Final position.

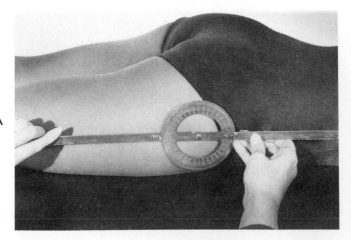

A

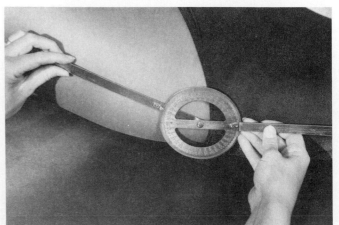

B

Fig. 6-42. Hip extension. **A,** Starting position. **B,** Final position.

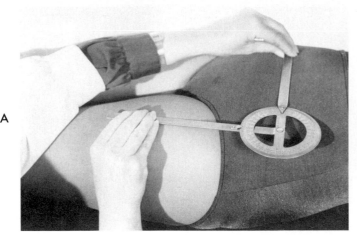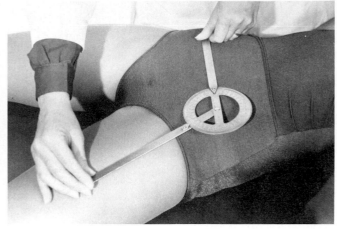

Fig. 6-43. Hip abduction. **A,** Starting position. **B,** Final position.

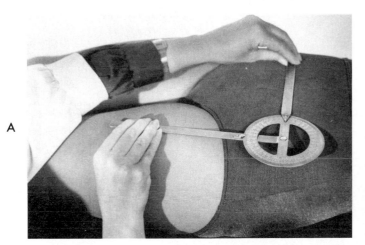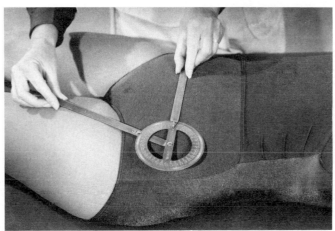

Fig. 6-44. Hip adduction. **A,** Starting position. **B,** Final position.

Abduction —0° to 40° (Fig. 6-43)

POSITION OF THE SUBJECT: Supine lying with legs extended.

POSITION OF GONIOMETER: Axis is placed on anterior superior iliac spine. Stationary bar is placed on a line between two anterior superior iliac spines, and movable bar is parallel to longitudinal axis of femur over anterior aspect of thigh. Note that starting position is at 90° for this measurement, and recording of measurement should be adjusted to accommodate to this exception to usual positioning of goniometer by subtracting 90° from total number of degrees obtained in arc of joint motion.

Adduction —0° to 35° (Fig. 6-44)

POSITION OF SUBJECT AND GONIOMETER: Supine lying with hip and knee of the leg to be tested in extension and neutral rotation. The leg not being tested should be in hip abduction with the knee flexed over the edge of the table. The goniometer is positioned same as for hip abduction.

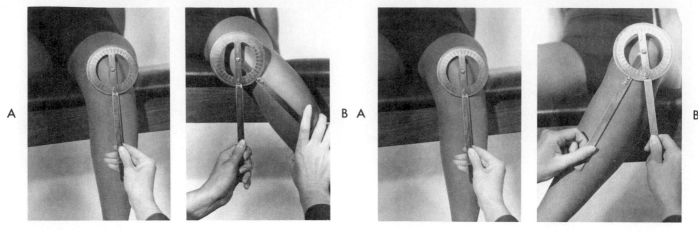

Fig. 6-45. Hip internal rotation. **A,** Starting position. **B,** Final position.

Fig. 6-46. Hip external rotation. **A,** Starting position. **B,** Final position.

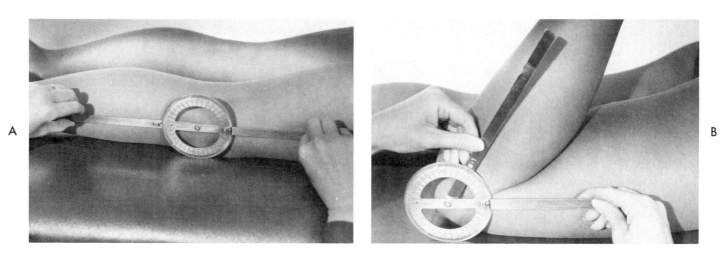

Fig. 6-47. Knee flexion. **A,** Starting position. **B,** Final position.

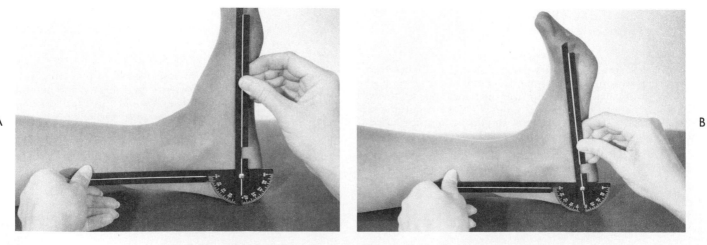

Fig. 6-48. Ankle dorsiflexion. **A,** Starting position. **B,** Final position.

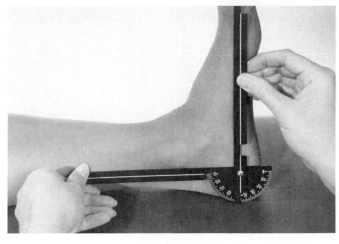
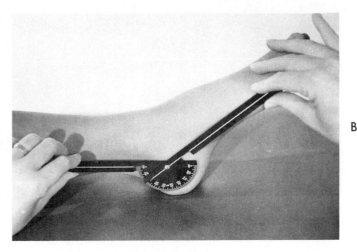

Fig. 6-49. Ankle plantar flexion. **A,** Starting position. **B,** Final position.

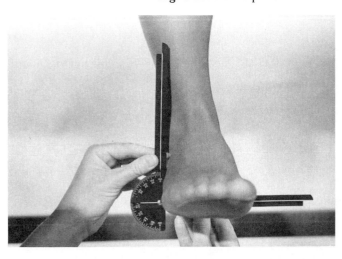
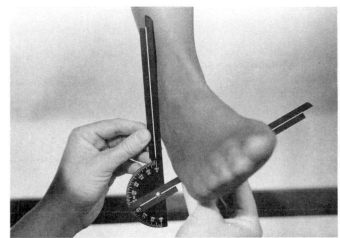

Fig. 6-50. Inversion. **A,** Starting position. **B,** Final position.

Internal rotation —0° to 45° (Fig. 6-45)

POSITION OF THE SUBJECT: Seated or supine with hip and knee flexed to 90°.

POSITION OF GONIOMETER: Axis is on center of patella of knee. Stationary and movable bars are parallel to longitudinal axis of tibia on anterior aspect of lower leg. Stationary bar remains in this position, perpendicular to floor, while movable bar follows tibia as hip is rotated.

External rotation —0° to 45° (Fig. 6-46)

POSITION OF SUBJECT AND GONIOMETER: Seated with hip and knee of leg to be tested flexed to 90°. The other leg should be (1) flexed at the knee so that the lower leg is back under the table or (2) flexed at the hip and knee so that the foot is resting on the table. This will allow the motion to take place without obstruction. The trunk should remain erect during the performance of the motion. The goniometer is positioned the same as for internal rotation.

Knee

Extension-flexion —0° to 135° (Fig. 6-47)

POSITION OF THE SUBJECT: Prone lying with legs extended.

POSITION OF GONIOMETER: Axis is centered on lateral aspect of knee joint at tibial condyle. Stationary bar is on lateral aspect of thigh to parallel longitudinal axis of femur.

Movable bar is parallel to longitudinal axis of tibia on lateral aspect of leg.

Ankle

Dorsiflexion —0° to 15° (Fig. 6-48)

POSITION OF THE SUBJECT: Supine lying or seated with knee flexed. Ankle is at 90° neutral position.

POSITION OF GONIOMETER: Axis is placed approximately 1 inch below medial malleolus. Stationary bar is parallel to midline of lower leg and movable bar parallel with first metatarsal. Note that measurement begins at 90° so that this must be subtracted when recording joint measurement.

Plantar flexion —0° to 50° (Fig. 6-49)

POSITION OF SUBJECT AND GONIOMETER: Same as for dorsiflexion.

Inversion —0° to 35° (Fig. 6-50)

POSITION OF THE SUBJECT: Sitting or supine with knee flexed and ankle in 90° neutral position.

POSITION OF GONIOMETER: Axis is placed at lateral border of foot near heel. Stationary bar is parallel to longitudinal axis of tibia on lateral aspect of leg. Movable bar is parallel to plantar surface of heel.

A 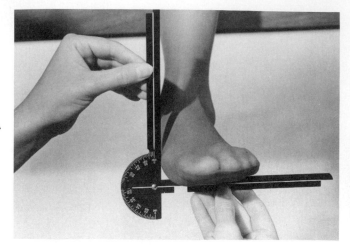 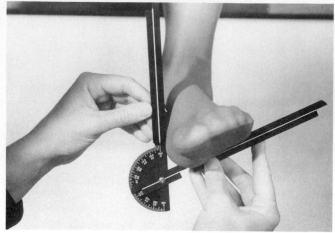 B

Fig. 6-51. Eversion. **A,** Starting position. **B,** Final position.

Eversion —0° to 20° (Fig. 6-51)

POSITION OF THE SUBJECT: Same as for inversion.

POSITION OF GONIOMETER: Axis is on medial border of foot just proximal to metatarsal-phalangeal joint. Stationary bar is parallel to longitudinal aspect of tibia on medial aspect of lower leg. Movable bar is parallel to plantar surface of sole. Note that measurements for inversion and eversion both begin at 90°. Therefore this amount must be subtracted from total when recording measurement.

REVIEW QUESTIONS

1. Describe general rules for positioning the goniometer when measuring joint ROM.
2. With which diagnoses would joint measurement be a primary evaluation procedure?
3. List and discuss four purposes of joint measurement.
4. Is formal joint measurement necessary for every patient? If not, how may ROM be evaluated?
5. Describe the steps in the procedure for joint measurement.
6. How is joint ROM measurement recorded on the evaluation form?
7. List the average normal ROM for elbow flexion, shoulder flexion, finger MP flexion, hip flexion, knee flexion, and ankle dorsiflexion.
8. Describe how to read the goniometer when using the 180° system of joint measurement.
9. List three common causes of joint limitation.
10. Define what is meant by "functional range of motion."
11. Discuss two approaches to treatment of joint limitation in occu-

pational therapy.
12. List six treatment methods that could be used by occupational and physical therapy to increase ROM.

EXERCISES

1. Measure all of the upper extremity joint motions of a normal subject. Record the findings on the form on page 64.
2. Repeat the first exercise, but the subject should play the role of someone with several joint limitations.

REFERENCES

1. American Academy of Orthopaedic Surgeons: Joint motion: method of measuring and recording, Chicago, 1965, American Academy of Orthopaedic Surgeons.
2. Baruch Center of Physical Medicine: The technique of goniometry, Lynchburg, VA, Medical College of Virginia. Unpublished.
3. Cole T: Measurement of musculoskeletal function: goniometry. In Kottke FJ, Stillwell GK, and Lehmann, JF: Krusen's handbook of physical medicine and rehabilitation, ed 3, Philadelphia, 1982, WB Saunders Co.
4. Esch D and Lepley M: Evaluation of joint motion: methods of measurement and recording, Minneapolis, 1974, University of Minnesota Press.
5. Hurt SP: Considerations of muscle function and their application to disability evaluation and treatment: joint measurement, Am J Occup Ther 1:69, 1947; 2:13, 1948.
6. Killingsworth A: Basic physical disability procedures, San Jose, 1987, Maple Press.
7. Norkin CC and White DJ: Measurement of joint motion: a guide to goniometry, Philadelphia, 1985, FA Davis Co.
8. Rancho Los Amigos Hospital: How to measure range of motion of the upper extremities, Downey, CA, Rancho Los Amigos Hospital. Unpublished.
9. Thomas CL, editor: Taber's cyclopedic medical dictionary, ed 13, Philadelphia, 1977, FA Davis Co.

7 Evaluation of muscle strength

LORRAINE WILLIAMS PEDRETTI

Many physical disabilities cause muscle weakness. Loss of strength places slight to significant limitations on the performance of occupational roles, depending on the degree of weakness and whether the weakness is permanent or temporary. Therefore the occupational therapist must assess the weakness and plan treatment that will improve strength or compensate for the loss of strength if it is not expected to improve.

Causes of Muscle Weakness

Disabilities in which a loss of muscle strength is a primary symptom or direct result of the disease or injury include (1) the lower motor neuron disorders, such as peripheral neuropathies and peripheral nerve injuries, spinal cord injury (since those muscles innervated at the level[s] of the lesion generally have a lower motor neuron paralysis), Guillain-Barré syndrome, and cranial nerve dysfunctions; (2) primary muscle diseases, such as muscular dystrophy and myasthenia gravis; and (3) neurological diseases in which the lower motor neuron is affected, such as in amyotrophic lateral sclerosis or multiple sclerosis. Disabilities in which a loss of muscle strength is caused by disuse or immobilization rather than by a direct effect of the disease process include burns, amputation, hand trauma (unless there is an accompanying nerve injury), arthritis, fractures, and a variety of other orthopedic conditions. In the final recovery stages of stroke or head injury when spasticity and synergy patterns have disappeared and the patient has achieved isolated control of voluntary muscle function, some underlying residual weakness may be detected. In these instances some assessment of strength can be of value in designing a treatment program.

Limitations Resulting from Muscle Weakness

Muscle weakness can restrict the performance of occupational roles and thus prevent pursuit of self-care, vocational, leisure, and social activities. These limitations are assessed through muscle testing combined with performance testing. Given good to normal endurance, the patient with good (G) to normal (N) muscle strength will be able to perform all ordinary activities of daily living (ADL) without undue fatigue.[8] (Ordinary ADL are considered here to be all self-maintenance tasks, mobility, and vocational roles except strenuous labor.) The patient with fair plus (F+) muscle strength usually has low endurance and will fatigue more easily than one with G to N strength. However, the patient will be able to independently perform many ordinary ADL but may require frequent rest periods. The patient with muscle grades of fair (F) will be able to move parts against gravity and perform light tasks requiring little or no resistance.[6,8] Low endurance is a significant problem and will limit the amount of activity that can be done. The patient can probably feed himself or herself finger foods and perform light hygiene if given the time and rest periods needed to reach the goals.[8] If muscle strength in the lower extremities is only F, ambulation will not be possible.[6] Poor (P) strength is considered below functional range, but the patient can perform some ADL with mechanical assistance and range of motion (ROM) can be maintained independently.[6] Patients with muscle grades of trace (T) and zero (0) are completely dependent and can perform no ADL without externally powered devices. Some activities are possible with special controls on equipment, such as electric wheelchair, communication devices, and hand splints.[8]

Purposes for Evaluating Muscle Strength

Muscle testing, particularly the evaluation of individual muscles, is essential for diagnosis in some neuromuscular conditions, such as peripheral nerve lesions and spinal cord injury. In peripheral nerve or nerve root lesions the pattern of muscle weakness may help determine which nerve or nerve roots are involved and whether the involvement is partial or complete. Careful evaluation can help determine the level or levels of spinal cord involvement.[7] Therefore muscle testing along with sensory evaluation can be an important diagnostic aid in neuromuscular conditions.

The purposes for evaluating muscle strength are (1) to determine the amount of muscle power available and thus establish a baseline for treatment; (2) to discern how muscle weakness is limiting performance of ADL; (3) to prevent deformities that can result from imbalances of strength; (4) to determine the need for assistive devices as compensatory measures; (5) to aid in the selection of activities within the patient's capabilities; and (6) to evaluate the effectiveness of treatment.[8]

Methods of Evaluation

Muscle strength can be evaluated in several ways. The most precise method is a test of individual muscles, as nearly as that is possible. In this procedure the muscle is carefully isolated through proper positioning, stabilization, and careful control of the movement pattern, and its strength is graded. This type of muscle testing is described by Kendall and McCreary.[7] Another and perhaps a more common method of manual muscle testing is to assess the strength of groups of muscles that perform specific motions at each joint. This type of testing was described by Daniels and Worthingham[6] and, for the most part, is the form that is presented later in this chapter.[6] Functional motion tests, functional muscle tests, or screening tests are also used to assess muscle strength. These tests are not as precise as manual muscle testing, and their purpose is to make a general evaluation of muscle strength and to determine areas of weakness and the need for more precise testing. Finally, muscle strength can be observed in the performance of ordinary activities.[6] During an ADL performance evaluation, for example, the therapist can observe for difficulties and movement patterns that may signal weakness, muscle imbalance, poor endurance for activity, and substitutions that are used for function. The performance evaluation should always be part of the assessment of strength.

Results of Evaluation as a Basis for Treatment Planning

When planning treatment for the maintenance or improvement of strength, the occupational therapist must consider several factors before determining treatment priorities, goals, and modalities. The results of the muscle strength assessment will suggest the progression of a strengthening program. What is the degree of weakness? Is it generalized or specific to one or more muscle groups? Are the muscle grades generally the same throughout, or is there significant disparity in muscle grades? If there is disparity, is there an imbalance of strength between the agonist and antagonist muscle that will require protection of the weaker muscles during treatment and ADL? Where there is significant imbalance between an agonist and antagonist muscle, treatment goals may be

directed toward strengthening the weaker group while maintaining the strength of the stronger group. Muscle imbalance may also suggest the need for orthoses to protect the weaker muscles from overstretching while recovery is in progress. Devices such as the bed footboard to prevent overstretching of the weakened ankle dorsiflexors and the wrist cock-up splint to prevent overstretching of weakened wrist extensors are examples. Muscle grades will suggest the level and type of therapeutic exercise and activity that can help to maintain or improve strength. Is the weakness mild (G range), moderate (F to F+), or severe (P to 0)?[8] Muscles graded F−, for example, could be strengthened by using active assisted exercise or activity against gravity. Muscles graded P likewise will require active exercise in the gravity-decreased plane with little or no resistance to increase strength. Further discussion of appropriate exercise and activity for specific muscle grades appears in Chapter 14.

The endurance of the muscles (how many repetitions of the muscle contraction are possible before fatigue sets in) is an important consideration in treatment planning. Frequently, one of the goals of the therapeutic activity program is to increase endurance as well as strength. Since the manual muscle test does not measure endurance, the therapist should assess it by engaging the patient in periods of exercise or activity graded in length to determine the amount of time that the muscle group can be used in sustained activity. There is usually a correlation between strength and endurance. Weaker muscles will tend to have less endurance than stronger ones. When selecting treatment modalities for increasing endurance, the therapist may elect not to tax the muscle to its maximal ability but rather to emphasize repetitive action at less than maximal contraction to increase endurance and prevent fatigue.[8]

Sensory loss, which often accompanies muscle weakness, complicates the ability of the patient to perform in an activity program. If there is little or no tactile or proprioceptive feedback from motion, the impulse to move is decreased or lost, depending on the severity of the sensory loss. Thus the movement may appear weak and ineffective even when strength is adequate for performance of a specific activity. With some diagnoses, a sensory stimulation program may be indicated to increase the patient's sensory awareness and feedback from the part. In other instances, the therapist may elect to help the patient compensate for the sensory loss through visual devices, such as mirrors, video playback, and biofeedback. These can be used as adjuncts to the strengthening program.

Another important consideration is the diagnosis and expected course of the disease. Is strength expected to increase, decrease, or remain about the same? If it is expected to increase, what is the expected recovery period? What effect will exercise or activity have on muscle function? Will too much activity delay the progress of the recovery? If muscle power is expected to decrease, how rapid is the progression? Are there factors to be avoided that can accelerate the decrease in strength, such as a vigorous exercise program? If strength is declining, is special equipment practical and necessary? How much muscle power is needed to operate the equipment? How long will the patient be able to operate a device before a decrease in muscle power makes it impracticable?[8]

The therapist should assess the effect of the muscle weakness on the ability to perform ADL. This can be observed during the ADL evaluation. Which tasks are most difficult to perform because of the muscle weakness? How does the patient compensate for the weakness? Which tasks are most important for the patient to be able to perform? Is special equipment necessary or desirable for the performance of some ADL, such as the mobile arm support for independence in eating?[8]

If the patient is involved in a total rehabilitation program and receiving several other health care services, the strengthening and activity programs must be synchronized and well balanced to meet the patient's needs rather than the needs of the professionals, their schedules, and possibly their competition. The occupational therapist needs to be aware of the nature and extent of the programs in which the patient is engaged in physical therapy, recreational therapy, and any other services being received. Ideally, the team should plan the exercise or activity program in concert to determine that the programs complement one another. Questions that may be asked are: What is the patient doing in each of the therapies? How long is each treatment session? Are the goals of all of the therapies similar or complementary, or are they divergent and conflicting? Is the patient being overfatigued in the total program? Are the various treatment sessions in rapid succession, or are they well spaced to meet the patient's need for rest periods?

On the basis of these considerations and of others pertinent to the specific patient, the occupational therapist can select enabling and functional activities designed to maintain or increase strength, improve performance of ADL, and enable the use of special equipment while protecting weak muscles from overstretching and overfatigue.

Relationship Between Joint ROM and Muscle Weakness

One criterion used to grade muscle strength is the excursion of the joint on which the muscle acts, that is, did the muscle move the joint through complete, partial, or no ROM. Another criterion is the amount of resistance that can be applied to the part once the muscle has moved the joint through the available ROM. In this context ROM is not necessarily the full average normal ROM for the given joint. Rather, it is the ROM available to the individual patient. When measuring joint motion, discussed in Chapter 6, it is the *passive* ROM that is the measure of the range available to the patient. Passive ROM, however, is no indication of muscle strength. When performing muscle testing, the occupational therapist must know what the patient's available passive ROM is to assign muscle grades correctly. It is possible that the passive ROM is limited or less than the average for that joint motion but that the muscle strength is normal. Therefore it is necessary for the therapist to have either measured joint ROM or to move the joint passively through its ROM to assess the available ROM before administering the muscle test. For example, the patient's passive ROM for elbow flexion may be limited to 0° to 110° because of an old fracture. If the patient can flex the elbow joint to 110° and hold against moderate resistance during the muscle test, the grade would be G. In such cases the examiner should record the limitation with the muscle grade, for example, 0-110°/G.[6] Conversely, if the patient's available ROM for elbow flexion was 0° to 140°, and he or she flexed the elbow against gravity through only 110°, the muscle would be graded F−, since the part moved through only partial ROM against gravity. When the therapist determines the patient's available ROM before performing the muscle test, the therapist is able to grade muscle strength on that basis rather than by using the average normal ROM as the standard.

MANUAL MUSCLE TESTING

The manual muscle test is a means of measuring the maximal contraction of a muscle or muscle group. It is used to determine amount of muscle power and to record gains and losses in strength. The muscle test is a primary evaluation tool for patients with lower motor neuron disorders, primary muscle diseases, and orthopedic dysfunction, as cited previously. The criteria used to measure strength are evidence of muscle contraction, amount of ROM through which the joint passes, and amount of resistance against which the muscle can contract, including gravity as a form of resistance.[6]

Limitations of the Manual Muscle Test

The limitations of the manual muscle test are that it cannot measure muscle endurance (number of times the muscle can contract at its maximum level), muscle coordination (smooth rhythmic interaction of muscle function), or motor performance capabilities of the patient (use of the muscles for functional activities).

The manual muscle test cannot be used accurately with patients who have spasticity caused by upper motor neuron disorders, such as a cerebrovascular accident or cerebral palsy. This is because in these disorders muscles are often hypertonic, muscle tone and ability to perform movements are influenced by primitive reflexes and the position of the head and body in space, and movements tend to occur in gross synergistic patterns that make it impossible for the patient to isolate joint motions, which is demanded in the manual muscle testing procedures.[2,3,9] Methods for measuring motor performance of persons with upper motor neuron dysfunction will be reviewed in subsequent chapters.

Knowledge and Skill of the Examiner

Validity of the manual muscle test depends on the examiner's knowledge and skill in using the correct testing procedure. Careful observation of movement, careful and accurate palpation, correct positioning, consistency of procedure, and experience of the examiner are critical factors in accurate testing.[6,7]

To be proficient in manual muscle testing, the examiner must have detailed knowledge about all aspects of muscle function. Joints and joint motions, muscle innervation, origin and insertion of muscles, action of muscles, direction of muscle fibers, angle of pull on the joints, and the role of muscles in fixation and substitution are important considerations. The examiner must be able to locate and palpate the muscles; recognize whether the contour of the muscle is normal, atrophied, or hypertrophied; and detect abnormal movements and positions. Knowledge and experience are necessary to detect substitutions and to interpret strength grades with accuracy.[7]

It is necessary for the examiner to acquire skill and experience in testing and grading muscles of normal persons of both sexes and of all ages. Some muscles in normal individuals may seem to be weak, but this may be normal for the particular person. Experience can help the examiner differentiate normal strength from slight muscle weakness if the age, sex, body build, and lifestyle of the subject are taken into account.[10]

General Principles of Manual Muscle Testing

PREPARATION FOR TESTING. When preparing to administer the muscle test, the examiner should observe contour of the part, comparative symmetry of muscle on both sides, and any apparent hypertrophy or atrophy. During passive ROM the examiner can estimate muscle tone. Is there lesser or greater than normal resistance to passive movement? During active ROM the examiner can observe quality of movement, such as movement speed, smoothness, rhythm, and any abnormal movements such as tremors.[10]

Correct positioning of the subject and the body part is essential to effective and correct evaluation. The subject should be positioned comfortably on a firm surface. Clothing should be arranged or removed so that the examiner can see the muscle or muscles being tested. If it is not possible for the subject to be placed in the correct position for the test, the examiner must adapt the test and use clinical judgment in approximating strength grades.[10] In addition to correct positioning, careful stabilization, palpation of the muscles, and observation of movement are essential to test validity.[6]

GRAVITY FACTORS INFLUENCING MUSCLE FUNCTION. Gravity is a form of resistance to muscle power.[7] It is used as a grading criterion in tests of the neck, trunk, and extremities, meaning that the muscle grade is based on whether or not a muscle can move the part against gravity.[7] Movements against gravity are in a vertical plane, that is, away from the floor or toward the ceiling and are used with grades F, G, and N. Movements against gravity and resistance are performed in a vertical plane with added manual or mechanical resistance and are used with F+ to N grades. Tests for the weaker muscles (O, T, P, and P+ grades) are often performed in a horizontal plane, that is, parallel to the floor, to reduce the resistance of gravity on the muscle power. This position has been referred to as the "gravity-eliminated," "gravity-decreased," or "gravity-lessened," test position.[6,7,10] Gravity-eliminated has been the commonly used term to designate this position.[10] However, because it is not possible to completely eliminate the effect of gravity on muscle function, gravity-decreased or gravity-lessened may be more accurate terms. The term gravity-decreased is used in this chapter.[6,7]

In many muscle tests the effect of gravity on the ability to perform the movement must be considered in grading muscle power. It is of lesser importance, however, in tests of the forearm, fingers, and toes because the weight of the part lifted against gravity is insignificant compared with the muscle strength.[6,7] Therefore the examiner may choose to do the tests for F to N in the gravity-decreased plane. In other tests, positioning for movements in the gravity-decreased position or the against-gravity position may not be feasible. For example, in the test for scapula depression, positioning to perform the movement against gravity would require the subject to assume an inverted position. In individual cases, positioning for movement in the correct plane may not be possible because of confinement to bed, generalized weakness, trunk instability, immobilization devices, and medical precautions. In these instances the examiner must adapt the positioning to the patient's needs and modify the grading using clinical judgment.

If tests of the forearm, fingers, and toes are done against gravity rather than in the gravity-decreased plane, the standard definitions of muscle grades can be modified when recording muscle grades. The partial ROM against gravity is graded P, and the full ROM against gravity is graded F.[6] Such modifications in positioning and grading should be noted by the examiner when recording results of the muscle test.

For consistency in procedure and grading, the gravity-decreased positions and against-gravity positions have been used in the muscle testing procedures described later, except where the positioning is not feasible or would be awkward or uncomfortable for the subject. Modifications in positioning and grading have been cited with the individual tests.

MUSCLE GRADES. Although the definitions of the muscle grades are standard, the assignment of muscle grades during the manual muscle test depends on clinical judgment, knowledge, and experience of the examiner.[6] This is especially true when determining "slight," "moderate," or "full" resistance. Age, sex, body type, occupation, and avocations all influence the amount of resistance that can be considered "slight," "moderate," or "full" for a subject.[6,7] "Normal" strength for an 8-year-old girl will be considerably less than for a 25-year-old man, for example. Additionally, strength tends to decline with age, and "full" resistance to the same muscle group will vary considerably from the 80-year-old man to the 25-year-old man.[7] Therefore the amount of resistance that can be applied to grade a particular muscle group as N or G varies from one individual to another.[6,7]

The amount of resistance that can be given also varies from one muscle group to another.[6] For example, the flexors of the wrist take much more resistance than the abductors of the fingers. The examiner must consider the size and relative power of the muscles and the leverage used when giving resistance.[8] The amount of resistance applied should be modified accordingly. When only one side of the body is involved in the dysfunction causing the muscle weakness, the examiner can establish the standards for strength by testing the unaffected side first.

Because weak muscles fatigue easily, results of muscle testing may not be accurate if the subject is tired. Pain, swelling, or muscle spasm in the area being tested may also interfere with the testing procedure and accurate grading. Such problems should be noted on the evaluation form.[10] Psychological factors must also be considered in interpreting muscle strength grades. The examiner must assess the motivation, co-

operation, and effort put forth by the subject when interpreting strength.[6]

In manual muscle testing, muscles are graded according to the following criteria[6,11]:

Number grade	Word/letter grade	Definition
0	Zero (0)	No muscle contraction can be seen or felt.
1	Trace (T)	Contraction can be felt, but there is no motion.
2−	Poor minus (P−)	Part moves through an incomplete ROM with gravity decreased.
2	Poor (P)	Part moves through a complete ROM with gravity decreased.
2+	Poor plus (P+)	Part moves through incomplete ROM (less than 50%) against gravity or through complete ROM with gravity decreased against slight resistance.[6]
3−	Fair minus (F−)	Part moves through an incomplete ROM (more than 50%) against gravity.[6]
3	Fair (F)	Part moves through complete ROM against gravity.
3+	Fair plus (F+)	Part moves through a complete ROM against gravity and slight resistance.
4	Good (G)	Part moves through a complete ROM against gravity and moderate resistance.
5	Normal (N)	Part moves through complete ROM against gravity and full resistance.

The purpose of using plus or minus designations with the muscle grades is to "fine grade" muscle strength. These designations are likely to be used by the experienced examiner. Two examiners testing the same individual may vary up to a half grade in their results, but there should not be a whole grade difference.[10]

SUBSTITUTIONS. The brain "thinks" in terms of movement and not contraction of individual muscles.[6] Thus a muscle or muscle group may attempt to compensate for the function of a weaker muscle to accomplish a movement. This is a substitution.[7] Substitutions can occur during the manual muscle test. To test muscle strength accurately, it is necessary to eliminate substitutions in the testing procedure by correct positioning, stabilization, palpation of the muscle being tested, and careful performance of the test motion without extraneous movements. The correct position of the body should be maintained and movement of the part performed without shifting the body or turning the part to allow substitutions.[7] The examiner must palpate contractile tissue (muscle fibers or tendon) to detect tension in the muscle group under examination. It is only through correct palpation that the examiner can be certain that the motion observed is not being performed by substitution.[6]

In the tests that follow, possible substitutions are described at the end of the directions. The examiner should be familiar with these so that possible substitutions can be detected and the procedure corrected. Detecting substitutions is a skill gained with time and experience.

PROCEDURE FOR MANUAL MUSCLE TESTING. Testing should be performed according to a standard procedure to ensure accuracy and consistency. The tests that follow are divided into (1) position, (2) stabilize, (3) palpate, (4) observe, (5) resist, and (6) grade.

First, the subject (S) should be *positioned* for the specific muscle test. The examiner (E) should position him or herself in relation to S. Then E *stabilizes* the part proximal to the part being tested to eliminate extraneous movements, isolate the muscle group, ensure the correct test motion, and eliminate substitutions. E should then demonstrate or describe the test motion to S and ask S to perform the test motion and return to the starting position. E makes a general *observation* of the form and quality of movement, looking for substitutions or difficulties that may require adjustments in positioning and stabilization. E then places fingers for *palpation* of one or more of the prime movers, or its tendinous insertion, in the muscle group being tested and asks S to repeat the test motion. E again *observes* the movement for possible substitution and the amount of range completed. When S has moved the part through the available ROM, S is asked to hold the position at the end of the available ROM. E removes the palpating fingers and uses this hand to *resist* in the opposite direction of the test movement. E usually must maintain stabilization when resistance is given. These muscle tests use the "break test," that is, the resistance is applied *after* S has reached the end of the available ROM.

Muscles exert different amounts of force at various points in the ROM. In the "break" test, the resistance is applied near the weakest point in the ROM. However, if the examiner is consistent and always uses the same procedure, this will not affect reliability of the results. Functional interpretation of the muscle grade may be not as accurate, however.[6]

S should be allowed to establish a maximal contraction (set the muscles) before the resistance is applied.[6,8] E applies the resistance after preparing S by giving the command to "hold." Resistance should be applied gradually in a direction opposite to the line of pull of the muscle or muscle group being tested. The "break test" should not evoke pain, and resistance should be released immediately if pain or discomfort occurs.[6] Finally, E *grades* the muscle strength according to the preceding standard definitions of muscle grades. This procedure is used for the tests of strength of grades F and above. Resistance is not applied for tests of muscles from P to 0. Slight resistance is sometimes applied to a muscle that has completed the full available ROM in the gravity-decreased plane to determine if the grade is P+. Fig. 7-1 is a sample form for recording muscle grades.

SEQUENCE OF MUSCLE TESTING. To avoid frequent repositioning of the subject, the test can be given in the sequence outlined so that all tests are performed in order of backlying position, facelying position, sidelying position, and, finally, sitting position.

Backlying (supine)

Grades N to F
Scapula abduction and upward rotation
Shoulder horizontal adduction
All tests for forearm, wrist, and fingers can be given in the backlying position if necessary

Grades P to 0
Shoulder abduction
Elbow flexion
Elbow extension
Hip abduction
Hip adduction
Hip external rotation
Hip internal rotation
Foot inversion
Foot eversion

Facelying (prone)

Grades N to F
Scapula depression
Scapula adduction
Scapula adduction and downward rotation
Shoulder extension
Shoulder external rotation
Shoulder internal rotation
Shoulder horizontal abduction
Elbow extension
Hip extension
Knee flexion
Ankle plantar flexion

Grades P to 0
Scapula elevation
Scapula depression
Scapula adduction

Sidelying

Grades N to F
Hip abduction
Hip adduction
Foot inversion
Foot eversion

Grades P to 0
Shoulder flexion
Shoulder extension
Hip flexion
Hip extension
Knee flexion
Knee extension
Ankle plantar flexion
Ankle dorsiflexion

Sitting

Grades N to F
Scapula elevation
Shoulder flexion
Shoulder abduction
Elbow flexion
All forearm, wrist, finger, and thumb movements
Hip flexion
Hip external rotation
Hip internal rotation
Knee extension
Ankle dorsiflexion with inversion

Grades P to 0
All forearm, wrist, finger, and thumb movements
Ankle dorsiflexion with inversion

LIMITATIONS OF INSTRUCTIONS FOR PROCEDURES. The following directions do not include tests for the face, neck, and trunk. Refer to Kendall and McCreary or Daniels and Worthingham for these tests.[6,7]

MUSCLE EXAMINATION

Patient's name_____ Chart no._____

Date of birth_____ Name of institution_____

Date of onset_____ Attending physician_____ MD

Diagnosis:

LEFT   RIGHT

			Examiner's initials				
			Date				
			NECK Flexors	Sternocleidomastoid			
			Extensor group				
			TRUNK Flexors	Rectus abdominis			
			Rt. ext. obl. Rotators Lt. int. obl.	Lt. ext. obl. Rt. int. obl.			
			Extensors	Thoracic group Lumbar group			
			Pelvic elev.	Quadratus lumb.			
			HIP Flexors	Iliopsoas			
			Extensors	Gluteus maximus			
			Abductors	Gluteus medius			
			Adductor group				
			External rotator group				
			Internal rotator group				
			Sartorius				
			Tensor fasciae latae				
			KNEE Flexors	Biceps femoris Inner hamstrings			
			Extensors	Quadriceps			
			ANKLE Plantar flexors	Gastrocnemius Soleus			
			FOOT Invertors	Tibialis anterior Tibialis posterior			
			Evertors	Peroneus brevis Peroneus longus			
			TOES MP flexors	Lumbricales			
			IP flexors (first)	Flex. digit. br.			
			IP flexors (second)	Flex. digit. l.			
			MP extensors	Ext. digit. l. Ext. digit. br.			
			HALLUX MP flexor	Flex. hall. br.			
			IP flexor	Flex. hall. l.			
			MP extensor	Ext. hall. br.			
			IP extensor	Ext. hall. l.			

Measurements:

Cannot walk	Date	Speech	
Stands	Date	Swallowing	
Walks unaided	Date	Diaphragm	
Walks with apparatus	Date	Intercostals	

KEY

5	N	Normal	Complete range of motion against gravity with full resistance.
4	G	Good*	Complete range of motion against gravity with some resistance.
3	F	Fair*	Complete range of motion against gravity.
2	P	Poor*	Complete range of motion with gravity eliminated.
1	T	Trace	Evidence of slight contractility. No joint motion.
0	0	Zero	No evidence of contractility.
S or SS			Spasm or severe spasm.
C or CC			Contracture or severe contracture.

*Muscle spasm or contracture may limit range of motion. A question mark should be placed after the grading of a movement that is incomplete from this cause.

Fig. 7-1. Muscle examination. Adapted with the express permission and authority of the March of Dimes Birth Defects Foundation.

LEFT   RIGHT

				Examiner's initials					
				Date					
				SCAPULA	Abductor	Serratus anterior			
					Elevator	Upper trapezius			
					Depressor	Lower trapezius			
					Adductors	Middle trapezius			
						Rhomboids			
				SHOULDER	Flexor	Anterior deltoid			
					Extensors	Latissimus dorsi			
						Teres major			
					Abductor	Middle deltoid			
					Horiz. abd.	Posterior deltoid			
					Horiz. add.	Pectoralis major			
				External rotator group					
				Internal rotator group					
				ELBOW	Flexors	Biceps brachii			
						Brachioradialis			
					Extensor	Triceps			
				FOREARM	Supinator group				
				Pronator group					
				WRIST	Flexors	Flex. carpi rad.			
						Flex. carpi uln.			
					Extensors	Ext. carpi rad.			
						l. & br.			
						Ext. carpi uln.			
				FINGERS	MP flexors	Lumbricales			
					IP flexors (first)	Flex. digit. sub.			
					IP flexors (second)	Flex. digit. prof.			
					MP extensor	Ext. digit. com.			
					Adductors	Palmar interossei			
					Abductors	Dorsal interossei			
				Abductor digiti quinti					
				Opponens digiti quinti					
				THUMB	MP flexor	Flex. poll. br.			
					IP flexor	Flex. poll. l.			
					MP extensor	Ext. poll. br.			
					IP extensor	Ext. poll. l.			
					Abductors	Abd. poll. br.			
						Abd. poll. l.			
				Adductor pollicis					
				Opponens pollicis					
				FACE					

Additional data:

Fig. 7-1, cont'd. Muscle examination.

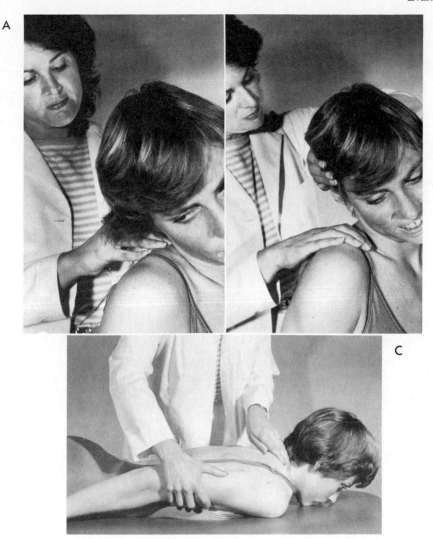

Fig. 7-2. Scapula elevation. **A,** Palpate and observe **B,** Resist. **C,** Gravity-decreased position.

MANUAL MUSCLE TESTING OF THE UPPER EXTREMITY

Motion:

Scapula Elevation, Neck Rotation, and Lateral Flexion

Muscles[6]	Innervation (Nerve, Nerve Roots)[6,7]
Upper Trapezius	Accessory N., (Cr. 11), C2,3,4
Levator Scapula	Dorsal Scapular N., C3,4,5

Procedure for Testing Grades Normal (N) to Fair (F)

POSITION: S is seated erect with arms resting at sides of body. E stands behind S toward the side to be tested.

STABILIZE: Chair back can offer stabilization to the trunk, if necessary.

PALPATE: The upper trapezius parallel to the cervical vertebrae, near the shoulder-neck curve.[6]

OBSERVE: Elevation of the scapula as S shrugs the shoulder toward the ear, rotates and laterally flexes the neck toward the side being tested at the same time (Fig. 7-2, *A*).[7]

RESIST: With one hand on top of the shoulder toward scapula depression and with the other hand on the side of the head toward derotation and lateral flexion to the opposite side (Fig. 7-2, *B*).[7]

Procedure for Testing Grades Poor (P), Trace (T), and Zero (0)

POSITION: S lying prone with the head in midposition. E stands opposite the side being tested.

STABILIZE: Weight of the trunk on the supporting surface is adequate stabilization.

PALPATE: The upper trapezius as described above while observing S shrug the shoulder being tested. Because of the positioning, the neck rotation and lateral flexion components are omitted for these grades (Fig. 7-2, *C*).

GRADE: According to standard definitions of muscle grades.

SUBSTITUTIONS: Rhomboids and levator scapula can elevate the scapula if the upper trapezius is weak or absent. In the event of substitution, some downward rotation of the acromion would be observed during the movement.[4,8,11]

E refers to examiner or therapist, *S*, is subject or patient. Normal (5) to Fair (3) tests are performed so muscle moves part in vertical plane or against gravity. Poor (2) to Zero (0) tests move part in horizontal plane or gravity-decreased position.

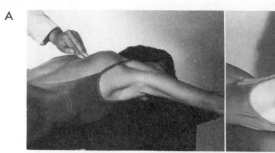
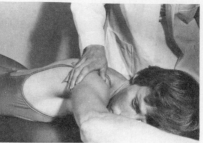
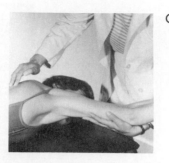

Fig. 7-3. Scapula depression. **A,** Palpate and observe. **B,** Resist. **C,** Test for Grades P to O.

Motion:
Scapula Depression, Adduction, and Upward Rotation

Muscles[1,4]	Innervation[6]
Lower Trapezius	Accessory N., Spinal Portion
Middle Trapezius	Accessory N., Spinal Portion
Serratus Anterior	Long Thoracic N., C5,6,7

Procedure for Testing Grades Normal (N) to Fair (F)

POSITION: S lying prone with arm positioned overhead in approximately 120° to 130° of abduction and resting on the supporting surface. E stands next to S on the opposite side.[6]

STABILIZE: Weight of the body is adequate stabilization. This test is given in the gravity-decreased position because it is not feasible to position S for the against-gravity movement (head down). If deltoid is weak, arm may be supported and passively raised by E while S attempts the motion.[6]

PALPATE: The lower trapezius distal to the medial end of the spine of the scapula and parallel to the thoracic vertebrae approximately at the level of the inferior angle of the scapula.[6]

OBSERVE: S lift the arm up off the supporting surface. During this movement, there is strong downward fixation of the scapula by the lower trapezius (Fig. 7-3, *A*).[6]

RESIST: At the lateral angle of the scapula toward elevation and abduction (Fig. 7-3, *B*).[6] Resistance may be given on the dorsum of the forearm in a downward direction if shoulder and elbow strength is adequate.[7]

Procedure for Testing Grades Poor (P), Trace (T), and Zero (0)

POSITION AND STABILIZE: As described above. No stabilization is required unless it is necessary for E to support S's arm because of weak posterior deltoid and triceps.

PALPATION AND OBSERVATION: Same as described above (Fig. 7-3, *C*).

GRADE: According to modified grading criteria.
Full ROM for F
P if 50% ROM was achieved[6]

SUBSTITUTIONS: Rhomboids may substitute. Rotation of the inferior angle of the scapula toward the spine is evidence of substitution.[11]

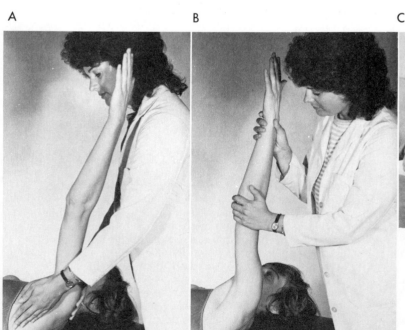
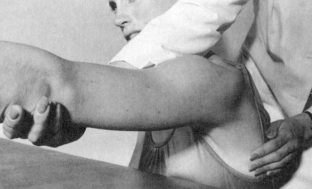

Fig. 7-4. Scapula abduction. **A,** Palpate and observe. **B,** Resist. **C,** Gravity-decreased position.

Motion:
Scapula Abduction and Upward Rotation

Muscles[6,7]	**Innervation**[6,7]
Serratus Anterior	Long Thoracic N., C5,6,7

Procedure for Testing Grades Normal (N) to Fair (F)

POSITION: S lying supine with the shoulder flexed to 90° and slightly abducted, elbow extended.[6] E stands next to S on the side being tested.

STABILIZE: Over the shoulder.

PALPATE: The digitations of the origin of the serratus anterior on the ribs, along the midaxillary line and just distal and anterior to the axillary border of the scapula.[6] Note that muscle contraction may be difficult to detect in women and overweight subjects.

OBSERVE: S reach upward as if pushing the arm toward the ceiling, abducting the scapula (Fig. 7-4, *A*).[6]

RESIST: Over the elbow with one hand and at the distal end of the forearm with the other and push arm directly downward toward scapula adduction (Fig. 7-4, *B*).[6]

Procedure for Testing Grades P, T, and 0.

POSITION: S seated at a high table with the arm resting on it in 90° of shoulder flexion.[6] E supports S's arm slightly above the table surface to eliminate resistance from friction and the weight of the arm.

STABILIZE: Over the shoulder to be tested.

PALPATE: The digitations of the serratus anterior on the ribs along the midaxillary line just distal and anterior to the axillary border of the scapula.

OBSERVE: For abduction of the scapula as the arm moves forward (Fig. 7-4, *C*).[6]

GRADE: Graded according to standard definitions of muscle grades.

SUBSTITUTIONS: Pectoralis major may pull scapula forward into abduction at its insertion on humerus. E observes for humeral horizontal adduction followed by scapula abduction.[8]

Motion:
Scapula Adduction

Muscles[6,7]	**Innervation**[6]
Middle Trapezius	Spinal Accessory N., C3,4
Rhomboids	Dorsal Scapular N., C5

Procedure for Testing Grades Normal (N) to Fair (F)

POSITION: Lying prone with the shoulder abducted to 90° and elbow flexed to 90°, humerus resting on the supporting surface. E stands on the side being tested.[6,7]

STABILIZE: Weight of the trunk on the supporting surface is usually adequate stabilization or over the midthorax to prevent trunk rotation, if necessary.

PALPATE: The middle trapezius between the spine of the scapula and the adjacent vertebrae in alignment with the abducted humerus.

OBSERVE: Movement of the vertebral border of the scapula toward the thoracic vertebrae as the arm is lifted off the supporting surface (Fig. 7-5, *A*).

RESIST: At the vertebral border of the scapula toward abduction (Fig. 7-5, *B*).[6]

Procedure for Testing Grades Poor P, T, and 0

POSITION AND STABILIZE: As described above, but E now supports the weight of the arm by cradling under the humerus and forearm.[8] S may also be positioned sitting erect with arm resting on a high table and the shoulder midway between 90° flexion and abduction.[6] E stands behind S in this instance.

PALPATE AND OBSERVE: The middle trapezius. Ask E to "bring the shoulders together" as if assuming an erect posture. Observe movement of the scapula toward the vertebral column (Fig. 7-5, *C*).

GRADE: According to standard definitions.

SUBSTITUTIONS: Posterior deltoid can act on the humerus and produce scapula adduction. Observe for humeral extension being used to initiate scapula adduction. Rhomboids may substitute but scapula will rotate downward.[8,11]

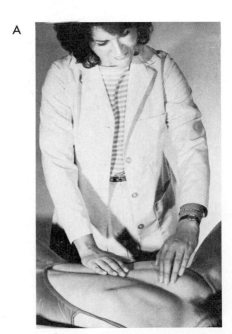
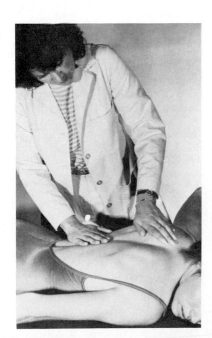
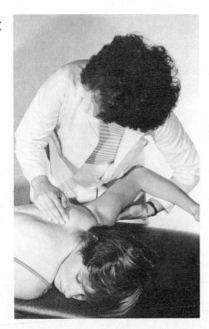

Fig. 7-5. Scapula adduction. **A,** Palpate and observe. **B,** Resist. **C,** Test for Grades P to O.

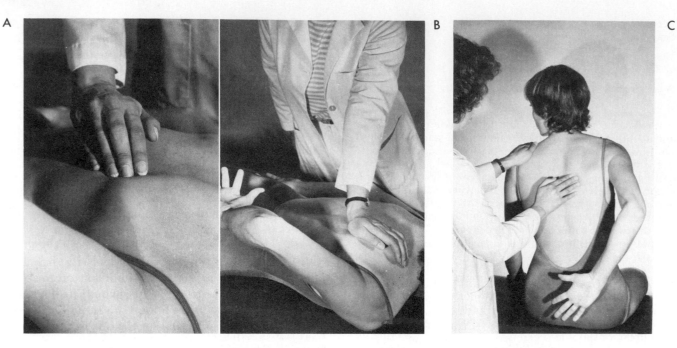

Fig. 7-6. Scapula adduction and downward rotation. **A,** Palpate and observe. **B,** Resist. **C,** Gravity-decreased position.

Motion:

Scapula Adduction and Downward Rotation

Muscles[6,7]	Innervation[6,7]
Rhomboids Major and Minor	Dorsal Scapular N., C5
Levator Scapula	Dorsal Scapular N., C3,4,5
Middle Trapezius	Spinal Accessory N., C3,4

Procedure for Testing Grades Normal (N) to Fair (F)

POSITION: S lying prone with the head rotated to the opposite side; arm on the side being tested is placed in shoulder adduction and internal rotation with the elbow slightly flexed and the dorsum of the hand resting over the lumbosacral area of back. E stands opposite the side being tested.[6]

STABILIZE: Weight of the trunk on the supporting surface offers adequate stabilization.[7]

PALPATE: Rhomboid muscles between the vertebral border of the scapula and the 2nd to 5th thoracic vertebrae.[6,7] (They may be more easily discerned toward the lower half of the vertebral border of the scapula, since they lie under the trapezius muscle.)

OBSERVE: As S raises the hand up off the back. During this motion the anterior aspect of the shoulder must lift from the table surface. Observe scapula adduction and downward rotation while the shoulder joint is in some extension (Fig. 7-6, *A*).[6]

RESIST: On the vertebral border of the scapula toward abduction and upward rotation (Fig. 7-6, *B*).

Procedure for Testing Grades P, T, and 0

POSITION: S sitting erect with the arm positioned behind the back in the same manner described above. E stands behind S a little opposite the side being tested.[6]

STABILIZE: Trunk by placing one hand over the shoulder opposite the one being tested to prevent trunk flexion and rotation.

PALPATE: The rhomboids.

OBSERVE: Scapula adduction and downward rotation as S lifts the hand away from the back (Fig. 7-6, *C*).

GRADE: According to standard definition.

SUBSTITUTIONS: Middle trapezius, but the movement will not be accompanied by downward rotation. Posterior deltoid acting to perform horizontal abduction or glenohumeral extension can produce scapula adduction through momentum. Scapula adduction would be preceded by extension or abduction of the humerus.[8,11]

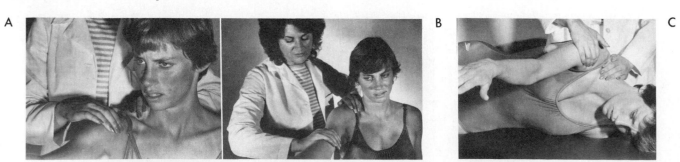

Fig. 7-7. Shoulder flexion. **A,** Palpate and observe. **B,** Resist. **C,** Gravity-decreased position.

Motion:
Shoulder Flexion

Muscles[6]	Innervation[6]
Anterior Deltoid	Axillary N., C5,6
Coracobrachialis	Musculocutaneous N., C6,7

Procedure for Testing Grades Normal (N) to Fair (F)

POSITION: S seated with the arm relaxed at the side of the body with the hand facing backward. A straightback chair may be used to offer trunk support. E stands on the side being tested and slightly behind S.[6,11]

STABILIZE: Over the shoulder being tested, but allow the normal abduction and upward rotation of the scapula that occurs with this movement.[6]

PALPATE: The anterior deltoid just below the clavicle on the anterior aspect of the humeral head.

OBSERVE: S flex the shoulder joint by raising the arm horizontally to 90° of flexion (parallel to the floor) (Fig. 7-7, A).[6]

RESIST: At the distal end of the humerus downward toward shoulder extension (Fig. 7-7, B).

Procedure for Testing Grades Poor (P), Trace (T), and Zero (0)

POSITION: S in sidelying. Side being tested is superior. If S cannot maintain weight of the arm against gravity, it can be supported on a smooth board placed under it or by E. E stands behind S.[6,11] If the sidelying position is infeasible, S may remain seated, and the test procedure described above can be performed with grading modified.[6]

PALPATE AND OBSERVE: Same as described above. The arm is moved forward toward the face to 90° of shoulder flexion (Fig. 7-7, C).

GRADE: According to standard definitions of muscle grades. If the seated position was used for the tests of grades Poor to Zero, partial ROM against gravity should be graded Poor.[6]

SUBSTITUTIONS: Pectoralis major, clavicular fibers, can perform flexion through partial ROM while performing horizontal adduction. Biceps brachii may flex the shoulder, but the humerus will first be rotated externally for the best mechanical advantage. The upper trapezius will assist flexion by elevating the scapula. Observe for flexion accompanied by horizontal adduction, external rotation, or scapula elevation.[8,11]

Motion:
Shoulder Extension

Muscles[4,6,7]	Innervation[6]
Latissimus Dorsi	Thoracodorsal N., C6,7,8
Teres Major	Inferior Subscapular N., C5,6
Posterior Deltoid	Axillary N., C5,6

Procedure for Testing Grades Normal (N) to Fair (F)

POSITION: S prone lying with the shoulder joint adducted and internally rotated so that the palm of the hand is facing up. E stands on the opposite side.

STABILIZE: Over the scapula on the side being tested.

PALPATE: The teres major along the axillary border of the scapula. The latissimus dorsi may be palpated slightly below this point or closer to its origins parallel to the thoracic and lumbar vertebrae.[6] The posterior deltoid may be found over the posterior aspect of the humeral head.

OBSERVE: As S lifts the arm up off the table extending the shoulder joint (Fig. 7-8, A).

RESIST: At the distal end of the humerus in a downward and outward direction, toward flexion and slight abduction (Fig. 7-8, B).[6,7]

Procedure for Testing Grades Poor (P), Trace (T), and Zero (0)

POSITION: S in the sidelying position; E stands behind S.

STABILIZE: Over the scapula. If S cannot maintain weight of the part against gravity, E should support S's arm or place a smooth board between the arm and the trunk.[6] If the sidelying position is infeasible, S may remain in the prone lying position and the test may be performed as described above with modified grading.[6]

PALPATE: The teres major as described above.

OBSERVE: S move the arm backward in a plane parallel to the floor (Fig. 7-8, C).

GRADE: According to standard definitions of muscle grades. If the test for grades Poor to Zero were done in the prone lying position, completion of partial ROM should be graded poor.[6]

SUBSTITUTIONS: Scapula adduction will effect some shoulder extension. Observe for flexion of the shoulder or adduction of the scapula preceding extension of the humerus.[8]

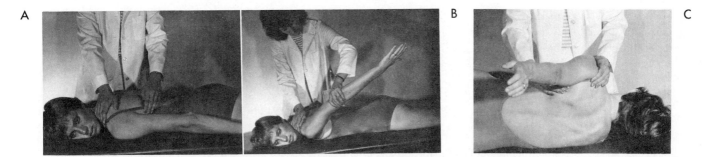

Fig. 7-8. Shoulder extension. **A,** Palpate and observe. **B,** Resist. **C,** Gravity-decreased position.

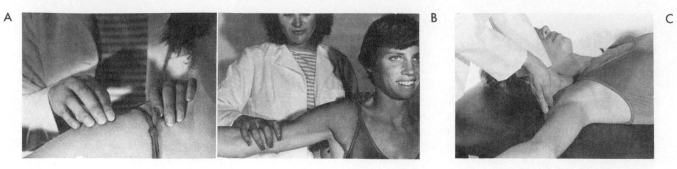

Fig. 7-9. Shoulder abduction. **A,** Palpate and observe. **B,** Resist. **C,** Gravity-decreased position.

Motion:
Shoulder Abduction

Muscles[6,7]	Innervation[6]
Middle Deltoid	Axillary N., C5,6
Supraspinatus	Suprascapular N., C5

Procedure for Testing Grades Normal (N) to Fair (F)

POSITION: S seated with the arms relaxed at sides of body. The elbow on the side to be tested should be slightly flexed and the palms facing toward the body. E stands behind S.

STABILIZE: Over the scapula on the side to be tested.[6,7]

PALPATE: The middle deltoid over the middle of the shoulder joint from the acromion to the deltoid tuberosity.[6-8]

OBSERVE: S abduct the shoulder to 90°. During the movement S's palm should remain down and E should observe that there is no external rotation of the shoulder or elevation of the scapula.[6-8] The supraspinatus may be difficult to palpate because it lies under the trapezius muscle, but it may be palpated in the supraspinatus fossa (Fig. 7-9, *A*).[6]

RESIST: At the distal end of the humerus as if pushing the arm down toward adduction (Fig. 7-9, *B*).

Procedure for Testing Grades Poor (P), Trace (T), and Zero (0)

POSITION: S in supine lying with the arm to be tested resting at the side of the body, palm facing in and the elbow slightly flexed. E stands in front of the supporting surface toward the side to be tested.

STABILIZE: Over the shoulder to be tested.

PALPATE AND OBSERVE: Same as described above. E asks S to bring the arm out and away from the body, abducting the shoulder to 90° (Fig. 7-9, *C*).

GRADE: Grade according to standard definitions of muscle grades.

SUBSTITUTIONS: The long head of the biceps may attempt to substitute. Observe for elbow flexion and external rotation accompanying the movement. The anterior and posterior deltoids can act together to effect abduction. The upper trapezius may attempt to assist. Observe for scapula elevation preceding the movement.[8,11]

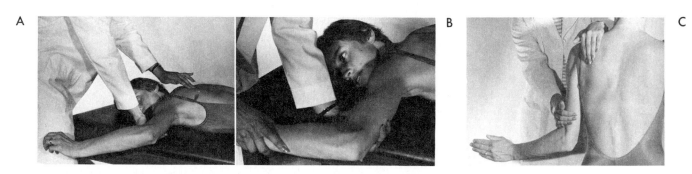

Fig. 7-10. Shoulder external rotation. **A,** Palpate and observe. **B,** Resist. **C,** Gravity-decreased position.

Motion:
Shoulder External Rotation

Muscles[4,6-8]	Innervation[4,6,7]
Infraspinatus	Suprascapular N., C5,6
Teres Minor	Axillary N., C5,6

Procedure for Testing Grades Normal (N) to Fair (F)

POSITION: S lying prone with the shoulder abducted to 90° and the humerus in neutral (0°) rotation, elbow flexed to 90°. Forearm is in neutral rotation, hanging over the edge of the table, perpendicular to the floor. E stands in front of the supporting surface toward the side to be tested.[6,7]

STABILIZE: At the distal end of the humerus by placing a hand under the arm on the supporting surface.[7]

PALPATE: The infraspinatus muscle just below the spine of the scapula on the body of the scapula or the teres minor along the axillary border of the scapula.[6]

OBSERVE: Rotation of the humerus so that the back of the hand is moving toward the ceiling (Fig. 7-10, *A*).[6,7]

RESIST: On the distal end of forearm toward the floor in the direction of internal rotation (Fig. 7-10, *B*).[6,7]

Procedure for Testing Grades Poor (P), Trace (T), and Zero (0)

POSITION: S seated with arm adducted and in neutral rotation at the shoulder. The elbow is flexed to 90° with the forearm in neutral rotation. E stands in front of S toward the side to be tested.

STABILIZE: Arm against the trunk at the distal end of the humerus to prevent abduction and extension of the shoulder and over the shoulder to be tested.[5,11] This hand can be used to palpate the infraspinatus simultaneously.

PALPATE: The infraspinatus and teres minor as described.

OBSERVE: Movement of the forearm away from the body by rotating the humerus while maintaining neutral rotation of the forearm (Fig. 7-10, *C*).[11]

GRADE: According to standard definitions of muscle grades.

SUBSTITUTIONS: If the elbow is extended and S supinates the forearm, the momentum could aid external rotation of the humerus. Scapular adduction can pull the humerus backward and into some external rotation. E should observe for scapula adduction and initiation of movement with forearm supination.[8,11]

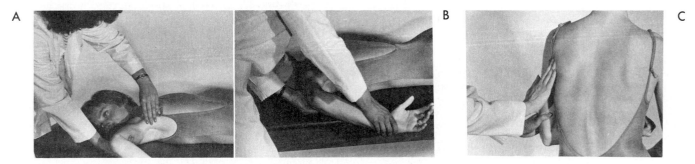

Fig. 7-11. Shoulder internal rotation. **A**, Palpate and observe. **B**, Resist. **C**, Gravity-decreased position.

Motion:
Shoulder Internal Rotation

Muscles[6,7,8]	Innervation[4,5,6]
Subscapularis	Subscapular N., C5,6
Pectoralis Major	Anterior Thoracic N., C5 through T1
Latissimus Dorsi	Thoracodorsal N., C6,7,8
Teres Major	Subscapular N., C5,6

Procedure for Testing Grades Fair (F) to Normal (N)

POSITION: S lying prone with the shoulder abducted to 90° and the humerus in neutral rotation. The forearm is perpendicular to the floor. E stands on the side to be tested just in front of S's arm.

STABILIZE: At the distal end of the humerus by placing a hand under the arm and on the supporting surface as for external rotation.[6,7]

PALPATE: The teres major and latissimus dorsi along the axillary border of the scapula toward the inferior angle.

OBSERVE: Movement of the palm of the hand upward toward the ceiling, internally rotating the humerus (Fig. 7-11, *A*).[6]

RESIST: At the distal end of the volar surface of the forearm anteriorly toward external rotation (Fig. 7-11, *B*).[6,7]

Procedure for Testing Grades Poor (P), Trace (T), and Zero (0)

POSITION: S seated with the shoulder adducted and in neutral rotation, elbow flexed to 90° with the forearm in neutral rotation. E stands on the side to be tested.[11]

STABILIZE: Arm at the distal end of the humerus against the trunk to prevent abduction and extension of the shoulder.

PALPATE: The teres major and latissimus dorsi as described above.

OBSERVE: S move the palm of the hand toward the chest, internally rotating the humerus (Fig. 7-11, *C*).

SUBSTITUTIONS: If the trunk is rotated, gravity will act on the humerus, rotating it internally. If the arm is in extension, pronation of the forearm can substitute. E should observe for trunk rotation during the test in sitting.[8,11]

Motion:
Shoulder Horizontal Abduction

Muscles[4,6,8]	**Innervation**[6]
Posterior Deltoid	Axillary N., C5, 6
Infraspinatus	Suprascapular N., C5, 6

Procedure for Testing Grades Normal (N) to Fair (F)

POSITION: S prone with the shoulder abducted to 90° and in slight external rotation, elbow flexed to 90°, and forearm perpendicular to the floor. E stands on the side being tested.[7,8]

STABILIZE: Over the scapula.[6]

PALPATE: The posterior deltoid below the spine of the scapula and distally toward the deltoid tuberosity on the posterior aspect of the shoulder.[6]

OBSERVE: Movement of the arm as it is lifted toward the ceiling, horizontally abducting the humerus (Fig. 7-12, *A*).

RESIST: Just proximal to the elbow obliquely downward toward adduction and horizontal adduction (Fig. 7-12, *B*).[7]

Procedure for Testing Grades Poor (P), Trace (T), and Zero (0)

POSITION: S seated with the arm in 90° abduction, the elbow flexed to 90°, and the palm down, supported on a high table or by E. If a table is used, powder may be used on the surface to reduce friction.

PALPATE: Posterior deltoid as described above.

OBSERVE: As the arm is pulled backward into horizontal abduction (Fig. 7-12, *C*).

GRADE: According to standard definitions of muscle grades.

SUBSTITUTIONS: Latissimus dorsi and teres major may assist the movement if the posterior deltoid is very weak.

Movement will occur with more shoulder extension rather than at the horizontal level. Scapula adduction may produce slight horizontal abduction of the humerus, but trunk rotation and shoulder retraction would occur.[8,11]

Motion:
Shoulder Horizontal Adduction

Muscles[4,8]	**Innervation**[4,6]
Pectoralis Major	Medial and Lateral Anterior Thoracic Ns, C5, 6, 7, 8, T1
Anterior Deltoid	Axillary N., C5, 6
Coracobrachialis	Musculocutaneous N., C6, 7

Procedure for Testing Grades Normal (N) to Fair (F)

POSITION: S supine with the shoulder abducted to 90°, elbow flexed or extended. E stands next to S on the side being tested or behind S's head.[4,6]

STABILIZE: The trunk by placing one hand over the shoulder on the side being tested to prevent trunk rotation and scapula elevation.

PALPATE: Over the insertion of the pectoralis major at the anterior aspect of the axilla.

OBSERVE: S move the arm toward the opposite shoulder, horizontally adducting the humerus to a position of 90° of shoulder flexion.[7] If S cannot maintain elbow extension, E may guide the forearm to prevent the hand from hitting S's face (Fig. 7-13, *A*).

RESIST: At the distal end of the humerus in an outward direction toward horizontal abduction (Fig. 7-13, *B*).[6]

Procedure for Testing Grades Poor (P), Trace (T), and Zero (0)

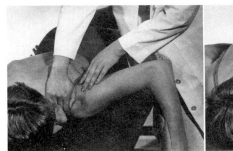 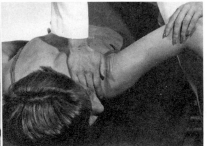 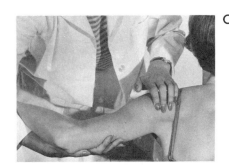

Fig. 7-12. Shoulder horizontal abduction. **A,** Palpate and observe. **B,** Resist. **C,** Gravity-decreased position.

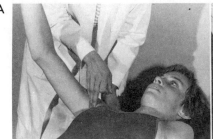 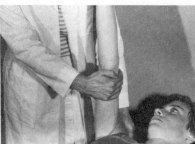 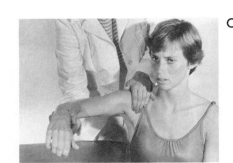

Fig. 7-13. Shoulder horizontal adduction. **A,** Palpate and observe. **B,** Resist. **C,** Gravity-decreased position.

A 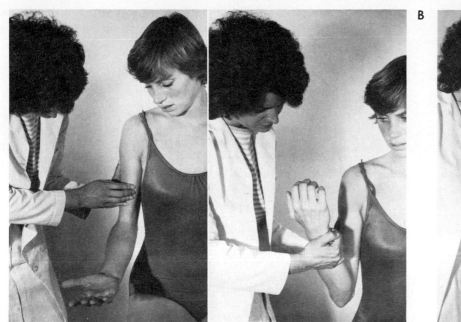 B 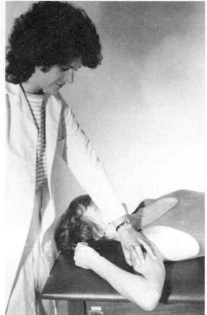 C

Fig. 7-14. Elbow flexion. **A,** Palpate and observe. **B,** Resist. **C,** Gravity-decreased position.

POSITION: S seated next to a high table with the arm supported in 90° of shoulder abduction and slight flexion at the elbow.[4,11] Powder may be sprinkled on the supporting surface to reduce the effect of resistance from friction during the movement, or E may support the arm.

STABILIZE: Over the shoulder on the side being tested, using the stabilizing hand to simultaneously palpate the pectoralis major muscle.

PALPATE: Pectoralis major as described above.

OBSERVE: S move the arm toward the opposite shoulder, horizontally adducting it in a plane parallel to the floor (Fig. 7-13, C).

SUBSTITUTIONS: Muscles may substitute for one another. If the pectoralis major is not functioning, the other muscles will perform the motion, but it will be considerably weakened.[8]

Motion:
Elbow Flexion

Muscles[6,7,8]	Innervation[7]
Biceps Brachii	Musculocutaneous N., C5, 6
Brachialis	Musculocutaneous N., C5, 6
Brachioradialis	Radial N., C5, 6

Procedure for Testing Grades Normal (N) to Fair (F)
POSITION: S sitting with the arm adducted at the shoulder and extended at the elbow, held against the side of the trunk. The forearm is supinated to test for the biceps, primarily. (Forearm should be positioned in pronation to test for the brachialis, primarily and in midposition to test for brachioradialis primarily).[6] E stands next to S on the side being tested or directly in front of S.

STABILIZE: Humerus in adduction.

PALPATE: The biceps brachii over the muscle belly on the middle of the anterior aspect of the humerus. Its tendon may be palpated in the middle of the antecubital space.[6] (Brachioradialis is palpated over the upper third of the radius on the lateral aspect of the forearm just below the elbow. Brachialis may be palpated lateral to the lower portion of the biceps brachii, if the elbow is flexed and in the pronated position.)[8]

OBSERVE: Elbow flexion, movement of the hand toward the face. E should observe for maintenance of forearm in supination (when testing for biceps) and for relaxed or extended wrist and fingers (Fig. 7-14, A).[8]

RESIST: At the distal end of the volar aspect of the forearm, pulling downward toward elbow extension (Fig. 7-14, B).[6,7]

Procedure for Testing Grades Poor (P), Trace (T), and Zero (0)
POSITION: S supine with the shoulder abducted to 90° and externally rotated, elbow extended and forearm is supinated. E stands at the head of the table on the side being tested.

STABILIZE: The humerus. The stabilizing hand can be used simultaneously for palpation here.

PALPATE: The biceps as described above.

OBSERVE: Elbow flexion, movement of the hand toward the shoulder.[6] Watch for maintenance of forearm supination and relaxation of the fingers and wrist (Fig. 7-14, C).[8]

GRADE: According to standard definitions of muscle grades.

SUBSTITUTIONS: Brachioradialis will substitute for biceps, but the forearm will move to midposition during flexion of the elbow. Wrist and finger flexors may assist elbow flexion, which will be preceded by finger and wrist flexion.[6,8] Pronator teres may assist. Forearm pronation during the movement may be evidence of this substitution.[8]

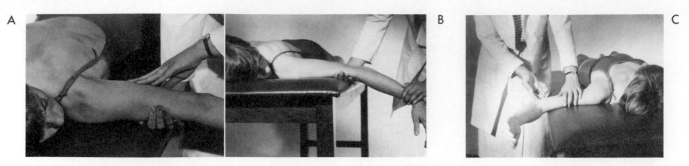

Fig. 7-15. Elbow extension. **A,** Palpate and observe. **B,** Resist. **C,** Gravity-decreased position.

Motion:
Elbow Extension

Muscles[6,7]	Innervation[6,7]
Triceps	Radial N., C7, 8
Anconeus	Radial N., C7, 8

Procedure for Testing Grades Normal (N) to Fair (F)

POSITION: S prone with the humerus abducted to 90° and in neutral rotation, elbow flexed to 90°, and the forearm, which is perpendicular to the floor, in neutral rotation. E stands next to S just behind the arm to be tested.[7,11]

STABILIZE: The humerus by placing one hand for support under it, between S's arm and the table.[7]

PALPATE: The triceps over the middle of the posterior aspect of the humerus or the triceps tendon just proximal to the elbow joint on the dorsal surface of the arm.[6,8]

OBSERVE: Extension of the elbow to just less than maximum range. The wrist and fingers remain relaxed (Fig. 7-15, A).

RESIST: In the same plane as the forearm motion at the distal end of the forearm, pushing toward the floor or elbow flexion. Before resistance is given, be sure that the elbow is not locked. Resistance to a locked elbow can cause joint injury (Fig. 7-15, B).[6]

Procedure for Testing Grades Poor (P), Trace (T), and Zero (0)

POSITION: S supine with the humerus abducted to 90° and in external rotation, elbow fully flexed, and forearm supinated. E is standing next to S just behind to the arm to be tested.[6]

STABILIZE: The humerus by holding one hand over the middle or distal end of it to prevent shoulder motion.

PALPATE: The triceps as described above.

OBSERVE: Extension of the elbow or movement of the hand away from the head (Fig. 7-15, C).

GRADE: According to standard definitions of muscle grades.

SUBSTITUTIONS: Finger and wrist extensors may substitute for weak elbow extensors. Observe for finger and wrist extension preceding elbow extension. When upright, gravity and eccentric contraction of the biceps will effect elbow extension from the flexed position.[8]

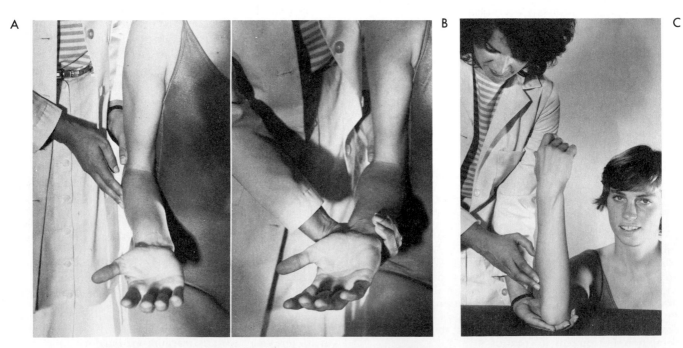

Fig. 7-16. Forearm supination. **A,** Palpate and observe. **B,** Resist. **C,** Gravity-decreased position.

Motion:
Forearm Supination

Muscles[4,6,8]	Innervation[6]
Biceps Brachii	Musculocutaneous N., C5, 6
Supinator	Radial N., C6

Procedure for Testing Grades Normal (N) to Fair (F)
POSITION: S seated with the humerus adducted, the elbow flexed to 90°, and the forearm in full pronation. E stands next to S on the side to be tested.[6]

STABILIZE: The humerus just proximal to the elbow.[6,9]

PALPATE: Over the supinator muscle on the dorsal-lateral aspect of the forearm, below the head of the radius. The muscle can be best felt when the radial muscle group (extensor carpi radialis and brachioradialis) are pushed up out of the way.[4] E may also palpate the biceps on the middle of the anterior surface of the humerus.

OBSERVE: Supination, turning the hand palm up. Gravity may assist the movement after the 0° neutral position is passed (Fig. 7-16, *A*).

RESIST: By grasping around the dorsal aspect of the distal forearm with the fingers and heel of the hand, turning the arm toward pronation (Fig. 7-16, *B*).

Procedure for Testing Grades Poor (P), Trace (T), and Zero (0)
POSITION: S seated, shoulder flexed to 90° and the upper arm resting on the supporting surface. Elbow flexed to 90° and the forearm in full pronation in a position perpendicular to the floor.[11] E stands next to S on the side to be tested.

STABILIZE: The humerus just proximal to the elbow.

PALPATE: The supinator or biceps as described above.

OBSERVE: Supination, turning the palm of the hand toward the face (Fig. 7-16, *C*).

GRADE: According to standard definitions of muscle grades.

SUBSTITUTIONS: With the elbow flexed, external rotation and horizontal adduction of the humerus will effect forearm supination. With the elbow extended, shoulder external rotation will place the forearm in supination. The brachioradialis can bring the forearm from full pronation to midposition. Wrist and thumb extensors, assisted by gravity, can initiate supination. E should observe for external rotation of the humerus, supination to midline only, and initiation of motion by wrist and thumb extension.[8,11]

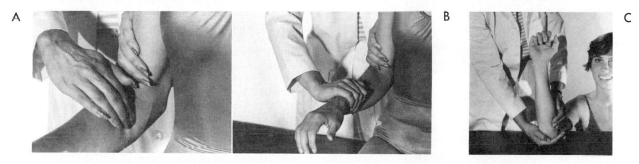

Fig. 7-17. Forearm pronation. **A,** Palpate and observe. **B,** Resist. **C,** Gravity-decreased position.

Motion:
Forearm Pronation

Muscles[4,8]	Innervation[7]
Pronator Teres	Median N., C6, 7
Pronator Quadratus	Median N., C8, T1

Procedure for Testing Grades Normal (N) to Fair (F)
POSITION: S seated with the humerus adducted, elbow flexed to 90° and the forearm in full supination. E stands beside S on the side to be tested.[6]

STABILIZE: The humerus just proximal to the elbow to prevent shoulder abduction.[6,7]

PALPATE: The pronator teres on the upper part of the volar surface of the forearm, medial to the biceps tendon and diagonally from the medial condyle of the humerus to the lateral border of the radius.[6-8]

OBSERVE: Pronation, turning the hand palm down (Fig. 7-17, *A*).[6]

RESIST: By grasping over the dorsal aspect of the distal forearm using the fingers and heel of the hand and turn toward supination (Fig. 7-17, *B*).

Procedure for Testing Grades Poor (P), Trace (T), and Zero (0)
POSITION: S seated, shoulder flexed to 90°, elbow flexed to 90° and the forearm in full supination. The upper arm is resting on the supporting surface and the forearm is perpendicular to the floor.[11] E stands next to S on the side to be tested.

PALPATE: Palpate the pronator teres as described above.

OBSERVE: Pronation, turning the palm of the hand away from the face (Fig. 7-17, *C*).

GRADE: According to standard definitions of muscle grades.

SUBSTITUTIONS: With the elbow flexed, internal rotation and abduction of the humerus will produce apparent forearm pronation. With the elbow extended, internal rotation can place the forearm in a pronated position. Brachioradialis can bring the fully supinated forearm to midposition. Wrist flexion, aided by gravity, can effect pronation.[6,8,11]

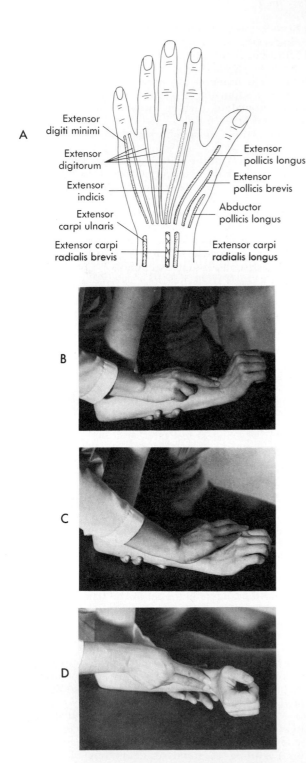

A, Extensor digiti minimi, Extensor digitorum, Extensor indicis, Extensor carpi ulnaris, Extensor carpi radialis brevis, Extensor pollicis longus, Extensor pollicis brevis, Abductor pollicis longus, Extensor carpi radialis longus

Motion:
Wrist Extension with Radial Deviation

Muscles[6,7,8]	Innervation[8]
Extensor Carpi Radialis Longus	Radial N., C5, 6, 7, 8
Extensor Carpi Radialis Brevis	Radial N., C5, 6, 7, 8
Extensor Carpi Ulnaris	Radial N., C6, 7, 8

Procedure for Testing Grades Normal (N) to Fair (F)

POSITION: S seated or supine with the forearm resting on the supporting surface in pronation, the wrist at neutral, and the fingers and thumb relaxed. E sits opposite S or next to S on the side to be tested.[6,7]

STABILIZE: Over the volar aspect of the mid- to distal forearm (Fig. 7-18, A).[6,7]

PALPATE: The extensor carpi radialis longus and brevis tendons on the dorsal aspect of the wrist at the bases of the 2nd and 3rd metacarpals respectively.[6,8] The tendon of the extensor carpi ulnaris may be palpated at the base of the 5th metacarpal, just distal to the head of the ulna.[4,6,8]

OBSERVE: Wrist extension and radial deviation, lifting the hand up from the supporting surface and moving it medially (to the radial side) simultaneously. The movement should be performed without finger extension, which could substitute for the wrist motion (Fig. 7-18, B).[6,8]

RESIST: Over the dorsum of the 2nd and 3rd metacarpals toward flexion and ulnar deviation (Fig. 7-18, C).[6,7]

Procedure for Testing Grades Poor (P), Trace (T), and Zero (0)

POSITION: As described above, except that the forearm is resting in midposition on its ulnar border.[6,11]

STABILIZE: At the ulnar border of the forearm, supporting it slightly above the table surface.[6]

PALPATE: Radial wrist extensors as described above.

OBSERVE: Extension of the wrist with movement of the hand away from the body (Fig. 7-18, D).

GRADE: According to standard definitions of muscle grades.

SUBSTITUTIONS: Wrist extensors can substitute for one another. In the absence of the extensor carpi radialis muscles, the extensor carpi ulnaris will extend the wrist but in an ulnar direction. The combined extension and radial deviation will not be possible. The extensor digitorum communis muscle and the extensor pollicis longus can initiate wrist extension, but finger and/or thumb extension will precede wrist extension.[8,11]

Fig. 7-18. **A,** Arrangement of extensor tendons at wrist. **B,** Wrist extension with radial deviation. Palpate and observe. **C,** Resist. **D,** Gravity-decreased position.

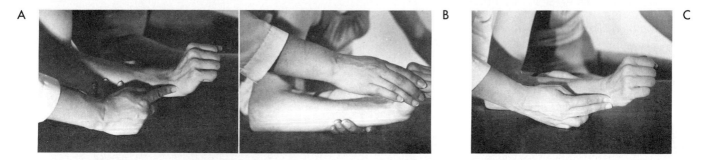

Fig. 7-19. Wrist extension with ulnar deviation. **A,** Palpate and observe. **B,** Resist. **C,** Gravity-decreased position.

Motion:

Wrist Extension with Ulnar Deviation

Muscles[6, 7, 8]	Innervation[7]
Extensor Carpi Ulnaris	Radial N., C6, 7, 8
Extensor Carpi Radialis Longus	Radial N., C5, 6, 7, 8
Extensor Carpi Radialis Brevis	Radial N., C5, 6, 7, 8

Procedure for Testing Grades Normal (N) to Fair (F)

POSITION: S seated, forearm in pronation, wrist neutral, fingers and thumb relaxed. E sits opposite or next to S on the side to be tested.

STABILIZE: Over the volar aspect of the mid- to distal forearm.[6,7]

PALPATE: Extensor carpi ulnaris tendon at the base of the 5th metacarpal, just distal to the head of the ulna, and the extensor carpi radialis longus and brevis tendons at the bases of the 2nd and 3rd metacarpals.

OBSERVE: S bring the hand up from the supporting surface and move it laterally (to the ulnar side) simultaneously. E should observe that the movement is not preceded by thumb or finger extension (Fig. 7-19, A).[6,8]

RESIST: Over the dorsal-lateral aspect of the 5th metacarpal toward flexion and radial deviation (Fig. 7-19, B).[6,7]

Procedure for Testing Grades Poor (P), Trace (T), and Zero (0)

POSITION: As described above, except that the forearm is in 45° of pronation.

STABILIZE: Arm at the volar aspect of the forearm, supporting it slightly above the supporting surface.[6,7]

PALPATE: Extensor tendons as described above.

OBSERVE: S bring the hand away from the body and move it ulnarly at the same time (Fig. 7-19, C).

GRADE: According to standard definitions of muscle grades.

SUBSTITUTIONS: In the absence of the extensor carpi ulnaris muscle, the extensor carpi radialis longus and brevis muscle can extend the wrist but will do so in a radial direction. The ulnar deviation component of the test motion will not be possible. Long finger and thumb extensors can initiate wrist extension, but the movement will be preceded by finger and/or thumb extension.[8,11]

Motion:
Wrist Flexion with Radial Deviation

Muscles[7]	Innervation[5,6,7]
Flexor Carpi Radialis	Median N., C6, 7, 8
Flexor Carpi Ulnaris	Ulnar N., C8, T1
Palmaris Longus	Median N., C7, 8, T1

Procedure for Testing Grades Normal (N) to Fair (F)
POSITION: S seated or supine with the forearm resting in nearly full supination on the supporting surface, fingers and thumb relaxed.[8] E is seated next to S on the side to be tested.

STABILIZE: Over the volar aspect of the mid-forearm.[6,7]

PALPATE: Muscle tendons. The flexor carpi radialis tendon can be palpated over the wrist at the base of the second metacarpal bone. The palmaris longus tendon is at the center of the wrist at the base of the 3rd metacarpal, and the flexor carpi ulnaris tendon can be palpated at the ulnar side of the volar aspect of the wrist at the base of the 5th metacarpal (Fig. 7-20, A).[4]

OBSERVE: S bring the hand up from the supporting surface toward the face, deviating the hand toward the radial side simultaneously. E should observe that the fingers remain relaxed during the movement (Fig. 7-20, B).

RESIST: In the palm at the radial side of the hand over the 2nd and 3rd metacarpals toward extension and ulnar deviation (Fig. 7-20, C).

Procedure for Testing Grades Poor (P), Trace (T), and Zero (0)
POSITION: S seated with the forearm in midposition with the ulnar border of the hand resting on the supporting surface.[6,11] E sits next to S on the side to be tested.

STABILIZE: At the ulnar border of the forearm, slightly above the supporting surface.

PALPATE: Wrist flexor tendons as described above.

OBSERVE: S move the hand toward the body and in a radial direction, flexing the wrist. Movement should not be initiated with finger flexion (Fig. 7-20, D).

GRADE: According to standard definitions of muscle grades.

SUBSTITUTIONS: Wrist flexors can substitute for one another. If flexor carpi radialis is weak or nonfunctioning in this test, flexor carpi ulnaris will produce wrist flexion, but in an ulnar direction, and the radial deviation will not be possible. The finger flexors can assist wrist flexion, but finger flexion will occur before the wrist is flexed. The abductor pollicis longus, with the assistance of gravity, can initiate wrist flexion.[8]

Motion:
Wrist Flexion with Ulnar Deviation

Muscles[6]	Innervation[5,6,7]
Flexor Carpi Ulnaris	Ulnar N., C8, T1
Palmaris Longus	Median N., C7, 8, T1
Flexor Carpi Radialis	Median N., C6, 7, 8

Procedure for Testing Grades Normal (N) to Fair (F)
POSITION: S seated or supine with the forearm resting in nearly full supination on the supporting surface, fingers and thumb relaxed. E is seated opposite or next to S on the side to be tested.[6,7]

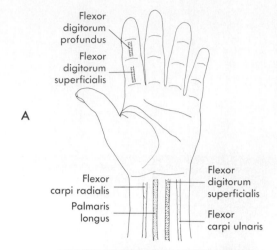

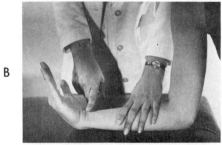

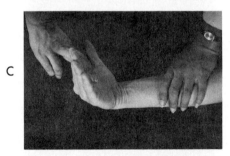

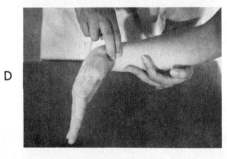

Fig. 7-20. A, Arrangement of flexor tendons at wrist. **B,** Wrist flexion with radial deviation. Palpate and observe. **C,** Resist. **D,** Gravity-decreased position.

STABILIZE: Over the volar aspect of the middle of the forearm.[6,7]

PALPATE: Flexor tendons on the volar aspect of the wrist, the flexor carpi ulnaris at the base of the 5th metacarpal, the flexor carpi radialis at the base of the 2nd metacarpal, and the palmaris longus at the base of the 3rd metacarpal.[4]

OBSERVE: S bring the hand up off the supporting surface, flexing the wrist and deviating it ulnarly simultaneously (Fig. 7-21, *A*).

RESIST: In the palm of the hand over the hypothenar eminence toward extension and radial deviation (Fig. 7-21, *B*).[7]

Procedure for Testing Grades Poor (P), Trace (T), and Zero (0)

POSITION: S seated with the forearm resting in 45° of supination on the ulnar border of the arm and hand.[8,11] E sits opposite S or next to S on the side being tested.

STABILIZE: At the dorsal-medial aspect of the forearm to prevent elbow and forearm motion. S's arm can be supported slightly above the supporting surface.

PALPATE: Wrist flexor tendons as described above.

OBSERVE: S bring the wrist toward the body, flexing and deviating it ulnarly simultaneously (Fig. 7-21, *C*).

GRADE: According to standard definitions of muscle grades.

SUBSTITUTIONS: Wrist flexors can substitute for one another. If flexor carpi ulnaris is weak or absent, flexor carpi radialis can produce wrist flexion in a radial direction and the ulnar deviation will not be possible. The finger flexors can also assist wrist flexion, but the motion will be preceded by flexion of the fingers.[8,11]

Motion:
Metacarpophalangeal (MP) Flexion with Interphalangeal (IP) Extension

Muscles[1,4]	Innervation[6]
Lumbricals 1 & 2	Median N., C6, 7
Lumbricals 3 & 4	Ulnar N., C8, T1
Dorsal Interossei	Ulnar N., C8, T1
Palmar Interossei	Ulnar N., C8, T1

Procedure for Testing Grades Normal (N) to Fair (F)

POSITION: S seated with forearm in supination, wrist at neutral, resting on the supporting surface.[6] The MP joints are extended and the IP joints are flexed.[11] E sits next to S on the side being tested.

STABILIZE: Over the palm to prevent wrist motion.

PALPATE: The first dorsal interosseous muscle just medial to the distal aspect of the 2nd metacarpal on the dorsum of the hand. The remainder of these muscles are not easily palpable because of their size and deep location in the hand.[8,11]

OBSERVE: S flex the MP joints and extend the IP joints simultaneously (Fig. 7-22, *A*).[7]

RESIST: Each finger separately by grasping the distal phalanx and pushing downward on the finger into the supporting surface toward MP extension and IP flexion, or apply pressure first against the dorsal surface of the middle and distal phalanges toward flexion, followed by application of pressure to the volar surface of the proximal phalanges toward extension (Fig. 7-22, *B*)[7]

Procedure for Testing Grades Poor (P), Trace (T), and Zero (0)

POSITION: S seated or supine with the forearm and wrist in midposition and resting on the ulnar border on the supporting surface.[6] MP joints are extended and IP joints are flexed. E sits next to S on the side being tested.

STABILIZE: The wrist and palm of the hand.

PALPATE: As described above.

OBSERVE: S flex the MP joints and extend the IP joints simultaneously (Fig. 7-22, *C*).

GRADE: According to standard definitions of muscle grades.

SUBSTITUTIONS: Flexor digitorum profundus and superficialis may substitute for weak or absent lumbricals. If this is the case, MP flexion will be preceded by flexion of the distal and proximal interphalangeal joints.[8,11]

A
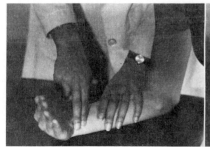
B
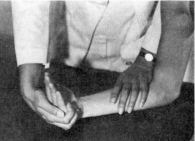
C
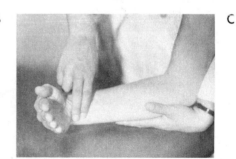

Fig. 7-21. Wrist flexion with ulnar deviation. **A,** Palpate and observe. **B,** Resist. **C,** Gravity-decreased position.

A
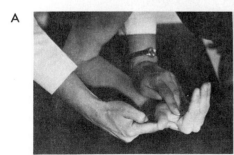
B
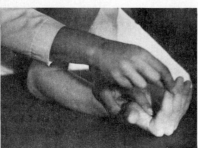
C
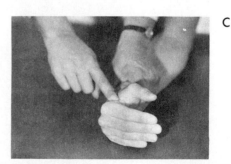

Fig. 7-22. MP flexion with IP extension. **A,** Palpate and observe. **B,** Resist. **C,** Gravity-decreased position.

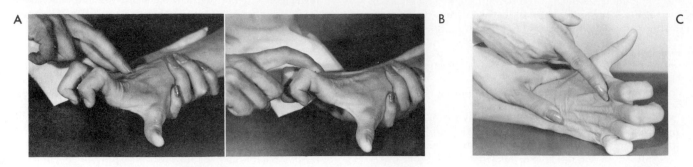

Fig. 7-23. MP extension. **A,** Palpate and observe. **B,** Resist. **C,** Gravity-decreased position.

Motion:

MP Extension

Muscles[6, 7, 8]	Innervation[6]
Extensor Digitorum Communis	Radial N., C6, 7, 8
Extensor Indicis Proprius	
Extensor Digiti Minimi	

Procedure for Testing Grades Normal (N) to Fair (F)

POSITION: S seated with the forearm pronated and the wrist in the neutral position, MP and IP joints partially flexed.[6] E sits opposite or next to S on the side to be tested.

STABILIZE: The wrist and metacarpals slightly above the supporting surface.[6,7]

PALPATE: The extensor digitorum tendons where they course over the dorsum of the hand.[6] In some individuals, the extensor digiti minimi tendon can be palpated or visualized just lateral to the extensor digitorum tendon to the 5th finger. The extensor indicis proprious tendon can be palpated or visualized just medial to the extensor digitorum tendon to the first finger.

OBSERVE: S raise the fingers away from the supporting surface, extending the MP joints but maintaining the IP joints in some flexion (Fig. 7-23, *A*).

RESIST: Each finger individually over the dorsal aspect of the proximal phalanx toward MP flexion (Fig. 7-23, *B*).[6,7]

Procedure for Testing Grades Poor (P), Trace (T), and Zero (0)

POSITION: Same as described above, except that S's forearm is in midposition and the hand and forearm are supported on the ulnar border.[6]

STABILIZE: Same as described above.

PALPATE: Same as described above.

OBSERVE: S move the fingers backward, extending the MP joints while keeping the IP joints somewhat flexed. (Fig. 7-23, *C*).

GRADE: According to standard definitions of muscle grades.

SUBSTITUTIONS: With the wrist stabilized, no substitutions are possible. When the wrist is not stabilized, wrist flexion with tendon action can produce MP extension.[8,11]

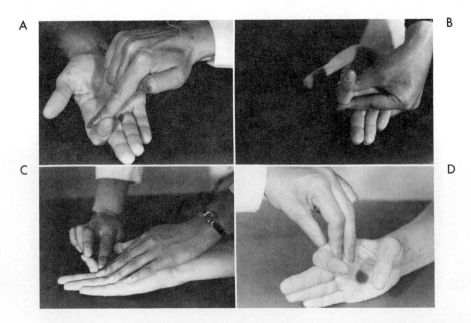

Fig. 7-24. PIP flexion. **A,** Palpate and observe. **B,** Position to assist with isolation of PIP joint flexion. **C,** Resist. Therapist checks for substitution by flexor digitorum profundus. **D,** Gravity-decreased position.

Motion:
PIP Flexion, 2nd through 5th Fingers

Muscles[6, 7]	**Innervation**[6, 7]
Flexor Digitorum Superficialis (FDS)	Median N., C7, 8, T1

Procedure for Testing Grades Normal (N) to Fair (F)

POSITION: S seated with the forearm in supination, wrist at neutral, fingers extended, and hand and forearm resting on the dorsal surface.[6] E sits opposite or next to S on the side being tested.

STABILIZE: MP joint and proximal phalanx of the finger being tested.[6,7]

PALPATE: The FDS tendon on the volar surface of the proximal phalanx. A stabilizing finger may be used palpate in this instance.[8] The tendon supplying the 4th finger may be palpated over the volar aspect of the wrist between the flexor carpi ulnaris and the palmaris longus tendons, if desired.[4]

OBSERVE: S flex the PIP joint while maintaining the DIP joint in extension (Fig. 7-24, *A*). If isolating PIP flexion is difficult, hold all of the fingers not being tested in MP hyperextension and PIP extension by pulling back over the IP joints. This maneuver inactivates the flexor digitorum profundus so that S cannot flex the distal joint (Fig. 7-24, *B*).[4,11] Most individuals cannot perform isolated action of the PIP joint of the 5th finger even with this assistance.[8]

RESIST: With one finger at the volar aspect of the middle phalanx toward extension.[6,7] If the index finger is used to apply resistance, the middle finger may be used to move the DIP joint to and fro to verify that the flexor digitorum profundus (FDP) is not substituting (Fig. 7-24, *C*).

Procedure for Testing Grades Poor (P), Trace (T), and Zero (0)

POSITION: S seated with the forearm in midposition and the wrist at neutral, resting on the ulnar border.[11] E sits opposite or next to S on the side to be tested.

STABILIZE: The MP joint and proximal phalanx of the finger.[6,7] If stabilization during the motion is difficult in this position, the forearm may be returned to full supination, since the effect of gravity on the fingers is not significant.

PALPATE AND OBSERVE: The same as described above, except that the movement is performed in a plane parallel to the floor (Fig. 7-24, *D*).

GRADE: According to standard definitions of muscle grades. In the test for grades Poor and below is done with the forearm in full supination; partial ROM against gravity may be graded Poor.[6]

SUBSTITUTIONS: The FDP may substitute for the FDS. DIP flexion will precede PIP flexion. Tendon action of the long finger flexors accompanies wrist extension and can produce an apparent flexion of the fingers through partial ROM.[8,11]

Motion:
DIP Flexion, 2nd through 5th Fingers

Muscles[6]	**Innervation**[6]
Flexor Digitorum Profundus	Median and Ulnar N., C8, T1

Procedure for Testing Grades Normal (N) to Fair (F)

POSITION: S seated with the forearm in supination, the wrist at neutral, and the fingers extended. E sits opposite or next to S on the side being tested.[6]

STABILIZE: The wrist at neutral and the PIP joint and middle phalanx of the finger being tested.[11]

PALPATE: Use the finger stabilizing the middle phalanx to simultaneously palpate the FDP tendon over the volar surface of the middle phalanx.[6,8]

OBSERVE: S bring the fingertip up away from the supporting surface, flexing the DIP joint (Fig. 7-25, *A*).

RESIST: With one finger at the volar aspect of the distal phalanx toward extension (Fig. 7-25, *B*).[6,7]

Procedure for Testing Grades Poor (P), Trace (T), and Zero (0)

POSITION: S seated with the forearm in midposition and with wrist at neutral resting on the ulnar border.[11] S may be positioned with the forearm supinated, if necessary.

STABILIZE: Same as described above.

PALPATE: The same as described above.

OBSERVE: S flex the DIP joint (Fig. 7-25, *C*).

GRADE: According to standard definitions of muscle grades except that if the test for the grades Poor and below was done with the forearm in full supination, movement through partial ROM may be graded Poor.[6]

SUBSTITUTIONS: None possible during the testing procedure if the wrist is well stabilized, since the FDP is the only muscle that can act to flex the DIP joint when it is isolated. However, during normal hand function, wrist extension with tendon action of the finger flexors can produce partial flexion of the DIP joints.[8,11]

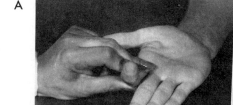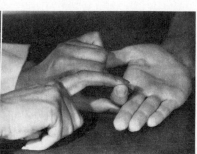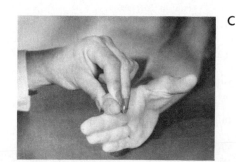

Fig. 7-25. DIP flexion. **A,** Palpate and observe. **B,** Resist. **C,** Gravity-decreased position.

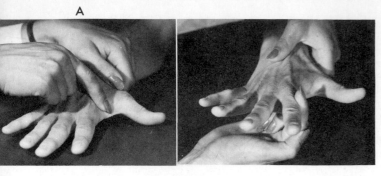

Fig. 7-26. Finger abduction. **A,** Palpate and observe. **B,** Resist.

Motion:
Finger Abduction

Muscles[6]	Innervation[6]
Dorsal Interossei	Ulnar N., C8, T1
Abductor Digiti Minimi	Ulnar N., C8, T1

Procedure for Testing Grades Normal (N) to Fair (F)

POSITION: S seated or supine with the forearm pronated, wrist at neutral, and fingers extended and adducted. E is seated opposite or next to S on the side to be tested.[6]

STABILIZE: The wrist and metacarpals slightly above the supporting surface.

PALPATE: The 1st dorsal interosseous muscle on the lateral aspect of the second metacarpal or of the abductor digiti minimi on the ulnar border of the 5th metacarpal.[6] The remaining interossei are not palpable.

OBSERVE: S spread the fingers apart, abducting them at the MP joints (Fig. 7-26, *A*).

RESIST: The first dorsal interosseous by applying pressure on the radial side of the distal end of the proximal phalanx of the 2nd finger in an ulnar direction (Fig. 7-26, *B*); the 2nd dorsal interosseous on the radial side of the proximal phalanx of the middle finger in an ulnar direction; the 3rd dorsal interosseous on the ulnar side of the proximal phalanx of the middle finger in a radial direction; the 4th dorsal interosseous on the ulnar side of the proximal phalanx of the ring finger in a radial direction: the abductor digiti minimi on the ulnar side of the proximal phalanx of the little finger in a radial direction.[7]

Procedure for Testing Grades P, T, and 0

The tests for these muscle grades are the same as described above. Because the test motions were not performed against gravity, some judgment of the examiner must be used in grading. For example, partial ROM in gravity-decreased position may be graded Poor and full ROM graded Fair.[6]

SUBSTITUTIONS: Extensor digitorum communis can assist weak or absent dorsal interossei, but abduction will be accompanied by MP extension.[8,11]

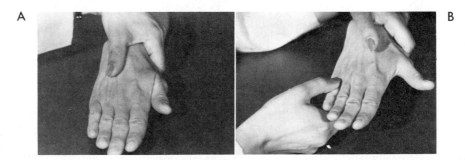

Fig. 7-27. Finger adduction. **A,** Therapist observes movement of fingers into adduction. Palpation of these muscles is not possible. **B,** Resist.

Motion:
Finger Adduction

Muscles[6,7]	Innervation[6]
Palmar Interossei, 1, 2, 3	Ulnar N., C8, T1

Procedure for Testing Grades Normal (N) to Fair (F)

POSITION: S seated with forearm pronated, wrist in neutral, and fingers extended and abducted.[6]

STABILIZE: The wrist and metacarpals slightly above the supporting surface.

PALPATE: Not palpable.

OBSERVE: S adduct the 1st, 4th and 5th fingers toward the middle finger (Fig. 7-27, *A*).

RESIST: The index finger at the proximal phalanx by pulling it in a radial direction, the ring finger at the proximal phalanx in an ulnar direction, and the little finger likewise (Fig. 7-27, *B*).[7] These muscles are very small and resistance will have to be modified to accommodate to their comparatively limited power.

Procedure for Testing Grades Poor (P), Trace (T), and Zero (0) The test for these muscle grades is the same as described above. The examiner's judgment must be used in determining degree of weakness. Achievement of full ROM may be graded Fair and partial ROM graded Poor.[6]

SUBSTITUTIONS: Flexor digitorum profundus and superficialis can substitute for weak palmar interossei, but IP flexion will occur with finger adduction.[8,11]

Motion:
Thumb MP Extension

Muscles[6,7]	Innervation[6,7]
Extensor Pollicis Brevis	Radial N., C6, 7, 8

Procedure for Testing Grades Normal (N) to Fair (F)

POSITION: S seated or supine, forearm in midposition, wrist at neutral, and hand and forearm resting on the ulnar border.[6] The thumb is flexed into the palm at the MP joint and the IP is extended, but relaxed. E sits opposite or next to S on the side to be tested.

STABILIZE: The wrist and the thumb metacarpal.

PALPATE: The extensor pollicis brevis (EPB) tendon at the base of the 1st metacarpal on the dorsoradial aspect. It lies just medial to the abductor pollicis longus tendon on the radial side of the "anatomical snuff box," which is the hollow space created between the EPL and EPB tendons when the thumb is fully extended and radially abducted.[4]

OBSERVE: S extend the MP joint. The IP joint remains relaxed (Fig. 7-28, A). It is difficult for many individuals to isolate this motion.

RESIST: On the dorsal surface of the proximal phalanx toward MP flexion (Fig. 7-28, B).[6,7]

Procedure for Testing Grades (P), (T), and (0)

POSITION AND STABILIZE: Positioning and stabilizing are the same as described above, except that the forearm is fully pronated and resting on the volar surface.[11] E may stabilize the 1st metacarpal, holding the hand slightly above the supporting surface. The test may also be performed in the same manner as for grades Normal to Fair, with modification in grading.[6]

PALPATE AND OBSERVE: Palpation is the same as described above. MP extension is performed in a plane parallel to the supporting surface (Fig. 7-28, C).

GRADE: According to standard definitions of muscle grades. If midposition of forearm was used, partial ROM is graded Poor and full ROM is graded Fair.[6]

SUBSTITUTIONS: Extensor pollicis longus may substitute for extensor pollicis brevis. IP extension will precede MP extension.[8,11]

Motion:
Thumb IP Extension

Muscles[6-8]	Innervation[6,7]
Extensor Pollicis Longus	Radial N., C6, 7, 8

Procedure for Testing Grades Normal (N) to Fair (F)

POSITION: S seated or supine, forearm in midposition, wrist at neutral, and hand and forearm resting on the ulnar border.[6] The MP joint of the thumb is extended or slightly flexed, and the IP is flexed fully into the palm. E sits opposite or next to S on the side being tested.

STABILIZE: The wrist at neutral, 1st metacarpal and the proximal phalanx of the thumb.

PALPATE: The extensor pollicis longus tendon on the dorsal surface of the hand medial to the EPB tendon, between the head of the 1st metacarpal and the base of the 2nd on the ulnar side of the anatomical snuff box.[4,6]

OBSERVE: S bring the tip of the thumb up, out of the palm, extending the IP joint (Fig. 7-29, A).

RESIST: On the dorsal surface of the distal phalanx, down toward IP flexion (Fig. 7-29, B).[6,7]

Procedure for Testing Grades (P), (T), and (0)

POSITION AND STABILIZE: Positioning and stabilizing are the same as described above, except that the forearm is fully pronated.[11] E may stabilize so that S's hand is held slightly above the supporting surface. The test may also be performed in the same position as for grades Normal to Fair with modification in grading.

PALPATE AND OBSERVE: Palpation is the same as described above. IP extension is performed in the plane of the palm, parallel to the supporting surface (Fig. 7-29, C).

GRADE: According to standard definitions of muscle grades. If the test was performed with the forearm in midposition, partial ROM is graded Poor.[6]

SUBSTITUTIONS: A quick contraction of the flexor pollicis longus followed by rapid release will cause the IP joint to rebound into extension. IP flexion will precede IP extension.[8] Abductor pollicis brevis, flexor pollicis brevis, the oblique fibers of the adductor pollicis, and the 1st palmar interossous can extend the IP joint because of their insertions into the extensor expansion of the thumb.[7,11]

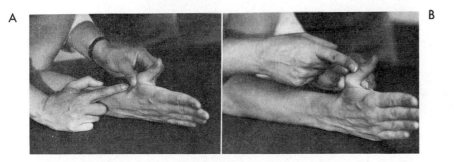
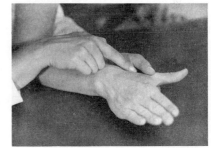

Fig. 7-28. Thumb MP extension. **A,** Palpate and observe. **B,** Resist. **C,** Gravity-decreased position.

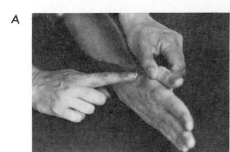
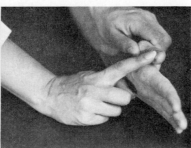
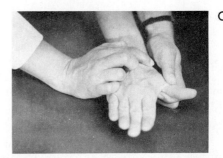

Fig. 7-29. Thumb IP extension. **A,** Palpate and observe. **B,** Resist. **C,** Gravity-decreased position.

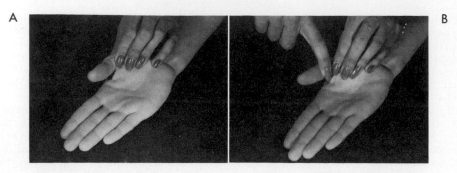

Fig. 7-30. Thumb MP flexion. **A,** Palpate and observe. **B,** Resist.

Motion:
Thumb MP Flexion

Muscles[6,7]	**Innervation**[6,7]
Flexor Pollicis Brevis	Median and Ulnar N., C6, 7, 8, T1

Procedure for Testing Grades Normal (N) to Fair (F)

POSITION: S seated or supine, the forearm fully supinated, the wrist in the neutral position, and the thumb in extension and adduction. E is seated next to or opposite S.[6,7]

STABILIZE: The 1st metacarpal and the wrist.

PALPATE: Over the middle of the palmar surface of the thenar eminence just medial to the abductor pollicis brevis muscle.[6] The hand that is used to stabilize may also be used for palpation.

OBSERVE: S flex the MP joint while maintaining extension of the IP joint (Fig. 7-30, A). It may not be possible for some individuals to isolate flexion to the MP joint. In this instance, both MP and IP flexion may be tested together as a gross test for thumb flexion strength and graded according to the examiner's judgment.

RESIST: On the palmar surface of the first phalanx toward MP extension (Fig. 7-30, B).[6,7]

Procedure for Testing Grades Poor (P), Trace (T), and Zero (0) Positioning, stabilizing and palpating are the same as described above.

OBSERVE: S flex the MP joint so that the thumb moves over the palm of the hand.

GRADE: Full ROM is graded Fair; partial ROM is graded Poor.[6]

SUBSTITUTIONS: Flexor pollicis longus can substitute for flexor pollicis brevis. If this is the case, isolated MP flexion will not be possible and MP flexion will be preceded by IP flexion.[8,11]

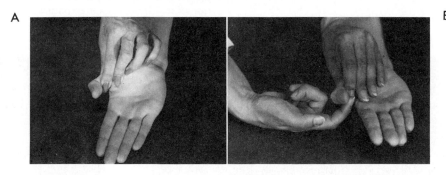

Fig. 7-31. Thumb IP flexion. **A,** Palpate and observe. **B,** Resist.

Motion:
Thumb IP Flexion

Muscles[6-8]	**Innervation**[7]
Flexor Pollicis Longus	Median N., C7, 8, T1

Procedure for Testing Grades Normal (N) to Fair (F)

POSITION: S seated with the forearm fully supinated, wrist in neutral position, and thumb in extension and adduction.[6] E is seated next to or opposite S.

STABILIZE: The 1st metacarpal and the proximal phalanx of the thumb in extension.[6,7]

PALPATE: The flexor pollicis longus tendon on the palmar surface of the proximal phalanx. In this instance, the palpating finger may be the same one used for stabilizing the proximal phalanx.

OBSERVE: S flex the IP joint in the plane of the palm. (Fig. 7-31, A).[6]

RESIST: On the palmar surface of the distal phalanx, toward IP extension (Fig. 7-31, B).[6,7]

Procedure for Testing Grades Poor (P), Trace (T), and Zero (0) The test for these muscle grades is the same as described above. The examiner's judgment must be used in determining degree of weakness. Achievement of full ROM may be graded Fair and partial ROM graded poor.[6]

SUBSTITUTIONS: A quick contraction and release of the extensor pollicis longus may cause an apparent flexion of the IP joint. E should observe for IP extension preceding IP flexion.[8,11]

Motion:
Thumb Palmar Abduction

Muscles[7, 8]	**Innervation[7]**
Abductor Pollicis Brevis	Median N., C6, 7, 8, T1

Procedure for Testing Grades Fair (F) to Normal (N)

POSITION: S seated or supine, forearm in supination, wrist at neutral, thumb extended and adducted, and CMC joint rotated so that the thumb is resting in a plane perpendicular to the palm. E sits opposite or next to S on the side to be tested.[6,7]

STABILIZE: The metacarpals and wrist.

PALPATE: The abductor pollicis brevis muscle on the lateral aspect of the thenar eminence, lateral to the flexor pollicis brevis muscle.[6]

OBSERVE: S raise the thumb away from the palm in a plane perpendicular to the palm (Fig. 7-32, A).[7]

RESIST: At the lateral aspect of the proximal phalanx, downward toward adduction (Fig. 7-32, B).[7]

Procedure for Testing Grades Poor (P), Trace (T), and Zero (0)

POSITION: As described above, except that the forearm and hand are resting on the ulnar border.[11]

STABILIZE: The wrist and metacarpals.

PALPATE: The abductor pollicis brevis muscle on the lateral aspect of the thenar eminence.

OBSERVE: S move the thumb away from the palm in a plane at right angles to the palm of the hand and parallel to the supporting surface (Fig. 7-32, C).

GRADE: According to standard definitions of muscle grades.

SUBSTITUTIONS: Abductor pollicis longus can substitute for abductor pollicis brevis. However, abduction will take place more in the plane of the palm rather then perpendicular to it.[8,11]

Motion:
Thumb Radial Abduction

Muscles[7]	**Innervation[7]**
Abductor Pollicis Longus	Radial N., C6, 7, 8

Procedure for Testing Grades Normal (N) to Fair (F)

POSITION: S seated or supine, forearm in neutral rotation, wrist at neutral, thumb adducted and slightly flexed across the palm. Hand and forearm are resting on the ulnar border.[7] E sits opposite or next to S on the side being tested.

STABILIZE: The wrist and metacarpals of the fingers.[6,7]

PALPATE: The abductor pollicis longus tendon on the lateral aspect of the base of the first metacarpal. It is the tendon immediately lateral (radial) to the extensor pollicis brevis tendon.[4,6]

OBSERVE: S move the thumb out of the palm of the hand, abducting it in the plane of the palm (Fig. 7-33, A).

RESIST: At the lateral aspect of the distal end of the 1st metacarpal toward adduction (Fig. 7-33, B).[6,7]

Procedure for Testing Grades Poor (P), Trace (T), and Zero (0)

POSITION: As described above, except that the forearm is in full supination and the forearm and hand are resting on the dorsal surface.[6]

STABILIZE: The wrist and palm of the hand.

PALPATE: Same as described above.

OBSERVE: S move the thumb out away from the palm of the hand in the plane of the palm, parallel to the supporting surface (Fig. 7-33, C).

GRADE: According to standard definitions of muscle grades.

SUBSTITUTIONS: Abductor pollicis brevis can substitute for abductor pollicis longus. However, abduction will not take place in the plane of the palm, but rather in a more ulnarward direction.[8,11]

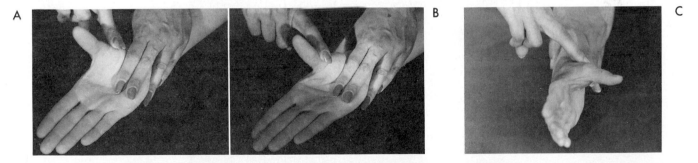

Fig. 7-32. Thumb palmar abduction. **A,** Palpate and observe. **B,** Resist. **C,** Gravity-decreased position.

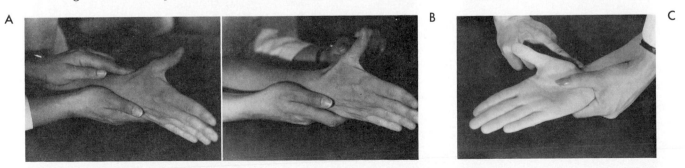

Fig. 7-33. Thumb radial abduction. **A,** Palpate and observe. **B,** Resist. **C,** Gravity-decreased position.

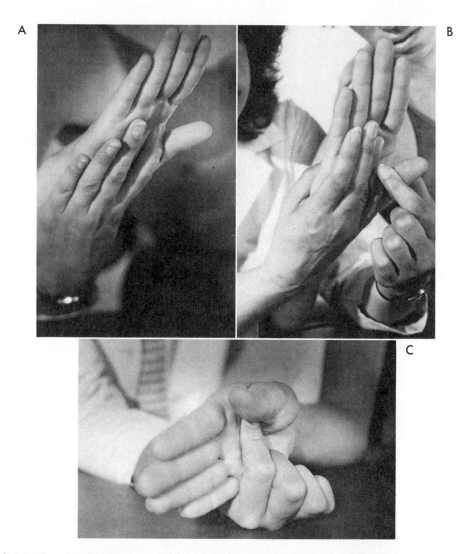

Fig. 7-34. Thumb adduction. **A,** Palpate and observe. **B,** Resist. **C,** Gravity-decreased position.

Motion:

Thumb Adduction

Muscles[6,7]	Innervation[6,7]
Adductor Pollicis	Ulnar N., C8, T1

Procedure for Testing Grades Fair (F) to Normal (N)

POSITION: S seated or supine, forearm pronated, wrist at neutral, thumb opposed and abducted.[6,11] E is sitting opposite or next to S on the side to be tested.

STABILIZE: The wrist and metacarpals, supporting the hand slightly above the resting surface.[6]

PALPATE: Adductor pollicis on the palmar side of the thumb web space.[8]

OBSERVE: S bring the thumb up to touch the palm (Fig. 7-34, A).[6] (The palm is turned up in the illustration to show the palpation point.)

RESIST: By grasping the proximal phalanx of the thumb near the metacarpal head and pull downward, toward abduction (Fig. 7-34, B).[6]

Procedure for Testing Grades Poor (P), Trace (T), and Zero (0)

POSITION: Same as described above, except that the forearm is in midposition and the forearm and hand are resting on the ulnar border.[11]

STABILIZE: Over the wrist and palm of the hand.

PALPATE: Same as described above.

OBSERVE: S bring the thumb in to touch the radial side of the palm of the hand or the 2nd metacarpal (Fig. 7-34, C).

GRADE: According to standard definitions of muscle grades.

SUBSTITUTIONS: Flexor or extensor pollicis longus muscles may assist weak or absent adductor pollicis. If one substitutes, adduction will be accompanied by thumb flexion or extension preceding adduction.[8,11]

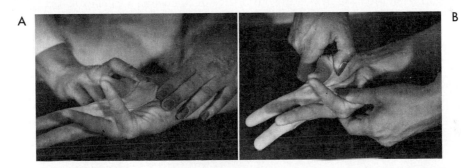

Fig. 7-35. Thumb opposition. **A,** Palpate and observe. **B,** Resist.

Motion:

Opposition of the Thumb to the 5th Finger

Muscles[6,7]	Innervation[6,7]
Opponens Pollicis	Median N., C6, 7, 8, T1
Opponens Digiti Minimi	Ulnar N., C8, T1

Procedure for Testing Grades Normal (N) to Fair (F)

POSITION: S seated or supine with forearm in full supination, wrist at neutral, thumb and 5th finger extended and adducted.[6,7] E sits opposite or next to S on the side to be tested.

STABILIZE: The forearm and wrist.

PALPATE: The opponens pollicis along the radial side of the shaft of the first metacarpal, lateral to the abductor pollicis brevis. The opponens digiti minimi cannot be easily palpated.[6,8]

OBSERVE: S bring the thumb out and across the palm to touch the thumb pad to the pad of the 5th finger (Fig. 7-35, A).

RESIST: At the distal ends of the 1st and 5th metacarpals toward derotation of these bones and flattening of the palm of the hand (Fig. 7-35, B).[6]

Procedure for Testing Grades Poor (P), Trace (T), and Zero (0) The same procedure described above may be used for these grades, if grading is modified to compensate for the movement of the parts against gravity. For example, movement through full ROM would be graded Fair and through partial ROM would be graded Poor.[6]

SUBSTITUTIONS: Abductor pollicis brevis will assist with opposition by flexing and medially rotating the CMC joint, but the IP joint will extend. The flexor pollicis brevis will flex and medially rotate the CMC joint, but the thumb will not move away from the palm of the hand. The flexor pollicis longus will flex and slightly rotate the CMC joint, but the thumb will not move away from the palm and the IP joint will flex strongly.[8,11]

MANUAL MUSCLE TESTING OF THE LOWER EXTREMITY

Motion:
Hip Flexion

Muscles[4, 6-8]	Innervation[4, 6-8]
Psoas Major	Lumbar Plexus, L1, 2, 3, 4
Iliacus	Femoral N., L2, 3
Rectus Femoris	Femoral N., L2, 3, 4
Tensor Fascia Latae	Superior Gluteal N.,
Sartorius	Femoral N., L2, 3, 4, 5, S1
Pectineus	Femoral N., L2, 3

Procedure for Testing Grades Normal (N) and Fair (F)

POSITION: S seated with knees flexed over the edge of the table and feet above the floor. E stands next to S on the side being tested.

STABILIZE: The pelvis at the iliac crest on the side being tested. S may hold onto the edge of the table or fold arms across chest.[6,7]

PALPATE: The psoas and iliacus are difficult to palpate. The rectus femoris may be palpated on the middle anterior aspect of the thigh just lateral to the sartorius muscle.[4,8]

OBSERVE: S lift the leg up from the table flexing the hip through the remainder of the ROM. Observe for internal rotation, external rotation, and abduction accompanying the flexion as signs of substitution or muscle imbalance in this muscle group (Fig. 7-36, *A*).[7]

RESIST: Just proximal to the knee on the anterior surface of the thigh, down toward the table into hip extension (Fig. 7-36, *B*).[6,7]

Procedure for Testing Grades Poor (P), Trace (T), and Zero (0)

POSITION: S sidelying. E stands behind S, supporting the upper leg in neutral rotation and slight abduction, with the knee extended.[6] The lower leg (to be tested) is extended at the hip and knee.

STABILIZE: Weight of the trunk may be adequate stabilization, or E may stabilize the pelvis.[6]

PALPATE: Same as described above.

OBSERVE: S bring the lower leg up toward the trunk, flexing the hip and knee (Fig. 7-36, *C*).[6]

GRADE: According to standard definitions of muscle grades.

SUBSTITUTIONS: The hip flexors can substitute for one another. If the iliacus and psoas major muscles are weak or absent, hip flexion will be accompanied by other movements: abduction and external rotation (sartorius), abduction and internal rotation (tensor fascia latae), adduction (pectineus).[6,8] If the anterior abdominal muscles do not stabilize the pelvis, it will flex on the thighs and the hip flexors may hold against resistance, but not at maximum ROM.[7]

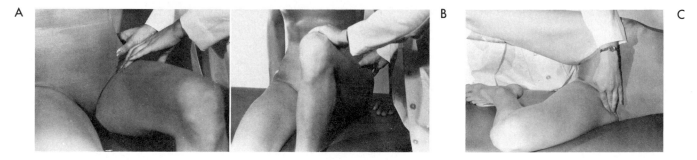

Fig. 7-36. Hip flexion. **A,** Palpate and observe. **B,** Resist. **C,** Gravity-decreased position.

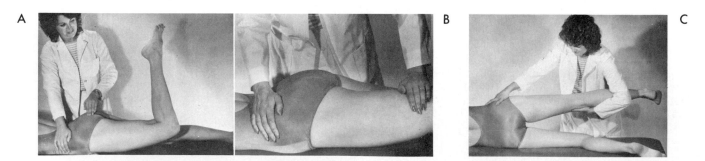

Fig. 7-37. Hip extension. **A,** Palpate and observe. **B,** Resist. **C,** Gravity-decreased position.

Motion:
Hip Extension

Muscles[6,7]	Innervation[6]
Gluteus Maximus	Inferior Gluteal N., L5, S1, 2

Procedure for Testing Grades Normal (N) to Fair (F)

POSITION: S lying prone with the hip at neutral and the knee flexed to about 90°. E stands next to S on the opposite side.[7]

STABILIZE: Over the iliac crest on the side being tested.[6]

PALPATE: The gluteus maximus on middle posterior surface of the buttock.[8]

OBSERVE: S lift the leg from the supporting surface, extending the hip while keeping the knee flexed to minimize action of the hamstring muscles on the hip joint (Fig. 7-37, A).

RESIST: At the distal end of the posterior aspect of the thigh, downward, toward flexion (Fig. 7-37, B).[6,7]

Procedure for Testing Grades Poor (P), Trace (T), and Zero (0)

POSITION: Sidelying. E stands in front of S, supporting the upper leg in extension and slight abduction.[6] The lower leg (to be tested) is flexed at the hip and knee.

STABILIZE: The pelvis over the iliac crest.[6]

PALPATE: Same as described above.

OBSERVE: S bring the lower leg backward, extending the hip but maintaining flexion of the knee (Fig. 7-37, C).

GRADE: According to standard definitions of muscle grades.

SUBSTITUTIONS: Elevation of the pelvis and extension of the lumbar spine can produce some hip extension. In supine, gravity and eccentric contraction of the hip flexors can return the flexed hip to extension.[8]

Motion:
Hip Abduction

Muscles[6-8]	Innervation[6,7]
Gluteus Medius	Superior Gluteal N., L4, 5, S1
Gluteus Minimus	Superior Gluteal N., L4, 5, S1
Tensor Fascia Latae	Superior Gluteal N., L4, 5, S1

Procedure for Testing Grades Normal (N) to Fair (F)

POSITION: S sidelying, upper leg (to be tested) has the knee extended and hip extended slightly beyond the neutral position; lower leg is flexed at the hip and knee to provide a wide base of support. E stands in front of S.[6,7]

STABILIZE: The pelvis over the iliac crest.[6,7]

PALPATE: The gluteus medius on the lateral aspect of the ilium above the greater trochanter of the femur.[6]

OBSERVE: S lift the leg upward, abducting the hip (Fig. 7-38, A).

RESIST: Just proximal to the knee in a downward direction, toward adduction (Fig. 7-38, B).[6]

Procedure for Testing Grades Poor (P), Trace (T), and Zero (0)

POSITION: S lying supine with both legs extended and in neutral rotation. E stands next to S on the opposite side.[6]

STABILIZE: The pelvis at the iliac crest on the side to be tested and the opposite limb at the lateral aspect of the calf.[6]

PALPATE: Use the hand stabilizing over the pelvis to palpate the gluteus medius muscle simultaneously by adjusting the position of the hand so that the fingers are touching the lateral aspect of the ilium, above the greater trochanter, as described above.

OBSERVE: S move the free leg sideward, abducting the hip as far as possible and maintaining neutral rotation during this movement (Fig. 7-38, C).[6]

GRADE: According to standard definitions of muscle grades.

SUBSTITUTIONS: Lateral muscles of the trunk may contract to bring the pelvis toward the thorax, effecting partial abduction at the hip.[6] If the hip is externally rotated, the hip flexors may assist in abduction.[6,8]

A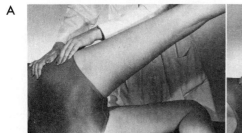 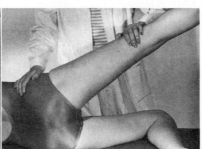B 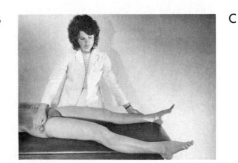C

Fig. 7-38. Hip abduction. **A,** Palpate and observe. **B,** Resist. **C,** Gravity-decreased position.

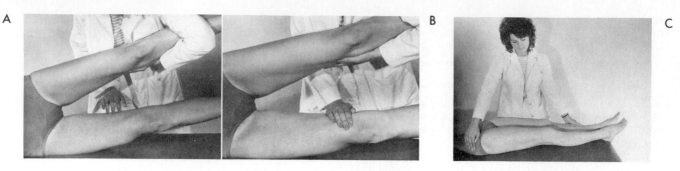

Fig. 7-39. Hip adduction. **A,** Palpate and observe. **B,** Resist. **C,** Gravity-decreased position.

Motion:

Hip Adduction

Muscles[4,6-8]	Innervation[1,6,7]
Adductor Magnus	Obturator and Sciatic N., L2, 3, 4, 5, S1
Adductor Brevis	Obturator, L2, 3, 4
Adductor Longus	Obturator, L2, 3, 4
Gracilis	Obturator, L2, 3, 4
Pectineus	Femoral and Obturator, L2, 3, 4

Procedure for Testing Grades Normal (N) to Fair (F)

POSITION: S sidelying on right for test of right leg or on left side for test of left leg; body in a straight line with legs extended. E stands behind S.

STABILIZE: Support S's upper leg in partial abduction while S holds on to the supporting surface for stability.[5-7]

PALPATE: Any of the adductor muscles as follows: adductor magnus at the middle of the medial surface of the thigh; adductor longus at the medial aspect of the groin; gracilis on the medial aspect of the posterior surface of the knee, just anterior to the semitendinosus tendon.[8]

OBSERVE: S raise the lower leg up from the supporting surface, keeping the knee extended. Observe that there is no rotation, flexion, or extension of the hip or pelvic tilting (Fig. 7-39, *A*).[7]

RESIST: Over the medial aspect of the leg, just proximal to the knee, downward toward abduction (Fig. 7-39, *B*).[6,7]

Procedure for Testing Grades Poor (P), Trace (T), and Zero (0)

POSITION: S supine; limb to be tested is abducted to 45°. E stands next to S on the opposite side.

STABILIZE: Over the iliac crest on the side to be tested.[6]

PALPATE: Same as described above.

OBSERVE: S adduct the leg toward midline (Fig. 7-39, *C*).

GRADE: According to standard definitions of muscle grades.

SUBSTITUTIONS: Hip flexors may substitute for adductors. S will internally rotate the hip and tilt the pelvis backward. Hamstrings may be used to substitute for adduction. S will externally rotate the hip and tip the pelvis forward.[7,8]

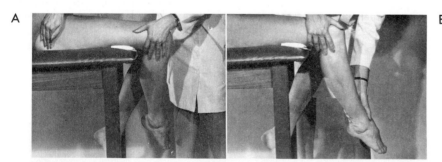 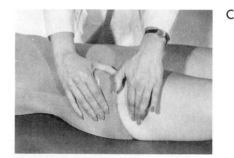

Fig. 7-40. Hip external rotation. **A,** Palpate and observe. **B,** Resist. **C,** Gravity-decreased position.

Motion:

Hip External Rotation

Muscles[6-8]	Innervation[6,7]
Quadratus Femoris	Sacral Plexus, L4,5,S1
Piriformis	Sacral Plexus, L5,S1,2
Obturator Internus	Sacral Plexus, L5, S1, 2
Obturator Externus	Obturator N., L3, 4
Gemellus Superior	Sacral Plexus, L5, S1, 2
Gemellus Inferior	Sacral Plexus, L4, 5, S1

Procedure for Testing Grades Normal (N) to Fair (F)

POSITION: S seated with knees flexed over the edge of the table. A small pad or folded towel is placed under the knee on the side to be tested. E stands in front of S toward the side to be tested.[6,7]

STABILIZE: On the lateral aspect of the knee on the side to be tested. S may grasp the edge of the table to stabilize the trunk and pelvis.[6,7]

PALPATE: Difficult or impossible to palpate these deep muscles. Action of the external rotators may be detected by palpating deeply posterior to the greater trochanter of the femur.[6]

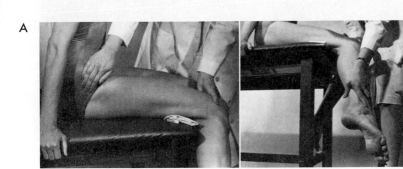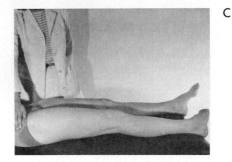

Fig. 7-41. Hip internal rotation. **A,** Palpate and observe. **B,** Resist. **C,** Gravity-decreased position.

OBSERVE: S rotate the thigh outwardly, moving the foot medially (Fig. 7-40, *A*).

RESIST: At the medial aspect of the ankle in a lateral direction, toward internal rotation.[6,7] Resistance should be given carefully and gradually, since the use of the long lever arm can cause joint injury if sudden forceful resistance is given (Fig. 7-40, *B*).[6]

Procedure for Testing Grades Poor (P), Trace (T), and Zero (0)

POSITION: S lying supine with hips and knees extended; hip to be tested is internally rotated. E is standing next to S on the opposite side.[6]

STABILIZE: The pelvis on the side to be tested.

PALPATE: Action of the external rotators may be detected by palpating deeply posterior to the greater trochanter of the femur.[6]

OBSERVE: S roll the thigh outward (laterally). Gravity may assist this motion once S has passed the neutral position. E may use one hand to palpate and the other to offer slight resistance during the second half of the movement to compensate for the assistance of gravity. If the range can be completed with slight resistance, a grade of Poor can be given (Fig. 7-40, *C*).[6]

GRADE: According to standard definitions of muscle grades for Fair to Normal muscles. Muscles are graded Poor if ROM in the gravity-decreased position can be achieved against slight resistance during the second half of the ROM. A grade of Trace can be assigned if contraction of external rotators can be detected by the deep palpation, described above, when the movement is attemped in the gravity decreased position.[6]

SUBSTITUTIONS: Gluteus maximus may substitute for the deep external rotators when the hip is in extension. Sartorius may substitute, but external rotation will be accompanied by hip abduction and knee flexion.[8]

Motion:

Hip Internal Rotation

Muscles[4, 6-8]	Innervation[6, 7, 8]
Gluteus Minimus	Superior Gluteal N., L4, 5, S1
Gluteus Medius	Superior Gluteal N., L4, 5, S1
Tensor Fascia Latae	Superior Gluteal N., L4, 5, S1

Procedure for Testing Grades Normal (N) to Fair (F)

POSITION: S seated on a table with the knees flexed over the edge with small pad placed under the knee. E stands next to S on the side to be tested.[6] (E is shown on the opposite side in the illustration so that the palpation and stabilization will be apparent.)

STABILIZE: At the medial aspect of the knee. S may grasp the edge of the table to stabilize the pelvis and trunk.[6,7]

PALPATE: The gluteus medius between the iliac crest and the greater trochanter.[4]

OBSERVE: S rotate the thigh inwardly, moving the foot laterally. E should observe that S does not lift the pelvis on the side being tested (Fig. 7-41, *A*).[6]

RESIST: At the lateral aspect of the lower leg, pushing the leg medially and thus the thigh toward external rotation (Fig. 7-41, *B*).[6,7]

Procedure for Testing Grades Poor (P), Trace (T), and Zero (0)

POSITION: S supine with hips and knees extended; hip to be tested in external rotation. E stands on the opposite side.[6]

STABILIZE: Over the iliac crest on the side to be tested.[6]

PALPATE: Same as described above.

OBSERVE: S rotate the thigh inwardly or medially. As in external rotation, gravity may assist the motion once the neutral position is passed. However, this will not be as significant as in the test for external rotation (Fig. 7-41, *C*).

GRADE: According to standard definitions of muscle grades.

SUBSTITUTIONS: The tensor fascia latae may substitute for the gluteus minimus, but the movement will be accompanied by some hip flexion. Trunk medial rotation may also effect some internal rotation of the hip.[8]

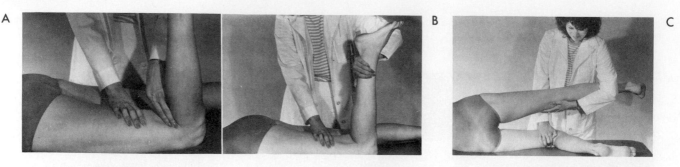

Fig. 7-42. Knee flexion. **A,** Palpate and observe. **B,** Resist. **C,** Gravity-decreased position.

Motion:
Knee Flexion

Muscles[4, 6-8]	Innervation[4, 6, 7]
(Hamstrings)	
Biceps Femoris	Sciatic N., L5, S1, 2, 3
Semitendinosus	Sciatic N., L4, 5, S1, 2
Semimembranosus	Sciatic N., L4, 5, S1, 2

Procedure for Testing Grades Normal (N) to Fair (F)

POSITION: S lying prone with knees and hips in extension and neutral rotation.[5-7] E stands next to S on the opposite side, toward the lower end of the supporting surface.[6]

STABILIZE: Firmly over the posterior aspect of the thigh, above the tedinous insertion of the knee flexors.[7]

PALPATE: For the biceps femoris tendon on the lateral aspect of the posterior surface of the knee as it nears its insertion on the head of the fibula or for the semitendinosus tendon in the middle of the posterior surface of the knee.[4,8] It is the most prominent tendon on the back of the knee.[1]

OBSERVE: S flex the knee to slightly less than 90° (Fig. 7-42, *A*).[8]

RESIST: By grasping S's leg over the posterior aspect of the ankle and pushing downward toward knee extension.[6] Note that not as much resistance can be applied to knee flexion in this position as when tested with the hip flexed as in sitting (Fig. 7-42, *B*).[7]

Procedure for Testing Grades Poor (P), Trace (T), and Zero (0)

POSITION: S sidelying with knees and hips extended and in neutral rotation. E stands next to S and supports the upper leg in slight abduction to allow testing of the lower leg.[6]

STABILIZE: Over the medial aspect of the thigh.

PALPATE: The semitendinosus as described above.

OBSERVE: S flex the knee of the lower leg. (Fig. 7-42, *C*).

GRADE: According to standard definitions of muscle grades.

SUBSTITUTIONS: Sartorius may substitute or assist the hamstrings, but hip flexion and external rotation will occur simultaneously.[6,8] Gracilis may substitute, causing hip adduction with knee flexion. Gastrocnemius may assist or substitute if strong plantar flexion of the ankle occurs during knee flexion.[6]

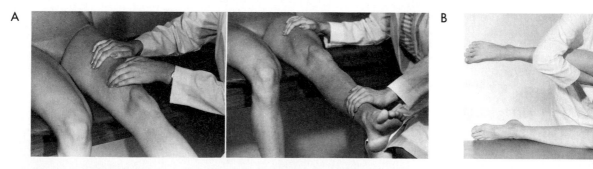

Fig. 7-43. Knee extension. **A,** Palpate and observe. **B,** Resist. **C,** Gravity-decreased position.

Motion:
Knee Extension

Muscles[6]	Innervation[6]
Quadriceps Femoris Group	Femoral N., L2, 3, 4
Rectus Femoris	
Vastus Intermedius	
Vastus Medialis	
Vastus Lateralis	

Procedure for Testing Grades Normal (N) to Fair (F)

POSITION: S sitting with knees flexed over the edge of the table, feet suspended off the floor. S may lean backward slightly to release tension on the hamstrings and grasp the edge of the table for stability.[6] E stands next to S on the side to be tested.

STABILIZE: Thigh by holding hand firmly over it, or place one hand under S's knee to cushion it from the edge of the table.[6,7]

PALPATE: Any of the muscles in the quadriceps femoris

group as follows: rectus femoris on the anterior aspect of the thigh; vastus medialis on the "anteromedial aspect of the lower third of the thigh"; vastus lateralis on the "anterolateral aspect of the lower third of the thigh."[8] Vastus intermedius cannot be palpated.[8]

OBSERVE: S raise the leg toward the ceiling, extending the knee to slightly less than full ROM. Observe for hip movements as evidence of substitutions (Fig. 7-43, A).

RESIST: On the anterior surface of the leg, just above the ankle, with downward pressure toward knee flexion.[6,7] S should not be allowed to "lock" the knee joint at the end of the ROM when full extension is achieved. Maintenance of a slight amount of knee flexion will prevent this. Resistance to a locked knee can cause joint injury (Fig. 7-43, B).[6]

Procedure for Testing Grades Poor (P), Trace (T), and Zero (0)

POSITION: S sidelying on the side to be tested. The lower leg is positioned with the hip extended and the knee flexed to 90°. E stands behind S.

STABILIZE: The upper leg in slight abduction with one hand and with the other over the anterior aspect of the thigh on the leg to be tested.[6]

PALPATE: Any of the muscles, as described above, with the same hand used to stabilize S's thigh. Then ask S to straighten the leg, extending the knee. Observe for hip movements as signs of substitution (Fig. 7-43, C).

GRADE: According to standard definitions of muscle grades.

SUBSTITUTIONS: Tensor fascia latae may substitute for or assist weak quadriceps. In this case, hip internal rotation will accompany knee extension.[6,7]

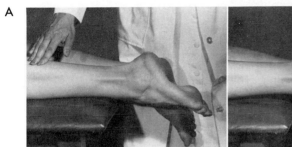 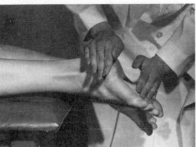 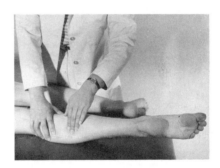

Fig. 7-44. Ankle plantar flexion. **A,** Palpate and observe. **B,** Resist. **C,** Gravity-decreased position.

Motion:
Ankle Plantar Flexion

Muscles[4,6-8]	Innervation[7]
Gastrocnemius	Tibial N., S1, 2
Soleus	Tibial N., L5, S1, 2
Plantaris	Tibial N., L4, 5, S1

Procedure for Testing Grades Normal (N) to Fair (F)

POSITION: S lying prone with the hips and knees extended and the feet projecting beyond the edge of the table. E stands at the lower end of the table facing S's feet.[5,7]

STABILIZE: Weight of the leg is usually adequate stabilization.

PALPATE: The gastrocnemius on the posterior aspect of the calf of the leg, or the soleus, slightly lateral to and beneath the lateral head of the gastrocnemius.[8] The gastrocnemius tendon above the calcaneus may also be palpated.[6]

OBSERVE: S pull the heel upward, plantar flexing the ankle. Observe for flexion of the toes and forefoot prior to movement of the heel as evidence of substitutions (Fig. 7-44, A).[7,8]

RESIST: On the posterior aspect of the calcaneus as if pulling downward and on the forefoot as if pushing forward. If there is significant weakness, pressure to the calcaneus may be sufficient (Fig. 7-44, B).[7]

Procedure for Testing Grades Poor (P), Trace (T) and Zero (0)

POSITION: S lying on the side to be tested; hip and knee of the lower limb are extended and the ankle is in midposition. The upper limb may be flexed at the knee to keep it out of the way. E stands at the lower end of the table.[6]

STABILIZE: Over the posterior aspect of the calf.[6]

PALPATE: As described above.

OBSERVE: S pull the heel upward, pointing the toes down. Observe for toe flexion, inversion, or eversion of the foot as evidence of substitutions (Fig. 7-44, C).

GRADE: According to standard definitions of muscle grades.

SUBSTITUTIONS: Flexor digitorum longus and flexor hallucis longus can substitute for plantar flexors, producing toe flexion and flexion of the forefoot, with incomplete movement of the calcaneus. Substitution by the peroneus longus and brevis will cause foot everion and substitution by the tibialis posterior will cause foot inversion. Substitution by all three will effect plantar flexion of the forefoot, with limited movement of the calcaneus.[6,8]

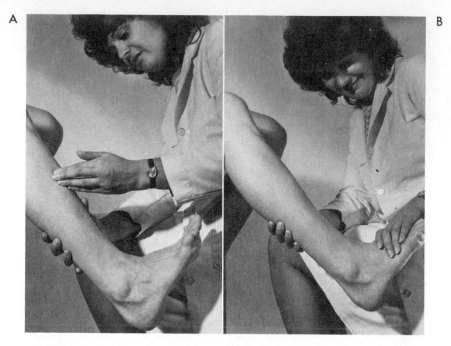

Fig. 7-45. Ankle dorsiflexion with inversion. **A,** Palpate and observe. **B,** Resist.

Motion:

Ankle Dorsiflexion with Inversion

Muscles[6,7]	**Innervation**[6,7]
Tibialis Anterior	Peroneal N., L4,5,S1

Procedure for Testing Grades Normal (N) to Fair (F)

POSITION: S seated with the legs, flexed at the knees, over the edge of the table. E sits in front of S, slightly to the side to be tested. S's heel can rest in E's lap.[6,7]

STABILIZE: The leg just above the ankle.

PALPATE: The tibialis anterior tendon on the anterior medial aspect of the ankle.[6] Muscle fibers may be palpated on the anterior surface of the leg, just lateral to the tibia.[8]

OBSERVE: S pull the forefoot upward and inward, keeping the toes relaxed, dorsiflexing and inverting the foot. Watch for extension of the great toe preceding the ankle motion as a sign of muscle substitution (Fig. 7-45, *A*).[6]

RESIST: On the medial dorsal aspect of the foot, toward plantar flexion and eversion (Fig. 7-45, *B*).[6,7]

Procedure for Testing Grades Poor (P), Trace (T), and Zero (0) The same position and procedure described above may be used with modified grading. The test may also be performed with S in the supine position.[6]

GRADE: If the against-gravity position is used in the procedure for grades Poor to Zero, clinical judgment of the examiner must be used to determine muscle grades. Partial ROM against gravity can be graded Poor. If the test is performed in the supine position for these grades, standard definitions of muscle grades may be used.[6]

SUBSTITUTIONS: Peroneus tertius, a foot everter, can assist for foot dorsiflexion. However, dorsiflexion will be accompanied by foot eversion.[8] Extensor hallucis longus and extensor digitorum longus may also assist or substitute. Movement will be preceded by extension of the great toe or by all of the toes.[6-8]

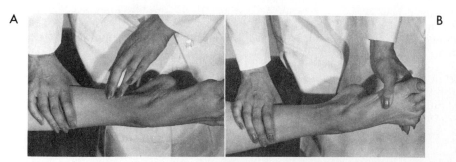
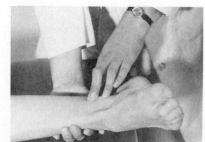

Fig. 7-46. Foot inversion. **A,** Palpate and observe. **B,** Resist. **C,** Gravity-decreased position.

Motion:
Foot Inversion

Muscles[6,7]	Innervation[6,7]
Tibialis Posterior	Tibial N., L5,S1

Procedure for Testing Grades Normal (N) and Fair (F)

POSITION: S lying, on the side to be tested, with the hip in neutral rotation, knee extended, and ankle in slight plantar flexion.[6] The upper leg may be flexed at the knee to keep it out of the way. E stands at the end of the table, facing S's feet.

STABILIZE: Leg to be tested above the ankle joint on the dorsal surface of the calf, being careful not to put pressure on the tibialis posterior muscle.[6]

PALPATE: The tendon of the tibialis posterior muscle between the medial malleolus and navicular bone or above and just posterior to the medial malleolus.[6]

OBSERVE: S move the foot upward (medially), and in-

verting it, keeping the toes relaxed. There normally will be some plantar flexion as well (Fig. 7-46, A).[6,7]

RESIST: On the medial border of the forefoot toward eversion (Fig. 7-46, B).[6,7]

Procedure for Testing Grades Poor (P), Trace (T), and Zero (0)

POSITION: S lying supine with the hip extended and in neutral rotation, knee extended, and the ankle in midposition.

STABILIZE: Same as described above.

PALPATE: Same as described above.

OBSERVE: S move the foot inward (medially), inverting it while keeping the toes relaxed (Fig. 7-46, C).

GRADE: According to standard definitions of muscle grades.

SUBSTITUTIONS: Flexor hallucis longus and flexor digitorum longus can substitute for tibialis posterior. Movement will be accompanied by toe flexion, or toes will flex when resistance is applied.[6-8] Tibialis anterior may assist in inversion if there is simultaneous dorsiflexion.[1-9]

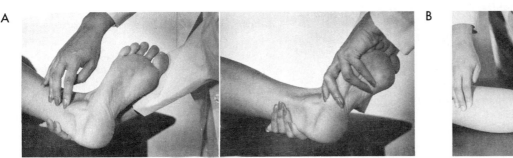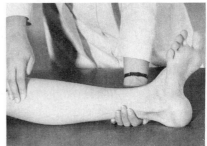

Fig. 7-47. Foot eversion. **A,** Palpate and observe. **B,** Resist. **C,** Gravity-decreased position.

Motion:
Foot Eversion

Muscles[6,7]	Innervation[6,7]
Peroneus Longus	Peroneal N., L4,5,S1
Peroneus Brevis	
Peroneus Tertius	

Procedure for Testing Grades Normal (N) and Fair (F)

POSITION: S sidelying with the lower leg to be tested in hip extension and neutral rotation, knee in extension, and ankle in midposition. The upper leg is flexed at the knee to keep it out of the way.[6,7]

STABILIZE: Above the ankle on its medial suface, supporting the foot slightly above the table surface.[6,7]

PALPATE: The peroneus longus over the upper half of the lateral aspect of the calf, just distal to the head of the fibula.[6,8] Its tendon can be palpated on the lateral aspect of the ankld, above and behind the lateral malleolus. Peroneus brevis tendon may be palpated on the lateral border of the foot, proximal to the base of the 5th metatarsal.[6,8] Its muscle fibers can be found on the lower half of the lateral surface of the leg, ove the fibula.[6]

OBSERVE: S turn the sole of the foot outward, everting it. (Note that this movement is normally accompanied by some degree of plantar flexion.)[7,8] Observe for dorsiflexion or toe extension as evidence of substitutions (Fig. 7-47, A).

RESIST: Against the lateral border and the plantar surface of the foot toward inversion and dorsiflexion (Fig. 7-4, B).[7]

Procedure for Testing Grades Poor (P), Trace (T), and Zero (0)

POSITION: S lying supine, hip extended and in neutral rotation.[6] The knee is extended and ankle is in midposition.

STABILIZE: The leg under the calf.

PALPATE: The same as described above.

OBSERVE: S move the foot in a sideward or lateral direction, thus everting it (Fig. 7-47, C).

GRADE: Grade according to standard definitions of muscle grades.

SUBSTITUTIONS: Peroneus tertius, while everting the foot, also dorsiflexes it. If it is substituting for peroneus longus and peroneus brevis, dorsiflexion will accompany eversion. Extensor digitorum longus can also substitute for the peroneals, and toe extension will precede or accompany eversion.[8]

FUNCTIONAL MUSCLE TESTING

The functional muscle test is a useful tool when screening muscles for normal strength.[10] It is used by occupational therapists in some health care facilities where the specific muscle testing is the responsibility of the physical therapy service. To avoid duplication of services, the occupational therapist may wish, then, to perform a functional muscle test to assess the strength and motion capabilities of the patient. In dysfunctions in which muscle weakness is not a primary or significant symptom, it may not be important to perform discrete muscle testing, but a general estimate of strength is desirable and adequate to plan tretment and measure progress. In still other instances, a quick functional muscle test may be performed to identify areas of significant weakness that deserve more discrete testing. Thus the functional muscle test may serve as a screening tool.

Such a screening test may be used to conserve the examiner's time and the subject's energy. Various screening tests have been devised. In one, the examiner places the part passively in the position used for the normal test, without considering gravity, and asks the subject to hold the position against resistance. Still another method tests both sides simultaneously while the subject is in the sitting position. If the subject cannot hold against resistance in the screening test, the more careful manual muscle test should be administered. Observation of the subject performing ordinary ADL can also be used as a screening test of baseline strength for function.[6]

The following functional muscle test should be performed while the subject is comfortably seated in a sturdy chair or wheelchair.

The subject is asked to perform the test motion against gravity or in the gravity decreased position, if the former is not feasible.

In all of the tests the subject is allowed to complete the test motion before the examiner applies resistance. The resistance is applied at the end of the ROM while the subject maintains the positon and resists the force applied by the examiner. The examiner may make modifications in positioning to suit individual needs. As in the manual muscle tests, the examiner should stabilize proximal parts and attempt to rule out substituions. It is assumed that the reader is familiar with joint motions, their prime movers, manual muscle testing, and muscle grades before performing this test.

Functional muscle test

Scapular elevation (upper trapezius and levator scapula): S elevates shoulders, and E pushes down on shoulders into depression.

Scapular abduction (serratus anterior): With S's arms positioned in 90° of elbow and shoulder flexion, E pushes at shoulder into scapular adduction.

Scapular adduction (middle trapezius and rhomboids): S extends shoulder and flexes elbow fully, producing scapular adduction. E pushes at shoulder joint into scapular abduction.

Scapular depression (lower trapezius, latissimus dorsi): S extends arm down at side of body as if reaching to floor. E attempts to push arm up at a point just proximal to elbow joint. Muscles act to stabilize scapula and prevent elevation.

Shoulder flexion (anterior deltoid and coracobrachialis): With S's shoulder flexed to 90° and elbow flexed or extended, E pushes down on arm proximal to elbow into extension.

Shoulder extension (latissimus dorsi and teres major): S moves shoulder into full extension. E pushes from behind at a point proximal to elbow into flexion.

Shoulder abduction (middle deltoid and supraspinatus): S abducts shoulder to 90° with elbow flexed or extended. E pushes down on arm just proximal to elbow into adduction.

Shoulder horizontal adduction (pectoralis major, anterior deltoid): S crosses arms in front of chest. E reaches from behind and attempts to pull arms back into horizontal abduction at a point just proximal to elbow.

Shoulder horizontal abduction (posterior deltoid, teres minor, infraspinatus): S moves arms from full horizontal adduction as described above to full horizontal abduction. E pushes forward on arms just proximal to elbow into horizontal adduction.

Shoulder external rotation (infraspinatus and teres minor): S holds arm in 90° of shoulder abduction and 90° of elbow flexion, then externally rotates shoulder through available ROM. E supports or stabilizes upper arm proximal to elbow and pushes from behind at dorsal aspect of wrist into internal rotation.

Shoulder internal rotation (subscapularis, teres major, latissimus dorsi, pectoralis major): S begins with arm as described for external rotation but performs internal rotation. E supports or stabilizes upper arm as before and pulls up into external rotation at volar aspect of wrist.

Elbow flexion (biceps, brachialis): With forearm supinated S flexes elbow from full extension. E sits opposite subject and stabilizes upper arm against trunk while attempting to pull forearm into extension at volar aspect of wrist.

Elbow extension (triceps): With S's upper arm supported in 90° of abduction (gravity-decreased position) or 160° shoulder flexion (against-gravity position), elbow is extended from full flexion. E pushes forearm into flexion at dorsal aspect of wrist.

Forearm supination (biceps, supinator): Upper arm is stabilized against trunk by S or E. Elbow is flexed to 90°, and forearm is in full pronation. S supinates forearm. E grasps distal forearm and attempts to rotate it into pronation.

Forearm pronation (pronator teres, pronator quadratus): S is positioned as described for forearm supination except that forearm is in full supination. S pronates forearm. E grasps distal forearm and attempts to rotate it into supination.

Wrist flexion (flexor carpi radials, flexor carpi ulnaris, palmaris longus): S's forearm is supported on its dorsal surface on a tabletop or armrest. Hand is moved up from tabletop, using wrist flexion. E is seated next to or opposite S and pushes on palm of hand, giving equal pressure on radial and ulnar sides into wrist extension or down toward tabletop.

Wrist extension (extensor carpi radialis longus and brevis, extensor carpi ulnaris): S's forearm is supported on a tabletop or armrest, resting on its volar surface. Hand is lifted from tabletop, using wrist extension. E sits next to or opposite S and pushes on dorsal aspect of palm, giving equal pressure at radial and ulnar sides into wrist flexion or down toward tabletop.

Finger MP flexion and IP extension (lumbricales and interossei): With forearm and hand supported on tabletop on dorsal surface, E stabilizes palm and S flexes MP joints while maintaining extension of IP joints. E pushes into extension with index finger across proximal phalanges or pushes on tip of each finger into IP flexion and MP extension.

Finger IP flexion (flexors digitorum profundus and sublimis): S is positioned as described for MP flexion. IP joints are flexed while maintaining extension of MP joints. E attempts to pull fingers back into extension by hooking fingertips with those of S.

Finger MP extension (IP joints flexed) (extensor digitorum communis, extensor indicis proprius, extensor digiti minimi): S's forearm and hand are supported on a table surface, resting on ulnar border. Wrist is stabilized by E in 0° neutral position. S moves MP joints from flexion to full extension (hyperextension) while keeping IP joints flexed. E pushes fingers at PIP joints simultaneously into flexion.

Finger abduction (dorsal interossei, abductor digiti minimi): S's forearm is resting on volar surface on a table. E may stabilize wrist in slight extension so that hand is raised slightly off supporting surface. S abducts fingers. E pushes two fingers at a time together at the proximal phalanges into adduction. First, index finger and middle fingers are pushed together, then, ring finger and middle fingers, and finally, little finger and ring fingers. Resistance is modified to accommodate small muscles.

Finger adduction (palmar interossei): S is positioned as described for finger abduction. Fingers are adducted tightly. E attempts to pull fingers apart, one at a time at the proximal phalanges. First, index finger is pulled away from middle finger, then, ring finger is pulled away from middle finger, and finally, little finger is pulled away from ring finger. In normal hand adducted finger "snaps" back into adducted position when E pulls it into abduction and lets go quickly. An alternate method would be for examiner to place index finger between two of S's fingers. S should adduct against it, thus estimating amount of force or pressure that S is exerting.

Thumb MP and IP flexion (flexor pollicis brevis and flexor pollicis longus): S's forearm should be supported on a firm surface, with elbow flexed at 90° and forearm in 45° supination. Thumb is flexed across palm. E pulls on tip of thumb into extension.

Thumb MP and IP extension (extensor pollicis brevis and extensor pollicis longus): S is positioned as for thumb MP and IP flexion. Thumb is extended away from palm. E pushes on tip of thumb into flexion.

Thumb palmar abduction (abductor pollicis longus and abductor pollicis brevis): S is positioned as described for thumb flexion and extension. Thumb is abducted away from palm in a plane perpendicular to palm. S resists movement at metacarpal head into adduction.

Thumb adduction (adductor pollicis): S is positioned as for all other thumb movements. Thumb is adducted to palm. E attempts to pull thumb into abduction at metacarpal head or proximal phalanx.

Opposition of thumb to 5th finger (opponens pollicis, opponens digiti minimi): S is positioned with elbow flexed to 90° and dorsal surface of forearm and hand resting on a tabletop or armrest. Thumb is opposed to 5th finger, making pad-to-pad contact. E attempts to pull fingers apart, applying force at metacarpal heads of both fingers.

Functional Muscle Test of the Lower Extremities
All of these tests can be performed with S sitting with legs flexed over edge of supporting surface and feet slightly above floor, except for hip extension test.

Hip flexion (psoas major, iliacus): S flexes hip, bringing leg up from seat, E pushes down on distal apsect of the thigh.

Hip extension (gluteus maximus): S lying prone and lifts leg from supporting surface. E pushes down on posterior distal aspect of thigh. Test can be done with knee flexed to 90°.

Hip abduction (gluteus medius): S moves leg to be tested away from other leg. Leg is supported by E from posterior aspect of knee to reduce effect of resistance from friction on supporting surface. E pushes inward at distal lateral aspect of thigh.

Hip adduction (adductor group): E places palm of hand at medial aspect of distal thigh of leg to be tested and asks S to bring legs together, knees touching. E pulls outward on leg.

Hip external rotation (obturators, gemelli, piriformis, quadratus femoris): S moves foot medially by rotating hip externally. E pushes at medial aspect of ankle in lateral direction, while stabilizing at lateral aspect of thigh, just above knee.

Hip internal rotation (gluteus minimus): S moves foot laterally by internally rotating hip. E pushes at lateral aspect of ankle in medial direction while stabilizing at medial aspect of thigh, just above knee.

Knee flexion (hamstrings): S flexes knee so that leg is flexed under seat of supporting surface. E pushes forward at posterior aspect of ankle.

Knee extension (quadriceps femoris group): S extends knee, straightening leg in seated position. E pushes downward on anterior distal aspect of ankle. To avoid injury, S should not lock knee but should maintain a slight amount of knee flexion during resistance.[6] E can assist by stabilizing with one hand under knee being tested.

Ankle plantar flexion (gastrocnemius, soleus): S is asked to point foot downward. E places hand on metatarsal heads and pushes upward toward dorsiflexion.

Ankle dorsiflexion with inversion (tibialis anterior): S points foot upward and inward simultaneously. E pushes on medial dorsal aspect of foot in downward and lateral direction.

Foot inversion (tibialis posterior): S turns sole of foot medially while maintaining neutral position between plantar flexion and dorsiflexion of ankle. E pushes on medial border of forefoot in outward direction.

Foot eversion (peroneal group): S turns sole of foot laterally while maintaining neutral position of ankle, as above. E pushes on lateral border of foot in inward direction.

SUMMARY

Manual muscle testing evaluates the level of strength in a muscle or muscle group. It is a primary evaluation tool for patients with lower motor neuron dysfunction, orthopedic conditions, and muscle diseases. It does not measure muscle endurance or coordination nor used accurately if spasticity is present.

Accurate assessment of muscle strength depends on the knowledge, skill, and experience of the examiner. Although there are standard definitions of muscle grades, clinical judgment is important in accurate evaluation.

Muscle test results are used to plan treatment strategies to increase strength and/or compensate for weakness. Functional muscle tests are can be used to assess the general level of strength available for ADL and to screen for patients who need specific manual muscle testing.

REVIEW QUESTIONS

1. List three general classifications of physical dysfunction in which muscle weakness is a primary symptom.
2. Given F + muscle strength and low endurance, in which kinds of activities can the patient be expected to participate?
3. List at least three purposes for evaluating muscle strength.
4. Discuss five considerations and their implications in treatment planning that are based on the results of the muscle strength evaluation.
5. Define "endurance" and discuss its correlation with muscle strength.
6. How can muscle weakness be differentiated from joint limitation?
7. If there is joint limitation, can muscle strength be measured accurately? How is strength recorded when available ROM is less than normal?
8. What does the manual muscle test measure?
9. What does the manual muscle test *not* measure about motor function?
10. What are the criteria used to determine muscle grades?
11. In relation to the floor as a horizontal plane, describe or demonstrate what is meant by "with gravity assisting," "with gravity decreased," "against gravity," and "against gravity and resistance."
12. List five factors that can influence the amount of resistance against which a muscle group can hold?
13. Define the muscle grades: N (5), G (4), F − (3−), F (3), P (2), P − (2−), T (1), and zero (0).
14. Define what is meant by "substitution."
15. How are substitutions most likely to be ruled out in the muscle testing procedure?
16. List the steps in the muscle testing procedure.
17. Is it always necessary to perform the manual muscle test to determine level of strength? If not, what alternative may be used to make a general assessment of strength? Generally describe the procedure.
18. Describe or demonstrate the muscle testing procedures for testing grades of normal to fair for the following muscle groups: scapula adduction, shoulder flexion, elbow extension, forearm pronation, wrist flexion, opposition, hip extension, knee flexion, and ankle dorsiflexion.
19. List the purposes of functional muscle testing.

REFERENCES

1. Basmajian JF: Muscles alive, ed 4, Baltimore, 1978, Williams & Wilkins.
2. Bobath B: Adult hemiplegia: evaluation and treatment, ed 2, London, 1978, William Heinemann Medical Books Ltd.
3. Brunnstrom S: Movement therapy in hemiplegia, New York, 1970, Harper & Row, Inc.
4. Brunnstrom S: Clinical kinesiology, Philadelphia, 1972, FA Davis Co.
5. Chusid J: Correlative neuroanatomy and functional neurology, ed 19, Los Altos, Ca, 1985, Lange Medical Publications.
6. Daniels L and Worthingham C: Muscle testing, ed 5, Philadelphia, 1986, WB Saunders Co.
7. Kendall FP and McCreary EK: Muscles: testing and function, ed 2, Baltimore, 1983, Williams & Wilkins.
8. Killingsworth A: Basic physical disability procedures, San Jose, 1987, Maple Press.
9. Landen B, Amizich A: Functional muscle examination and gait analysis, J Amer Phys Ther Assoc 43:39, 1963.
10. Pact V, Sirotkin-Roses M, and Beatus J: The muscle testing handbook, Boston, 1984, Little, Brown & Co.
11. Rancho Los Amigos Hospital, Department of Occupational Therapy: Guide for muscle testing of the upper extremity, Downey, Ca, 1978, The Professional Staff Association of the Rancho Los Amigos Hospital, Inc.

8 Evaluation of muscle tone and coordination

BARBARA ZOLTAN
LORRAINE WILLIAMS PEDRETTI

MUSCLE TONE

Normal muscle tone is a component of a normal postural reflex mechanism. It is a continuous state of mild contraction of muscle and is dependent on the integrity of peripheral and central nervous system (CNS) mechanisms and the properties of muscle, such as contractility, elasticity, ductility, and extensibility. A normal muscle at rest is not entirely atonic. It has a certain amount of resilience; when stretched passively, it offers a small amount of involuntary resistance. It allows movement to proceed smoothly and without interruption. The loss of normal muscle tone will interfere with normal selective movement. The facilitation of its return is crucial to the patient's ultimate recovery of function.[5]

The maintenance of normal muscle tone is dependent on normal function of the cerebellum, motor cortex, basal ganglia, midbrain, vestibular system, spinal cord functions, neuromuscular system, and a normally functioning stretch reflex.[4] The stretch reflex can produce increased tension in certain muscle groups to provide a background of increased postural tone from which voluntary movement can proceed.[7] The stretch reflex is mediated by the muscle spindle, a sophisticated sensory receptor continuously reporting sensory information from muscles to the CNS.

For a more complete discussion of the anatomy of the muscle spindle and other proprioceptors that influence muscle tone, the reader is referred to Chapter 17.

Normal Muscle Tone

The estimation of muscle tone can only be made in relation to normal muscle tone. Although normal tone varies from one individual to another and is dependent on factors such as age, sex, and occupation, normal muscle tone is characterized by:

1. Effective cocontraction (stabilization) at proximal joints
2. Ability to move against gravity and resistance
3. Ability to maintain the position of the limb if it is placed passively by the examiner and then released[4,10]
4. Balanced tone between agonist and antagonist muscles
5. Ease of ability to shift from stability to mobility and vice versa as needed
6. Ability to use muscles in groups or selectively, if necessary[10]
7. Resilience or slight resistance in response to passive movement[7]

GENERAL PRINCIPLES OF MUSCLE TONE/ MOVEMENT EVALUATION

The specific objective evaluation of muscle tone is difficult due to its continuous fluctuation and its real relationship to the remaining components of the postural reflex mechanism.[4,12] The release of primitive reflexes and associated reactions will alter postural tone, depending on the patient's body or head position or on exteroceptive stimulation such as touch or pressure. The stroke patient, for example, may exhibit a moderate level of upper-extremity spasticity when lying down and severe spasticity when sitting. The level and distribution of spasticity changes as the position of the patient's head in space and its relation to the body changes.[4]

Many clinicians believe that the close association of abnormal tone with the abnormal postural patterns of the patient with CNS dysfunction necessitates the simultaneous evaluation of these two factors.[4] Assessing tone in conjunction with posture and selective movement will generate valuable information about the patient's overall function. Normal motor function requires selective movement and a variety of motor patterns supplied by a normal postural background that support these movements and patterns.[4] Muscle tone deficits can include flaccidity, spasticity, and/or rigidity depending on the specific diagnosis and level of motor recovery. Each type of deficit has its own characteristics, which the therapist must understand in order to differentiate among them. This differentiation is crucial because treatment techniques for the spastic patient, for example, are quite different from those for the patient with rigidity.

Once the therapist has established the type of muscle tone deficit, he or she examines the degree of deficit that is present, depending on the patient's position and attempted movement. Fluctuations in tone are examined when the patient is lying down, rolling, moving into a sitting position, sitting, and, if appropriate, when standing and walking. The quality of the patient's movements is examined in conjunction with how abnormal tone interferes with these movements.

Flaccidity

Flaccidity is hypotonicity of muscle, that is, a decrease of normal muscle tone. Hypotonicity is usually the result of damage to the proprioceptive innervation of muscle, a disruption of the reflex arc, or cerebellar disease and is seen temporarily in the "shock" phase after cerebral or spinal insult.[17] It may also result from muscle disuse and prolonged immobilization.[3]

CHARACTERISTICS OF FLACCIDITY. Hypotonic muscles feel soft and flabby and offer less resistance to passive movement than does a normal muscle.[8] Because of the laxity of the muscle, there may be an unusually wide range of motion (ROM) possible.[23] If the flaccid limb is placed passively in a given position and is then released, the patient cannot maintain the limb in the position. Rather, it is likely to drop heavily, because the muscles are unable to resist gravity.[3] Cocontraction of proximal joints is weak or absent.[10] Deep tendon reflexes are diminished or absent.[8,17] The patient with hypotonicity may be unable to posturally fixate an extremity.[23]

OCCURRENCE OF FLACCIDITY. Flaccidity or hypotonicity of muscle occurs in primary muscle diseases, lower motor neuron disorders (such as peripheral neuropathies and polyneuritis), and cerebellar lesions and follows stroke or spinal cord injury during the shock phase. In these latter conditions the flaccidity usually gives way to increasing spasticity as the shock phase passes.

METHOD OF EVALUATION. Flaccidity is estimated by performing passive movements. The movements must be gentle. Without telling the patient what to expect, the therapist may take the patient's hand and gently move the fingers backward and forward from tip to wrist to produce slow undulating flexion and extension movements of fingers and wrist, thus estimating the tone in the flexors and extensors of the wrist and fingers. Similar movements can be performed at the larger joints of the upper and lower

extremities, with the examiner noting the degree of resistance to passive movement and any unusually wide ROM.[3]

SCALE OF SEVERITY OF FLACCIDITY. The following scale is suggested in estimating the degree of flaccidity.

Mild flaccidity. Mild flaccidity is characterized by:
1. Decreased muscle tone; weak cocontraction of agonist and antagonist muscles in stabilizing joints
2. Ability of the limb to resist gravity briefly if placed in position and released
3. Decreased muscle strength; functional motion still possible

Moderate to severe flaccidity. Moderate to severe flaccidity is characterized by:
1. Significantly decreased or absent muscle tone
2. Absence of cocontraction
3. Limb dropping immediately if placed against gravity and released[10]
4. Minimal or lack of ability to move against gravity
5. Significant loss of strength; no functional motion possible

Spasticity

Upper motor neuron systems control fusimotor neurons to keep them inhibited. Damage to these upper motor neuron systems can cause a release or disinhibition of fusimotor neurons from central control. This results in their increased firing, which in turn causes the muscle spindle to become more sensitive and to produce more firing of Ia afferent fibers. The final result is increased stimulation of the lower motor neurons with a resultant increased alpha motor activity called spasticity.[11]

Spasticity is associated with the release of an abnormal postural reflex mechanism that results in static versus dynamic postural control. Any neurologic condition changing upper motor neuron pathways that directly or indirectly inhibit or facilitate alpha motor neuron activity may result in spasticity.[12]

CHARACTERISTICS OF SPASTICITY. Spasticity is characterized by hypertonic muscles, hyperactive deep tendon reflexes, clonus, and abnormal spinal reflexes.[19] The hypertonicity usually occurs in definite patterns of flexion or extension.[4,13,19] Typically, the pattern of spasticity occurs in the antigravity muscles of the upper and lower extremities. In the upper extremity the flexor pattern usually dominates. It includes adduction (retraction) and depression of the scapula, internal rotation and adduction at the shoulder joint, elbow flexion with forearm pronation, wrist flexion, and finger flexion with adduction. In the lower extremity the antigravity muscles are the extensors, and the spastic pattern is elevation and retraction of the pelvis, external rotation and extension at the hip, and knee extension with inversion of the foot and plantar flexion at the ankle.[13]

Cerebral and spinal spasticity differ. Spasticity associated with stroke or head trauma is often seen in combination with other residual motor deficits such as rigidity or ataxia. It is influenced by position change and labyrinthine and tonic neck reflexes.[12] Spinal cord spasticity that is generally seen in patterns of flexion or in flexion/extension is often violent in nature, with severe episodic muscle spasms.[12,20] The degree of spasticity in incomplete spinal lesions varies, depending on the degree and direction of remaining supraspinal influences.[20]

In spasticity there is increased resistance to passive movement. After the initial resistance there may be a sudden relaxation of muscle known as the clasp-knife phenomenon.[7,12] This is thought to be a result of the function of the Ib sensory afferent fibers from the Golgi tendon organs (GTO). The GTO are sensitive to both passive stretch and active contraction of the muscle. When applying passive stretch to a spastic muscle, the sudden relaxation or clasp-knife phenomenon is thought to be the result of inhibition of the Ib fibers preventing the firing of the overactive lower motor neurons so that the muscle will not be damaged because of the excessive resistance of the spastic muscle.[11]

OCCURRENCE OF SPASTICITY. Spasticity is commonly seen in upper motor neuron disorders, such as multiple sclerosis, cerebral palsy, spinal cord injury and disease, cerebrovascular accident, head injury, and brain tumors or infections.

FACTORS INFLUENCING SPASTICITY. The degree and patterns of spasticity are influenced by several factors including functions of the postural reflex mechanism, such as the righting and equilibrium reactions, and the presence of primitive postural reflexes, such as the tonic neck reflexes, tonic labyrinthine reflexes, and associated reactions. Therefore the position of the body and head in space and the head in relation to the body influence the degree and distribution of abnormal muscle tone.[4] Extrinsic factors that also have an influence on the degree of spasticity include the presence of contractures, anxiety, fear, environmental temperature extremes, painful physical conditions, infection, urinary tract obstruction, heterotopic ossification, sensory overload, and upsetting emotional experiences.[11,12] Conversely, relaxation, rest, good health, and satisfying life experiences tend to minimize the aversive influence of spasticity.[19]

Because of these internal and external influences, spasticity is changeable and fluctuating; it is not possible to measure it accurately and with certainty.[4,19]

Bobath proposes that a specific evaluation of spasticity is not necessary; rather, assessment of the distribution of abnormal tone should be part of a comprehensive evaluation of the postural reflex mechanism, including selective movement.[3] However, criteria have been suggested for estimating the severity of spasticity.[3,6] Using these criteria and being aware of spasticity's changing character and the factors that influence muscle tone, the therapist can estimate the degree and pattern of spasticity.

METHOD OF EVALUATION. Spasticity is usually evaluated by estimating the degree of resistance to passive motion of a given muscle group or pattern of movement. The therapist should grasp the part gently but firmly and move it briskly through the desired motion or movement pattern. When spasticity is first developing (for example, following the flaccid stage after stroke), it is necessary to move the part more quickly in an effort to detect mild stretch reflex activity, a sign of developing spasticity.

There are no standardized methods of evaluating muscle tone with absolute objectivity. When reporting the results of a spasticity evaluation, the occupational therapist should make note of the position in which the testing was done and of any known internal and external environmental factors that may have influenced muscle tone. In addition, abnormal reflex influences on muscle tone should be observed and noted. Methods of testing reflexes are described in Chapter 9.

An alternative evaluation method recommended by Bobath and used by many clinicians assesses muscle tone as part of the evaluation of the postural reflex mechanism.[4] This includes evaluation of righting reactions, equilibrium reactions, and automatic adaptation of muscles to changes in posture. The latter is tested by "placing" and is an excellent way to detect resistance to passive movement and the failure of muscles to adapt quickly to postural change. The therapist moves the patient's body or limbs, using specific movement patterns that should be learned or performed later in treatment. Normally, muscle tone adapts quickly to changes in position. If the therapist's hands are removed, the limb does not fall, and there is no resistance to the movement as the limb is placed in the given position. Conversely, if spasticity is influencing the passive movement during placing, resistance is felt if the movement is in a direction opposite to the pattern of spasticity; uncontrolled assistance to the passive movement is felt if the movement is performed toward the pattern of spasticity. Bobath provides an extensive evaluation with the specific movement patterns to be tested.[4]

The effect of spasticity on performance of functional activities should be of particular concern to the occupational therapist. During activities such as bed mobility, transferring, dressing, and toileting, the therapist should observe how and where spasticity interferes with righting and equilibrium reactions, protective reactions, weight shifting, weight bearing, position changing, movement speed, and coordination.

The use of the manual muscle test described in Chapter 7 is inappropriate for assessing spasticity because the relative tone and "strength" of spastic muscles are influenced by the position of the head and body in space, failures in reciprocal innervation, abnormal cocontraction, and deficits in tactile and proprioceptive sensation. Therefore muscle tone and ability to hold against resistance are variable when there is spasticity.[4]

SCALE OF SEVERITY OF SPASTICITY. The following scale is suggested as a guide for estimating the degree of spasticity.

Mild spasticity. Mild spasticity is characterized by:
1. Mild or weak stretch reflexes evoked during passive movement and often not until late in the ROM
2. A slight decrease in balance of tone between agonist and antagonist muscles[10]
3. A mild increase of resistance to passive stretch; but it is possible for the therapist to move the part through the complete ROM with relative ease[10]
4. A slight decrease in mobility; gross movements are performed with fairly normal coordination[4,10]
5. A decreased ability to perform selective motion; fine movement is impossible or performed clumsily[4]

Moderate spasticity. Moderate spasticity is characterized by:
1. Moderately strong stretch reflexes evoked during passive motion and often earlier in the ROM than is seen in slight spasticity
2. A marked imbalance of tone between agonist and antagonist muscles[10]
3. Considerable resistance to passive stretch that is felt throughout the ROM; but it is possible for the therapist to move the part through the complete ROM with some effort
4. Some gross movements can be performed slowly and with much effort but with abnormal coordination.[4]

Severe spasticity. Severe spasticity is characterized by:
1. Strong stretch reflexes evoked during passive motion and often in the initial segment of the ROM
2. Marked resistance to passive movement[10]
3. Inability to complete the ROM passively because of the "strength" or severity of the spasticity

4. Presence of joint contractures because severe spasticity makes effective ROM exercises nearly impossible, and the spasticity may not respond well to techniques for relaxation[10]
5. Severely decreased mobility and lack of any active movement[4,10]

Rigidity

Rigidity is an increase of muscle tone of agonist and antagonist muscles simultaneously. Both groups of muscles contract steadily, resulting in increased resistance to passive movement in any direction and throughout the ROM.[9,17] Rigidity is a sign of involvement of the extrapyramidal pathways in the circuitry of the basal ganglia, diencephalon, and brainstem.[9]

CHARACTERISTICS OF RIGIDITY. A feeling of constant resistance occurs throughout the ROM when the part is moved passively in any direction. This is called "plasticity" or lead pipe rigidity because of the similarity to the feeling of bending solder or a lead pipe. In rigidity the deep tendon reflexes are normal or only moderately increased.[9,17] Another type of rigidity in the cogwheel type in which there is a rhythmic "give" in the resistance throughout the ROM, much like the feeling of turning a cogwheel.[17] The clasp-knife phenomenon seen in spasticity is *not* characteristic of rigidity. It is crucial for the therapist to differentiate between the two types of rigidity in evaluation, documentation, and treatment.

OCCURRENCE OF RIGIDITY. Rigidity occurs as a result of lesions of the extrapyramidal system, such as in Parkinson's disease, some degenerative diseases, encephalitis, and tumors.[7] Cogwheel rigidity occurs in some types of parkinsonism and also after administration of high doses of reserpine or chlorpromazine and its derivatives. It can occur after carbon monoxide poisoning as well.[2] Frequently, there are lesions of both the pyramidal and the extrapyramidal systems, and rigidity and spasticity of muscle may occur together.[9]

UPPER EXTREMITY SELECTIVE MOVEMENT/ TONE EVALUATION

Abnormal muscle tone should not be evaluated in isolation but in conjunction with the patient's overall motor control and level of recovery. Postural tone, the integration of primitive reflexes, the presence of righting and equilibrium reactions, and the degree of selective movement are all examined. One specific evaluation that the occupational therapist performs along with the tone evaluation is of upper extremity selective movement and control. The therapist identifies where and how much the patient's motor control is dominated by static abnormal patterns of movement and where some isolated movement may be present. The degree to which abnormal tone intereferes with selective control and the severity of the tonal problem are identified.

Although the therapist is focusing on upper extremity movement, related areas that will influence this movement must be examined. For example, the beginning of the evaluation should include a general observation of the patient in the sitting position. When appropriate, upper extremity movement should also be evaluated with the patient supine, standing, or both. Areas such as trunk symmetry, weight bearing, and head, upper extremity, and lower extremity positions should be noted. The presence of synergistic patterns and the influence of abnormal postural reflexes should be described.

Once the patient has been observed in the sitting position, the therapist asks the patient to perform some simple arm movements such as placing the hand on the knee or touching the nose or behind the back. Alternatively, the therapist places the limb in position and evaluates the patient's ability to hold that position. Bobath identifies three grades or levels of difficulty of evaluation tasks.[4] The following are examples of each grade:

Grade 1: Can the patient hold the extended arm in elevation after having it placed there? With internal rotation? With external rotation?

Grade 2: Can the patient bend the elbow with the arm in elevation to touch the top of the head? With pronation? With supination?

Grade 3: Can the patient pronate the forearm without adduction of the arm at the shoulder?

Once the therapist has observed the patient's response and identified abnormalities, the movements are repeated while the therapist handles the part. The therapist feels for abnormal tone and determines how it is interfering with the required movement. In addition, tone inhibition and handling techniques are introduced, and their effect on the patient's tone and movement are noted. The therapist is evaluating and treating simultaneously, that is, constantly altering intervention depending on the patient's response. The reader is referred to Fig. 8-1 for a sample upper extremity tone and selective movement evaluation worksheet.

Results of evaluation as a basis for treatment planning

An evaluation of muscle tone should suggest some directions of treatment for the therapist. If muscle tone is low, that is, if there is flaccidity, a manual muscle test to determine the exact degree of muscle weakness is indicated. If recovery of muscle function is expected, enabling exercise and therapeutic activities for improving strength may be selected for the treatment program. In addition, bed and chair positioning, splints, and other positioning devices such as wheelchair arm trough may be necessary to protect weak muscles from overstretching and stronger antagonist muscles from becoming contracted. Strengthening exercise and activity must be directed toward the weaker muscle groups to effect a balance of strength and tone between agonist and antagonist muscles. Temporarily (or permanently if recovery of strength is not expected), the occupational therapist may have to assist the patient in managing activities of daily living (ADL) in spite of mild to severe weakness. Some of the methods and devices for ADL described in Chapter 15 are useful for patients with muscle weakness.

If muscle tone is above normal, that is, hypertonic (rigid or spastic), treatment methods that use techniques of inhibition, such as the sensorimotor approaches described in Chapters 18 through 21 may be appropriate, depending on the disability, severity and distribution of the hypertonicity, and concomitant problems. Application of cold is used to inhibit spasticity in some approaches.

Cold will inhibit gamma spasticity; however, the duration of its action is short, lasting approximately 20 minutes.[9] Since it can affect circulation, application of cold must be used cautiously (especially at proximal joints of the upper extremities) if there is cardiac involvement or reduced blood supply to the brain.[13] Inhibition of spasticity is necessary for maintaining joint ROM and for learning more normal movement patterns. If spastic agonist muscles can be inhibited, antagonist muscles may be facilitated, and performance of movement may be made possible, using one of the sensorimotor approaches to treatment.

In many cases spasticity is severe enough to require spasticity-reduction splints or progressive inhibition casting.[2,15,18,22] Casting provides the necessary circumferential pressure that will prevent soft tissue contractures.[9] In addition, it can maintain the normal length of the muscle for functional ROM.

Serial casting is most successful when a contracture has been present for less than 6 months. The cast may be bivalved for skin protection; however, many clinicians believe a non–bivalved cast is more effective and actually causes less skin breakdown.[2] Another alternative treatment option is a dropout cast, which will allow therapy to progress in spite of a rigid cast. A combination of peripheral nerve blocks and casting or splinting is often used.[2,14] Lidocaine blocks administered prior to casting can alter spasticity to a manageable level for easier limb positioning.[14]

SANTA CLARA VALLEY MEDICAL CENTER
OCCUPATIONAL THERAPY DEPARTMENT

Name: _____ Chart #: _____

Date(S) Tested: _____

Testing Position: Supine/sitting/standing (circle appropriate choice(s)

RESTING POSTURE (Describe prior to handling)

Trunk:

Head:

Scapula and Upper Extremities:

Lower Extremities:

UPPER EXTREMITY MUSCLE TONE: Spasticity/Flaccidity/Rigidity

(Circle appropriate choice/choices. Describe fluctuations in tone with position change as well as the grade or degree of abnormal tone)

UPPER EXTREMITY SELECTIVE MOVEMENT (Describe the qualilty of movement without and with intervention)

1. Lower extended arm from elevation to horizontal and back to elevation.
2. Lift arm to touch opposite shoulder.
3. Shrug shoulders
4. Touch back of head; small of back
5. Touch nose, then knee, back to nose
6. Place flat hand on table
7. Grasp/Release object: elbow extended, elbow flexed
8. Oppose fingers and thumb

UPPER EXTREMITY FUNCTION: Non functional/stabilizing assist/gross motor assist/good functional use (circle appropriate choice/choices)

What can the patient do?

What can't the patient do?

What is interfering with function? Why isn't the patient moving normally?

RESPONSE TO INTERVENTION
What treatment methods are the most beneficial to increasing function?

How long is a response maintained?

Is movement more successful in one position versus another?

How much assistance is required to produce normal movement? Where is the assistance given?

Fig. 8-1. Upper extremity muscle tone and selective movement evaluation. Adapted and reproduced with permission from Occupational Therapy Dept., Santa Clara Valley Medical Center, San Jose, CA.

ASSOCIATED DEFICITS
What abnormal reflex activity is interfering with upper extremity function?

Are there any associated reactions? Can these reactions be decreased or eliminated with an activity of lesser difficulty or with increased therapist assistance?

Are there other deficits which are impacting the evaluation (i.e. pain, decreased sensation, emotional status?)

TREATMENT STRATEGIES/RECOMMENDATIONS:
Short Term Goals/Plan:

Long Term Goals/Plan:

Fig. 8-1, cont'd. Upper extremity muscle tone and selective movement evaluation. Adapted and reproduced with permission from Occupational Therapy Dept., Santa Clara Valley Medical Center, San Jose, CA.

Patients with severe spasticity accompanied by severe pain may require drug therapy as part of the treatment approach. The three drugs most commonly used are diazepam, dantrolene, and baclofen.[2,14] Diazepam is a centrally acting, habituating drug, and its sudden discontinuance may cause seizures. Dantrolene is a peripherally acting drug that can cause weakness lasting up to a week and liver damage. Baclofen is a centrally acting drug that is more effective with spinal cord injuries than with cerebral injuries. Its potential side effects are confusion, hallucination, and increased seizures. No matter what drug is used, it is crucial for the occupational therapist to communicate to the medical staff any noted side effects that interfere with the patient's overall function.

Positioning and movement of parts in patterns opposite to spastic patterns are an important part of the neurodevelopmental treatment (Bobath) approach.[4] In this approach the reduction of spasticity is integrated with the development of a more normal postural reflex mechanism. Such positioning and movement are applied during ADL, crafts, games, and work activities for a total approach to treatment.

Whether spasticity is temporary or persistent, severe, and unchangeable, the patient must learn techniques to maintain ROM and to perform essential ADL under the circumstances of his or her motor function. Self-ROM techniques described in Chapter 34 and one-handed dressing techniques described in Chapter 15 are examples.

The patient must also be aware of his or her reflex patterns of spasticity and of environmental stimuli that set them off.[20] The patient should be taught how to inhibit the abnormal tone or how to instruct others to do so.

COORDINATION

Coordination is the ability to produce accurate, controlled movement. Such movement is characterized by smoothness, rhythm, appropriate speed, refinement to the minimum number of muscle groups necessary to produce the desired movement, and appropriate muscle tension, postural tone, and equilibrium.

To effect coordinated movement, all of the elements of the neuromuscular mechanism must be intact. Coordinated movement is dependent on the contraction of the correct agonist muscles with simultaneous relaxation of the correct antagonist muscles together with the contraction of the joint fixator and synergist muscles. In addition, proprioception, body schema, and the ability to accurately judge space and to direct body parts through space with correct timing to the desired target must be intact.[3]

Occurrence of Incoordination

Coordination of muscle action is under the control of the cerebellum and influenced by the extrapyramidal system. However, intact proprioception and knowledge of the body schema and body-to-space relationships are essential to the production of coordinated movement. Therefore, many types of lesions can produce disturbances of coordination.[3] Disturbances of movement not caused by cerebellar lesions that can interfere with coordination include diseases and injuries of muscles and peripheral nerves, lesions of the posterior columns of the spinal cord, and lesions of the frontal and postcentral cerebral cortex. Paralysis of the limbs caused by a peripheral nervous system lesion prevents carrying out tests for coordination even though CNS mechanisms are intact.[17]

Cerebellar dysfunction can cause incoordination that can affect any body region and cause a variety of clinical symptoms. For example, the patient may have postural difficulties that include slouching or leaning positions (bilateral lesions) or spinal curvature (unilateral lesions) and wide-based standing.[23] Eye movements, both voluntary and reflexive, may be affected as well as the resting position of the eye.[23] The following are common signs of cerebellar dysfunction that the therapist may encounter[6,12,16,23]:

Ataxia: This literally means lack of order. It results in staggering, wide-based gait with reduced or no arm swing. Step length may be uneven, and the patient may have a tendency to fall to the side of the lesion. Ataxia will result in a lack of postural stability with patients tending to fixate to compensate for their instability.

Adiadochokinesis: Inability to perform rapidly alternating movements, such as pronation and supination or elbow flexion and extension.

Dysmetria: Inability to estimate the ROM necessary to reach the target of the movement, such as when touching the finger to the nose or an object on a table, or in placing limbs in voluntary movement.

Dyssynergia: In effect, a "decomposition of movement" in which voluntary movements are broken up into their component parts and appear jerky. It can cause problems in articulation and phonation.

Tremor: An intention tremor that is associated with cerebellar disease occurs during voluntary movement, is often intensified at the termination of the movement, and is often seen in multiple sclerosis. The patient with intention tremor may have trouble performing tasks that require accuracy and precision of limb placement (for example, drinking from a cup or inserting a key in a door).

Stewart-Holmes sign: Lack of a "check reflex," or the inability to quickly stop a motion to avoid striking something, so that if the patient's arm is flexed against the resistance of the examiner and the resistance is released suddenly and unexpectedly, the patient's hand will hit his or her face or body.

Nystagmus: An involuntary movement of the eyeballs in an up-and-down, back-and-forth, or rotating direction. Nystagmus will interfere with head control and fine adjustments required for balance.

Hypotonia: Decreased resistance to passive movement and floppiness of the limbs.

Dysarthria: Explosive or slurred speech caused by an incoordination of the speech mechanism. The patient's speech may also vary in pitch, appear nasal and tremulous, or both.

Signs of extrapyramidal disease that produce incoordination include[4,10]:

Tremors: Resting tremors, such as the pill-rolling tremor seen in parkinsonism.

Choreiform movements: Irregular, purposeless, coarse, quick, jerky, and dysrhythmic movements of variable distribution that may also occur during sleep.

Athetoid movements: Continuous, slow, wormlike, arrhythmic movements that primarily affect the distal portions of the extremities, occur in the same patterns in the same subject, and are not present during sleep.

Spasms: Involuntary contraction of large groups of muscles of the arm, leg, or neck.

Dystonia: Bizarre twisting movements of the trunk and proximal muscles of the extremities. Torsion spasms are included, with spasmodic torticollis being the most common. Dystonic movements tend to involve large portions of the body and produce grotesque posturing with bizarre writhing movements.

Ballism: A rare symptom that is produced by continuous, gross, abrupt contractions of the axial and proximal musculature of the extremity, it causes the limb to fly out suddenly, occurs on one side of the body (hemiballism), and is caused by lesions of the opposite subthalamic nucleus.

Clinical Evaluation of Coordination

Incoordination consists of errors in rate, range, direction, and force of movement. Therefore, observation is an important element of the evaluation. The neurologic examination for incoordination may include the nose-finger-nose test, the finger-nose test, the heel-knee test, the knee pat (pronation-supination) test, hand pat and foot pat tests, finger wiggling, and drawing a spiral.[3,17] Such tests can reveal dysmetria, dyssynergia, adiadochokinesis, tremors, and ataxia. Usually these examinations have been performed by the neurologist.

Occupational Therapy Evaluation of Coordination

Because occupation is the hallmark of occupational therapy, the occupational therapist should seek to translate the clinical evaluation to a functional one. Selected activities and specific performance tests can reveal the effect of incoordination on function—the primary concern of the occupational therapist. The occupational therapist can observe for coordination difficulties during the ADL evaluation. The therapist can prepare simulated tasks that require coordinated muscle function, such as stacking blocks, stringing beads, writing, placing tiles, placing objects into containers, tossing and catching a bean bag, and playing a board game.[21] The therapist should observe for irregularity in the rate of movement, excessive ROM and force of movement, incorrect sequence of movement, and sudden corrective movements in an attempt to compensate for incoordination. Thus, movement during the performance of various activities may appear irregular and jerky and overreach the mark.[17]

The following general guidelines and questions can be used when evaluating incoordination, more specifically, ataxia:

1. Assess the patient's tone and joint mobility as described in this chapter and in Chapter 6.
2. Observe the patient in the sitting position. Look for fixation and locate any overdeveloped muscle bulk.
3. Observe for ataxia proximally to distally in all planes of upper-extremity movement. Are movements away from or toward the body more difficult for the patient? Where, within the range of movement, is ataxia most prevalent?
4. Establish at which joint or joints ataxia is located. Stabilize joints proximally to distally during the functional task and note differences in patient performance as compared with performance without stabilization.
5. Check for fluctuating ataxia. Is resting or intention tremor present? Are the eyes and speech affected?
6. Apply manual resistance throughout the entire ROM during the functional task to establish if weighting will be an effective treatment option. Note the amount of resistance provided.
7. Does patient's emotional status affect ataxia?
8. How does the patient's ataxia affect function?

Several standardized tests of motor function and manual dexterity outlined by Smith[21] are available and can be used to evaluate coordination. Some of these include:

1. The Purdue Pegboard, available from Science Research Associates, Inc., 259 East Erie St., Chicago, Ill. 60611
2. Minnesota Rate of Manipulation Test, available from American Guidance Service, Inc., Publisher's Bldg., Circle Pines, Minn. 55014

3. Lincoln-Oseretsky Motor Development Scale, available from C.H. Stoelting Co., 424 N. Hohman Ave., Chicago, Ill. 60624
4. The Pennsylvania Bi-Manual Work Sample, available from Educational Test Bureau, American Guidance Service, Inc., Publisher's Bldg., Circle Pines, Minn. 55014
5. The Crawford Small Parts Dexterity Test, available from the Psychological Corporation, 304 East 45th St., New York, N.Y. 10017[13]

Results of Evaluation as a Basis for Treatment Planning

Admittedly, treatment of incoordination is difficult, and several approaches may be used. Incoordination arising from lesions of the pyramidal system may be improved using one of the sensorimotor approaches directed to the normalization of muscle tone and the development of more normal movement patterns. Specific sensory input is used to change muscle tone and evoke adaptive motor responses. Activities graded on the basis of normal motor development may be helpful in attaining proximal stability and then mobility. Therapy directed toward the integration of primitive reflexes and the enhancement of higher cortical control mechanisms, such as the righting and equilibrium reactions, can help to improve coordination. Weight-bearing, joint approximation, placing and holding techniques, and fixed points of stability (table-top) can be helpful.[6] Begin with small ranges of movement and gradually increase as the patient progresses. Work initially in the plane and direction of movement that are easiest for the patient, and progress toward more difficult areas.

Some of the involuntary movements of cerebellar or extrapyramidal origin are difficult to manage or change. Pharmacological agents or surgical intervention may be employed by the physician in an effort to control tremors or other involuntary movements. Therapists have used weights on the extremities and proximal fixation in an effort to help the patient gain an improvement in motor control. These are sometimes of some help but often not practical in day-to-day activities. Methods and devices to compensate for incoordination may be necessary to make ADL safer, more possible, and more satisfying. Some of these are described in Chapter 15.

REVIEW QUESTIONS
1. Define "muscle tone."
2. Describe the characteristics of "normal muscle tone."
3. Describe the characteristics of "hypotonicity" (flaccidity).
4. In which diagnoses do flaccidity usually occur?
5. Describe the characteristics of "spasticity."
6. In which diagnoses do spasticity usually occur?
7. How is rigidity unlike spasticity, and how is it like spasticity?
8. List five factors that can influ-

ence spasticity negatively?

9. Why should the evaluation of muscle tone be performed in conjunction with the patient's overall motor function?

10. List the components of and procedure for an upper extremity muscle tone evaluation and a selective movement evaluation.

11. Define "coordination."

12. List several factors on which normal coordination is dependent.

13. Which types of disabilities produce incoordination.

14. How is coordination evaluated?

15. What should the therapist observe for when evaluating coordination using performance of ordinary activities?

REFERENCES

1. Anderson TP: Rehabilitation of patients with completed stroke. In Kotke FJ, Stillwell GK, and Lehman JF, editors: Krusen's handbook of physical medicine and rehabilitation, Philadelphia, 1982, WB Saunders Co.

2. Berrol S: Models of brain injury rehabilitation, Kent, England, publication in press, Croom and Relm.

3. Bickerstaff ER: Neurological examination in clinical practice, ed 3, London, 1973, Blackwell Scientific Publications, Ltd.

4. Bobath B: Adult hemiplegia: evaluation and treatment, ed 2, London, 1978, William Heineman Medical Books, Ltd.

5. Carr JH and Shepherd RB: A motor relearning programme for stroke, Rockville, MD, 1983, Aspen Publications.

6. Charness A: Stroke/head injury: a guide to functional outcomes in physical therapy management, Rockville, MD, 1986, Aspen Publications.

7. Chusid JG: Correlative neuroanatomy and functional neurology, ed 18, Los Altos, CA, 1982, Lange Medical Publications.

8. Davies PM: Steps to follow, New York, 1985, Springer-Verlag.

9. De Myer W: Technique of the neurologic examination: a programmed text, ed 2, New York, 1974, McGraw-Hill Book Co.

10. Farber S: Neurorehabilitation: a multisensory approach, Philadelphia, 1982, WB Saunders Co.

11. Felten DL and Felten SY: A regional and systemic overview of functional neuroanatomy. In Farber S: Neurorehabilitation: a multisensory approach, Philadelphia, 1982, WB Saunders Co.

12. Griffith ER: Spasticity. In Rosenthal M and others, editor: Rehabilitation of the head injured adult, Philadelphia, 1983, FA Davis Company.

13. Johnstone M: Restoration of motor function in the stroke patient, ed 2, New York, 1983, Churchill Livingstone, Inc.

14. Keenan MA: The orthopedic management of spasticity, J Head Trauma Rehabil 2(2):62, 1987.

15. King TI: Plaster splinting as a means of reducing elbow flexor spasticity: a case study, Am J Occup Ther 36:671, 1982.

16. Marsden CD: The physiological basis of ataxia, Physiotherapy 61:326, 1975.

17. Mayo Clinic and Mayo Clinic Foundation: Clinical examinations in neurology, ed 5, Philadelphia, 1981, WB Saunders Co.

18. McPherson JJ and others: A comparison of dorsal and volar resting hand splints in the reduction of hypertonus, Am J Occup Ther 36:664, 1982.

19. Okamoto GA: Physical medicine and rehabilitation, Philadelphia, 1984, WB Saunders Co.

20. Schneider F: Traumatic spinal cord injury. In Umphred DA, editor: Neurological rehabilitation, St Louis, 1985, CV Mosby Co.

21. Smith HD: Assessment and evaluation: specific evaluation procedures. In Hopkins HL and Smith HD: Willard and Spackman's occupational therapy, ed 7, Philadelphia, 1988, JB Lippincott Co.

22. Snook JH: Spasticity reduction splint, Am J Occup Ther 33:648, 1979.

23. Urbscheit NL: Cerebellar dysfunction. In Umphred DA, editor: Neurological rehabilitation, St Louis, 1985, CV Mosby Co.

9 Evaluation of reflexes and reactions

BARBARA ZOLTAN

Normal motor control is accomplished through a normal postural reflex mechanism. A normal postural reflex mechanism provides postural control that, in turn, provides an appropriate level of stability and mobility.[3] This level of motor control is mastered primarily in the first 3 years of life both through the integration of brain stem-level reflexes and through the development of higher-level righting and equilibrium reactions.[3,5] The balanced interaction of postural reactions allows for trunk control and mobility, head control, midline orientation of self, weight-bearing and weight-shifting in all directions, dynamic balance, and controlled voluntary limb movement.[2,3]

The paramount importance of a normal postural reflex mechanism for functional competency becomes evident in observing the motor behavior of patients in whom this system has been disrupted. The cerebrovascular accident (CVA) or head injury patient, for example, moves in awkward stereotypical patterns and lacks the equilibrium and stability required for even basic daily tasks. The patient's movements are no longer smooth, controlled, and selective but are dominated by abnormal tone and mass patterns. It is crucial, therefore, for the occupational therapist to evaluate the integrity of the postural reflex mechanism for those patients with central nervous system (CNS) trauma or disease.

The components of a normal postural reflex mechanism include normal postural tone, integration of primitive reflexes and mass patterns, righting reactions, protective reactions, selective voluntary movement, postural control, and equilibrium reactions.[1-3] The results of this evaluation are used to design a motor relearning program associated with improving the patient's functional competency. The information provided in this chapter focuses on the postural reflex mechanism components of primitive reflexes and mass patterns, righting reactions, protective reactions, postural control, and equilibrium reactions. Information related to the evaluation and treatment of postural tone and selective movement is presented in Chapter 8.

GENERAL PRINCIPLES OF TESTING

The evaluation of postural tone, reflexes, and reactions must be viewed in conjunction with associated sensory, perceptual, cognitive, and joint mobility deficits. For example, patients with sensory deficits may lack the urge or motivation to move and may not know how to move. The patient may no longer have a postural sense or may be unable to appreciate passive movements. Perceptual motor problems such as apraxia will alter the patient's ability to move effectively. The evaluation of sensory, perceptual, and cognitive deficits is presented in Chapters 11, 12, and 13. The evaluation of range of motion (ROM) and muscle tone and coordination is addressed in Chapters 6 and 8. The reader is referred to these chapters for detailed information.

SPECIFIC REFLEXES AND REACTIONS

Normal motor development encompasses the integration of primitive reflexes and the subsequent development of righting and equilibrium reactions that are present throughout life. Due to decreased cortical inhibition resulting from brain damage, previously integrated reflexes and reactions may dominate the motor performance of the adult brain-damaged patient. Research and clinical experience have shown that not all reflexes reappear but that there are several common reflexes that relate to the movement difficulties of the adult brain-damaged patient.[4] These reflexes and reactions include the asymmetrical tonic neck reflex (ATNR), symmetrical tonic neck reflex (STNR), tonic labyrinthine reflex (TLR), positive supporting reaction, crossed extension reflex, associated reactions, and the grasp reflex.[2,4] Although discussion of reflexes and reactions is presented separately, the reader should be aware that clinically these reflexes and reactions are rarely seen in isolation. Motor behavior is accomplished through the interaction of a number of reflexes.[2]

REFLEX/REACTION: Asymmetrical tonic neck reflex (ATNR)

DESCRIPTION: The ATNR is a released tonic reflex without higher cortical control. It is elicited by a proprioceptive response from the muscles and joints of the neck and is

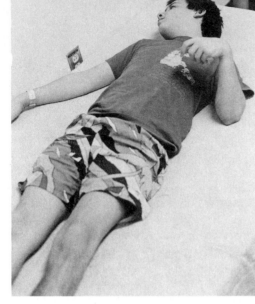

Fig. 9-1. The asymmetric tonic neck reflex (ATNR).

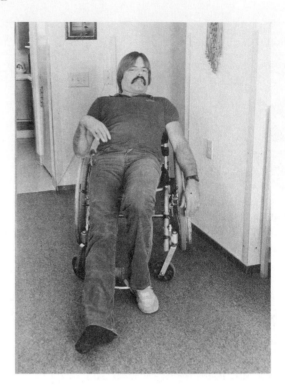

Fig. 9-2. Functional influence of the TLR on sitting up in a wheelchair.

stimulated by rotation of the head.[1,4,5] This rotation causes extension of the extremities toward which the head is rotated and increased flexion of the extremities on the opposite side (Fig. 9-1). Some patients may exhibit only tonal changes, with the predominant reaction present in the arms.

FUNCTIONAL IMPLICATIONS: The patient may have difficulty maintaining the head in midline and moving the eyes toward or past midline.[1] The patient may be unable to extend an arm without turning the head or to flex the arm by turning the head the other way.[1,4] The patient may be unable to move either or both arms to midline (especially when in the supine position), which makes it difficult or impossible to bring an object to the mouth, hold an object in both hands, or grasp an object in front of the body while looking at it.

REFLEX/REACTION: Symmetrical tonic neck reflex (STNR)

DESCRIPTION: The STNR is a brain stem–level reflex caused by flexion or extension of the head.[4] It is a proprioceptive reflex usually seen with the ATNR.[1] When the neck is extended, there is increased extension of the arms and increased flexion of the legs.[1,4,5] When the neck is flexed, there is increased flexion in the arms and increased extension in the legs.[1,4,5]

FUNCTIONAL IMPLICATIONS: The patient with a dominant STNR will be unable to support the body weight on hands and knees, maintain balance in quadruped, and/or crawl normally.[2] The patient will have difficulty moving from lying to sitting because when the head is lifted to initiate the task, increased hip extension resists the movement. As the patient struggles to sit up, increased leg extension may also interfere.[4] The patient will have difficulty with bed-to-wheelchair transferring because as the arms and head are extended to initiate the transfer, one or both legs may show increased flexion, which may cause the patient to slide under

the bed. Additionally, the affected leg may actually lift off the floor, causing an inability to bear weight.[4]

REFLEX/REACTION: Tonic labyrinthine reflex (TLR)

DESCRIPTION: The supine or prone position is the stimulus for the brain stem–level TLR.[1,5] The supine position causes severe extensor tone, with most patients also showing rigid adduction of the legs.[1,4,5] As the head pushes back and the spine extends, the shoulders retract and the extremities extend.[4] The prone position, on the other hand, causes severe flexion throughout the body and extremities.

FUNCTIONAL IMPLICATIONS: The patient with a dominant or poorly integrated TLR will be severely limited in the ability to move. A few examples of functional limitations are the inability to lift the head in supine, sit up independently, and roll or sit in a wheelchair for long periods.[2,4] In attempting to move from a supine to sitting position, the patient will experience domination of extensor tone until half way up when flexor tone begins to take over. Flexor tone continues until full sitting is reached, resulting in the head falling forward, the spine flexing, and the patient falling forward.[1] Sitting in a wheelchair for extended periods can result in increased extensor tone as the patient extends the head to view the environment.[4] The knee is extended, the foot is pushed forward off the foot-plate, and eventually the patient may slip or remain in a half-lying asymmetrical position (Fig. 9-2).[4]

REFLEX/REACTION: Positive supporting reaction

DESCRIPTION: The positive supporting reaction is a brain stem–level reaction elicited by exteroceptive stimulation to the toe pads and ball of the foot. The reaction often begins when these parts of the foot touch the ground. This results in increased extensor tone throughout the leg with contraction of the antagonist muscles for joint stability and weight-bearing (Fig. 9-3).[3]

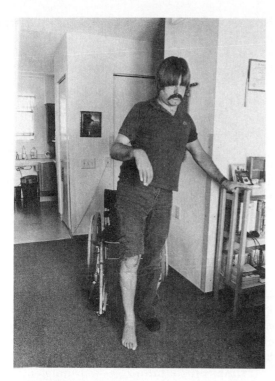

Fig. 9-3. The positive supporting reaction.

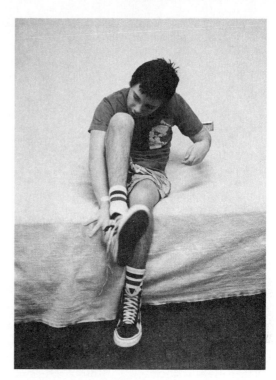

Fig. 9-4. Associated reaction elicited during lower extremity dressing.

FUNCTIONAL IMPLICATIONS: The patient with a positive supporting reaction will have difficulty placing the heel on the ground for standing, putting the heel down first in walking, and having normal body weight transference in walking.[2,4] The patient will have difficulty getting up from or sitting down in a chair and walking down steps because it is not possible to move the joints in weight-bearing (leg remains stiff in extension).[1] The rigid leg will be able to carry the patient's body weight but is unable to contribute to any balance reactions. All balance reactions, therefore, are compensatory from other parts of the body.[1]

REFLEX/REACTION: Crossed extension reflex

DESCRIPTION: This spinal level reflex causes increased extensor tone in one leg when the other leg is flexed.[1,4,5] It is augmented by and often seen in conjunction with the positive supporting reaction.

FUNCTIONAL IMPLICATIONS: The patient with a crossed extension reflex will be unable to bridge in bed and transfer body weight over the affected leg to initiate walking and will have difficulty with balance.[1,4]

REFLEX/REACTION: Associated reactions

DESCRIPTION: Associated reactions are abnormal reflex movements or an increase in spasticity of some parts of the body produced by forceful activity of other parts, or both.[1,2,4] The reaction can be seen with any difficult activity the patient experiences including those that evoke emotional responses such as fear of falling and new or strange situations.[2]

FUNCTIONAL IMPLICATIONS: The presence of associated reactions makes most functional activities more difficult. For example, putting on a shirt or dressing the lower extremities while sitting may elicit a reaction (Fig. 9-4). Writing, yawning, or maintaining balance are just a few examples of tasks that can cause an associated reaction. The constant reinforcement of abnormal associated reactions during functional tasks, which are difficult for the patient to do, can lead to joint deformities and adversely affect motor recovery.[1]

REFLEX/REACTION: Grasp reflex

DESCRIPTION: The grasp reflex is elicited by tactile and proprioceptive stimuli to the palm of the hand and palmar aspects of the fingers.[4] This stimulus causes a grasp response, with the fingers flexing and adducting.[1,4]

FUNCTIONAL IMPLICATIONS: Any object placed in the patient's hand will increase flexor tone. It will not be possible to clasp hands for self-exercise or to release objects even if active finger extension is present.[4]

AUTOMATIC REACTIONS

REFLEX/REACTION: Righting reactions

DESCRIPTION: Righting reactions are automatic reactions that ". . . maintain and restore the normal position of the head in space and its normal relationship with the trunk together with the normal alignment of trunk and limbs."[2] Righting reactions become integrated into equilibrium reactions and selective voluntary movement.[2] The movements associated with righting reactions are supine to prone and back, raising the head from either the supine or prone position, getting on hands and knees, and standing.[1,2,5]

FUNCTIONAL IMPLICATIONS: The patient who has not reestablished effective righting reactions following brain injury or disease will have difficulty getting up from the floor, getting out of bed, sitting up, and kneeling.[2]

REFLEX/REACTION: Equilibrium reactions

DESCRIPTIONS: Equilibrium reactions, which are elicited by stimulation of the labyrinths, maintain and regain balance in all activities.[1,2,7] These reactions ensure sufficient postural alignment when the body's supporting surface is changed, altering the center of gravity.[1,7] Equilibrium reactions overlap developmentally with righting reactions and can only be functional when postural tone is normal.[1,2]

FUNCTIONAL IMPLICATIONS: The patient with poorly established or inadequate equilibrium reactions will have difficulty maintaining and recovering balance in all positions and activities.

RELFEX/REACTION: Protective extension (Parachute)

DESCRIPTION: The protective extension reaction is an automatic reaction that is closely associated with equilibrium reactions.[2,5] This reaction consists of protective extension of the arms and hands, which are used to protect the head and face when one is falling.[2]

FUNCTIONAL IMPLICATIONS: The patient without an adequate protective extension reaction, for example, the spastic hemiplegic, will be reluctant to bear weight on the affected side in sitting, standing, and walking.[2] The patient's fear of falling may interfere with general balance reactions and function.

TREATMENT PLANNING

In order to develop an effective treatment approach for the patient with abnormal motor behavior, the therapist must have a thorough understanding of the components of normal movement. This is accomplished through assessment techniques described in this chapter and in Chapters 8 and 20. Although specific reflex testing is feasible for some adult patients, the primary mode of evaluation is through clinical observation and patient handling during functional activities. The therapist identifies how pathological reflexes are interfering with specific functional competency. Similar information is gathered on the impairment or absence of higher-level righting and equilibrium reactions. Once the movement assessment has been completed, the primary aim of treatment is to accomplish the inhibition of primitive reflexes and to encourage subsequent facilitation of higher-level righting and equilibrium reactions.[1-3] This is achieved primarily through positioning and handling techniques by the therapist, which allow the patient to experience the sensation of moving normally.[2] The therapist's ultimate goal is to have the patient gain control over abnormal postural reflex activity. Intrinsic to these treatment techniques are several underlying concepts related to normal development and to the use of feedback. Charness summarized the following related developmental treatment principles[3]:

1. Motor development proceeds cephalocaudally and proximodistally.
2. Mobility is first established, followed by stability, and, ultimately, by controlled mobility. The end result is distal skilled movement with proximal stabilization.
3. Mass patterns are replaced by selective voluntary movement.
4. Gross motor development precedes fine motor development.
5. Vertical movement is followed by horizontal movement, which is followed by rotary movement.
6. Isometric contraction precedes isotonic movement.
7. Symmetrical movement precedes asymmetrical movement.
8. Midrange movements precede end-of-range movements.
9. Support on the extremities is a requirement for integrating primitive reflexes and movement patterns.

Each of these principles can be effectively applied in treatment. For example, the patient may have abnormal reflex activity that affects the trunk and all extremities. In applying the principle of proximodistal development, the therapist would work to gain normal trunk control prior to establishing controlled mobility in the extremities. In many patients, the establishment of normal trunk control will automatically improve distal control, at least to some degree.

The effective use of both internal and external feedback is crucial to reestablishing normal motor control. Internal feedback is provided by proprioceptors, the receptors of touch, stretch, and pressure of the joints and the vestibular system.[3] The therapist ensures that the patient experiences internal feedback of normal movement through handling and positioning techniques. External feedback occurs when the patient decides that the objective of a particular movement is completed.[4] The therapist gives the patient external feedback by identifying when and why a movement is correct or incorrect.

The normalization of the postural reflex mechanism is accomplished through repeated practice, with the therapist gradually withdrawing support.[4] Through repeated environmental interactions, especially by way of the tactile-kinesthetic system, motor relearning can occur.[4] Just as a child learns to maintain balance and posture in a number of positions, so too can the adult with brain damage. Without the integration of primitive reflexes and the development of righting and equilibrium reactions, normal motor behavior and function cannot be expected.

REVIEW QUESTIONS

1. What are the components of a normal postural reflex mechanism?
2. What are the most commonly observed abnormal reflexes in the brain-damaged adult?
3. Describe the asymmetrical tonic neck reflex (ATNR).
4. What are the functional implications of a dominant symmetrical tonic neck reflex (STNR)?
5. What are the stimuli for the tonic labyrinthine reflex? What are related functional implications?
6. Describe the positive supporting reaction and the functional implications of its presence in motor behavior.
7. Name three activities that can cause an associated reaction.
8. What is the major goal of treatment for the patient with an abnormal postural reflex mechanism?

REFERENCES

1. Bobath B: Abnormal postural reflex activity caused by brain lesions, ed 2, London, 1975, William Heinemann Medical Books Limited.
2. Bobath B: Adult hemiplegia: evaluation and treatment, ed 2, London, 1978, William Heinemann Medical Books Limited.
3. Charness A: Stroke/head injury: a guide to functional outcomes in physical therapy management, Rockville, MD, 1986, Aspen Publications.
4. Davies PM: Steps to follow: a guide to the treatment of adult hemiplegia, New York, 1985, Springer-Verlag.
5. Fiorentino MR: Reflex testing methods for evaluating CNS development, Springfield, IL, 1973, Charles C Thomas Publishers.
6. Fisher AG, Wietlishbach SE, and Wilbarger JL: Adult performance on three tests of equilibrium, Am J Occup Ther, 42(1):30, 1988.
7. Jewell MJ: Neuroanatomical correlation of reflexes, reactions, and behaviors with levels of central nervous system organization. In Umphred DA: Neurological rehabilitation, St Louis, 1985, CV Mosby Company.

10 Dysphagia: Evaluation and treatment

KAREN NELSON

Eating is the most basic activity of daily living (ADL), necessary for survival from birth and throughout the life span. Dysphagia is traditionally defined as the inability to eat.[32] Eating includes the ability to reach for food, place it in the mouth, chew it, and swallow it.

The occupational therapist is trained to evaluate and treat all components of dysphagia. These components are motor control; muscle tone, and positioning of the trunk, head, and upper and lower extremities; inhibition of primitive reflexes; oral and pharyngeal function; and the treatment of sensory, perceptual, and cognitive dysfunction, which may interfere with the eating process.

This chapter provides the occupational therapist with a foundation for the evaluation and treatment of the patient with an acquired dysphagia. Anatomic and developmental dysphagias are not discussed. Some of the conditions that can result in an acquired dysphagia are CVA, head injury, brain tumor, anoxia, Guillain-Barré syndrome, multiple sclerosis, amyotrophic lateral sclerosis, Parkinson's disease, myasthenia gravis, poliomyelitis, and quadriplegia.[32]

ANATOMY AND PHYSIOLOGY OF NORMAL SWALLOW

Deglutition, the normal consumption of solids or liquids, is a complex process involving the brain stem, six cranial nerves, the first three cervical nerve segments, and 48 muscles.[8,18,31] A normal swallow requires all the above-mentioned structures to be intact (Fig. 10-1). Therefore the occupational therapist treating the dysphagic patient must have a thorough understanding of the anatomy and physiology of swallowing (Fig. 10-2). The swallowing process can be divided into four stages: (1) oral preparatory phase, (2) oral phase, (3) pharyngeal phase, and (4) esophageal phase[22] (Table 10-1).

I would like to acknowledge Pamela Hope Dent, OTR, and Annette van Boldrik, OTR, for the time and effort each provided to read and contribute input to this chapter. I also wish to thank Meadowbrook Neurological Care Center colleagues for their support, encouragement, and coffee.

Oral Preparatory Phase

The oral preparatory phase of swallowing begins with the act of looking at and reaching for food.[6] Visual and olfactory information stimulates salivary secretions. Salivation plays an important role as a triggering mechanism for the entire swallowing process.[31] As tactile contact is made with the food, the jaw comes forward to open. The lips close around a glass or utensil to remove the food. The labial musculature forms a seal to prevent any material from leaking out of the oral cavity.

As chewing begins, the mandible moves in a strong, combined, rotary, and lateral direction. The upper and lower teeth shear and crush the food. The tongue moves laterally to push the food between the teeth. The buccinator muscles of the cheeks contract to act as lateral retainers to prevent food particles from falling into the sulcus between the jaw and cheek. The tongue sweeps through the mouth, gathering food particles and mixing them with saliva to shape a bolus. The tongue carries sensory information of taste, texture, and temperature of the bolus or liquid through the seventh and ninth cranial nerves to the brain stem. The chewing action of the mandible and tongue is repeated rhythmically until a cohesive bolus is formed.

When liquids are introduced into the oral cavity, the tongue moves anteriorly, stopping behind the incisors and forming a groove. The shape of this groove along the dorsal surface of the tongue funnels the liquid toward the pharynx.[12]

In preparation for the next stage, the bolus, having been formed into a cohesive mass, is held between the anterior tongue and palate. The tongue cups around the bolus to seal it against the hard palate. The larynx and the pharynx are at rest during this phase of the swallowing process.

Oral Phase

The oral phase of swallowing begins when the tongue moves the bolus toward the back of the mouth.[2] The tongue elevates to squeeze the bolus up against the hard palate. A central groove is formed by the tongue to funnel the food posteriorly. The oral

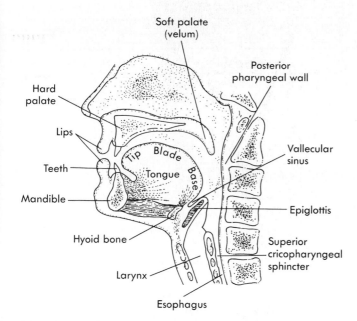

Fig. 10-1. Oral structures. From Sister Kenny Institute, Publication #706, Minneapolis, 1980.

stage of the swallow is voluntary, requiring the person to be alert.[28] A normal voluntary swallow is necessary to elicit a strong swallow reflex during the pharyngeal stage that follows. Overall, the oral sequence takes approximately 1 second to complete.

Pharyngeal Phase

The pharyngeal phase of swallowing begins when the bolus passes through the anterior faucial arch and into the pharynx. This marks the start of the reflexive component of the swallow. After the swallow response has been triggered, it continues with no pause in bolus movement until the total act is completed. The swallow response is controlled by the medulla oblongata of the brain stem. Within the medulla oblongata, the medullary reticular formation is responsible for screening out all extraneous sensory patterns and for responding only to those patterns that indicate the need to swallow. The reticular formation also assumes control of all motor neurons and related muscles

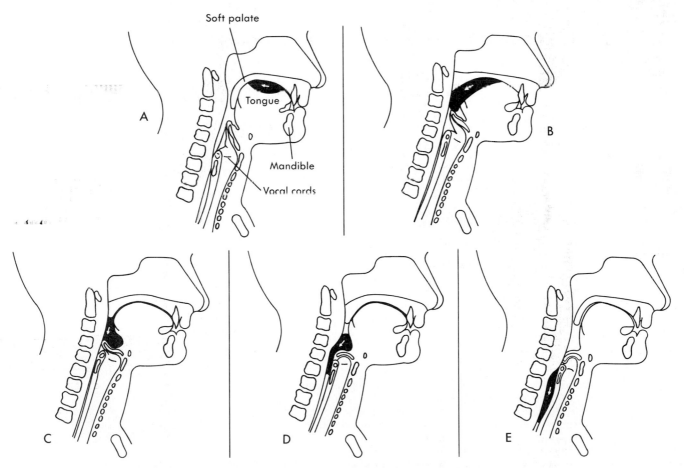

Fig. 10-2. The normal swallow. **A,** Voluntary initiation of swallow. **B,** Swallow reflex. **C,** Bolus passage through the pharynx. **D,** Bolus begins to enter the esophagus. **E,** Completion of the pharyngeal stage as entire bolus moves into the esophagus. From Logeman J: Evaluation and treatment of swallowing disorders, San Diego, 1983, College-Hill Press.

Table 10-1 Swallowing Process*

Structure	Muscle	Movement	Cranial nerve	Sensation
Oral preparatory stage				
Jaw	Pterygoideus medialis	Opens jaw	Trigeminal (V)	Face, temple, mouth, teeth, mucus
	Pterygoideus medialis and lateralis	Protrudes lower jaw; moves jaw laterally		
	Masseter	Closes jaw		
	Digastricus; mylohyoideus; geniohyoideus	Depresses lower jaw		
Mouth	Orbicularis oris	Compresses and protrudes lips	Facial (VII)	
	Zygomaticus minor	Protrudes upper lip		
	Zygomaticus major	Raises lateral angle of mouth upward and outward (smile)		
	Levator anguli oris	Moves angle of mouth straight upward		
	Risorius	Draws angle of mouth backward (grimace)		
	Depressor labii inferioris	Draws lower lip downward and outward		
	Mentalis	Protrudes lower lip (pouting)		
	Depressor anguli oris	Draws down angles of mouth		
Tongue	Superior longitudinal	Shortens tongue; raises sides and tip of tongue	Facial (VII) →	Taste, anterior two thirds of tongue
	Transverse	Lengthens and narrows tongue	Glossopharyngeal (IX)	Taste, posterior third of tongue
	Vertical	Flattens and broadens tongue	←Hypoglossal (XII)	
	Inferior longitudinal	Shortens tongue Turns tip of tongue downward		
Oral Stage				
Tongue	Styloglossus	Elevates and pulls tongue posteriorly	Accessory (XI)	
	Palatoglossus	Elevates and pulls tongue posteriorly; narrows fauces		
	Genioglossus	Depresses, protrudes and retracts tongue; elevates hyoid	Hypoglossal (XII)	
	Hyoglossus	Depresses and pulls tongue posteriorly		
Soft palate	Tensor veli palatini	Tenses soft palate	←Trigeminal (V)→	Mouth
	Levator veli palatini	Elevates soft palate	←Accessory (XI)	
	Uvulae	Shortens soft palate		
Pharyngeal stage				
Fauces	Palatoglossus	Narrows fauces	←Vagus (X)→	Membranes of pharynx
	Palatopharyngeus	Elevates larynx and pharynx		
Hyoid	Suprahyoideus	Elevates hyoid anteriorly, posteriorly	←Trigeminal (V)	
	Stylohyoideus			
	Sternothyroideus	Depresses thyroid cartilage	←Cervical segments 1, 2, 3	
	Omohyoideus	Depresses hyoid		
Pharynx	Salpingopharyngeus	Pharynx elevation	←Glossopharyngeal (IX)	
	Palatopharyngeus	Pharynx elevation		
	Stylopharyngeus	Pharynx and larynx elevation		

*See references 5, 9, 21.

Continued.

Table 10-1 Swallowing Process—cont'd

Structure	Muscle	Movement	Cranial nerve	Sensation
Pharyngeal stage				
Pharynx	Constrictor pharyngeus superior	Sequentially constricts the nasopharynx, oropharynx, laryngopharynx	←Vagus (X)→	Membranes of pharynx
	Constrictor pharyngeus medius			
	Constrictor pharyngeus inferior			
	Cricopharyngeus	Relaxes during swallow; prevents air from entering esophagus		
Larynx	Aryepiglotticus	Closes inlet of larynx	←Vagus (X)→	Membranes of larynx
	Thyroepiglotticus			
	Thyroarytenoideus	Closes glottis; shortens vocal cords		
	Arytenoid—oblique, transverse	Adducts arytenoid cartilages		
	Lateral cricoarytenoid	Adducts and rotates arytenoid cartilage		
	Vocalis	Controls tension of vocal cords		
	Postcricoarytenoideus	Widens glottis		
	Cricothyroideus—straight, oblique	Elevates cricoid arch		
Esophageal Stage				
Esophagus	Smooth	Peristaltic wave	Vagus (X)	

needed to complete the swallow. Higher brain functions such as speech, in addition to the respiratory reflex center are preempted.[32]

When the swallow reflex is triggered, several physiologic functions occur simultaneously. The velum elevates and retracts, closing the velopharyngeal port to prevent regurgitation of material into the nasal cavity. The entire pharyngeal tube elevates, initiating a peristaltic wave, which carries the bolus into and through both sides of the pharynx to the cricopharyngeal sphincter located at the top of the esophagus. This movement must be rapid and efficient so that respiration is interrupted only briefly.

Concurrently, the larynx elevates beneath the back of the tongue base, protecting the airway. Three sphincters facilitate closure of the larynx: the epiglottis, and the true and false vocal folds. Food is now prevented from entering the airway. As the bolus reaches the cricopharyngeal sphincter, the sphincter relaxes, allowing food to pass from the pharynx into the esophagus. If the swallow reflex does not trigger, none of the above physiologic functions occurs, thus preventing a safe, normal swallow.[22,32]

The entire pharyngeal phase of the swallow takes about 1 second to complete. It is important to note that both voluntary and reflexive components are needed in a normal swallow. Neither mechanism alone is sufficient to produce an immediate, consistent swallow necessary for normal feeding.[22]

Esophageal Phase

The esophageal phase of the swallow starts when the bolus enters the esophagus through the cricopharyngeal juncture. The esophagus is a straight tube, 10 inches in length, which runs from the pharynx to the stomach. The upper third of the esophagus is composed of both striated and smooth muscle. The lower two thirds of the tube is made up of smooth muscle. The food is transported through the esophagus by peristaltic wave contractions. The overall transit time needed for the bolus to reach the stomach varies from 8 to 20 seconds.

EVALUATION

Upon receiving a physician's referral, a thorough dysphagia evaluation must be completed. The occupational therapist needs to review the patient's medical history and to assess the patient's mental status, physical control of head, trunk, and extremities, and oral structures.

Medical Chart Review

Review of the patient's medical chart prior to the actual evaluation reveals important information. The therapist should take note of the patient's diagnosis, pertinent medical history, prescribed medications, and current nutritional status.

The medical diagnosis may help to indicate the cause or type of swallowing problem that the patient may be experiencing. For example, the presence of a neurologic disorder should alert the therapist that dysphagia problems may exist. It is important to learn whether the dysphagia was of sudden or gradual onset. The therapist should seek out information regarding the onset and duration of the patient's swallowing difficulties. The therapist also should note whether previous surgeries have been mentioned involving the head, neck, and gastrointestinal tract that affect deglutition.

Particular attention should be paid to reported episodes of pneumonia or aspiration (entry of material into the airway).[22] Aspiration pneumonia is a complication that occurs when food enters the lungs. Spiking temperatures may indicate that a patient is aspirating.

Information regarding the patient's current nutritional status may be found in the dietary section of the chart or in the nursing progress notes. Consideration should be given to prescribed medications that may alter the patient's alertness, orientation, and muscle control. The manner in which the patient is receiving food is important, for example, whether the patient is receiving food orally or through a nasogastric or gastrostomy tube, is able to take all nutrients orally, or is receiving supplemental tube feedings. The nurses notes may indicate whether the patient has difficulty managing certain food or liquid consistencies and whether the patient coughs or chokes during eating.

A review of the patient's intake and output (I & O) record provides additional information about hydration status.

Mental Status

It is necessary to assess a patient's ability to actively participate in a feeding evaluation or treatment program. The therapist should establish whether the patient is alert, oriented to name, day, and date, and able to follow simple directions—either verbally or with guidance. The patient who exhibits confusion, dementia, or a poor level of awareness may not be a good candidate for eating, because chewing and swallowing require voluntary control.[2,34]

Physical Status

Head and trunk control are important components for a safe swallow. To evaluate head control, the therapist asks the patient to turn the head from side to side and up and down. Assessment should include the quality of head movement, whether it is smooth and coordinated and whether it is adequate to allow the patient to maintain control with assistance. The therapist also should move the head passively from side to side and up and down to look for stiffness or abnormal muscle tone. Poor head control may be indicative of decreased strength, decreased or increased muscle tone, or decreased awareness. Head control is important because it develops first, jaw movement follows, and last, quality tongue movement occurs.

In evaluating the patient's trunk control the therapist observes whether the patient is sitting in midline with equal weight-bearing on both hips. Thus, the therapist can establish whether the patient can maintain the midline position when provided with postural supports such as wheelchair trunk supports or a lap board and whether a return to midline is possible if loss of balance occurs.

To participate in a feeding training program, the patient must maintain an upright position, with head and trunk in midline to provide sufficient alignment of the swallowing structures.[4] If the patient has poor head or trunk control, the therapist may assist the patient during evaluation and treatment.

Oral Evaluation

OUTER ORAL STATUS. The face and mouth are sensitive areas to evaluate. Most adults are cautious about or even threatened by having another person touch their face. Therefore, as the outer oral structures are evaluated, including the facial musculature and mobility of the cheeks, jaw, and lips, each step of the process should be carefully explained, using terms that are understood by the patient. The therapist also should give the patient an indication of how long he or she will be touching the face, for example, "for a count of three." Working within the patient's visual field, the therapist moves his or her hand(s) slowly toward the patient's face. This allows the patient time to process and acknowledge the approach. If the patient is hypersensitive or resistant to the therapist's touch, guiding the patient's own hand to the area to be evaluated and in the manner needed to evaluate that area can be done initially.

It is important for the patient to feel comfortable with the therapist's touch during evaluation. If a patient is not comfortable with the face or lips being touched, he or she will certainly be less inclined to allow the therapist's hand inside the mouth.

Sensation. Indications of poor oral sensation are drooling, food on the mouth, or food falling out of the mouth without the patient's awareness. To evaluate the patient's awareness of touch, the vision is occluded and a cotton-tipped swab is used to touch the patient gently with a quick stroke to different areas of the face. The patient is asked to point to where he or she was touched. If pointing is difficult for the patient, the patient is asked to nod "yes" or "no" when touched. The patient with intact sensation responds accurately and quickly.

Ability to sense hot and cold should be evaluated. The therapist may use two test tubes filled with hot and cold water or a laryngeal mirror that is heated and cooled with hot and cold water. The patient is touched on the face or lips in several places and is asked to indicate whether the touch was hot or cold. An aphasic patient may have difficulty correctly answering. In this instance, the therapist has to make an assessment from clinical observations.

Poor sensory awareness affects the patient's ability to move facial musculature appropriately. The patient's self-esteem also may be affected, especially in social situations, if decreased awareness causes the patient to ignore food or liquids remaining on the face or lips.

Musculature. Evaluation of the facial muscles provides the therapist with information regarding the movement, strength, and tone available to the patient for chewing and swallowing.

First, the patient's face is observed at rest, and visible asymmetry is noted. If a facial droop is obvious, the therapist should observe whether the muscles feel slack or taut and whether the patient's face has a *mask* appearance, with little change in facial expression. The therapist observes whether the patient appears to be frowning or grimacing, with jaw clenched and mouth pulled back. Information obtained through clinical observations should be compared with that which is seen during actual movement.

To test the facial musculature, the patient is asked to perform the movements listed in Table 10-2. The therapist should note how much assistance that the patient requires to perform these movements. As the patient moves through each task, bilateral symmetry is assessed. Asymmetry may indicate weakness or increased tone. Musculature is palpated for abnormal resistance to the movement. Resistance feels as if the patient is fighting the movement. This is caused by hypertonicity in the antagonist muscle group.

If the patient is able to hold the position at the end of the movement, pressure is applied against the muscle to determine the muscle's strength. The patient with normal strength is able to hold the position throughout the applied resistance. The patient who is able to hold the position briefly against pressure may have adequate strength for chewing and swallowing with assistance. The patient who is unable to move into the testing position independently or with assistance will have difficulty with eating and with facial expression.

Oral reflexes. A patient with a clearly documented

Table 10-2 Outer Oral Motor Evaluation

Function	Instruction to patient	Testing procedure*
Facial expression	Lift your eyebrows as high as you can.	Place one finger above each eyebrow. Apply downward pressure.
	Bring your eyebrows toward your nose in a frown.	Place one finger above each eyebrow. Apply pressure outward.
	Wrinkle your nose.	Place one finger on tip of nose and apply downward pressure.
	Suck in your cheeks.	Apply pressure outward against each inside cheek.
Lip control	Smile.	Observe for symmetric movement. Palpate over each cheek.
	Press your lips together tightly.	Place one finger above and one finger below lips. Apply pressure, moving fingers away from each other.
	Pucker your lips as in a kiss.	Apply pressure inwardly against lips (toward teeth).
Jaw control	Open your mouth as far as you can.	Assist patient to maintain head control. Apply pressure from under chin upward and forward.
	Close your mouth tightly. Don't let me open it.	Assist patient to maintain head control. Apply pressure on chin downward.
	Push your bottom teeth forward	Place two fingers against chin and apply pressure backward.
	Move your jaw from side to side.	Place one finger on left cheek and apply pressure to right.

*Apply resistance only in the absence of abnormal muscle tone.

neurologic involvement may display primitive oral reflexes that interfere with a dysphagia retraining program. The rooting, bite, and suck-swallow reflexes, normal from 0 to 5 months of age, reappear in adults when higher cortical structures are damaged. The gag, palatal, and cough reflexes, which should be present in adults and act to protect the airway, may be disturbed. Specific evaluation techniques can be found in Table 10-3. Persistence of these primitive oral reflexes interferes with the patient's development of isolated motor control needed for chewing and swallowing.

INNER ORAL STATUS. Evaluation of the patient's inner oral status includes an examination of oral structures, tongue musculature, palatal function, and swallowing. By preceding the inner oral evaluation with the outer oral status evaluation, the therapist has established a rapport and trust with the patient. Each procedure is first explained to the patient. The therapist works within the patient's visual field and gives the patient time to process the instructions.

It is important to place only a wet finger or tongue blade into the patient's mouth, because the mouth is normally a wet environment and because a dry finger or tongue blade is uncomfortable.[6] After a count of three, the therapist removes the finger and allows the patient to swallow the saliva. The therapist should wear latex gloves for protection from infections. Appropriate hand washing techniques are also necessary.

Dentition. Because the adult uses teeth to shear and grind food during bolus formation, the therapist needs to evaluate the condition and quality of the patient's teeth and gums.

For evaluation purposes, the mouth is divided into four quadrants: right upper, right lower, left upper, and left lower. Each quadrant is evaluated separately, and each side separately, that is, right upper side, then right lower side. First, the therapist slides a wet fifth finger under the patient's upper lip and moves it back toward the cheek, rubbing the gums three times.[6] The therapist notes whether the patient's gums are bleeding, tender or inflamed and whether the gums feel spongy or firm. The presence of loose teeth and sensitive or missing teeth is also noted. The therapist should take caution to avoid placing his or her finger between the patient's teeth until it has been determined that the patient does not have a bite reflex.

After assessing the gums, the therapist turns over

Table 10-3 Oral Reflexes*

Reflex	Evaluation	Functional implications
Rooting (0–4 months)	*Stimulus*: touch patient on right or left corner of mouth	Limits isolated motor control of lip muscles
	Response: patient moves lips in direction of stimulus.	Moves head out of midline altering alignment of swallowing mechanism
Bite (4–7 months)	*Stimulus*: touch crowns of teeth with unbreakable object.	Prevents normal forward, lateral, and rotary movements of jaw necessary for chewing
	Response: patient involuntarily clamps teeth shut.	
Suck-swallow (0–4 months)	*Stimulus*: introduction of food/liquid.	Prevents development of normal voluntary swallow
	Response: sucking	
Tongue thrust (abnormal)	*Stimulus*: introduction of food/liquid.	Interferes with ability to keep lips and mouth closed.
	Response: tongue comes forward to front of teeth.	Prevents tongue from propelling food to back of mouth in preparation for swallow. Prevents formation of bolus, loss of tongue lateralization.
Gag (0–adult)	*Stimulus*: pressure on back of tongue.	Protects airway (not always present in normal adult). Hypersensitive gag reflex can interfere with chewing, swallowing.
	Response: tongue humping, pharyngeal constriction, grimacing	
Palatal (0–adult)	*Stimulus*: stroke along faucial arches	Protects airway, closes off nasal passages, triggers swallow response
	Response: constriction of faucial arches, elevation of uvula	

*See references 12, 31.

his or her finger, sliding the pad against the inside of the patient's cheek and gently pushing cheek outward to feel the tone of the buccal musculature. He or she notes whether the cheek is firm with an elastic quality, too easy to stretch, or tight without any stretch. At this point, the therapist should remove the finger from the patient's mouth. Allow or assist the patient to swallow saliva. Assist the patient to move the lip and cheek musculature into the normal resting position. This procedure is repeated for each quadrant. The therapist should avoid moving the finger from right to left side across the patient's gums because this can be annoying.

If the patient has dentures, the therapist must discern whether the fit is adequate for chewing. Because dentures are held in place and controlled by normal musculature and sensation, changes in these areas, or marked weight loss, affect the patient's ability to effectively use dentures.[9] The dentures should fit over the gums without slipping or sliding during eating or talking. Because the patient needs to wear dentures throughout the dysphagia training period, necessary corrections or repairs should be completed quickly.[31] A dental consultation may be needed to ensure appropriate denture fit if dentures cannot be held firmly with commercial adhesive creams or powders. Patients who have gum or dental problems require appropriate follow-up and good oral hygiene to participate in a feeding program. Loose dentures or teeth may necessitate changes in food consistencies that the patient may have otherwise managed.

Tongue movement. The tongue is an intricate part of the normal chewing and swallowing process. Controlled tongue movement is necessary for moving and shaping food in the mouth. The tongue propels the food back in preparation for swallowing; therefore, a thorough evaluation of the tongue's strength, range of motion, control, and tone are needed.[6,23,32]

The patient is asked to open the mouth, and the therapist, with a flashlight, can assess the appearance of the tongue and note whether the tongue is pink and moist, angry red, or heavily coated white. A heavily coated tongue may decrease the patient's sensations of taste, temperature, and texture and may be indicative of poor tongue movement.

In examining the shape of the tongue, the therapist notes whether it is flattened out, bunched up, or rounded. Normally, the tongue is slightly concave with a groove running down the middle. The position of the tongue is observed. The examiner should determine whether it is at midline, resting just behind the front teeth in the normal position, retracted or pulled back away from the front teeth, or deviated to the right or left side. A retracted tongue indicates an

increase of abnormal muscle tone. The patient displaying tongue deviation with protrusion, may have a muscle weakness on the affected side, causing the tongue to deviate toward the unaffected side, because the stronger muscles dominate. The patient also may have abnormal tone, which results in the tongue deviating toward the affected side.

Grasping the tongue gently between the forefinger and thumb, the therapist can pull the tongue slowly forward. A wet gauze square wrapped around the tip of the tongue may help the therapist to grip it.[6] Next, the therapist walks a wet finger along the tongue from front to back, to determine whether the tongue feels hard, firm, or mushy. The right side is compared with the left side of the tongue. An abnormally hard tongue may be due to increased muscle tone.

While continuing to grip the tongue between forefinger and thumb, the therapist can evaluate the patient's available range of motion by moving the tongue forward, side to side, and up and down. The tongue with normal range moves freely in all directions without resistance.[6] Moving the tongue through its range, the therapist can simultaneously evaluate tone. As the therapist pulls the tongue forward, he or she determines whether it comes easily or whether resistance feels as if the tongue were pulling back against the movement, indicating increased tone. A tongue that seems to stretch too far beyond the front teeth is indicative of decreased tone. When moving the tongue side to side it is noted whether it is easier to move in one direction or the other. The presence of increased abnormal tone makes it difficult for the therapist to move the tongue in any direction without feeling resistance against the movement. The amount of assistance required to reduce or increase tone to within normal limits should be noted.

To evaluate the tongue's motor control (strength and coordination), the patient is asked to elevate, stick out, and move the tongue laterally (Table 10-4). If the patient has difficulty following verbal directions, the therapist can use a wet tongue blade to guide the patient through the desired movements. The patient is asked to place the tongue against the tongue blade and to keep it there. The therapist then moves the tongue blade slowly, guiding the patient's tongue in the testing direction.[6] Ease of movement, strength of movement, and coordination of movement are assessed for each direction.

Poor muscle strength or abnormal tone decreases the ability of the tongue to sweep the mouth and gather particles to form a cohesive bolus. If the tongue loses even partial control of the bolus, food may fall into the valleculae, the pyriform sinuses, or the airway, possibly leading to aspiration before the actual swal-

Table 10-4 Inner Oral Motor Evaluation*

Function	Instruction to patient	Testing procedure†
Tongue		
Protrusion	Stick out your tongue.	Apply slight resistance toward the back of the throat with tongue blade after patient exhibits full ROM.
Lateralization	Move your tongue from side to side.	Apply slight resistance in opposite direction of motion with tongue blade.
	Touch your tongue to your inside cheek—right, left; move it up and down.	Using finger on outside of cheek, push against tongue inwardly.
Tipping	Touch your tongue to your upper lip.	With tongue blade between tongue tip and lip, apply downward pressure.
	Open your mouth. Touch your tongue behind your front teeth.	With tongue blade between tongue and teeth, apply downward pressure on tongue.
	Touch your tongue behind your bottom teeth.	With tongue blade between tongue and bottom teeth, apply upward pressure.
Humping	Say "ng"; say "ga."	Observe for humping of tongue against hard palate. Tongue should flow from front to back.
	Run your tongue along the roof of your mouth, front to back.	Observe for symmetry and ease of movement.
Swallow		
Hard palate	Open your mouth and hold it open.	Using flashlight, gently examine for sensitivity by walking finger from front to back.
Soft palate	Say "ah" for as long as you can (5 seconds).	Observe for tightening of facial arches, elevation of uvula. Using laryngeal mirror, stroke juncture of hard and soft palate to elicit palatal reflex. Observe for upward and backward movement of soft palate.
Hyoid elevation (base of tongue)	Can you swallow for me?	Place finger at base of patient's tongue underneath the chin, and feel for elevation just prior to movement of the larynx.
Laryngeal		
ROM	I am going to move your Adam's apple back and forth.	Grasp larynx by placing fingers and thumb along sides. Move larynx gently back and forth, evaluate for ease and symmetry of movement
Elevation	Can you swallow for me?	Place fingers along larynx; 1st finger at hyoid, 2nd finger at top of larynx, and so on. Feel for quick and smooth elevation of larynx as patient swallows.
Cough		
Voluntary	Can you cough?	Observe for ease and strength of movement, loudness of cough.
Reflexive	Take a deep breath.	As patient holds breath, using palm of hand, push downward (toward stomach) on the sternum. Evaluate strength of reaction.

*References 8, 16, 18.
†Apply resistance in absence of abnormal muscle tone.

low.[22] The back of the tongue must also elevate quickly and strongly to propel the bolus past the faucical arch into the pharynx to trigger the swallow reflex.[6] The therapist must carefully assess the tongue's function. The patient with poor tongue control may not be a candidate for eating. The therapist first has to nor-malize tone and improve tongue movement before attempting to feed the patient. The correct selection of appropriate foods also facilitates motor control when the patient is ready for eating.

Clinical evaluation of swallowing. Because aspiration is of primary concern in swallowing, the occupational therapist must carefully evaluate the patient's ability to have a safe swallow. Before presenting the patient with material to swallow, the ability of the patient to protect the airway is assessed. To effectively protect the airway, the patient needs an intact palatal reflex, elevation of the larynx, and a reflexive cough.[32] Directions for evaluating all the components of the swallow are described in Table 10-4. The therapist should make note of the speed and strength of each component. The patient with intact cognitive skills may accurately report to the therapist, where and when there is difficulty with the swallow.[22]

The occupational therapist must assimilate all the information obtained during the entire evaluation process. Clinical judgment plays an important role in the accurate assessment of dysphagia.[6,34] Questions that must be asked are: Is the patient alert enough to follow through with bolus formation and an immediate swallow when presented with food? With assistance, does the patient maintain adequate trunk and head control, normalizing tone and facilitating quality movement? Does the patient display adequate tongue control to form a partially cohesive bolus and to regulate the speed in which the bolus enters into the pharynx? Is the larynx mobile enough to elevate quickly and strongly? Can the patient handle his or her saliva with minimal drooling? Does the patient have a cough reflex strong enough to expel any material that may enter the airway? If the answer is yes to all of the above questions, the therapist may evaluate the patient's oral and swallow control with a variety of food consistencies.

The therapist should request an evaluation tray from dietary services consisting of a sample of puréed food, soft food such as a banana or macaroni and cheese, melba toast, and ground tuna with mayonnaise or chopped meat with gravy. The tray also should include a thickened drink such as nectar blended with one half banana for a 7-ounce drink, a thick drink such as fruit nectar or a yogurt drink, and a thin liquid such as water.[1]

Puréed foods are chosen for patients with decreased motor control because the thickness of this consistency helps prevent material from entering the pharynx before the swallow reflex is triggered. Soft foods are easily formed into a bolus and require less chewing than ground meat for patients who have poor oral motor control. Soft foods also stay together in a cohesive bolus. Ground foods allow the therapist to assess a patient's ability to chew, form a cohesive bolus, and move it in the mouth. Thickened liquids move more slowly from front to back, giving the patient with a delayed swallow more time to control the liquid until the reflex is triggered. Thin liquids are the most

difficult to control, because they require a normal swallow to prevent aspiration.

The safest sequence to present material to the patient is to start with puréed and soft foods and then moving to introduce solid materials if the patient is doing well.[6,31] The following procedures should be completed after each swallow of food or liquid.

Using a fork, the therapist places a small amount—⅓ teaspoon—at a time on the middle of the tongue. A fork allows the therapist greater control of food placement in the mouth.[6,23] This is repeated for each substance for two or three bites to check for fatigue.

The therapist palpates for the swallow by placing the index finger at the hyoid notch, the 2nd finger at the top of the larynx, and the third finger along the midlarynx. The therapist can feel the strength and smoothness of the swallow.[6] The therapist also can evaluate the oral transit time by making note of when food entered the mouth and when tongue movement was initiated, to when the elevation of the hyoid notch is felt, indicating the beginning of the swallow process. The therapist can time the swallow from the time that hyoid movement begins to when laryngeal elevation occurs, indicating triggering of the swallow reflex.[22] A normal swallow takes only 1 second to complete.

The therapist asks the patient to open the mouth, to check for remaining food. Common areas in which food is seen are in the lateral sulci, under the tongue, on the base of the tongue and against the hard palate.[23] Food remaining in the mouth indicates decreased or poor oral transit skills. The patient who exhibits oral motor deficits has increasing difficulty with chewing, shaping a bolus, and channeling food backward as harder consistencies of food are introduced.[6]

The therapist asks the patient to say "ah." By listening carefully, the therapist can assess the patient's voice quality and classify the sound production as strong, clear or gurgly.[6,23] A gurgly voice may result from a delayed swallow reflex, which allows material to collect in the larynx. The therapist asks the patient to take a second "dry" swallow to clear any pooling of material. Asking the patient to say "ah" again, enables the therapist to assess whether the voice quality remains gurgly for any length of time after the dry swallow. If the voice is still gurgly, the therapist should be concerned with the possibility that material has been aspirated into the larynx, coming into contact with the vocal cords.[22] In this instance, a videofluoroscopy may be considered.

If the patient has significant coughing episodes, particularly before the therapist feels the initiation of the swallow (elevation of hyoid notch) with any consistency, the procedure should not be continued. If the patient has coughing from food with a puréed consistency, the therapist may try a soft food such as a banana if the patient has good anterior to posterior tongue movement.[6] A neurologically impaired patient with poor sensation may have difficulty with a puréed consistency, because it does not stay together as a bolus. The weight of soft foods may adequately trigger the swallow reflex. If the patient continues to cough even with soft foods, the swallow evaluation should be discontinued. A patient who is having difficulty at this level can only be considered appropriate for a prefeeding treatment program.

A patient who has difficulty handling solid consistencies may or may not have difficulty with liquids. To evaluate the patient's swallow with liquids, the assessment is started with a thickened nectar, then a pure nectar, and finally a thin liquid such as water. Small amounts of the liquid are placed with either a spoon or straw, on the middle of the patient's tongue. The therapist proceeds by following the same sequence used with solids. The therapist evaluates the patient's skill at moving material from front to back, the time of oral transit and swallow, and the voice quality after each swallow. Each liquid consistency is assessed for two or three swallows to check for fatigability. A patient with a poor swallow may aspirate directly or pool liquids in the pyriform sinuses, which, when full, overflow into the larynx and down into the

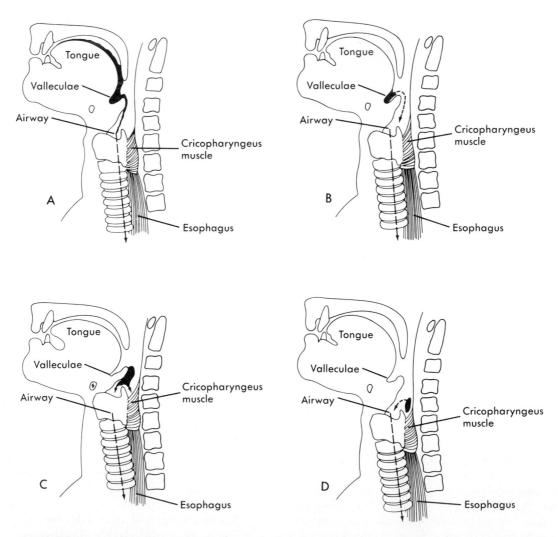

Fig. 10-3. Types of aspiration. **A,** Aspiration before the swallow due to reduced tongue control. **B,** Aspiration before the swallow due to absent swallow reflex. **C,** Aspiration during the swallow due to reduced laryngeal closure. **D,** Aspiration after the swallow due to pooled material in the pyriform sinuses overflowing into the airway. From Logeman J: Evaluation and treatment of swallowing disorders, San Diego, 1983, College-Hill Press.

trachea. If a patient continues to have a gurgly voice after a second dry swallow or to have significant coughing with any of the liquid consistencies, the evaluation should be discontinued (Fig. 10-3).

A patient with a tracheostomy tube in place can be evaluated by the therapist in the same manner as previously described. The same criteria described previously must be met before assessing the patient's swallow with food or liquids. The therapist must have a thorough understanding of the types of tracheostomy tubes and varied functions.

There are two major types of tracheostomy tubes: fenestrated or nonfenestrated.[22,30] A fenestrated tube is designed with an opening in the middle of the tube to allow for increased air flow. A fenestrated tube is frequently used for patients being weaned from a tube. By placing an inner cannula piece into the tracheostomy tube, the fenestrated opening can be closed off. This allows a patient to breathe nasally for periods of time as he or she relearns a normal breathing pattern. With the inner cannula in place, a trachea button also may be used to allow the patient to talk. A nonfenestrated tube has no opening. A fenestrated tube is preferred when treating a dysphagia patient.

A tracheostomy tube, fenestrated or nonfenestrated, may also be cuffed or uncuffed. A cuffed tube has a balloonlike cuff surrounding the bottom of the tube.[22] When inflated, the cuff comes into contact with the trachea wall, preventing the aspiration of secretions into the airway. A cuffed tube is used in cases in which aspiration has occurred. The therapist should consult with the patient's attending physician to see whether the patient is still at risk of aspirating.

Before presenting the "trached" patient with any materials, the inner cannula is inserted, and the cuff is slowly deflated. The patient needs to be suctioned orally and through the tracheostomy to ensure that all secretions have been cleared.[22] The suctioning procedure can be performed by the nursing staff or a therapist who has been trained and is considered competent.

After presenting food or liquids, the therapist should check for oral transit skills and swallow. Blue food coloring added to food or liquids can aid the therapist in identifying material in the trachea. If the tracheostomy tube is cuffed, the cuff is slowly deflated. The patient is suctioned through the tracheostomy tube to determine whether any material entered the airway. The swallow evaluation should not be continued if material is found in the trachea. The presence of a tracheostomy tube may affect a patient's swallow as secretions are increased and laryngeal mobility is decreased. When evaluation is complete, the patient is thoroughly suctioned. The inner cannula is

removed, and the cuff inflated to the level prescribed by the physician.[15]

The patient's performance on the swallowing evaluation determines whether he or she is able to participate in a feeding program and at which food and liquid consistencies he or she is able to function efficiently. The therapist must decide which consistency is the safest for the patient. The safest consistency is that which the patient is able to chew, move through the oral cavity, and swallow with the smallest health risk.

The indicators of swallowing dysfunction include coughing before, during, or after the swallow, gurgly voice quality, delayed or absent swallow reflex, poor cough, and reflux of food after meals.[6,22,34] The presence of any swallowing dysfunction can lead to aspiration pneumonia. Acute symptoms of aspiration occurring immediately after the swallow are any change in the patient's color, particularly if the airway is obstructed, gurgly voice, and extreme breathiness or loss of voice.[15] Over the next 24 hours the therapist and medical staff must observe the patient for other signs of aspiration, such as nasal drip, an increase to profuse drooling of a clear liquid, and temperatures of 100° or greater, which may not have been evident during the clinical examination.[17,22] A patient who develops aspiration pneumonia needs to be reevaluated for a change in diet levels or taken off the feeding program, if necessary. An alternative feeding method is required.

Evaluation with videofluoroscopy. An important technique that can be used to evaluate a patient's swallow is videofluoroscopy. A videofluoroscopy is a radiographic procedure, using a modified barium swallow recorded on videotape. This technique allows the therapist to actually see the patient's jaw and tongue movement, to measure the transit times of the oral and pharyngeal stages, the swallow, any residue in the valleculae and the pyriform sinuses, and any aspiration. With a videofluoroscopy the therapist can determine the etiology of any aspiration. A videofluoroscopy also may be used to determine which treatment techniques may be effective in assisting the patient to achieve a safe swallow.

Aspiration can occur before the swallow because of poor tongue control, or a delayed or absent swallow reflex or both. Poor laryngeal closure can result in aspiration during the swallow. Aspiration after the swallow is the result of pooled material in the pyriform sinuses overflowing into the trachea. Knowing the reason why a patient is aspirating can aid the occupational therapist in the treatment.[22]

To perform a radiographic study a fluoroscopy machine is needed, which has three components: a fluoroscopy tube, a monitor to view the picture, and an elevation table or platform. A TV videocassette recorder is set up to record the image. Other necessary equipment normally available in a radiology department are lead-lined aprons, lead-lined gloves, and foam positioning wedges.[24] Because the fluoroscopy machine may not lower enough to view a patient seated in a wheelchair, a special plywood seat system or wheelchair platform with a ramp may be required.

A videofluoroscopy is necessary to rule out silent aspiration. Forty percent of dysphagia patients are silent aspirators during the clinical evaluation.[22,25] It is important to rule out the occurrence of aspiration. Other indicators for a videofluoroscopy are difficulties with liquid consistencies and a need to identify specific pharyngeal problems. Some clinicians, however, advocate that all patients should be evaluated by videofluoroscopy regardless of the above indicators. Contraindications to performing a videofluoroscopy include rapid progress of the patient, poor level of awareness or poor cognitive status, oral stage problems only, and the physical inability of the patient to undergo the test.[34]

To perform a videofluoroscopy, three people are involved: the radiologist, the occupational therapist, and the person who sets up and runs the video equipment. The patient should be positioned to allow for a lateral view, with the fluoroscopy tube focused on the lips, hard palate, and posterior pharyngeal wall. The lateral view is most frequently used because it allows the therapist to evaluate all four stages of the swallow. This view clearly shows the presence of aspiration. An anteroposterior view also may be needed to evaluate asymmetry in the vocal cords.

During a videofluoroscopy evaluation, the therapist presents the patient with food or liquid to which barium paste has been added. The most commonly used barium paste is Esophatrast.[5,22] Squeezing Esophatrast from its tube, the therapist mixes or spreads small amounts onto each food or liquid consistency. Premixing the consistencies with the barium paste prior to starting prevents time-consuming interruptions during the actual evaluation.

Food and liquids are presented in the same sequence used for the clinical evaluation. Starting with puréed foods, the patient is given 1/3 teaspoon at a time of each consistency and asked to swallow when instructed. Liquids are evaluated separately, beginning with the thickened substance. Small amounts of material are given to reduce the risks of aspiration, if it occurs. An experienced dysphagia therapist may choose to evaluate only foods or liquids that the patient had difficulty with during the clinical examination, rather than to proceed through the entire sequence. The therapist continues to evaluate each consistency until aspiration occurs.

If the patient aspirates during the swallow, allowing material to fall directly into the airway, the therapist should discontinue the evaluation of that consistency. If aspiration occurs before the swallow, secondary to poor tongue control or a delayed swallow reflex, a thicker or denser substance should be tried because it is easier for the patient to control. When evaluating liquids, if the patient aspirates after the swallow because of pooling in the valleculae or pyriform sinuses, the evaluation with that consistency is discontinued. The solid and liquid consistency that the patient handles without aspiration is selected as the starting point for feeding training. A patient aspirating on puréed or soft foods is not suited to an oral program. The patient who is aspirating thickened liquids is not a candidate for liquid intake.

In addition, the videofluoroscopy procedure can be used to observe for fatigue. The patient is asked to take repeated or serial swallows of solids and liquids. The therapist should evaluate the patient's ability to control mixed consistencies of solids and liquids such as soups, and to alternate between solids and liquids.

A videofluoroscopy is a valuable tool to be used in conjunction with the clinical examination. It can provide the therapist with additional information regarding the patient's difficulties. By identifying silent aspirators, the therapist can feel comfortable with the decisions made in determining a course of treatment. Because videofluoroscopy is a radiographic procedure, exposing the patient to radiation, the therapist should exercise good clinical judgment when deciding that a videofluoroscopy is needed. The therapist must keep in mind that a videofluoroscopy records the patient's performance in an isolated instance and is not a conclusive indicator of the patient's potential ability in a feeding program. If a patient continues to progress without difficulty, a second videofluoroscopy is not necessary. A second videofluoroscopy may be needed, however, to reevaluate a patient who shows signs of readiness to participate in a feeding program or to determine whether a patient can progress to thin liquids.[6,34]

When documenting the results of a videofluoroscopy test, foods that were presented, problems that occurred at each stage, and the number of swallows taken to clear the food or liquid are noted. The therapist also should document any facilitation techniques used during the procedure that worked efficiently.[5]

The results of a thorough evaluation determine the course of treatment to increase a patient's ability to eat. Upon completion of the entire dysphagia evaluation, the therapist should clearly document the patient's major problems, treatment recommendations and plan, and goals. The documentation should be concise and measurable. The treatment plan should include the type of diet needed, the training and facilitation that the patient requires, positioning techniques to be used during feeding, and the type of supervision that must be provided (Fig. 10-4). The treatment recommendations should be communicated to the appropriate nursing and medical staff.

TREATMENT

Because a patient may display one or more than one problem at each stage of deglutition, the intervention and treatment of dysphagia are multifaceted. The treatment of the dysphagic patient includes trunk and head positioning and control, hand-to-mouth skills, oral motor skills, and swallowing. Perceptual and cognitive deficits that interfere with eating also are addressed. To treat the dysphagic patient, the occupational therapist needs to devote 35% to 45% of the patient's total daily treatment time to oral motor and swallowing retraining.[17] A patient with severe problems can require up to 6 months of intense intervention before reaching optimal recovery. In preparing a treatment plan for the patient with acquired dysphagia, the therapist must identify the symptoms and causes of the patient's deficits.[6,9,34]

Goals

The overall goals of occupational therapy in the treatment of dysphagia are[2,6,12,22]:

1. To facilitate appropriate positioning during eating
2. To improve motor control at each stage of swallow through normalization of tone and the facilitation of quality movement
3. To maintain an adequate nutritional intake
4. To prevent aspiration
5. To reestablish oral eating to the safest, optimum level

Team Management

Due to the complex nature of dysphagia treatment, the development of a team approach facilitates the patient's optimal progress. The dysphagia team should consist of the patient's attending physician, the occupational therapist, the dietitian, the nurse, the physical therapist, the speech-language pathologist, the radiologist, and the patient's family. Each professional contributes his or her own expertise toward patient improvement. It is important that all members of the dysphagia team have a thorough working knowledge of treating patients with dysphagia. Interdepartmental inservice is frequently required so that team members have a similar frame of reference.

The occupational therapist's role is to evaluate the patient and to implement the appropriate course of treatment. He or she is also responsible for coordinating the team effort. This includes the evaluation and obtaining physician's orders as needed, communicating with all other team members and staff, and family education to ensure proper follow-through, and selecting the appropriate diet. The occupational therapist initiates changes in the patient's program whenever necessary.[31,34]

The attending physician's role involves the medical management of the patient's health and safety. The physician oversees all decisions regarding treatment for diet level selection, oral/nonoral feeding procedures, and progression of the patient as recommended by the team. The physician should reinforce the course of treatment with the patient and the family.[17,22,31,34]

The dietitian is responsible for monitoring the patient's caloric intake. He or she makes recommendations to ensure that the patient receives a balanced nutritional diet in accordance with the medical condition. The dietitian is involved in suggesting types of feeding formulas for the nonoral patient. Diet supplements to augment oral intake may be recommended. In conjunction with the occupational therapist, the dietitian ensures that the proper food and liquid consistencies are served to the patient. Additional inservice training may be necessary for the dietary staff because dysphagia diets vary from traditional medical diets.

The patient's treating physical therapist is involved in muscle reeducation and tone normalization techniques of the trunk, neck, and face. The patient receives treatment in balance, strength, and control. The physical therapist is involved in increasing the patient's pulmonary status for breath support, chest expansion, and cough.[1]

The role of the speech-language pathologist involves the reeducation of the oral and laryngeal musculature used in speaking and voice production. Because these muscles also are used in swallowing, a therapist with dysphagia experience may participate in oral motor and swallowing training during prefeeding and feeding sessions.[17]

The nurse is another key member of the dysphagia team. The nursing staff is responsible for monitoring the patient's medical and nutritional status. The nurse usually is the first to notice changes in the patient's condition, such as an elevated temperature and an increase in secretions indicating swallowing dysfunction. The nurse then informs the physician and occupational therapist of these changes. The patient's oral and fluid intake is recorded in the nursing notes

Dysphagia Evaluation

Pt: _____

Dx: _CHI_____

Onset: _4/13/88_____

Medical hx: _Pt. is a 20 y.o. male who was involved in a single car accident resulting in bihemispheric cerebral damage, brainstem contusion, & subcortical damage to the reticular activating system._

Current nutritional status: _gastrostomy tube, NPO_

	WNL	Adequate—without assistance	Unable	Comments
Mental status:				
Alert/oriented		c̄ assist		oriented to name, max assist for date
Direction following		c̄ assist		appropriate c̄ guiding
Physical status (symmetry, control, tone):				
Head control		c̄ assist		slight ↑'d tone c̄ head turning
Trunk control		c̄ assist		ataxic, TLR present
Endurance		c̄ assist		fatigues after 30 min.
Respiratory				
Suctioning required	✓			
Tracheostomy	✓			
Outer oral status:				
Facial expressions		c̄ assist		flat affect 2° ↑'d tone to moderate degree
Jaw movement			✓	poor rotary chew, poor jaw glide, pt. uses up & down movt.
Lip movement		c̄ assist		unable to purse & retract, poor lip compression
Sensation		c̄ assist		delayed 2° ↓'d attention
Abnormal reflexes		c̄ assist		suck-swallow present, others absent
Inner oral status (symmetry, control, tone):				
Dentition	✓			good, slightly inflamed gums
Tongue				
Appearance		c̄ assist		slight white coating & mid ® tongue laceration
Tone		c̄ assist		↑'d c̄ retraction
Movement: Protrusion		c̄ assist		deviated to ®
Lateralization		c̄ assist		mild weakness
"n → ga"			✓	poor anterior to posterior
Soft palate/gag reflex:	✓			uvula rises symmetrically
Cough (reflexive/voluntary):	✓			
Swallow:				
Spontaneous	✓			intact
Voluntary	✓			delayed 2° to tone
Laryngeal movement				
Tongue		c̄ assist		requires tone reduction
Elevation		c̄ assist		delayed fatigue factor after serial swallows
Food management:				Overall pt. shows ↓'d cognitive awareness of food in mouth & requires cueing
Puree		c̄ assist		pt. uses suck-swallow
Mechanical soft		c̄ assist	}	pocketing assist
Chopped/ground		c̄ assist	}	needed c̄ rotary chew
Regular diet			N/A	
Liquids: Thickened		c̄ assist		c̄ straw, 5 sec. delay, ∅ cough
Thick		c̄ assist		c̄ straw, 5 sec. delay, coughing
Thin			N/A	

Dysphagia Evaluation

Major problems:

① ↓'d cognition for attention awareness of food in mouth c̄ cueing.

② ↑'d jaw & facial tone resulting in poor rotary chew.

③ Poor isolated tongue movements for lateralization, humping.

④ ↑'d laryngeal tone resulting in delayed swallow.

Recommendations/treatment plan:
(positioning, diet level, environment, techniques)

① Positioning - upright on solid seating surface, slight forward lean.

② Tone reduction techniques for jaw, tongue, & larynx before & during meal.

③ Diet level - pureed & mechanical soft foods, thickened liquids 2x daily c̄ therapist only.

④ Therapeutic feeding in quiet setting.

⑤ No food or liquid in pts. room.

⑥ Monitor patient for signs of aspiration.

Long-term goals:

① Independent trunk and head control.

② ↑ attention and awareness of food in mouth to WFL.

③ ↑ isolated motor control of facial expression to WNL.

④ ↑ isolated motor control of jaw, tongue, & larynx to WFL.

⑤ ↑ oral intake for solids from pureed to regular diet.

⑥ ↑ oral intake for liquids from thickened to thin.

⑦ Family education.

Fig. 10-4. Dysphagia evaluation. See p. 157 for indicators regarding the need to evaluate through video fluoroscopy.

and the dysphagia team is notified by the nurse when the patient's nutritional status is adequate or inadequate. Supplemental tube feedings that have been ordered by the physician are administered by the nursing staff, which also provides oral hygiene, tracheostomy care, and supervision for appropriate patients during meals.[17,22,27]

The patient's family is included as a team member to act as a program supporter. The family frequently underestimates the danger of aspiration; therefore it is important to educate the family and the patient from the first day of evaluation. The family and patient should understand which food consistencies are safe to eat and which foods must be avoided.

Although the roles just described may vary from facility to facility, those designated roles must be clearly defined to ensure a coordinated team approach.

Positioning

Proper positioning is essential for treating the dysphagia patient. The patient should be positioned symmetrically with a normal alignment between the head, neck, trunk, and pelvis. To achieve this goal, the patient is seated on a firm surface, such as a chair, with feet flat on the floor, knees at 90° flexion, equal weight-bearing on both ischial tuberosities of the hips, trunk flexed slightly forward (100° hip flexion) with a straight back, both arms placed forward on the table, and head erect in midline with slightly tucked chin.[3,9] Fig. 10-5 *A* and *B* illustrates two hand-hold techniques that allow the therapist to assist the patient in maintaining head control. Correct positioning normalizes tone, thereby facilitating quality motor control and function of the facial musculature, jaw and tongue movement, and the swallow process, all of which minimize the potential for aspiration. A patient who has difficulty moving into the correct position or maintaining the position, presents a challenge to the occupational therapist. A more careful analysis of the patient is required to determine the major problem preventing good positioning. Poor positioning may be due to decreased control or balance secondary to hypertonicity or hypotonicity or poor body awareness in space secondary to perceptual dysfunction (Fig. 10-6).[3,6,9] After the cause is identified, the therapist can treat it accordingly. Specific treatment suggestions can be found in Table 10-9.

To assist in maintaining trunk position, the therapist may consider the use of an adaptive lateral trunk support. Forward trunk support is provided by seating the patient at a table.

Oral Hygiene

Oral care by nursing and therapy team members prevents gum disease, the accumulation of secretions, the development of plaque, and the aspiration of food particles that remain after eating. To begin the oral hygiene process, the patient is positioned upright and symmetrically. The patient who is apprehensive or who displays a hypersensitive oral cavity may first require preparation by the therapist. Preparation steps may include firmly stroking outside the patient's mouth or lips with the patient's or therapist's finger. Sensitive gums can also be firmly rubbed, preparing the patient for the toothbrush.

For cleaning purposes, the mouth can be divided into four quadrants. A toothbrush with a small head and soft bristles is used to clean each quadrant, starting with the top teeth and moving from front to back. When brushing the bottom teeth, the therapist brushes from back to front. Next, holding the toothbrush at a vertical angle, the inside teeth are brushed

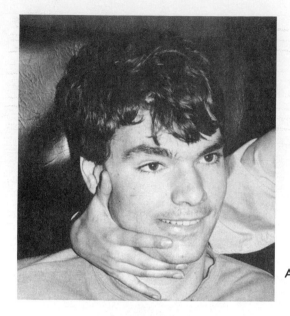

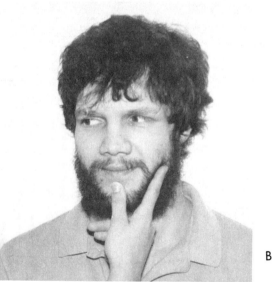

Fig. 10-5. Head control. **A,** Side hold position for patients requiring maximum-moderate assistance. **B,** Front hold position for patients requiring minimal assist. From Meadowbrook Neurological Care Center, San José, CA, 1988.

in a downward fashion from gums to teeth. Finally, the cutting surfaces of the teeth are brushed. An electric toothbrush is more effective if it can be tolerated by the patient.

After each procedure, the patient is allowed to dispose of his or her secretions. After brushing, the patient is carefully assisted in rinsing the mouth. If the patient can tolerate thin liquids, small amounts of water can be given. Having the patient flex the chin slightly toward the chest helps to prevent the water from being swallowed. The therapist can assist the patient to expel the water by placing one hand on

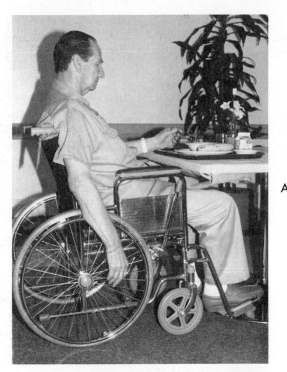

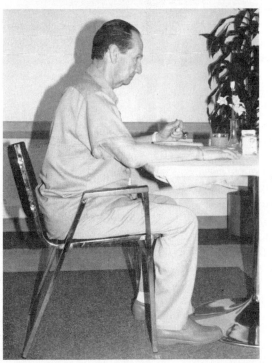

Fig. 10-6. Positioning of the dysphagia patient. **A,** Incorrect positioning. **B,** Correct positioning. From Meadowbrook Neurological Care Center, San José, Ca, 1988.

apist and nursing staff also can consider using small amounts of baking soda instead of toothpaste, because it is easier to rinse out.[6,9]

Oral hygiene for the nonoral or oral patient can be used as an effective treatment for sensory stimulation of touch, texture, temperature, and taste, and can be used to facilitate beginning jaw and tongue movement and encourage an automatic swallow.[6] Lack of oral stimulation over a prolonged period of time leads to hypersensitivity within the oral cavity. Patients who display poor tongue movement and are eating frequently have food remaining on their teeth or dentures or between the cheek and gum. A patient with decreased sensation is not even aware of the remaining food. A thorough cleaning should occur each time the patient eats.

Nonoral Feedings

A patient who is aspirating more than 10% of food or liquid consistencies or whose combined oral and pharyngeal transit time is more than 10 seconds, regardless of positioning or facilitation techniques, is inappropriate for oral eating.[6,22] This patient needs a nonoral nutritional method until he or she is again capable of eating or drinking. Patients who lack the endurance to take in sufficient calories also may require nonoral feedings or supplements.

The two most common procedures for nonoral feedings are a nasogastric tube and a gastrostomy tube.[30] A nasogastric tube is passed through the nostril, through the nasopharynx, and down through the pharynx and esophagus to rest in the stomach.[15] The nasogastric (NG) tube is a temporary measure, which should not be used for longer than 3 months.[22] The advantages of using a NG tube are (1) it can be inserted and removed nonsurgically, if necessary; (2) it allows the physician to choose between continuous or bolus feedings (a feeding which runs no more than 40 minutes); and (3) it allows the therapist to begin prefeeding and feeding training while the tube is in place. The disadvantages of the NG tube are that it can desensitize the swallow reflex, that it can interfere with a positioning program (the patient needs to be elevated to 30° during feeding), and that it decreases the patient's self-esteem.

Placement of a gastrostomy (G) tube is a minor surgical procedure. The patient receives a local anesthetic, and a small skin incision is made to make an external opening in the abdominal wall. A latex tube is passed through the opening into the stomach. The advantages of using a gastrostomy tube are (1) it allows the physician to choose between continuous or bolus feedings, (2) it allows the therapist to begin a prefeeding or feeding program while the tube is in place,

each cheek and, simultaneously, pushing inward on the cheeks while the chin remains slightly tucked. If the patient has no ability to manipulate liquids, a dampened sponge toothette can be used. The ther-

(3) it carries less risk of reflex and aspiration, (4) it does not irritate or desensitize the swallowing mechanisms, (5) it does not interfere with a positioning program, and (6) it can be removed when the patient no longer requires supplemental feedings or liquids.

The disadvantages of a gastrostomy tube are that the stoma site can become irritated or inflamed and that the tube can be perceived as permanent by the family.[30] A gastrostomy tube is the ideal choice for the involved dysphagic patient who may require tube feeding or supplemental feedings for longer than 3 months.[22]

A commercially prepared liquid formula that provides complete nutrition usually is used for tube feedings. Many types and brands can be used. The physician and dietitian determine which formula is best suited to the patient. The feedings are administered either by a bolus or a continuous method. A bolus feeding takes 20 to 40 minutes to run through either the NG tube or the G tube. It can be gravity-assisted, or it can run through a feeding pump. Bolus feedings can be scheduled at numerous times throughout a 24-hour period. Continuous feedings, which may be better tolerated by the patient, are smaller amounts that are administered continuously by a feeding pump. The feeding pump can be set to regulate the rate that the formula is dripped into the tube. A disadvantage of continuous feedings is that the patient is less mobile, because the pump always accompanies the patient.

While the patient is on a nonoral program, the occupational therapist concentrates efforts on retraining the patient in oral motor control and swallowing. The prefeeding retraining can occur whether the patient is on bolus or on continuous feedings. However, as a patient begins to eat enough to require an adjustment in the intake amount of formula, bolus feedings become the preferred method.[34] A bolus feeding allows the therapist to work with the physician to wean the patient from formula feeding. A bolus feeding can be held back prior to a feeding session, and the number of bolus feedings per day can be decreased as the patient improves. If satisfied by the tube feedings, the patient will not have an appetite and will have decreased motivation to eat. As the patient improves, oral intake can be increased and the formula feeding can be used to supplement the patient's caloric intake. An accurate calorie count, determined by recording the percentage of oral intake, assists the physician in decreasing the calories received through the tube feedings as the patient begins to meet nutritional needs orally. If the patient has progressed only enough to handle solids, the NG or G tube can be used to meet the patient's total or partial fluid

requirements. Either tube can be removed when the patient is safely able to eat and drink enough to meet caloric and fluid needs.[27]

Oral Feedings

To determine whether a patient is an appropriate candidate for oral feeding, several criteria must be met. The same criteria to evaluate a patient's swallow with foods or liquids can be used. To participate in an oral feeding program, a patient must be alert, able to maintain adequate trunk and head positioning with assistance, have beginning tongue control, manage his or her secretions with minimal drooling, and have a reflexive cough. The therapist needs to identify the food or liquid consistency that is the most appropriate for the patient. The safest consistency with which to initiate the oral program is one that enables the patient to complete the oral and pharyngeal stages combined in less than 10 seconds and to swallow with minimal aspiration (10% or less)[22]. The overall goal of an oral feeding program is for the patient to achieve swallowing without any aspiration.

Diet Selection

A dysphagia diet must be carefully selected to reflect the needs of the patient. In general, foods chosen for dysphagia diets should have the following properties: uniformity in consistency and texture, provide sufficient density and volume, remain cohesive, provide pleasant taste and temperature, and be easily removed or suctioned when necessary.[6,34] Foods that exhibit the following properties are contraindicated for dysphagia diets. They are foods with multiple textures such as vegetable soup and salads, fibrous and stringy vegetables, meats and fruits, crumbly and flaky textures, foods that liquefy such as gelatin and ice cream, and foods with skins and seeds.[34] Garnishes, such as lettuce and parsley, also should be avoided because they may be unsafe for the confused patient.

The occupational therapist needs to work closely with the dietitian to develop dysphagia diet levels. Specific dysphagia diets facilitate ordering appropriate foods consistently. Once developed, the medical, nursing, and therapy staff should be educated as to which foods are in each level to ensure the patient's safety. Liquid diet levels also should be established. When requesting a dysphagia diet, the therapist should specify both levels desired, liquid and solid, because a patient may handle each differently.

Diet Progression

Tables 10-5 through 10-7 are samples of three dysphagia levels stated in order of progression.[27,29] After a patient has mastered the stage III food items, he or

Table 10-5 Dysphagia, Stage I Food Level*

Food groups	Foods allowed	Foods to avoid
Cereals/breads	Cooked refined cereals, cream of wheat/rice, malt-o-meal	All others
Eggs	Custard, puréed egg salad (without onions or celery)	All others
Fruits	Puréed fruit, applesauce	Whole fruits, juicy fruits; all others
Potatoes or substitutes	Mashed (white or sweet) potatoes mixed with thick gravy	All others
Vegetables	Puréed asparagus, beets, carrots, green beans, peas, spinach, squash	All others
Soups	Thickened, strained cream soups—consistency of a puréed vegetable	All others
Meat, fish, poultry, cheese	Puréed meat, puréed poultry	All others
Fats	Butter, margarine, cream mixed with puréed foods	All others
Desserts	Plain puddings, smooth yogurt without fruit, custard	Any with nuts, coconut, seeds, all others
Sugars/sweets	Honey, sugar, syrup, jelly mixed in with puréed food	All others

*Reprinted with permission from Meadowbrook Neurological Care Center, 1987, San José, CA.

Table 10-6 Dysphagia, Stage II Food Level*

Food groups	Foods allowed	Foods to avoid
Cereals/Breads	Cooked refined cereals, cream of wheat/rice, malt-o-meal, oatmeal; white, wheat, or rye bread (without crust or seeds); graham crackers, soft french toast without crust	Hard rolls, bread with nuts, seeds, coconut, and fruit. Bread with cracked wheat particles, sweet rolls, waffles, melba toast, English muffins, popcorn, cereals, such as Rice Krispies, corn flakes, puffed rice
Eggs	Custard, boiled, poached, and scrambled eggs, minced egg salad (without onions or celery)	All others
Fruits	Puréed fruit, applesauce, ripe banana and avocado; soft, canned, and cooked fruits such as peaches, pears, apricots, pitted plums, stewed prunes, grapefruit, and orange sections (no membrane), baked apple (no skin), cranberry sauce	Fruits with seeds, coarse skins, and fibers, fruits with pits, all raw fruit except those listed as allowed; raisins, grapes, fruit cocktail
Potatoes or substitutes	Mashed potatoes (white or sweet), baked potatoes (no skin), soft noodles, spaghetti, and macaroni, finely chopped.	Fried potatoes, potato or corn chips, rice
Vegetables	Cooked or canned artichoke hearts, asparagus tips, beets, carrots, mushrooms, squash, pumpkin, green beans, tomato purée and paste (no skins or seeds)	All other raw, stringy, fried, and dried vegetables; pickles
Soups	Thickened, strained cream soups made with puréed allowed vegetables	All others
Meat, fish, poultry, cheese	Finely ground meat, poultry, tuna (without celery or onions); soft casseroles, soft sandwiches (without crust); cream or cottage cheese, American cheese	Fish (due to bones); meat—any consistency other than finely ground; bacon; all other cheeses
Fats	Butter, margarine, cream, mayonnaise mixed with food; thick gravy, thick cream sauce	Nuts, olives; all others
Desserts	Plain puddings, custard, tapioca, fruit whip, smooth yogurt, soft cake, cream pie with graham cracker crust	Cookies, cake with nuts, seeds, raisins, dates, coconuts, and fruits not on allowed list; all others
Sugars/sweets	Honey, sugar, syrup, jelly; plain soft milk chocolate bars	Marmalade, coconut; all others

*Reprinted with permission from Meadowbrook Neurologic Care Center, 1987, San José, CA.

Table 10-7 Dysphagia, Stage III Food Level*

Food groups	Foods allowed	Foods to avoid
Cereals/breads	Cooked cereals, ready-to-eat cereals† such as Rice Krispies, corn flakes, puffed rice; pancakes, French toast, white, wheat, and rye bread (with crust), salt crackers, soda and graham crackers; sweet rolls, English muffins, melba toast, donuts	Hard rolls, bread with nuts, seeds, coconut, and fruit, coarse cereals such as granola, Grapenuts; popcorn
Eggs	Soft- and hard-boiled, poached, fried, scrambled eggs; egg salad (without onions and celery)	All others
Fruits	Banana, avocado; soft, canned and cooked fruit, ripe fruit	Fruits with seeds, coarse skins and fibers, pits; fruit cocktail
Potatoes or substitutes	Mashed potatoes (white or sweet), creamed potatoes, baked potatoes (with skin), noodles, spaghetti, and macaroni	Fried potatoes, potato and corn chips, rice without gravy
Vegetables	Cooked and canned vegetables (without skins, seeds, and stringy fibers)	All raw, stringy, fried, and dried vegetables
Soups	Thickened creamed soups made with puréed or whole allowed vegetables only	All others
Meat, fish, poultry, cheese	Finely diced/minced meat, poultry, tuna (without onions or celery), flaked fish, fish sticks; soft casseroles, sandwiches, and cheeses	Bacon; fish with bones; poultry with skin
Fats	Butter, margarine, cream, mayonnaise, gravy, cream sauces	Nuts; all others
Desserts	Soft cookies, cakes, pies, puddings, custard, yogurt	Cookies, cake with nuts, seeds, coconuts, and fruits not on allowed list; hard pies, crusts/pastries; all others
Sugars/sweets	Honey, sugar, syrup, jelly; plain soft milk chocolate bars	Marmalade, coconut; all others

*Reprinted with permission from Meadowbrook Neurologic Care Center, 1987, San José, CA.
†Allowed only if thin liquids are appropriate.

she may progress to a regular diet. Stage I foods are puréed. This food group is best for patients with little or no jaw or tongue control, a moderately delayed swallow, and a decreased pharyngeal peristalsis, resulting in a pooling in the valleculae.[6,22,34] Puréed foods move more slowly past the faucial arches and into the pharynx, allowing time for the swallow reflex to trigger. Because puréed foods cannot be formed into an adequate bolus, they offer little opportunity for increasing oral motor control.[6] Stage I foods are best used only to increase the patient's oral intake. The patient should be progressed to the next level as soon as possible.

Stage II items are soft foods that stay together as a cohesive bolus; thus, the possibility of particles spilling into the airway is decreased. Stage II foods are best for patients with a beginning rotary chew, enough tongue control with assistance to propel food back toward the pharynx, and a minimally delayed swallow.[6] Soft foods reduce the risk of aspiration in patients who have both a motor and a sensory loss affecting the triggering of the swallow reflex.[2,16] Soft foods with a density provide increased proprioceptive input throughout the mouth. These foods also stay

as a cohesive bolus rather than crumbling and falling uncontrolled into the airway. Because the patient at this diet stage displays improved tongue control, the swallow reflex is triggered faster as the back of the tongue elevates toward the hard palate. For the patient who is just beginning to chew, mashing the food with a fork enhances the patient's ability to keep it together as a bolus.[6]

Stage III food items require chewing, controlled bolus formation, and a fair swallow. This food group offers a wider variety of consistencies. Meats should be finely cut to facilitate a controlled swallow. Smaller particles are less likely to obstruct the airway and are less of a health risk than large pieces, if minimal aspiration occurs. These foods are safer than items found on a regular diet, yet require work on the part of the patient. Stage III foods work well for patients who have minimal problems with jaw or tongue control, and an intact swallow reflex. The patient who has reached a stage III level needs to be concerned with a delayed swallow only when fatigued.

When a patient is ready to progress to the next diet level, the therapist can adjust the meals by requesting one or two items from the higher group, enabling assessment at the new level. This technique is also appropriate for patients who fatigue. The patient is thus able to work with the therapist on the harder food item first, then continue the meal with foods that are easier. The therapist also may consider arranging several small meals throughout the day for the patient who fatigues, rather than three traditional meals.

A patient should be progressed to a regular diet when oral motor control is within functional limits, allowing the patient to chew and form any consistency into a bolus and propel it back toward the faucial arches. The patient at this level should be able to swallow any food or liquid consistency with only occasional coughing. Continuing dietary precautions for a patient with a history of dysphagia include avoiding raw vegetables, stringy foods, and foods containing nuts or seeds.[27,34]

Because a patient may exhibit a difference in ability to handle liquids, a progression of liquid levels, separate from the solid levels, should be developed. The liquid progression is divided into three groups: thickened, thick, and thin liquids.[1,27,29] Examples of these levels are found in Table 10-8.

Thickened liquids are made by adding thickening agents such as banana, puréed fruit, yogurt, dissolved gelatin, baby cereal, and cornstarch. A dietitian can provide the occupational therapist with specific recipes. These substances are usually added to the liquids and power-blended for smoothness. The thickened drink or soup should stay blended and not be allowed to separate or liquefy. Thickened liquids are the appropriate choice for patients with markedly delayed swallow. A thickened liquid moves more slowly through the faucial arches, giving some time for the swallow reflex to trigger. Thick liquids such as fruit nectars, buttermilk, tomato juice, and yogurt drinks are used with patients who have a moderate swallow

delay of 3 to 5 seconds.[6,22] Thin liquids, the highest liquid level, require an intact swallow.

Principles of Oral Feeding

The therapist should incorporate certain principles into the oral feeding program. First, an important aspect of the oral preparation stage is looking at and reaching for food. To achieve this, the patient must actively participate in the eating process. Food presented should be within the patient's visual field. For the patient with a severe field deficit or unilateral neglect, the therapist needs to assist him or her to visually scan the plate or tray. When physically possible, the patient should be allowed self-feeding. If the patient does not have a normal hand-to-mouth movement pattern, the therapist must assist the patient to achieve one by guiding the extremity in the correct pattern. Abnormal movement of the upper extremity facilitates abnormal movement in the trunk, head, face, tongue, and pharynx, and causes a decrease in the patient's functioning. If the patient is not capable of self-feeding, the therapist can keep the patient actively involved by having him choose which food or liquid he would like for each bite. During feeding of the patient, food is presented by moving the utensil slowly from the front toward the mouth so that the patient can see the food for the entire time. The utensil should not be brought in from the side because the patient will have less preparation time. The patient should be allowed as much control of the situation as possible.

The patient should eat in a normal setting, if possible, while participating in oral feeding training. For adults, eating is a social activity shared with friends and family. The patient can be redirected if distracted and can use environmental cuing when eating in a dining room with others. Adjustments, such as eating

---

Table 10-8 Liquids*

Thin liquids	Thick liquids	Thickened liquids
Water	Extra thick milkshake	Nectar thickened with banana
Coffee, tea	Extra thick eggnog	Nectar with puréed fruit
Decaffeinated coffee	Strained creamed soup	Regular applesauce with juice
Milk	Tomato juice, V-8 juice	Eggnog with baby cereal
Hot chocolate	Plain nectars	Creamed soup thickened with mashed potatoes
All fruit juices	Yogurt and milk	
Broth/consommé	blended	
Gelatin dessert		
Ice cream		
Sherbet		

*Reprinted with permission from Meadowbrook Neurologic Care Center, 1987, San José, CA.

in the dining room but at a separate table, can be made to facilitate patient concentration. The therapist needs to be conscious of how the patient appears to others and help the patient to eat in a normal manner.

The occupational therapist must continually assess the patient's positioning, upper extremity movement, muscle tone, oral control, and swallow while the patient is eating, whether it is one food item or an entire meal. The therapist assists the patient to perform the task correctly and does not allow eating while the patient exhibits an abnormal pattern. If the patient displays poor oral motor skills, the therapist evaluates for food pocketing after every few bites. The rate of the patient's intake is monitored. The therapist should determine when too much food is in the mouth and when the patient puts food into the mouth before the previous bite has been cleared. The therapist feels for the swallow with a finger at the hyoid notch if the patient displays abnormal laryngeal tone or a delayed swallow.[6] He or she also assesses voice quality upon completion of the swallow.

The frequency with which the therapist must check each component depends on the skill level and performance of the patient. The more difficulty that the patient exhibits, the more frequent the assessment. The therapist may find it necessary to assess after each bite or drink or after a few bites or drinks or after each food item. Use of good observational skills allows the therapist to make the appropriate clinical decision. Specific techniques for evaluation during feeding trials can be found in the swallowing evaluation section of this chapter. After completing the feeding process, the patient should remain in an upright position for 30 minutes to reduce the risk of refluxing food back-up and to reduce the risk of aspirating small food particles that may remain in the throat.[2]

The therapist also must continue to monitor the patient for signs of aspiration while eating and for the development of aspiration pneumonia over a period of time. Although a conservative estimate of aspiration is 10% of material swallowed, it is difficult to measure this while a patient eats. Patients vary in the amount of aspiration that they can tolerate before developing aspiration pneumonia according to age, health, and pulmonary status. The signs of acute and chronic aspiration were outlined previously.

When a patient is participating in oral feedings, careful monitoring of the nutritional status must occur. The caloric needs for each patient are determined by the dietitian and the physician and depend on height, weight, activity level, and medical condition.[27] A patient's fluid intake is monitored by having the physician order a calorie count. Each person who supervises or works with the dysphagia patient should record, in percentages, the caloric amount of each item that the patient eats or drinks. The dietitian converts the percentages into a daily calorie total. In addition to monitoring a patient's intake through calorie counts, the patient should be monitored for physical signs of nutritional deficiency and dehydration. These symptoms are weakness, irritability, decreased alertness, change in eating habits, hunger, thirst, decreased turgor, and changes in amounts or color of urine.[31] If a patient is not able to take in the necessary calories (75% of the determined total), supplemental feedings are necessary to make up the difference.[18] The number of supplemental feedings is decided by the physician and the dietitian.

Treatment Techniques for the Management of Dysphagia

Tables 10-9 through 10-12 show examples of treatment techniques that the occupational therapist may use in the management of the dysphagia patient. They are not intended to be used as a recipe for all situations. Each patient presents a different clinical picture. A patient may display one deficit or a combination of deficits. After careful assessment, the therapist must determine the primary cause of the patient's deficits and treat accordingly. The patient must be assessed and treated as a whole person rather than treated as a person with a single deficit.

Treating a patient with dysphagia requires a logical and consistent approach.[6] Abnormal tone, for example, should be normalized before the therapist can expect good motor control. Motor control must be improved before a patient can shape food into a cohesive bolus and achieve an effective swallow. Individualized prefeeding techniques can be used to adequately prepare the patient for eating. The therapist should strive toward facilitating the return of normal eating patterns in each patient.

Continual assessment of treatment by the therapist is essential. The therapist must continually evaluate the patient's response, which should reflect the desired change that the therapist is seeking. Therefore, it is necessary for the therapist to develop good observational skills.[6] The clinician needs to adapt treatment to reflect the patient's performance and progress. For difficult patients, the clinician should seek a consultation with an experienced dysphagia therapist. To develop expertise in dysphagia management, it is recommended that the therapist continue education in this area.

Table 10-9 Dysphagia Treatment

Structure	Symptoms	Problem	Prefeeding technique	Feeding technique
Oral preparatory stage*				
Trunk	Leaning to one side	Decreased trunk tone Ataxia	Facilitate trunk strength Exercise	Assist patient to hold correct position; assist with head control also (see Fig. 10-5)
		Increased trunk tone, Poor body awareness in space	Have patient clasp hands. Patient leans down and touch foot, middle, other foot to decrease tone Patient with hands clasped and arms raised to 90° shoulder flexion move arms, turning from trunk, side to side	Assist patient to hold correct feeding position; provide with perceptual boundary; consider use of lateral trunk supports.
	Hips sliding forward out of chair	Increased tone in hip extensors Poor body awareness in space	See above Provide firm seating surface	Adjust correct positioning so that patient leans slightly forward at hips, arms forward on table.
Head	Inability to hold head in midline	Decreased tone	Facilitate strength through neck and head exercises; flexion, extension, lateral flexion	Assist with head control (see Fig. 10-5)
	Inability to move head	Increased tone	Tone reduction of head, shoulders, and trunk; facilitate normal movement	See above.
UE†	Spillage of food from utensils	Decreased tone Apraxia Decreased coordination	Facilitate increased tone through weight-bearing, sweeping, or tapping muscle belly of desired muscle	Guide patient through correct movement pattern; adaptive equipment; provide adaptive utensils as needed.
	Inability to self-feed	Increased tone Synergy patterns	Proximal tone reduction from scapula mobilization, weight-bearing through arm	
Face	Drooling, food spillage from mouth	Decreased lip control Poor lip closure 2°, decreased tone, poor sensation	Place a wet tongue blade between patient lips; ask patient to hold tongue blade while therapist tries to pull it out. Vibrate lips with back of electric toothbrush down cheek and across lips; Lip exercises (movements described in the outer oral motor evaluations are used); patient performs repetitions 2–3 times daily. Blow bubbles into glass of liquid with straw.	Using side handgrip for head control, the therapist approximates lip closure by guiding and assisting with jaw closure. Have patient use a straw when drinking liquids until control improves.
		Decreased sensation	Fan lips so that patient feels drool or wetness on lips or chin to increase awareness.	Teach patient to "mop" vs wipe mouth and chin every few bites.

*See references 3, 6, 9, 12.
†UE = upper extremities.

Continued.

Table 10-9 Dysphagia Treatment—cont'd

Structure	Symptoms	Problem	Prefeeding technique	Feeding technique
Oral preparatory stage Face— cont'd				
	Mask appearance; Inability to change facial expression; Facial droop	Poor facial motor control 2°; decreased tone; apraxia	Facial muscle exercises, (movements described in the outer oral evaluation; repetitions 2–3 times daily Facilitate desired movement by Guiding patient in correct movement Vibrate with electric toothbrush or sweeping with hand in the direction of desired movement.	Reduce tone as needed during meal or training sessions Give patient frequent breaks
	See above Facial grimace	Increased tone	Using both hands, slowly stretch tight muscle in opposite direction to normalize tone. Place finger inside cheek to slowly stretch and vibrate tight buccal musculature. Tone reduction for neck, if needed	Correct positioning Head control as needed to maintain head in midline
Jaw	Difficulty chewing	Poor rotary jaw movement 2° increased tone; Apraxia	Vibrate masseters, provide quick stretch to masseters, place fruit or marshmallows in wet gauze; using hand hold in Fig. 10-5, assist patient to chew, moving gauze from side to side. Jaw exercises; use movements described in outer oral motor evaluation.	Guide rotary chew movements using side hand hold Fig. 10-5
	Retracted jaw Deviated jaw at rest Assymetric jaw opening Lateral chew	Increased tone	Position patient's head with forward flexion chin slightly tucked. Have patient open mouth. Place 2 fingers on each mandibular angle and gently assist patient to slide jaw forward. Position patient as mentioned above. Hook thumb over patient's bottom teeth. Gently assist patient to slide jaw forward. For deviated jaw, normalize tone bilaterally, work for symmetry.	Reduce tone prior to and during feeding; guide rotary chew movements using side hand hold as in Fig. 10-5.

Continued.

Table 10-9 Dysphagia Treatment—cont'd

Structure	Symptoms	Problem	Prefeeding technique	Feeding technique
Oral preparatory stage				
Tongue	Pocketing of food in cheeks or sulci Poor bolus formation	Poor tongue control for lateralizaton, and/or tipping 2°; decreased tone Poor sensation	Tongue exercises; use movements described in inner oral motor evaluation Oral hygiene Concentrate on motor control within oral cavity to increase functional isolated skills.	Avoid crumbling foods Stroke patient's outside cheek where pocketing occurs with index finger back and up toward patient's ear.
	Retracted tongue	Increased tone Retracted jaw	Tongue ROM, wrap tip of tongue in wet gauze; gently pull tongue forward, side to side and up and down; move slowly. Pull tongue wrapped in wet gauze forward past front teeth, using index and middle finger to vibrate tongue back and forth sideways to decrease tone and facilitate protrusion. Normalize neck tone Normalize jaw tone	Avoid crumbly foods Reduce tone as needed during meal. Correct positioning; see Fig. 10-6.

Table 10-10 Dysphagia treatment

Structure	Symptoms	Problem	Prefeeding Technique	Feeding Technique
Oral stage*				
Tongue	Slow oral transit Inability to make a "ng-ga" sound	Poor anterior to posterior movement 2° decreased tone, poor sensation		
	Tongue retraction Inability to make a "ng-ga" sound	Increased tone	Practice "ng-ga" sounds. Grasping tongue wrapped in gauze, pull it forward past front teeth; use finger or tongue blade to vibrate base of tongue back and forth sideways Tongue ROM (previously described)	Position food posteriorly Avoid crumbly foods Cold/hot foods vs warm Correct positioning Place index finger at base of tongue under chin. Stroke up and forward.
	Slow oral transmit time Inability to channel food back toward larynx	Inability to form central groove in tongue; apraxia	Grasping tongue wrapped in gauze, pull forward to front teeth; stroke firmly down middle of tongue with edge of tongue blade.	See above.
	Repetitive movement of tongue; food is pushed out front of mouth.	Tongue thrust	Facilitate tongue retraction to bring tongue back into normal resting position; vibrate on either side of the frenulum found inside the mouth, under the tongue with finger. Increase jaw control; teach isolated tongue movements (described in Table 10-4).	Correct positioning Place food away from midline of tongue toward back of mouth Provide pressure to base of tongue with spoon after food placement.
	Food falls off tongue into sulci, or food remains on tongue without patient awareness.	Poor sensation	Ice tongue; ice tongue in gauze to prevent ice chips from slipping into the pharynx; brush tongue with toothbrush to stimulate receptors.	Use foods with high density Alternate presentation of foods—cold, warm during meal.
	Slow oral transit time; food remains on hard palate; coughing before swallow	Poor tongue elevation; decreased tone	Ask patient to practice k, g, n, d, t sounds Lightly touch tongue blade or soft toothbrush to roof of mouth at back of tongue, instruct patient to press spot with tongue; resist movement with blade or brush to increase strength Vibrate tongue at base below chin; provide quick stretch by pushing down on base of tongue.	Correct positioning. See Fig. 10-6. With finger under chin at base of tongue, move finger upward and forward to facilitate elevation. Avoid crumbly foods.
	Slow oral transmit time. Food remains on back of tongue as patient is unable to elevate tongue to push food to hard palate. Coughing before swallow; retracted tongue	Increased tone Decreased LOA	Tone reduction; grasping tongue with gauze wrapped around tip, pull tongue forward with finger or tongue blade. Vibrate base of tongue back and forth sideways. Grasping base of tongue under chin between two fingers, move it back and forth to decrease tone.	Adjust correct positioning by increasing forward flexion at hips, arms forward to decrease tone. Reduce tone as needed; give patient breaks because tone increases with effort. With finger under chin at base of tongue, move finger upward and forward to facilitate elevation.

*See references 6, 9, 12, 22, 31.

Table 10-11 Dysphagia Treatment

Structure	Symptoms	Problem	Prefeeding technique	Feeding technique
Pharyngeal stage* Soft palate	Tight voice; nasal regurgitation Air felt through nose or mist seen on mirror when patient says "ah" Decreased tone nasal speech	Inadequate soft palate movement 2° increased tone; rigidity; decreased tone	Facilitate normal head/neck positioning Have patient tuck chin into therapist's cupped hand then push into hand as therapist applies resistance. Patient says "ah" afterward. Speed and height of uvula elevation should increase. Follow by thermal stimulation.	Facilitate normal head/neck positioning. With head/neck in midline, have patient tuck chin slightly to decrease rate of food entering into pharynx before elevation of faucial arches and triggering of reflex occurs.
	Delayed swallow	Decreased triggering of swallow reflex	Thermal stimulation; using a laryngeal mirror #00 after being placed in ice water or chips for 10 seconds, touch base of faucial arch. Repeat up to 10 times. Process can be repeated several times a day.	Alternate presentation of food; start very cold substance, then warm. Cold substance can increase sensitivity of faucial arches. Tuck chin slightly forward to decrease vallecular space.
Hyoid	Delayed elevation of hyoid bone Poor tongue elevation	Delayed swallow	Increase tongue humping (see Table 10-10) as elevation of tongue and hyoid stimulates triggering of reflex.	Place index finger under chin at base of tongue and push up and forward to facilitate tongue elevation.
	Tongue retraction	Abnormal tongue tone	Tone reduction (see Table 10-10)	
Pharynx	Coughing after swallow	Decreased pharyngeal peristalsis	None	If appropriate, alternate presentation of liquid with stage II or stage III solids. Liquid material moves solids through pharynx.
	Coating of pharynx seen on video-fluroscopy Gurgly voice			Have patient take a second dry swallow to clear valleculae

*See references 4, 9, 22, 23.

Table 10-11 Dysphagia Treatment—cont'd

Structure	Symptoms	Problem	Prefeeding technique	Feeding technique
Pharyngeal stage*				
Pharynx—cont'd				
	Seen on video-fluoroscopy, AP view. Material residue seen on one side. Weak or hoarse voice	Unilateral pharyngeal peristalsis	None	Compensatory technique for patients with low tone: Have patient turn head toward affected side during swallow, to prevent pooling in affected pyriform sinuses. Evaluate technique against its effect on patient positioning and tone in trunk, upper extremities
Larynx	Coughing, choking after swallow	Decreased laryngeal elevation 2°; decreased tone	Quick ice up sides of larynx; ask patient to swallow. Assist movement by guiding larynx upward. Vibrate laryngeal musculature from under chin, downward on each side to sternal notch.	Teach patient to clear throat immediately after swallow to move residual.
	Noisy swallow	Increased tone Rigidity	ROM—place fingers and thumb along both sides of larynx and gently move it back and forth until movement is smooth and easy, tone decreased. Using chipped ice, form pack in washcloth and place around larynx for 5 min	Placing fingers and thumb along both sides of larynx, assist patient with upward elevation prior to swallow.
Trachea	Continuous coughing before, during, after swallow	Aspiration—before 2° poor tongue control; during 2° delayed swallow reflex; after 2° decreased pharyngeal peristalsis	Teach patient how to produce a voluntary cough. Ask patient to take a deep breath and cough while breathing out; therapist uses palm of hand to push downward (toward stomach) on the sternum. Blocked airway: None	Encourage patient to keep coughing; facilitate reflexive cough. Push downward on sternum as patient breathes out. Suction patient if problem increases. Push into patient's sternal notch to assist with cough. Seek medical assistance.

*See references 6, 9, 22, 23.

Continued.

Table 10-12 Dysphagia Treatment

Structure	Symptoms	Problem	Prefeeding technique	Feeding technique
Esophageal stage*				
Esophagus	Frequent regurgitation of food or liquid and coughing or choking after the swallow; 2° material collecting in a side pocket either in pharynx or esophagus.	Esophageal diverticulum	Requires a medical diagnosis; Problem can be seen through traditional barium x-ray study. Surgical correction is needed.	Report symptoms to medical staff. (Therapist cannot treat.)
	Regurgitation of food, coughing, or choking on food after the swallow 2° inability of food to pass through the pharynx or esophagus	Partial or total obstruction of the pharynx or esophagus	See above.	See above.

*See references 6, 9, 22, 23.

REVIEW QUESTIONS

1. List the components of dysphagia.
2. List the four stages of swallowing and the characteristics of each.
3. List the physiologic functions that occur when the swallow reflex triggers and explain why these functions are necessary.
4. Why is it necessary to assess a patient's mental status during a dysphagia evaluation?
5. Describe what the therapist should look for when evaluating the trunk and head during the dysphagia evaluation.
6. What information can be gained by the therapist when evaluating the patient's facial motor control?
7. How does poor tongue control contribute to aspiration?
8. Name the three components required to effectively protect the airway.
9. What is the safest food sequence to follow for a swallowing evaluation?
10. Describe the finger placement that a therapist can use to feel the strength and smoothness of the swallow.
11. Why should the therapist assess voice quality after a swallow?
12. Will a patient who has difficulty handling solids also have difficulty with liquids?
13. What options does the occupational therapist have when a patient displays significant coughing?
14. List the indicators of swallowing dysfunction.
15. List the acute symptoms of aspiration.
16. When is a videofluoroscopy necessary?
17. List the elements in treatment of the dysphagia patient.
18. Describe the position in which a patient should be treated, and give the rationale for this position.
19. What are the indications for placing a patient on a nonoral treatment program?
20. Name five important criteria that a patient must meet to participate in an oral feeding program.
21. List the properties of food preferred for dysphagia diets.
22. Describe the effect that poor hand-to-mouth movements have on the patient's swallow.
23. Why is it important to involve the patient in the eating process?
24. What are the symptoms of nutritional deficiency?
25. Describe two possible treatment techniques used for a patient who displays a masked appearance.
26. Name three treatment techniques that the occupational therapist can use for poor rotary jaw movement and increased tone.
27. Describe two ways in which a therapist can decrease abnormally high tone in the tongue.
28. Describe thermal stimulation as a treatment technique. For which problem is it used?
29. When is use of the "dry swallow" technique appropriate?
30. How can the therapist facilitate a cough?

REFERENCES

1. Alta Bates Hospital Rehabilitation Services; Dysphagia evaluation and treatment protocol, 1982, Berkeley, CA.

2. Asher I: Management of neurologic disorders—the first feeding session. In Groher M, editor: Dysphagia: diagnosis and management, Stoneham, MA, 1984, Butterworth Publishers.

3. Bobath B: Adult hemiplegia: evaluation and treatment, ed 2, London, 1978, William Heinemann Medical Books Limited.

4. Buchholz D, Bosma J, and Donner M: Adaption, compensation, and decompensation of the pharyngeal swallow, Gastrointest Radiol 10:235, 1985.

5. Community Hospital Los Gatos—Saratoga, Rehabilitation Services, Dysphagia protocol, Los Gatos, CA, 1986.

6. Coombes K: Swallowing dysfunction in hemiplegia and head injury. Four day course presented by International Clinical Educators, 1986 and 1987, Los Gatos, CA.

7. Curtis D, Cruess D, and Wilgress E: Normal solid bolus swallowing erect position: Dysphagia, 1:63, 1986.

8. Daniels L and Worthington C: Muscle testing, ed 5, Philadelphia, PA, 1986, WB Saunders Co.

9. Davies P: Steps to follow, New York, 1985, Springer-Verlag.

10. Doble R: Rehabilitation of swallowing disorders, Am Fam Phys 27:84, 1978.

11. Donner M, Bosma J, and Robertson B: Anatomy and physiology of the pharynx, Gastrointest Radiol 10:196, 1985.

12. Farber S: Neurorehabilitation, a multisensory approach, Philadelphia, 1982, WB Saunders Co.

13. Griffen J and Tollison J: Dysphagia, Am Fam Phys 22:154, 1980.

14. Griffin K: Swallowing training for dysphagic patients, Arch Phys Med Rehabil 55:467, 1974.

15. Griggs B: Nursing management of swallowing disorders. In Groher M, editor: Dysphagia: diagnosis and management, Stoneham, MA, 1984, Butterworth Publishers.

16. Groher M: Bolus management and aspiration pneumonia with pseudobulbar dysphagia, Dysphagia 1:215, 1987.

17. Groher M and Asher I: Establishing a swallowing program. In Groher M, editor: Diagnosis and management, Stoneham, MA, 1984, Butterworth Publishers.

18. Huxley E et al: Pharyngeal aspiration in normal adults and patients with depressed consciousness, Am J Med 64:April, 1978.

19. Kendall H, Kendall F, and Wadsworth G: Muscles, testing and function, Baltimore, MD, 1971, Williams & Wilkins Co.

20. Lazzara G, Lazarus C, and Logeman J: Impact of thermal stimulation on the triggering of the swallow reflex, Dysphagia 1:73, 1986.

21. Liebman M: Neuroanatomy made easy and understandable, Rockville, MD, 1986, Aspen Publishers, Inc.

22. Logemann J: Evaluation and treatment of swallowing disorders, San Diego, CA, 1983, College Hill Press.

23. Logemann J: Evaluation and treatment of swallowing disorders. Symposium presented at Mills Hospital, San Mateo, CA, February, 1985.

24. Logemann J: Manual for the videofluorographic study of swallowing. Boston, MA, 1986, College Hill Press, Inc.

25. Logemann J: Treatment for aspiration related to dysphagia: an overview, Dysphagia 1:34, 1988.

26. Lowe A: The neural regulation of tongue movement, Prog Neurobiol 15:295, 1981.

27. Meadowbrook Neurologic Care Center, Rehabilitation Services: Dysphagia protocol (unpublished), 1986, San Jose, CA.

28. Miller A: Neurophysiological basis of swallowing, Dysphagia 1:91, 1986.

29. Mills Memorial Hospital: Dietary guidelines for swallowing dysfunctions, 1980, San Mateo, CA.

30. Pillsbury H and Buckwalter J: Surgical intervention in dysphagia. In Groher M, editor: Dysphagia: diagnosis and management, Stoneham, MA, 1984, Butterworth Publishers.

31. Silverman and Elfant IL: Dysphagia: an evaluation and treatment program for the adult, Am J Occup Ther 33:382, 1979.

32. Sister Kenny Institute: Dysphagia, Publication #706 Minneapolis, 1980.

33. Stone M and Shawker T: An ultrasound examination of tongue movement during swallowing, Dysphagia 1:78, 1986.

34. Van Boldrick A and Godfrey M: Treatment of the dyphagic patient: positioning, feeding and facilitation techniques. One day course presented at OTAC Conference, November 1987, San Jose, CA.

35. Williams H: Treating dysphagia, J Gerontol Nurs 9(12):December, 1983.

Chapter

11

Evaluation of sensation and treatment of sensory dysfunction

LORRAINE WILLIAMS PEDRETTI

Motor performance in purposeful activity is profoundly dependent on sensory function.[19] Without sensation, the conscious perception of peripheral sensory stimuli is lost, and the affected part may be virtually paralyzed, even when there is adequate recovery of muscle function.[8] Adaptive motor behavior frequently occurs in response to external sensory stimuli. For example, striking the keys of a typewriter in touch typing provides touch, pressure, and proprioceptive feedback into the central nervous system (CNS), which enables the typist to determine correct pressure and finger position and location on the keyboard without the aid of vision. Because adequate sensation is essential for effective movement, it is necessary to understand the patient's sensory status to fully appreciate the motor dysfunction and to plan appropriate treatment goals and methods.

Sensation and "sensibility" are terms found in the literature that refer to the reception, transmission, and interpretation of sensory stimuli. The terms are sometimes used interchangeably, or they may be differentiated.[5,8,17] Callahan defined sensation as the sensory stimuli conveyed to the central interpretive centers by the afferent nerves and sensibility as the ability to perceive or interpret the sensory stimuli.[5] For the purposes of this chapter, the terms "sensation" and "sensory" are used.

Occupational therapists frequently need to evaluate sensation. Any patient with CNS or peripheral nervous system (PNS) dysfunction should be routinely evaluated for sensory loss. Patients with CNS dysfunction will tend to show loss of many sensory modalities over generalized areas, whereas those with PNS disorders will tend to have loss of specific sensory modalities in circumscribed areas. Sensory testing may also be indicated in patients with burns, in whom sensory receptors in the skin are destroyed, patients with arthritis, in whom joint swelling may cause compression of a peripheral nerve, and patients with traumatic hand injuries, in whom skin, muscles, tendons, ligaments, and nerves may be involved.

Examples of other diagnoses that require sensory testing are peripheral nerve injuries and diseases, spinal cord injuries and diseases, brain injuries and diseases, and fractures, when there is peripheral nerve involvement, or to help determine if there is peripheral nerve involvement.

Sensory Supply to Specific Areas

The sensory distribution of the major peripheral nerves of the body and limbs is shown in Fig. 11-1 *A* and *B*. When evaluating for peripheral nerve dysfunction, it is important to test the area supplied by the given nerve or nerves that are affected. The sensory distribution of the dermatomes that correspond to spinal cord segments is also shown here. It is important in patients with spinal cord injury or disease to test according to this dermatomal distribution. This can be helpful in determining the level or levels of spinal cord lesion and any sparing of spinal cord function.

Purposes of Testing

By performing a sensory test, it is possible to carefully outline areas of intact, impaired, or absent sensation. This information is sometimes of diagnostic or prognostic value to the physician and provides a baseline for progress. Results of the sensory evaluation can also be used to determine the need to teach the patient how to protect against injury, how to use compensatory techniques such as visual guidance for movement during activities, and whether a sensory retraining program is feasible. Sensory loss may affect the use of splints and braces, since the patient may be unaware of pressure points during use. Sensory loss may also affect controlled use of a dynamic splint because the patient's sensory feedback is faulty.

Tests of sensory function do not always accurately predict functional use of the hand. Moberg, cited by Dellon, studied patients with median nerve injury to determine if there was a correlation between results of clinical sensory tests and hand function.[8] He used a series of everyday activities that required several different types of grip and prehension and a test of picking up small objects and placing them in a con-

PERIPHERAL DISTRIBUTION

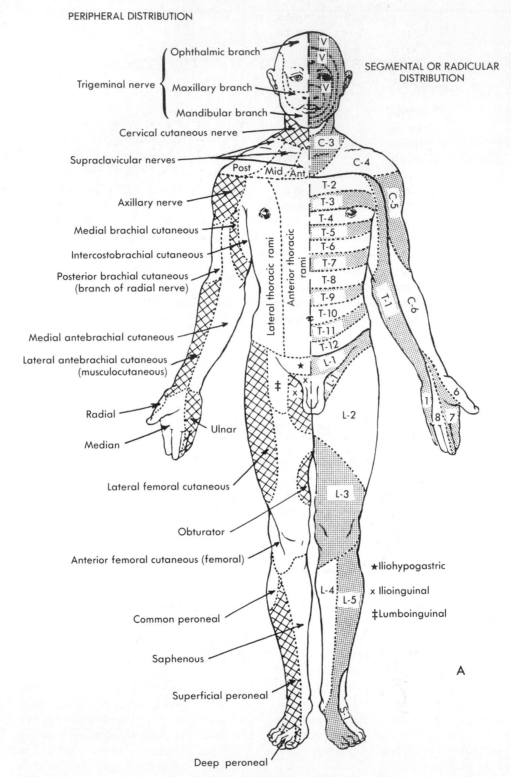

Fig. 11-1. A, Sensory distribution of the major peripheral nerves and dermatomes corresponding to spinal cord segments, anterior view. Reproduced with permission from Chusid JG: Correlative neuroanatomy & functional neurology, ed. 19. Copyright Lange Medical Publications, 1985.

Continued.

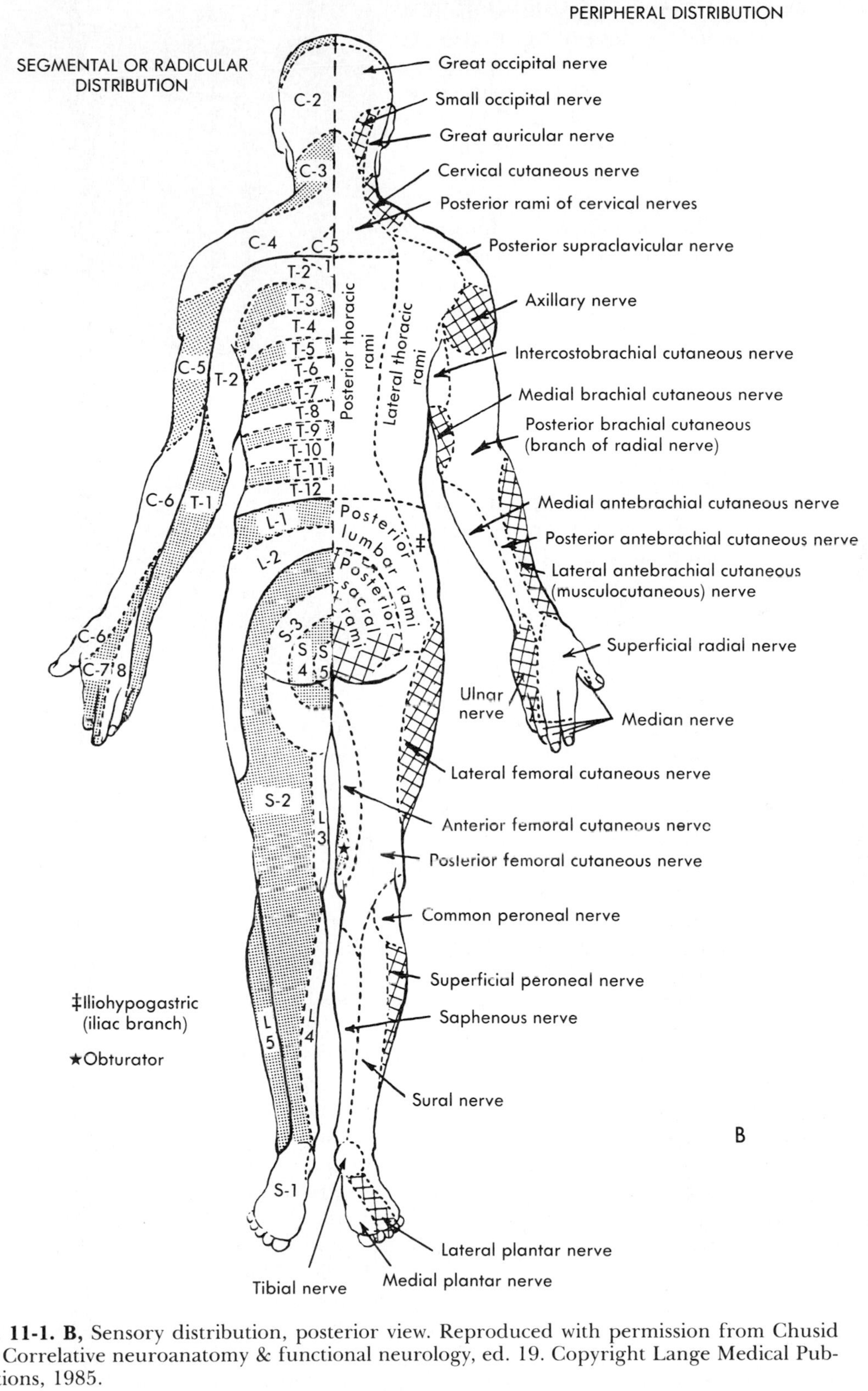

PERIPHERAL DISTRIBUTION

SEGMENTAL OR RADICULAR
DISTRIBUTION

Fig. 11-1. B, Sensory distribution, posterior view. Reproduced with permission from Chusid JG: Correlative neuroanatomy & functional neurology, ed. 19. Copyright Lange Medical Publications, 1985.

tainer (Moberg Picking Up Test) to evaluate hand function. Moberg concluded that tests of touch, pain, temperature, and vibration did not correlate with hand function. There was some correlation between two-point discrimination and hand function.[8] The results of his work are significant to occupational therapy because it underscores a primary purpose and principle of occupational therapy practice: to evaluate function or performance. Thus it is important for the occupational therapist not only to evaluate the sensory modalities but to evaluate function as well. This can be done by using one of the several hand function tests available to observe hand use under simulated conditions, and more reliably still, to observe for spontaneous use of the affected part in bilateral activities of daily living (ADL).

Occluding Vision During Testing

All of the sensory tests described below require that the patient's vision be occluded so that the test stimuli cannot be seen. Use of a blindfold or keeping the eyes shut are the *least* desirable methods of occluding vision.

A blindfold can be a source of sensory distraction and can be very anxiety-provoking to patients with sensory, perceptual, and balance disturbances.[10] It is difficult for many individuals with CNS dysfunction to maintain eye closure because of apraxia and motor impersistence, in addition to the above stated reasons.

There are several alternative methods for occluding vision. A small screen made by suspending a curtain between two posts is convenient and effective (Fig. 11-3). If such a device cannot be constructed, something similar can be made by folding in the sides of a corrugated box and draping a cloth over one side (Fig. 11-2, *A*), or a file folder can be held over the area being tested (Fig. 11-2, *B*).

TESTS FOR SENSATION

The following tests are based on evaluation tools of clinical neurology and are designed to test gross sensation of adults with CNS or PNS dysfunction.[3,18]

The reader is referred to the references [5, 8, and 25] for additional sensory tests and tests of discrete sensation. Tests of moving touch, constant touch, vibration sense, and two-point discrimination are described in Chapter 28.

Procedure

It is important for the examiner (E) to orient the subject (S) to the test procedures and to the rationale for administering the tests. The examiner should be sure that the subject understands how to respond. The subject's vision can be occluded by shielding the parts to be tested from view.

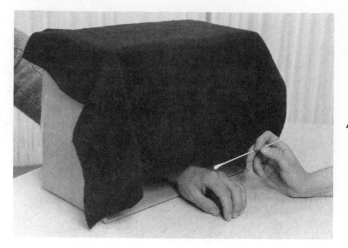

A

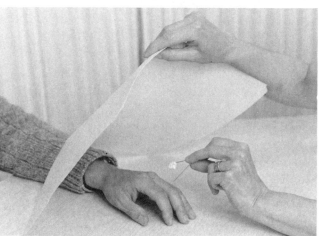

B

Fig. 11-2. A, Device for occluding vision during sensory testing: box with cloth drape. **B,** File folder can be used to occlude vision during sensory testing.

Superficial Pain Sensation

The ability to detect painful stimuli is critical to the avoidance of injury during performance of daily activities and to the prevention of skin breakdown while wearing splints and braces and using wheelchairs, crutches, and other adaptive devices. In normal circumstances, the onset of pain sensation warns the individual to move quickly, as when withdrawing a finger from a hot surface, or to adjust the position of clothing, as when an elastic legband is binding, or to remove an offending article of apparel, as when a shoe is rubbing a blister on the foot. The patient who lacks the ability to detect such painful stimuli is more likely to be injured. If there is absent or impaired pain sensation, it will be important to teach sensory compensation and safety awareness in the treatment program.

The following test uses a safety pin to apply light pain stimuli. The examiner should be aware that atrophic skin is particularly susceptible to injury and that a pinprick stimulus, which would not break normal skin, could produce a tiny break in atrophic skin. Skin atrophy occurs after peripheral nerve injury. The interruption of nerve supply interferes with normal tissue nutrition and causes the atrophy.[5] If this possibility is a concern, the end of an unbent paper clip may be used for the test.

Test for superficial pain[3,14,18,19]

PURPOSE: To make a gross evaluation of superficial pain sensitivity.

LIMITATIONS: Persons with receptive aphasia cannot be validly tested.

MATERIALS: A small curtain between two posts or a manila folder to occlude S's vision. A large safety pin or unbent paper clip, cotton balls, and rubbing alcohol.

CONDITIONS: A nondistracting environment where S is seated at a narrow table. Affected hand and forearm should rest comfortably on table. E sits opposite S on other side of table. If it is not possible to position S in this manner, the test may be administered while S is in bed or sitting in the wheelchair with arms resting on the lapboard.

METHOD: S's hand and forearm are hidden from S's view by placing them under curtain or by E holding a manila folder over them. The safety pin is swabbed with alcohol before the test begins. Affected hand and forearm are touched lightly at random locations, using sharp and dull stimuli in random order (Fig. 11-3). A few trial stimuli should be conducted with S watching to be sure that S understands test and knows how to respond. Test may be conducted entirely on an unaffected area first to establish a standard and determine that instructions are understood. If spasticity is a problem, E may support hand on dorsal surface and hold thumb in radial abduction and extension to secure relaxation for palmar testing. Each stimulus should be applied with same degree of pressure.

NOTES: Calloused or toughened areas (for example, palms) may be normally less sensitive than other areas. If S is fearful of a safety pin, the unbent paper clip may be used.

RESPONSES: S should be asked to say "sharp" or "dull" in response to each stimulus. If S is aphasic or dysarthric, E should ask S to indicate a response by pointing to appropriate side of an open safety pin in S's view.

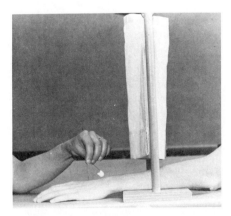

Fig. 11-3. Test for superficial pain sensation.

SCORING: E marks a plus at stimulus point on scoring chart for a correct response, a minus for an incorrect or unduly delayed response, and a zero for no response. Space for recording results of evaluation is presented in Fig. 11-4.

Light Touch and Pressure Sensation

Tactile sensitivity is critical to performance of all ADL. For example, to know that there is an object in the hand or to feel clothes on the body and know whether or not they are correctly adjusted is dependent on intact touch sensitivity. Pressure sensation is also important in ADL because it is continuously received in activities such as sitting, pushing drawers and doors, crossing the knees, wearing belts and collars, and a host of other activities that stimulate pressure receptors. It is possible for a patient to have intact pressure sensation when touch is impaired or absent. It is important to know this because pressure sensation can aid in performance of ADL and substitute for touch feedback in some activities.

Various tools have been used to apply stimuli for the light touch and pressure tests. These include a cotton ball, cotton swab, the finger tip, or a pencil eraser. All of these objects can provide a gross or cursory evaluation of light touch or pressure sensation. More discrete and accurate testing of cutaneous pressure thresholds of light touch to deep pressure can be performed by using the Semmes-Weinstein monofilaments described in Chapter 28.[8,24]

Test for light touch sensation[3,14,18]

PURPOSE: To determine S's ability to recognize and localize light touch stimuli.

LIMITATIONS: Patients with receptive aphasia cannot be validly tested.

MATERIALS: A small curtain between two posts or a manila folder to occlude vision. A cotton swab.

CONDITIONS: A nondistracting environment where S is seated at a narrow table or as described previously for superficial pain if sitting at a table is not possible. Affected hand and forearm rest comfortably on table. E sits opposite S.

METHOD: S's hand and forearm are hidden from S's view by placing them under curtain or by E holding manila folder over them. Hand and forearm are touched lightly with a cotton swab at random locations. A few trial stimuli should be administered while S is watching to be sure S understands procedure and how to respond. Test may be administered on an uninvolved area first to establish a standard. If spasticity is a problem, E may support hand on dorsal surface and hold thumb in radial abduction and extension to secure relaxation of fingers for palmar testing (Fig. 11-5).

RESPONSES: After each stimulus, E asks if S was touched (recognition). S responds by nodding or saying "yes" or "no." Curtain or folder is removed after each stimulus, and S is asked to point to place where S was touched, using unaffected hand if possible. If this cannot be done, S is asked to describe location, and E should select locations that are easy to name (for example, over proximal interphalangeal joint).

FORM FOR RECORDING SCORES ON
TESTS OF SENSATION

Department of Occupational Therapy

Name____________________ Age________ Sex____________

Diagnosis____________________ Disability__________________

Date____________________

TEST FOR SUPERFICIAL PAIN — LEFT — RIGHT

Use a large safety pin and touch random locations with sharp and dull ends on anterior and posterior surfaces.
Indicate on diagram:
Intact: +
Impaired: -
Absent: 0

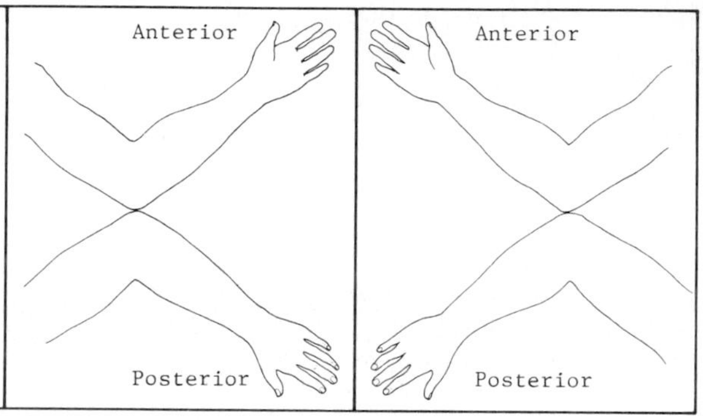

TEST FOR LIGHT TOUCH SENSITIVITY — LEFT — RIGHT

Use a cotton swab and touch random locations on anterior and posterior surfaces.
Indicate on diagram:
Intact: +
Impaired: -
Absent: 0

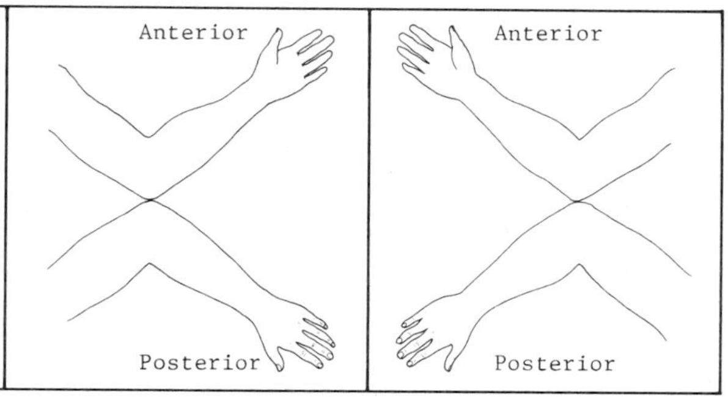

Fig. 11-4. Form for recording scores on tests of sensation.

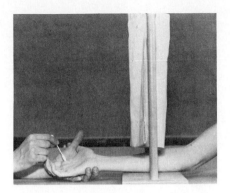

Fig. 11-5. Test of light touch sensation.

SCORING: On scoring chart E marks a plus for ability to recognize and localize touch stimuli, a minus for ability to recognize only, and a zero for inability to recognize or localize a stimulus. Fig. 11-5 includes space for recording scores on test for touch sensitivity.

STANDARDS: Deviations of ⅗ to 1⅕ inches (1.5 to 3 cm) from the point of application of the stimulus are normal, depending on an area of hand or arm touched. Responses should be more accurate on hand than on forearm and more accurate on forearm than on upper arm.

Test for pressure sensation

Pressure sensitivity may be tested in exactly the same manner as described for light touch, except that E should press hard enough with the cotton swab to dent and blanch the skin. If light touch sensitivity is severely impaired or absent, pressure sensitivity may be intact and may provide important sensory feedback to compensate and enhance function. Normally, pressure stimuli can be localized on the hand from 2.44 to 2.83 mg of pressure.[24]

Thermal Sensation

The ability to detect temperatures, especially extremes in temperature, is essential for the prevention of injury in many ADL such as bathing, cooking, ironing, and using a curling iron. The ability to detect temperature also contributes to the enjoyment of food and to the detection of uncomfortable environmental temperatures. If the patient lacks accurate thermal discrimination, it will be necessary to teach precautions against injury and to structure ADL to prevent burns. As in the other sensory tests, the results can serve as a baseline for progress, and changes in sensory status may be used to measure recovery or deterioration, depending on the diagnosis.

Tests for thermal sensitivity have used techniques such as touching the area to be tested with test tubes filled with hot and cold water, immersing the fingers or hand into hot or cold water, or touching small hot or cold compresses to the area being tested. A recent development is the Hot/Cold Discrimination Kit by Rolyan.* This kit includes two metal temperature

---
*Smith & Nephew Rolyan, Inc., Menomonee Falls, WI

probes with a thermometer at the head of each, two thermal cups, and a single stem thermometer. One thermal cup is filled with ice and water, and the other is filled with hot tap water. The single thermometer is inserted in the thermal cup. When the desired temperature is reached, the probe is inserted into the thermal cup and allowed to reach the desired testing temperature. The metal probes, which look much like test tubes, are then put in contact with the skin surface to be tested. This kit makes is possible to control temperatures accurately and to maintain constant temperature stimuli for the duration of the test.

Test for thermal sensation[3,9,14]

PURPOSE: To determine S's ability to discriminate between extremes of hot and cold and to detect variations in temperature at four levels.

LIMITATIONS: Persons with receptive aphasia cannot be validly tested.

MATERIALS: Four test tubes (¾-inch or 2-cm diameter) with stoppers.

CONDITIONS: A nondistracting environment where S is seated comfortably at a table with both hand and forearm resting on table or alternatives described for previous tests.

METHOD:

Subtest I: Two test tubes are used, one filled with very cold water and one with very hot water. Ice water may be used for cold and hottest tap water tolerable to normal touch used for hot. Stoppers are placed in tubes. E touches sides of test tubes to skin surfaces to be tested in random order and at random locations, being sure to cover test area thoroughly (Fig. 11-6).

Subtest II: Four test tubes are used, one filled with very cold water, one with tepid water, one with warm water, and one with hot water. E should color code stoppers as follows: yellow—hot, green—warm, orange—tepid, and red—cold. Place stoppers in tubes. E asks S to touch or hold test tubes with affected hand(s) in random order. If S is unable to hold tubes, E may touch each one to S's palm and fingertips.

RESPONSES:

Subtest I: S responds "hot" or "cold" in response to each stimulus. If S is aphasic, E should work out an alternate nonverbal response before beginning tests.

Subtest II: S is asked to arrange test tubes on table from hottest to coldest in order from left to right. E checks cor-

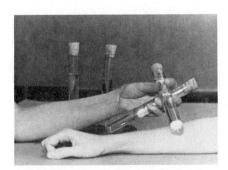

Fig. 11-6. Test for thermal sensation.

```
TEST FOR THERMAL SENSITIVITY
    SUBTEST I.
        Test site (fill in location tested)            Score (+, 0)
                                        Dates
```

Use diagram to record scores on test of arms

```
    SUBTEST II.                                    Date    Date    Date

        Arrange test tubes in correct order       ____    ____    ____
        Arrange test tubes in wrong order         ____    ____    ____

        Indicate arrangement of test tubes by filling in spaces below with
        H for hot, W for warm, T for tepid, and C for cold.

        Date:_____  _____  _____  _____  _____
             _____  _____  _____  _____  _____
```

```
    SUBTEST III.                                   Date    Date    Date

        Temperature feels the same to both hands   ____    ____    ____
        Temperature feels different to each hand   ____    ____    ____

            All feel warmer to affected hand       ____    ____    ____
            All feel cooler to affected hand       ____    ____    ____
            All feel warmer to unaffected hand     ____    ____    ____
            All feel cooler to unaffected hand     ____    ____    ____

            Hottest is intolerably hot to affected hand   ____    ____    ____
            Coldest is intolerably cold to affected hand  ____    ____    ____
```

Fig. 11-7. Form for recording scores on test of thermal sensation.

rectness of order by color-coded stoppers and/or feeling tubes.

SCORING (Fig. 11-7):

Subtest I: E marks a plus on form if temperature is correctly identified and marks a zero if S cannot distinguish hot from cold. Subtests II is not administered if S cannot succeed at subtest I.

Subtest II: E marks appropriate blanks on form with a check and the appropriate letter to indicate S's responses.

STANDARD: Normal adults should be able to complete all items on this test successfully.

Olfactory Sensation

A loss of the sense of smell is known as anosmia. It may result from local chronic or acute inflammatory nasal disease or from intracranial lesions that may be the result of cerebral vascular accident, head injury, tumors, and infections.[3]

Anosmia interferes with function, for example, if the patient has an occupation where the sense of smell is critical to safety or for detection of household gas, chemicals, smoke, car exhaust, and noxious environmental odors.

In some disturbances in which the sense of smell is distorted, pleasant odors are perceived as noxious (parosmia). The disturbance may interfere with the perception and enjoyment of food odors.

A decreased sense of smell affects the ability to taste.[11]

Test for olfactory sensation

PURPOSE: To determine if the sense of smell is intact, impaired, or lost and whether the loss is unilateral or bilateral.

LIMITATIONS: Persons with receptive aphasia cannot be validly tested. Persons with expressive aphasia who cannot communicate using symbols, such as pictures or words, to indicate responses cannot be validly tested. Test is quite subjective and E must rely on S's report.

MATERIALS: Five small opaque or dark-colored bottles containing essences, powders, or crystalline material of familiar odors. Coffee, almond, chocolate, lemon oil, and peppermint are some that are suitable.[3] Ammonia or other irritating chemical odors should *not* be used in a test of olfaction, since they stimulate all receptors of the mucous membranes and tend to be irritating.[9] If S cannot respond verbally, small cards with the word or a picture for each odor on them will be needed.

CONDITIONS: A nondistracting environment where no strong odors are present with S seated or semireclining.

METHOD: The cork of the bottle or a cotton swab moistened with essence is held under S's nostril; in the case of solid substances the container may be held under S's nostril. S is asked to compress one nostril or this may be done by E. S is then asked to take a breath to demonstrate that the remaining nostril is open. With vision occluded, if the substances could be recognized from their appearance, the cotton swab, cork, or bottle is then held under the open nostril, and S is asked to take two moderate sniffs. Each of the substances is tried with a short delay between them, and the nostrils are tested alternately using the same and different substances.[3,18]

RESPONSES: E asks S to (1) detect an odor, (2) identify the odor, (3) distinguish if the odors are the same or different to both nostrils.[3,18]

SCORING (Fig. 11-8). E marks a plus on the form if the odor is detected and correctly identified, a minus if an odor is detected, and a zero if no odor is detected. Whether or

RECORDING SCORES OF OLFACTORY AND GUSTATORY SENSATION

Name: _____

Age: _____ Diagnosis: _____

Date: _____

Key: + = Can detect and identify odor
     − = Can detect odor, cannot identify odor
     O = Cannot detect or identify odor
     S = Can detect same odors, both nostrils
     D = Can detect different odors, both nostrils

OLFACTORY SENSATION

	Left nostril		Right nostril		Comparisons	
Dates						
Coffee						
Almond						
Chocolate						
Lemon						
Peppermint						

GUSTATORY SENSATION

Key: + = Identifies taste correctly
     − = Cannot identify taste

			Remarks
Dates			
Sweet			
Salt			
Sour			
Bitter			

Fig. 11-8. Form for recording scores on olfactory and gustatory sensation.

not the same odors are perceived as the same by both nostrils and whether S can differentiate between different odors presented to each nostril should be noted on the form.

STANDARD: Ability to detect and identify odors quickly, ability to detect odor without identification, and ability to detect and differentiate odors without identification may all be regarded as normal responses.[3] Distortion of the odor (parosmia) and inability to detect odors are regarded as dysfunction. If test responses are vague and variable, the results are unreliable, and it is best to postpone the test to a more favorable time.[3]

Gustatory Sensation (Taste)

Taste is subserved by the facial and glossopharyngeal nerves (cranial nerves VII and IX). Disturbances of taste may be caused by PNS or CNS lesions.[18] Taste is not only basic to the enjoyment of food but is one of the sensory stimuli that triggers salivation and swallowing. Therefore taste sensation may be of concern to the occupational therapist as part of a comprehensive evaluation of oral-motor mechanisms and for planning feeding training programs.[21]

Test for gustatory sensation

PURPOSE: To determine if the sense of taste is intact, impaired, or absent.

LIMITATIONS: The same limitations as cited for the test of olfaction apply here. The most accurate method of administering the test requires that S keep the tongue extended.[6,21] Therefore S must respond by pointing to a word or picture. In instances where S has speech but cannot recognize words or pictures, a verbal response should be allowed. If S is aphasic, E should observe for aversive responses to the sour and bitter stimuli.[21] The appreciation of taste depends on an intact sense of smell.[3,11]

MATERIALS: Sugar, salt, lemon or vinegar, and quinine in small containers to test the four basic tastes: sweet, salt, sour, and bitter. Cotton swabs.

CONDITIONS: A nondistracting environment where S is seated or semireclining. E should sit directly in front of S. S's vision should be occluded. The oral cavity should be clean and free of residual food tastes.

METHOD: S is instructed to protrude the tongue and a small amount of the test substance on the tip of a wet cotton swab is applied to the appropriate place on the tongue: sweet—side/front of tongue; salt—all areas of tongue; sour—side/middle of tongue; and bitter—side/back of tongue.[21] If this is not effective, rubbing the substance along the side of the protruded tongue should be tried.[3,18] The tongue should be irrigated with plain water between each stimulus.[11]

RESPONSES: S is instructed to point to the response card before withdrawing the tongue and diffusing the taste to all areas of the tongue.[3,18]

SCORING (Fig. 11-8): E should record a plus if the taste is correctly identified and a minus if it cannot be identified.

STANDARD: Normal adults should be able to recognize all tastes accurately.

Position and Motion Sense

Kinesthesia is the conscious awareness of joint position and movement. Proprioception refers to unconscious information about joint position and motion that arises from receptors in the muscles, joints, ligaments, and bone.[1] These senses make it possible to detect joint motion and position of the body or any of its parts. Sensation that is evoked from movement is essential to being able to move effectively. Feedback about the motion and position of the body and its parts in space help human beings to maintain erect posture, make adjustments in posture, and know where the limbs, trunk, and head are at any moment. This sensory information, combined with touch and stereognosis, makes it possible to write without looking at the pencil, type without looking at the keys, and button clothes behind the back.

The awareness of motion and position is on a subcortical level and normally does not require conscious effort. To test position and motion sense, however, it is necessary to raise the sensation to a conscious level so that the patient can make appropriate responses. A partial or complete loss of position and motion senses will seriously impair movement, even if muscle function is within normal limits. Therefore it is important for the occupational therapist to know if the patient has the sensory loss so that the motor dysfunction can be more fully understood. Results of the evaluation will help to plan treatment by using compensatory methods or through a sensory retraining program.

Test of position and motion sense[3,7,14-16,19]

PURPOSE: To evaluate S's senses of motion and position.

MATERIALS: Curtain on posts shown on test for light touch sensitivity (Fig. 11-6) or a manila folder. For testing elbow and shoulder, if space and equipment permit, a curtained screen high and wide enough to conceal S's arm when held overhead or out in front when in a seated position. Curtain on screen should be full, continuous, and attached at top only. If such a screen is not available, an assistant can shield S's vision with a manila folder.

CONDITIONS: Test should be conducted in privacy in a nondistracting environment. When fingers and wrist are being tested, S should be seated at a table with screen in front in a position to accommodate affected hand and forearm comfortably. E should sit opposite S on other side of screen in a position comfortable to accommodate S's hand for conducting test. When elbow and shoulder are being tested, S should be seated, and curtain screen placed at S's affected side. Curtain should be draped over the shoulder in such a manner that S is unable to see the affected arm. If this position is not feasible, test may be conducted with S seated or reclining in bed or seated in a wheelchair.

RESPONSES: To determine appreciation of direction of movement, S should be instructed to respond "up" (away from floor) and "down" (toward floor) or "out" (away from body) and "in" (toward body) as soon as he or she perceives direction of movement. Aphasic subjects may respond by pointing in appropriate direction. If there is one unaffected extremity, as in hemiplegia, S should be asked to imitate with unaffected extremity final position in which part rests after E has ceased movement to determine appreciation of position.

METHOD:

Test of fingers: Test positions are index finger flexion, middle finger extension, thumb extension, and little finger flexion. These should be presented in random order. No range should be carried to such an extreme as to elicit pain or a stretch reflex. S's hand and forearm should be placed under curtain, resting on dorsal surface. When testing a right hand, E should support S's hand with the left palm and hold thumb out of way with the left thumb if necessary. This position should induce relaxation of fingers if S has flexor spasticity. With the right hand, E should grasp finger to be tested on each side at distal phalanx to avoid giving pressure cues with E's thumb and index finger. Finger being tested should be separated from others and should be kept from touching palm to avoid cues from contact. Position of E's hands is reversed when testing a left hand (Fig. 11-9).

Test of wrist: Test positions are wrist flexion and extension. The ranges should not be carried to such an extreme as to elicit tendon action or a stretch reflex. E's and S's hands are positioned as for testing fingers. However, E makes a somewhat firmer grasp at sides of S's hand, reducing contact between E's palm and back of S's hand.

Test of elbow and shoulder: Starting position for all motions is with S's arm at side, shoulder supported in 20° to 30° of abduction, elbow supported at 90° of flexion, and wrist stabilized at neutral. Test positions are elbow extension, shoulder flexion, shoulder internal rotation, and shoulder flexion-abduction (halfway between 90° of flexion and 90° of abduction). Test positions should be presented in random order. Ranges should not be carried to such an extreme as to elicit a stretch reflex or cause pain if there is joint tightness. S should be seated away from table. Curtained screen should be arranged at S's test side. E should stand at S's test side and guide limb passively through test positions. When testing a right arm, E's right hand should be placed along ulnar border of S's hand and wrist, stabilizing wrist at neutral. E's left hand should be placed on dorsal surface of upper arm just proximal to elbow. Position is reversed when testing left arm. E may carry out all test positions for elbow and shoulder without changing position of hands (Fig. 11-10).

SCORING (Fig. 11-11):

Appreciation of direction of movement: E records plus if direction is correctly perceived or zero if direction is not perceived.

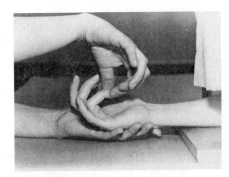

Fig. 11-9. Motion and position sense test of fingers.

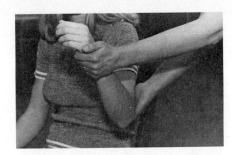

Fig. 11-10. Motion and position sense test of elbow and shoulder.

Appreciation of position: E records plus if correct response is given, minus if response is delayed or nearly correct, and zero if response is obviously incorrect or no response is given.

Remarks: On the recording form, E comments on S's reactions, unusual statements, observations, and individual variations in test procedure adapted for specific dysfunctions.

STANDARD: Normal individuals can detect movements of 1 or 2 mm in a joint.[11] A grade of intact was given by Kent if movement could be detected in the first 15 degrees of the ROM.[16]

TACTILE PERCEPTION
Stereognosis

Stereognosis is the perceptual skill that makes it possible to identify common objects and geometric shapes through tactile perception without the aid of vision. It results from the integration of the senses of touch, pressure, position, motion, texture, weight, and temperature and is dependent on intact parietal cortical function.[14]

This perceptual function is essential to daily living because the ability to "see with the hands" is critical to most everyday activities. It is the skill that makes it possible to reach into a pocket or purse and find keys and to reach into a dark room and find the light switch. Stereognosis, along with proprioception, enables the use of all hand tools and performance of hand activities without the need to visually concentrate on the implements being used. Examples are knitting while watching television, sawing wood while focusing on the wood rather than the saw, and using a fork while conversing.

Test for stereognosis[2,7,15,16]

PURPOSE: To evaluate S's ability to perceive tactile properties and identify common objects.

MATERIALS: Curtain described in test for light touch. Pencil, fountain pen, sunglasses, key, nail, large safety pin, metal teaspoon, quarter, and small leather coin purse.

CONDITIONS: Test should be conducted in privacy in a nondistracting environment. S should be seated at a table with curtain in front in a position that accommodates affected hand and forearm comfortably. E should sit opposite S. If S is unable to manipulate test objects because of motor

FORM FOR RECORDING TESTS OF POSITION/MOTION SENSE AND STEREOGNOSIS

Department of Occupational Therapy

Name _____ Age _____ Sex _____ Onset _____

Diagnosis/disability _____

Date _____

Test of Motion/Position Sense	Shoulder flexion-abduction	Shoulder internal rotation	Shoulder flexion	Elbow extension	Wrist extension	Wrist flexion	Little finger flexion	Thumb extension	Middle finger extension	Index finger flexion
Appreciation of direction of movement										
Appreciation of position										
Remarks:										

TEST OF STEREOGNOSIS

COMMON OBJECTS	+ − 0	DESCRIPTION
Pencil		
Fountain pen		
Sunglasses		
Key		
Nail		
Safety pin		
Teaspoon		
Quarter		
Leather coin purse		

Remarks:

Fig. 11-11. Form for recording the scores on tests of motion/position sense and stereognosis.

weakness, E should assist S to manipulate them in as near normal a manner as possible.

METHOD: S's hand is under curtain, resting on dorsal surface on table. Objects are presented in random order. Manipulation of objects is allowed and encouraged. Manipulation of objects may be assisted by E if S's hand is partially or completely paralyzed.

RESPONSES: S should be asked to name object or describe its properties if unable to name it. Aphasic patients may view a duplicate set of test objects after each trial and point to a choice.

SCORING: E marks plus if object is identified quickly and correctly and minus if there is a long delay before identification of object or if S can only describe properties (for example, size, texture, material, and shape) of object. E marks a zero if S cannot identify object or its properties (Fig. 11-11).

Test for graphesthesia[6,14,19]

An additional test of discriminative sensation that measures parietal lobe function is the test for graphesthesia. This is the ability to recognize numbers, letters, or forms written on the skin.[6,14,19] The loss of this ability is called agraphesthesia.[19] To apply the test, the vision is occluded, and letters, numbers, or geometric forms are traced on the fingertips or palm with a dull pointed pencil or similar instrument. The subject tells the examiner which symbol was written.[19] If the subject is aphasic, pictures of the symbols may be used for the subject to indicate a response after each test stimulus.

SENSORY DYSFUNCTION

Sensory disturbances can result from CNS or PNS dysfunction or from cranial nerve disorders. In peripheral and cranial nerve lesions, the sensory disturbance is localized to the area supplied by the affected nerve. Sensory disorders of nerve root origin are localized to the dermatome supplied by the affected nerve root. Sensory dysfunction of CNS origin is more generalized and affects the contralateral side of the body after stroke or head injury, resulting in hemiplegia.[6] Some of the terms associated with sensory disturbances are *anesthesia* (complete loss of sensation); *paresthesia* (abnormal sensation such as tingling or crawling); *hypesthesia* (decreased sensation); *hyperesthesia* (increased tactile sensitivity); *analgesia* (complete loss of pain sensation); *hypalgesia* (diminished pain sensation); and *astereognosis* (the inability to identify common objects by touch alone).[6]

Because correct interpretation of sensory stimuli is critical to effective movement and feedback from movement, sensory loss may have a profound effect on the patient's ability to function in everyday activities. It is important to facilitate sensory recovery or reeducation to the extent possible.

Treatment of Sensory Dysfunction

Before treatment of sensory dysfunction can be initiated, a sensory evaluation and an evaluation of functional use of the affected part should be completed. The therapist must have knowledge of the diagnosis, the cause of the sensory dysfunction, the prognosis for return of sensation, and the current progression of recovery. This information may help to determine whether the treatment approach should be remedial, compensatory, or both.

The patient who is to begin a sensory reeducation program should be motivated and able to concentrate. Cognitive ability should be adequate to understand the purpose of the training, to persevere in daily sessions, and to make every effort to use the affected part in ADL.[4,10]

Central Nervous System Dysfunction

EFFECTS OF SENSORY LOSS. Following cerebral vascular accident (CVA) and other CNS disorders such as head injury, sensory loss can be a significant problem. Sensory loss inhibits motor function, even when there is good motor return. The inclination to move is based on sensory input and feedback. Persons with poor sensation have little urge to move. Movement that is attempted may be clumsy or incoordinated. Sensory loss may contribute to, but is not the only cause of, neglect of the affected extremity so often seen in these patients. The possibility of injury is a serious concern, and the dependence on visual control negates carrying out many activities such as reaching into a purse or pocket to retrieve an item and fastening clothing at the side or back.[10]

COMPENSATORY TREATMENT. A first concern is safety and ensuring that the patient is not injured by bumping, burning, or becoming snagged in furniture or equipment during performance of ADL. If the loss of sensation is permanent, compensation will facilitate rehabilitation. Examples of compensation are using the less affected hand to perform activities such as cooking, eating, and ironing; using vision to observe motion and location of body parts; testing bath water with the less affected hand or a bath thermometer; and using adaptive devices such as the one-handed cutting board.[22]

The stroke (CVA) patient needs to be made aware of his or her sensory deficits. Safety factors during performance of everyday activities must be continuously brought to the patient's attention and reinforced. To compensate for sensory loss, it may be possible to train the patient to check the position of the limbs by looking at them. Patients must be evaluated for safety awareness and trained to consider safety in hazardous activities. The patient who wishes to return to home management should demonstrate good judgment, safety awareness, and the ability to use visual compensation for sensory loss.[20] Frequent repetition of instructions and cueing by the therapist are often necessary with the patients. Cognitive disturbances such as poor memory, perseveration, poor judgment, and inability to see cause and effect relationships make it difficult for some patients to learn and attend effectively to compensatory techniques. In such instances, supervision is required.

REMEDIAL TREATMENT. The use of sensory bombardment involving as many of the senses as possible has been found to be useful for sensory retraining in some CVA patients. During regular therapeutic activities and handling, the therapist can touch or stroke the affected parts, encourage the patient to look at them and to see the movement and touch stimulation. Weight-bearing on legs, arms, and trunk increases proprioceptive feedback.[22]

Eggers advocates integrating sensory retraining with motor retraining, using the Bobath approach (see Chapter 20).[10] Bobath described a sensory retraining program that focuses primarily on tactile and kinesthetic reeducation. A prerequisite to sensory retraining is for the therapist to normalize the patient's muscle tone and to find the optimal position for the sensory reeducation activities. The therapist must find ways to stimulate sensation without increasing spasticity. Sufficient time must be allowed for the patient to make responses because many patients exhibit delayed processing of sensory information. Other deficits such as hemianopsia, aphasia, and visual perceptual deficits must be considered when retraining tactile-kinesthetic functions. Repetition and variation of sensory stimuli are necessary with CNS patients if they are to relearn sensation.[10]

A graded treatment program for sensory deficits is described by Eggers.[10] Initially, the patient is allowed to see and hear an object as it is being felt, for the benefit of intersensory facilitation; then vision is occluded during the tactile exploration; and, finally, a pad is placed on the table top so that both auditory and visual clues are eliminated and the patient relies on tactile-kinesthetic input alone. The program for tactile-kinesthetic reeducation begins with gross discrimination of objects that are very dissimilar, for example, smooth and rough textures or round and square shapes. Next, the patient is asked to estimate quantities (such as quantity of marbles in a box) through touch. Then the patient must discriminate between large and small objects hidden in sand and progresses to discriminate between two- and three-dimensional objects. Finally, the patient is required to pick a specific small object from among several objects. The reader is referred to the original source for a detailed description of specific training activities.[10]

Fox studied the effect of cutaneous stimulation on selected tests of perception with CVA patients.[13] She applied a corduroy-covered, padded, wooden stimulator to any or several areas of the patient such as the dorsum of the forearm, the hand and fingers, and the ventral surface of the hand. The patients grasped a rough-surfaced cardboard cone for pressure stimulation of the volar surface of the hand. The results of the study were somewhat favorable, particularly for the treatment of finger agnosia (inability to recognize the pattern of the fingers). The author noted that more research is needed in this area.[13]

Farber described a treatment approach to retrain stereognosis in adults and children with CNS dysfunction.[11] First, the patient is allowed to examine the training object visually as it is rotated by the therapist. The patient is then allowed to handle the object in the less affected hand while observing the hand. In the next step, the patient is allowed to manipulate the object with both hands while looking. Then the object is placed in the affected hand to be manipulated while looking at it. The patient may place the hand in a mirror-lined, three-sided box during these manipulations to increase visual input. This sequence is then repeated with the vision occluded. Once several objects can be identified consistently, two of the objects may be hidden in a tub of sand or rice. The patient is then asked to reach into the tub and retrieve a specific object. If the sensation of the sand or rice is overstimulating or disturbing, the objects can be placed in a bag.[11]

Vinograd, Taylor, and Grossman described a similar program.[23] However, they included objects for discrimination of shape, size, weight, and texture, as well as common objects, in the training. Wooden blocks were included for shape recognition, sandbags and cotton bags for weight recognition, and different grades of sandpaper and smooth leather for texture discrimination.[23]

The effect of intensive stereognostic training on spastic, cerebral, palsied adults was studied by Ferreri, with some favorable results for improving stereognosis. Training sessions of 20 minutes, three to four times a week for a period of 5 weeks were held. The training program consisted of comparing two different objects or forms using the uninvolved hand, then the involved hand. The subjects were assisted with manipulation of the objects, if there was motor paralysis. The examiner talked about the qualities of the objects or forms and emphasized the hand and finger positions. A particular training item was used for each session until five consecutive correct responses were given in the testing portion of the session before a new training item was introduced.[12]

Sensory reeducation for those with CNS dysfunction focuses on both general sensory stimulation to enhance sensory perception and the use of repetitive sensory stimulation with shapes, textures, weights, and common objects. The training programs use intermodal reinforcement through visual, auditory, and tactile senses to confirm the sensory experience.

Peripheral Nervous System Dysfunction

COMPENSATORY TREATMENT. A compensatory approach for patients with PNS dysfunction is similar to that described above for patients with CNS dysfunction. The patient must be made aware of the specific sensory deficits and taught safety awareness for ADL. It may be necessary to avoid use of the affected limb during bilateral activities which are potentially hazardous.

Callahan proposed the following guidelines for patients with PNS dysfunction who lack protective sensation[4]:

1. Avoid exposure of the involved area to heat, cold, and sharp objects.
2. When gripping a tool or object, be conscious of not applying more force than necessary.
3. Beware that the smaller the handle, the less distribution of pressure over gripping surfaces. Avoid small handles by building up the handle or using a different tool whenever possible.
4. Avoid tasks that require use of one tool for long periods of time, especially if the hand is unable to adapt by changing the manner of grip.
5. Change tools frequently at work to rest tissue areas.
6. Observe the skin for signs of stress, that is, redness, edema, and warmth, from excessive force or repetitive pressure, and rest the hand if these signs occur.
7. If blisters, lacerations, or other wounds occur, treat them with the utmost care to avoid further injury to the skin and possible infection.
8. To keep skin soft and pliant, follow a daily routine of skin care, including soaking and oil massage to lock in moisture.

The patient with PNS dysfunction may be more capable of learning and attending to the compensatory techniques than the patient with CNS dysfunction, since cognitive skills are intact.

REMEDIAL TREATMENT. Following nerve injury repair and recovery, the neural impulses received in the sensory cortex from sensory stimulation of the injured hand are altered. The new pattern of neural impulses may be so different as to preclude correct interpretation of the stimulus. Thus, although sensory information is received, it cannot be interpreted correctly. The purpose of sensory reeducation is to assist the patient to reinterpret the sensory impulses reach-

ing his or her consciousness. The patient's potential for functional recovery following nerve repair will be enhanced by a sensory reeducation program.[8]

Dellon described a sensory reeducation program that is divided into early and late phases, and progression of the program is based on the recovery process.[8] The nerve recovery is determined by giving specific sensory tests. In the early phase of the program, the focus is on reeducating moving touch, constant touch, pressure, and touch localization. For moving touch, a pencil eraser or fingertip is used to move up and down the area being treated. The patient observes the stimulus. Vision is occluded the patient concentrates on the stimulus, then opens the eyes to verify what is happening. The patient verbalizes what is being felt, such as "I feel a soft object moving down the palm of my hand." A similar procedure is followed for constant touch. A pencil eraser is used to press down on one place on the finger or palm in an area where constant touch is recovered. The patient is encouraged to practice these reeducation techniques four times a day for at least 5 minutes each but is directed not to stimulate one hand with the other because this would send two sets of sensory stimuli to the brain.[8]

Late phase sensory reeducation is initiated as soon as moving and constant touch are perceived at the fingertips. This is often 6 to 8 months after nerve repair at the wrist. The goal in this phase is to facilitate the recovery of stereognosis. The exercises involve a series of tactile discrimination tasks. These begin with identification of large objects that are significantly different from one another and progress to objects with finer and more subtle differences. Familiar household objects are used at the outset. The process is to grasp the object while looking at it, then to occlude the vision and concentrate on the perception, and, finally, to look again at the object for reinforcement. The next set of objects are those that differ in texture and then objects that are smaller and require more discrete discrimination. Manipulation of the training objects also contributes to motor recovery. Ultimately, the therapist can incorporate activities that simulate those of the patient's occupational roles.[8]

Wynn Parry described a sensory retraining program for patients with PNS injuries affecting the hand.[25] The rationale underlying the technique is that the patient can learn to "lay down a new code" in the CNS. It has been shown that in nerve regeneration following traumatic lesions, there is a marked disturbance of cortical representation of sensory nerve fibers in the hand. The training program works best with patients who are cooperative, well motivated, and need to use their sensation for everyday activities.[25]

The training program begins when the patient has sensation in the fingers, about 6 to 8 months after a nerve suture at the wrist, with the use of large wood blocks of different shapes. The patient's vision is occluded, and a block is placed in the affected hand. The patient is asked to feel it and describe its shape and to compare its weight with a block placed in the unaffected hand. If an incorrect response is given, the patient is allowed to look at the blocks and repeat the manipulation, integrating visual and tactile information. The patient then compares the sensory experience with that of the normal hand. The procedure continues with various shaped blocks, and when these have been mastered, blocks with textures—such as sandpaper or velvet—on some surfaces are used. The patient is asked to differentiate textured surfaces from wood surfaces.[25]

In the next phase of training, the patient is asked to identify several textures such as sheepskin, leather, silk, canvas, rubber, plastic, wool, carpet, and sandpaper. These are all presented with the vision occluded. Finally, common objects are used in training, and the patient is asked to identify them without the aid of vision. If there are incorrect responses for texture and object identification, the patient is allowed to perform the manipulations while looking at the training objects and to relate what is felt to what is seen. Objects are graded from large to small. Training sessions may be varied by burying objects in a bowl of sand and asking the patient to retrieve a specific object, using a form board in which to place specific forms, or identifying wooden letters for spelling out words. Training is done in two to four 10-minute sessions a day.[25]

To train touch localization, Wynn Parry recommends the following procedure.[25] Vision is occluded and the therapist touches several places on the volar surface of the hand. The patient is asked to locate each stimulus with the index finger of the unaffected hand. If the response is incorrect, the patient is directed to look at the place where the hand was touched and to relate where the touch was felt to where the stimulus was actually applied.[25]

To evaluate effectiveness of retraining, reevaluation is done at 1 month, 3 months, and 6 months after the initial examination. Criteria used to evaluate treatment effectiveness are time to recognize objects, time to recognize textures, and time for correct localiza-tion. To avoid a training effect, different objects and some new textures are used in testing than those used in the training program.[25]

Turner described a sensory reeducation program for patients with peripheral nerve lesions.[22] Retraining is initiated when there is return of protective sensation (deep pressure and pin prick) and touch perception. The retraining activities consist of having the patient identify objects, shapes, and textures with the vision occluded. If the response is incorrect, the patient is allowed to look at the object and compare its sensation in the normal hand. This is to allow the integration of tactile sensation and vision. Activities such as using textured dominoes or checkers, cut-out shapes, and large to small common objects that may be hidden in rice or lentils may be helpful. Training with these objects is carried out three or four times a day for ¾ of an hour. The training periods are alternated with periods of general bilateral activity such as pottery, bread-kneading, weaving, and macramé. The patient is encouraged to use the affected hand in bilateral activities and to compare the feelings of the tools and materials as compared in the affected hand with those in the unaffected hand.[22]

A program of sensory reeducation following nerve injury was described by La Croix and Helman.[17] The purpose of the program is to help the patient correctly interpret different sensory impulses. A series of graded stimuli is used in treatment such as constant pressure, movement, light touch, and vibration. The least stressful stimuli are presented first. The patient does the training exercises several times a day for short periods. The exercises are done on the unaffected side and then on the affected side, with the aid of vision and then with vision occluded. Areas of hypersensitivity are noted. Sensory stimulation such as stroking, deep pressure, rubbing and maintained touch, using different textures and shapes, are used to reduce hypersensitivity.[17]

Sensory reeducation for PNS disorders focuses on applying graded stimuli according to the progression of nerve recovery. Sensory stimuli such as touch localization, moving touch, and constant touch are followed by exercises for tactile discrimination of shape, size, texture, and object identification. Intermodal reinforcement through visual, auditory, and tactile senses is an important part of the reeducation program.

REVIEW QUESTIONS

1. Why is sensory and perceptual evaluation necessary and important to occupational therapy?
2. What types of disabilities should be routinely given sensory evaluation?
3. Describe how light touch sensitivity is evaluated.
4. If the patient recognizes that he or she was touched but cannot localize the stimulus, what grade would be given on the test for light touch?
5. What are the alternatives for responses in the position sense test?
6. Why is it important to grasp the fingers and wrist laterally during the test for position sense?
7. What are some methods for occluding the patient's vision? What are the alternatives to blindfolding or asking the patient to keep eyes closed?
8. Define "stereognosis," and describe how it can be evaluated.
9. Describe two methods for testing thermal sensation.
10. How are olfactory and gustatory sensations related?
11. What is the functional significance of olfactory sensation?
12. Define graphesthesia and paresthesia.
13. Discuss two approaches to the treatment of sensory dysfunction and the purposes of each.
14. Describe one approach to sensory reeducation for the patient with CNS dysfunction and one for the patient with PNS dysfunction.
15. What is the neurophysiological principle on which sensory education for PNS dysfunction is based?

REFERENCES

1. Ayres AJ: Sensory integration and learning disorders, Los Angeles, 1972, Western Psychological Services.
2. Benton AL and Schultz LM: Observations of tactual form perception (stereognosis) in preschool children, J. Clin. Psychol. 5:359, 1949.
3. Bickerstaff ER: Neurological examination in clinical practice, ed 3, London, 1973, Blackwell Scientific Publications, Ltd.
4. Callahan AD: Sensibility testing: clinical methods. In Hunter JM, et al, editors: Rehabilitation of the hand, ed 2, St Louis, 1984, CV Mosby Co.
5. Callahan AD: Methods of compensation and reeducation for sensory dysfunction. In Hunter JM, et al editors: Rehabilitation of the hand, ed 2, St Louis, 1984, CV Mosby Co.
6. Chusid JG: Correlative neuroanatomy and functional neurology, ed 19, Los Altos, CA, 1985, Lange Medical Publications.
7. De Jong R: The neurologic examination, New York, 1958, Paul B Hoeber, Inc.
8. Dellon AL: Evaluation of sensibility and re-education of sensation in the hand, Baltimore, 1981, Williams and Wilkins.
9. De Myer W: Technique of the neurologic examination: a programmed text, ed 2, New York, 1974, McGraw-Hill Book Co.
10. Eggers O: Occupational therapy in the treatment of adult hemiplegia, Rockville, MD, 1984, Aspen Systems Corp.
11. Farber SD: Neurorehabilitation, a multisensory approach, Philadelphia, 1982, WB Saunders Co.
12. Ferreri JA: Intensive stereognostic training, Am J Occup Ther 16:3(141), 1962.
13. Fox JVD: Cutaneous stimulation, Am J Occup Ther, 18:2(53), 1964.
14. Gilroy J and Meyer JS: Medical neurology, London, 1969, The Macmillian Co.
15. Head H, et al: Studies in neurology, London, 1920, Oxford University Press.
16. Kent BE: Sensory-motor testing: the upper limb of adult patients with hemiplegia, Phys Ther J Am Phys Ther Assoc, 45:550, 1965.
17. La Croix E and Helman J: Upper extremity orthopedics. In Logigian MK, editor: Adult rehabilitation: a team approach for therapists, Boston, 1982, Little, Brown & Co.
18. Mayo Clinic and Mayo Foundation: Clinical examinations in neurology, Philadelphia, 1981, WB Saunders Co.
19. Occupational Therapy Department, Rancho Los Amigos Hospital: Upper extremity sensory evaluation: a manual for occupational therapists, Downey, CA, 1985.
20. Ruskin A: Understanding stroke and its treatment. In Ruskin A, editor: Current therapy in physiatry, Philadelphia, 1984, WB Saunders Co.
21. Silverman EH and Elfant IL: Dysphagia: an evaluation and treatment program for the adult, Am J Occup Ther 33:382, 1979.
22. Turner A: The practice of occupational therapy, ed 2, New York, 1987, Churchill Livingstone.
23. Vinograd A, Taylor E, and Grossman S: Sensory retraining of the hemiplegic hand, Am J Occup Ther 16:246, 1962.
24. Werner JL and Omer GE: Evaluating cutaneous pressure sensation of the hand, Am J Occup Ther 24:347, 1970.
25. Wynn Parry CB: Rehabilitation of the hand, London, 1981, Butterworths.

12 Evaluation of visual, perceptual, and perceptual motor deficits

BARBARA ZOLTAN

Perception can be viewed as an individual's awareness of experiences and objects within the environment. This awareness, developed through the registration and integration of sensations, serves as a foundation for higher level cognitive skills, which are described in Chapter 13. Components of the overall concept of perception include auditory perception, visual perception, and sensory perception. The material presented in this chapter deals solely with visual, visual perceptual, and perceptual motor dysfunction. Deficit areas are defined, along with sample evaluation procedures and general principles of evaluation and treatment.

GENERAL PRINCIPLES OF EVALUATION

Prior to the administration of the visual or perceptual evaluation, the therapist must have a clear understanding of the patient's sensory, language, and motor picture as well as the overall level of awareness. All of these areas will affect the patient's performance on the perceptual evaluation and must be considered in the interpretation of results. The evaluation of visual, perceptual, and perceptual motor dysfunction should follow a hierarchy of testing. Vision, for example, is an intricate process that both contributes and leads to the development of visual perception and, therefore, should be evaluated first. Motor planning, or praxis, serves as a foundation for the development of an individual's body scheme and affects the patient's performance on any test items with a motor component. Thus praxis should be evaluated prior to the evaluation of body scheme and higher level visual discrimination skills.

The patient's age and premorbid status should be considered in the interpretation of performance in perceptual testing. For example, the majority of patients who have sustained a cerebral vascular accident (CVA) will also be elderly. Numerous changes in visual, auditory, perceptual, and cognitive functions are associated with the natural aging process. Similarly, many head injured patients have documented perceptual problems, learning problems, or both prior to the sustained head injury. In order to accurately interpret test results and establish realistic treatment goals, the therapist should have a clear picture of the patient's premorbid status. If the patient is unable to supply the necessary information, family, friends, and educators should be consulted.

VISUAL DEFICITS

Visual system dysfunction can range from acuity or binocular deficits to attentional or oculomotor problems. The majority of patients with visual deficits have sustained brain damage and are unaware of a visual sensory loss and, therefore, visual problems may go undiagnosed or unrecognized.[23] Alternatively, a referral is made to an ophthalmologist who performs a physiological evaluation rather than an examination of the function of the entire visual system.[21] The occupational therapist, working in conjunction with the optometrist, should assess the integrity of the visual system. The primary areas of specific assessment performed by the optometrist are acuity, binocularity, eye health, strabismus, field of vision, and oculomotor function. The occupational therapist should perform specific clinical assessments of visual attention, pursuits and saccades, visual fields, visual neglect or imperception, and depth of vision. In addition, clinical observation of acuity problems, double vision, and nystagmus during functional tasks such as reading, driving, or writing should be noted and communicated to the optometrist prior to the evaluation.[22] A checklist of vision problems can be used to assist in clinical observation (Fig. 12-1).

Evaluation of Visual Deficits

ACUITY. It is the role of the optometrist, ophthalmologist, or vision specialist to perform a comprehensive evaluation of acuity. If, however, these specialists are inaccessible or unavailable to the patient, an acuity screening by the occupational therapist may be indicated. The visual assessment should begin with distance and near acuities testing because the patient's acuity status will impact on the results of subsequent tests.[18] An acuity measurement of 20/20 is normal, and a measurement of 20/40 is required for a valid

CHECKLIST: Vision Problems

Name _____ Date _____ Therapist _____

Rating Codes: Typ = typical pattern
Obs = observed
NO = not observed
IO = insufficient opportunity to observe

	Typ	Obs	NO	IO
1. APPEARANCE OF EYES:				
One eye turns in or out at any time	—	—	—	—
Reddened eyes or lids	—	—	—	—
Eyes tear excessively	—	—	—	—
Encrusted eyelids	—	—	—	—
Frequent styes on lids	—	—	—	—
2. COMPLAINTS WHEN USING EYES FOR CLOSE WORK:				
Headaches in forehead or temples	—	—	—	—
Burning or itching after reading or close work	—	—	—	—
Nausea or dizziness	—	—	—	—
Print blurs after reading a short time	—	—	—	—
3. BEHAVIORAL SIGNS OF VISUAL PROBLEMS:				
A. *Eye Movement Abilities (Ocular Motility):*				
Head turns while scanning, e.g. as reads across page	—	—	—	—
Loses place often during reading	—	—	—	—
Needs finger or marker to keep place	—	—	—	—
Displays short attention span, e.g. in reading or copying	—	—	—	—
Too frequently omits words	—	—	—	—
Repeatedly omits "small" words	—	—	—	—
Writes up or down hill on paper	—	—	—	—
Rereads or skips lines unknowingly	—	—	—	—
Orients drawings poorly on page	—	—	—	—
B. *Eye Teaming Abilities (Binocularity):*				
Complains of seeing double (diplopia)	—	—	—	—
Repeats letters within words	—	—	—	—
Omits letters, numbers or phrases	—	—	—	—
Misaligns digits in number columns	—	—	—	—
Squints, closes or covers one eye	—	—	—	—
Tilts head extremely while doing close work	—	—	—	—
Consistently shows gross postural deviations in close work activities	—	—	—	—
C. *Eye-Hand Coordination Abilities:*				
Must feel things to assist in any interpretation required	—	—	—	—
Eyes not used to "steer" hand movements (extreme lack of orientation, placement of words or drawings on page)	—	—	—	—
Writes crookedly, poorly spaced, cannot stay on ruled lines	—	—	—	—
Misaligns both horizontal and vertical series of numbers	—	—	—	—
Uses his hands or fingers to keep his place on the page	—	—	—	—
Uses other hand as "spacer" to control spacing or alignment on page				
Repeatedly confuses left-right directions	—	—	—	—
D. *Visual Form Perception (Visual Comparison, Visual Imagery, Visualization)*				
Mistakes words with same or similar beginnings	—	—	—	—
Fails to recognize same word in next sentence	—	—	—	—
Reverses letters and/or words in writing and copying	—	—	—	—
Confuses likenesses and minor differences	—	—	—	—

Fig. 12-1. Behavioral checklist of symptoms of visual system dysfunction.

Continued.

Confuses same word in same sentence   — — — —
Repeatedly confuses similar beginnings and endings of words   — — — —
Fails to visualize what is read either silently or orally   — — — —
Whispers to self for reinforcement while reading silently   — — — —
Returns to "drawing with fingers" to decide likes and differences

E. *Refractive Status (Nearsightedness, Farsightedness, Focus Problems, etc.)*

Comprehension reduces as reading continues; loses interest too quickly   — — — —

Mispronounces similar words as reading continues   — — — —

Blinks excessively at near vision tasks (i.e., reading) and not elsewhere   — — — —

Holds book too closely; face too close to desk surface/computer screen   — — — —

Avoids near-point tasks or close up work   — — — —

Complains of discomfort in tasks that demand visual interpretation   — — — —

Closes, covers, or squints one eye while reading or doing close work   — — — —

Makes errors in copying information from the distance to paper (e.g., copying a sign from the wall)   — — — —

Makes errors copying from reference book to notebook   — — — —

Squints (e.g., to read signs on the wall) or requests to move nearer   — — — —

Rubs eyes during or after short periods of visual activity   — — — —

Fatigues easily; after doing close work blinks to clarify distance information (e.g., sign on the wall)   — — — —

OBSERVER'S COMMENTS

Fig. 12-1, cont'd. Behavioral checklist of symptoms of visual system dysfunction. Reproduced with permission. Gianutsos R and Ramsey G: Enabling rehabilitation optometrists to help survivors of acquired brain injury, J Vision Rehabil 2(1)37: 1988.

day and night driver's license. The patient should wear glasses during testing, if normally worn. Distance acuity testing requires the use of a distance acuity chart, occluder, tape measure, and corrective lenses, if normally used.[18] Near acuity testing requires a near point test and occluder and corrective lenses, if necessary.[18] For specific testing procedures, the reader is referred to the references.[18]

An established distance acuity deficit will affect the patient's spatial judgments, depth perception, and facial recognition. Decreased near vision will affect all functional activities requiring near vision such as reading and writing. If either problem is suspected by the occupational therapist, a referral to the optometrist should be made for corrective lenses and visual retraining as appropriate.

GROSS VISUAL SKILLS. Elements included in the evaluation of gross visual skills are attention, oculomotor skills (scanning and convergence), saccadic eye movements, visual fields, and visual neglect or imperception. The inability to visually attend, a voluntary function for the normal adult, may occur as an isolated deficit or in association with a spatial or body neglect or inattention. The patient who has sustained frontal lobe damage is likely to have difficulty obtaining and sustaining fixation.[39] Visual attention can be evaluated simply by asking the patient to look at a bright object for approximately 20 seconds. In addition, the therapist should observe for the patient's attentional abilities during functional activities. Oculomotor skills consist of visual scanning or pursuits, saccadic eye movements, and convergence. Visual scanning deficits can range from decreased conjugate eye movements to ocular disorders in all planes of movement, depending on the lesion site.[5] All six muscles that move the eye, therefore, should be tested as follows:

***Direction of gaze*[13]**
MUSCLES TESTED: Superior, inferior, medial, and lateral rectus muscles and superior and inferior oblique muscles
DIRECTIONS: The patient is asked to look to one side and then the other without moving the head. When the patient is looking to one side, he or she is then asked to look up and down. This same sequence is repeated on the other side.

Alternatively, ocular pursuit skills can be evaluated by having the patient follow with his eyes a bright object or ball that the therapist moves in all directions. No matter which test is used, the therapist observes for jerky or incomplete movements and signs of nystagmus. Saccadic eye movements are rapid sequenced eye movements that refer to the patient's ability to localize stimuli.[42] Saccadic eye movements can be observed in function primarily through reading skills. In addition, tools such as the King-Devick Test and a clinical test requiring gaze shifting on command between two objects can be used.[18,28] No matter which test is used, the therapist observes for consistency and accuracy and overshooting or undershooting the target. Treatment of impaired saccadic eye movements can include functional, table top, and movement-based or sensory integrative techniques.

Convergence involves the process of directing the visual axis of the two eyes to a near point. Convergence can be evaluated clinically by asking the patient to watch a ball or bright object as the therapist moves it in closer to the patient's face.[18,41]

Visual field deficits will vary, depending on the size and location of the brain lesion, and may be seen in isolation or accompanied by a visual neglect or imperception.[27] Visual field deficits are evaluated through confrontation testing.[16,36] During confrontation testing, the examiner and patient sit opposite each other and the patient is asked to fixate on the examiner's nose. The examiner alternately brings a target forward from the right or left periphery. The patient is instructed to state when and where one or both targets are seen.

General Principles of Treatment

Treatment of visual deficits should follow a structured sequence. Visual attention, for example, should be treated before higher level skills. Oculomotor therapy should start at the monocular level, or one eye at a time, progressing to the biocular level and finally to the binocular level.[31] The use of tactile feedback by the hand to assist tracking is recommended as needed initially, progressing to the more dominant eye.[31] Treatment of specific deficit areas can range from prisms or lenses to clinical exercises, depending on the identified problem.[14,31] Clinical exercises may include the use of worksheets with the adaptive techniques of anchoring or pacing to Marsden Ball training (patient identifies letters on a suspended ball as it comes into vision) or use of alphabet pencils (patient calls out letters that are written on two pencils held 12 inches apart).[17,31] Many clinicians also use computer programs specifically designed for visual retraining.[27] In addition to these specific techniques, the occupational therapist incorporates the remediation of visual deficits into the functional approach.

No matter what approach or technique is used, the occupational therapist should have ongoing communication with the optometrist and other team members relative to the patient's progress.

APRAXIA

Apraxia is an inability to perform purposeful movement even though there is no loss of motor power, sensation, or coordination.[27] Included in the category of praxis is ideational and ideomotor praxis, constructional praxis, verbal praxis, and dressing praxis. Any one or a combination of motor planning deficits can be seen in an individual patient. Because all aspects of activities of daily living (ADL) require the effective planning and carrying out of skilled purposeful movement, the apraxic patient is faced with a frustrating and devastating residual deficit of brain injury.

Clinical Evaluation of Apraxia

IDEOMOTOR AND IDEATIONAL APRAXIA. Full test batteries of ideational and ideomotor apraxia have been developed by Brown, Goodglass and Kaplan, and Solet.[11,24,35] Each of these evaluations differentiates praxis abilities with certan body parts (that is, buccal-facial, unilateral limb, bilateral limb, and total body movements) and by level of concreteness (that is, command, imitation, object usage, nonrepresentational movements, and so on). In addition, many occupational therapists use the Imitation of Postures Subtest of the Southern California Sensory Integration Test with adults. Fig. 12-2 describes a sample praxis evaluation developed at Santa Clara Valley Medical Center.[41] This screening evaluation, which has established interrater reliability with head injury patients (r = 0.99), is used as an indicator for the need of a more complete praxis evaluation.

CONSTRUCTIONAL APRAXIA. Constructional apraxia is the inability to copy, draw, or construct a design, whether on command or spontaneously.[42] Research has demonstrated its strong correlation with body scheme, dressing, daily living skills, and the ability to use objects purposefully.[6,25,29,38] Traditional tests of constructional praxis have included paper and pencil tasks, matchstick designs, and block designs.[8,9,24,37,42] Recent research, however, has identified a strong correlation between matchstick and block designs, indicating that the use of both tests is unnecessary duplication.[5,6]

DRESSING APRAXIA. Dressing apraxia, or the inability to dress oneself, has been linked with problems of spatial orientation, constructional apraxia, spatial dysgraphia, dyslexia, and dyscalculia.[32] Clinically, the patient may have difficulty initiating dressing or may make errors in orientation by putting the clothes on the wrong side of the body, upside down, or inside out.[2]

PRAXIS (MOTOR PLANNING)

Procedure:

The examiner sits directly in front of the patient. The examiner asks the patient to demonstrate or copy actions in the following sequence. First the examiner asks the patient to demonstrate each verbal command listed below. If the patient is unable to perform the action, the examiner demonstrates the action and asks the patient to imitate it. After all items are completed to command and imitation, items 1 through 5 are repeated with the examiner asking the patient to use the real object.

Time: 10 seconds for each item (the examiner times the patient from the start of the gesture to the end of the gesture).

Directions:

"I AM GOING TO ASK YOU TO TRY SOME DIFFERENT ACTIONS. IN SOME OF THEM, I WILL ASK YOU TO DEMONSTRATE OR COPY MY MOVEMENTS, AND IN SOME I WILL ASK YOU TO USE OBJECTS."

To Command:

1. "SHOW ME HOW YOU BLOW OUT A MATCH."
2. "SHOW ME HOW YOU DRINK A GLASS OF WATER."
3. "SHOW ME HOW YOU BRUSH YOUR TEETH WITH A TOOTHBRUSH."
4. "SHOW ME HOW YOU CUT PAPER WITH SCISSORS."
5. "SHOW ME HOW YOU THROW A BALL."
6. "SHOW ME HOW YOU SALUTE."
7. "SHOW ME HOW YOU WASH YOUR HANDS."
8. "SHOW ME HOW YOU ACT LIKE A BOXER."

To imitations: The examiner carries out the actions for each test item stating "I AM BLOWING OUT A MATCH, NOW YOU SHOW ME HOW YOU . . .

With the object: The examiner presents the real object for items 1-5 and states "SHOW ME HOW YOU . . ."

Note: During this portion of the test, the examiner should insure the patient's safe handling of the objects. For bilateral tasks (command 4), the examiner may assist by holding the paper.

Observe for:
1.   type of apraxia indicated

Test Item	Apraxia
1. Blowing out match	Buccal-facial
2. Drinking from glass	Buccal-facial
	Unilateral limb kinetic
3. Brushing teeth	Buccal-facial
	Unilateral limb kinetic
4. Cutting with scissors	Unilateral limb kinetic
5. Throwing a ball	Unilateral or bilateral limb kinetic
6. Saluting	Cultural apraxia
	Unilateral limb kinetic
7. Washing hands	Bilateral limb kinetic
8. Boxing	Bilateral limb kinetic

2. use of body part as the object (BPO).
3. performance in the correct place of movement (PLM)
4. which body parts the patient uses to carry out verbal/imitation commands?

Fig. 12-2. Praxis (motor planning). Reproduced with permission. Zoltan B et al: Perceptual motor evaluation for head injured and other neurologically impaired adults, rev ed, San Jose, Calif, 1987, Santa Clara Valley Medical Center.

Continued.

5. which movements are easier toward or away from the body?
6. differences in performance: unilateral vs. bilateral, objects vs. no object, veral vs. imitation?

Scale

Rate each item separately:
3—Unable to perform—unable to attempt response
2—Severely impaired—poor approximation of accurate response, uses trial and error and response is greater than allotted time
1—Impaired—able to approximate accurate response for majority of the task, quality of response is compromised or response is greater than allotted time
0—Intact—response is accurate and within allotted time

Fig. 12-2, cont'd. Praxis (motor planning).

General Principles of Treatment

Understanding the underlying mechanisms and pinpointing where there is a breakdown in a particular action or task is crucial to the effective treatment of apraxia.[32] Activity analysis will, for example, identify not only that a patient is unable to put on his pants but also when and how performance breaks down. Additional task analysis for other motor planning deficits will identify which deficits generalize to several functional areas. For example, the patient may have difficulty manipulating objects in certain planes of movement no matter what the task.[40] Several treatment approaches have been proven successful for the treatment of the apraxic patient. The transfer of training approach is widely used for constructional problems. A functional approach combined with a tactilely based or neurodevelopmental approach is effective for the patient with dressing apraxia. Although there may be occasions when a single approach is indicated, more often a combination of techniques or approaches is most effective.[6]

BODY SCHEME

An individual's body scheme is a postural model related to how one perceives the position of the body and the relationship of the body parts.[5] It is an individual's body scheme that is considered to be the foundation for future skills in the perception of environmental space.[41] Body scheme disorders are associated with parietal lobe damage and can include somatognosia, unilateral neglect, impaired right/left discrimination, and finger agnosia.[1,15,16,33,42]

Somatognosia is usually evaluated by having the patient point to body parts on command and/or by imitation.[30,34,41,42] In addition, many clinicians use the draw-a-person test and body and face puzzles.[30,41,42] The clinician, however, must rule out constructional deficits as the cause of poor performance for these tests.

Right/left discrimination deficits can occur in extrapersonal space, intrapersonal space, or body scheme-related disorientation. Right/left discrimination deficits can be seen in isolation or linked with acalculia, finger agnosia, and writing disability, to form Gerstmann's Syndrome.[41] The most basic testing of right/left discrimination abilities is to have the patient point to a lateral body part on his or her body or, on a more advanced level, identify body parts on the examiner.[10]

Unilateral neglect relates to the inability to integrate perceptions from the left side of the body or the left side of the environment.[42] The patient may exhibit a body neglect with or without associated visual and sensory impairments. The evaluation of unilateral neglect is often done through table top tasks such as body or face puzzles, scanning worksheets, or the draw-a-person test.[41] When using these tests, however, deficits such as constructional apraxia and/or visual field deficits must be ruled out as causes of poor performance. The most effective evaluation of unilateral neglect as it relates to a body scheme disorder is direct observation during dressing and other ADL.

The patient with finger agnosia will have difficulty naming fingers on command or identifying which finger has been touched.[25] The evaluation of finger agnosia is accomplished through finger localization, or naming on command, or having the patient imitate finger movements made by the therapist.[30,34]

General Treatment Principles

The treatment of body scheme disorders can include a sensorimotor, transfer of training, functional, or neurodevelopmental approach or a combination of these. Unilateral body neglect, for example, can be treated by applied sensory input (rubbing patient's arm or leg) prior to dressing. Alternatively, bilateral weight-bearing with handling techniques (neurodevelopmental approach) can be used to facilitate total body awareness.[42] Finally, a repetitive functional approach with cuing can be effective for the patient with a body neglect.

VISUAL DISCRIMINATION SKILLS

Visual discrimination skills include form perception, depth perception, figure-ground perception, and perception of position in space.

Form Perception

Form perception relates to the ability to differentiate between different forms. The evaluation of form constancy or perception can include table top tasks such as the Frostig Form Constancy Test in which the patient is required to trace circles and squares on a page of similar shapes.[19] A popular and universally accepted method of evaluation is through the use of form boards.[7,41] The treatment of form constancy deficits can include the transfer of training and functional approaches. The use of computer activities that focus on form discrimination can also be effective.[42]

Depth Perception

Depth perception (stereopsis) involves the ability to use visual cues to determine the distance of objects from each other and from the individual. Difficulties in depth perception can result from both brain stem and cortical damage.[41] The evaluation of depth perception can include stereograms (pictures representing objects with the impression of solidity) or basic functional tests.[26,42] Treatment of depth perception can be accomplished through a functional approach, clinical visual retraining approach, or both. The patient and family are also educated regarding potential functional safety problems such as managing stairs.

Figure/Ground Perception

Figure/ground perception is the ability to distinguish between foreground and background. The patient with parietal lobe dysfunction or a large lesion anywhere in the brain is likely to have difficulty with figure/ground perception.[3] This deficit is generally tested by hidden geometric figures, ambiguous figures on embedded or hidden pictures.[16] One of the most effective figure/ground tests used by occupational therapists is the Ayres Figure-Ground Test.[4] Although initially designed for use with children, recent research has indicated that it can be a useful, reliable tool with adults suffering from brain damage.[5] In addition to the administration of embedded picture tests, the occupational therapist should evaluate figure/ground perception functionally. The therapist should observe whether the patient has difficulty with tasks such as retrieving an item from a cluttered drawer or grocery store shelf.

The transfer of training and functional approaches can be used to treat a figure/ground deficit. The patient can be taught to compensate for the problem through systematic scanning, and the environment can be adapted, that is, kept uncluttered.

Position in Space

The perception of position in space is the ability to perceive the position of two or more objects in relation to one another and to self.[20] The patient with poor position-in-space perception will have difficulty with concepts such as up-down, in-out, and front-behind.[42] The evaluation of position in space is accomplished through placement or positioning of objects or blocks or through the use of geometric figures.[4,12,42] The position-in-space subtest of the Southern California Sensory Integration Tests, although originally designed for use with children, is commonly used with adults. Interrater reliability for this test has been established with adult patients with head trauma.[5] Treatment of position-in-space deficits can include table top activities requiring the patient to discriminate different orientations, a functional approach, or both.

SUMMARY

Visual, visual perceptual, and perceptual motor deficits will affect the patient's overall function. Problems will vary in intensity and diversity depending on the patient's diagnosis and area of brain damage. A systematic comprehensive evaluation of these areas, therefore, is crucial to the patient reaching his or her highest functional potential. The information provided in this chapter is meant to be an overview of the evaluation of key deficit areas. The reader should seek additional resources for specific evaluation techniques and procedures.

REVIEW QUESTIONS

1. Which should be evaluated first, praxis or body scheme? Why?
2. List seven behavioral signs of visual problems.
3. What are the areas included in a gross visual skills evaluation?
4. Define apraxia.
5. List and define the four potential areas of a body scheme disorder.
6. How can figure/ground perception affect function?
7. How do you test for a position-in-space deficit?

REFERENCES

1. Anderson E and Choy E: Parietal lobe syndromes in hemiplegia: a program for treatment, Am J Occup Ther 24(1):13, 1970.
2. Archibald YM and Wepman JM: Language disturbance and non-verbal cognitive performance in eight patients following injury to the right hemisphere, Brain 91:117, 1968.
3. Ayres AJ: Sensory integration and learning disorders, Los An-

geles, 1980, Western Psychological Services.

4. Ayres AJ: Southern California sensory integration tests, Los Angeles, 1972, Western Psychological Services.

5. Baum B: The establishment of reliability and validity of a perceptual evaluation on a sample of adult head trauma patients, thesis, University of Southern California, December 1981.

6. Baum B and Hall K: Relationship between constructional praxis and dressing in the head injured adult, Am J Occup Ther 35(7):438, 1981.

7. Bender M and Feldman M: The so-called "visual agnosias," Brain 95:173, 1972.

8. Benton A: Revised visual retention test, New York, 1974, Psychological Corporation.

9. Benton AL and Fogel ML: Three-dimensional constructional praxis: a clinical test, Arch Neurol 7:347, 1962.

10. Boone P and Landes B: Right-left discrimination in hemiplegic patients, Arch Phys Med Rehabil 49:533, 1968.

11. Brown J: Aphasia, apraxia, agnosia, Springfield, Ill, 1972, Thomas Publishers.

12. Butters N and Barton M: Effect of parietal lobe damage on the performance of reversible operations in space, Neuropsychologia 8:205, 1970.

13. Chusid JG: Correlative neuroanatomy and functional neurology, 19 ed, Los Altos, California, 1985, Lange Medical Publications.

14. Cohen AH and Soden R: An optometric approach to the rehabilitation of the stroke patient, Am Optom Assoc 52(9), September 1981.

15. Critchley M: The parietal lobes, London, 1953, Edward Arnold Co.

16. DeRenzi E and Scotti G: Autopagnosia: fiction or reality, Arch Neurol 23:221, 1970.

17. Diller L and Gordon W: Interventions for cognitive deficits in brain-injured adults, J Consult Clin Psychol 49(6):822, 1981.

18. Efferson L: Vision screening test manual, IHC Rehabilitation Services, rev ed, March 1987.

19. Frostig M: Developmental test of visual perception, Palo Alto, 1966, Consulting Psychologists Press.

20. Frostig M and Horne D: Frostig program for the development of visual perception, rev ed, Chicago, 1973, Follett Publishing Co.

21. Gianutsos R and Matheson P: The rehabilitation of visual perceptual disorders attributable to brain injury. In Meier MJ, Benton AL, and Diller L, editors: Neuropsychological rehabilitation, New York, 1987, Churchill Livingstone.

22. Gianutsos R and Ramsey G: Enabling rehabilitation optometrists to help survivors of acquired brain injury, J Vision Rehabil 2(1):37, 1988.

23. Gianutsos R, Ramsey G, and Perlin R: Rehabilitative optometric services for survivors of traumatic brain injury, Arch Phys Med Rehabil, 1988.

24. Goodglass H and Kaplan E: Assessment of aphasia and related disorders, ed 2, Philadelphia, 1972, Thomas Publishers.

25. Gregory ME and Aitkin JA: Assessment of parietal lobe function in hemiplegia, Occup Ther 34:9, 1971.

26. Instructo-Clinic: a psychophysical testing apparatus, Bumpa-Tel, Inc, PO Box 611, Cape Gir, MO.

27. Kadet TS: Visual rehabilitation in traumatic brain injury. Paper presented at the National Head Injury Foundation 6th Annual National Symposium, December 1987.

28. Lieberman S, Cohen AH, and Rubin J: NYSOA K-D test, J Am Optom Assoc 54(7):631, 1983.

29. Lorenze EJ and Cancro R: Dysfunction in visual perception with hemiplegia, its relationship to activities of daily living, Arch Phys Med Rehabil 43:514, 1962.

30. Macdonald J: An investigation of body scheme in adults with cerebral vascular accident, Am J Occup Ther 14:72, 1960.

31. Maino DM: Out of office oculomotor and hand-eye therapy, Cognitive Rehabil, November/December 1986.

32. Miller N: Dyspraxia and its management, Rockville, Md, 1986, Aspen Publishers.

33. Mountcastle VB: The view from within: pathways to the study of perception, Johns Hopkins Med J, 136:109, 1975.

34. Sauget J, Benton AL, and Hacaen H: Disturbances of the body scheme in relation to language impairment and hemispheric locus of lesion, J Neurol Neurosurg Psychiat 34:496, 1971.

35. Solet J: The Solet test for apraxia, Copyright by author, 1975.

36. Wall N, et al: Hemiplegic evaluation, Boston, 1979, Spaulding Rehabilitation Hospital.

37. Warrington E, James M, and Kinsborne M: Drawing ability in relation to laterality of lesion, Brain 89:53, 1966.

38. Williams N: Correlations between copying ability and dressing activities in hemiplegia, Am J Phys Med 46:1332, 1967.

39. Young F: Early experience and visual information processing in perceptual and reading disorders, Washington, DC, 1970, National Academy of Sciences.

40. Zoltan B: Remediation of visual, perceptual and perceptual motor deficits, ed 2, Philadelphia, 1989, FA Davis Co.

41. Zoltan B, et al: Perceptual motor evaluation for head injured and other neurologically impaired adults, rev ed, San Jose, Ca, 1987, Santa Clara Valley Medical Center.

42. Zoltan B, Siev E, and Freishtat B: Perceptual and cognitive dysfunction in the adult stroke patient, ed 2, Thorofare, N.J., 1986, Charles B Slack, Inc.

13 Evaluation and treatment of cognitive dysfunction

BARBARA ZOLTAN

Cognitive deficits are perhaps the most devastating residual problems following a cerebral vascular accident (CVA), traumatic head injury, or acquired disease resulting in brain damage. Although many clinicians tend to think of "cognitive/perceptual" deficits as a single entity, a more accurate analysis necessitates separation of these areas. As described in Chapter 12, perception can be viewed as an awareness of environmental objects and experiences developed through both physical sensations and mental processes. Cognition, on the other hand, includes the skills of understanding and knowing, the ability to judge and make decisions, and an overall general environmental awareness.[9] Cognition allows individuals to use and process the information perceived in order to think and act.

The identification and clinical evaluation of discrete cognitive deficits are far from easy to make and are somewhat arbitrary. Deficit areas are rarely seen in isolation, and the interpretation of a patient's behavior is difficult at best. There are, however, several categories of cognitive deficits that can and should be identified and treated by the occupational therapist along with other allied health professionals. These areas include attention, memory, initiation, planning and organization, mental flexibility, abstraction, insight, problem solving, and calculation abilities. The material in this chapter outlines the evaluation of these deficit areas and related theoretical principles and gives a description of additional factors that influence cognitive function and treatment application.

UNDERLYING PRINCIPLES OF COGNITIVE EVALUATION

Several theoretical principles should be incorporated into the administration and interpretation of the clinical cognitive evaluation. First, cognition should always be seen in relation to other potential deficit areas. Intact cognitive processes and skills are dependent on the integrity of the patient's sensory, language, visual, and perceptual systems. For example, the patient may be unable to attend to and concentrate on a particular task primarily caused by an underlying deficit in visual scanning. Because of this interrelationship, it is crucial that the occupational therapist administer the sensory, visual, and perceptual evaluations prior to initiating cognitive testing. In addition, communication with the speech pathologist concerning the patient's language and auditory abilities is essential. Without prior knowledge of all these areas, interpretation of the cognitive evaluation will be inaccurate and invalid. The therapist should always look at the total picture when interpreting patient behavior.

A second principle of testing relates to environment. The testing environment will influence the results of the cognitive evaluation. The concept of environment includes not only the physical features to time of day but also the amount of structure and feedback provided by the examiner. For example, the patient's ability to attend to tasks may be very different early in the morning while lying in bed compared with taking a structured test while in a wheelchair with cuing provided by the examiner. Controversy among health team members over the patient's cognitive status often occurs when, in fact, discrepancies are merely the result of environmental differences in the administration of testing. Instead of being alarmed by these differences in test results, the more constructive approach is to analyze and use the information in designing the most effective remediation plan.

The final principle of cognitive evaluation relates to the patient with brain damage who is also elderly. Research has clearly identified normal age-related problems with memory, abstraction and mental flexibility, and problem-solving ability.[1,2,13,14,17] In addition, research has indicated that the elderly are more easily distracted than younger individuals.[12] It is therefore crucial that before testing the elderly patient with brain damage, the therapist have a clear picture of the patient's premorbid cognitive functioning. This information can usually be provided by the patient's family and friends.

Specific Deficit Evaluation

Just as cognitive function is interdependent with clinical areas such as perception and sensation, specific cognitive skills are also interdependent. For example, an individual will be unable to display effective problem-solving skills when he or she cannot attend to or remember a particular task. It is therefore indicated that a specific progression of testing be followed that reflects a hierarchy of cognitive skills. Following is the recommended progression of testing.

ATTENTION. Attention is an active process that assists the individual in deciding which environmental information and sensations are relevant at a particular time. Attention includes the three components of alertness, selectivity, and effort. Attention, which can be focused or divided, can vary in intensity and duration.[5,13]

The two types of information processing relevant to attention are automatic processing and controlled processing. Automatic processing is used by the individual at a subcortical level, whereas controlled processing is used when new information is being considered.[33] Two disorders—focused attentional deficit and divided attentional deficits—are related to these two types of information processing.[35] A focused attentional deficit occurs when an automatic response is replaced by a controlled response.[33] An example of this deficit familiar to many clinicians is the stroke patient concentrating on trying to walk. A divided attentional deficit, on the other hand, occurs when the function of controlled processing is inadequate for the individual to process all the information required for task completion.[33] This deficit results in the patient becoming "overloaded."

Examples of standardized tests of attention include the Random Letter Test and Digit Repetition Test.[27] (The reader is referred to the references for additional information on these and other standardized tests of attention.[27,35]) The occupational therapist's evaluation of attention should include structural clinical observation and activity analysis during functional tasks. The following are guidelines for this evaluation.

General guidelines for evaluation of attention*

1. Identify the components of attention (for example, alertness, selectivity, effort) that are intact and those that are impaired.
2. Observe the patient in a number of settings and activities at different times during the day. Position changes (lying, sitting) can also affect attention.
3. Establish functional baseline measures. Consider the frequency and severity of the problem. Select relevant functional tasks as the basis for the evaluation and reassessment.

Specific questions to consider and evaluate*

1. Which sensory systems are affected? Visual? Auditory?
2. What are the duration and frequency of the patient's attentional abilities?
3. Under what environmental conditions can the patient attend to a task? When does attention begin to break down?
4. What are some behavioral indications of the patient's inattention?
5. Does the patient have memory problems? Does he or she have problem-solving difficulties? Decreased processing? Are these or related problems caused in part by decreased attention?
6. Are there any tasks or areas that seem to particularly interest the patient and therefore increase his attention?
7. Is processing occurring only at a conscious level compared with a normal combination of automatic and conscious levels?

MEMORY. Memory is a dynamic process that includes several components related to learning and perception.[22] Memory requires environmental input, central nervous system (CNS) change, maintenance of that change, and related behavioral or informational output.[13] The memory process is summarized in Fig. 13-1. There are several types and components of memory that the therapist must understand before beginning a memory evaluation. These components are summarized in Table 13-1. Structured tests that evaluate memory include the Wechsler Memory Scale[30,31] and questionnaires such as the Subjective Memory Questionnaire.[3,30,31] (For detailed information on these tests the reader is referred to references 30, 31, and 35.)

The following are guidelines and questions for structured clinical observation and activity analysis related to memory evaluation.

General guidelines for evaluation*

1. Identify the aspects of memory that are impaired and those that are relatively intact.
2. Observe the patient in a number of settings.
3. Consider the amount of structure versus nonstructure within the environment.
4. Consider the interval between stimulus and recall (that is, immediate, short term, and long term).
5. Establish functional baseline measures. Consider the frequency and severity of the problem as it relates to function. Select relevant functional areas or tasks as the basis for evaluation and reassessment.

---

*From Zoltan B and others: Perceptual and cognitive dysfunction in the adult stroke patient, Thorofare, NJ, 1986, Charles B Slack, Inc.

THE MEMORY PROCESS

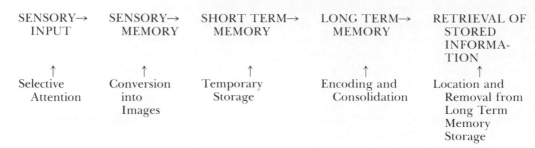

Fig. 13-1. The memory process.

Specific areas and questions to consider and evaluate*

1. Which sensory system is affected? For instance, immediate recall can be tested for different sensory systems as follows[8,29,34]:
   a. *Visual.* The patient is asked to reproduce simple geometric figures that are presented for 5 to 10 seconds and then covered. (Note: If the patient's perceptual abilities are impaired, it is likely that this will affect memory for visual material and the ability to use visually based strategies to assist in memory problems.)
   b. *Kinesthetic.* The patient is asked to reproduce a series of hand positions presented to him or her.[8]
2. Is nonverbal memory impaired? Verbal memory?
3. Is memory loss global or modality-specific?
4. Is it a learning or performance problem? Can the patient improve with practice?
5. Is it a problem of learning new information or recalling old information?
6. Which memory processes are affected? Does the patient have trouble identifying and reproducing (recall versus recognition)?
7. Is it a semantic memory loss? Is it episodic?
8. Does the patient have difficulty with free recall?
9. Does the patient have difficulty with serial learning (that is, remembering sequences)?
10. Does the patient have difficulty with paired associates (that is, remembering relationships)?

INITIATION. Frontal lobe lesions generally result in the residual deficit of poor initiation. Most therapists have little difficulty observing behavioral manifestations often linked with decreased initiation. For example, the patient may demonstrate apathy, indifference, or decreased spontaneity. The patient may also exhibit a slowness of response or absence of initiative. The therapist must remember, however, that similar behaviors may be related to other clinical deficits such as poor comprehension or apraxia. Ongoing close observation and evaluation will ensure correct interpretation of patient behavior.

Initiation can be evaluated through clinical observation and activity analysis as follows:

General guidelines for evaluation*

1. Observe the patient in a number of settings.
2. Consider the amount of structure and cuing required for initiation of activity by the patient.
3. Establish functional baseline measures. Consider the frequency and severity of the problem as it relates to function. Select relevant functional areas or tasks as the basis for evaluation and reassessment.

Specific areas and questions to consider and evaluate*

1. Are there any associated behavioral problems such as flat or blunted affect? Behavioral outbursts? Disinhibition?
2. Is the patient's behavior generally passive? Does he or she respond passively to questions or suggestions?
3. What does the patient do during the day? Does someone have to organize activity for him or her?
4. What, if any, activities can the patient initiate by him or herself without cuing or structure?
5. What cuing method or sensory modality appears to be the most effective? For example, do tactile or kinesthetic cues work better than visual or auditory cues?
6. Is the patient aware that he or she has an initiation problem? Does he or she accept it when it is pointed out?
7. Is an associated attentional or memory problem affecting initiation abilities?

PLANNING AND ORGANIZATION. An additional potential residual problem of frontal lobe damage is the patient's poor ability to plan and organize. This poor planning ability and insufficient organizational skills prevent the patient from achieving a specific goal. Planning and organizational deficits will vary in degree and may involve one or more task components.[10,17] Specific components of planning and or-

Table 13-1 Memory (Types, Description and Associated Lesion Site)

Types and components of memory	Definition and description	Associated lesion site
1. Recognition	A factor inherent in recall; a primitive memory function that serves to alert one to the surroundings by focusing shifting attention	Thalamus
2. Iconic	Sensory memory; the initial processing of the information after the input sensation has been received by sense organs	Predominantly a retinal phenomenon mediated by rod vision
3. Short term (also called immediate, primary span, short term store, recent)	Length is only 20 to 40 seconds; 5 to 10 items can be held in short-term memory; retention span of events, objects, or ideas in immediate awareness constitutes consciousness, since people are aware of cognitive processes that are not automatic	Frontal lobe: Verbal—left hemisphere Nonverbal—right hemisphere
4. Long term (also called secondary, delayed, distant)	Represents permanent record of learned material; has three stages—consolidation, storage, and retrieval of stored memory	
a. Consolidation	Involves transfer of material into long-term memory and its consolidation; strengthens memory trace to facilitate permanence; material is coded during the transfer process	Hippocampus: Verbal—left hippocampus Nonverbal—right hippocampus Limbic system (thalamus)
b. Storage	Relatively permanent storage of materials that have been consolidated; two categories of long term memory storage are: 1. Episodic-information related to events with temporal and spatial components (when and where)	Lateral surface of temporal lobe
	2. Semantic-memory with no temporal or spatial content (e.g., words, symbols)	Anterior portion of right or left temporal lobe
c. Retrieval (recall)	Higher level cognitive function is dependent upon lower functioning recognition; permits creativity and planning; takes two forms—direct verbatim access or access to a general idea of the original material; successful retrieval requires the availability of information in storage and access to that information at the desired time	Temporal lobe Hippocampus Thalamus

From Zoltan B, and others: Perceptual and cognitive dysfunction in the adult stroke patient, Thorofare, NJ, 1986, Charles B Slack, Inc.

ganizational skills are described in the material on specific questions and areas to evaluate.

Clinical observation and activity analysis*
General guidelines for evaluation

1. Determine whether the patient is aware that he or she has a planning deficit. Defective planning often can be revealed by asking the patient what he or she intends to do.
2. Observe the patient in a number of settings and activities during the day. Can the patient plan for activities requiring two-step operations? Three-step operations? More complex operations?
3. Establish functional baseline measures. Consider the duration and frequency of the problem. Select relevant functional tasks as the basis of evaluation and reassessment.
4. Can the patient conceptualize change (as evidenced through verbal or other means of com-

munication) from the present?
5. Can the patient present alternatives to an established plan?
6. Can the patient weigh these alternatives and make a choice based on his or her judgments?
7. Does the patient appear to have a framework for the plan or a direction he or she is demonstrating for task completion?

MENTAL FLEXIBILITY AND ABSTRACTION. Conceptual thinking is necessary even for the most basic functional tasks in life. Patients with frontal lobe damage will often lose this ability and think only in the most concrete, literal manner. This literal thinking is often paired with poor mental flexibility, resulting in perseverative or stimulus-bound behavior. These cognitive deficits and resultant behaviors create difficulty in knowledge generalization and problem-solving.[35]

Mental flexibility can be evaluated by simple cross-out tasks that tests the patient's ability to shift from one task to another. This is accomplished with a visual search worksheet and the therapist's alternative instructions to cross out odd and even numbers. Abstraction and conceptual thinking can be evaluated in a number of ways. Testing can include definitions, object comparisons, logical relationships, opposites, categorization, and interpretation of proverbs.[8,27,35] The therapist should also evaluate mental flexibility and abstraction through close clinical observation. The aforementioned perseverative or stimulus-bound behavior should be noted, both as it relates to a specific environment and to particular tasks.

DECREASED INSIGHT AND IMPULSIVITY. Most therapists are familiar with the patient with brain damage who falls out of bed trying to walk to the bathroom despite paralysis. This and other behaviors are the result of a lack of awareness or blatant denial of the limitations related to brain damage. This limited insight results in impulsive and unsafe behavior. The patient with this deficit will be unable to monitor, correct, and regulate the quality of his behavior.[35]

The evaluation of poor insight is easily accomplished through structured clinical observation as follows.

Evaluation of decreased insight*
General guidelines for evaluation
1. Determine whether the patient is aware of and responsive to his or her environment. One measure of the patient's awareness is the ability to use feedback.
2. Observe the patient in a number of settings and activities during the day. His or her limited insight, poor safety awareness, and impulsiveness can vary depending on the setting and the task.
3. Establish functional baseline measures. Consider the degree and frequency of the problem. Select relevant functional tasks as the basis of evaluation and reassessment.

Specific areas and questions
to consider and evaluate*
1. Can the patient perceive and verbalize (or somehow communicate) the extent and type of problems he or she is having?
2. Is the patient willing to try to understand and accept his or her problems when they are pointed out?
3. Once he or she admits to a specific problem, can the patient then perceive how it will affect overall function beyond a specific task?

---

*Adapted and reproduced with permission from Bourne LE, Dominowski RL, Loftus EF: Cognitive Processes. Englewood Cliffs, New Jersey, 1979, Prentice-Hall Inc.

4. How does the environment affect the patient's awareness and behavior? Does a quiet structured environment decrease impulsivity and increase insight? In which environments does safety become an issue, for example, in the kitchen; in the community?
5. Does verbal, visual, or tactile cuing improve insight or decrease impulsiveness?
6. What are the duration and frequency of the patient's impulsiveness and decreased insight or safety awareness?
7. Is there a task or tasks that are particularly helpful in illustrating a specific problem to the patient?

PROBLEM-SOLVING. Problem-solving is a complex process involving many cognitive skills. It requires attention, memory, planning and organization, and the ability to make judgments.

The patient must be able to process complex information in order to plan strategies and to evaluate established strategies.[4,24] The evaluation of problem-solving is conducted during selected functional tasks, as follows[5,35]*:

Preparation and understanding the problem (problem analysis)
1. Can the patient identify the elements of the problem?
2. Can the patient identify solution criteria?
3. Can the patient identify limitations related to potential attempts at problem-solving?
4. Can the patient describe how the problem compares with those he or she has already solved?
5. Can the patient divide the problem into parts or segments?
6. Can the patient construct a simpler problem by ignoring some information?

Production: generating possible solutions
1. Can the patient retrieve necessary information from long-term memory?
2. Does the patient scan the environment for available information?
3. Does the patient act on the content in short-term memory?
4. Does the patient store information in long-term memory for later use?
5. Can the patient generate a potential solution?

Judgment: evaluating the solutions generated
1. Does the patient compare the solution with the initial solution components?
2. Does the patient decide either that the problem has been solved or that more work is needed?

ACALCULIA. The inability to perform simple calculations is associated with right or left hemisphere damage. It can occur with parietal, temporal, or occipital lobe damage and may be seen in isolation or in association with other deficits. The major standardized test of acalculia is the Arithmetic Subscale of the Wechsler Adult Intelligence Scale (WAIS).[31] This test consists of a series of simple to complex word problems. However, the occupational therapist should evaluate acalculia because it relates to function. This is easily accomplished through the development of a test that includes number recognition and simple to complex operations. Functionally oriented items that should be included are calculating change, recognition of coins, and budgeting.

Treatment

The treatment of cognitive deficits should follow the same principles outlined above. These principles include (1) consideration of cognition in relation to other deficit areas, (2) environmental influence on patient performance, (3) evaluation and treatment of cognitive deficits in a logical progression, and (4) the effects of aging on cognition. (For detailed information on specific treatment techniques for individual cognitive deficits, the reader is referred to reference 35.)

The concept of environment as it relates to cognition includes not only physical features but also structure and feedback. Examples of the use of the physical environment in treatment are the treatment of an inattentive patient in a quiet, uncluttered environment or the treatment of the patient with poor memory in the same environment every day.

Environmental feedback, or "cuing", refers to the alteration of specific instructions or facets of a task to facilitate improved skill and performance.[13] Feedback or cuing can be provided by the therapist through any sensory mode or, using a behavioral approach, through tokens or rewards. Cuing can include both internal cuing, performed by the patient, or external cuing, provided by the therapist. An example of internal cuing is the use of rehearsal techniques when the patient silently repeats the information he or she has been asked to remember.[13] An example of external cues for this same patient includes diaries, alarm clocks, and lists. The therapist must always be aware that the ultimate goal of treatment is the internalization of cues or reduction of need for environmental cuing for successful performance.[35]

The aging process affects an individual's cognitive abilities. It is important for the therapist to keep this in mind when treating the elderly patient with brain damage. Repetition and practice are important, as well as limiting distractions and extraneous information.[2,26] In addition, the therapist should always allow enough time for the patient to respond and use appropriate sensory cuing whenever possible.

The Use of Computers in Cognitive Retraining

The use of computers by occupational therapists for cognitive rehabilitation has increased significantly in recent years.[23] As with any new treatment modality, its efficacy remains unclear. Documented research studies are few, with those that are available consisting primarily of program descriptions.[6,20] Despite the limited research, many clinicians believe computer use offers a definite benefit as a treatment tool for cognitive rehabilitation. For successful application, the therapist must keep up with state-of-the-art software and critically analyze what is currently available.

Before the clinician selects a computer system, the available software for that particular system should be explored.[19] Most cognitive rehabilitation software will run on the Apple II + /IIe/IIc series.[19] Available software includes games, educational programs, and software specifically designed for cognitive rehabilitation.[15,20] Specific software for cognitive rehabilitation that is available for use with the Apple II computer includes programs for remediation of arithmetic, attention and concentration, concept formation, nonverbal memory, reasoning, association, categorization, cause and effect, problem-solving, organization, generalization, level of abstraction, judgment of safety, spatial orientation sequencing, and verbal memory. (For additional information on specific software used to treat these and other related areas, the reader is referred to the references 7, 15, and 16. The reader is also referred to references 18, 21, and 28 for general computer resources with the disabled.)

One final area to consider in computer-assisted cognitive rehabilitation is the input device. Patients with brain damage may require an oversized joystick, a light pen, or touch screen to compensate for specific motor deficits. These and other adaptive input devices may also require additional custom adaptations by the occupational therapist.

SUMMARY

Basic, underlying principles of cognitive evaluation and treatment, specific deficit evaluation through structured clinical observation and activity analysis, and general guidelines for treatment application have been presented. The area of cognitive dysfunction is complex and requires that the therapist develop astute observational skills and attain knowledge and understanding of underlying principles of evaluation and treatment techniques. The reader is encouraged to seek additional sources and experiences as needed to refine therapeutic skill in dealing with patients with cognitive dysfunction.

REVIEW QUESTIONS

1. Why is it important for the occupational therapist to differentiate between perception and cognition?
2. List the areas of cognition that the occupational therapist should evaluate through structured clinical observation and activity analysis.
3. What are the major underlying principles of cognitive evaluation that the therapist must consider?
4. Describe the memory process.
5. What are some behavioral manifestations of poor initiation?
6. Describe three specific areas and questions to consider in evaluating the patient with a planning and organization deficit.
7. What behaviors will the patient with poor mental flexibility and abstraction display?
8. What are the three major stages of problem-solving?
9. What tasks should a functional test of acalculia include?
10. What is environmental feedback or "cuing"?

REFERENCES

1. Arenberg D: A longitudinal study of problem solving in adults, J Gerontol 29:656, 1974.
2. Arenberg D and Robertson-Tchabo E: Learning and aging. In Birren J and Schame K, editors: Handbook of the psychology of aging, New York, 1977, Von Reinhold Co.
3. Bennett-Levy J and Powell G: The subjective memory questionnaire (SMQ): an investigation into the self-reporting of "real life" memory skills, Br J Soc Clin Psychol 19:177, 1980.
4. Bolger J: Cognitive retraining: a developmental approach, Clin Neuropsychol 4:66, 1982.
5. Bourne LE, Dominowski RL, and Loftus EF: Cognitive processes, Englewood Cliffs, N.J., 1979, Prentice-Hall, Inc.
6. Bracy O: Computer-based cognitive rehabilitation, Cognitive Rehabil 1:(1)7, 1983.
7. Bracy O: Program for cognitive rehabilitation, catalog, Indianapolis Software Services, 1985.
8. Christenson AL: Luria's neuropsychological investigation, New York, 1975, Spectrum Publications.
9. Craine JF: Principles of cognitive rehabilitation. In Trexler LE: Cognitive rehabilitation: conceptualization and intervention, New York, 1982, Plenum Press.
10. Craine JF: The retraining of frontal lobe dysfunction. In Trexler LE: Cognitive rehabilitation: conceptualization and intervention, New York, 1982, Plenum Press.
11. Craine JF, Gudeman HE: The rehabilitation of brain functions: principles, procedures and techniques of neurotraining, Springfield, Ill, 1981. Charles C Thomas Publishers.
12. Crook T: Psychometric assessment in the elderly. In Raskin A and Jawick L: Psychiatric symptoms and cognitive loss in the elderly, New York, 1979, Hemisphere Publishing Co.
13. Filskov S and Boll T: Handbook of clinical neuropsychology, New York, 1981, John Wiley and Sons, Inc.
14. Kramer N and Farbik L: Assessment of intellectual changes in the elderly. In Raskin A and Jabik L: Psychiatric symptoms and cognitive loss in the elderly, New York, 1979, Hemisphere Publishing Co.
15. Kreutzer J, Hill M, and Morrison C: Cognitive rehabilitation resources for the Apple II Computer, Indianapolis, In, 1987, NeuroScience Publishers.
16. Kreutzer J and Morrison C: A guide to cognitive rehabilitation software for the Apple IIe/IIC computer, Cog Rehabil 4(3):6, 1986.
17. Lezak M: Neuropsychological assessment, New York, 1983, Oxford University Press.
18. Lynch W: Adaptive devices for microcomputers, Part 1, J head trauma Rehabil 1(4):80, 1986e.
19. Lynch W: Microcomputer technology in the rehabilitation of brain disorders. Advances in clinical rehabilitation, Springer Publishing Co, in press.
20. Lynch WJ: The use of electronic games in cognitive rehabilitation. In Trexler LE, editor: Cognitive rehabilitation—a conceptualization and intervention, New York, 1982, Plenum Press.
21. Marks C, Parente R, and Anderson J: Retention of gains in outpatient cognitive rehabilitation therapy, Cognitive Rehabil 4(3):20, 1986.
22. Meltzer M: Poor memory: a case report, J Clin Psychol 39(1):3, 1983.
23. Milner D: Use of microcomputers in the treatment of patients with physical disabilities. Physical Disability Special Interest Section Newsletter, American Occupational Therapy Association, 7(2):1, 1984.
24. Rabbit P: Changes in problem solving ability in old age. In Birren J and Schaie K: Handbook of psychology of aging, New York, 1977, Von Nostrand Reinhold Co.
25. Kahmani L: The intellectual rehabilitation of brain damaged patients, Clin Neuropsychol 4:44, 1982.
26. Riege WH, Klane LT, Melter EJ, and Hanson WR: Decision speed and bias after unilateral stroke, Cortex 18:345, 1982.
27. Strub RL, Black FW: The mental status examination in neurology, Philadelphia, 1977, FA Davis Co.
28. Smith M: Microcomputer programs for cognitive rehabilitation, catalog, Dimondale, Mi, Hartley Courseware 1984.
29. Wall N, et al: Hemiplegic evaluation, Boston, 1979, Massachusetts Rehabilitation Hospital.
30. Wechsler D: A standardized memory scale for clinical use, J Psychol 19:87, 1945.
31. Wechsler D: Manual for the Wechsler adult intelligence scale, New York, 1955, The Psychology Corporation.
32. Wilson PG: Software selection and use in language and cognitive retraining, Cognitive Rehabil 1(1):9, 1983.
33. Wood RL: Management of attention disorders following brain injury. In Wilson BA and Moffat

N: Clinical management of memory problems, Rockville, Md, 1984, Aspen Publishers.

34. Zoltan B, Jabri J, Panikoff L, and Ryckman D: Perceptual motor evaluation for head injured and other neurologically impaired adults, San Jose, 1987, Santa Clara Valley Medical Center.

35. Zoltan B, Siev E, and Frieshtat E: Perceptual and cognitive dysfunction in the adult stroke patient: a manual for evaluation and treatment, rev ed, Thorofare, New Jersey, 1986, Charles B Slack, Inc.

Chapter

14 Therapeutic activity

LORRAINE WILLIAMS PEDRETTI

In this text therapeutic activity is defined as arts, crafts, recreational, sports, leisure, self-care, home management, and work-related activities that may be used or adapted for use to meet one or more of the following therapeutic objectives: (1) to develop or maintain strength, endurance, work tolerance, range of motion (ROM), and coordination; (2) to practice and use voluntary, automatic movement in goal-directed tasks; (3) to provide for purposeful use of and general exercise to affected parts; (4) to explore vocational potential or train in work adjustment skills; (5) to improve sensation, perception, and cognition; and (6) to improve socialization skills and enhance emotional growth and development.

PURPOSEFUL ACTIVITY

One of the first principles of occupational therapy, stated by Dunton in 1918, is that there must be some useful end to occupation for it to be effective in the treatment of mental and physical disability.[19] This principle implies that the activity or occupation has a purpose and that purposeful activity has an autonomous or inherent goal beyond the motor function required to perform the task.[1] Conversely, nonpurposeful activity has been defined as activity in which there is no inherent goal other than the motor function used to perform the activity.[19] By this definition, methods such as therapeutic exercise, sanding wood, stacking blocks, and hammering nails for no purpose other than to perform the associated movement patterns cannot be considered purposeful activity. This does not imply, however, that such enabling methods do not have a place in the treatment continuum.

Purposeful activity is the "cornerstone of occupational therapy," and it is one of its primary modalities.[19,20] Much is written about it in the professional literature, but it has not been defined to the satisfaction and agreement of all members of the profession.[2,5,7,16,17,20]

Hinojosa and others defined purposeful activity as "tasks or experiences in which the person actively participates" and that elicit coordination between physical, emotional, and cognitive systems.[4]

The uniqueness of occupational therapy lies in its emphasis on the extensive use of purposeful activity. This emphasis gives occupational therapy the theoretical foundation for its broad application to both psychosocial and physical dysfunction as well as to health maintenance.[4]

During performance of purposeful activity, attention is directed to the task itself "rather than to the internal processes required for achievement of the task."[4] Purposeful activity has both inherent and therapeutic goals. For example, sawing wood may have the inherent goal of securing parts for construction of a bookshelf, whereas the therapeutic objectives may be to strengthen shoulder and elbow musculature and to provide for release of aggression. Therefore purposeful motor function is the use of the neuromuscular system to accomplish the inherent or autonomous goal of the activity being performed. The conscious effort of the patient performing the activity is focused on the ultimate objective of the movement and not on the movement itself.[1] The patient directs and is in control of the movement. As the patient becomes absorbed in the performance of the activity, it is assumed that the affected parts are used more naturally and with less fatigue.[21] It has been postulated that concentration on motion has a detrimental effect on that motion and that muscles controlled by conscious attention and focused effort fatigue rapidly. Therefore it is more sound to focus attention on the activity and its inherent goal than on the muscles or motions being used to accomplish the activity.[1]

Studies have been done that attempt to prove the efficacy of purposeful activity. The results of a study by Steinbeck supported the assumption that patients performing purposeful activity are motivated to perform for a longer period than when they are performing nonpurposeful activity.[19]

A study of motivation for product-oriented versus non-product-oriented activity by Thibodeaux and Ludwig indicated the need to determine the patient's level of interest in the process and in the end product of the activity and his or her liking of the activity in treatment planning.[20] The importance of keeping or not keeping the activity product was studied by Rocker and Nelson.[17] They found that not being allowed to keep an activity product can elicit hostile feelings in normal subjects. Their studies suggest that in developing a treatment plan, the inherent goals of the activity, the patient's level of interest in the activity, and the meaning of the activity product are important factors in the ultimate effectiveness of the media and methods selected for treatment.

Therapeutic Modalities

Traditionally, occupational therapy was associated with the use of arts and crafts as therapeutic modalities. Arts and crafts are still in use as treatment methods and constitute an effective and substantial portion of many occupational therapy programs. But occupational therapy is not restricted to the use of arts and crafts, and the scope of its treatment methods has changed and broadened considerably over the years.

Media and methods used in professional practice are influenced by many factors at any given time. Reed defined medium as "the means by which a therapeutic effect is transmitted." For example, a loom or vestibular ball is a medium.[16] Methods are defined as "the steps, sequence or approach used to activate the therapeutic effect of a medium." Examples are one-handed dressing techniques and joint protection techniques.[16]

Reed also identified eight factors that influence the selection and discarding of media and methods in occupational therapy.[16] They are cultural practices, social acceptance or nonacceptance, economics of health care, available technology, influences of a given theoretical model, historical influences, and research. An analysis of these factors would yield information for educators and therapists about why particular media and methods are used in occupational therapy and whether they are consistent with occupational therapy philosophy.

Purposeful activities, other than arts and crafts, used in treatment programs today include activities of daily living (ADL) such as self-care, travel, communications, and home management activities; simulated work activities or actual job samples; and leisure activities.

In addition to purposeful, goal-oriented activities, therapists have become increasingly skillful in the use of therapeutic exercise and in sensorimotor approaches to treatment, both of which traditionally belong to the field of physical therapy. These methods are used by some occupational therapists because they enable the development of the individual's ability to perform activities that will increase the level of in-

dependent functioning, a primary aim of occupational therapy. Occupational therapists also apply the principles of therapeutic exercise and of the sensorimotor approaches to treatment to activities for the greatest therapeutic benefit. The sensorimotor approaches and their application to purposeful activity are discussed in Chapters 18 through 21. Therapeutic exercise and its application to purposeful activity are outlined in the following sections.

THERAPEUTIC EXERCISE

Early in the history of occupational therapy the psychological effects of the performance of purposeful activity were considered primary in the treatment of persons with physical dysfunction.[7] It was later recognized that physical benefits accrued from the performance of activity and kinesiological considerations were also applied in the selection of appropriate therapeutic activities. In order to apply kinesiologic considerations to purposeful activity, it was necessary to understand the principles of therapeutic exercise.

Therapeutic exercise is the prescription of bodily movement or muscle contraction to correct an impairment, improve musculoskeletal function, and maintain a state of well-being.[8] Many of its principles are applicable to therapeutic activity, and many occupational therapists use it in treatment programs. If used by occupational therapists, its purposes should be to prepare the patient for performance of functional activities and to augment therapeutic activity and performance skills phases of the occupational therapy program.

General Principles

After partial or complete denervation of muscle and during inactivity or disuse, muscle strength decreases. When strength is inadequate, substitution patterns or "trick movements" are likely to develop.[22] A substitution is the attempt to achieve a functional goal by using muscle groups and patterns of motion not ordinarily used because of loss or weakness of the muscles normally used to perform the movements.[22] An example is using shoulder abduction to achieve a hand-to-mouth movement if elbow flexors cannot perform against gravity (Fig. 14-1). When muscle loss is permanent, some substitution patterns may be desirable as a compensatory measure to improve performance of functional activities. However, many are not desirable, and it is often the aim of therapeutic exercise to prevent or correct substitution patterns.[22]

A muscle must contract to its maximal capacity to effect an increase in strength. Therefore strengthening exercises are not effective if the contraction is insufficient. Excess strengthening, on the other hand,

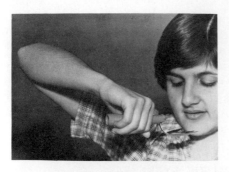

Fig. 14-1. Shoulder abduction is used to compensate for weak elbow flexion.

may result in muscle fatigue, pain, and temporary reduction of strength.[10] If a muscle is overworked, it becomes fatigued and is not able to contract. Selection of the type of exercise must suit the muscle grade and the patient's fatigue tolerance level. Fatigue level varies from individual to individual, and the threshold for muscle fatigue decreases in pathological states.[10] Many patients may not be sensitive to fatigue or may push themselves beyond tolerance in the belief that this hastens recovery. This means that the therapist must make a careful assessment of the patient's muscle power and capacity for exercise. The therapist must also supervise the patient closely and observe for signs of fatigue. These signs may be slowed performance, distraction, perspiration, increase in rate of respiration, performance of exercise pattern through a decreased ROM, and inability to complete the prescribed number of repetitions.

Purposes

The general purposes of exercise are (1) to develop awareness of normal movement patterns and improve voluntary, automatic movement responses; (2) to develop strength and endurance in patterns of movement that are acceptable and necessary and do not produce deformity; (3) to improve coordination, regardless of strength; (4) to increase specific power of desired isolated muscles or muscle groups; (5) to aid in overcoming ROM deficits; (6) to increase strength of muscles that will power hand splints, mobile arm supports, and other devices; (7) to increase work tolerance and physical endurance through increased strength; and (8) to prevent or eliminate contractures developing as a result of imbalanced muscle power by strengthening the antagonistic muscles.[15]

Prerequisites for Use

For therapeutic exercise to be effective, the patient must meet certain criteria. Therapeutic exercise is most effective in the treatment of orthopedic disorders, such as fractures and arthritis, and lower motor neuron disorders that produce weakness and flaccidity. Examples of these are peripheral nerve injuries and diseases, poliomyelities, Guillain-Barre syndrome, infectious neuronitis, and spinal cord injuries and diseases.

Therapeutic exercise is contraindicated for patients who have poor general health or inflamed joints or who have had recent surgery.[14] As defined and described here, it cannot be used effectively with those who have spasticity and lack voluntary control of isolated motion or those who cannot control dyskinetic movement. The latter conditions are likely to occur in upper motor neuron disorders. It may not be useful where there is severely limited joint ROM as a result of well-established, permanent contractures.

The candidate for therapeutic exercise must be medically able to participate in the exercise regimen, be able to understand the directions for the exercise and its purposes, and be interested and motivated to perform the exercise. The patient must have available motor pathways, as demonstrated by muscle power or muscle testing, and the potential for recovery or improvement of strength, ROM, coordination, or movement patterns, as applicable. It is important that some sensory feedback is available to the patient. This means that sensation must be at least partially intact so that the patient can perceive motion and position of the exercised part and have some sense of superficial and deep pain. Muscles and tendons must be intact, stable, and free to move. Joints must be able to move through an effective ROM for those types of exercise that use joint motion as part of the procedure. The patient should be relatively free of pain during motion and should be able to perform isolated, coordinated movement. If there is any dyskinetic movement, the patient should be able to control it so that the exercise procedure can be performed as prescribed.[14]

Types of Muscle Contraction Used[6,10]

ISOMETRIC CONTRACTION. During an isometric contraction there is no joint motion, and the muscle length remains the same. A muscle and its antagonist may be contracted at any point in the ROM to stabilize a joint. This may be without resistance or against some outside resistance, such as the therapist's hand or a tabletop. An example of isometric exercise of triceps against resistance is pressing against the tabletop with the ulnar border of the forearm while the elbow remains at 90°.

ISOTONIC OR CONCENTRIC CONTRACTION. During an isotonic contraction there is joint motion, and the muscle shortens. This may be done with or without resistance. Isotonic contractions may be performed in positions with gravity assisting or gravity decreased or against gravity, according to the patient's muscle grade and the goal of the exercise. An example of isotonic contraction of the biceps is lifting a fork to the mouth during eating. If a filled cup is lifted to the mouth, the biceps contracts against resistance.

ECCENTRIC CONTRACTION. When muscles contract eccentrically, the tension in the muscle increases or remains constant while the muscle lengthens. This may be done with or without resistance. An example of an eccentric contraction performed against no resistance is the slow lowering of the arm to the table. The biceps is contracting eccentrically in this instance. An example of eccentric contraction against resistance is the controlled return of a pail of sand lifted from the ground. Here, the biceps is contracting eccentrically to control the rate and coordination of the elbow extension in setting the pail on the ground.

Exercise Classification

The type of exercise selected depends on muscle grade, muscle endurance, joint mobility, diagnosis and physical condition, treatment goals, position of the patient and desirable plane of movement.

RESISTIVE EXERCISE. Resistive exercise uses isotonic muscle contraction. It is also possible to use eccentric contraction. Resistive exercise is primarily for increasing strength of fair plus to normal muscles but may also be helpful for producing relaxation of the antagonistic muscles of the contracting muscles. This latter purpose can be useful if increased range is desired for stretching or relaxing spastic muscles.

The patient performs muscle contraction against resistance and moves the part through the full ROM. The resistance applied should be the maximum against which the muscle is capable of contracting. Resistance may be applied manually or by weights, springs, elastic bands, sandbags, or special exercise devices. It is graded by progressively increasing the amount of resistance (Fig. 14-2).[6,10] The number of repetitions that are possible will depend on the patient's general physical endurance and the endurance of the specific muscle.

One specialized type of resistive exercise is the DeLorme method of progressive resistive exercise (PRE).[3,18] Progressive resistive exercise is based on the overload principle (increasing the load on the muscle), the principle that muscles perform more efficiently if given a "warm-up" period, and the principle that muscles must be taxed beyond usual daily activity to improve in performance.[3]

During the exercise procedure small loads are used initially. These are increased gradually after each set

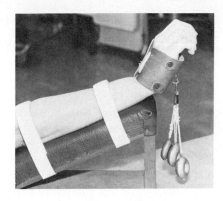

Fig. 14-2. Resistive exercise to wrist extensors, using forearm stabilizer and handcuff to compensate for inadequate grasp.

of 10 repetitions of the desired movement. The muscle is thus warmed up to prepare to exert its maximal power for the final 10 repetitions. The exercise procedure consists of three sets of 10 repetitions each, with resistance applied as follows: (1) first set, 10 repetitions at 50% of maximal resistance; (2) second set, 10 repetitions at 75% of maximal resistance; and (3) third set, 10 repetitions at maximal resistance. The patient is instructed to inhale during the shortening contraction and exhale during the relaxation or eccentric contraction.[3,18]

An example of a PRE is a triceps extending the elbow against a 12-pound maximal resistance, performing 10 repetitions against 6 pounds of resistance, 10 repetitions against 9 pounds, and the final 10 repetitions against 12 pounds.

Maximal resistance, the amount of resistance the muscle can lift through the ROM 10 times, is determined by contracting the muscle and moving the part through the full ROM against progressively increasing loads for sets of 10 repetitions until the maximal load that can be lifted 10 times is reached.

At the beginning of the treatment program it is often difficult for the therapist to determine the maximal resistance that the patient is capable of taking. This may be because (1) the patient may not know how to exert maximal effort, (2) the patient may be reluctant to exercise strenuously for fear of pain or reinjury, (3) the patient may be unwilling or unable to endure discomfort, and (4) the patient may have difficulty with timing of exercises.

The experience of the therapist and trial and error aid in determining maximal resistance when this is difficult. The therapist should estimate the amount of resistance the patient can take and then add or subtract resistance (for example, weight or tension) until the patient can perform the sets of repetitions adequately.

The exercises should be performed once daily four or five times weekly and rest periods of 2 to 4 minutes should be allowed between each set of 10 repetitions. Modifications of the exercise procedure may be made to suit individual needs. Some possibilities are 10 repetitions at 25% of maximal resistance, 10 repetitions at 50%, 10 repetitions at 75%, and 10 repetitions at maximal resistance. Another possibility is 5 repetitions at 50% and 10 repetitions at maximal resistance. Still another possibility is to omit the second set of exercises. Adjustments in the first two sets of exercises may be made to suit the capacity of the individual.

Another approach is the "Oxford" technique, essentially a reverse of the DeLorme method. The exercise sequence begins with 100% resistance and decreases to 75% and then to 50% on subsequent sets of 10 repetitions each.[3,18] The greatest gains may be made in the early weeks of the treatment program, with smaller increases occurring at a slower pace in the subsequent weeks or months. During performance of the exercise, the therapist should be aware of joint alignment of exercise device; proper fit and adjustment of device; ruling out substitute movements; and clear instruction of speed, ROM, and proper breathing.[15]

APPLICATION TO ACTIVITY. Many purposeful activities lend themselves well to resistive exercise. For instance, leather lacing is an activity that can be performed in a way to offer slight resistance to the anterior deltoid if it is pulled in an upward direction. Sanding with a weighted sandblock is an activity that can be done to offer significant resistance to the same muscle if done on an inclined plane sanding board.

ACTIVE EXERCISE. Isotonic muscle contraction is used in active exercise. Eccentric contraction may also be used. Active exercise is done when the patient moves the joint through its available ROM against no outside resistance.

Active motion through the complete ROM with gravity decreased or against gravity may be used for poor to fair muscles for the purpose of improving strength, with the added benefit of maintaining ROM. It may be used with higher muscle grades for the maintenance of strength and ROM when resistance is contraindicated. Active exercise is *not* used to increase range of motion because this purpose requires added force not present in this exercise.

In active exercise the patient moves the part through the complete ROM independently. If the exercise is performed in a gravity-decreased plane, a powdered surface, skateboard, deltoid aid, or free-moving suspension sling may be used to reduce the resistance produced by friction. It is graded by adding resistance as strength improves.[6,10]

APPLICATION TO ACTIVITY. Activities that offer little or no resistance can be used as active exercise. A needlework activity performed in the gravity-decreased plane can provide active exercise to the wrist extensors or elbow extensors. When a grade of Fair or 3 is reached, the wrist can be moved against gravity in an activity such as picking up and placing tiles.

ACTIVE-ASSISTED EXERCISE. In active-assisted exercise, isotonic muscle contraction is used. The patient moves the joint through partial ROM, and the range is completed by the therapist (Fig. 14-3) or a mechanical device. Mechanical asistance may be supplied by slings, pulleys, weights, springs, or elastic bands (Fig. 14-4).[18] The goal of active-assisted exercise is to increase strength of trace to poor muscles while maintaining ROM. In the case of trace muscles the patient merely contracts the muscle, and the therapist completes the entire ROM. This exercise is graded by decreasing the amount of assistance until the patient can perform active exercises.[6,10]

APPLICATION TO ACTIVITY. If assistance is required to complete the movement, an activity must be structured so that it can be offered by the therapist, the patient's other arm or leg, or a mechanical device.

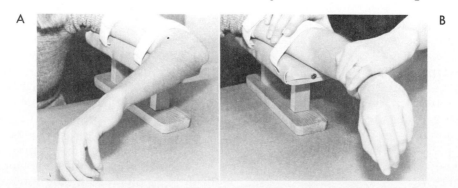

A   B

Fig. 14-3. A, Patient extends elbow from full flexion toward extension in gravity-decreased plane to degree possible actively. **B,** Therapist assists patient to complete ROM.

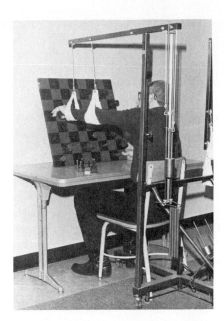

Fig. 14-4. Active-assisted exercise with deltoid aid assisting shoulder in reaching activity.

For example, in a weaving activity, the patient pushes the beater bar away by extending the affected elbow through partial ROM but completes the movement with the other hand. Various bilateral activities lend themselves well to active-assisted exercise. The bicycle jig saw, bilateral sanding, bilateral sponge wiping, using a sweeper, and sawing are some examples. In these activities, the unaffected arm or leg can perform the major share of the work and the affected arm or leg can perform to the extent possible.

PASSIVE EXERCISE. In passive exercise there is *no* muscle contraction. Therefore it is of no use for increasing strength. It is not useful to increase ROM because no force is applied to the joint.

In passive exercise, the joint is moved through its ROM by the therapist or a mechanical device. The purpose of passive exercise is to maintain ROM, thereby preventing contractures and adhesions and deformity.

To achieve these goals, it should be performed for at least three repetitions, twice daily.[8] It is used when absent or minimal muscle strength (grades O-T) precludes the active motion or when active exercise is contraindicated because of the patient's physical condition. During the exercise procedure the joint or joints to be exercised are moved through their normal ranges manually by the therapist or patient or mechanically by an external device, such as a pulley or counterbalance sling. The joint proximal to the joint being exercised should be stabilized during the exercise procedure[6] (Fig. 14-5).

APPLICATION TO ACTIVITY. It is often possible

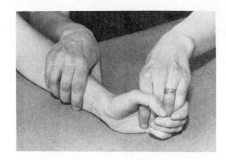

Fig. 14-5. Therapist is performing passive exercise of wrist.

to include a passive limb in a bilateral activity if the contralateral limb is unaffected. Several of the activities described above for active-assisted exercise can be used for passive exercise as well.

Stretching or Forced Exercise

PASSIVE STRETCH. When doing passive stretching, the therapist moves the joint through the available ROM and holds momentarily, applying a gentle but firm force at the point of maximal stretch. There should be no residual pain when the stretching is discontinued. Passive stretch or forced exercise is to increase ROM. It is used when there is a loss of joint ROM, and stretching is not contraindicated.

If the patient's muscle grades are adequate, the patient can move the part actively through the available ROM, and the therapist can take it a little further, thus forcing or stretching the soft structures around the joint.

Passive stretching requires a good understanding of joint anatomy and muscle function. It should be carried out cautiously under good medical supervision and with medical approval. Muscles to be stretched should be in a relaxed state.[10] The therapist should never force muscles when pain is present unless ordered by the physician to work through pain. Gentle, firm stretching held for a few seconds is more effective and less hazardous than quick, short stretching. The parts around the area being stretched should be stabilized, and compensatory movements should be prevented. Incorrect stretching procedures can produce muscle tearing, joint fracture, and inflammatory edema.[8]

APPLICATION TO ACTIVITY. Passive stretching may be incorporated into an activity if an unaffected part guides the movement of the affected part and forces it slightly beyond the available ROM. One example is the passive stretch of wrist flexors during a block printing activity if the block is pressed down with the open hand while the patient is standing.

Active Stretch

The purpose of active stretch is the same as the purpose of passive stretch, that is, to increase joint ROM. In active stretching, the patient uses the force of the antagonist muscle to increase the length of the agonist. It requires good to normal strength of the antagonist, good coordination, and motivation of the patient. Because the exercise may produce discomfort, there will be a natural tendency to avoid the stretching component of the movement. For example, forceful contraction of the triceps to stretch the biceps muscle can be performed.

APPLICATION TO ACTIVITY. Many activities can be used to incorporate active stretching. Slowly sawing wood, for example requires a forceful contraction of the triceps with a concomitant stretch of the biceps.

Isometric Exercise

ISOMETRIC WITH NO RESISTANCE. Isometric exercise uses isometric contractions of a specific muscle or muscle group. In isometric exercises a muscle or group of muscles is actively contracted and relaxed without producing motion of the joint that it ordinarily mobilizes.

The purpose of isometric exercise with no resistance is to maintain muscle strength when active motion is not possible or is contraindicated. It may be used with any muscle grade above trace. It is especially useful for patients in casts or with arthritis or burns.

The patient is taught to "set" or contract the muscles voluntarily and to hold the contraction for 5 or 6 seconds. The therapist's fingers may be placed distal to the joint, without offering resistance, to help the patient learn to set the muscle. If passive motion is allowed, the therapist may move the joint to a point in the ROM and ask the patient to hold the position.

ISOMETRIC WITH RESISTANCE. Isometric exercise with applied resistance uses isometric muscle contraction performed against some outside resistance. Its purpose is to increase muscle strength of muscles graded Fair+ or 3+ to Normal or 5. The patient sets the muscle or muscle group while resistance is applied and holds the contraction for 5 or 6 seconds. Isometric exercises should be performed for one exercise session per day, 5 days a week. Besides manual resistance, the patient may hold a weight or push up under a table top, depending on the muscle group being exercised. A small weight held in the hand requires isometric contractions of the wrist flexors and extensors.

Muscle strength is graded by increasing the amount of outside resistance or the degree of force the patient holds against. A tension gauge should be used to accurately monitor the amount of resistance applied. It has been shown that daily single, brief isometric exercises are at least as effective and sometimes more effective than isotonic exercises for increasing strength. Isometric exercises also increase the endurance to a higher level than isotonic resistive exercises. However, brief isometric exercises performed at resting length are not always superior to isotonic exercises. There are many situations in which movement through complete ROM is a desirable aspect of the exercise program, for example, to maintain joint ROM, prevent contracture, and prepare for use of prosthetic devices. Isometric exercise has several specific applications, as in arthritis, when joint motion may be contraindicated but muscle strength must be increased or maintained.[6,8,15]

APPLICATION TO ACTIVITY. Any activity that requires holding, or static, posture incorporates isometric exercise. Holding tool handles or holding the arm in elevation while painting are examples. This type of exercise, if contraction is sustained, can be very fatiguing.

Coordination Exercises[9]

Coordination is the combined activity of many muscles into smooth patterns and sequences of motion. Coordination is an automatic response monitored primarily through proprioceptive sensory feedback. Kottke differentiated neuromuscular control from coordination.[9] He defined control as "the conscious activation of an individual muscle or the conscious initiation of a preprogrammed engram." Control involves conscious attention to and guidance of an activity.

An *engram* is a preprogrammed pattern of muscular activity as it is represented in the central nervous system (CNS). An engram is formed only if there are many repetitions of a specific motion or activity. With repetition, conscious effort of the patient is decreased, and the motion becomes more and more automatic. Ultimately, the motion can be carried out with little conscious attention. When an engram is excited, the same pattern of movement is produced automatically.

Procedures for the development of neuromuscular control and neuromuscular coordination are briefly outlined in the following section. The reader is referred to the original source for a full discussion of the neurophysiologic mechanisms underlying these exercises. Neuromuscular education or control training involves teaching the patient to control individual muscles or motions through conscious attention. Coordination training is used to develop preprogrammed multimuscular patterns or engrams.[9]

Training Neuromuscular Control

It may be desirable to teach control of individual prime movers when they are so weak that they cannot be used normally. The purpose of the exercise is to improve muscle strength and muscle coordination into normal motor patterns. To achieve these ends, the person must learn precise control of the muscle. This is an essential step in the development of optimal coordination for persons with neuromuscular disease.

Requirements for Training

To participate successfully in this type of exercise the patient must be rational and be able to learn and follow instructions, cooperate, and concentrate on the muscular retraining. Before beginning, the patient should be comfortable and securely supported. The exercises should be carried out in a nondistracting environment. It is important that the patient be alert, calm, and rested. There should be an adequate pain-free arc of motion of the joint on which the muscle acts and good proprioception. Visual and tactile sensory feedback may be used to compensate or substitute for limited proprioception, but the coordination achieved will never be as great as when proprioception is intact.

PROCEDURE. The patient's awareness of the desired motion and the muscles that effect it is first increased by passive lengthening and relaxing of the muscle to stimulate the proprioceptive stretch reflex. This passive movement may be repeated several times. The patient's awareness may be enhanced if the therapist also demonstrates the desired movement and if the movement is performed by the analogous unaffected part. The skin over the muscle belly and tendon insertion may be stimulated to enhance the effect of the stretch reflex. Stroking and tapping over the muscle belly may also be used to facilitate muscle action.[9]

The therapist should explain the location and function of the muscle, its origin and insertion, line of pull, and action on the joint. The therapist should then demonstrate the motion, and instruct the patient to think of the pull of the muscle from insertion to origin. The skin over the muscle insertion can be stroked in the direction of the pull while the patient concentrates on the sensation of the motion during the passive movement performed by the therapist.

The exercise sequence then begins with instructing the patient to think about the motion while the therapist carries it out passively and strokes the skin over the insertion in the direction of the motion. The patient is then instructed to assist by contracting the muscle while the therapist performs passive motion and stimulates the skin as before. Next the patient moves the part through the ROM with assistance and cutaneous stimulation while the therapist emphasizes contraction of the prime mover only. Finally the patient carries out the movement independently, using the prime mover.

Coordination exercises must be initiated against minimal resistance if activity is to be isolated to prime movers. If the muscle is very weak (Trace to Poor), the procedure may be carried out entirely in an active-assisted manner, so that the muscle contracts against no resistance and can function without activating synergists.

Progression from one step to the next depends on successful performance of the step without substitutions. Each step is carried out three to five times per training session for each muscle to be exercised, depending on the patient's exercise tolerance.

Training Coordination

The goal of coordination training is to develop the ability to perform multimuscular motor patterns that are faster, more precise, and stronger than those performed when only control of individual muscles is used. The development of coordination depends on repetition. Initially in training, the movement must be simple and slow so that the patient can be consciously aware of the activity and its components. Good coordination does not develop until repeated practice results in a well-developed activity pattern that no longer requires the conscious effort and attention of the performer.

PROCEDURE. Training should take place in an environment in which the patient can concentrate and perform the given exercise correctly. The exercise is divided into components that the patient can perform correctly. Kottke calls this *desynthesis*.[9] It is important to keep the effort low by reducing speed and resistance to prevent the spread of excitation to muscles that are not part of the desired movement pattern.

When the motor pattern is divided into units that the patient can perform successfully, each unit is trained by practicing it under voluntary control as described above for training of control. The therapist instructs the patient in the desired movement and uses sensory stimulation and passive movement. The patient must observe and voluntarily modify the motion. Slow practice is imperative to make this monitoring possible. The therapist must offer enough assistance to ensure precise movement and patient concentration on the sensations produced by the movements. With concentration on movement, fatigue occurs rapidly and the patient should be given frequent short rests. As the patient masters the components of the pattern and performs them precisely and independently, the exercise sequence is graded to subtasks or several components that are practiced repetitively. As the engrams for the subtasks are perfected, they are chained progressively until the movement pattern can be performed.

The exercise can be graded for speed, force, or

complexity, but the therapist must be aware that this increases the effort put forth by the patient and may result in incoordinated movement. Therefore the grading must remain within the patient's capacity to perform the precise movement pattern. It is important that the motor pattern not be performed incorrectly in order to avoid the development of faulty engrams.

If CNS impulses irradiate to muscles not involved in the movement pattern, incoordinated motion results. Constant repetition of an incoordinated pattern reinforces it, resulting in a persistent incoordination. Factors that increase incoordination are fear, poor balance, too much resistance, pain, fatigue, strong emotions, and prolonged inactivity.[9]

APPLICATION TO ACTIVITY. Occupational therapy can be used to develop coordination, strength, and endurance. Activities in occupational therapy have the advantage of engaging the patient's attention and interest. Activities should be structured to enable the patient to use the precise movement pattern and to work at speeds consistent with the maintenance of precision.

Occupational therapists, often in conjunction with physical therapists, may initiate coordination training with neuromuscular education and progress to repetitious activities requiring desired coordinated movement patterns. Examples of exercise-like activities that demand repetitious patterns of nonresistive movement are placing small blocks, marbles, cones, paper cups, or pegs. These can later be translated to more purposeful activities such as leather lacing, mosaic tile work, needlecrafts, and repetitive household tasks such as wiping, sweeping, and dusting.

Summary

Several types of exercises have been described. These may be applied by the occupational therapist to purposeful activity. Therapeutic exercise is more expertly applied by the physical therapist, who is extensively trained in its use. In many treatment facilities, the physical therapist is responsible for the formal exercise program, and the occupational therapist helps the patient apply newly gained strength, range, and coordination in therapeutic activities and daily living skills. The respective therapists' roles may not be sharply defined, with each sharing in exercise and activity aspects of the treatment program according to their skills, interests, and agreed-on division of labor.

THERAPEUTIC ACTIVITY
Theory of Activity

Occupational therapy was founded on the concept that human beings have an "occupational nature,"

that is, it is natural for humans to be engaged in activity, and the process of being occupied contributes to the health and well-being of the organism.[1,7] Activity is valuable for the maintenance of health in the healthy person and for the restoration of health after illness and disability. By engaging in relevant, meaningful, and purposeful activity, a person is able to effect changes in behavior and performance from dysfunctional toward more functional patterns. The occupational therapist acts as facilitator of the change process.[2] Therefore physical dysfunction can be ameliorated when the patient participates in goal-directed activity.[1] The value of purposeful activity lies in the patient's mental and physical involvement in an activity that provides the exercise needed to help develop purposeful use of the affected parts and an opportunity to meet emotional, social, and personal gratification needs.[1,21]

Cynkin, in *Occupational Therapy: Toward Health Through Activities,* maintains that occupational therapy deals with the activities of everyday life.[2] The activities that form the pattern to one's life are taken for granted until some dysfunction occurs to disrupt the activities pattern. Occupational therapy was founded on the premise that performance of activities promotes physical and mental well-being. From this idea came the use of activities as therapeutic media for persons with mental or physical dysfunction. This implies that dysfunction can be modified, altered, or reversed toward function through engagement in activities. Cynkin stated,

The uniqueness of occupational therapy rests with activities, in the belief (1) that activities are characteristic of and essential to human existence; (2) that culturally specific activities patterns can be detected and described by studying the manifest activities, values, and norms of different sociocultural groups; (3) that acceptable or unacceptable idiosyncratic variations can be found by studying the individual activities patterns of those groups; (4) that the individual leads a most satisfying way of life if able to carry out a set of activities approved by the group but also fulfilling personal needs and wants; (5) that such activity patterns can be equated with function; and (6) that activities themselves, systematically selected and combined in patterns tailored to each individual, are means for the development or restoration of function.*

Cynkin makes several assumptions about activities that relate to their nature, human nature, and change; these are summarized here. Activities fulfill many of a person's needs and wants, and they are essential to physical and psychosocial growth and development and the achievement of mastery and competence. Activities are socioculturally regulated by the values and

---

*From Cynkin, S.: Occupational therapy: toward health through activities, Boston, 1979, Little, Brown & Co.

beliefs of the culture that defines acceptable behavior for groups of people in the culture. A society may be rigid or flexible in its interpretation of acceptable behaviors for various groups. In either case, there is a point at which deviations in behavior or activities patterns are deemed unacceptable. Changes in activities patterns can move or change from dysfunctional toward more functional. Persons can change and desire change. Change takes place through motor, cognitive, and social learning.

Cynkin concludes from these assumptions that activities must be analyzed for "their inherent properties, socioculturally acquired characteristics, their meaning to individuals, and their potential as instruments of change."[2] A careful analysis by the occupational therapist is essential to use activities for therapeutic purposes. An analysis should yield information about the usefulness and application of purposeful activities as intervention strategies for physical dysfunction and health maintenance.

Principles of Activity Analysis

If activities are to be used as the core of occupational therapy, their usefulness as therapeutic modalities must be defined, analyzed, and classified.[2] Activities selected for therapeutic purposes should (1) be goal-directed; (2) have some significance and meaning to the patient to meet individual needs in relation to social roles; (3) require the mental or physical participation of the patient; (4) be designed to prevent or reverse dysfunction; (5) develop skills to enhance performance in life roles; (6) relate to the patient's interests; (7) be adaptable, gradable, and age appropriate; and (8) be selected through knowledge and professional judgment of the occupational therapist in concert with the patient.[5]

Analysis for the Biomechanical Approach

The biomechanical approach to treatment is likely to be used in lower motor neuron and orthopedic dysfunctions. Improvement of strength, ROM, and muscle endurance is the goal of occupational therapy for such dysfunctions. Thus the emphasis of activity analysis is on muscles, joints, and motor patterns required to perform the activity. This is usually done by observation, palpation, joint measurement, and knowledge of kinesiology.

An activity should be analyzed under the specific circumstances that it is to be performed. Steps of the activity must be identified and broken down into the motions required to perform each step. Range of motion, degree of muscle strength, and type of muscle contraction to perform each step should be identified. The activity analysis model that follows is based on the biomechanical approach.

ANALYSIS FOR SENSORIMOTOR APPROACHES. Sensorimotor approaches to treatment are likely to be used for upper motor neuron disorders such as cerebral palsy, stroke, and head injury. Activity analysis for these dysfunctions should focus on the movement patterns required in the particular treatment approach. The therapist must also consider the effect of the activity on balance, posture, muscle tone, and the facilitation or inhibition of primitive or abnormal reflexes and movements. For example, if using the Proprioceptive neuromuscular facilitation (PNF) approach, it will be important to incorporate PNF patterns in the activity or to select activities that naturally use these patterns. For the neurodevelopmental (Bobath) approach, postures and movements that inhibit abnormal reflexes and tone are important. These and other sensorimotor approaches and their applications to activity are discussed in Chapters 18 through 21.

Analysis of the perceptual and cognitive requirements of the activity is particularly important for patients with upper motor neuron disorders, because these functions are often disturbed. It is important for the therapist to select activities that not only meet the requirements for motor performance but that also can be performed with some success.

ACTIVITY CONFIGURATION. Selecting appropriate and meaningful activities for the patient should begin with obtaining and analyzing the individual's activity configuration.[20] This model, adapted from Cynkin, includes information about the patient's values, educational history, work history, leisure interests and activities, and vocational interests and plans.[2] It concludes with a daily schedule, described in Chapter 3, a list of life roles, an analysis of the activity balance, and an assessment of developmental tasks (Fig. 14-6). If the patient is an outpatient and is in the advanced stages of the rehabilitation program, a daily schedule for the present and a schedule reflecting activity prior to the injury or illness can be constructed and compared. If the patient is acutely ill or in the early stages of rehabilitation, a daily schedule reflecting activity prior to the injury or illness should be made. This information may be obtained from interviews with the patient and significant friends and family members.

Requirements of funding sources and budget regulations may not permit the occupational therapist to spend time with a patient for the sole purposes of this lengthy interview. It is possible to obtain much of this information gradually during treatment sessions for specific physical problems. It is not necessary to gather the information all at once or through a formal interview.

Patient's Name _____ Age _____ Sex _____

Life Stage _____

Educational History

  1. Highest educational level achieved
  2. Location and type of schools (public, private, parochial)
  3. Subjects of greatest interest
  4. Subjects of least interest
  5. Average grades achieved
  6. Likes/dislikes about school
  7. Leisure interests during school years
  8. Social groups to which subject belonged
  9. Educational level of parents, siblings
 10. Future educational plans
 11. Career aspirations

Work History

  1. Most recent work/job performed
  2. Previous jobs
  3. Special job training—past, present
  4. Likes and dislikes about jobs, past and present
  5. Most preferred jobs—real or imagined
  6. Preferences for working alone or with others
  7. Works alone or with others?
  8. Socializes with co-workers?—on the job? off the job?
  9. Who is job supervisor?
 10. Type of supervision received—close, distant?
 11. Most effective/desireable type of supervision
 12. Future plans for work or job changes

Leisure Interests and Activities

  1. Interests in sports, games, hobbies—specify
  2. Participation in sports, games, hobbies
     When? How long?
  3. Other leisure interests which would be pursued given adequate time
  4. Are leisure skills considered important to life? Why? Why not?

Values and Cultural Influences

  1. Cultural group with which the patient identifies
  2. Describe cultural customs which are important? (e.g. celebrations, holiday festivals, foods, religious practices, garments, family traditions.
  3. Health practices which are unique to this culture. Special beliefs about health and illness. Respective roles of ill and well members of family. If raised in another country, attitudes towards health care system in USA. Experiences with health care system in USA.
  3. Describe things (concrete and abstract) which are most valued. Why are they valuable? (e.g. cars, jewels, toys, pictures, family traditions, honesty, integrity, fairness)

Daily Schedule

Construct a daily schedule for a typical weekday and typical weekend day in the patient's life. Give detail for hour by hour activities.

Life Roles

List all of the occupational roles of the patient (e.g. worker, father, brother, sportsman, gardener, etc.)

Continued.

Fig. 14-6. Activity configuration/daily schedule. Outline for interview.

Life Balance

Approximate percent of time spent by the patient in each of the performance areas of self maintenance, home and child management, work, and play/leisure.

Life Tasks

Review the patient's life stage and adaptive tasks in progress during this stage. Consider how these tasks influence the use of time and choice of activities.

*Adapted from Cynkin, Simme: Occupational therapy: toward health through activities, Boston, 1979, Little, Brown and Co.

Fig. 14-6, cont'd. Activity configuration/daily schedule. Outline for interview.

Adaptation and Gradation of Activity

It may be necessary to adapt activities to suit the special needs of the patient or the environment. An activity may need to be performed in an unusual way to accomodate the patient's residual abilities. Eating with one hand with the aid of a special splint could be considered such an adaptation. An activity may need to be adapted to the positioning of the patient or to the environment. Setting up a special reading stand and the use of prism glasses to enable a patient to read while in a supine position in bed would be an example of this type of adaptation. Such adaptations require the therapist to analyze the patient's needs, abilities, the environment, and positioning in relation to the goals of the activity and of the treatment program.

GRADATION. Activities may also be adapted for purposes of gradation. Gradation of activity means that the activity should be appropriately paced and modified to demand the patient's maximal capacities at any point in the treatment process.

For example, if the required movement patterns or degree of resistance cannot be obtained when the activity is performed in the usual manner, simple adaptations or modifications may be made. These are usually accepted by the patient if they are not complex and do not require motions that are strained and unnatural to the performance of the activity. The novice is cautioned that the value of the activity to the patient may be diminished if it is designed to be performed with artificial movements or excessive resistance. Such methods discourage participation and interfere with the development of coordination.[9,21] They also require that the patient focus on movements rather than on the process or end product. This reduces satisfaction and defeats one of the primary purposes and benefits of purposeful activity described at the beginning of this chapter.

There are many ways in which activities may be graded to suit the patient's needs and the treatment objectives. Activities can be graded for increasing strength; ROM; endurance and tolerance; coordination; and perceptual, cognitive, and social skills.

STRENGTH. Strength may be graded by increasing resistance. This is accomplished by changing the plane of movement from gravity-decreased to against-gravity and by adding weights to the equipment or to the patient, using tools of increasing weight, grading the texture of the materials from soft to hard, or fine to rough, or changing to another more or less resistive activity. For example, a wrap sandbag with a Velcro fastener attached to the wrist could be used to increase resistance to arm movements during macrame or weaving. A pulley and weight system can be attached to the beater of the floor loom to increase resistance to the biceps or triceps, depending on whether the weight is attached to the back or the front of the loom (Fig. 14-7). Springs may be used to increase resistance on a small table loom or block printing press. When grasp strength is inadequate, grasp mitts may be used

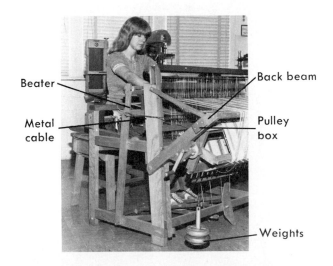

Fig. 14-7. Floor loom adapted with metal cable attached from beater through pulley on back beam from which weights are hung. Weights provide resistance to elbow flexors and shoulder extensors, as arranged.

to hold onto a tool or equipment handle, allowing arm motion.

RANGE OF MOTION (ROM). Activities for increasing or maintaining joint ROM may be graded by positioning materials and equipment to demand greater reach or excursion of joints or adapting equipment with lengthened handles.

An example of a simple adaptation is positioning a large checkerboard in a vertical position to achieve the desired range of shoulder flexion while playing the game (Fig. 14-8). Positioning an object, such as a mosaic tile project, at increasing or decreasing distances from the patient on the tabletop can affect the range needed to reach the materials. Handles may be extended to effect increased range, such as on a loom (Fig. 14-9). Tool handles may be increased in size by using a larger dowel or by padding the handle with foam rubber to accommodate limited ROM or to facilitate grasp.

ENDURANCE AND TOLERANCE. Endurance may be graded by moving from light to heavy work and increasing the length of the work period. Standing and walking tolerance may be graded by increasing the length of time spent standing to work, perhaps at first at a stand-up table (Fig. 14-10), and increasing the time and distance spent in activities requiring walking. These may include home management and workshop activities.

COORDINATION. Coordination and muscle control may be graded by decreasing the amount of gross resistive movements and increasing the fine controlled movements required in the purposeful activities. An

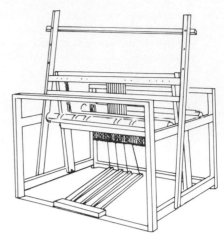

Fig. 14-9. Floor loom with adjustable vertically extended beater bar to require increasing ranges of shoulder flexion.

example is progressing from sawing wood with a crosscut saw to using a coping saw to using a jewelers' saw to using chip-carving tools. Dexterity and speed of movement may be graded by practice, at increasing speeds, once movement patterns have been mastered through coordination training and neuromuscular education.

Perceptual, Cognitive, and Social Skills

Grading activity for increasing cognitive demands requires an analysis of those demands in the given activity. For example, in grading cognitive skills, the treatment program can begin with simple one- or two-step activities that require little judgment, decision

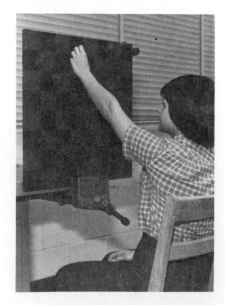

Fig. 14-8. Checkerboard is positioned vertically to increase ROM of shoulder flexion while playing game.

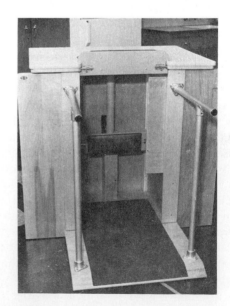

Fig. 14-10. Stand-up table with sliding door, padded knee support, and backrest.

making, or problem solving and progress to activities with several steps that require some judgment or problem-solving processes. A patient in a lunch preparation group may be assigned the task of buttering bread that has already been lined up on the work surface. This could be graded to lining up the bread, then buttering it and placing a slice of lunch meat on it, and, ultimately, to making sandwiches.

Similarly, for grading social interaction, the treatment program may be initiated with an activity that demands sole interaction with the therapist. The patient can progress to activities requiring dyadic interaction with another patient and, ultimately, to small group activities. The therapist can facilitate the patient's progression from the role of observer to that of participant and then to leader. Concomitantly, the therapist would decrease his or her supervision, guidance, and assistance to facilitate more independent functioning in the patient.

Adaptation of activity can be a challenge to the creativity and ingenuity of the occupational therapist. The therapist should remember that for the adaptations to be used effectively, the patient must be able to use them in a good, comfortable position. The patient must understand the need and purpose of the activity and the adaptations and be willing to perform the activity with the simple modifications. Peculiar and complicated adaptations that require frequent adjustment and modification should be avoided.[21]

Selection of Activity

In the treatment of physical dysfunction, activities are usually selected for their potential to improve physical performance skills and their potential psychosocial benefits. Activities selected for improvement of physical performance should provide desired exercise or purposeful use of affected parts. They should enable the patient to transfer the motion, strength, and coordination gained to useful, normal daily activities.

If activities are to meet requirements for physical restoration, they must meet the following three basic criteria.

1. Activities should provide action rather than position of involved joints and muscles; that is, they should allow alternate contraction and relaxation of the muscles being exercised and allow the joints to course through their available ROM.
2. Activities should provide repetition of motion. This means that activities should allow for an indefinite but controllable number of repetitions of the desired movement patterns sufficient to be of benefit to the patient.
3. Activities should allow for one or more kinds of

gradation, such as for resistance, range, coordination, endurance, or complexity.[5,21]

The type of exercise that is needed must be considered. Active and resistive exercises are most often used in the performance of purposeful activity.[21] Requirements for passive and assistive exercise are less easily applied to purposeful activities, although not impossible.

Other important considerations in the selection of activity are (1) properties of the materials and equipment; (2) safety factors; (3) preparation and completion time; (4) complexity; (5) type of instruction and supervision required; (6) structure and controls in the activity; (7) learning requirements; (8) independence, decision-making, and problem-solving required; (9) social interaction potential; (10) communication skills required, and (11) potential gratification to the person.

Prevocational activities must be selected for their ability to evaluate or develop work-related skills. Crafts, job samples, or work simulations may be selected for their similarities to skills required in the

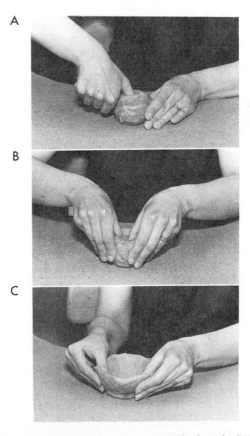

Fig. 14-11. A, Opening pinch pot with thumb. **B,** Walls of pot are gradually spread with pinching motion of fingers. **C,** Pinching continues in circular direction until desired size of pot is reached.

actual job. Physical skills required, work speed, concentration, ability to follow instructions and accept supervision, and work habits and attitudes may be assessed or developed through the use of such activities.[5]

It is assumed that if the therapist selects an activity in which the patient has an interest, the patient will experience enough satisfaction to sustain performance of the activity. This satisfaction is an important characteristic of intrinsic motivation. Thus it is believed that purposeful activity provides intrinsic motivation to sustain performance.[19]

Therapy must be individualized for each patient. The means of doing this are evaluative tools such as the interest checklist, activity configuration, occupational history, interview, and activity analysis.[20]

ACTIVITY ANALYSIS

An activity analysis model and a completed sample activity analysis follow, which offer the student or therapist a systematic approach to looking at activities for their therapeutic potential. This model includes the important factors that must be considered in the selection of activity that have been outlined.

Summary

Therapeutic activity is the core of occupational therapy practice. Its value lies in its health-giving and remedial nature. The selection of appropriate therapeutic activities is based on the patient's activity configuration and on careful activity analysis. Appropriate therapeutic activity is individualized and designed to be meaningful and interesting to the patient while meeting therapeutic objectives.

Therapeutic activity may be adapted to meet special needs of the patient or the environment. It may be graded for physical, perceptual, cognitive, and social purposes to keep the patient functioning at maximal potential at any point in the treatment program. The uniqueness of occupational therapy lies in its extensive use of goal-directed purposeful activity as treatment media and methods.

REVIEW QUESTIONS

1. Define "therapeutic exercise."
2. What is meant by "substitution patterns"? Why do they occur?
3. What demand must be made on a muscle for its strength to increase?
4. What happens to a muscle that is fatigued?
5. List four signs of fatigue from excess exercise.
6. List at least four purposes of therapeutic exercise.
7. With which types of disabilities would you use therapeutic exercise? Which disabilities is it less useful for? Why?
8. To participate in a therapeutic exercise program the patient must possess certain characteristics. List and discuss at least four of these requirements.
9. List four precautions or contraindications to therapeutic exercise, and explain why each can preclude the use of therapeutic exercise.
10. Define three types of muscle contraction, and give an example of how each occurs in daily activity.
11. What type of exercise should be used if muscle grades are Fair + to Good? Why?
12. If a patient has joint pain and inflammation with good muscle strength, what type of exercise should be used? Why?
13. How is passive stretching different from passive exercise?
14. Describe the procedure and precautions for passive stretching.
15. When beginning PRE, how is the patient's maximal resistance determined?
16. Describe the procedure for PRE to strengthen Fair + wrist extensors.
17. Describe the steps in coordination exercises.
18. List four objectives of therapeutic activities.
19. Name four classifications of activities that could be used for therapeutic objectives.
20. Discuss Cynkin's premises about activities in occupational therapy.
21. List at least five requirements that activities need to meet if they are to be used for therapeutic purposes.
22. How can activities be adapted to meet specific therapeutic objectives and allow for gradation of the therapeutic program?
23. List four ways in which activities may be graded.
24. What are the three criteria an activity must meet to be useful for exercise purposes?
25. Name and discuss at least five factors that should be considered in the selection of activities.
26. Can therapeutic activity and therapeutic exercise be used simultaneously in a treatment program? How and why?
27. Select one of the following activities, and complete an activity analysis according to the model provided.
    a. Sawing wood
    b. Placing mosaic tiles
    c. Sanding a vertical surface
    d. Pulling leather lacing
    e. Rolling out dough
    f. Using a push broom

Activity analysis model

A. Activity or process under analysis:
  1. Describe the activity and its component steps
  2. Describe the necessary equipment and materials and positioning of the worker in relation to the equipment and materials.

B. Criteria for use of the activity as an exercise.
  1. Action rather than position of muscles and joints.
      a. To which joints is movement localized?
      b. Which joints are in static or holding positions?
      c. Which muscle groups are used to perform the movements of the joints in motion? What types of muscle contraction are used?
      d. How much muscle strength is required to perform the activity/parts of activity (indicate muscle groups and estimated muscle grade needed for each).
      e. Estimate amount of normal ROM that moving joints are coursing through. List and indicate minimal, moderate, and full.
  2. Repetition of motion.
      a. Is the same movement/movement pattern performed repeatedly? Describe patterns.
      b. Is the number of repetitions controllable; that is, can the activity be stopped at any time without negating the goal of the activity or ruining the end product?
      c. Is the number of repetitions sufficient to effect the desired treatment goals?
  3. Gradation.
      a. Is the activity gradable? How?
      b. How can the activity be graded if increased/decreased ROM is desired?
      c. How can the activity be graded if increased/decreased strength (resistance) is desired?
      d. How can the activity be graded if increased coordination (gross to fine movement patterns) is desired?
      e. What other types of gradation are possible?

C. Sensory-perceptual-cognitive demands of the activity.
  1. Sensory input from materials and performance.
      a. Tactile
      b. Proprioceptive
      c. Vestibular
      d. Visual
      e. Olfactory
      f. Gustatory[12]
      g. Pain
      h. Thermal
      i. Pressure
      j. Visceral[11]
  2. Sensory integration processes.
      a. Tactile-proprioceptive-vestibular functions.
          (1) Equilibrium and protective reactions: What are the sitting and standing balances required?[12]
          (2) Postural and bilateral integration: Are postural adjustments and coordinated use of both body sides required?[12]
          (3) Does the activity require tactile discrimination? Describe.
          (4) How essential is proprioceptive feedback to adequate performance?
          (5) Are the required motor planning skills simple or complex?

  b. Visual functions.
      (1) Does the activity require visual scanning? How much? Describe.
      (2) What types of differentiation and recognition are required?
          (a) Color
          (b) Size
          (c) Shape and form.[12]
      (3) Does the activity require simple or complex perception of position in space and spatial relationship?[12] Describe.
          (a) Fitting parts
          (b) Matching, fitting shapes or forms
          (c) Differentiating patterns
          (d) Observing, changing positions of parts
      (4) Is the figure-background perception required simple or complex? Describe.
      (5) Does the activity require gross or fine visual-motor coordination? Describe.
      (6) Does the activity require simple or complex sequencing or ordering of visual patterns (for example, arranging from top to bottom, left to right, or first to last)? Describe.
  c. Auditory functions.
      (1) Is hearing essential to the performance of the activity; that is, could activity be performed if one could not hear?
      (2) Is sound discrimination essential to adequately perform the activity? Why? Describe.
  d. Cognitive demands of the activity.
      (1) How critical is long-term memory (more than 2 days) to the performance of the activity?[12]
      (2) How critical is short-term memory (1 hour to 2 days) to the performance of the activity?[12]
      (3) Does the activity require the logical sequencing or ordering of steps or stages?[11] Does the completion of one step depend on the anticipation of the next step and readiness for it?
      (4) Does the activity require analysis of problems and problem-solving skills (for example, recognizing errors, analyzing problems, determining solutions, and using the correct procedures to effect the solutions)?
      (5) Does the activity require the ability to do any of the following?
          (a) Read
          (b) Write
          (c) Speak
          (d) Comprehend oral instructions
          (e) Comprehend written instructions
          (f) Comprehend demonstrated instructions.
          (g) Comprehend diagrams
          (h) Learn another system of symbols
      (6) What level of concentration does the activity require?
      (7) Does the activity require generalization of learning from past experience or for future use?

Continued.

Activity analysis model—cont'd

D. **Safety factors.**
   1. Is there danger of cutting, piercing, or burning the skin?
   2. Is there danger of losing control of tools or machinery?

E. **Interpersonal aspects of the activity.[2]**
   1. What is the number of people required or possible for participation?
   2. What is the nature of interpersonal transactions?
      a. Dependent
      b. Independent
      c. Cooperative
      d. Collaborative
      e. Competitive

F. **Sociocultural symbolism of the activity.**
   1. What does the activity symbolize in the culture?
   2. What does the activity symbolize in any specific subgroup within the culture?
   3. Does the activity connote sex-role identification in the culture or to most individuals?

G. **Psychological-emotional responses to the activity.**
   1. What feelings does the activity evoke in the worker (for example, aggression, peace, boredom, fear, pleasure, indifference).[12]
   2. Does the worker derive personal gratification from the performance of the activity?

H. **Therapeutic use of the activity.**
   1. List the autonomous or inherent objectives of the activity.
   2. List the possible therapeutic objectives.
      a. Physical
      b. Sensory integrative
      c. Psychosocial
      d. Vocational

SAMPLE ACTIVITY ANALYSIS

A. **Activity or process under analysis:**
   Pinch process in pinch pottery.
   1. A hole is made with the thumb in a ball of clay 3 to 4 inches in diameter (Fig. 14-11, *A*). The thumb and first two fingers then pinch around and around the hole from base to top of the ball of clay to gradually thin and spread the walls of the clay to produce a small, round clay pot (Fig. 14-11, *B* and *C*).
   2. The activity requires a ball of soft ceramic clay and a wooden table surface or a wooden work board on a metal or formica table. The table should be 30 to 32 inches high or a comfortable height for the worker when the worker is in an erect, sitting position at the table.

B. **Criteria for use of the activity as an exercise.**
   1. Action rather than position of muscles and joints.
      a. Movement is localized to flexion and extension of the metacarpophalangeal (MP) and interphalangeal (IP) joints of digits one and two, opposition and abduction of the carpometacarpal joint of thumb, and flexion and extension of the MP and IP joints of the thumb.
      b. Static or holding positions are maintained at the wrist during the pinch process. However, the wrist makes many minor adjustments into radial and ulnar deviation and flexion and extension as the hand moves around and up and down the pot. The back and neck are stabilized. There is only slight movement at the shoulder and elbow to make adjustments in the position of the hand as it moves around the pot.
      c. The opponens pollicis, flexors pollicis longus and brevis, and flexors digitorum profundis and superficialis are acting in concentric contraction. Palmar interossei are in isometric contraction to maintain adduction of the fingers. Lumbricales are acting concentrically to flex the MP joints and maintain extension of the IP joints of the fingers during the pinch process. The extensor digitorum communis, extensor indicis proprius, extensors pollicis longus and brevis, and abductor pollicis are in eccentric contraction, which accounts for their controlled lengthening during the pinch process and concentric contraction during the release from pinch.
      d. The muscle strength required in the flexor groups and the opponens pollicis is at least fair plus, because the muscles must overcome the slight resistance of the clay. Poor strength is adequate for the extensors and thumb abductors, because they act to release the pinch, and there is no resistance to these motions. Muscle endurance must be adequate to repeat the movement pattern around the pot at least once before a rest is required.
      e. Joints course through a minimal ROM. MP joints are in 60° to 90° of flexion, and IP joints are in nearly full extension during the pinch process.
   2. Repetition of motion.
      a. The pinching motion with the thumb in opposition to the first two digits is repeated until the pot has reached the desired height and thickness.

Continued.

Activity analysis model—cont'd

b. The number of repetitions is controllable, since the process may be stopped and the project damp-stored for future use at any time.

c. The number of repetitions is adequate for one or two treatment sessions. If more pinching activity is desirable, similar projects may be used.

3. Gradation. The activity cannot be graded for increasing ROM. It can be graded slightly for increasing strength by increasing the stiffness of the clay. It may also be graded for sitting tolerance by increasing the length of the work periods and for sitting balance by decreasing the amount of support for sitting.

C. **Sensory-perceptual-cognitive demands of the activity.**

1. Sensory input from materials and performance. There are tactile, proprioceptive, visual, slight olfactory, thermal, and pressure stimuli received from working with clay.

2. Sensory integration processes[11]

a. Tactile-proprioceptive-vestibular functions.

(1) The activity requires good sitting balance or trunk stabilization if balance is not adequate. Good head and neck control are required.

(2) The activity requires the ability to make slight postural adjustments of trunk and proximal upper extremity joints and the use of both hands, one for supporting and moving the pot and the other for the pinching process.

(3) Fine tactile discrimination is required to feel the texture, moisture content, and thickness of the clay. Visual functions may substitute to some extent.

(4) Proprioceptive feedback is necessary for adequate performance to determine position of hand and fingers and degree of strength of pinch, so as not to progress too

rapidly or break the clay by squeezing too hard.

(5) The motor planning skills required are relatively simple, because the same motor pattern and a familiar one already learned are repeated over and over. The motor pattern can be easily learned from visual or proprioceptive learning techniques.

b. Visual functions.

(1) The activity requires minimal visual scanning. Gaze is fixed on the object at the center of the work area.

(2) Differentiation and recognition.

(a) The activity does not require color differentiation.

(b) Size discrimination of the height and thickness of the walls is required. It can be obtained partially through tactile and proprioceptive feedback.

(c) Shape and form perception through visual and tactile feedback is required to maintain the round shape of the pot.

(3) Requirements for position in space and spatial relationships are simple, since there is only one object and no fitting, matching of parts or shapes, or differentiating patterns.

(4) Figure-background perception required is simple, since there is only one object on a significantly contrasting background.

(5) The activity requires moderate to fine visual-motor coordination, since fine muscles are acting in a controlled manner in response to visual, tactile, and proprioceptive information.

(6) Some simple visual sequencing is required to progress with the pinching in a circular manner and from bottom to top.

Continued.

Activity analysis model—cont'd

c. Auditory functions.
   (1) Hearing is not essential to the performance of pinch pottery except to receive instructions. Demonstrated and written/illustrated instructions may be substituted.
   (2) Sound discrimination is not required.
d. Cognitive demands of the activity.
   (1) Long-term memory is not required.
   (2) Short-term memory is essential if the project is to be completed in 2 to 3 days without reinstruction and continuous supervision.
   (3) The activity requires sequencing of steps, and the completion of one step is necessary before the next can be started.
   (4) The activity requires simple problem-solving skills for recognition of changes in shape and thickness of walls. Knowledge of the behavior of clay and its properties for analysis and when to seek assistance to correct problems is essential to the successful outcome of the end product.
   (5) The activity requires the ability to comprehend oral or demonstrated instructions.
   (6) The activity requires the ability to generalize from previous experience with pinch movements, soft materials, and round objects.

D. Safety factors.
1. There is no danger of cutting, piercing, or burning the skin.
2. There is no danger of losing control of tools or machinery, since none are used.

E. Interpersonal aspects of the activity.
1. The activity may be done alone or in a group of people performing the same or similar activities.
2. Interpersonal transactions may be independent if the worker is working alone or with others and needs little supervision and assistance; dependent if more assistance, supervision, prodding, or reassurance is required; and competitive if all group members are making the same or similar objects, and there is a sense of competition, for example,

for degree of attractiveness, use of the end product, speed of work, or admiration of supervisors.

F. Sociocultural symbolism of the activity.
1. The activity in American culture symbolizes the artistic or perhaps liberal or naturalistic groups of people in the society.
2. The activity is scen as a leisure rather than a work skill and may be associated with child's play by some persons.
3. The activity may have a more feminine than a masculine identification to the older or more conservative segments of the society.

G. Psychological-emotional responses to the activity.
1. The soft, moist, pliable, and plastic properties of the clay may evoke peace and pleasure in many persons. Others may regard it as "messy" and dirty.
2. The potential for gratification is good, because the end product is easy to achieve, is creative, is as personal as the worker's own fingerprints, and is useful.

H. Therapeutic use of the activity.
1. The inherent objectives of the activity are to derive pleasure and sense of worth from producing a creative object, produce a useful product, and interact with others with similar interests.
2. Therapeutic objectives.
   a. The physical objectives of the activity are to increase strength of opponens pollicis and flexor muscles of the fingers and thumb and improve coordination.
   b. The sensory-integrative objectives are to increase tactile, proprioceptive, and thermal sensory input to the hands and improve concentration and sequencing skills and form perception.
   c. The psychosocial objectives are to improve self-esteem and interaction skills, reduce anxiety, and provide an outlet for self-expression.
   d. There is little potential for vocationally related objectives in this activity.

REFERENCES

1. Ayres AJ: Occupational therapy for motor disorders resulting from impairment of the central nervous system, Rehabil. Lit. 21:302, 1960.
2. Cynkin, S: Occupational therapy: toward health through activities, Boston, 1979, Little, Brown & Co.
3. De Lateur BJ: Therapeutic exercise to develop strength and endurance. In Kottke FJ, Stillwell GK, and Lehmann JF, editors: Krusen's handbook of physical medicine and rehabilitation, ed 3, Philadelphia, 1982, WB Saunders Co.
4. Hinojosa J, Sabari J, and Rosenfeld, MS: Purposeful activities, Am J Occup Ther 37:805, 1983.
5. Hopkins HL, Smith HD, and Tiffany EG: The activity process. In Hopkins HL and Smith HD, editors: Willard and Spackman's occupational therapy, ed 5, Philadelphia, 1978, JB Lippincott Co.
6. Huddleston OL: Therapeutiic cxercises, Philadelphia, 1961, FA Davis Co.
7. Kielhofner G: A heritage of activity: development of theory, Am J Occup Ther 36:723, 1982.
8. Kottke FJ: Therapeutic exercise to maintain mobility. In Kottke FJ, Stillwell GK, and Lehmann JF, editors: Krusen's handbook of physical medicine and rehabilitation, ed 3, Philadelphia, 1982, WB Saunders Co.
9. Kottke FJ: Therapeutic exercises to develop neuromuscular coordination. In Kottke FJ, Stillwell GK and Lehmann JF, editors: Krusen's handbook of physical medicine and rehabilitation, ed 3, Philadelphia, 1982, WB Saunders Co.
10. Kraus H: Therapeutic exercise, Springfield, Ill, 1963, Charles C Thomas, Publisher.
11. Llorens L: Activity analysis for sensory integration (CPM) dysfunction, 1978. Unpublished.
12. Llorens LA: Activity analysis: agreement among factors in a sensory processing model, Am J Occup Ther 40:103, 1986.
13. Melvin JL: Rheumatic disease: occupational therapy and rehabilitation, ed 2, Philadelphia, 1982, FA Davis Co.
14. Rancho Los Amigos Hospital: Muscle reeducation, Downey, CA, 1963, Rancho Los Amigos Hospital. Unpublished.
15. Rancho Los Amigos Hospital: Progressive resistive and static exercise: principles and techniques, Downey, CA, Rancho Los Amigos Hospital. Unpublished.
16. Reed KL: Tools of practice: heritage or baggage? Am J Occup Ther 40:597, 1986.
17. Rocker JD and Nelson DL: Affective responses to keeping and not keeping an activity product. Am J Occup Ther 41:152, 1987.
18. Schram DA: Resistance exercise. In Basmajian JV, editor: Therapeutic exercise, ed 4, Baltimore, 1984, Williams & Wilkins.
19. Steinbeck TM: Purposeful activity and performance. Am J Occup Ther 40:529, 1986.
20. Thibodeaux CS and Ludwig FM: Intrinsic motivation in product-oriented and non–product-oriented activities. Am J Occup Ther 42:169, 1988.
21. Willard HS and Spackman CS, editors: Occupational therapy, ed 4, Philadelphia, 1971, JB Lippincott Co.
22. Wynn-Parry CB: Vicarious motions. In Basmajian, JV, editor: Therapeutic exercise, ed 3, Baltimore, 1982, Williams & Wilkins.

Chapter

15 Activities of daily living

LORRAINE WILLIAMS PEDRETTI

Activities of daily living (ADL) are tasks of self-maintenance, mobility, communication, and home management that enable an individual to achieve personal independence in his or her environment. Evaluation of and training in the performance of these important life tasks have long been important aspects of occupational therapy programs in virtually every type of health facility. Loss of ability to care for personal needs and to manage the environment can result in loss of self-esteem, a deep sense of dependence, and even feelings of infantilism and can profoundly affect the role and function of the caretakers of the person who has lost these performance skills.[17]

The role of occupational therapy in ADL is to assess ADL performance skills, determine problems that interfere with independence, determine treatment objectives, and provide training or equipment to enhance the achievement of a higher level of independence. The occupational therapist may also be involved in ameliorating physical, cognitive, social, and emotional barriers that are interfering with ADL performance. The need to learn new methods or use assistive devices to perform ADL may be temporary or permanent, depending on the particular dysfunction and the prognosis for recovery.

DEFINITION OF ADL

ADL include mobility, self-care, management of environmental hardware and devices, communication, and home management activities. These major classifications are further defined as follows: (1) mobility includes movement in bed, wheelchair mobility and transfers, indoor ambulation with special equipment, outdoor ambulation with special equipment, and management of public or private transportation; (2) self-care includes dressing, feeding, toileting, bathing, and grooming activities; (3) management of environmental hardware and devices includes the ability to use telephones, keys, faucets, light switches, windows, doors, scissors, and street control signals; (4) communication skills include the ability to write, operate a personal computer, read, type, or use the telephone, a tape recorder, or a special communications device;

(5) home management activities include marketing, meal planning and preparation, cleaning, laundry, child care, and operating household appliances, such as vacuum cleaners, can openers, ranges, refrigerators, electric mixers, and hand-operated utensils.

EVALUATION OF PERFORMANCE SKILLS

ADL or "self-care activities" is one of the major performance skills in the occupational performance frame of reference discussed in Chapter 1. A comprehensive evaluation of performance skills should include assessment of the patient's abilities and limitations in work and play/leisure activities and in self-care activities. A primary purpose of occupational therapy is to facilitate skill in performance of these essential tasks of living. It is important to help the patient to create a balance in the quantity of activity in each of these three performance areas, which is healthy for him or her in terms of personality, skills, limitations, needs, values, and life-style.

The therapist's evaluation of the patient's performance profile could begin with the charting of a daily or weekly schedule (see Chapter 3), an activities configuration, an interest checklist, or an occupational role history.[4,7,18,20,28] The activities configuration protocol can be used to gather data about the patient's values, educational history, and work history, including current or recent work experience, past work experience, and vocational interests and plans. The interest checklist can be used to determine degree of interest in five categories of activities: (1) manual skills, (2) physical sports, (3) social recreation, (4) activities of daily living (ADL), and (5) cultural and educational activities.[18] The occupational role history is used to gather data about past and current occupational roles and the balance between work and leisure roles.[7] Although the interest checklist and the occupational role history were developed for a psychiatric population, they can be adapted for application to patients with a physical dysfunction. In the practice of occupational therapy for physical dysfunction, occupational performance can be overlooked if therapists focus on remedying specific performance components and fail to integrate these with the development of occupational role performance.

An interview and performance evaluation can yield a well-rounded picture of the patient's occupational performance. Deficits and imbalances in occupational performance will be apparent. The performance evaluation is fundamental to the development of a comprehensive treatment plan, which deals with performance components that underlie those skills. The performance evaluations to be addressed in this chapter are ADL, home evaluation, and driving evaluation.

Work evaluation is assessment of specific work skills using a real or simulated work situation.[14] Work habits and attitudes are also observed and evaluated. Work evaluation may be carried out by the occupational therapist. (Work evaluation and work hardening programs are discussed in Chapter 16.)

FACTORS TO CONSIDER IN ADL EVALUATION AND TRAINING

Before commencing ADL performance evaluation and training, the occupational therapist must assess performance components and consider several factors about the patient and the individual environment. Physical resources, such as strength, range of motion (ROM), coordination, sensation, and balance, should be evaluated to determine potential skills and deficits in ADL performance and possible need for special equipment. Perceptual and cognitive functions should be evaluated to determine potential for learning ADL skills. General mobility in bed or wheelchair or ambulation should be assessed.

In addition to these relatively concrete and objective evaluations the occupational therapist should be familiar with the patient's culture and its values and mores in relation to self-care, the sick role, family assistance, and independence. The values of the patient and the patient's peer group and culture should be important considerations in selecting objectives and initial activities in the ADL program. The balance of activities in the patient's day, which demand time and energy, may influence how many ADL may be performed independently. The environment to which the patient will return is an important consideration. Will the patient live alone or with his or her family or a roommate? Will the patient be going to a skilled nursing facility or to a board and care home permanently or temporarily? Will the patient return to work and community activities? The type and amount of assistance available in the home environment must be considered if the appropriate caretaker is to receive orientation and training in the appropriate supervision and assistance required. The finances available for assistant care, special equipment, and home mod-

ifications are important considerations. For example, a wheelchair-bound patient who is wealthy may be willing and able to make major modifications in the home, such as installing an elevator, lowering kitchen counters, widening doorways, and replacing deep pile carpeting to accommodate a wheelchair life-style. A less well-off patient may need the assistance of an occupational therapist in making less costly modifications, such as removing scatter rugs and door sills, installing a plywood ramp at the entrance, replacing the bathroom door with a curtain, and attaching a hand-held shower head to the bathtub faucet.

The ultimate goal of any ADL training program is for the patient to achieve *his* or *her* maximal level of independence. It is important to note that the "maximal level of independence" is defined differently for each patient. For the patient with mild muscle weakness in one arm caused by a peripheral neuropathy, complete independence in ADL may be the "maximal," whereas for the high-level quadriplegic, feeding and oral hygiene activities with devices and assistance may be the maximal level of independence that can be expected. Therefore the potential for independence should be based on each patient's unique personal needs, values, capabilities, limitations, and environmental resources.

Independence is a strong value in the American culture. It should not be pursued solely on that basis or because it is a value of the rehabilitation personnel or family or friends of the patient. Achieving independence must be important to the patient and within the realm of possibility.

ADL EVALUATION
General Procedure

When some data have been gathered about the patient's physical, psychosocial, and environmental resources, the feasibility of ADL evaluation or training should be determined by the occupational therapist in concert with the patient, supervising physician, and other members of the rehabilitation team. In some instances ADL should be delayed because of limitations of the patient or in favor of more immediate treatment objectives that require the patient's energy and participation.

Evaluation of ADL performance is often initiated with an interview, using an ADL checklist as a guide for questioning the patient about individual capabilities and limitations. Several types of ADL checklists are available, but they all cover similar categories and performance tasks.[9]

The ADL interview may serve as a screening device to determine the need for further assessment by observation of performance. This is determined by the therapist's professional judgment based on knowledge of the patient, the dysfunction, and the results of previous evaluations. A partial or complete performance evaluation is invaluable in assessing ADL performance. The phrase "one look is worth a thousand words" applies well here. The ADL interview alone, as a measure of performance, can lead to inaccurate assumptions, because the patient may recall his or her performance before the onset of the dysfunction, may have some confusion or memory loss, and may overestimate or underestimate individual abilities, because he or she has had little opportunity to perform routine ADL after the onset of the physical dysfunction.

Ideally the occupational therapist should conduct the performance evaluation at the time and in the environment in which the activities to be evaluated usually take place. For example, a dressing evaluation could be arranged early in the morning in the treatment facility when the patient is dressed by nursing personnel or in the patient's home. Feeding evaluation should occur at regular meal hours. If this is not possible because of schedules, personnel, and environmental constraints in the treatment facility or the patient's home, the evaluation may be conducted during regular treatment sessions in the occupational therapy clinic under simulated conditions. This requires the patient to perform or reperform routine self-maintenance tasks at irregular times in an artificial environment and can contribute to a lack of carryover for those patients who have difficulty generalizing learning concepts.

The therapist should begin by selecting relatively simple and safe tasks from the ADL checklist for the patient to perform and should progress to more difficult and complex items. The evaluation should not be completed at one time, because this would cause fatigue and create an artificial situation. Those tasks that would be unsafe or very obviously cannot be performed should be omitted and the appropriate notation made on the evaluation form.

During the performance evaluation the therapist should observe the methods that the patient is using or attempting to use to accomplish the task and try to determine causes of performance problems. Some causes might be weakness, spasticity, involuntary motion, perceptual deficits, and low endurance. If problems and their causes can be identified, the therapist has a good foundation for establishing training objectives, priorities, and methods and need for assistive devices. Other very important aspects of this evaluation that should not be overlooked are the patient's need for respect and privacy and the ongoing interaction between the patient and the therapist. The pa-

tient's feelings about having his or her body viewed and touched should be respected. Privacy should be maintained for toileting, grooming, and dressing tasks. The therapist with whom the patient is most familiar and comfortable may be the appropriate person to conduct the ADL evaluation and training. As the therapist interacts with the patient during performance of ADL, it may be possible to elicit the patient's attitudes and feelings about the particular tasks, individual priorities in training, dependence and independence, and cultural, family, and personal values and customs about performance of daily living activities.

RECORDING RESULTS OF THE ADL EVALUATION. During the interview and performance evaluation the therapist makes the appropriate notations on the ADL checklists. These may include separate checklists for self-care, home management, mobility, and home environment evaluations. The information is then summarized succinctly for inclusion in the patient's permanent records so that interested professional coworkers can refer to it.

Home Management Evaluation

Home management tasks are evaluated similarly to self-care tasks. The patient should first be interviewed to elicit a description of the home and former and present home management responsibilities. Those tasks that the patient will need to perform when returning home, as well as those that he or she would like to perform, should be ascertained during the interview. If the patient has a communication disorders, aid from friends or family members may be enlisted to get the information needed. The patient may also be questioned about his or her ability to perform each task on the activities list. However, the evaluation is much more meaningful if this is followed by a performance evaluation in the ADL kitchen or apartment of the treatment facility or in the patient's home if possible.

The initial tasks should be simple one- or two-step procedures that are not hazardous, such as wiping a dish, sponging off a table, and turning the water on and off. As the evaluation progresses, tasks graded in complexity and involving safety precautions should be performed, such as making a sandwich and a cup of coffee and vacuuming the carpet. It is assumed that at this point the therapist has already evaluated motor, sensory, perceptual, and cognitive skills. Consequently the therapist should select tasks and exercise safety precautions consistent with the patient's capabilities and limitations.

Traditionally, home management skills were thought to apply primarily to women patients. However, they are appropriate for men and sometimes for children and adolescents as well. In modern society men are more often living independently or sharing home management responsibilities with their partners. In some homes it is necessary for a role reversal to occur after onset of a physical disability, and the woman partner may seek employment outside the home, while the disabled man remains at home. If he is going to be there alone, at the very least he needs to be able to prepare a simple meal, employ safety precautions, and get emergency aid if needed. The occupational therapist can evaluate potential for remaining at home alone through the activities of home management evaluation.

HOME EVALUATION

When discharge from the treatment facility is anticipated, a home evaluation should be carried out to facilitate the patient's maximal independence in the living environment. Ideally it should be performed by the physical and occupational therapists together on a visit to the patient's home with the patient and family members or house-mates present. Budgetary and time factors may not allow two professional workers to go to the patient's home, however. Therefore either the physical or occupational therapist should be able to perform the evaluation, or the evaluation may be referred to the home health agency that will be providing home care services to the patient. The patient and a family member should be interviewed to determine the patient's and family's expectations and the roles the patient will assume in the home and community. The cultural or family values regarding a disabled member may influence role expectations and whether or not independence will be encouraged. Willingness and financial ability to make modifications in the home can also be determined.[27]

Sufficient time should be scheduled for the home visit so that the patient can demonstrate the required transfer and mobility skills. The therapist may also wish to ask the patient to demonstrate selected self-care and home management tasks in the home environment. During the evaluation the patient should use the ambulation aids and any assistive devices that he or she is accustomed to use. The therapist should bring a device to measure width of doorways, height of stairs, and height of bed and others.

The therapist can begin by explaining the purposes and procedure of the home evaluation to the patient and others present, if not done before the visit. The therapist can proceed to take the required measurements while surveying the general arrangement of rooms, furniture, and appliances. It may be helpful to sketch the size and arrangement of rooms for later

reference and attach these to the home visit checklist (Fig. 15-1). After this is completed, the patient is involved in demonstrating his or her mobility and transfer skills as designated on the form and in demonstrating performance of essential self-care and home management tasks. The patient's ability to use the entrance to the home and to transfer to and from an automobile, if it is to be used, should be included in the home evaluation.

During the performance evaluation the therapist should be observing safety factors, ease of mobility and performance, and limitations imposed by the environment. If the patient requires assistance for transfers and other activities, the caretaker should be instructed in the methods that are appropriate.

At the end of the evaluation the therapist can make a list of problems. Additional safety equipment, assistive devices, home rearrangement, and alteration may be necessary to solve these. The most frequently needed changes are installation of a ramp or railings at the entrance to the home, removal of scatter rugs, extra furniture, and bric-a-brac, removal of door sills, addition of safety grab bars around the toilet and bathtub, rearrangement of furniture to accommodate a wheelchair, rearrangement of kitchen storage, and lowering of the clothes rod in the closet.[27]

When the home evaluation is completed, the therapist should write a report summarizing the information on the form and describing the patient's performance in the home. The report should conclude with a summary of the problems that the patient is encountering and recommendations for their solution that would facilitate independence. Any equipment or alterations that are recommended should be specific in terms of size, building specifications, costs, and sources.

These recommendations are carefully reviewed with the patient and his or her family. This is done with tact and diplomacy in a way that gives them options and freedom to refuse or consider alternative possibilities. Family finances may be a limiting factor in carrying out needed changes. The social worker may be involved in working out funding for needed equipment and alterations, and the patient should be made aware of this service when cost is discussed.[27]

The therapist should include recommendations regarding the feasibility of the patient's discharge to the home environment or remaining in or managing the home alone, if applicable.

If a home visit is not possible, much of the information can be gained by interviewing the patient and family member following a trial home visit. The family member or caretaker may be instructed to complete the home visit checklist and provide photographs or

HOME VISIT CHECKLIST

Name_____ Therapist _____

Address_____ Date_____

Diagnosis_____ Disability_____

Type of home   Apartment _____ Floor, if apt. _____

                 Private home ____ No. of rooms _____ No. of floors _____

ENTRANCE TO HOME
1. Elevator_____ Stairs _____
2. Number of stairs _____
3. Height of stairs _____
4. Is there a handrail? _____ Left _____ Right _____ (facing house)
5. Are there other entrances that can be used? Describe _____
    _____
    _____
6. Is construction of a ramp feasible?_____
7. Is addition of a handrail feasible?_____
    Comments _____
    _____
    _____

BEDROOM
1. Width of doorway _____
2. Is there a doorsill? _____
3. Height of bed_____
4. Is bed suitable for attachment of   side rails? _____ trapeze bar? _____
5. Can furniture be arranged more conveniently? _____
6. Can patient reach closets? _____ bureaus? _____
7. Is there room for a wheelchair to maneuver? _____
8. Is there room for additional furniture (e.g., commode seat)?_____

BATHROOM
1. Width of doorway _____
2. Is there a doorsill? _____
3. Type of bathtub: roll rim _____ square rim _____ wide square rim _____
4. Can wheelchair get close to   sink? _____ toilet? _____ bathtub? _____
5. Is tub enclosed by   shower curtain? _____ sliding doors? _____
6. Is there a separate shower stall? _____
7. Is bathroom on same floor as   bedroom? _____ living room? _____ kitchen? _____
8. Is it feasible to install handrails on   bathtub? _____ walls? _____ toilet? _____
9. Additional comments_____
    _____
    _____
    _____
    _____

Fig. 15-1. Home visit checklist. Adapted from the Hartford Easter Seal Rehabilitation Center, 1964, Hartford, CT.

Continued.

KITCHEN
1. Width of doors _____
2. Is there a doorsill? _____
3. Is there room for movement of wheelchair? _____
4. Are cupboards within reach? _____
5. Can patient use kitchen utilities? _____ (range, sink, refrigerator)
6. Is rearrangement of furniture feasible? _____
7. Additional comments _____
_____
_____

OTHER ROOMS
1. Width of doors _____
2. Are there doorsills? _____
3. Are light switches in easy reach? _____
4. Would furniture rearrangement be feasible? _____
5. Is telephone conveniently located? _____
6. If needed, is there suitable space for installation of parallel bars? _____

FUNCTIONAL ACTIVITIES OF PATIENT
1. Can patient enter and leave home independently? _____
    If not, what assistance is needed? _____
2. Can the patient move about the home freely? _____
    If not, comment on limitations. _____
_____
_____

3. Which transfer activities is patient unable to perform independently?
    Bed to wheelchair _____
    Chair to bed _____
    Toilet _____
    Bathtub _____
    Shower _____
    Automobile _____
4. Self-care activities: Comment on performance and limitations imposed by home
    environment, if any. _____
_____
_____

5. Home management activities _____
_____
_____

PROBLEM LIST _____
_____
_____
_____
_____

RECOMMENDATIONS FOR HOME MODIFICATION/SPECIAL EQUIPMENT _____
_____
_____
_____
_____
_____
_____

Fig. 15-1, cont'd. Home visit checklist. Adapted from the Hartford Easter Seal Rehabilitation Center, 1964, Hartford, CT.

sketches of the rooms and their arrangements. Problems encountered by the patient during the home visit should be discussed and the necessary recommendations for their solution made, as described earlier.[27]

DRIVING EVALUATION

Adaptive driving has become possible for an increasing number of disabled persons. Special devices and adaptations to motor vehicles along with special training of the disabled driver have made it possible for some severely disabled persons to drive. There are evaluation programs that can be obtained through some state Departments of Motor Vehicles and Licensing. Most large rehabilitation centers have driving evaluation programs.[21] Some having driving simulators for preroad testing.

The occupational therapist can play a vital role in determining the driving potential of a disabled person. Through various motor, sensory, perceptual, cognitive, and performance evaluations, pertinent information relevant to driving potential can be obtained and contributed by the occupational therapist. During evaluation and treatment of the patient, the therapist is observing and assessing functions that subserve driving skills. These include reaction time, visual acuity, peripheral vision, color, figure-ground, spatial and vertical-horizontal perception, ocular movements, hearing, and coordination. Cognitive and behavioral manifestations, such as attention, concentration, impatience, agitation, poor memory, confusion, problem-solving skills, safety awareness, and poor judgment can also be noted.[8,25]

Physical and performance skills that are necessary for driving are also evaluated by the occupational therapist. Muscle strength, joint range of motion, coordination, endurance, ability to use splints or other adapted devices, and transfer skills are some of these.[21,25]

Quigley and De Lisa described a program for assessing the driving potential of patients with cerebral vascular accident (CVA), which involved many members of the rehabilitation team in a comprehensive evaluation.[23] The responsibilities of the occupational therapist included gathering information on driving habits, assessing general knowledge of driving skills, and assessing selected visual functions and gross reaction time. In addition, the occupational therapist measured proprioception, range of motion, and coordination, and helped to determine the need for adapted equipment.

A driving simulator was used with some patients to observe visual memory and perception, laterality, directionality and cognitive tasks of following directions, sequencing, and learning new behaviors.

The occupational therapy evaluation also included use of the driver training car in which transfers, simple parking lot maneuvers, and reaction time and ability to use regular or adapted controls, to follow signs, to control speed, and to perceive hazards were assessed.

Programs describing driving evaluation for the patient with CVA or the brain-injured patient emphasize the importance of evaluating cognitive and perceptual deficits with these populations.[12,23] Problems such as left-right confusion, inadequate use of space, poor planning, limited ability to shift focus, figure-ground perception, and other visual, cognitive, perceptual, and behavioral functions may be limited and may interfere with adequate driving ability.

The occupational therapist is the most suitable health professional to administer selected parts of the driving assessment and to give driving instructions, especially in the early stages, to patients with brain damage or injury. The occupational therapist has access to the medical history and test results, has a good understanding of the patient's limitations, and is trained to predict and recognize the more abstract impairments that can hinder driving performance which would not be apparent to a non-medically trained driving instructor. The occupational therapist is trained to recognize and assess the need for adapted equipment, knows what kind of equipment is available, and can train the patient in its use.[12]

Candidates for Evaluation

The physician may play a primary role in facilitating the driving evaluation and certifying that the patient is a candidate for driving. Okamoto suggested the following criteria for selection of candidates:[21]

1. The patient wants to drive and is realistic about his or her limitations.
2. The patient's condition is stable or improving.
3. The patient is responsible and conscientious about taking medication. If there is a seizure disorder, drug compliance is excellent, and the patient has been free of symptoms for at least 6 months.
4. The patient has no history of drug or alcohol abuse.
5. The patient has been well motivated to achieve maximal function and is competent in necessary ADL.
6. The patient has adequate communication skills, visual-spatial perception, voluntary movement, and reasoning ability for safe driving.
7. The patient is rational and demonstrates predictable behavior. (Explosive, aggressive, hostile, paranoid, or suicidal behavior should not be present.)
8. The patient's family is supportive and firm.

Adaptive Devices

Standard modifications or specially designed assistive devices and custom modifications may be necessary to enable driving. Power steering, power brakes, and automatic transmission may be adequate adaptations for the less severely disabled person. Hand controls are required for the person with significant lower extremity disability and for the person with both lower and upper extremity disabilities. These hand controls may be push-pull, twist-push, or right angle−push types. The steering wheel may have a spinner or plain knob, latch, palm grip, tri-pin, driving ring, cuff, V-grip, or valve. Hooks or extensions may be used for brakes, turn signals, and gear selector. Pedals may be raised by attaching blocks or may need to be transferred to the opposite side. To facilitate transfers, sliding boards, bars, loops, straps, and floor boards are adaptive devices. For safe and comfortable seating, a cushion, safety belt, and chest harness may be used.[21] Special adaptations that are available for cars or vans include ramps and lifts for vans, car-top carriers for wheelchairs, and wheelchair locks that eliminate the necessity of transferring the person to the seat of the van and allow him or her to drive from the wheelchair.[25] The van that is fitted with lifts, wheelchair locks, and force-amplifying control systems has significantly increased the mobility of the severely disabled. The potential long-term benefits of such a van to the patient must be evaluated according to the high cost of the vehicle before it is obtained.[21]

The Unsafe Driver

The patient may be eager to return to driving in spite of deficits, unrecognized or denied, that make driving hazardous.[25] The patient may have a valid driver's license and commence driving against the advice of the physician and therapist. In such instances, Okamoto suggests that the physician discuss the medical and legal implications with the patient and the family; obtain a signed statement from the patient or a family member that the discussion took place, that risks were explained, and that driving is contraindicated; and consider writing a letter to an official in the state Department of Motor Vehicles if the patient refuses to follow recommendations. The physician must use good judgment and should consult a lawyer or officer of the state medical association if necessary.

ADL TRAINING

If, after evaluation, it is determined that ADL training is to be initiated, it is important to establish appropriate short- and long-term objectives, based on the evaluation and on the patient's priorities for independence. The following sequence of training for

self-care activities is suggested: feeding, grooming, continence, transfer skills, toileting, undressing, dressing, and bathing. This sequence is based on the normal development of self-care independence in children.[27]

This sequence provides a good guide but may have to be modified to accommodate the specific dysfunction and the capabilities, limitations, and personal priorities of the patient.

The occupational therapist should estimate which ADL are possible and which are impossible for the patient to achieve. The therapist should explore with the patient the use of alternate methods of performing the activities and the use of any assistive devices that may be helpful. He or she should determine for which tasks the patient requires assistance and how much should be given. It may not be possible to estimate these factors until training is underway.

The ADL training program may be graded by beginning with a few simple tasks and gradually increasing the number and complexity of tasks. Training should progress from dependent to assisted to supervised to independent, with or without assistive devices.[27] The rate at which grading can occur depends on the patient's recovery, endurance, skills, and motivation.

Methods of Teaching ADL

The methods of teaching the patient to perform daily living tasks must be tailored to suit each patient's learning style and ability. The patient who is alert and grasps instructions quickly may be able to perform an entire process after a brief demonstration and verbal instruction. Patients who have perceptual problems, poor memory, and difficulty following instructions of any kind will require a more concrete, step-by-step approach, reducing the amount of assistance gradually as success is achieved. For these persons it is important to break down the activity into small steps and progress through them slowly, one at a time. Slow demonstration by the therapist of the task or step in the same plane and in the same manner in which the patient is expected to perform is very helpful. Verbal instructions to accompany the demonstration may or may not be helpful, depending on the patient's receptive language skills and ability to process and integrate two modes of sensory information simultaneously.

Touching body parts to be moved, dressed, bathed, or positioned, passive movement of the part through the desired pattern to achieve a step or a task and gentle manual guidance through the task are helpful tactile and kinesthetic modes of instruction. These can augment or replace demonstration and verbal instruction, depending on the patient's best avenues of learning. It is necessary to perform a step or complete task repetitiously to achieve skill, speed, and retention of learning. Tasks may be repeated several times during the same training session, if time and the patient's physical and emotional tolerance allow, or they may be repeated on a daily basis until desired retention or level of skill is achieved. The process of "backward chaining" can be used in teaching ADL skills. In this method the therapist assists the patient until the last step of the process is reached. The patient then performs this step independently, which affords a sense of success and completion. When the last step is mastered, the therapist assists until the last two steps are reached and the patient then completes these two steps. The process continues with the therapist offering less and less assistance and the patient performing successive steps of the task, from last to first, independently. This method is particularly useful in training patients with brain damage.[27]

Before beginning training in any ADL the therapist must make some preparations by providing adequate space and arranging equipment, materials, and furniture for maximal convenience and safety. The therapist should be thoroughly familiar with the task to be performed and any special methods or assistive devices that will be used in its performance. The practitioner should be able to perform the task, as he or she expects the patient to perform it, skillfully. After the preparation the activity is presented to the patient, usually in one or more modes of guidance, demonstration, and verbal instruction described earlier. The patient then performs the activity either along with the therapist or immediately after being shown, with the amount of supervision and assistance required. Performance is modified and corrected as needed, and the process is repeated to ensure learning. In the final phase of instruction when the patient has mastered the task or several tasks, he or she is placed on his or her own to perform them independently. The therapist should follow up by checking on performance in progress and later arrange to check on adequacy of performance and carry-over of learning with nursing personnel, the caretaker, or the supervising family members.[11]

Recording Progress in ADL Performance

The ADL checklists used to record performance on the initial evaluation usually have one or more spaces for recording changes in abilities and results of reevaluation during the training process. The sample checklist given later in this chapter is so designed and filled out (see Fig. 15-2). Progress is usually summarized for inclusion in the medical record. The progress record should summarize changes in the patient's abilities and current level of independence and estimate the patient's potential for further independence, attitude, and motivation for ADL training, and future goals for the ADL program.

When describing levels of independence occupational therapists often use terms like *moderate independence, maximal assistance,* and *minimal skill.* These quantitative terms have little meaning to the reader unless they are defined or supporting statements are used in progress summaries to give specific meaning for each. It also should be specified whether the level of independence refers to a single activity, a category of activities such as dressing, or all ADL. In designating levels of independence an agreed-on performance scale should be used to mark the ADL checklist. General categories and their definitions might be the following:

1. Independent. Can perform the activity or activities without cueing, supervision, or assistance, with or without assistive devices, at normal or near normal speeds.
2. Partially dependent. Can perform at least 50% of the activity or activities independently, may be considerably slower than normal performance, use assistive devices, and require some level of assistance
   a. Minimal assistance: supervision, cueing, or less than 20% physical assistance
   b. Moderate assistance: supervision, cueing, and 20% to 50% physical assistance
   c. Maximal assistance: supervision, cueing, and 50% to 80% physical assistance
3. Dependent. Can perform only one or two steps of the activity or very few activities independently, may fatigue easily and perform very slowly, may require elaborate equipment and devices to perform basic skills such as feeding, needs more than 80% physical assistance

These definitions are broad and general. They can be modified to suit the program plan and approach of the particular treatment facility.

A sample case study, ADL and home management checklists, and summaries of an initial evaluation and progress report are included in Figs. 15-2 and 15-3. The reader should keep in mind that the evaluation and progress summaries relate to the ADL portion of the treatment program only.

SPECIFIC ADL TECHNIQUES

In many instances specific techniques to solve specific ADL problems are not possible. Rather the occupational therapist may have to explore a variety of methods or assistive devices to reach a solution. It is sometimes necessary for the therapist to design a spe-

Sample case study

J.V. is a 48-year-old married woman who suffered a cerebral thrombosis resulting in a CVA 6 months ago. She lives in a modest home with her husband and teenage daughter and was a full-time homemaker before the onset of her stroke. She was a cheerful and active woman who enjoyed cooking, baking, gardening, and visiting her neighbors and friends. The stroke resulted in the disturbance of cerebellar and brain stem functions. J.V. has a severe motor apraxia for speech, cannot close her mouth, drools, and walks with a broad-based ataxic gait. Since the onset of her disability J.V. has been very depressed, weeps frequently, is dependent for much of her self-care, and sits idly for long periods of time. She was referred to occupational therapy for evaluation and training in ADL, adjustment to disability, and development of drooling and swallowing control to facilitate feeding.

SAMPLE ADL PROGRESS REPORT

J.V. has attended occupational therapy 3 times weekly for 3 weeks since the initial evaluation. Further evaluation of self-care skills revealed that J.V. is capable of some hygiene skills, except a tub bath, nail care, hair care, and makeup application. However, at home she remains almost entirely dependent on Mr. V. for self-care, while crying and complaining of feeling weak.

Home management evaluation revealed considerable difficulty with most tasks except table setting, dusting, dishwashing, and sweeping, which she can perform if given cues and supervision. Performance of more complex tasks is limited by psychomotor retardation, incoordination, distractibility, inability to sequence a process, and apraxia for fine hand activities. It was necessary to supervise J.V. closely and give step-by-step instructions while she performed household tasks. A few simple homemaking tasks were performed for several training sessions, but performance did not improve.

J.V. appears to be very depressed and lacks intrinsic motivation. It was suggested to her family that they offer less assistance for self-care, and involve her with them in household tasks that she can perform, under their supervision, if possible.

The occupational therapy program will continue with greater emphasis on achieving control of mouth musculature, a primary goal of J.V. ADL training will be delayed until J.V. is moving toward the achievement of this primary goal.

OCCUPATIONAL THERAPY DEPARTMENT

ACTIVITIES OF DAILY LIVING EVALUATION

Name _J. V._ Age _48_ Diagnosis _CVA_ Dom. _Right_

Disability _Bilateral incoordination, ataxia, apraxia of mouth musculature_

Mode of ambulation _Independent_

Grading key:
- I = Independent
- MiA = Minimal assistance
- MoA = Moderate assistance
- MaA = Maximal assistance
- D = Dependent
- NA = Not applicable
- 0 = Not evaluated

TRANSFERS AND AMBULATION

	Date	Independent	Assisted	Dependent
Tub or shower	8/1			D
Toilet	8/1		MiA	
Wheelchair	NA			
Bed and chair		I		
Ambulation			MiA	
Wheelchair management	NA			
Car			MiA	

BALANCE FOR FUNCTION

	Adequate	Inadequate
Sitting	I	
Standing	I	
Walking		MiA

Fig. 15-2. ADL evaluation. Adapted from activities of daily living evaluation form 461-1, Hartford, CT, 1963, The Hartford Easter Seal Rehabilitation Center.   *Continued.*

ADL SKILLS

EATING	Date	8/1	8/25			REMARKS
		Grade				
Butter bread		I				
Cut meat		I				
Eat with spoon		I				
Eat with fork		I				
Drink with straw		D				Mouth apraxia
Drink with glass		D				prevents performance
Drink with cup		D				of these activities
Pour from pitcher		D				

UNDRESS	Date	8/1	8/25			REMARKS
Pants or shorts		I				Is physically
Girdle or garter belt		Mo A				capable of
Brassiere		Mi A				performing the
Slip or undershirt		I				activities as
Dress		I				indicated but
Skirt		I				Mr. V. reports
Blouse or shirt		I				that J.V. is
Slacks or trousers		I				dependent on him
Bandana or necktie		N A				for much assistance,
Stockings		Mo A				pleading fatigue,
Nightclothes		I				whining, and
Hair net		N A				crying for help
Housecoat/bathrobe		I				
Jacket		I				
Belt and/or suspenders		I				
Hat		I				
Coat		I				
Sweater		I				
Mittens or gloves		I				
Glasses		N A				
Brace		N A				
Shoes		Mo A				
Socks		Mo A				
Overshoes		Mo A				

DRESS	Date	8/1	8/25			REMARKS
Pants or shorts		Mi A				
Girdle or garter belt		Mo A				
Brassiere		Mo A				
Slip or undershirt		I				
Dress		I				
Skirt		I				
Blouse or shirt		I				
Slacks or trousers		I				
Bandana or necktie		N A				
Stockings		Mo A				
Nightclothes		I				
Hair net		N A				
Housecoat/bathrobe		I				
Jacket		I				
Belt and/or suspenders		I				
Hat		I				
Coat		I				
Sweater		I				
Mittens or gloves		I				
Glasses		N A				
Brace		N A				
Shoes		Mo A				
Socks		Mo A				
Overshoes		Mo A				

Continued.

Fig. 15-2, cont'd. ADL evaluation. Adapted from activities of daily living evaluation form 461-1, Hartford, CT, 1963, The Hartford Easter Seal Rehabilitation Center.

FASTENINGS	Date	8/1	8/25			REMARKS
		Grade				
Button		I				
Snap		MoA				
Zipper		MiA				
Hook and eye		MaA				
Garters		D				
Lace		D				
Untie shoes		D				
Velcro		MiA				

HYGIENE	Date	8/1	8/25			REMARKS
Blow nose		O	I			
Wash face, hands		O	I			
Wash extremities, back		O	MaA			
Brush teeth or dentures		O	I			
Brush or comb hair		O	I			
Set hair		O	D			
Shave or put on makeup		O	MiA			
Clean fingernails		O	I,D			
Trim fingernails, toenails		O	D			
Apply deodorant		O	I			
Shampoo hair		O	D			
Use toilet paper		O	I			
Use tampon or sanitary napkin		O	NA			

COMMUNICATION	Date	8/1	8/25			REMARKS
Verbal		D				
Read		I				
Hold book		I				
Turn page		I				
Write		I				Writes name and few words
Use telephone		D				
Type		D				

HAND ACTIVITIES	Date	8/1	8/25			REMARKS
Handle money		O				
Handle mail		O				
Use of scissors		O				
Open cans, bottles, jars		O				
Tie package		O				
Sew (baste)		O				
Sew button, hook and eye		O				
Polish shoes		O				
Sharpen pencil		O				
Seal and open letter		O				
Open box		O				

COMBINED PERFORMANCE ACTIVITIES	Date	8/1	8/25			REMARKS
Open-close refrigerator		O	I			
Open-close door		O	I			
Remove and replace objects		O	I			
Carry objects during locomotion		O	D			
		O				
Pick up object from floor		O	D			
Remove, replace light bulb		O	D			
Plug in cord		O	D			

OPERATE	Date	8/1	8/25			REMARKS
		Grade				
Light switches		O	I			
Doorbell		O	I			
Door locks and handles		O	D			
Faucets		O	I			
Raise-lower window shades		O	D			
Raise-lower venetian blinds		O	D			
Raise-lower window		O	D			
Open-close drawer		O	I			
Hang up garment		O	I			

Continued

Fig. 15-2, cont'd. ADL evaluation. Adapted from activities of daily living evaluation form 461-1, Hartford, CT, 1963, The Hartford Easter Seal Rehabilitation Center.

SUMMARY OF EVALUATION RESULTS

Date __8 / 1__

Intact	Impaired		REMARKS
		SENSORY STATUS	
X		Touch	
X		Pain	
X		Temperature	
	X	Position sense	More marked on left
	X	Olfaction	
	X	Stereognosis	More marked on left
	X	Visual fields (hemianopsia)	
		PERCEPTUAL/CONCEPTUAL TESTS	
X		Follow directions	Verbal
X		Visual spatial (form)	
	X	Visual spatial (block design)	Minimal impairment
X		Make change	
	X	Geometric figures (copy) square, circle, triangle, diamond	Some difficulty with triangle & diamond
	X	Praxis	Mild apraxia evident on fine hand activities
		FUNCTIONAL RANGE OF MOTION	
X		Comb hair—two hands	
X		Feed self	
X		Button collar button	
X		Tie apron behind back	
X		Button back buttons	
X		Button cuffs	
X		Zip side zipper	
	X	Tie shoes	Poor balance limits
	X	Stoop	Reach and bending for these activities
	X	Reach shelf	

Fig. 15-2, cont'd. ADL evaluation. Adapted from activities of daily living evaluation form 461-1, Hartford, CT, 1963, The Hartford Easter Seal Rehabilitation Center.

cial device, method, splint, jig, or piece of equipment to make a particular activity possible for the patient to perform. Many of the assistive devices available today through rehabilitation equipment companies were first conceived of and made by occupational therapists and patients. Many of the special methods used to perform specific activities also evolved through trial-and-error approaches of the therapists and their patients. Patients often have good suggestions for therapists, because they live with the limitation and are confronted regularly with the need to adapt the performance of daily tasks. The purpose of the following summary of techniques is to give the reader some general ideas about how to solve ADL problems for specific classifications of dysfunctions. The reader is referred to the references at the end of this chapter for more specific instruction in ADL methods.

Limited ROM

The major problem for persons with limited joint ROM is to compensate for the lack of reach and joint excursion through such means as environmental adaptation and assistive devices. Some adaptations and devices are outlined here.[16,19,22,27]

DRESSING ACTIVITIES. The following are general suggestions for facilitating dressing:

1. Use front-opening garments, one size larger than needed and made of fabrics that have some stretch.
2. Use dressing sticks with a garter on one end and a neoprene-covered coat hook on the other for pushing and pulling garments off and on feet and legs (Fig. 15-4). Use a pair of dowels with a cup hook on end of each to pull socks on if a loop tape is sewn to the tops of the socks.
3. Use larger buttons or zippers with a loop on the pull tab.
4. Replace buttons, snaps, hooks, and eyes with Velcro or zippers (for those patients who cannot manage traditional fastenings).
5. Eliminate the need to bend to tie shoelaces or to use finger joints in this fine activity by using elastic shoelaces or other adapted shoe fasteners.
6. Facilitate donning stockings without bending to the feet by using stocking aids made of garters attached to long webbing straps or by buying those that are commercially available (Fig. 15-5).
7. Use one of several types of commercially available buttonhooks if finger ROM is limited (Fig. 15-6).
8. Use reachers for picking up socks and shoes, ar-

ranging clothes, removing clothes from hangers, and picking up objects on the floor (Fig. 15-7).

FEEDING ACTIVITIES. The following are assistive devices that can facilitate feeding:

1. Built-up handles on eating utensils can accommodate limited grasp or prehension (Fig. 15-8).
2. Elongated or specially curved handles on spoons and forks may be needed to reach the mouth. A swivel spoon or spoon-fork combination can compensate for limited supination (Fig. 15-9).
3. Long plastic straws and straw clips on glasses or cups can be used if neck, elbow, or shoulder ROM limits hand-to-mouth motion or if grasp is inadequate to hold the cup or glass.
4. Universal cuffs or utensil holders can be used if grasp is very limited and built-up handles do not work (Fig. 15-10).
5. Plate guards or scoop dishes may be useful to prevent food from slipping off the plate.

HYGIENE AND GROOMING. Environmental adaptations that can facilitate bathing and grooming are:

1. A hand-held shower head on flexible hose for bathing and shampooing hair can eliminate the need to stand in the shower and offers the user

---

OCCUPATIONAL THERAPY DEPARTMENT

ACTIVITIES OF HOME MANAGEMENT

Name _J. V._   Date _8/25_

Address _Anytown, U.S.A._

Age _48_   Weight _135_   Height _5'5"_   Role in family _Wife, mother_

Diagnosis _CVA_   Disability _Bilateral ataxia, apraxia of mouth musculature_

Mode of ambulation _Independent, no aids, mild ataxic gait_

Limitations or contraindications for activity _____

DESCRIPTION OF HOME
1. Private house _✓_
    No. of rooms _6_ - kitchen, dining room, living room, 3 bedrooms
    No. of floors _2_
    Stairs _14_ - bedrooms on second floor
    Elevators _0_

2. Apartment house _____
    No. of rooms _____
    No. of floors _____
    Stairs _____
    Elevators _____

3. Diagram of home layout (attach to completed form)

Will patient be required to perform the following activities? If not, who will perform?

Meal preparation	_No_	_Daughter_
Baking	_No_	_Daughter (J.V. used to bake a lot)_
Serving	_Yes_	
Wash dishes	_Yes_	
Marketing	_No_	_Husband_
Child care (under 4 years)	_No_	
Washing	_Yes_	
Hanging clothes	_NA_	_Has dryer_
Ironing	_No_	_Daughter_
Cleaning	_Yes_	_Light cleaning_
Sewing	_No_	_Does not sew_
Hobbies or special interest	_Yes_	_Baking and gardening would be desirable activities_

Does patient really like housework? _No_

Sitting position: Chair _X_ Stool _X_ Wheelchair _NA_

Standing position: Braces _NA_ Crutches _NA_ Canes _NA_

Handedness: Dominant hand _Right_ Two hands _X_ One hand only _____ Assistive _____

Continued.

Fig. 15-3. Activities of home management. Adapted from Occupational Therapy Department, University Hospital, Ohio State University, Columbus, OH.

244
Part 2
Methods of evaluation and treatment for patients with physical dysfunction

Grading key:　I = Independent
MiA = Minimal assistance
MoA = Moderate assistance
MaA = Maximal assistance
D = Dependent
O = Not evaluated

CLEANING ACTIVITIES	Date	8/25				REMARKS
		Grade				
Pick up object from floor		D				
Wipe up spills		D				
Make bed (daily)		D				
Use dust mop		I				
Shake dust mop		D				
Dust low surfaces		I				
Dust high surfaces		D				
Mop kitchen floor		D				
Sweep with broom		I				
Use dust pan and broom		MiA				
Use vacuum cleaner		O				
Use vacuum cleaner attachments		D				
Carry light cleaning tools		I				
Use carpet sweeper		I				
Clean bathtub		D				
Change sheets on bed		D				
Carry pail of water		D				

MEAL PREPARATION	Date	8/25				REMARKS
Turn off water		I				
Turn off gas or electric range		I				
Light gas with match		D				
Pour hot water from pan to cup		D				
Open packaged goods		I				
Carry pan from sink to range		D				
Use can opener		D				
Handle milk bottle		I				
Dispose of garbage		D				
Remove things from refrigerator		D				
Bend to low cupboards		D				
Reach to high cupboards		D				
Peel vegetables		D				
Cut up vegetables		D				
Handle sharp tools safely		D				
Break eggs		D				
Stir against resistance		D				
Measure flour		D				
Use eggbeater		O				
Use electric mixer		D				
Remove batter to pan		D				
Open oven door		I				
Carry pan to oven and put in		D				
Remove hot pan from oven to table		O				
Roll cookie dough or piecrust		D				

Continued.

Fig. 15-3. Activities of home management. Adapted from Occupational Therapy Department, University Hospital, Ohio State University, Columbus, OH.

MEAL SERVICE	Date	8/25				REMARKS
Set table for four		I				
Carry four glasses of water to table		D				
Carry hot casserole to table		D				
Clear table		I				
Scrape and stack dishes		I				
Wash dishes (light soil)		I				
Wipe silver		I				
Wash pots and pans		MiA				
Wipe up range and work areas		MoA				
Wring out dishcloth		I				

LAUNDRY	Date	8/25				REMARKS
Wash lingerie (by hand)		D				
Wring out, squeeze dry		D				
Hang on rack to dry		I				
Sprinkle clothes		I				
Iron blouse or slip		D				
Fold blouse or slip						
Use washing machine						

SEWING	Date	8/25				REMARKS
Thread needle and make knot						
Sew on buttons						
Mend rip						
Darn socks						
Use sewing machine						
Crochet						
Knit						
Embroider						
Cut with shears						

HEAVY HOUSEHOLD ACTIVITIES. WHO WILL DO THESE?

	Date	8/25				REMARKS
Wash household laundry						
Hang clothes						
Clean range						
Clean refrigerator						
Wax floors						
Marketing						
Turn mattresses						
Wash windows						
Put up curtains						

WORK HEIGHTS

SITTING/STANDING
Wheelchair _____ Chair __X__ Stool __X__

Best height for	
Ironing	17½" seated
Mixing	26" on high stool at counter
Dish washing	26" on high stool at counter
General work	
Maximal depth of counter area (normal reach)	25"
Maximal useful height above work surface	33" if standing
Maximal useful height without counter surface	68" if standing
Maximal reach below counter area	20" if standing
Best height for chair	17½"-can be used at adjustable ironing board
Best height for stool with back support	24"-can be used at sink or food preparation counter

SUGGESTIONS FOR HOME MODIFICATION

Remove scatter rugs in bedroom
Install guard rail on both sides of toilet
Install grab bars on wall next to bathtub
Place nonskid strips on bottom of bathtub

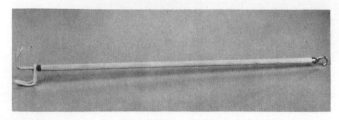

Fig. 15-4. Dressing stick or reacher. Reproduced with permission, Fred Sammons, Inc., A Bissell Healthcare Company, Box 32, Brookfield, IL.

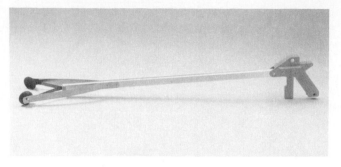

Fig. 15-7. Extended handled reacher.

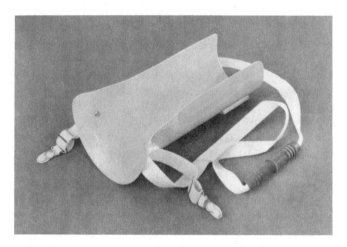

Fig. 15-5. Sock aid. Reproduced with permission, Fred Sammons, Inc., A Bissell Healthcare Company, Box 32, Brookfield, IL.

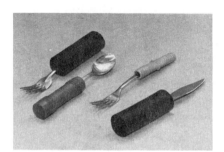

Fig. 15-8. Eating utensils with built-up handles.

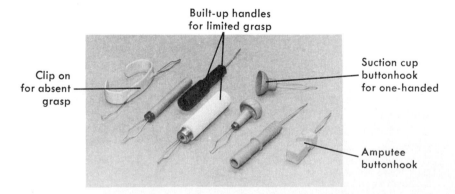

Fig. 15-6. Buttonhooks to accommodate limited or special types of grasp or amputation.

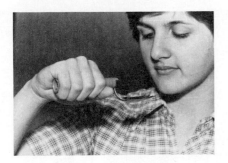

Fig. 15-9. Swivel spoon is used to compensate for limited supination.

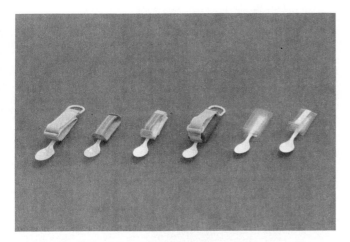

Fig. 15-10. Utensil holders/universal cuffs. Reproduced with permission, Fred Sammons, Inc., A Bissell Healthcare Company, Box 32, Brookfield, IL.

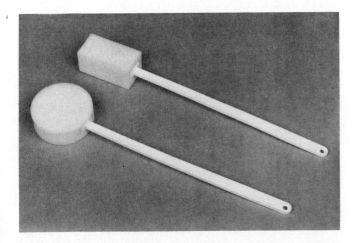

Fig. 15-11. Long-handled bath sponges. Reproduced with permission, Fred Sammons, Inc., A Bissell Healthcare Company, Box 32, Brookfield, IL.

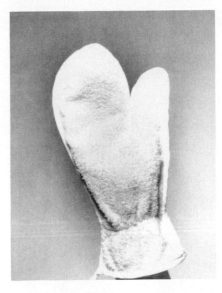

Fig. 15-12. Terry cloth bath mitt. Reproduced with permission, Fred Sammons, Inc., A Bissell Healthcare Company, Box 32, Brookfield, IL.

control of the direction of the spray. The handle can be built up or adapted for limited grasp.

2. A long-handled bath brush or sponge with a soap holder (Fig. 15-11) or long cloth scrubber can allow the user to reach legs, feet, and back. A wash mitt (Fig. 15-12) and soap on a rope can aid limited grasp.

3. A position-adjustable hair dryer described by Feldmeier and Poole may be helpful for those who prefer a hairstyle more elaborate than a simple hairstyle that can be airdried. This device is useful for patients with limited ROM, upper extremity weakness, incoordination, and use of only one upper extremity. The dryer is adapted from a desk lamp with spring-balanced arms and a tension control knob at each joint. The lamp is removed and the hair dryer is fastened to the spring-balanced arms. The device is mounted on a table or countertop and can be adjusted for various heights and direction of air flow. It frees the patient's hands to manage brushes or combs used to style the hair. The reader is referred to the original source for specifications for constructing this device.[6]

4. Long handles on comb, brush, toothbrush, lipstick, mascara brush, and safety or electric razor may be useful for limited hand-to-head or hand-to-face movements.

5. Spray deodorant, hair spray, and spray powder or perfume can extend the reach by the distance the material sprays. Special adaptations may be

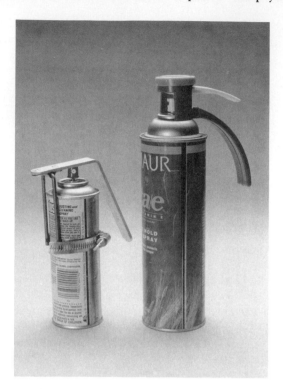

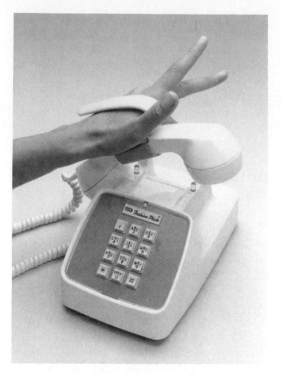

Fig. 15-13. Spray can adapter. Reproduced with permission, Fred Sammons, Inc., A Bissell Healthcare Company, Box 32, Brookfield, IL.

required by some persons to operate the spray mechanism (Fig. 15-13).

6. Electric toothbrushes and a Water-Pik may be easier to manage than a standard toothbrush.
7. A short reacher can extend reach for using toilet paper.
8. Dressing sticks can be used to pull garments up after using the toilet. An alternative is the use of a long piece of elastic or webbing with garters on each end that can be hung around the neck and fastened to pants or panties, preventing them from slipping to the floor during use of the toilet.
9. Safety rails can be used for bathtub transfers, and safety mats or strips can be placed in the bathtub bottom to prevent slipping.
10. A bathtub seat, shower stool, or regular chair set in the bathtub or shower stall can eliminate the need to sit on the bathtub bottom or stand to shower, thus increasing safety.

COMMUNICATION AND ENVIRONMENTAL HARDWARE ADAPTATIONS. The following are examples of environmental adaptations that can facilitate communication and hardware management:

1. Extended or built-up handles on faucets can accommodate limited grasp.
2. Telephones should be placed within easy reach. A clip-type receiver holder (Fig. 15-14), extended re-

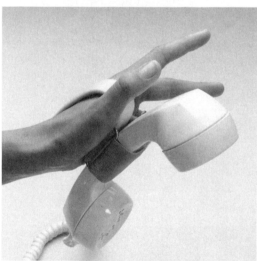

Fig. 15-14. Telephone clip holder. Reproduced with permission, Fred Sammons, Inc., A Bissell Healthcare Company, Box 32, Brookfield, IL.

ceiver holder, or speakerphone may be necessary. A dialing stick or push-button phone are other adaptations.

3. Built-up pens and pencils to accommodate limited grasp and prehension can be used. A wire stand pencil holder and several other commercially available or custom fabricated writing aids are possible (Fig. 15-15).
4. Electric typewriters or personal computers and

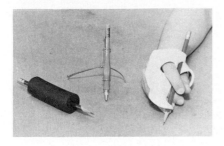

Fig. 15-15. Writing aids. **A,** Built-up pencil. **B,** Wire stand pencil holder. **C,** Thermoplastic custom-made writing device.

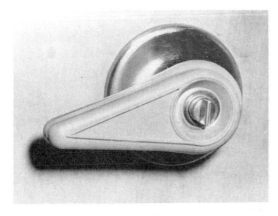

Fig. 15-16. Rubber door knob extension. Reproduced with permission, Fred Sammons, Inc., A Bissell Healthcare Company, Box 32, Brookfield, Il

book holders can facilitate communication for those with limited or painful joints.

5. Lever-type door knob extensions (Fig. 15-16), car door openers, and adapted key holders can compensate for hand limitations.

MOBILITY AND TRANSFER SKILLS. The individual who has limited ROM without significant muscle weakness may benefit from the following assistive devices:

1. A glider chair that is operated by the feet can facilitate transportation if hand and arm motion is limited.
2. Platform crutches can prevent stress on hand or finger joints and accommodate limited grasp.
3. Enlarged grips on crutches or canes can accommodate limited grasp.
4. A raised toilet seat can be used if hip and knee motion is limited.
5. A walker with padded grips and forearm troughs can be used if marked hand, forearm, or elbow joint limitations are present.
6. A walker or crutch bags can facilitate the carrying of objects.

HOME MANAGEMENT ACTIVITIES. Home management activities can be facilitated by a wide variety of environmental adaptations, assistive devices, energy conservation methods, and work simplification techniques.[15,22] The principles of joint protection are essential for those with rheumatoid arthritis. These are discussed in Chapter 27. The following are suggestions to facilitate home management for persons with limited ROM:

1. Store frequently used items on the fist shelves of cabinets just above and below counters or on counters where possible.
2. Use a high stool to work comfortably at counter height or attach a drop-leaf table to the wall for a planning and meal preparation area if a wheelchair is used.
3. Use a utility cart of comfortable height to transport several items at once.
4. Use reachers to get lightweight items (for example, cereal box) from high shelves.
5. Stabilize mixing bowls and dishes with nonslip mats.
6. Use lightweight utensils, such as plastic or aluminum bowls and aluminum pots.
7. Use electric can openers and electric mixers.
8. Use electric scissors.
9. Eliminate bending by using extended and flexible plastic handles on dust mops and brooms.
10. Facilitate sweeping by using dustpans and brushes with extended handles.
11. Eliminate bending by using wall ovens and countertop broilers.
12. Eliminate leaning and bending by using a top-loading automatic washer and elevated dryer. Wheelchair users can benefit from front-loading appliances.
13. Use an adjustable ironing board to make it possible to sit while ironing.
14. Elevate the playpen and diaper table and use a bathinette or a plastic tub on the kitchen counter for bathing to reduce the amount of bending and reaching for the ambulatory mother during child care. The crib mattress can be in a raised position until the child is 3 or 4 months old.
15. Use larger and looser fitting garments with Velcro fastenings on children.

Problems of Incoordination[1,16,27]

Incoordination in the form of tremors or ataxia or athetoid or choreiform movements can result from a variety of central nervous system (CNS) disorders, such as Parkinson's disease, multiple sclerosis, cerebral palsy, and head injuries. The major problems encountered in ADL performance are safety and adequate stability of gait, body parts, and objects to complete the tasks.

The degree of incoordinated movement may be influenced by fatigue, emotional factors, and fears. The patient must be taught appropriate energy conservation and work simplification techniques along with appropriate work pacing and safety methods to avoid the fatigue and apprehension that could increase incoordination and affect performance.

DRESSING ACTIVITIES. Potential dressing difficulties can be reduced by using the following adaptations:

1. Front-opening garments that fit loosely can facilitate donning and removing garments.
2. Large buttons, Velcro, or zippers with loops on the tab can facilitate opening and closing fasteners. A buttonhook with a large, weighted handle may be helpful.
3. Elastic shoelaces, other adapted shoe closures, and slip-on shoes eliminate the need for bow tying.
4. Trousers with elastic tops for women or Velcro closures for men are easier to manage than those with hooks, buttons, and zippers.
5. Brassieres with front openings or Velcro replacements for the usual hook and eye may facilitate donning and removing this garment. A slipover elastic-type brassiere or bra-slip combination also may eliminate the need to manage brassiere fastenings. Regular brassieres may be fastened in front at waist level, then slipped around to the back and the arms put into the straps, which are then worked up over the shoulders.
6. Clip-on ties can be used by men.
7. Dressing should be performed while sitting on or in bed or in a wheelchair or chair with arms to avoid balance problems.

FEEDING ACTIVITIES. For patients with problems of incoordination, eating can be a challenge. Lack of control during eating is not only frustrating but can cause embarrassment and social rejection. Therefore it is important to make eating safe, pleasurable, and as neat as possible. The following are some suggestions for achieving this goal:

1. Use plate stabilizers, such as nonskid mats, suction bases, or even wet dish towels.
2. Use a plate guard or scoop dish to prevent pushing food off the plate. The plate guard can be carried away from home and clipped to any ordinary dinner plate (Fig. 15-17).
3. Prevent spills during the plate-to-mouth excursion by using weighted or swivel utensils to offer stability. Weighted cuffs may be placed on the forearm to decrease involuntary movement (Fig. 15-18).

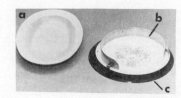

Fig. 15-17. A, Scoop dish. **B,** Plate with plate guard. **C,** Nonskid mat.

4. Use long plastic straws with a straw clip on a glass or cup with a weighted bottom to eliminate the need to carry the glass or cup to the mouth, thus avoiding spills. Plastic cups with covers and spouts may be used for the same purpose.
5. Use a resistance or friction-type arm brace similar to a mobile arm support, which was shown to help control patterns of involuntary movement during feeding activities of adults with cerebral palsy and athetosis by Holser and colleagues.[10] Such a brace may help many patients with severe incoordination to achieve some degree of independence in feeding.

HYGIENE AND GROOMING. Stabilization and handling of toilet articles may be achieved by the following suggestions:

1. Articles such as razor, lipstick, and toothbrush can be attached to a cord if frequent dropping is a problem. An electric toothbrush may be more easily managed than a regular one.
2. Weighted wrist cuffs may be helpful during the finer hygiene activities, such as applying makeup, shaving, and hair care.
3. The position-adjustable hair dryer described earlier for patients with limited ROM can be useful for patients with incoordination as well.[6]
4. An electric razor rather than a blade razor offers stability and safety.
5. A suction brush attached to the sink or counter can be used for nail or denture care (Fig. 15-19).

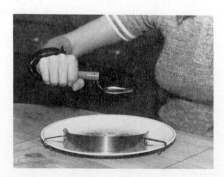

Fig. 15-18. Weighted wrist cuff and swivel utensil can sometimes compensate for incoordination or involuntary motion.

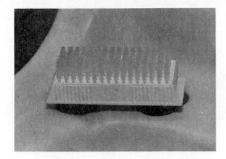

Fig. 15-19. Suction brush attached to bathroom sink.

6. Soap should be on a rope and can be worn around the neck or hung over a bathtub or shower fixture during bath or shower to keep it within easy reach.
7. An emery board or small piece of wood with fine sandpaper glued to it can be fastened to the tabletop for filing nails.
8. Large size roll-on deodorants are preferable to sprays or creams.
9. Sanitary pads that stick to undergarments may be easier to manage than tampons.
10. A bath mitt with a pocket to hold the soap can be used for washing and eliminates the need for frequent soaping and rinsing and wringing a washcloth.
11. Nonskid mats should be used inside and outside the bathtub during bathing. Their suction bases should be fastened securely to the floor and bathtub before use. Safety grab bars should be installed on the wall next to the bathtub or fastened to the edge of the bathtub. A bathtub seat or shower chair provides more safety than standing while showering or transferring to a bathtub bottom. Many uncoordinated patients require supervisory assistance during this hazardous activity. Sponge bathing while seated at a bathroom sink may substitute for bathing or showering several times a week.

COMMUNICATION AND ENVIRONMENTAL HARDWARE ADAPTATIONS. The following adaptations can facilitate communication for patients who have incoordination:
1. Doorknobs may be managed more easily if adapted with lever-type handles or covered with rubber or friction tape (Fig. 15-20).
2. Managing dials or push-buttons may be facilitated by using weighted cuffs or by stabilizing arms against body or on tabletop to control involuntary movement. A holder for a telephone receiver may be helpful.
3. Writing may be managed by using a weighted, enlarged pencil or pen. An electric typewriter with a

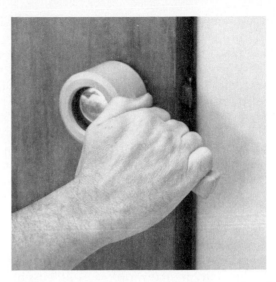

Fig. 15-20. Lever on door knob turner. Reproduced with permission, Fred Sammons, Inc., A Bissell Healthcare Company, Box 32, Brookfield, IL.

keyboard guard is a very helpful aid to communication.
4. Keys may be managed by placing them on an adapted key holder that is rigid and offers more leverage for turning the key. However, inserting the key in the keyhole may be very difficult unless the incoordination is relatively mild.
5. Extended lever-type faucets are easier to manage than knobs that turn and push-pull spigots. To prevent burns during bathing and kitchen activities, cold water should be turned on first and hot water added gradually.

MOBILITY AND TRANSFERS. Patients with problems of incoordination may use a variety of ambulation aids, depending on the type and severity of incoordination. In degenerative diseases it is sometimes necessary to help the patient recognize the need for and to accept ambulation aids. This may mean graduation from a cane to crutches to a walker and finally to a wheelchair for some persons. Patients with incoordination can improve stability and mobility by the following suggestions:
1. Instead of lifting objects, slide them on floors or counters.
2. Use suitable ambulation aids.
3. Use a utility cart, preferably a custom-made cart that is heavy and has some friction on the wheels.
4. Remove door sills, throw rugs, and thick carpeting.
5. Install banisters on indoor and outdoor staircases.
6. Substitute ramps for stairs wherever possible.

HOME MANAGEMENT ACTIVITIES.[15,16,27] It is important for the occupational therapist to make a careful assessment of homemaking activities performance to determine (1) which activities can be done safely, (2) which activities can be done safely if modified or adapted, and (3) which activities cannot be done adequately or safely and should be assigned to someone else. The major problems are stabilization of foods and equipment to prevent spilling and accidents and the safe handling of appliances, pots, pans, and household tools to prevent cuts, burns, bruises, electric shock, and falls. The following are suggestions for the facilitation of home management tasks:

1. Use a wheelchair and wheelchair lap board, even if ambulation is possible with devices. This saves energy and increases stability if balance and gait are unsteady.
2. If possible, use convenience and prepared foods to eliminate as many processes as possible, for example: peeling, chopping, slicing, and mixing.
3. Use easy-open containers or store foods in plastic containers once opened. A jar opener is also useful.
4. Use heavy utensils, mixing bowls, and pots and pans to increase stability.
5. Use nonskid mats on work surfaces.
6. Use electrical appliances such as crock pots, electric fry pans, and toaster-ovens, because they are safer than using the range.
7. Use a blender and countertop mixer, because they are safer than hand held mixers and easier than mixing with a spoon or whisk.
8. If possible, adjust work heights of counters, sink, and range to minimize leaning, bending, reaching, and lifting, whether the patient is standing or using a wheelchair.
9. Use long oven mitts, which are safer than potholders.
10. Use pots, pans, casserole dishes, and appliances with bilateral handles, because they may be easier to manage than those with one handle.
11. Use a cutting board with stainless-steel nails to stabilize meats and vegetables while cutting. When not in use the nails should be covered with a large cork. The bottom of the board should have suction cups or should be covered with stair tread, or the board should be placed on a nonskid mat to prevent slippage when in use (Fig. 15-21).
12. Use heavy dinnerware, which may be easier to handle, because it offers stability and control to the distal part of the upper extremity. On the other hand, unbreakable dinnerware may be more practical if dropping and breakage are problems.
13. Cover the sink, utility cart, and countertops with protective rubber mats or mesh matting.

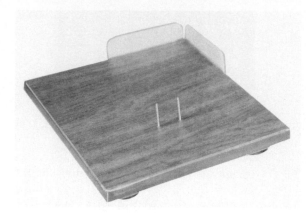

Fig. 15-21. Cutting board with stainless-steel nails, suction cup feet, and corner for stabilizing bread is useful for patients with incoordination or use of one hand. Reproduced with permission, Fred Sammons, Inc., A Bissell Healthcare Company, Box 32, Brookfield, IL.

14. Use a serrated knife for cutting and chopping, because it is easier to control.
15. Use a steamer basket or deep fry basket for preparing boiled foods to eliminate the need to carry and drain pots with hot liquids in them.
16. Use tongs to turn foods during cooking and to serve foods, because they may offer more control and stability than a fork, spatula, or serving spoon.
17. Vacuum with a heavy upright cleaner, which may be easier for the ambulatory patient. The wheelchair user may be able to manage a lightweight tank-type vacuum cleaner or electric broom.
18. Use dust mitts for dusting.
19. Eliminate fragile knickknacks, unstable lamps, and dainty doilies.
20. Eliminate ironing by using no-iron fabrics or a timed dryer or by assigning this task to other members of the household.
21. Use front-loading washers, a laundry cart on wheels, and premeasured detergents, bleaches, and fabric softeners.
22. Sit while working with an infant and use foam-rubber bath aids, an infant bath seat, and a wide, padded dressing table with safety straps with Velcro fastening to offer enough stability for bathing, dressing, and diapering an infant. (Child care may not be possible unless the incoordination is mild.)
23. Use disposable diapers with tape fasteners, because they are easier to manage than cloth diapers and pins.
24. Do not feed the infant with a spoon or fork unless the incoordination is very mild or does not affect the upper extremities. This task may need to be performed by another household member.

25. Provide clothing for the child that is large, loose, with Velcro fastenings, and made of nonslippery stretch fabrics.

Hemiplegia or Use of Only One Upper Extremity[1,15,16,27]

Suggestions for performing daily living skills apply to persons with hemiplegia, unilateral upper extremity amputations, and temporary disorders, such as fractures, burns, and peripheral neuropathy, which can result in the dysfunction of one upper extremity.

The hemiplegic patient requires specialized methods of teaching, and many have greater difficulty in learning and performing one-handed skills than those with orthopedic or lower motor neuron dysfunction. This is because the trunk and leg are involved, as well as the arm, and therefore ambulation and balance difficulties may exist. Also, sensory, perceptual, cognitive, and speech disorders may be present in a mild to severe degree. These disorders affect the ability to learn and retain learning and performance. Finally the presence of motor and ideational apraxia sometimes seen in this group of patients can have a profound effect on the potential for learning new motor skills and remembering old ones.

Therefore the patient with normal perception and cognition and the use of one upper extremity may learn the techniques quickly and easily. The hemiplegic patient needs to be evaluated for sensory, perceptual, and cognitive deficits to determine potential for ADL performance and to establish appropriate teaching methods (previously described) to facilitate learning.

The major problems for the one-handed worker are reduction of work speed and dexterity, stabilization to substitute for the role normally assumed by the nondominant arm, and, for the hemiplegic, balance and precautions relative to sensory loss.

DRESSING ACTIVITIES. If balance is a problem, dressing should be done while seated in a locked wheelchair or sturdy armchair. Clothing should be within easy reach. Reaching tongs may be helpful for securing articles and assisting in some dressing activities. Assistive devices should be minimal for dressing and other ADL.

One-handed dressing techniques.* Dressing techniques for the hemiplegic that employ neurodevelopmental (Bobath) treatment principles are discussed

*Summarized from Activities of daily living for patients with incoordination, limited range of motion, paraplegia, quadriplegia, and hemiplegia, Cleveland, 1968, Highland View Hospital, Cuyahoga County Hospitals, Division of Occupational Therapy. Mimeographed, unpublished.

in Chapter 20. The following one-handed dressing techniques can facilitate dressing for persons with use of one upper extremity.

Front-opening shirts may be managed by any one of three methods. The fist method can be used for jackets, robes, and front-opening dresses.

METHOD I
Donning shirt (Fig. 15-22)

1. Grasp shirt collar with normal hand and shake out twists (a).
2. Position shirt on lap with inside up and collar toward chest (b).
3. Position sleeve opening on affected side so it is as large as possible and close to affected hand, which is resting on lap (c).
4. Using normal hand, place affected hand in sleeve opening and work sleeve over elbow by pulling on garment (d_1, d_2).
5. Put normal arm into its sleeve and raise up to slide or shake sleeve into position past elbow (e).
6. With normal hand, gather shirt up middle of back from hem to collar and raise shirt over head (f).
7. Lean forward, duck head, and pass shirt over it (g).
8. With normal hand, adjust shirt by leaning forward and working it down past both shoulders. Reach in back and pull shirttail down (h).
9. Line shirt fronts up for buttoning and begin with bottom button (i). Button sleeve cuff of affected arm. Sleeve cuff of unaffected arm may be prebuttoned if cuff opening is large. Button may be sewn on with elastic thread or sewn onto a small tab of elastic and fastened inside shirt cuff. A small button attached to crocheted loop of elastic thread is another alternative. Slip button on loop through button-hole in garment so that elastic loop is inside. Stretch elastic loop to fit around original cuff button. This simple device can be transferred to each garment and positioned before shirt is put on. Loop stretches to accommodate width of hand as it is pushed through end of sleeve.[26]

Removing shirt

1. Unbutton shirt.
2. Lean forward.
3. With normal hand, grasp collar or gather material up in back from collar to hem.
4. Lean forward, duck head, and pull shirt over head.
5. Remove sleeve from normal arm and then from affected arm.

METHOD II
Donning shirt

Method II may be used by patients who get shirt twisted or have trouble sliding the sleeve down onto normal arm.

1. Position shirt as described in method I, steps 1 to 3.
2. With normal hand place involved hand into shirt sleeve opening and work sleeve onto hand, but do *not* pull up over elbow.
3. Put normal arm into sleeve and bring arm out to 180° of abduction. Tension of fabric from normal arm to wrist of affected arm will bring sleeve into position.

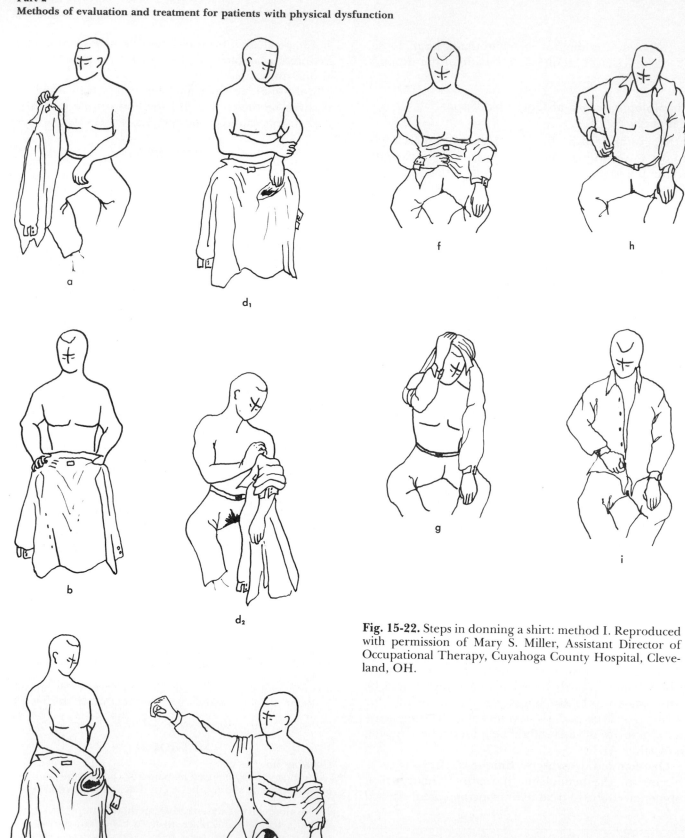

a

d₁

f

h

b

d₂

g

i

c

e

Fig. 15-22. Steps in donning a shirt: method I. Reproduced with permission of Mary S. Miller, Assistant Director of Occupational Therapy, Cuyahoga County Hospital, Cleveland, OH.

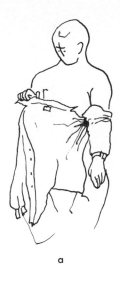

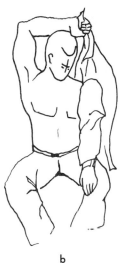

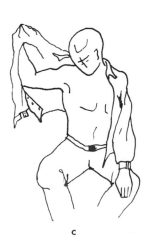

Fig. 15-23. Steps in donning a shirt: method III. Reproduced with permission of Mary S. Miller, Assistant Director of Occupational Therapy, Cuyahoga County Hospital, Cleveland, OH.

4. Lower arm and work sleeve on affected arm up over elbow.
5. Continue as in steps 6 through 9 of method I.

Removing shirt

1. Unbutton shirt.
2. With normal hand, push shirt off shoulders, first on affected side, then on normal side.
3. Pull on cuff of normal side with normal hand.
4. Work sleeve off by alternately shrugging shoulder and pulling down on cuff.
5. Lean forward, bring shirt around back, and pull sleeve off affected arm.

METHOD III

Donning shirt (Fig. 15-23)

1. Position shirt and work onto arm as described in method I, steps 1 to 4.
2. Pull sleeve on affected arm up to shoulder (a).
3. With normal hand, grasp tip of collar that is on normal side, lean forward, and bring arm over and behind head to carry shirt around to normal side (b).
4. Put normal arm into sleeve opening, directing it up and out (c).
5. Adjust and button as described in method I, steps 8 and 9.

Removing shirt

The shirt may be removed using the same procedure described previously for method II.

Variation—donning pullover shirt. Pullover shirts can be managed by the following procedure:

1. Position shirt on lap, bottom toward chest and label facing down.
2. With normal hand, roll up bottom edge of shirt back up to sleeve on affected side.
3. Position sleeve opening so it is as large as possible and use normal hand to place affected one into sleeve opening. Pull shirt up onto arm past elbow.
4. Insert normal arm into sleeve.
5. Adjust shirt on affected side up and on to shoulder.
6. Gather shirt back with normal hand, lean forward, duck head, and pass shirt over head.
7. Adjust shirt.

Variation—removing pullover shirt. Pullover shirts are removed by the following procedure:

1. Gather shirt up with normal hand, starting at top back.
2. Lean forward, duck head, and pull gathered back fabric over head.
3. Remove from normal arm and then affected arm.

Trousers may be managed by one of the following methods. These may be adapted for shorts and women's panties as well. It is recommended that trousers have a well-constructed button fly front opening. This may be easier to manage than a zipper. Velcro may be used to replace buttons and zippers. Trousers should be worn in a size slightly larger than worn previously and should have a wide opening at the ankles. They should be put on after the socks have been put on but before the shoes are put on.

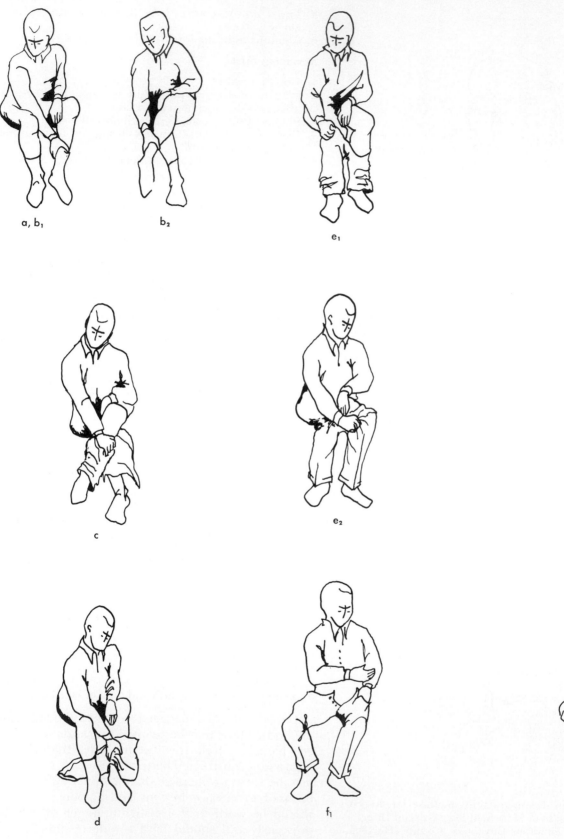
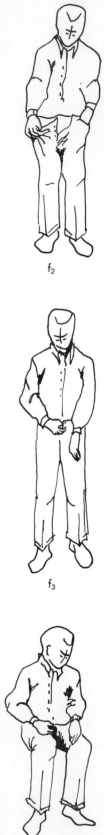

Fig. 15-24. Steps in donning trousers: method I. Reproduced with permission of Mary S. Miller, Assistant Director of Occupational Therapy, Cuyahoga County Hospital, Cleveland, OH.

METHOD I

Donning trousers (Fig. 15-24)

1. Sit in sturdy armchair or in locked wheelchair *(a)*.
2. Position normal leg in front of midline of body with knee flexed to 90 degrees. Using normal hand reach forward and grasp ankle of affected leg or sock around ankle *(b₁)*. Lift affected leg over normal leg to crossed position *(b₂)*.
3. Slip trousers onto affected leg up to position where foot is completely inside of trouser leg *(c)*. Do *not* pull up above knee or difficulty will be encountered in inserting normal leg.
4. Uncross affected leg by grasping ankle or portion of sock around ankle *(d)*.
5. Insert normal leg and work trousers up onto hips as far as possible *(e₁, e₂)*. If wheelchair is used, place footrests in an up position.
6. If able to do so safely, stand and pull trousers over hips. To prevent trousers from dropping, place affected hand in pocket or place one finger of affected hand into belt loop *(f₁, f₃)*.
7. Sit down to button front *(g)*. If standing balance is good, remain standing to pull up zipper or button *(f₃)*.

Removing trousers

1. Unfasten trousers and work down on hips as far as possible while seated.
2. Stand, letting trousers drop past hips or work them down past hips.
3. Sit and cross affected leg over normal leg, remove trousers, and uncross leg.
4. Remove trousers from normal leg.

METHOD II

Donning trousers

Method II is used for patients who are in wheelchairs with brakes locked or are in sturdy straight armchairs positioned with back against wall and for patients who cannot stand independently.

1. Position trousers on legs as in method I, steps 1 through 5.
2. Elevate hips by leaning back against chair and pushing down against the floor with normal leg. As hips are raised, work trousers over hips with normal hand.
3. Lower hips back into chair and fasten trousers.

Removing trousers

1. Unfasten trousers and work down on hips as far as possible while sitting.
2. Lean back against chair, push down against floor with normal leg to elevate hips, and with normal arm work trousers down past hips.
3. Proceed as in method I, steps 3 and 4.

METHOD III

Donning trousers

Method III is for patients who are in a recumbent position. It is more difficult to perform than those methods done sitting. If possible, bed should be raised to semireclining position for partial sitting.

1. Using normal hand, place affected leg in bent position and cross over normal leg, which may be partially bent to prevent affected leg from slipping.
2. Position trousers and work onto affected leg, first, up to the knee. Then uncross leg.
3. Insert normal leg, and work trousers up onto hips as far as possible.
4. With normal leg bent, press down with foot and shoulder to elevate hips from bed and with normal arm pull trousers over hips or work trousers up over hips by rolling from side to side.
5. Fasten trousers.

Removing trousers

1. Hike hips as in putting trousers on in method III, step 4.
2. Work trousers down past hips, remove unaffected leg, and then remove affected leg.

Clothing items, such as brassieres, neckties, socks, stockings, and braces, may be difficult to manage with one hand. The following methods are recommended.

BRASSIERE

Donning

1. Tuck one end of brassiere into pants, girdle, or skirt waistband, and wrap other end around waist. Hook brassiere in front at waist level and slip fastener around to back (at waistline level).
2. Place affected arm through shoulder strap, and then place normal arm through other strap.
3. Work straps up over shoulders. Pull strap on affected side up over shoulder with normal arm. Put normal arm through its strap and work up over shoulder by directing arm up and out and pulling with hand.
4. Use normal hand to adjust breasts in brassiere cups.

NOTE: It is helpful if brassiere has elastic straps and is made of stretch fabric. If there is some function in affected hand, a fabric loop may be sewn to back of brassiere near fastener. Affected thumb may be slipped through this to stabilize brassiere while normal hand fastens it. All elastic brassieres, prefastened or without fasteners, may be put on adapting method I for shirts described previously.

Removing

1. Slip straps down off shoulders, normal side first.
2. Work straps down over arms and off hands.
3. Slip brassiere around to front with normal arm.
4. Unfasten and remove.

NECKTIE

Donning

Clip-on neckties are attractive and convenient. If conventional tie is used, the following method is recommended:

1. Place collar of shirt in up position and bring necktie around neck and adjust so that smaller end is at desired length when tie is completed.
2. Fasten small end to shirt front with tie clasp or spring clip clothespin.
3. Loop long end around short end (one complete loop) and bring up between V at neck. Then bring tip down through loop at front and adjust tie, using ring and little fingers to hold tie end and thumb and forefingers to slide knot up tightly.

Removing

Pull knot at front of neck until small end slips up enough for tie to be slipped over head. Tie may be hung up in this state and replaced by slipping it over head, around upturned collar, and knot tightened, as described in step 3 of donning necktie.

SOCKS OR STOCKINGS

Donning

1. Sit in straight armchair or in wheelchair with brakes locked.
2. With normal leg directly in front of midline of body, cross affected leg over it.
3. Open top of stocking by inserting thumb and first two fingers near cuff and spreading fingers apart.
4. Work stocking onto foot before pulling over heel. Care should be taken to eliminate wrinkles.
5. Work stocking up over leg. Shift weight from side to side to adjust stocking around thigh.
6. Fasten stocking to garter. Velcro tabs may be substituted for garters.

NOTE: Stockings should be seamless and of soft, stretch-type-fabric.

Removing

1. While sitting, unfasten garters.
2. Work socks or stockings down as far as possible with normal arm.
3. Cross affected leg over normal one as described in step 2 of putting on socks or stockings.
4. Remove sock or stocking from affected leg. Dressing stick may be required by some patients to push sock or stocking off heel and off foot.
5. Lift normal leg to comfortable height or to seat level and remove sock or stocking from foot.

SHORT LEG BRACE

Donning (Fig. 15-25)

1. Sit in straight armchair or wheelchair with brakes locked *(a)*.
2. Bring normal leg to body midline. Cross hemiplegic leg over normal leg *(b)*.
3. Pull tongue of shoe through laces and tuck under bottom part of lace, so that it does not push down into shoe as brace is donned *(c)*.
4. Fold Velcro mesh flap back and hold back with calf band. With normal hand, swing brace back and then forward so heel is between uprights. Swing shoe far enough forward so that toes can be inserted into shoe *(d₁)*. Still holding onto upright bar of brace, turn shoe inward so that toes go in at a slight angle, preventing catching toes at sides of shoe *(d₂)*.
5. Pull brace up onto leg as far as possible *(e₁)*. If difficulty is encountered in getting brace up far enough on leg, raise affected leg by pulling up on crossbar, making foot easier to slip into shoe. Brace can now be held in position by pressure against crossbar between affected leg and normal leg, while shoehorn is inserted under heel in back *(e₂)*. If brace is difficult to keep on while inserting shoehorn, raise affected leg by pulling up on crossbar to position at which ankle of affected leg is resting against knee of normal leg, with uprights on each side *(e₃)*.

6. By holding uprights, uncross affected leg and position at 90-degree angle to floor *(f₁, f₂)*. Shoehorn is now in position where heel is pressing on it. Alternately, direct pressure downward on the knee and move shoehorn back and forth, using normal hand, until foot slips into shoe *(f₃–f₅)*.
7. Fasten laces and straps. One of many methods of one-handed bow tying may be used. Elastic shoelaces or other commercially available shoe fasteners may be required if unable to tie shoes *(g)*.

Removing
Variation I

1. While seated as for donning a brace, cross affected leg over normal leg.
2. Unfasten straps and laces with normal hand.
3. Push down on brace upright until shoe is off foot.

Variation II

1. Unfasten straps and laces.
2. Straighten affected leg by putting normal foot behind heel of shoe and pushing affected leg forward.
3. Push down on brace upright with hand and at same time push foward on heel of brace shoe with normal foot.

NOTE: Shoes may be donned by crossing legs, as described for stockings. Long-handled shoehorn may be helpful. Shoe tongue can have holes punched at top and shoelaces threaded through it to prevent tongue from being pushed into shoe when foot is forced in. Elastic shoelaces, buckles, and other adapted shoe closures are recommended for hemiplegic patients. Method for one-handed shoe tying is illustrated in Fig. 15-26 for those patients who prefer standard tie oxford.

FEEDING ACTIVITIES. The only real problem encountered by the one-handed individual is managing a knife and fork simultaneously for meat cutting. This problem can be solved by the use of a rocker knife for cutting meat and other foods (Fig. 15-27). It cuts with a rocking motion rather than a slicing back and forth action. Use of a rocking motion with a standard table knife or a sharp paring knife may be adequate to accomplish cutting tender meats and foods. If such a knife is used, the patient is taught to hold the knife handle between the thumb and the third, fourth, and fifth fingers, and the index finger is extended along the top of the knife blade. The knife point is placed in the food in a vertical position, and then the blade is brought down to cut the food. The rocking motion, using wrist flexion and extension, is continued until the food is cut.

The occupational therapist should keep in mind that one-handed meat cutting involves learning a new motor pattern and may be difficult for patients with hemiplegia and apraxia.

HYGIENE AND GROOMING ACTIVITIES. With some assistive devices and the use of alternate methods, hygiene and grooming activities can be accomplished by those with the use of one hand or one side

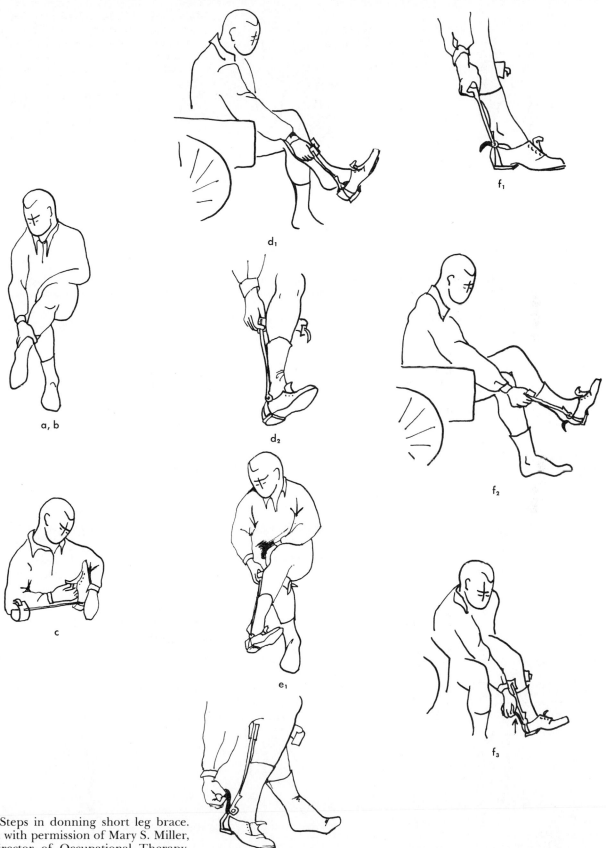

Fig. 15-25. Steps in donning short leg brace. Reproduced with permission of Mary S. Miller, Assistant Director of Occupational Therapy, Cuyahoga County Hospital, Cleveland, OH.

Continued

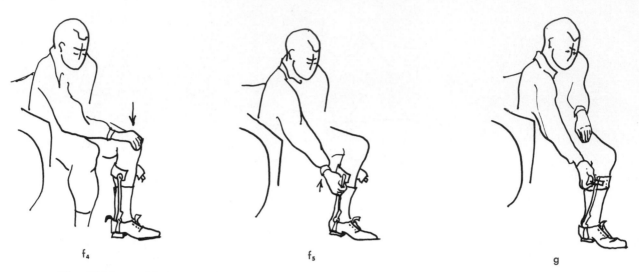

f₄   f₅   g

Fig. 15-25, cont'd. Steps in donning short leg brace. Reproduced with permission of Mary S. Miller, Assistant Director of Occupational Therapy, Cuyahoga County Hospital, Cleveland, OH.

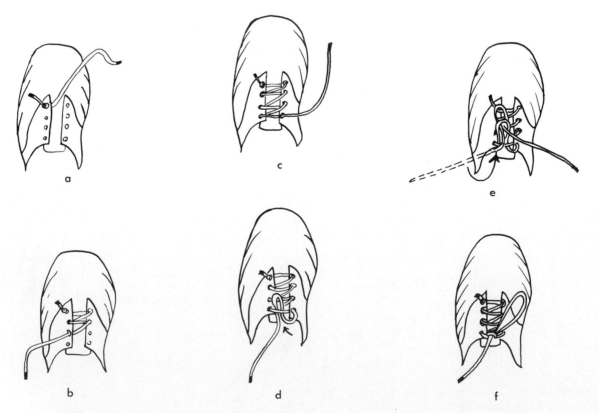

a   c   e

b   d   f

Fig. 15-26. One-hand shoe-tying method. Reproduced with permission of Mary S. Miller, Assistant Director of Occupational Therapy, Cuyahoga County Hospital, Cleveland, OH.

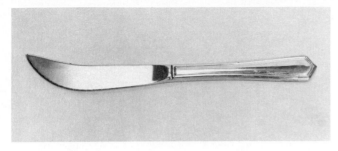

Fig. 15-27. One-handed rocker knife. Reproduced with permission, Fred Sammons, Inc., A Bissell Healthcare Company, Box 32, Brookfield, IL.

of the body. The following are suggestions for achieving hygiene and grooming with one hand:
1. Use an electric razor rather than a safety razor.
2. Use a bathtub seat or chair in the shower stall, wash mitt, long-handled bath sponge, safety rails on the bathtub or wall, soap on a rope or suction soap holder, and suction brush for fingernail care.
3. Sponge bathe while sitting at the lavatory, using the wash mitt, suction brush, and suction soap holder. The uninvolved forearm and hand may be washed by placing a soaped washcloth on the thigh and rubbing the hand and forearm on the cloth.
4. Use the position-adjustable hair dryer previously described. Such a device frees the unaffected upper extremity to hold a brush or comb to style the hair during blow-drying.[6]
5. Care for fingernails as described previously for patients with incoordination.
6. Use spray deodorants rather than creams or roll-ons, because they can be applied more easily to the uninvolved underarm.
7. Use a suction denture brush for care of dentures (Fig. 15-28). The suction fingernail brush may also serve this purpose.

COMMUNICATION AND ENVIRONMENTAL HARDWARE. The following are suggestions to facilitate writing, reading, and using the telephone:
1. The primary problem in writing is stabilization of the paper or tablet. This can be overcome by using a clipboard or paperweight or by taping the paper to the writing surface. In some instances the affected arm may be positioned on the tabletop to stabilize the paper passively.
2. If dominance must be shifted to the nondominant extremity, writing practice may be necessary to improve speed and coordination. One-handed writing and typing instruction manuals are available.
3. Book holders may be used to stabilize a book while reading or holding copy for typing and writing practice.

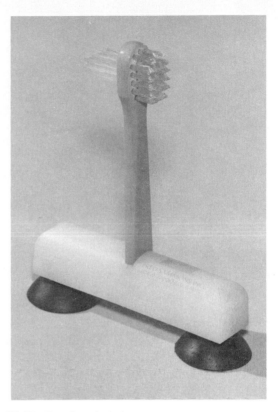

Fig. 15-28. One-handed denture brush. Reproduced with permission, Fred Sammons, Inc., A Bissell Healthcare Company, Box 32, Brookfield, IL.

4. The telephone is managed by lifting the receiver to listen for the dial tone, setting it down, dialing or pressing the buttons, then lifting the receiver to the ear. To write while using the telephone, a telephone receiver holder that is on a stand or that rests on the shoulder must be used.

MOBILITY AND TRANSFERS. Specific transfer techniques for clients with hemiplegia are described in Chapter 22.

HOME MANAGEMENT ACTIVITIES. A variety of assistive devices is available to facilitate home management activities.[15] Whether the patient is disabled by the loss of function of one arm and hand, as in amputation or peripheral neuropathy, or whether both arm and leg are affected along with possible visual, perceptual, and cognitive dysfunctions, as in hemiplegia, are the determining factor regarding how many home management activities can realistically be performed, which methods can be used, and how many assistive devices can be managed. The reader is referred to the references listed at the end of this chapter for details of home management with one hand. The following are some suggestions for one-handed homemakers:[15]
1. Stabilization of items is a major problem for the

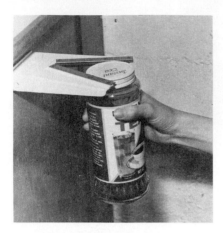

Fig. 15-29. Zim jar opener.

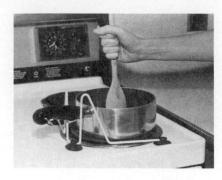

Fig. 15-30. Pan stabilizer.

one-handed homemaker. Stabilize foods for cutting and peeling by using a board with two stainless-steel or aluminum nails in it. A raised corner on the board stabilizes bread while making sandwiches or spreading butter. Suction cups or a rubber mat under the board will keep it from slipping. Rubber stair tread may be glued to the bottom of the board.

2. Use sponge cloths, non-skid mats pads, wet dishcloths, or suction devices to keep pots, bowls, and dishes from turning or sliding during food preparation.

3. To open a jar, stabilize it between the knees or in a partially opened drawer while leaning against it, or use a Zim jar opener (Fig. 15-29).

4. Open boxes, sealed paper, and plastic bags by stabilizing between the knees or in a drawer, as just described, and cutting open with a household shears.

5. Open an egg by holding it firmly in the palm of the hand, hitting it in the center against the edge of the bowl, and then using the thumb and index finger to push the top half of the shell up and the ring and little finger to push the lower half down. Separate whites from yolks by using an egg separator or a funnel.

6. Eliminate the need to stabilize the standard grater by using a grater with suction feet.

7. Stabilize pots on counter or range for mixing or stirring by using a pan holder with suction feet (Fig. 15-30).

8. Eliminate the need to use hand-cranked or electric can openers requiring two hands by using a one-handed electric can opener.

9. Use a utility cart to carry items from one place to another. A cart that is weighted or constructed of wood may be used as a minimal support during ambulation for some patients.

10. Transfer clothes to and from the washer or dryer by using a clothes carrier on wheels.

11. Use electrical appliances, such as a lightweight electrical hand mixer, blender, and food processor, which can be managed with one hand and save time and energy. Safety factors and judgment need to be evaluated carefully when electrical appliances are considered.

12. Floor care becomes a greater problem if ambulation and balance, as well as one arm, are affected. For those patients with involvement of one arm only, a standard dust mop, carpet sweeper, or upright vacuum cleaner should present no problem. A self-wringing mop may be used if the mop handle is stabilized under the arm and the wringing lever operated with the normal arm. Patients with balance and ambulation problems may manage some floor care from a sitting position. Dust mopping or using a carpet sweeper may be possible if gait and balance are fairly good without the aid of a cane.

These are just a few of the possibilities to solve home management problems for one-handed individuals. The occupational therapist must evaluate each patient to determine how the dysfunction affects performance of home-making activities. One-handed techniques take more time and may be difficult for some patients to master. Activities should be paced to accommodate the patient's physical endurance and tolerance for one-handed performance and use of special devices. Work simplification and energy conservation techniques should be employed.

New techniques and devices should be introduced on a graded basis as the patient masters one technique and device and then another. Family members need to be oriented to the patient's skills, special methods used, and work schedule. The therapist with the family and patient may facilitate the planning of home-making responsibilities to be shared by other family members and the supervision of the patient, if that is needed.

If special equipment and assistive devices are needed for ADL, it is advisable to acquire these through the health agency, if possible. The therapist can then train the patient in their use and demonstrate to a family member before these items are used at home.

ADL for Wheelchair-Bound Individuals with Good to Normal Arm Function (Paraplegia)

Patients who are confined to a wheelchair need to find ways to perform ADL from a seated position, to transport objects, and to adapt in an environment designed for standing and walking. Given normal upper extremity function, the wheelchair ambulator can probably perform independently.

DRESSING ACTIVITIES.* It is recommended that wheelchair-bound patients put on clothing in this order: stockings, undergarments, braces (if worn), trousers or slacks, shoes, shirt, or dress.

TROUSERS

Donning

Trousers and slacks are easier to fasten if they button or zip in front. If braces are worn, zippers in side seams may be helpful. Wide bottom slacks of stretch fabric are recommended. Procedure for putting on trousers, shorts, slacks, and underwear is as follows:

1. Use side rails or trapeze to help pull up to sitting position.
2. Sit on bed and reach forward to feet or sit on bed and pull knees into flexed position.
3. Holding top of trousers flip pants down to feet.
4. Work pant legs over feet and pull up to hips. Crossing ankles may help get pants on over heels.
5. In semireclining position roll from hip to hip and pull up garment.
6. Reaching tongs may be helpful to pull garment up or position garment on feet.

Removing

Remove pants or underwear by reversing procedure for putting on. Dressing sticks may be helpful to push pants off feet.

SOCKS OR STOCKINGS

Donning

1. Put on socks or stockings while seated on bed.
2. Pull one leg into flexion with one hand.
3. Use other hand to slip sock or stocking over foot and pull it on.

NOTE: Soft stretch socks or stockings are recommended. Panty hose that are slightly large may be useful. Elastic garters or stockings with elastic tops should be avoided. Dressing sticks or a stocking device may be helpful to some patients.

---

*Summarized from Activities of daily living for patients with incoordination, limited range of motion, paraplegia, quadriplegia, and hemiplegia, Cleveland, 1968, Highland View Hospital, Cuyahoga County Hospitals, Division of Occupational Therapy. Mimeographed, unpublished.

Removing

Remove socks or stockings by flexing leg as described for donning, pushing sock or stocking down over heel. Dressing sticks may be needed to push sock or stocking off heel and toe and to retrieve it.

SLIPS AND SKIRTS

Donning

1. Sit on bed, slip garment over head, and let it drop to waist.
2. In semireclining position, roll from hip to hip and pull garment down over hips and thighs.

NOTE: Slips and skirts slightly larger than usually worn are recommended. A-line, wraparound, and full skirts are easier to manage and look better on a person seated in a wheelchair than narrow skirts.

Removing

1. In sitting or semireclining position, unfasten garment.
2. Roll from hip to hip, pulling garment up to waist level.
3. Pull garment off over head.

SHIRTS

Donning

Shirts, pajama jackets, robes, and dresses opening completely down front may be put on while patient is seated in wheelchair. If it is necessary to dress while in bed, the following procedure can be used:

1. Balance body by putting palms of hands on mattress on either side of body. If balance is poor, assistance may be needed or bed backrest may be elevated. (If backrest cannot be elevated, one or two pillows may be used to support back.) With backrest elevated, both hands are available.
2. If difficulty is encountered in customary methods of applying garment, open garment on lap with collar toward chest. Put arms into sleeves and pull up over elbows. Then hold on to shirttail or back of dress, pull garment over head, adjust, and button.

NOTE: Fabrics should be wrinkle-resistant, smooth, and durable. Roomy sleeves and backs and full skirts are more suitable styles than closely fitted garments.

Removing

1. Sitting in wheelchair or bed, open fastener.
2. Remove garment in usual manner.
3. If this is not feasible, grasp collar with one hand while balancing with other hand. Gather material up from collar to hem.
4. Lean forward, duck head, and pull shirt over head.
5. Remove sleeve from supporting arm and them from working arm.

SHOES

Donning

Shoes may be applied by one of the following variations.
Variation I

1. In sitting position on bed pull one knee at a time into flexed position with hands.
2. While supporting leg in flexed position with one hand, use free hand to put on shoe.

Variation II

1. Sit on edge of bed or in wheelchair for back support.
2. Bend one knee up to flexed position, supporting leg with arm, and with free hand slip shoe on.

Variation III

1. Sit on edge of bed or in wheelchair for back support.
2. Cross one leg over other and slip shoe on.
3. Put foot on footrest and push down on knee to push foot into shoe.

Removing

1. Flex or cross leg as described for appropriate variation.
2. For variations I and II remove shoe with one hand while supporting flexed leg with other hand.
3. For variation III remove shoe from crossed leg with one hand while maintaining balance with other hand, if necessary.

FEEDING ACTIVITIES. Eating activities should present no special problem for the wheelchair-bound person with good to normal arm function. Wheelchairs with desk arms and swing-away footrests are recommended so that it is possible to sit close to the table.

HYGIENE AND GROOMING. Face and oral hygiene and arm and upper body care should present no problem. Reachers may be helpful to secure towels, washcloths, makeup, deodorant, and shaving supplies from storage areas, if necessary. Tub baths or showers require some special equipment. Transfer techniques for toilet and bathtub will be discussed in Chapter 22. The following are suggestions for facilitating bathing activities:

1. Use a hand-held shower head and keep a finger over the spray to determine sudden temperature changes in water.
2. Use long-handled bath brushes with soap insert for ease in reaching all parts of the body.
3. Use soap bars attached to a cord around the neck.
4. For sponge bath in wheelchair, cover the chair with a sheet of plastic.
5. Use shower chairs or bathtub seats.
6. Increase safety during transfers by installing grab bars on wall near bathtub or shower and on bathtub.
7. Fit bathtub or shower bottom with nonskid mat or adhesive material.

COMMUNICATION AND ENVIRONMENTAL HARDWARE. With the exception of reaching difficulties in some situations, use of the telephone should present no problem. Short-handled reachers may be used to grasp the receiver from the cradle. Dialing could be accomplished with a short, rubbertipped, 1/4-inch dowel stick. Use of writing implements, typewriter, tape recorder, and personal computer should be easily possible for these patients.

Managing doors may present some difficulties. If the door opens toward the person, opening it can be managed by the following procedure:

1. If doorknob is on right, approach door from right, and turn doorknob with left hand.
2. Open door as far as possible and move wheelchair close enough so that it helps keep door open.
3. Holding door open with left hand, turn wheelchair with right hand and wheel through door.
4. Start closing door when halfway through.

If the door is very heavy and opens out or away from the person, the following procedure is recommended:

1. Back up to door so knob can be turned with right hand.
2. Open door and back through so that big wheels keep it open.
3. Also use left elbow to keep door open.
4. Wheel backward with right hand.[3]

MOBILITY AND TRANSFERS. Specific transfer techniques will be discussed in Chapter 22.

HOME MANAGEMENT ACTIVITIES.[15] When performing homemaking activities from a wheelchair, the major problems are work heights, adequate space for maneuverability, access to storage areas, and transfer of supplies, equipment, and materials from place to place. If funds are available for kitchen remodeling, lowering counters and range to a comfortable height for wheelchair use is recommended. However, such extensive adaptation is often not feasible. Suggestions for home management are as follows:

1. Remove cabinet doors to eliminate the need to maneuver around them for opening and closing. Frequently used items should be stored toward the front of easy-to-reach cabinets above and below the counter surfaces.
2. If entrance and inside doors are not wide enough, use a wheelchair narrower or make doors slightly wider by removing strips along the door jambs.
3. Increase the user's height with a wheelchair cushion so that standard counters may be used.
4. Use detachable desk arms and swing-away detachable footrests to allow the wheelchair user to get as close as possible to counters and tables and also to stand at counters, if that is possible (Fig. 15-31).
5. Transport items safely and easily by using a wheelchair lapboard. The lapboard may also serve as a work surface for preparing food and drying dishes. It also protects the lap from injury from hot pans and prevents utensils from falling into the lap (Fig. 15-32).
6. Fasten a drop-leaf-type board to a bare wall or slide-out board under a counter to give the wheelchair homemaker one work surface that is a com-

fortable height in a kitchen that is otherwise standard.

7. Fit cabinets with custom- or ready-made lazy Susan devices to eliminate need to reach to rear space (Fig. 15-33).
8. Ranges ideally should be at a lower level than standard height. If this is not possible, place the controls at the front of the range, and hang a mirror angled at the proper degree over the range so that the homemaker can see contents of pots.
9. Substitute small electric cooking units for the range if it is not safely manageable.
10. Use front-loading washers and dryers.
11. Vacuum carpets with a carpet sweeper or tank-type cleaner that rolls easily and is lightweight or self-propelled. A retractable cord may be helpful to prevent tangling of cord in wheels.

ADL for the Wheelchair-Bound Individual with Upper Extremity Weakness (Quadriplegia)

In general, persons with muscle function from spinal cord levels C7 and C8 can follow the methods just described for paraplegia. Individuals with muscle function from C6 can be relatively independent with adaptations and assistive devices, whereas those with muscle function from C4 and C5 will require a considerable amount of special equipment and assistance. Patients with muscle function from C6 may benefit from the use of a wrist-driven flexor hinge splint. Externally powered splints and arm braces or mobile

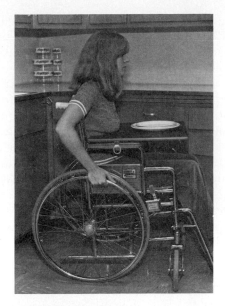

Fig. 15-32. Wheelchair lapboard is used to transport items.

arm supports are recommended for C3, C4, and C5 levels of muscle function.[1]

DRESSING ACTIVITIES

Criteria. Training in dressing can be commenced when the spine is stable.[2,24] Minimal criteria for upper extremity dressing are (1) fair to good muscle strength in deltoids, upper and middle trapezii, shoulder rotators, rhomboids, biceps, supinators, and radial wrist extensors; (2) ROM of 0° to 90° in shoulder flexion and abduction, 0° to 80° in shoulder internal rotation,

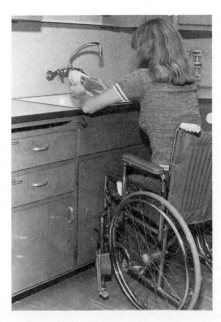

Fig. 15-31. Wheelchair footrests are swung away to allow close access to sink.

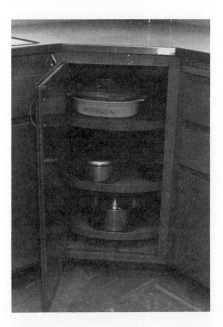

Fig. 15-33. Lazy Susan-type kitchen storage cabinet.

0° to 30° in external rotation, and 15° to 140° in elbow flexion; (3) sitting balance in bed or wheelchair, which may be achieved with the assistance of bed rails or wheelchair safety belt; and (4) finger prehension achieved with adequate tenodesis grasp or wrist-hand orthosis (formerly the flexor-hinge splint). Additional criteria for dressing the lower extremities are (1) fair to good muscle strength in pectoralis major and minor, serratus anterior, and rhomboid major and minor; (2) ROM of 0° to 120° in knee flexion and 0° to 110° in hip flexion; (3) body control for transfer from bed to wheelchair with minimal assistance; (4) ability to roll from side to side, balance in side lying, or turning from supine position to prone position and back; and (5) vital capacity of 50% or better.[24]

Contraindications. Dressing is contraindicated if any of the following factors are present: (1) unstable spine at site of injury, (2) pressure sores or tendency for skin breakdown during rolling, scooting, and transferring, (3) uncontrollable muscle spasms in legs, and (4) less than 50% vital capacity.[2,24]

Sequence of dressing. The recommended sequence for training to dress is to put on underwear and trousers while still in bed, then transfer to a wheelchair and put on shirts, socks, and shoes.[24] Some patients may wish to put the socks on before the trousers, because they may help the feet to slip through the trouser legs more easily.

Expected proficiency. Total dressing, which includes both upper and lower extremity dressing skills, can be achieved by patients with spinal cord lesions at C7 and below. Total dressing can be achieved by patients with lesions at C6, but lower extremity dressing may be difficult or impracticable in terms of time and energy for these patients. Upper extremity dressing can be achieved by patients with lesions at C5 to C6 with some exceptions. It is difficult or impossible for these patients to put on a brassiere, tuck a shirt or blouse into a waistband, and fasten buttons. Factors such as age, physical proportions, coordination, concomitant medical problems, and motivation will affect the degree of proficiency in dressing skills that can be achieved by any patient.[2]

Types of clothing. Clothing should be loose and have front openings. Trousers need to be a size larger than usually worn to accommodate the urine collection device or leg braces if worn. Wraparound skirts and rubber pants are helpful for women. The fasteners that are easiest to manage are zippers and Velcro closures. Because the quadriplegic patient often uses the thumb as a hook to manage clothing, loops attached to zipper pulls, undershorts, and even the back of the shoes can be helpful. Belt loops on trousers are used for pulling and should be reinforced. Brassieres should have stretch straps and no boning in them. Front-opening brassiere styles can be adapted by fastening loops and adding Velcro closures; back-opening styles can have loops added at each side of the fastening. Shoes can be one-half to one size larger than normally worn to accommodate edema and spasticity and to avoid pressure sores. Shoe fasteners can be adapted with Velcro, elastic shoe laces, large buckles, or flip-back tongue closure. Loose woolen or cotton socks without elastic cuffs should be used initially. As skill is gained, nylon socks, which tend to stick to the skin, may be possible. If neckties are used, the clip-on type or a regular tie that has been preknotted and can be slipped over the head may be manageable for some patients.[2,24]

The following dressing techniques can facilitate dressing for persons with upper extremity weakness.

TROUSERS AND UNDERSHORTS
Donning

1. Sit on bed with bed rails up. Trousers are positioned at foot of bed with trousers legs over end of bed and front side up.[24]
2. Sit up and lift one knee at a time by hooking right hand under right knee to pull leg into flexion, then put trousers over right foot. Return right leg to extension or semiextended position while repeating procedure with left hand and left knee.[2] If unable to maintain leg in flexion by holding with one arm or through advantageous use of spasticity, dressing band may be used. This is a piece of elasticized webbing that has been sewn into a figure-eight pattern, with one small loop and one large loop. The small loop is hooked around foot and the large hoop is anchored over knee. Band is measured for individual patient so that its length is appropriate to maintain desired amount of knee flexion. Once the trousers are in place, knee loop is pushed off knee and dressing band is removed from foot with dressing stick.[5]
3. Work trousers up legs, using patting and sliding motions with palms of hands.
4. While still sitting with pants to midcalf height, insert dressing stick in front belt loop. Dressing stick is gripped by slipping its loop over wrist. Pull on dressing stick while extending trunk, returning to supine position. Return to sitting position and repeat this procedure, pulling on dressing sticks and maneuvering trousers up to thigh level.[24] If balance is adequate, an alternative is for patient to remain sitting and lean on left elbow and pull trousers over right buttock, then reverse process for other side. Another alternative is for patient to remain in supine position and roll to one side; throw opposite arm behind back; hook thumb in waistband, belt loop, or pocket; and pull trousers up over hips. These maneuvers can be repeated as often as necessary to get trousers over buttocks.[2]
5. Using palms of hands in pushing and smoothing motions, straighten the trouser legs.
6. In supine position, fasten trouser placket by hooking thumb in loop on zipper pull, patting Velcro closed, or using hand splints and button hooks if there are buttons.[2,24]

Removing

1. Lying supine in bed with bed rails up, unfasten belt and placket fasteners.
2. Placing thumbs in belt loops, waist band, or pockets, work trousers past hips by stabilizing arms in shoulder extension and scooting body toward head of bed.
3. Use arms as described in step 2 and roll from side to side to get trousers past buttocks.
4. Coming to sitting position and alternately pulling legs into flexion, push trousers down legs.[24]
5. Trousers can be pushed off over feet with dressing stick or by hooking thumbs in waistband.

CARDIGANS OR PULLOVER GARMENTS

Cardigan and pullover garments include blouses, vests, sweaters, skirts, and front-opening dresses.[2,24] Procedure for putting on these garments is as follows:

Donning

1. Garment is positioned across thighs with back facing up and neck toward knees.
2. Place both arms under back of garment and in armholes.
3. Push sleeves up onto arms past elbows.
4. Using a wrist extension grip, hook thumbs under garment back and gather material up from neck to hem.
5. To pass garment over head, adduct and externally rotate shoulders and flex elbows while flexing head forward.
6. When garment is over head, relax shoulders and wrists, and remove hands from back of garment. Most of material will be gathered up at neck, across shoulders, and under arms.
7. To work garment down over body, shrug shoulders, lean forward, and use elbow flexion and wrist extension. Use wheelchair arms for balance if necessary. Additional maneuvers to accomplish task are to hook wrists into sleeves and pull material free from underarms or lean forward, reach back, and slide hand against material to aid in pulling garment down.
8. Garment can be buttoned from bottom to top with aid of button hook and wrist-hand orthosis if hand function is inadequate.

Removing

1. Sit in wheelchair and wear wrist-hand orthosis. Unfasten buttons (if any) while wearing splints and using button hook. Remove splints for remaining steps.
2. For pullover garments, hook thumb in back of neckline, extend wrist, and pull garment over head while turning head toward side of raised arm. Maintain balance by resting against opposite wheelchair armrest or pushing on thigh with extended arm.
3. For cardigan garments, hook thumb in opposite armhole and push sleeve down arm. Elevation and depression of shoulders with trunk rotation can be used to get garment to slip down arms as far as possible.
4. Hold one cuff with opposite thumb while elbow is flexed to pull arm out of sleeve.

BRASSIERE (Back opening)

Donning

1. Place brassiere across lap with straps toward knees and inside facing up.
2. Using a right-to-left procedure, hold end of brassiere closest to right side with hand or reacher and pass brassiere around back from right to left. Lean against brassiere at back to hold it in place, while hooking thumb of left hand in a loop that has been attached near brassiere fastener. Hook right thumb in a similar loop on right side and fasten brassiere in front at waist level.
3. Hook right thumb in edge of brassiere and using wrist extension, elbow flexion, shoulder adduction, and internal rotation, brassiere is rotated around body so that front of brassiere is in front of body.
4. While leaning on one forearm, hook opposite thumb in front end of strap and pull strap over shoulder, then repeat procedure on other side.[2,24]

Removing

1. Hook thumb under opposite brassiere strap, and push down over shoulder while elevating shoulder.
2. Pull arm out of strap, and repeat procedure for other arm.
3. Push brassiere down to waist level, and turn around as described previously to bring fasteners to front.
4. Unfasten brassiere.

SOCKS

Donning

1. Sit in wheelchair or on bed if balance is adequate in cross-legged position with one ankle crossed over opposite knee.
2. Pull sock over foot with wrist extension grip and patting movements with palm of hand.[2,24]
3. If trunk balance is inadequate and cross-legged position cannot be maintained, prop foot on stool, chair, or open drawer while opposite arm is around upright of wheelchair for balance. Wheelchair safety belt or leaning against wheelchair armrest on one side are alternatives to maintain balance.
4. Use stocking aid or sock cone (see Fig. 15-4) to assist in putting on socks while in this position. Powder sock cone and apply sock to it by using thumbs and palms of hands to smooth sock out on cone. Powder inside of cone to reduce friction against cone.
5. Place cord loops of sock cone around the wrist or thumb and cone is thrown beyond foot.
6. Maneuver cone over toes by pulling cords using elbow flexion. Insert foot as far as possible into cone.
7. To remove cone from sock after foot has been inserted, move heel forward off wheelchair footrest using wrist extension of hand not operating sock cone behind knee and continue pulling cords of cone until it is removed and sock is in place on foot. Use palms to smooth sock with patting and stroking motion.[24]

Removing

1. While sitting in wheelchair or lying in bed, use dressing stick or long-handled shoe horn to push sock down over heel. Cross legs if possible.
2. Use dressing stick with cuphook on end to pull sock off toes.[3]

SHOES

Donning

1. Use same position for donning socks as for putting on shoes.

2. Use extended-handle dressing aid and insert it into tongue of shoe; then place shoe opening over toes. Remove dressing aid from shoe, and dangle shoe on toes.
3. Using palm of hand on sole of shoe, pull shoe toward heel of foot. One hand is used to stabilize leg while other is pushing against sole of shoe to work shoe onto foot. Use thenar eminence and sides of hand for this pushing motion.
4. With feet flat on floor or on wheelchair footrest and knees flexed 90°, place a long-handled shoe horn in heel of shoe and press down on flexed knee.
5. Fasten shoes.[24]

Removing

1. Sitting in wheelchair with legs crossed as described previously, unfasten shoes.
2. Use shoe horn or dressing stick to push on heel counter of shoe, dislodging it from heel; then shoe will drop or can be pushed to floor with dressing stick.[24]

FEEDING ACTIVITIES. Eating may be assisted by a variety of devices, depending on the level of muscle function.[1] Levels C5 and above require mobile arm supports or externally powered splints and braces. A wrist splint and universal cuff may be used together if a wrist-hand orthosis (flexor hinge splint) is not used. The univeral cuff holds the eating utensil, and the splint stabilizes the wrist. A nonskid mat and a plate with plate guard may provide adequate stability of the plate for pushing and picking up food (Fig. 15-34). The spoon-plate is an option for independent feeding for patients with high spinal cord injuries. It is a portable device that can be adjusted in height to the level of the patient's mouth. The plate is made of a high-temperature thermoplastic and is formed over a mold that has a rim bowled to the approximate depth and length of a spoon. The patient rotates the device with mouth and neck control. Food is removed from the rim of the plate with the mouth. Successful use of the device depends on adequate oral control, head and trunk control, and motivation. The reader is referred to the original source for information on making or obtaining this device.[29]

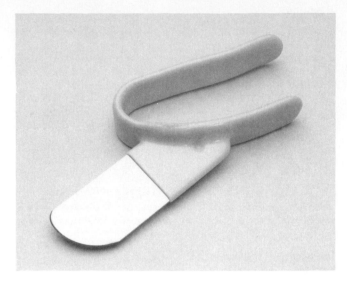

Fig. 15-35. Quad-quip knife.

A regular or swivel spoon-fork combination can be used when there is minimal muscle function (C4 to C5). A long plastic straw with a straw clip to stabilize it in the cup or glass eliminates the need for picking up these drinking vessels. A bilateral or unilateral clip-type holder on a glass or cup makes it possible for many persons with hand and arm weakness to manage liquids without a straw.

Built-up utensils may be useful for those with some functional grasp or tenodesis grasp. Cutting food may be managed with a quad quip knife if arm strength is adequate to manage the device (Fig. 15-35).

HYGIENE AND GROOMING.[1] General suggestions to facilitate hygiene and grooming are as follows:

1. Use a shower or bathtub seat and transfer board for transfers.
2. Extend reach by using long-handled bath sponges with loop handle or built-up handle.
3. Eliminate need to grasp washcloth by using bath mitts.
4. Hold comb and toothbrush with a universal cuff.[1]

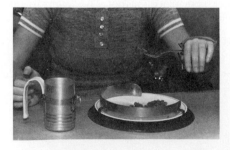

Fig. 15-34. Feeding with aid of universal cuff, plate guard, nonskid mat, and clip-type cup holder to compensate for absent grasp.

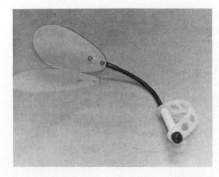

Fig. 15-36. Skin inspection mirror.

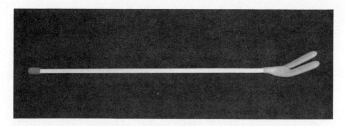

Fig. 15-37. Wand mouthstick. Reproduced with permission, Fred Sammons, Inc., A Bissell Healthcare Company, Box 32, Brookfield, IL.

5. Use the position-adjustable hair dryer previously described.[6] Use a universal cuff to hold brush or comb for hair styling while using this mounted hair dryer.
6. Use a clip-type holder for electric razor.
7. Suppository inserters for quadriplegics who can manage bowel care independently with this aid can be used.
8. Use skin inspection mirror with long stem and looped handle for independent skin inspection (Fig. 15-36). Devices selected and methods must be adapted to the degree of weakness for each patient.

COMMUNICATION AND ENVIRONMENTAL HARDWARE. The following are suggestions for facilitating communication:

1. Turn pages with an electric page turner, mouth stick, or head wand if hand and arm function are inadequate (Fig. 15-37).
2. Insert pen, pencil, typing stick, or paintbrush in a universal cuff that has been positioned with the

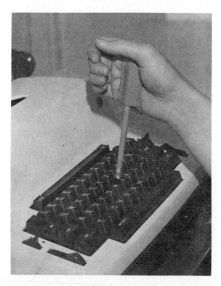

Fig. 15-38. Typing with aid of universal cuff and typing stick.

opening on the ulnar side of the palm for typing, writing, operating a tape recorder, and painting (Fig. 15-38).
3. Dial the telephone with the universal cuff and a pencil positioned with eraser down or with mouth stick or head wand if hand and arm function are absent. The receiver may need to be stationed in a telephone arm and positioned for listening. Special adaptations are available to substitute the need to replace the receiver in the cradle.
4. Use electric typewriters, which are easier to use than standard ones, or personal computers.
5. Built-up pencils and pens or special pencil holders are needed for patients with hand weakness.
6. Sophisticated electronic communications devices operated by mouth, suck and blow, and head control are available for patients with no upper extremity function.[27]
7. Kelly described two mouthsticks and a cassette tape holder that allow C3, C4, or C5 quadriplegic patients to operate a tape recorder or radio independently.[13] The first mouthstick, a rod about 19.7 inches (50 cm) long with a friction tip, is used to depress the operating buttons and adjust the volume and selector dials of the radio. The second mouthstick is a metal rod that separates into two prongs at its end. These prongs are 4 inches (10.1 cm) apart, and the mouthstick is used to place the cassettes from the cassette holder to the tape recorder and remove the cassettes from the recorder. The cassette tape stand has eight levels and is designed to hold eight tapes. It is a vertical stand made of metal and tilted backward to a 70° angle. The reader is referred to the original source for specifications on construction of these devices.[13]

MOBILITY AND TRANSFERS. Wheelchair transfer techniques for the individual with quadriplegia will be described in Chapter 22. Mobility depends on degree of weakness. Electric wheelchairs operated by hand or mouth controls have greatly increased the mobility of persons with severe upper and lower extremity weakness. Vans fitted with wheelchair lifts and stabilizing devices have made it possible for such patients to be transported to pursue community, vocational, educational, and avocational activities with an assistant.

Adaptations for hand controls have made it possible for many patients with function of at least C6 level to drive independently.

HOME MANAGEMENT ACTIVITIES. Many individuals with upper extremity weakness who are bound to wheelchair ambulation are dependent or partially dependent for homemaking activities. Patients with muscle function of C6 or better may be independent for light homemaking with appropriate devices, adaptations, and safety awareness. Many of the suggestions for wheelchair maneuverability and environmental adaptation outlined for the paraplegic apply here as well. In addition, the patient with upper extremity weakness needs to use lightweight equipment and special devices. The *Mealtime Manual for People With Disability and the Aging* compiled by Judith Lannefeld Klinger contains many excellent and specific suggestions that apply to the homemaker with weak upper extremities.[15]

REVIEW QUESTIONS

1. Define "activities of daily living" (ADL) and list four classifications of tasks that may be considered in ADL.
2. What is the role of occupational therapy in restoring ADL independence?
3. List at least three activities that are considered self-care skills, three mobility skills, three communication skills, and three home management skills.
4. List three factors that the occupational therapist must consider before commencing ADL performance evaluation and training. Describe how each could limit or effect ADL performance.
5. What is the ultimate goal of the ADL training program?
6. Discuss the concept of maximal independence, as defined in the text.
7. List the general steps in the procedure for ADL evaluation.
8. Describe how the occupational therapist can use the ADL checklist.
9. List the steps in the activities of home management evaluation.
10. What is the purpose of the home evaluation?
11. List the steps in the home evaluation.
12. Who should be involved in a comprehensive home evaluation?
13. What kinds of things are assessed in a home evaluation?
14. How does the therapist record and report results of the home evaluation and make the necessary recommendations?
15. Describe the role of the occupational therapist in the driving evaluation.
16. List eight criteria that can be used to select potential candidates for driving.
17. List six physical and performance skills that can help to determine driving potential.
18. How does the occupational therapist, with the patient, select ADL training objectives after the ADL evaluation?
19. Describe three approaches to teaching ADL skills to a patient with perception or memory deficits.
20. List the important factors to include in an ADL progress report.
21. Define three general levels of independence, as defined in the text.

EXERCISES

1. Demonstrate the use of at least three assistive devices mentioned in the text.
2. Teach another person to don a shirt, using one hand.
3. Teach another person how to don and remove trousers, as if hemiplegic.
4. Teach another person how to don and remove trousers, as if the legs were paralyzed.

REFERENCES

1. Activities of daily living for patients with incoordination, limited range of motion, paraplegia, quadriplegia, and hemiplegia, Cleveland, 1968, Highland View Hospital, Cuyahoga County Hospitals, Division of Occupational Therapy. Unpublished.
2. Bromley I: Tetraplegia and paraplegia: a guide for physiotherapists, ed 2, London, 1981, Churchill Livingstone.
3. Buchwald E: Physical rehabilitation for daily living, New York, 1952, McGraw-Hill, Inc.
4. Cynkin S: Occupational therapy: toward health through activities, Boston, 1979, Little, Brown & Co.
5. Easton LW and Horan AL: Dressing band, Am J Occup Ther 33:656, 1979.
6. Feldmeier DM and Poole JL: The position-adjustable hair dryer, Am J Occup Ther 41:246, 1987.
7. Florey LL and Michelman SM: Occupational role history: a screening tool for psychiatric occupational therapy, Am J Occup Ther 36:301, 1982.
8. Gurgold GD and Harden DH: Assessing the driving potential of the handicapped, Am J Occup Ther 32:41, 1978.
9. Hays CA et al, editors: Sample forms for occupational therapy, Rockville, MD, 1980, American Occupational Therapy Association.
10. Holser P, Jones M, and Ilanit T: A study of the upper extremity control brace, Am J Occup Ther 16:170, 1962.
11. Hopkins HL, Smith HD, and Tiffany EG: Therapeutic application of activity. In Hopkins HL, and Smith HD, editors: Willard and Spackman's occupational therapy, ed 6, Philadelphia, 1983, JB Lippincott Co.
12. Jones R, Giddens H, and Croft D: Assessment and training of brain damaged drivers, Am J Occup Ther 37:754, 1983.
13. Kelly SN: Adaptations for independent use of cassette tape recorder/radio by high-level quadriplegic patients, Am J Occup Ther 37:766, 1983.
14. Kester DL: Prevocational and vocational assessment. In Hopkins HL and Smith HD, editors: Willard and Spackman's occupational therapy, ed 6, Philadelphia, 1983, JB Lippincott Co.
15. Klinger JL: Mealtime manual for people with disabilities and the aging, Camden, NJ, 1978, Campbell Soup Co.
16. Malick MH and Almasy BS: Activities of daily living and homemaking. In Hopkins HL and Smith HD, editors: Willard and Spackman's occupational therapy, ed 6, Philadelphia, 1983, JB Lippincott Co.

17. Malick MH and Almasy BS: Assessment and evaluation: life work tasks. In Hopkins HL and Smith HD, editors: Willard and Spackman's occupational therapy, ed 6, Philadelphia, 1983, JB Lippincott Co.
18. Matsusuyu J: The interest checklist, Am J Occup Ther 23:323, 1969.
19. Melvin JL: Rheumatic disease: occupational therapy and rehabilitation, ed 2, Philadelphia, 1982, FA Davis Co.
20. Moorhead L: The occupational history, Am J Occup Ther 23:329, 1969.
21. Okamoto GA: Physical medicine and rehabilitation, Philadelphia, 1984, WB Saunders Co.
22. The Professional Manual Subcommittee of the Educational Committee, Allied Health Professional Section of the Arthritis Foundation: Arthritis manual for allied health professionals, New York, 1973, The Arthritis Foundation.
23. Quigley FL and DeLisa JA: Assessing the driving potential of cerebral vascular accident patients, Am J Occup Ther 37:474, 1983.
24. Runge M: Self-dressing techniques for patients with spinal cord injury, Am J Occup Ther 21:367, 1967.
25. Spencer EA: Functional restoration: theory, principles and techniques. In Hopkins HL and Smith HD: Willard and Spackman's occupational therapy, ed 6, Philadelphia, 1983, JB Lippincott Co.
26. Sokaler R: A buttoning aid, Am J Occup Ther 35:737, 1981.
27. Trombly CA, editor: Occupational therapy for physical dysfunction, ed 2, Baltimore, 1983, Williams & Wilkins.
28. Watanabe S: Activities configuration, regional institute on the evaluation process, Final Rep. RSA-123-T-68, New York, 1968, American Occupational Therapy Association.
29. Wykoff E and Mitani M: The spoon plate: a self-feeding device, Am J Occup Ther 36:333, 1982.

Chapter

16 Work hardening

PATRICIA SMITH

In American society, feelings of personal identity and self-worth are closely tied to a person's role as a competitive wage earner. Abrupt loss of the worker role due to injury frequently leads to forced role reversal within the family, life-style changes due to economic hardship, forced inactivity and dependence, and depression and maladaptive psychosocial responses. Particularly when recovery from injury is prolonged or compounded by individual maladaptive coping techniques, the worker may slip into a mire of discouragement, lowered self-esteem, lost confidence, chronic pain syndromes, and a host of other disabling cycles, ultimately leading to low motivation for return to work.

Injuries to workers sustained in the course of performance of job duties are receiving increased attention from employers, insurance carriers, medical personnel, and the public in general. With the costs of industrial injuries reaching astronomical proportions in terms of monetary costs and lost productivity, employers and their industrial insurance carriers (Worker's Compensation) are continually looking for cost-controlling measures. Paramount among work-related injuries are low back injuries followed by injuries to the upper extremities. Although 90% of persons who have acute episodes of low back pain recover in 3 months, in 10% the condition becomes chronic, lasting for many months or even years. These persons account for $.80 of every $1.00 spent for treatment and disability compensation.[12] Their injuries, though costly in terms of lost wages, lost time on the job, medical treatment, and ancillary treatment, also extract a heavy personal toll for the worker and the worker's family.

Work hardening is a restorative and reconditioning treatment process which has been described in various ways but must incorporate the goals of expeditious and physically appropriate return to employment. Work hardening uses work, defined as real or simulated job tasks, as the treatment modality. These tasks may be combined with injury-specific, graded, strengthening and flexibility training, support, and reinforcement to renew and build behavioral characteristics necessary to successful competitive employment.

Interest in work hardening concepts is increasingly gaining acceptance as a "new service" in the vocational rehabilitation arena to assist in return to work. In reality work hardening is far from new and has roots deep in occupational therapy theory and practice. Formal involvement of occupational therapy in the vocational rehabilitation movement can be traced to the federal Vocational Rehabilitation Act of 1923, which required inclusion of occupational therapy in general hospitals serving persons with industrial accidents and illnesses. Amendments to the Act in 1954 increased the prominence of the profession in the vocational rehabilitation field through provisions for establishment of prevocational services within facilities. The role of occupational therapy was further enhanced with amendments in 1978 to the Vocational Rehabilitation Act.[1]

HISTORY OF OCCUPATIONAL THERAPY INVOLVEMENT
Review of Literature

Work therapy, as it was often called, dates far back in occupational therapy literature. In the mid-1800s tuberculosis patients were prescribed graded exercise and work tolerance activities as part of a medical regimen of good food and fresh air. Activities such as woodworking and clerical tasks of a progressively demanding nature were added to the treatment protocol as the final stage to prepare the patient for return to work and to estimate resistance to breakdown from physical effort and emotional upsets.[11]

In 1919 Barton stated that the purpose of work was to divert the mind, to exercise some part of the anatomy, and to relieve the monotony and boredom of illness. Work did not, he suggested, have to be of practical value beyond its immediate purpose. World War I reconstruction workers, the first occupational therapists, taught crafts in military hospitals as "work cure." Crafts were used as therapy and were seen as legitimate work used to foster a sense of intrinsic productivity and fulfillment rather than to rehabilitate the patient for the work force.[5] In the early 1920s, programs of "habit training" were described, with the goal of developing the habits of industry that had been impaired by disease or accident.

In the psychiatric literature of the 1940s, work hardening was described as a program to prepare the patient for return to competitive life after the sheltered environment of the hospital. Realistic work environments were used, including the hospital laundry, barber shop, and carpentry shop. The patient was also observed for personality traits such as cooperation and friendliness, characteristics felt to be important for harmonious working.

The physical disability literature of the same era also stressed real work experiences designed to make the worker aware of the relationship of his work hardening program to a job which might support his family. Work speed was variable, but quality standards were not altered during the treatment program.[11]

In the 1950s a program at Massachusetts General Hospital was described that used the nonmedical departments of the hospital to aid in evaluation of progress. A progressive-resistive exercise component was added. By measuring strength increases in pounds, it was possible to track changes. By adding this new component, principles of objective and quantified outcome measures were incorporated.[13]

Lillian Wegg, a leader in the field of work hardening and work therapy during the late 1950s, described a multidisciplinary program combining an occupational therapist, vocational counselor, physiatrist, and industrial engineer. Work hardening activities included use of work samples (in early stages of development), work tests, and job simulations. At program conclusion, a list of recommendations were given, including assistive equipment, length of work day and job classifications that should be considered for placement.[14] Several years later Wegg described important changes in the program. Work hardening had moved away from a medical model to a vocational model. A physician's prescription was no longer needed. Instead, approval for patient participation was required. Work hardening was seen as a distinct program to follow more vocationally oriented evaluation since the purpose of work hardening was to develop work habits and improve work assets that had been identified in the evaluated process.[15]

In other programs of the era, an emphasis on real work was maintained. Patients produced items for sale and worked in hospital or community settings to build a sense of self-worth and repertoires of acceptable behaviors, as well as physical work tolerances.

CURRENT MODELS OF PRACTICE

Work hardening program models currently being used by occupational therapists clearly draw on concepts from past experiences while adding present day technology and theory from developmental models, systems models, occupational and career development models, models of medical intervention and ergonomic and anthropomorphic principles.[11] The occupational therapy process in provision of services incorporates an orderly sequence of services designed to prepare the person for vocational evaluation, on-the-job or formal training, and, eventually, employment at the highest possible level of independent functioning.[1]

In some settings work hardening is considered a work adjustment activity. Work adjustment is primarily focused on acquisition of work habits and skills necessary for successful functioning in training and competitive employment. These habits and skills include punctuality, appropriate receptivity to supervision, interpersonal communication, work-specific grooming and dress, ability to maintain focus on task, and ability and willingness to ask for assistance when needed. Because of individual psychological responses to injury, prolonged inactivity, and residual disability, a previously competent worker may need these special remedial services to regain appropriate worker behaviors and habits.[1]

The basic principles and responsibilities of occupational therapy practice in provision of work hardening services have been summarized by the American Occupational Therapy Association in the Work Hardening Guidelines (Fig. 16-1). These guidelines provide basic structure for services provided in a variety of settings, encompassing several theoretical models and frames of reference represented in occupational therapy practice.

Occupational therapy intervention through work hardening services can occur at any of several points in the process of return to work. Traditionally, occupational therapists have focused their efforts in the early intervention model by entering the rehabilitation process during the medical phase of treatment, perhaps during a hospital stay for acute care of an injury. For the person injured on the job, occupational therapy intervention may begin during acute care, for example, with splinting and ADL evaluation and training, and quickly progress to energy conservation training, pain control methods, and pacing. As soon as it is medically feasible, this same injured worker may begin work hardening sessions as an outpatient, which often coincides with and is coordinated with physical therapy and on-going visits to the treating physician. Work hardening services in this early in-

Work Hardening Guidelines

Approved by the Representative Assembly of the American
Occupational Therapy Association, April, 1986

Screening

Occupational therapists have the responsibility to perform an initial screening to determine appropriateness for assessment.

Screening methods include the following:

- Review of pertinent records, which may include educational, legal, employment, medical, and other related records;

- Intake interview identifying life-style, work history, and educational background;

- Observation of motor, sensorimotor, visual perceptual, interpersonal, and cognitive skills;

- Communication of the findings to the appropriate source with recommendations for services and/or referral to other more appropriate programs.

Referral

Typical referral sources for work hardening may include

physicians

attorneys

rehabilitation personnel

employers

educational personnel

human service agency personnel

insurance representatives

self-referrals

Under federal, state, or private worker's compensation systems and/or professional licensing requirements, the following may be required:

- The physician's referral

- The physician's written consent and statement of medical restrictions;

- The physician's final report with permanent medical contra-indications and the extent of disability identified;

- Written authorization from the referral source if other than a physician;

- A statement of referral questions to be answered and/or anticipated goals.

Assessment

Components of the occupational therapy work hardening assessment often include the following:

1. A physical evaluation that is related to work with a baseline measurement of the client's current or demonstrated physical abilities, including mobility, strength, endurance, sensation, hand function, and gross and fine motor coordination;

2. Evaluation procedures that include measures of sensorimotor, cognitive, and psychosocial skills with respect to the client's interests, motivation, age, education, culture, and ethnic background;

3. An evaluation of work behaviors, including the client's response to supervision, attendance, punctuality, initiative, and interpersonal relations, and the ability to follow policies and procedures;

4. A functional evaluation of the client's body mechanics and ability to work under pressure and over time;

5. An evaluation of the client's cardiopulmonary responses to work and ability to work under stress, including an analysis of the client's knowledge of appropriate body mechanics, work simplification techniques, and methods of symptom control;

6. An evaluation of the client's knowledge and use of common and specific tools, if required for job performance;

7. A job analysis, including an on-site evaluation when necessary to develop a step-by-step breakdown of specific job tasks and critical job demands to identify program areas as they relate to the client's condition;

8. An analysis of the need for modification of the equipment or workplace that would help the client perform with greater efficiency, effectiveness, and safety.

Program Planning

Occupational therapists use the results of the assessment to develop an individualized work hardening program that involves selection of the media, methods, environment, and personnel needed to accomplish goals and objectives that are (a) stated in measurable terms appropriate to the client's level of functioning, limitations, referral restrictions, and expected prognosis for program results or competitive employment and (b) consistent with current principles, practices, and concepts of occupational therapy considering ethical practices and legal requirements.

The planning process includes collaborating with the client, the referral source, and other related personnel to determine short- and long-term goals that often include

- Establishing an appropriate productivity level for homebound, sheltered, modified, or competitive work;

- Increasing physical and psychological tolerances, such as cardiopulmonary endurance and stress tolerance;

- Improving functional ability to perform self-care and self-paced work-related tasks;

- Facilitating interpersonal communication in employer/employee relations;

- Developing work behavior traits and attitudes, such as attention to task, punctuality, response to supervision, and self-confidence;

- Minimizing or controlling pain or the effects of pain;

- Determining the frequency and duration of work hardening services;

- Participating in a case conference to discuss assessment findings, to review goals and objectives, to formulate recommendations, and to coordinate program implementation.

Program Implementation

1. Work hardening services are implemented according to the program plan.

2. Occupational therapists formulate modifications in the work hardening program when changes occur in the client's

Fig. 16-1. Work hardening guidelines.

Continued

performance that are consistent with program goals.

3. Occupational therapy personnel document the results of the program and the frequency of the services provided according to regulations and procedures established by facilities, government agencies, and accrediting bodies.

4. Case conferences are conducted to report the client's status and change. Written reports are regularly submitted to the referral source and other professionals related to the case.

Discontinuation of Services

1. Occupational therapists discontinue services when the client has achieved the goals or has demonstrated an inability to benefit from work hardening services.

2. Occupational therapists prepare written reports that include

• Results and an interpretation of standardized and nonstandardized tests administered;

 • Statements of program goals and objectives;

 • Comparisons between initial assessment and discharge status;

 • Recommendations and effect on performance of adaptive devices/modifications;

• Client behaviors and attitudes applicable to the work environment;

• Recommendations and conclusions.

3. Occupational therapy personnel participate in case conferences to outline progress, modifications or adaptations, physical and psychological tolerances, recommendations, and any other information pertinent to the referral source for work-related planning.

Quality Assurance

Occupational therapy personnel conducting work hardening programs shall periodically and systematically review all aspects of individual programs provided and total services offered for effectiveness, efficiency, and quality by using predetermined criteria that reflect professional consensus, research, and theory.

Fig. 16-1, cont'd. Work hardening guidelines.

tervention model are guided by the physician and are usually provided on a prescription basis. The goal is expeditious return to the waiting job or perhaps a temporarily modified job that eases the transition back to full employment. Although the cost of work hardening in this medical model is high when several medical providers may be involved simultaneously, time off the job is usually shortened, ultimately saving dollars that would be spent on disability or income replacement benefits (Fig. 16-2).

When return to the original job and original employer is not feasible either because of medical preclusions or other factors, the worker enters the vocational rehabilitation phase. The goals of work hardening remain the same in this late intervention model—rapid and safe return to employment. However the program in the vocational model must consider and allow for additional difficulties and constraints. Among these are the worker's fears and anxieties about a forced career change, unrealistic expectations of the vocational rehabilitation/legal system, and other real and imagined barriers and disappointments experienced by the displaced worker.

PROGRAM GOAL PLANNING
Overall Goals

The goals of work hardening are always individually designed to maximize employability through achievement of a level of productivity acceptable in the labor market. Employability is an individual's ability to be employed in a particular labor market, both

geographically and with respect to ability to meet the demands of specific jobs. Work hardening improves employability in several ways. By improving physical work tolerances, the worker becomes eligible for a greater number of jobs. Better understanding of tolerance, assessed over time, is achieved in the work hardening process with resulting improved definition of appropriate job fit to the individual. Abilities of the worker are established on the basis of actual demonstrated performance rather than supposition. With the ability to accurately predict appearance of symptoms, symptom control measures such as pacing, proper body mechanics, posture, and compensatory techniques can be used to prevent or circumvent symptomatic limitations. Finally, with a more complete understanding of limitations and abilities, appropriate modifications of the task, tool, and/or worker can be designed.[8]

Within the overall goal of preparing the worker to reenter the labor market at the highest level of functioning possible, there are several subgoals. These are (1) attaining optimal physical reconditioning, (2) increasing confidence for resumption of productive work, (3) identification of problems that may require selection of an alternative job, (4) maintaining or reintroducing appropriate worker behaviors, and (5) providing optimal cognitive and psychosocial reconditioning.[7]

Activities and real or simulated job tasks, are tailored to replicate the requirements of a specific job. Critical to the success of work hardening is the work-

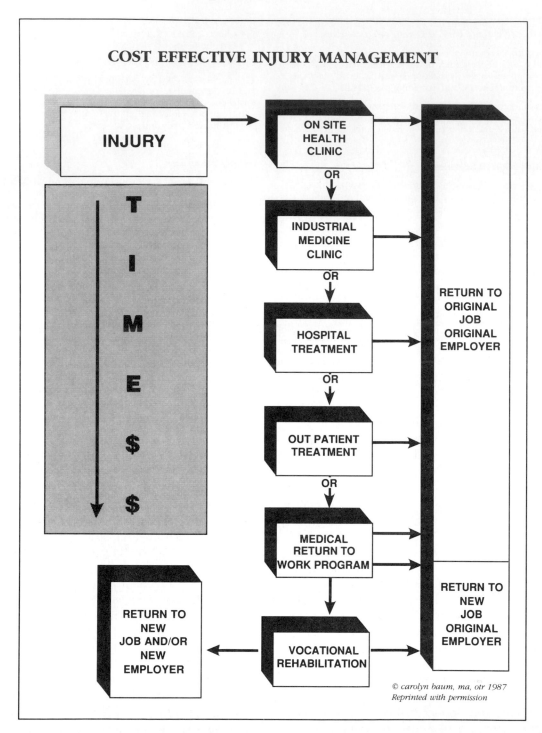

Fig. 16-2. Cost-effective injury management.

er's involvement in an active, doing, program that encourages individual responsibility and participation and discourages a disabled mindset. As in programs of former years, it is important that the work hardening program requires what is real and believable to the person so that it has face validity and encourages participation and motivation.

Individualized Goals

In order to plan a program for an injured worker that is meaningful, relevant, and measurable, the worker's job requirements must be understood. This information is gathered through task analysis of the physical and cognitive demands of the worker's former job, when return to the accustomed job is expected or analysis of the new job when this is antici-pated. Because design of program activities is based on job demands and because job placement decisions are made on the basis of successful performance of these activities, it is necessary to have an accurate de-scription of all pertinent job demands. The job may have been analyzed previously by the employer, in-surance carrier, rehabilitation nurse or counselor, or other professional involved in the case. The analysis should include detailed information about the de-mands placed on the worker for the following: walk-ing, balancing, climbing, standing, crouching, bend-ing, sitting, reaching, lifting, carrying, pushing/pull-ing, handling, hearing, and others. Also considered are environmental conditions such as noise, cold, and vibration.

When this information has not been provided to the therapist, it can be sought through various chan-nels depending on procedures governing various state workers' compensation systems. Pertinent informa-tion is necessary at program outset; however, a more formal analysis of tasks is not always essential. For some jobs a formal analysis may be unnecessary be-cause the information is readily available, for exam-ple, the job of a nursing assistant in the worker's own facility. Frequently a sufficiently comprehensive job description can be obtained from the worker who may be able to explain with clarity the weights and items to be lifted, distances traveled, and other tasks critical to the job and relevant in terms of the type of injury being treated.

When a job analysis is unavailable or when accuracy of the reported information is in question, an analysis is made through on-site observation and measure-ment. Occupational therapists by their basic training are qualified to perform these on-site analyses of phys-ical and cognitive demands; however, additional ex-perience and training is usually required for the ther-apist to translate the obtained information into the form needed for medical/legal documentation. Sev-eral government publications can be used as refer-ences to assist in development of the document: *Dic-tionary of Occupational Titles, Handbook for Analyzing Jobs,* and *A Guide to Job Analysis.*[6]

Equally as important as job analysis in individual program planning is determination of the worker's current level of functioning. Assessment of functional status is undertaken through a screening of all per-tinent physical and cognitive factors. A factor is per-tinent if it is a requirement of the job and is subject to impairment as a result of the injury. Also consid-ered are relevant nonindustrial conditions such as di-abetes, hearing loss, and hypertension, which may not be sequelae of the work injury but must be considered because of their impact on job performance.

Establishing Baseline Function

A screening of physical function and work toler-ances is usually the initial step in a work hardening program. The worker is evaluated for ability to per-form the activities addressed in the job analysis (e.g., reaching, lifting, carrying) that are the demands of the job for which the worker hopes to qualify. A worker with a low back injury would most likely be evaluated for lifting, carrying, standing, and climbing but may not be evaluated for grip or pinch strength in the absence of reasonable expectation of limitations in these abilities. If the physician has restricted the worker from performing certain activities these re-strictions are, of course, adhered to at all times. The worker is also encouraged to monitor activities and avoid any breach of medically recommended precau-tions (Figs. 16-3 and 16-4).

The screening of physical tolerances usually occurs on the initial day of work hardening. Occasionally this information accompanies the worker when the refer-ral is made. Baseline values may have been established by another professional or estimated by the physician. Work hardening program personnel may wish to quickly verify this information to identify any gains or losses that may have occurred, especially if some time has elapsed since measurements of function were made. Losses can occur very rapidly because of delays or intervening medical treatment or complications.

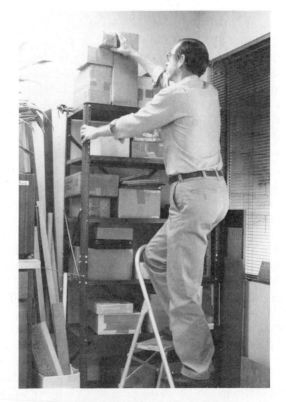

Fig. 16-3. Reaching and climbing.

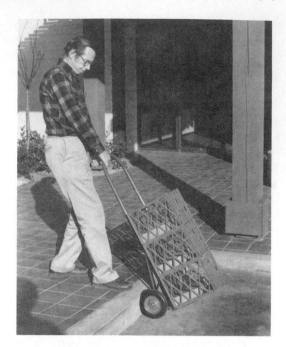

Fig. 16-4. Pushing and pulling.

Assessment of other factors, such as worker behaviors, safety awareness and stressors may be extended over a longer period of time to permit sufficient observation and evaluation. The purpose of the screening is to establish areas of deficit that are amenable to treatment and improvement through the work hardening process.

Individual Work Hardening Plan

When current functional abilities are thoroughly defined and requirements of the desired job are adequately determined an Individual Work Hardening Plan is developed that details how the goals of the worker's program shall be met. The plan can be thought of as an agreement between the worker and the therapist, which lists in measurable terms the graded activities to be used and the mutually agreed upon desired outcomes. Included in the plan may be hours of participation, work tasks, units of work to be completed in a given period of time, strengthening and flexibility activities, number and duration of work breaks, and specific goals suggested by the referral source. The plan is developed with the cooperation and collaboration of the injured worker. Areas of deficit and outcomes must be mutually agreed on if the program is to be successful.

When work hardening is conducted in a vocational model rather than an earlier intervention-type model, there frequently are goals in the plan such as development and maintenance of appropriate attendance and specific hours of participation. Often the worker

has been off the job for many months or even years and has adopted a pattern of sleeping late and needs encouragement to adjust to regular work hours.

Considering the severity of the injury, stage of medical recovery, motivation, and degree of discrepancy between current functional capabilities and necessary levels of function, predictions are now possible regarding expectations for improvement and success as well as program length. If reasonable progress and improvement are not anticipated, serious consideration is given to discontinuation of the program or recommending referral to other services that may be more beneficial. In a climate of strict cost management and accountability, program personnel must be diligent in preventing unnecessary costs and delays.

WORK TASKS AND ACTIVITIES

Much of the guidance for program development and treatment processes comes from literature on back injury, prevention, and research. Back injuries represent the major disability condition referred to centers treating a full range of injuries. These injuries also represent the greatest loss of work time and treatment dollars. Training in proper techniques for working while protecting the body from further injury is therefore frequently incorporated in the work hardening program. This training is also helpful for the person who does not have a history of back pain but who is engaged in heavy work or work performed in awkward or static postures. Education for back pro-

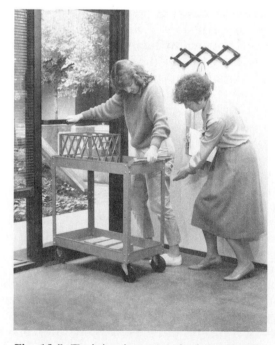

Fig. 16-5. Training in proper body mechanics.

tection and safety principles is taught in a manner consistent with the worker's level of education and background. The principles taught are applied to the person's job demands and are practiced consistently while performing job tasks so that responses become automatic and are integrated (Fig. 16-5).

The worker is encouraged to be aware of activities that create discomfort. Proper methods of working with safe techniques and pacing are demonstrated. The worker is urged to use problem solving and apply new solutions to the identified problems. The work hardening setting becomes a supportive atmosphere and work environment in which the worker can test increasing skills and reduce the risk of reinjury by using principles of proper movement to diminish fear of activity.[2]

Fear of movement because of pain can lead to bracing (guarding) and other dysfunctional pain behaviors. Acute back pain often leads to increased muscle tension, which is a normal physiologic response to pain and to the memory of painful previous episodes of pain. The resulting tension leads to increases in pain, which leads to more tension and so on in a cycle that is difficult to interrupt.

The worker's perception of pain can be compared with objective medical findings. The presence of a significant discrepancy suggests potential for development of chronic pain syndromes.[3] Because reporting pain is subjective, occupational therapists focus on observable graded activity levels as an indicator of improvement.[4] For reasons of sound treatment principles and also because of liability issues while the worker is in the program, care must be taken to remove all reasonable risk factors. The worker must not be permitted to use unsafe methods whatever the presenting injury may be. Assuring a safe work environment in the work hardening setting is the responsibility of all program personnel involved in client care.

Along with back safety and injury prevention principles, the worker is engaged in a program of activities and simulated or actual work tasks. Activities are selected to be compatible with the worker's beginning level of function and to advance toward increased capability, at the same time reducing discomfort or maintaining symptoms at a manageable level. Although it may not be possible to eliminate all residual physical symptoms associated with the injury, the worker must still be capable of productive efforts with acceptably competitive results.

The selection of work tasks and activities, as previously mentioned, is based on the worker's individual job demands and limitations in abilities to meet these demands. It is not always possible to duplicate all tasks of a job. When this is the case, activities are chosen

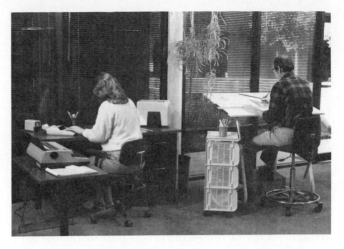

Fig. 16-6. Work is performed in realistic work stations.

that require similar body motions and skills. If it is not feasible for a worker to replace automobile mufflers, it may be possible to design an activity requiring prolonged tool use and reaching overhead. Individual program design is limited only by the therapist's creativity and resources at hand.

A work hardening facility replicates a realistic work environment with a variety of work station configurations and "raw material" from which can be constructed a variety of job simulations or actual work tasks (Figs. 16-6 and 16-7).

With the use of work that is relevant and meaningful the worker is helped to face the reality of the situation and come to a better understanding and acceptance of possible limitations and a realization of abilities and vocational strengths. The therapist's presence is vital to offer support when needed, make suggestions for compensation and modification when appropriate, and to encourage internalization of new learning.

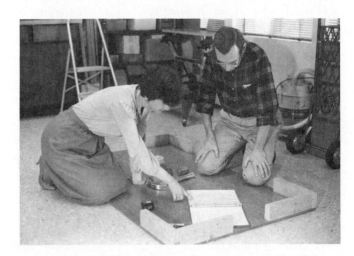

Fig. 16-7. Actual or simulated job tasks.

Work hardening is usually a group process with a number of workers present, who may be experiencing similar difficulties and fears. The desire to be competitive with one's peers can be invaluable as is an atmosphere of peer understanding and support. All these features should be fostered by the therapist.

Depending on constraints of the referring agency, work hardening services may be continued as long as the worker makes steady gains toward meeting program goals. Services are usually terminated when goals are substantially met in order to permit a return to work, when improvement has reached a plateau, or when sufficient progress is not demonstrated and does not appear to be reasonably attainable. Pressure to achieve results more rapidly is part of the growing climate of accountability and cost containment that is evident in all areas of health care, including vocational rehabilitation.

REPORTING RESULTS

In accordance with facility protocols, governing procedures and accrediting requirements results of the program are reported at agreed-upon intervals. Case conferences are held periodically for all persons involved to discuss progress and concerns. Written reports document program goals and results. Reports are submitted in a timely manner to the referring agency and are often reviewed by a number of persons who may not be medically trained. Language used is therefore clear, concise, and free of jargon.[10]

If the program continues beyond the initial period, subsequent progress reports list new goals to be attained. At program termination, a final report is submitted that may include recommendations based on information gathered in the work hardening process. An example might be recommendation of a specific tool handle design that proved helpful in promoting optimal productivity and minimizing symptoms.

CASE STUDY

KL, a 36-year-old man, was injured in a fall from a ladder while working as a carpenter. He sustained a lumbar strain superimposed on degenerative disk disease. He was referred for work hardening to improve tolerances or full-time participation in a computer repair training program scheduled to begin in 3 weeks.

At first, KL demonstrated ability to lift 15 pounds in a full range of body postures. He was able to carry this weight and place it on a table. He sat comfortably for only a few minutes and performed all movements stiffly and slowly while rigidly holding his body erect. His Individual Work Hardening Plan addressed his goals of gradually increasing tolerances for lifting and working with tools at a workbench while seated and while standing. Additional goals concerned improving his pattern of spontaneous movement without unnecessary bracing or fear of reinjury. Specific tasks were assigned to simulate his training requirements for working continuously with small tools and parts at workbench level. Twice-daily stretching and conditioning activities were assigned to promote more natural movements. He was given frequent coaching and support to promote proper body mechanics while diminishing his anxiety about anticipated pain.

KL made steady gains toward meeting all of his goals while maintaining his commitment to enter training. His work hardening program was concluded after 3 weeks so that he could enter training. After the program conclusion, he continued to be active by attending an evening swimming program at a local spa and walking each day to maintain flexibility and a feeling of well being.

REVIEW QUESTIONS

1. What are the benefits of work hardening in an early intervention model?
2. What are the special factors that must be considered in a work hardening program conducted in a vocational rehabilitation model (late intervention model)?
3. What, if any, is the role of work adjustment concepts in a work hardening program?
4. Why is it important for work hardening to use a "real work" approach and have a worklike environment?
5. At what point(s) in the treatment process is the worker assessed for physical tolerances and limitations?
6. What factors are considered when making a decision to terminate a work hardening program?

REFERENCES

1. Ad Hoc Committee of the Commission on Practice: The role of occupational therapy in the vocational rehabilitation process: official position paper, Am J Occup Ther 34(13):881, 1980.
2. Bettencourt CM and Carlstrom P: Using work simulations to treat adults with back injuries, Am J Occup Ther 40(1):12, 1986.
3. Caruso LA and Chan DE: Evaluation and management of the patient with acute back Pain, Am J Occup Ther 40(5):347, 1986.
4. Flower A et al: An occupational therapy program for chonic back pain, Am J Occup Ther 35(4):243, 1981.
5. Harvey-Krefting L: The concept of work in occupational therapy: a historical review, Am J Occup Ther 39(5):301, 1985.
6. Heck C: Job-site analysis for work capacity programming, Physical Disabilities Special Interest Section Newsletter, Am Occup Ther Assoc 10:2, 1987.
7. Jacobs K: Occupational therapy: work-related programs & assessment, Boston, 1985, Little, Brown & Co.

8. Matheson L et al: Work hardening: occupational therapy in industrial rehabilitation, Am J Occup Ther 39(5):314, 1985.

9. Phelan LB: Role of manual arts therapy in a neuropsychiatric hospital, J Rehabil 14:3, 1949.

10. Smith PC and Bohmfalk JS: Work-related programs in occupational therapy, New York, 1985, The Haworth Press.

11. Smith PC and McFarlane B: A work hardening model for the 80's, Proceedings of the National Forum on Issues in Vocational Assessment, Menomonie, Wisconsin, 1984, Materials Development Center.

12. Vermont Rehabilitation Engineering Center for Low Back Pain: Report of progress (activity period 10/1/85 - 10/14/86), Burlington, VT.

13. Watkins AL: Prevocational evaluation and rehabilitation in a general hospital, JAMA 171:4, 1959.

14. Wegg L: Role of the occupational therapist in vocational rehabilitation, Am J Occup Ther 11:4, 1957.

15. Wegg L: Essentials of work evaluation, Am J Occup Ther 14(2):65, 1960.

17 Neurophysiology of sensorimotor approaches to treatment

GUY L. McCORMACK

Occupational therapy is an ever-expanding field. To treat patients who have neurologic dysfunctions the therapist should have an operational understanding of neurophysiology. With this knowledge the therapist can help patients achieve the ability to perform purposeful activities and understand why certain motor disturbances exist. This chapter will review the basic neurophysiologic rationale for the therapeutic approaches that are described in subsequent chapters.

DIVISIONS OF THE NERVOUS SYSTEM

The nervous system is often subdivided into the peripheral, autonomic, and central nervous systems.

Peripheral Nervous System

The peripheral nervous system begins in the skin and in the special sense organs. It carries information along 31 pairs of spinal nerves, related ganglia, and 12 pairs of cranial nerves.[40,74] The receptors in the skin possess the ability to discharge when stimulated by certain kinds of mechanical energy. The receptors (end organs) in the skin transmit sensory impulses along specific fibers. These nerve fibers vary greatly in their diameter, degree of myelination, and conduction velocity.[75] Generally speaking, the greater the diameter of the fiber and the thicker the myelin sheath, the faster the rate of conduction.[25] There is no universal method of classification of the nerve fibers. Two classifications of nerve fibers are presently in use. One is an electrophysiologic classification based on the speed of conduction of sensory and motor fibers. This classification uses an alphabetical system consisting of three groups: A, B, and C. The A and B fibers are thicker in diameter and myelinated, whereas C fibers are thin and unmyelinated.[40] The A fibers are further divided into subgroups called alpha, beta, gamma, and delta. The A fibers contain two motor components: alpha fibers, which supply skeletal (extrafusal) muscle, and gamma fibers, which innervate muscle spindle (intrafusal) muscle.

The second classification pertains only to sensory fibers and uses Roman numerals to designate fiber size and fiber origin. This includes group Ia for the primary ending of the muscle spindle; group Ib for the Golgi tendon organs; group II for secondary sensory ending from muscle spindles; group III for touch, pressure, pain, and temperature receptors; and group IV for nonspecific unmyelinated pain and temperature fibers. Table 17-1 summarizes the two classifications and differentiates the major modalities. Table 17-2 compares proprioception with pain and temperature.

Once the sensory impulse reaches the spinal cord, it may cross to the opposite side, ascend the spinal cord, or connect directly with a motor neuron. This transfer of coded information from one neuron to another constitutes a synaptic transmission, which is largely a chemical phenomenon.

When the sensory neuron synapses directly with a motor neuron in the spinal cord and carries that impulse back out to activate a muscle, it is called a monosynaptic reflex arc[48] (Fig. 17-1). This reflex arc is a basic neuronal circuit that causes stereotyped reactions to stimuli from the environment. To remain intact the reflex arc must have a complete receptor unit, sensory fiber, synapse within the spinal cord, motor neuron, and viable myoneural connection.[21] If any of these components are destroyed, the reflex arc is abolished. Reflex arcs enable the nervous system to react to stimuli that may be potentially harmful without exerting conscious effort. Thus touching the cornea of the eye results in a blink, touching a hot object results in a withdrawal reflex, or foreign objects in the windpipe produce coughing. The reflex arc is also used to examine the integrity of the nervous system or to elicit crude components of movement.[41]

Alpha motor neurons are the largest of the anterior horn cells. They can be stimulated through the reflex arc by the Ia primary afferents and group II secondary afferents of the muscle spindles.[91] Alpha motor neurons are also influenced by higher centers and by fibers from the corticospinal, raphe spinal, reticulospinal, and lateral vestibulospinal tracts.[105] Whenever a motor act is elicited, either voluntary or reflexive,

Table 17-1 Nerve Fiber Classification

Letter	Roman numeral	Functional component	Fiber diameter (μm)*
A alpha	Group I		
	Ia	Primary muscle spindle ending (stretch)	12-22
	Ib	Golgi tendon organ (contraction)	
A beta	Group II	Secondary sensory ending from muscle spindle (maintained stretch) Encapsulated endings Cutaneous afferents from skin and joints (joint position-pressure)	6-13
A gamma		Motor to muscle spindle (static-dynamic)	—
B		Motor—branch of alpha motor neuron Preganglionic autonomic efferents	—
A delta	Group III	Bare nerve endings, cutaneous mechanoreceptors; cold and nociceptors	1-6
C fibers	Group IV	Unmyelinated, nonspecific sensory reception; cold, warm, and nociceptors	1-1.5

*Micron millimeters.

Table 17-2 Comparison of Proprioception with Pain and Temperature

Proprioception		Pain and temperature	
A alpha (I)	*A alpha (III)*	*A delta (III)*	*C (IV)*
Muscle stretch Muscle contraction	Muscle stretch Position sense Vibration Velocity detection Pressure		
		Cold Light touch Pain	Cold Touch Pain Warmth

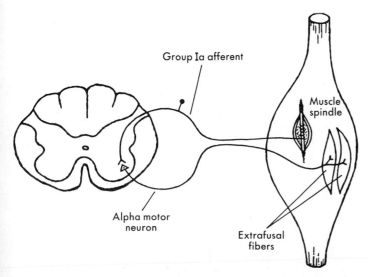

Group Ia afferent

Muscle spindle

Alpha motor neuron

Extrafusal fibers

Fig. 17-1. Monosynaptic stretch reflex (reflex arc).

the impulse must travel to the muscle by way of an alpha motor neuron. Because the alpha motor neuron is the last remaining connection between the spinal cord and extrafusal muscle, it is called the "final common pathway."[24] If the cell body or axon of the alpha motor neuron is destroyed, the reflex arc is abolished, and the muscle becomes hypotonic. This constitutes a lower motor neuron dysfunction, and efforts to activate that muscle through sensory stimulation are nonproductive unless some regeneration of the reflex arc has occurred.

The gamma loop or the fusimotor system plays a very important role in sensorimotor treatment techniques. Gamma motor neurons innervate the intrafusal muscle fibers within the muscle spindles of skeletal muscle.[3,75] The intrafusal muscle fibers align themselves parallel with the extrafusal (skeletal) fi-

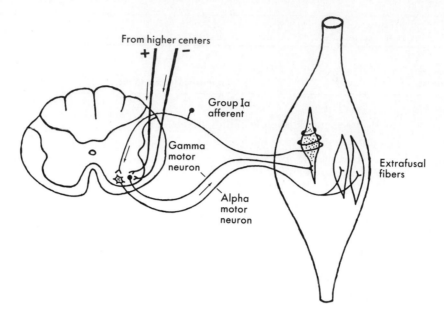

Fig. 17-2. Gamma loop (added gamma neuron to reflex arc).

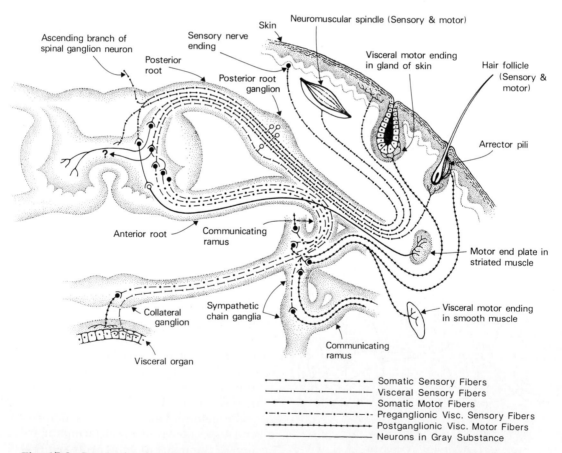

Fig. 17-3. Composite drawing showing a transverse section of the spinal cord, spinal nerve roots, posterior root ganglia, sympathetic ganglia, and various end organs. Redrawn and expanded from Schaffer G, editor: Morris' human anatomy, New York, 1953, The Blakiston Company.

bers. Any change in the length of the muscle also modifies the length of the intrafusal fibers. The motor fibers supplying the intrafusal muscles are smaller than the thinly myelinated gamma fibers. Their cell bodies are found in the anterior horn of the spinal cord along with the alpha motor neuron.[63,87]

The static gamma motor neurons terminate primarily on the nuclear chain fibers but also branch to nuclear bag fibers. The static gamma motor neurons are regulated by nuclei in the cerebellum, reticular system, basal ganglia, and vestibular system. The static gamma motor neurons are involved during a maintained shortening or contraction of muscle[91] (see Fig. 17-3).

The principal function of the gamma motor neuron is to adjust the length of the intrafusal fibers during contraction of the muscle, which enables the muscle spindle to automatically reinforce the power of contraction.[75]

Gamma and alpha motor neurons work in a collaborative fashion. The gamma motor neuron serves the muscle spindle by changing its length so that its sensory endings are in a constant state of readiness to discharge as the length of the extrafusal fibers are changed.[69]

The gamma loop is described as a servoassistance mechanism that aids in the production and control of movement (Fig. 17-2). This collaborative effort between alpha and gamma motor neurons is known as coactivation.[87] The anatomic and sensory aspects of the muscle spindle are discussed in the forthcoming section on receptors.

Autonomic Nervous System

The autonomic nervous system regulates glands, smooth muscles, cardiac muscle, and reflexive mechanisms in the skin.[1,12,24] This system functions predominantly at the subconscious level but is connected with conscious emotional states and influenced by events in the environment.[48,72,76] Functionally, the autonomic nervous system consists of two branches, the sympathetic and the parasympathetic systems.

Sympathetic Nervous System

The sympathetic nervous system expends energy and is known to be a catabolic system. The cell bodies of the preganglionic sympathetic neurons exit the spinal cord at levels T1 to L2 (thorax-lumbar outflow) and enter the paravertebral ganglion chain that runs adjacent to either side of the spinal column.[25,34] The sympathetic chain extends from the top to the bottom of the spinal column so that impulses can travel up or down the chain for considerable distances. To activate glands or internal organs the sympathetic im-

pulse must travel through a two-neuron chain. The preganglionic neurons arise from the intermediate gray column of the spinal cord. The postganglionic neuron is located in the paravertebral ganglia and innervates the smooth muscles of all the organs. Each spinal nerve receives a branch from the sympathetic trunk ganglia that are distributed to the blood vessels, erector pili muscles of hair, and secretory organs of the skin throughout the distribution of the nerve.[87] The viscera of the pelvic and abdominal cavities are innervated by sympathetic branches of the splanchnic nerves.[13] The sympathetic nervous system liberates neurotransmitters that are norepinephrinelike substances classified as adrenergic[40] (Fig. 17-3).

The nervous system is stimulated when a person experiences strong emotions, such as fear and rage, and when he or she is exposed to cold or pain. This stimulation produces a generalized physiologic response, allowing the adrenal glands to liberate substances into the bloodstream that reinforce the effects of sympathetic neurons. As a result, the blood vessels in the skin and digestive systems constrict, whereas the blood vessels in the cardiac and skeletal muscles dilate. The bronchioles of the lungs and pupils of the eyes also dilate. Heart rate and force of contraction increase. The sweat, lacrimal, and salivary glands increase secretions. Last, the spleen may release extra red blood cells into the bloodstream in case of blood loss. These reactions are part of the organism's biologic response to situations that are perceived as potentially dangerous. When faced with tangible situations that are a real threat to survival, the fight or flight response is appropriate. However, modern society produces many intangible stressors.

In actuality, many circumstances that cause no immediate harm can activate the autonomic nervous system, which, in turn, does not differentiate between psychological and physical stressors. As a result, the biologic responses to psychological and physical circumstances are the same.

Unfortunately, social structures prevent the natural responses to fight or flight by inhibiting their expression, resulting in anxiety and deleterious stress reactions. In recent years, much has been written about the harmful effects of prolonged stress and anxiety.[2,16,20,23,50,77] Many pathologic conditions such as high blood pressure, heart disease, gastrointestinal disorders, arthritis, tumors, cancer, and reduced immune responses all have been associated with sustained fight or flight responses.

In summary, the major function of the sympathetic nervous system is to mobilize the body during stress or emergency situations. Modern society has created psychological stress situations that have generated prolonged sympathetic nervous system responses that cannot be acted upon through overt aggression.

Parasympathetic Nervous System

In contrast, the parasympathetic nervous system conserves energy and is known to be an anabolic system.[42] The preganglionic cell bodies arise from the craniosacral regions of the central nervous system. The cranial portion consists of cranial nerves III, VII, IX, and X. Cranial nerve X (vagus nerve) supplies the organs of the thorax. The sacral portion arises from spinal segments S2, S3, and S4. The sacral division communicates with pelvic splanchnic nerves and supplies muscular walls of the colon, rectum, and urinary and reproductive organs. The postganglionic terminals of the parasympathetic system liberate acetylcholine and are classified as cholinergic.[40]

The parasympathetic system can act simultaneously with the sympathetic system during the fight or flight situation. During exaggerated fear the sacral segment may produce involuntary emptying of the bladder and rectum. In contrast to the sympathetic response, the parasympathetic system acts to dilate blood vessels in the skin and digestive tract, constrict bronchial tubes, contract the pupils of the eyes, and increase motility of the gastrointestinal tract. During sexual arousal the parasympathetic system controls penile and clitoral erection, and the sympathetic branch mediates ejaculation.[34]

Much is yet to be learned about the autonomic nervous system. For instance, there appears to be complex synaptic connections joining skin efferents and visceral afferents with the autonomic neurons. Thus sensory stimulation to some areas of the skin can influence the action of certain internal organs. Several reflex arcs have been identified, but the interneuronal pathways have not been clearly delineated.[87,98]

In recent years it has been found that the autonomic nervous system can be manipulated through facilitory and inhibitory techniques. Research has shown that various relaxation techniques, visualization, and biofeedback can reduce the activity level of the sympathetic branch of the autonomic nervous system.[2,16,19,23,31,60,79,83,107] One technique does not seem to work for all patients. Patients more receptive to visual stimulation respond well to visualizations and metaphors. Patients responding to auditory input may respond better to guided imagery and background music. Patients who are more physically or kinesthetically oriented, respond well to progressive relaxation in which muscles are actively contracted and relaxed. Furthermore, the autonomic nervous system cannot be suppressed by an explosion of physical activity.[8,102]

Gellhorn has described anatomic and physiologic factors contributing to states of stress and relaxation on a continuum.[37] The fight or flight state combines increased sympathetic activity, arousal of the cortex, and increased muscle tone. Gellhorn termed this the ergotropic response. The other end of the continuum is a state that combines increased parasympathetic activity, cortical relaxation, and decreased muscle tone. This state has been termed the trophotropic end of the continuum.

In the process of using facilitory or inhibitory activities the therapist should determine where the patient's capabilities fall along this ergotropic-trophotropic continuum. If the goal is to reduce spasticity, the patient should be toward the trophotropic (parasympathetic) end. However, if the goal is to promote learning or increase tonicity in muscles, the activities should be stimulating and compatible with the ergotropic (sympathetic) response.

Research has revealed that the nervous system and the endocrine system respond simultaneously to stressful situations.[28,51,76,79,102] In fact, the endocrine glands have been described as massively developed nerve endings that produce hormones that are transmitted through the bloodstream to all areas of the body.[28,37,50,61] The autonomic nervous system and the endocrine system are regulated by the hypothalamus. The endocrine system also plays an important role in the fight or flight response. For example, the adrenal glands release adrenalin (epinephrine) and noradrenalin (norepinephrine) resulting in increased metabolic rate, cardiac output, and rapid respiration. The pancreas secretes insulin and glucagon to control levels of blood sugars for energy. The pituitary regulates the quantity of hormones that the endocrine glands release. The pineal glands act as the body's clock, regulating menstrual cycles and the onset of maturation. The thymus gland stimulates the production of white blood cells. The thyroid glands regulate the amount of calcium that is deposited in the bones and reduces it in the blood. The parathyroid glands remove calcium from bones and increase it in the bloodstream. Therefore, the endocrine system and the autonomic nervous system affect the internal functions of the entire body.[1,12,34,67,76]

Central Nervous System

THE SPINAL CORD. The central nervous system (CNS) consists of the spinal cord, brainstem, cerebellum, subcortical nuclei, and the cerebral cortex.[34,53] The spinal cord is phylogenetically old and less complex than other structures in the CNS. The spinal cord is less than an inch (2.54 cm) in diameter with enlargements in the lower cervical and in the lower lumbar regions to accommodate the outflow to the extremities. The spinal cord begins at the foramen magnum and extends caudally to vertebrae level L1 or L2.[75,106] The spinal cord is subdivided into segments. The spinal segments do not align opposite the corresponding vertebrae because the cord is about 9⅘ inches (25 cm) shorter. There are 31 pairs of spinal nerves: 8 cervical, 12 thoracic, 5 lumbar, 5 sacral, and 1 coccygeal. Each spinal nerve has dorsal and ventral roots that form the sensory and motor components. All the sensory (afferent), somatic, and visceral fibers enter the spinal cord by way of the dorsal roots. All motor fibers (efferent) exit the spinal cord via the ventral roots. In a transverse section the spinal cord appears to have a butterfly-shaped area of gray substance surrounded by white matter. The white matter is composed of longitudinal ascending and descending fiber tract systems. The cell bodies of the efferent fibers are located in the gray matter. The gray matter can be further subdivided into 10 laminae, each extending the length of the cord. The white matter of the spinal cord is divided into three pairs of funiculi (anterior, lateral, and dorsal).[74,91] Some generalizations may be made about the sensory and motor tracts of the spinal cord. In respect to the motor tracts the older phylogenetic systems are located in the anterior and anterolateral quadrants of the cord. Efferent impulses are transmitted along these tracts to be excitatory to extensor motor neurons and inhibitory to flexor motor neurons. The anterolateral quadrant of the spinal cord contains the phylogenetically newer motor systems. These neurons tend to be excitatory to flexors and inhibitory to extensors.[105]

A similar relationship exists in the sensory tracts. The anterolateral tracts (spinothalamic) are phylogenetically old and mediate pain, temperature, and touch along small diameter fibers. This is felt to be a primitive protective system. Conversely, the dorsal columns of the spinal cord (lemniscal system) represent a newer sensory system conveying discriminative sensory information from the skin and deep structures to the cerebral cortex. This system is rapidly conducting because the fibers are large and well myelinated and undergo few synapses en route to the cortex.[4,105]

BRAIN STEM. The brain stem has been regarded by Ayres as the center of sensory integration.[4] That is, all perceptual processes basic to learning are dependent on sensory integration at the brainstem level. The brain stem consists of the medulla oblongata, pons, midbrain, and thalamus.[87] The brain stem contains the 12 cranial nerves, reticular system, major nuclei, and ascending and descending tract systems. The lowest portion of the brainstem, the medulla, contains nuclei for five cranial nerves, the reticular formation, the vestibular system, and the respiratory and cardiac functions. All the major ascending and descending tracts pass through the medulla.[42] The pons is a large mass that lies above the medulla. The pons plays an important role as a relay station between the cerebellum and the cerebral cortex. The pons contains four cranial nerves, pontine nuclei, and major fiber tracts.[12,40]

The midbrain is a relatively short section of the brain stem but contains several important structures. Some of these structures are the corpora quadrigemina (superioinferior colliculi), red nucleus, substantia nigra, crura cerebri, and cranial nerves III and IV.[40,74] Two major motor tracts arising from the midbrain are the rubrospinal and tectospinal tracts. A lesion to the midbrain region results in strong extensor tone or rigidity.[21]

The cerebellum is located in the posterior cranial fossa. It is attached to the pons, medulla, and midbrain by the cerebellar peduncles. The cerebellum is divided into three lobes. The flocculonodular lobe (archicerebellum) located in the posteroinferior region communicates with the vestibular system. The anterior lobe (paleocerebellum) receives proprioceptive information via the spinocerebellar tracts; the posterior lobe (neocerebellum) is located between the other two lobes and communicates with the motor cortex.[1,24,48]

THALAMUS. The thalamus is a complex structure that makes up the rostral portion of the brain stem. With the exception of the olfactory system, all sensory information passes through the thalamus en route to the cortex.[88,105] For this reason the thalamus has been regarded as a sensory relay station. In the past it was believed that the thalamus participated in the realization of crude sensation. However, recent evidence suggests that the thalamus participates in refining or consolidating sensory information before it reaches the cortex.[88] The thalamus may also play a role in emotion and behavior through its connections with the limbic system. Cerebrovascular accidents may cause destruction to parts of the thalamus resulting in the so-called thalamus syndrome. This condition can cause exaggerated pain or unpleasant sensations to nonnoxious stimuli.[21]

HYPOTHALAMUS. The hypothalamus lies inferior to the thalamus and forms the ventral floor of the third ventricle. Although the hypothalamus is only about the size of a fingernail, it exerts a direct or indirect influence on every function of the body.[76] Through widespread connections the hypothalamus coordinates the activities of the autonomic nervous system, the endocrine system, and the limbic system.[1,12,34,74,91]

In short, it regulates emotions, sexual drive, hormones, eating, drinking, body temperature, sleeping and waking states, heart rate, and chemical balances.[87,88] In recent years, regulation of weight has been attributed to the hypothalamus.[76] It appears to have an automatic setting similar to that of a thermostat. Therefore, for some persons dieting may be ineffective because the hypothalamus is set to retain body fat. It has also been postulated that certain kinds of exercises, such as walking, jogging, and Tai Chi help to gauge the metabolic setting of the hypothalamus.[2,71,73,87,99]

LIMBIC SYSTEM. The limbic system, sometimes called the visceral brain, is a collection of interconnected structures contributing to emotional responses, affective behavior, and survival of the organism.[31] According to Moore, the limbic system integrates the newest cognitive structures in the cortex with the older reticular formation, sensorimotor systems and primitive visceral structures.[72]

The principle structures of the limbic system are the cingulate gyrus, septal area, insula, parahippocampal gyrus, amygdala, and hippocampal formation.[1,40] Although the limbic system is not directly related to motor systems, its emotional and behavioral components affect autonomic and somatic responses.

Studies have shown that the limbic system is rich in neuropeptides.[11,28,61] The highest concentrations of neuropeptides are found in the amygdala and the hypothalamus, which are part of the limbic brain.[93] These neuropeptides play a prominent role in the brain and throughout the body. Neuropeptides are very potent and regarded as the neurotransmitters of emotions. Neuropeptides link the nervous system, endocrine system, and immune systems into a complex communication network.[18,27,50,60,102]

Moore has expounded on the importance of the limbic system in rehabilitation techniques.[69] This system governs feeding, fighting, and reproductive behaviors.

BASAL GANGLIA. The major structures of the basal ganglia are the caudate nucleus, putamen, and globus pallidus. The basal ganglia may also be functionally related to the amygdaloid nucleus, claustrum, subthalamic nucleus, and substantia nigra.[1,25] The basal ganglia receive much input from the cerebral cortex and transmit it into many circuits and feedback loops. Attempts to delineate the functions of the basal ganglia have credited it with the refinement of complex movement, automatic movement patterns, associated movements, and regulation of postural tone in antigravity muscles.[21,34]

CEREBRAL CORTEX. The cortex makes up the outermost region of the cerebrum. It has been attributed to intellectual functions, memory storage, language, consciousness, perception, and complex motor activities.[25] The cortex is composed of six layers of densely packed neuron cell bodies. The cortex has been anatomically divided into four lobes and 52 distinct areas, based on types of cell groupings.[75] Clinically, some of the most significant areas include the primary motor strip (area 4) supplementary motor area (area 6), prefrontal cortex (areas 9 through 12), Broca's area (areas 44 and 45), Wernicke's area (area 22), sensory strip (areas 1, 2, and 3), and supramarginal gyrus (area 40). Lesions to the areas just mentioned result in profound sensory or motor dysfunction.[13,24]

In an article in the *American Journal of Occupational Therapy*, Moore described the new technology that allows scientists to see the brain as it has never been seen before.[71] In the past the brain was mapped out by defining boundaries, structures and functional units.[24,78] New techniques in computerized tomography and metabolic mapping have revealed considerable overlap of structural and functional capacities of the brain.[11,29,35,46,80,81] The functional overlap is particularily evident in the area called the sensory and motor strip (homunculus) and the visual system.

BASIS FOR RATIONALE OF THE SENSORIMOTOR APPROACHES TO TREATMENT
The Neuron

The neuron is unique among all cells in the body because of its ability to transmit coded information for long distances. The neuron varies in form and structure, depending on its role in the transport of information. Each neuron has a cell body containing a nucleus, dendrites that receive stimuli, an axon that conducts impulses away from the cell body, and axon terminals.[12] To convey information the neuron must have two properties, conductivity of electrical impulses and neurotransmission of a chemical substance.[31,48] These two properties are briefly described in the following text.

The neuron has an excitable membrane that is activated by the difference between the interior of the cell and the fluid surrounding it. If there is an ionic balance existing between the cytoplasm of the neuron and the extracellular fluid, the cell is in a state of resting potential (expressed in voltage as -70 mV).[73] This balance is achieved by the permeability of the cell membrane to sodium (Na^+) and potassium (K^+) ions. The interior of the nerve cell contains high concentrations of potassium and low concentrations of sodium and chloride (Cl^-), whereas the extracellular fluid contains low potassium and high concentrations of sodium and chloride. When a neuron membrane is excited by an outside stimulus, changes in potential occur along the cell membrane.[87] If the stimulus is strong enough, the cell reaches its threshold and discharges an *action potential* (nerve impulse). The impulse then travels along the axon with a constant rate of electrical energy until it reaches the terminal ending. A *graded potential* is a small change in resting potential and membrane voltage. It is not sufficient to discharge impulses along the axon but is carried by dendrites and cell bodies.[87] Under some circumstances, several weak stimuli (subthreshold) may impinge on the neuron (spatial summation) to cause an action potential to develop. This phenomenon is called *summation*.[31] This is a very important concept in therapy because it means neurons can be stimulated to action potential by increasing the sensory input. If, for example, a traumatic lesion has destroyed neuronal circuits that normally stimulate a group of neurons to discharge, alternative pathways can be developed by consistent sensory stimulation. Bach-y-Rita[5,6] has used the analogy of the telephone line to describe this process. If a phone line were damaged between two cities on the east and west coasts, messages could be rerouted through less direct lines. The new network would be slower and as efficient but would nevertheless transmit messages that would improve over time. Neurons have the ability to adapt and change the direction of impulses through axon collaterals.[86] Synaptic transmissions get stronger and more efficient with use.[73]

NEUROTRANSMISSION. Neurotransmission represents the chemical aspect of interneuronal communication. It occurs between the presynaptic and postsynaptic membranes of two nerve cells. Normally there is a space or cleft between two communicating neurons called a *synapse*. A synapse can occur between the dendrite, axon, or cell body of a receiving neuron. The transmission of information is propagated by a release of a chemical substance (neurotransmitter) that is capable of either producing or preventing electrical changes in the postsynaptic neuronal membrane.[74] If the neurotransmitter traverses the synapse and causes an action potential in the subsequent neuron, it is facilitory. However, if the neurotransmitter causes a hypopolarization of the postsynaptic cell membrane, it is called inhibitory.[91] Synaptic junctions between neurons vary considerably throughout the nervous system. The average motor neuron may have about 6000 axon collateral synapses. Thus each neuron is capable of receiving several thousand messages from different sources. Generally speaking, sensory neurons conduct impulses in only one direction, away from the area in which the stimulus originated.[12]

The latest findings suggest that neurons work co-operatively in networks requiring hundreds of millions of synapses between nerve cells at any given time. The complexity of these networks of neurons depends on the sophistication of the messages being transmitted. Neuronal networks feed information forward into higher level assemblies of neurons in various centers in the central nervous system. This allows neuronal pathways versatility to feed into a variety of feedback loops, allowing new information to go forward while sending back newly integrated information to locations where the original signals were produced. Moore suggests that this system allows neurons to anticipate, modify and dampen synapses at each juncture.[71,72] The intensity of the stimulus may determine the action potential, yet the distance the impulse travels is dependent on the neuronal assembly receiving the communication.[40] Impulses can travel along several different circuits. Some neurons have many collateral branches that synapse with many neurons and form a *divergent circuit* to several regions of the nervous system. On the other hand, a single neuron may receive synaptic messages from several other neurons. This process is called *convergence*.[87] In this case the neuron must process both the excitatory and inhibitory impulses converging on it and decide to fire or inhibit the transmission. When the excitatory synapses predominate, action potentials are discharged and facilitation has occurred. Another facilitory circuit is called positive feedback or *reverberating excitation*. Hypothetically, this occurs in a circuit in which neurons further down the chain feed back excitation to the preceding neurons. Reverberating excitation occurs through axon collaterals and forms a continuous feedback loop, causing the neuron to discharge for a long time.[88] Reverberating circuits have been associated with short-term memory or arousal states generated within the reticular system.[48] It has been postulated that cutaneous stimulation (icing or brushing) may also initiate reverberating excitation.[52]

Neurons may also transmit through inhibitory circuits, which automatically suppress too much excitation. Typical inhibitory circuits include reciprocal inhibition through interneurons (Renshaw cells) or through groups of inhibitory neurons occupying parallel positions to excitatory neurons (surrounded inhibition).[87] Within the CNS there are regions in which inhibitory circuits play a greater role in suppressing excitatory impulses.[25] These neuronal circuits help to smooth out or prevent unwanted actions during movement. When the CNS is damaged, there is an imbalance between the excitatory and inhibitory circuits.[86] Consequently, patients may exhibit degrees of paralysis, alterations of reflex patterns, and changes in muscle tone.[41] When the inhibitory circuits are damaged, their dampening effects on excitatory neurons are "released." This phenomenon is called *disinhibition*. Clinically, it may be seen as spasticity, rigidity, tremors, or athetosis.

In summary, the concept of a single neuron conveying a message to a second single neuron has been questioned by many investigators.* However, a single neuron can have more than one type of neurotransmitter.[11,61,93] Thus, the single neuron does have some capacity to accept or inhibit a chemical transmission.

Guyton has described another phenomenon called *rebound*, which is related to fatigue of spinal level reflexes.[48] Rebound occurs immediately after a reflex response has been evoked. Following the reflex response there is a period of fatigue, and the same reflex becomes more difficult to elicit. Strangely enough, reflexes of the antagonist muscles can be elicited more briskly. This is a manifestation of reciprocal innervation and is a contributing factor to rhythmical movements. The term *rebound* has also been used to describe generalized reciprocal responses to prolonged use of thermal stimuli. For instance, if a patient stays in a heated therapeutic swimming pool too long, his biologic thermoregulatory system (posterior hypothalamus) may work as a thermostat and increase the activity in the parasympathetic nervous system, causing a state of relaxation. An hour later the autonomic nervous system can generate a sympathetic response, and the patient may become agitated and excitable and have an increase in muscle tone. This mechanism is not well understood and may be due to imbalances in types of chemotransmitters reactive to changes in body temperatures. Serotonin and norepinephrine levels have been associated with temperature, agitation and changes in moods.[28,61,67]

The therapist must weigh the value of certain sensorimotor techniques with respect to long-term or short-term gains. Some inhibitory techniques, if used too long, can trigger a reciprocal sympathetic response. It should also be noted that high-intensity cutaneous stimulation can cause similar rebound phenomenon.

Myelination

Myelin is a spirally deposited, fatlike substance that wraps around the axons of rapidly conducting nerve fibers.[12] It is produced by Schwann's and oligodendroglial cells. The myelin sheath is important to the function of the nervous system because it increases the velocity of the impulses up to 100 times.[7,71] Myelination begins relatively late in development—not

until the end of the third fetal month. Many of the tracts in the nervous system myelinate at different times. The vestibulospinal tract, tectospinal tract, and reflex arc begin myelination by the end of the fifth month.[31] The corticospinal tracts, which are responsible for voluntary skilled movements, continue myelination into the second year. Some areas of the reticular formation and the cerebellum continue to myelinate into early adulthood. The association fibers of the cortex may continue to myelinate throughout life.

Most myelinated nerve fibers exist predominately in the cranial and spinal nerves. Therefore unmyelinated fibers are more abundant in the autonomic nervous system.[106] Evidence suggests that sensory stimulation during the developmental years may improve the myelination process.[98]

Dendritic Growth

Dendrites are the small branches (spines) projecting from the cell body of a neuron. Dendrites form synaptic connections with other neurons. Greenough[45] has conducted definitive animal studies to demonstrate the importance of environmental stimuli on the developing brain.[45] The studies have shown that sensory stimulation promotes dendritic growth.[29] It is postulated that the proliferation of dendrites contributes to intelligence and adaptive behavior in humans.[73]

Current studies on the neurobiology of learning and memory continue to suggest that environmental stimuli contribute to the development of dendritic growth in specific regions of the brain.[5,6,11] Studies on the limbic system imply that both the dendrites in the hippocampus and the amygdala are associated with memory and learning.[96] This proposal that subcortical dendritic growth in the hippocampus contributes to procedural or emotional memory has been linked to the amygdala.

Dendritic growth also occurs before birth. Laboratory studies of animals found that when pregnant rats were exposed to an enriched environment, their offspring showed 10% to 16% greater dendritic growth in the cerebral cortex.[29]

Neuroplasticity

Recent neuroscientific studies have demonstrated that the CNS has some capacity to adapt or recover from traumatic injury.[6,86] The ability of neurons to adapt depends on (1) activation of latent neurons that may have been previously suppressed, (2) ability of neurons adjacent to the lesion to sprout collateral axons that form new synapses, and (3) changes in neurotransmitter sensitivity. For example, denervated muscles can develop increased sensitivity to neuro-

---

*References 17,29,35,71,93,96

transmitters through anatomic, physiologic, or biochemical changes. This phenomenon may be part of an adaptive process to compensate for loss of innervation.[5,6,98]

Research has shown that hormones influence neuroplasticity.[61,93] In animal studies the male sex hormones manufactured in the testes (androgens) have been shown to influence neuronal development. These hormones have also been found to influence the organization of spinal motor neurons. Thus, the ability of the nervous system to adapt to traumatic injury may depend on many chemical and physical changes in neuronal architecture.

To compensate for a lesion the damaged nervous system must be "forced" into recovery. Studies have shown that when the damaged system is forced into action, it recovers to a greater extent. For instance, animals with lesions and hemiparetic extremities have shown better recovery when the uninvolved limbs are restrained and the affected limbs are forced into use.[5,6]

Peripheral Control Hypothesis Versus Central Control Mechanism

Many sensorimotor theorists follow the assumption that the nervous system is stimulated and altered solely by stimuli that arise from the peripheral environment. Much scientific evidence supports this premise, but accumulating evidence also shows that nervous system has built-in internal control mechanisms.[79] These central control mechanisms may be compared with "printed circuits" or genetic programs for repetitive movements. For example, the so-called subcortical movements may be manifestations of innate movements passed down through evolutionary development. Animal studies and clinical observations on humans have shown that movements can be initiated both internally and externally. The central control hypothesis may have implications for rehabilitation techniques in the near future.

SOMATOSENSORY SYSTEM

The term *somatosensory* can be defined as the body's awareness of external stimuli. The body contains many types of sensory receptors (end organs) that provide information about changes in the immediate environment. These end organs can be viewed therapeutically as "portals" through which stimuli can be systematically programmed into the nervous system. Although this information on sensory receptors is incomplete, it is important for the occupational therapist to have a basic understanding of the characteristics that these receptors possess.

For the purposes of sensorimotor therapy, sensory receptors are classified into five categories in this discussion: (1) interoceptors, (2) exteroceptors, (3) proprioceptors, (4) kinesioceptors, and (5) acupoints.

Interoceptors

Interoceptors monitor events within the body and are located within the walls of the respiratory, cardiovascular, gastrointestinal, and genitourinary systems.[106] Interoceptors can detect a variety of stimuli, such as distention of a cavity wall, or monitor pH levels in the bloodstream. Many interoceptors are activated during therapeutic activities. The *carotid sinus* is a baroreceptor located in the walls of the carotid artery.[44] It is stimulated by blood pressure changes and linked to the parasympathetic nervous system. In therapy it is brought into action during inversion techniques.[31] Whenever the head approaches a position below the level of the shoulders, the increase in blood pressure distends the carotid sinus and fires impulses along the glossopharyngeal nerve (CN IX) to cardiovascular inhibitory centers of the vagus nerve, which in turn slows heart rate and reduces blood pressure. This is a negative feedback system that must be used with caution. Clinicians have used the carotid sinus to reduce hypertension and to produce a state of generalized inhibition.[21,31,105]

The process of lowering the head below the level of the shoulders may also affect the chemistry of the brain.[55,108] Persons practicing yoga claim that the inverted position enables them to reach higher levels of consciousness. Basketball players often lower the head below the shoulders before taking a foul shot. Swimmers have observed that lowering the head before the racing dive gets them off to a faster start. There may indeed be many neurophysiologic advantages to the inverted position. It alleviates the gravitational forces on the vertebral column, it increases blood flow to the brain and facial muscles, and it promotes postural drainage of the venous, lymphatic, and respiratory systems.[48,73,91]

The *mucous membranes* of the oral cavity provide another area in which interoceptors are used for therapeutic intervention. The gums around the teeth are rich in sensory innervation from the trigeminal nerve.[44,106] The mucous membranes contain receptors that are stimulated by several modalities, such as temperature, touch, stretch, and taste. Stimulation to this area discharges impulses to the brain stem via the sensory components of the trigeminal nerve (CN V), facial nerve (CN VII), glossopharyngeal nerve (CN IX), and vagus nerve.[15] Occupational therapists use oral stimulation primarily for functional activities of daily living that are related to feeding.

Therapists have used cutaneous stimulation and vibration to affect the interoceptors in the wall of the bladder or detrusor muscle to facilitate or inhibit the micturition reflex. Stimulation has been applied dermatomally or to the skin directly over the bladder.[31] Montagu describes the importance of sensory stimulation to the skin around the genitourinary organs in mammals.[68] Shortly after birth, the mother cleans the neonate by licking. The stimulus is important to the development of normal bowel and bladder evacuation. A similar phenomenon has been observed in human children. Cutaneous stimulation over dermatone S2 on children with delayed sphincter control seems to alleviate bed wetting and "accidents." These techniques should not be used without proper understanding of neurophysiology or supervision by a physician.

The use of temperature input is another way interoceptors are used in sensorimotor techniques. Neutral warmth and icing techniques not only influence cutaneous receptors but act on thermoregulatory centers in the spinal cord, brain stem, and hypothalamus.[14,88,106] Temperature input has been used primarily to reduce hypertonicity in skeletal muscles or for symptomatic pain. However, children exhibiting "tactile defensiveness" may benefit from a regimen that combines neutral warmth and skin exposure to cooler temperatures. The process needs further research but a systematic regimen of temperature changes should affect the receptors in the hypothalamus, causing an increased threshold level to cutaneous stimuli.[31,87,88]

Exteroceptors

Exteroceptors are found immediately under the skin in the external mucous membranes or in special sense organs.[75,106] These receptors respond to stimuli that arise outside the body. Exteroceptors vary tremendously in their structure, function, and reaction to mechanical stimuli. Following is a brief summary of the primary cutaneous exteroceptors.

FREE NERVE ENDINGS. The subcutaneous tissues are richly innervated by free nerve endings. These are unencapsulated receptors with projecting, unmyelinated branches for sensory detection. Free nerve endings are widely distributed in the skin and viscera. They are thought to be nonspecific receptors for pain, crude touch, and temperature.[1] The free nerve endings associated with pain outnumber all other receptors along the midline axis of the body.[73] Free nerve endings transmit impulses by way of unmyelinated "C" nerve fibers to the spinothalamic tracts.[15] In general the free nerve endings involved with touch are rapidly adapting. Those that are associated with chronic pain syndromes are slowly adapting.[14,33,73] For

therapeutic purposes free nerve endings are activated with thermal or brushing techniques and elicit primitive protective responses. Stimulation to free nerve endings can also cause states of arousal.[52] Also, some evidence supports the theory that forms of cutaneous stimulation such as ice packs and rubbing over the surface of the skin can alleviate acute pain. Melzack describes the process of applying a strong cutaneous stimulation to alleviate pain as a *counterirritation* technique.[33,65,66] The pain relief may be explained in two ways. A cutaneous stimulus strong enough to produce some pain can release endorphins and block pain impulses at the brain stem level. The second explanation involves the gate control theory, which suggests that counterstimulation overloads the synapses in the spinal cord at the substantia gelatinosa, thereby preventing the pain impulse from ascending to higher neurologic levels where pain is perceived. It is also believed that free nerve endings, along with other receptors, can synapse with gamma motor neurons and bias the muscle spindle.

HAIR END ORGANS. Hair end organs are actually a type of free nerve ending that wraps around the base of a hair follicle.[75] These receptor organs are activated by the bending or displacement of hair. They are rapidly adapting and transmit impulses predominately along A delta-size (group III) fibers.[73] In therapy hair receptors are stimulated during light touch or stroking of the skin. Although they are rapidly adapting, hair end organs discharge into neuron pools that reach the reticular system and probably bias the muscle spindle through the fusimotor system. Part of the more primitive nervous system, hair end organs were used by our ancestors as sensory receptors to alert them to stimuli in close proximity to the skin.[40] In addition, they are neurologically related to the autonomic nervous system. Because primitive man had much more hair on the surface of his body it acted as an insulator to the cold. When they were chilled, the arrector pili muscles attached to the hair follicles caused the hairs to fluff up and provide a thicker surface to contain body heat. Today the reminiscence of the hair follicles are seen as goose bumps when the body is exposed to cold.[76]

MEISSNER'S CORPUSCLES. Meissner's corpuscles are elongated, encapsulated end organs found just beneath the epidermis in hairless (glabrous) skin. They are particularly abundant in the skin of the fingertips, tip of the tongue, lips, and pads of the feet.[105] Histologic studies show that these receptors maintain a close relationship with the skin. They are abundant on the fingertips of the hand and are arranged on the ridges of skin that make up the fingerprints.[98,105,106] The corpuscles are primarily rapidly adapting receptors that transmit along the thicker A beta (group II) fibers. Meissner's corpuscles are largely responsible for fine tactile discrimination. They are very important in digital exploration and sensory substitution skills, such as reading braille. These receptors transmit discriminatory messages to the somatosensory cortex by way of the dorsal columns of the spinal cord.[75,105]

PACINIAN CORPUSCLES. Pacinian corpuscles are the largest encapsulated receptors and are almost as widely distributed as free nerve endings. They are located in the deep layers of the skin—in viscera, mesenteries, ligaments, and near blood vessels.[73] Pacinian corpuscles are probably the most rapidly adapting receptors in the body.[75] They respond to deep pressure but are amazingly sensitive to slight indentations in the skin.[98] Pacinian corpuscles also discharge with a steady train of impulses when exposed to vibration. Therefore with vibratory stimuli the pacinian corpuscle is a slowly adapting receptor. Although the pacinian corpuscle fires when vibrated, it has not been demonstrated to play a role in the tonic vibration reflex.[45,105]

The pacinian corpuscle has some interesting therapeutic features. It discharges along fast-conducting A beta (group II) fibers to the dorsal columns of the spinal cord. Stimulation to a single corpuscle in the skin can excite an area of the postcentral gyrus of the cortex.[31] Research has shown that the pacinian corpuscle can suppress pain perception at the cutaneous level.[63,73] It may also contribute to the inhibition of muscles when pressure is applied over tendinous insertions.[2] Furthermore, the pacinian corpuscle may play a role in the desensitization of hypersensitive skin in children who exhibit tactile defensiveness.[4]

Because the pacinian corpuscles transmit sensory impulses along thick fibers and synapse in the spinal cord at the substantia gelatinosa, they may indeed cause a condition of overload at this junction. According to the gate control theory, pain impulses travel along thin fibers and also synapse in the substantia gelatinosa. Also, increased sensory input carried along thick fibers can block the transmission of pain impulses that are carried along thin fibers.[65,66]

It is interesting to note that the hands, the soles of the feet and the mesentary of the abdomen contain an abundance of pacinian corpuscles. Thus the sole of the foot and hand might be an excellent target area when using vibratory stimuli for sensory stimulation. The stimulation should be done with low frequency vibration and light pressure so that the positive supporting reaction is not elicited.

It has been observed in sensory integrative therapy that deep pressure and vibratory stimuli have a calming effect on children with attention deficit disorders.[4] It also appears that the pacinian corpuscles play a major role in this calming effect because they transmit impulses into the dorsal columns, which send fewer impulses into the excitatory cells of the reticular activating system. The dorsal columns also terminate in the cerebral cortex where synapses are made with association fibers and inhibitory networks. An interesting therapeutic technique that uses the carotid sinus and the pacinian corpuscles is to invert the overactive child over a therapy ball in the prone position with the head positioned below the shoulders. The therapist can place a pillow over the child and apply gentle deep pressure so that the child is comfortably sandwiched between the pillow and the therapy ball. An electric vibrator can then be applied to the base of the therapy ball sending vibratory stimuli through the entire surface of the ball. This provides an inhibitory effect because of the combination of inversion, deep pressure, and vibratory stimuli. It may also be noted that the vibratory stimuli are transduced through the pacinian corpuscles in the mesentery underlying the abdominal muscles. Pressure over the abdomen is recommended as an inhibitory technique.[73,91]

MERKEL'S TACTILE DISKS. Merkel's tactile disks are nonencapsulated receptors found in the deepest layer of the epidermis in hairless skin. These receptors are located most abundantly on the volar surface of the fingers, lips, and external genitalia. Merkel's tactile disks are slowly adapting touch-pressure receptors. They transmit along A beta (group II) myelinated fibers.[73,105] These receptors are very sensitive to slow movements across the skin's surface. They have been related to the sense of tickle and pleasurable touch sensations.[98]

Proprioceptors

Proprioceptors monitor the awareness of position in space, posture, movement, and equilibrium reactions. These receptors are found in muscles, tendons, and joints. The process of proprioception can be conscious or subconscious. Conscious proprioceptors are discussed under kinesioceptors (joint receptors). Subconscious proprioception pertains to information received from muscle spindles, Golgi tendon organs, and the vestibular apparatus. Subconscious proprioception derived from Golgi tendon organs and muscle spindles transmits to the cerebellum. The vestibular apparatus may have connections to the cerebral cortex.[105]

GOLGI TENDON ORGANS. Golgi tendon organs (GTO) are spindle-shaped receptors found in the musculotendinous region of the proximal and distal insertions.[12] In the past the GTO was believed to be a high-threshold protective receptor designed to inform the nervous system when muscle tension was reaching damaging proportions. New evidence has shown that the GTO has a greater sensitivity to muscle contraction.[63,71] Therefore it more specifically monitors the tendon tension produced by muscle contraction rather than by muscle tension produced by stretch. In addition, GTO appears to complement the action of the muscle spindle. For example, during isometric contraction of the biceps brachii, tendon tension is developed, and the GTO discharges (action potential). In contrast, the muscle spindle remains relatively silent because muscle length has not changed. If the same muscle (biceps brachii) is completely relaxed and passively stretched (elbow extended), the muscle spindle fires, and the GTO remains relatively silent because little tension is put on the tendon. Therefore the GTO and muscle spindle work collaboratively to inform the nervous system about the muscle length and tension.[75]

The GTO transmits along A alpha (Ib) afferent fibers. It is a slowly adapting receptor that discharges at a rate nearly proportional to the tension of muscle contraction.[63] With respect to spinal reflexes the GTO is associated with autogenic inhibition.[48] In other words, it can cause inhibition of the primary muscle that is contracting against resistance. This occurs because the Ib fiber synapses with inhibitory interneurons in the spinal cord, which causes inhibition of the anterior horn cells that innervate the contracting muscle. Clinically, this is seen as a sudden lengthening reaction.[24,41] This phenomenon is commonly seen in patients with spasticity and is called the *clasp-knife reflex*.[25]

Golgi tendon organs are used to inhibit spasticity in adductors and superficial flexor muscles. This is accomplished by teaching the patient to produce very small range contractions of the spastic muscle and its antagonist. Gravity should be eliminated and small contractions should be done in several repetitions. A stimulus such as therapeutic vibration can be applied over the muscle bellies of the antagonistic abductor and extensor groups to promote isotonic contractions.[30] According to Moore, other joint receptors may also contribute to this phenomenon.[70]

MUSCLE SPINDLES. Muscle spindles are complex, encapsulated receptors that lie deep within skeletal muscle. Their principal function is to monitor changes in length of a muscle and the rate at which the length changes.[75]

Anatomically, the muscle spindle (Fig. 17-4) is a slender, encapsulated structure that houses four to six bundles of specialized muscle fibers called intra-

fusal muscles (Fig. 17-4). There are two types of intrafusal fibers: nuclear chain and nuclear bag fibers.[2] Nuclear bag fibers have an enlarged, noncontractile central region containing many nuclei and tapered, contractile (plate) endings. The nuclear chain fibers are smaller and contain a single row of nuclei in the equatorial region. As mentioned earlier, the muscle spindle receives motor innervation from gamma motor neurons.[56] The intrafusal fibers do not contribute to extrafusal muscle strength or joint movement but regulate the tension in the muscle spindle.[62] Hence, as the extrafusal fibers contract, the intrafusal fibers contract concurrently to maintain some tension in the equatorial region and restore its sensitivity to stretch. In summary, the gamma motor neurons regulate the tension of the intrafusal fibers so that their sensitivity remains constant as the extrafusal fibers change their length.[3,63,89]

The muscle spindle also contains two types of sensory endings. The first type is called the Ia primary fiber (annulospiral ending), which bifurcates within the spindle and wraps around the equatorial regions of both the nuclear bag and the nuclear chain. Because of this spiral arrangement, the Ia primary afferent is stretched like a spring when the equatorial region of the intrafusal muscle elongates. The Ia primary ending has a low threshold and is selectively sensitive to the onset of muscle stretch. Some authors have subdivided the Ia primary afferent into phasic and tonic functions.[52] Therefore whenever the muscle is put through a quick stretch within normal range, it fires the Ia phasic component. The Ia tonic component is believed to originate around the nuclear chain fiber. Therefore the Ia tonic component is less sensitive to quick stretch but fires when the stretch is maintained in the submaximal range.[3,63,89]

A second afferent fibers wraps around the nuclear bag and nuclear chain adjacent to the equatorial region (predominately on the nuclear chain fibers). This fiber was originally called the flowerspray ending because of its appearance. It is now called the secondary ending or group II fiber. The function of the secondary endings is not fully understood.[48] Classically, secondary endings are less sensitive to the onset of stretch but fire during maintained stretch, especially when the muscle is elongated to its maximal range.[40,75] The function of the secondary ending is controversial. However, in classical theory maintained stretch fires the secondary endings and produces facilitation of the flexor and inhibition of the extensor regardless of which muscle receives the stretch.[52] The problem with this principle is determining which muscles are the physiologic flexors and which are the anatomic flexors. For example, by definition a physiologic extensor

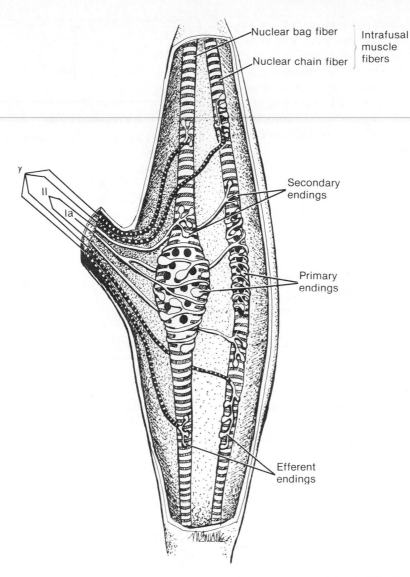

Nuclear bag fiber ⎤ Intrafusal
⎥ muscle
Nuclear chain fiber ⎦ fibers

Secondary
endings

Primary
endings

Efferent
endings

γ

II

Ia

Fig. 17-4. Muscle spindle (sensory and motor attachments). From Nolte J: The human brain: an introduction to its functional anatomy, St. Louis, 1981, The CV Mosby Company.

serves to elongate an extremity. Subsequently, if a person assumes the quadruped position with the palms of the hands flat on the floor and flexes the wrist, the forelimbs are elongated; physiologically, this represents extension. Kottke has suggested that the secondary endings feed into multisynaptic pathways to cause flexion or exension synergies.[55] Thus, if the extensors are stimulated, the secondary endings in extensors cause extensor synergies. If the flexors are stimulated, the secondary endings in flexors cause flexor synergies.

The primary spinal level reflex associated with the muscle spindle is reciprocal innervation. This is a basic stretch reflex in which one muscle group is facilitated and the opposing muscles are inhibited.[87] For example, when the biceps is stretched, it is facilitated, and the antagonist muscle (the triceps) is inhibited. This relationship is called reciprocal inhibition.[48,105] Therapists have used the reflex functions of the muscle spindle in a number of ways. Because the Ia primary ending has a low threshold, it can be fired by quick stretch, vibration, tapping over the muscle belly, or any action that causes elongation of the extrafusal fibers.[37] The results are usually the same. The muscle receiving the stimulus is facilitated and the antagonist inhibited. The properties of the muscle spindle have been described in isolation. Yet in reality whenever a muscle is stretched or contracted, a multitude of skin and joint receptors are firing concurrently.

In addition, the person's emotional state affects the resting threshold of the muscle spindle. Emotional tension increases spasticity in persons with neurologic impairments. Other factors affecting the resting threshold of the muscle spindle are pain syndromes, gravitational forces or position in space, cold environments, distention in the bowel or bladder, excessive auditory stimuli, and medications such as muscle relaxants.[24,30,32,89] Therefore, many factors can affect the muscle spindle. The therapist should eliminate as many variables as possible before applying inhibitory and facilitory techniques.

VESTIBULAR APPARATUS. The vestibular apparatus is classified as a proprioceptive organ.[25] It consists of three semicircular canals attached to a vestibule, which is further subdivided into the saccule and utricle (Fig. 17-5). The semicircular canal system is the kinetic labyrinth. This system is sensitive to head movement and rotatory acceleration or deceleration (spinning) (Fig. 17-6).[73,75] The vestibule (utricle and saccule) is regarded as the static labyrinth. This system is sensitive to head position and linear acceleration or deceleration.[88] The vestibular system acts as a complex relay center that influences many systems of the body. Thus vestibular stimulation has a profound influence on the development of the nervous system (Fig. 17-7).[4] However, as a proprioceptive organ, the vestibular system serves (1) to stabilize the position of the head in space, (2) to stabilize the position of the eyes in space during head movements, (3) to regulate posture and movement through tonic and phasic reflexes, and (4) to exert a powerful influence over the antigravity muscles of neck, trunk, and limbs.[73] The receptor organs in the semicircular canals are the crista ampullaris. In the vestibule, the receptor organ is called the

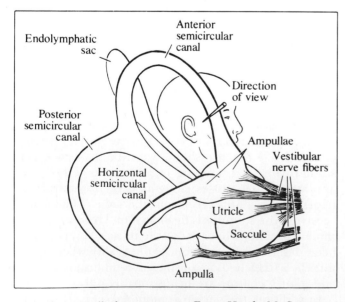

Fig. 17-5. Vestibular apparatus. From Hardy M: Structure of the vestibular apparatus, Anatomical record, New York, 1934.

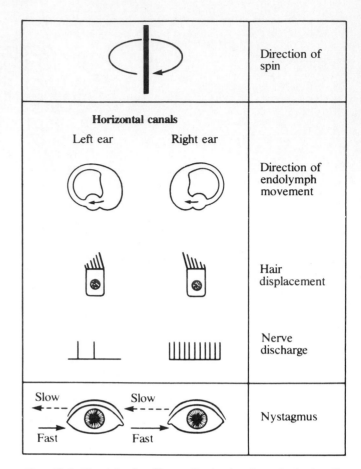

Fig. 17-6. Physiologic effects of spinning in a clockwise direction. The endolymph remains inert on acceleration causing the hair cells in the cristae ampularis to deflect to the left. The endolymph in the right ear is moving in the direction of the vestibule, and the endolymph in the left ear toward the semicircular canal. Nerve discharge is increased on the right and decreased below resting level on the left. After 20 seconds of continuous spinning, nerve discharge resumes the resting level of activity because the endolymph assumes the same rate of movement in relationship to the semicircular canals. When the spinning stops, the hair cells are deflected in the opposite direction. Acceleration and deceleration cause the greatest rate of nerve discharge. Reprinted with permission from Selkurt E: Basic physiology for the health sciences, ed, 2, Boston, 1982, Little, Brown & Company.

macula or otolith. The vestibular apparatus sends impulses to four nuclei in the upper medulla and disperses to centers throughout the nervous system. The descending tracts consist of the lateral and medial vestibulospinal tracts. Ascending fibers travel in the medial longitudinal fasciculus to extraocular muscles and other centers. Still other fibers connect with cranial nerves, the autonomic nervous system, and the cerebellum.[21,48,55]

The neurologic connections between the vestibular system and the cerebellum has many therapeutic im-

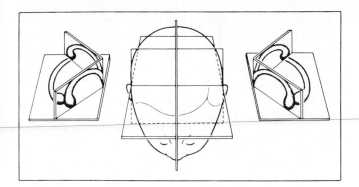

Fig. 17-7. The relationships of the horizontal, anterior, and posterior semicircular canals. They detect motions in the three dimensions of space and initiate the vestibulo-ocular reflexes. Reprinted with permission from Brown JL: Vestibular function. In Brobeck J, editor: Best and Taylor's physiological basis of medical practices, ed, 10, Baltimore, 1979, The Williams & Wilkins Company.

plications. Slow rocking and inversion can reduce hypertonicity in some patients. More accelerated rocking, spinning, and movement in various directions can be useful for stimulating vestibuloproprioceptors for normal postural activity and balance mechanisms.[30,31,73]

Kinesioceptors

Kinesioceptors are joint receptors that represent the conscious division of proprioception because they transmit to the cerebral cortex. Anatomically, joint receptors are located in joint capsules, ligaments, and tendons. These include Ruffini's end organs, Golgi-Mazzoni corpuscles, Vator-Pacini corpuscles, Golgi-type endings, and free nerve endings.

RUFFINI'S END ORGANS. Ruffini's end organs are exclusively joint receptors found only in fibrous joint capsules.[105] These receptors respond vigorously at the beginning of joint movement, but their discharge rate declines as the joint reaches a different position. Ruffini's end organs also fire when touch pressure is applied over the surface of the joint.[106]

GOLGI-MAZZONI CORPUSCLES. Golgi-Mazzoni corpuscles are similar in appearance to pacinian corpuscles. They are small, encapsulated receptors found in joint capsules and tendon surfaces.[105,106] It is interesting to note that the Golgi-Mazzoni receptors are abundant in the connective tissues of the hands. These are rapidly adapting receptors that detect rapid joint movements.[75] They also discharge under deep pressure or vibratory stimuli.[63]

VATER-PACINI CORPUSCLES. Vater-Pacini corpuscles are found in joint capsules and ligaments. They discharge at a greater rate as the joint reaches its maximal range of motion.[63] These receptors may

serve a protective function to inform the cortex when the joint has reached its end position of range.

GOLGI-TYPE ENDINGS. Golgi-type endings are a variation of the Golgi tendon organ found mostly in the joint ligaments. These receptors seem to monitor the rate of joint movement. They are slowly adapting and discharge most rapidly when joint movement is initiated.[15,105]

As previously mentioned, free nerve endings are widely distributed throughout all the soft tissues of the body. It appears that these receptors support the joint receptors by providing a crude awareness of joint movement. Free nerve endings also mediate touch, pain, and temperature sensations in the joint region.[106]

The major function of joint receptors is to inform the nervous system about joint position, velocity of movement, and perhaps the direction of movement. At this time there is no evidence that joint receptors contribute to the force of muscle contraction.[75] From this brief summary it appears that joint receptors supply the conscious awareness of joint position and joint movement.

As a group, joint receptors provide another means of sensory input. The therapist should incorporate activities that stress active range of motion and voluntary effort. Active movement generates much more neurologic activity. It requires a collaborative effort of receptors in the skin muscles and joints and sends a multitude of sensory stimuli to assemblies of neurons at the cortical level.

Myofascial Release

Fascia is a subcutaneous covering or sheet of connective tissue investing muscles and various body organs. Fascia is composed primarily of collagenous and elastic fibers that unite the skin with underlying tissue. It has also been regarded as a continuous laminated band of connective tissue covering the entire body. Normally, it permits free movement of the skin. Its collagenous fibers are pliable and tough and retain limited elasticity. According to Barnes, fascia contains both sensory and motor innervation.[11] Physical trauma to superficial and subcutaneous tissues may stretch fascia beyond its normal capacity, producing a reflex elastic contraction and the sensation of pain. Traumatic injury may result in loss of fascial mobility which results in abnormal physiologic motion. Myofascial release is a combination of procedures promoting mobilization of the whole body to evaluate and correct physical and structural dysfunction. Although myofascial release is in its infancy, it appears to provide another piece of the puzzle for restoring function and reducing pain. Until recently, the integrity of the fascia was not considered as a factor for mobilization in occupational therapy.[11]

Acupoints and Meridians

Eastern medicine has recognized acupressure and energy systems for more than 3,000 years.[95,104] Acupressure release procedures can (1) relieve pain by stimulating the circulation of endorphins, (2) reduce tone in skeletal muscles, (3) and produce a generalized relaxation response.[16,28,65,66] Acupressure is not a technique in and of itself but can be used as a precursor to neurophysiologic techniques.

In Eastern philosophy, meridians are described as channels through which bioelectric energy flows in a complex network throughout the body. In traditional Chinese medicine there are 12 to 14 major meridians, each corresponding to major organ systems or to other functions. According to the Eastern belief, disease or dysfunction results from imbalances or obstruction of the bioelectric energy flowing through these meridians. Manual light pressure applied to these points may set off a complex series of events that is not yet well understood by Western scientific medicine. However, there is mounting scientific evidence that some form of electrical energy exists in the soft tissues of the body.[17] Studies have shown that acupressure points found along the meridians possess either high electrical properties or, conversely, low electrical resistance.[33,65,66,95,104]

Nordinstrom, a Swedish radiologist has theorized that the human body is like a battery with electrical circuits composed of positively and negatively charged ions.[94] The balance or imbalances of these ions regulate many systems of the body. Injury to soft tissues results in an accumulation of positively charged ions. White blood cells are attracted to these positively charged ions, suggesting a natural healing mechanism in the tissues. Nordinstrom has developed an unconventional technique for treating tumors by inserting electrodes adjacent to the neoplasm to change the polarity of the skin. Preliminary procedures have shown that this process shrinks the tumors by dehydration. This approach defies the traditional canons of Western medicine and suggests the importance of biophysics and biochemistry in the health professions.

Smith has described the physics of bioelectric energy in the body and its relationships to Eastern and Western Medicine.[92] According to Smith, there are three energy flows in the body. The first is an outer field of energy surrounding and permeating the whole body. This enveloping energy field is very diffuse and sometimes is regarded as an aura. The second is a vertical energy flow passing through the less dense tissues conforming to the skin and connective tissues. The third bioelectric flow of energy conforms to the skeletal system and moves within the body. Many cultures have developed health care systems based on this bioelectric energy theory.[92] Specific regions of the body are believed to contain vortices of energy or pathways through which energy passes. In view of new findings in biophysics and biochemistry the energy theory is not too far-fetched. Because of the body's high metabolic rate, electrical discharges in the nervous system and physical movement through surrounding energy fields in the environment, the bioelectrical currents may indeed affect health and wellness.

There are two Americanized styles of acupressure release systems that are easy to learn to have great potential for inclusion in the occupational therapist's repertoire. One is called Jin Shin Do, developed by Teeguarden.[95] The second is called Jin Shin Juitsu or Family Therap/ease refined by Pendleton and Mahling[77] These systems are not interpreted as medical techniques but can be adjuncts to occupational therapy procedures.

Trigger Points

The origin of trigger points in the fascia and in muscles is somewhat controversial in rehabilitation medicine. Melzack has conducted much research on trigger points and their implication for pain management. Trigger points are not acupoints.[33,65,66,97] Travell and Margoles suggest that they are the result of trauma to muscles resulting in nodules formed from byproducts of lactic acid or carbon dioxide, and possibly calcium deposits on nerve endings.[97] On palpation, the trigger point feels like a knot in the muscle tissue; it is painful when touched and seems to contribute to muscle spasms. Trigger points are laid down in muscle tissue throughout life.[83] So called *satellite trigger points* also exist in myofascial tissue promoting pain syndromes remote from the trigger point location.

Occupational therapists see patients with a variety of pain syndromes secondary to their diagnoses. For example, the hemiplegic population has a high incidence of pain in the shoulder region. Van Leer reports that 72% of hemiparetic patients experience shoulder pain at least once during the course of recovery.[100]

Research has shown that injections into trigger points alleviate pain. A less invasive technique called *myotherapy* can obtain similar results.[83] The process entails finding the trigger points in the myofascial tissue of the painful area, then applying manual finger pressure over the trigger point for about 7 seconds. Following the application of pressure, the muscles are stretched through simple range-of-motion exercises.

The mechanism that produces the pain relief is not well understood. The pressure may dissipate the accumulation of lactic acid or calcium deposits. Because slight pain is induced by the pressure over the trigger point it may also cause a counterirritation phenomenon. No matter what the mechanism is, if the technique alleviates pain and the patient increases the ability to perform purposeful activities, it is well worth a try. Therapists should keep an open mind in looking at new theories to develop new techniques as information becomes available.

TRACT SYSTEM

Sensorimotor techniques are aimed at stimulating specific receptors and tract systems. From a sensory stimulation standpoint there are four tract systems through which sensory input travels.[15,73]

Sensory Tracts

SPINOTHALAMIC. The first system is called protopathic because it is phylogenetically old and serves a protective function.[4] Anatomically, this system constitutes the anterior and lateral spinothalamic tracts. The spinothalamic system contains fibers of the A delta (group III) and C fibers (group IV). This is a slowly conducting system because most of its fibers are unmyelinated and small in diameter. This system mediates pain, temperature, crude touch, and visceral pain. The first order neuron of this system enters the lateral portion of the dorsal horn of the spinal cord, synapses with interneurons, crosses to the opposite side of the cord, and ascends in an anterolateral spinothalamic tract. An important feature of this system is that it gives off numerous collaterals to the reticular-activating system.[4,88,105] The second order neuron continues its ascent to nonspecific nuclei of the thalamus. From there the third order neuron terminates with many areas of the cerebral cortex. In summary the spinothalamic system serves a protective function that is excitatory to the cortex because of its many collaterals in the reticular formation.

LEMNISCAL. The second system is phylogenetically advanced and is called epicritic because it has a high degree of specificity. Anatomically, this sensory tract system makes up the dorsal columns of the spinal cord and is called the lemniscal system.[21] The lemniscal system contains fibers from the A alpha (group I) and A beta (group II) classifications. Because this system contains well-myelinated, thick fibers with few collaterals, it is a fast conducting system. The lemniscal system carries impulses from the discriminative receptors (Meissner's corpuscles, pacinian corpuscles, and Ruffini's end organs). Therefore this system mediates stereognosis, 2-point discrimination, pressure, vibration, and other senses of fine recognition. The lemniscal system is well defined. The first order neuron enters the medial portion of the dorsal root and ascends in the dorsal columns of the cord on the same side it enters. This system gives off few collaterals to the reticular formation and synapses on the ventrobasal nuclei of the thalamus. The third order neuron terminates in areas 3, 1, and 2 of the somatosensory cortex.[4,88,105] To summarize, the lemniscal system has a high degree of specificity and carries discriminative information.

PROPRIOCEPTIVE. The proprioceptive tracts make up the third sensory pathway. Proprioception refers to the conscious or unconscious awareness of body position and movement of bodily segments. The proprioceptive pathways are of particular interest to the occupational therapist because they regulate movements toward purposeful activities.

Conscious proprioception is regulated by the lemniscal (dorsal column) system. This pathway begins in joint receptors and ends in the parietal lobe of the cerebral cortex where conscious awareness takes place. Conscious proprioception enables the cortex to refine voluntary movements for skillful activities.[24,34]

Unconscious proprioception is mediated by the spinocerebellar tracts. This pathway begins in the afferents of the muscle spindle and Golgi tendon organ and terminates in the cerebellum. Unconscious proprioception is concerned with muscle tension, muscle length, and speed of movement. The spinocerebellar tracts do not ascend to the cortex.[105] However, the cerebellum serves as a feedback mechanism for the motor cortex so it can modify or correct voluntary movements as they are being initiated.[24]

TRIGEMINAL. The trigeminal nerve (CN V) makes up the fourth and last division of the sensory tract systems. The trigeminal nerve is unique in many ways. It is responsible for direct transmission of tactile, proprioceptive, pain and temperature sensation in the skin of the facial region. The posterior of the head and neck is supplied by C2, C3, and C4 of the cervical spinal roots.[15,88,106] Therefore the trigeminal nerve transmits information directly to sensory nuclei that are connected to the reticular formation, cerebellum, and cerebral cortex. The sensory end organs and afferent fibers are separated into ophthalmic, maxillary, and mandibular divisions.

The trigeminal nerve is one of the earliest sensory roots to myelinate and respond to touch stimulation. Stimulation to the perioral area evokes a protective avoiding reaction at 7½ fetal weeks. The discriminative receptors begin their development and differentiation at about the fourth fetal month.[21] Because of the nerve's early ontogenetic development, some sensorimotor therapists begin cutaneous stimulation to the trigeminal nerve.

The motor branch of the trigeminal nerve supplies the muscles of mastication, tensor tympani muscle of the ear, and tensor veli palatini muscle of the soft palate.[25,53]

DERMATOMES

With the exception of the facial region the skin of the body receives its sensory innervation in a segmental fashion by nerve roots of the spinal cord. The area of skin supplied by a single dorsal root and its ganglion constitutes a dermatome.[70] The dermatomes are arranged on the surface of the body in a sequence corresponding to the related spinal cord segments. Cutaneously, the highest dermatomal level represents the posterior of the head, whereas the lowest is in the anal region.[15] Fig. 17-8 shows the segmental arrangement of dermatomes from the neck down to the anal region. There is much overlap in the segmental borders of the dermatomes, particularly in the trunk. It is important for the occupational therapist to have a fundamental understanding of dermatomal segments. The dermatomes are the skin areas that delineate the sensory regions of the skin. Each sensory dermatome that feeds into the spinal cord has a motor component for the respective segment. Also, all areas of the skin are not alike. For example, the facial area and the volar surface of the hands contain a greater number of discriminative receptors, whereas the central axis of the trunk contains more protective (protopathic) and autonomic afferents.

In many cases cutaneous stimulation is applied dermatomally in an effort to activate selected myotomes or muscle groups.[45] Dermatomes are also important in evaluating the integrity of peripheral nerves and the spinal cord segments.

CUTANEOUS REFLEX

An important concept in sensory stimulation is the existence of the cutaneous fusimotor reflex. This reflex was first demonstrated on polio patients by Kenny and later substantiated by Hagbarth.[49,55] In essence, studies have found that stimulation to certain areas of the skin can influence the specific muscles of the body. The cutaneous reflex is not a simple monosynaptic reflex arc. Instead, it is a polysynaptic system that entails cutaneous afferents, gamma motor neurons, and Ia afferents of the muscle spindle. Any stimulation to a dermatome discharges cutaneous receptors that synapse with gamma motor neurons at the same spinal segment in the ventral horn of the spinal cord. The gamma motor neurons cause intrafusal fibers to contract. This causes the Ia afferents to discharge, which in turn sends impulses back into the spinal cord where they synapse with alpha motor neurons. If the stimulus is strong enough to cause the alpha motor neuron to discharge, a reflexive contraction or increase in tone occurs in the muscle innervated at that segmental level. The activity of the cutaneous receptors and the gamma system is proportional to the intensity of the stimuli.[49,55] However, it should be emphasized that the cutaneous stimulus should be applied to the dermatome that corresponds to the muscles to be activated. This technique seems to work best on the dermatomes that overlie the muscles to be activated. In patients with spinal cord injury or with CNS lesions, the response may be exaggerated because the supraspinal centers are detached or the excitatory neurons are disinhibited.

HIERARCHICAL ORGANIZATION OF POSTURE AND MOVEMENT

Research on animal preparations and observations of human subjects with regional lesions suggest that neuromuscular function is based on reflex activity.[1,21]

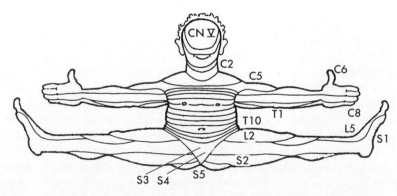

Fig. 17-8. Dermatomes (segmental levels). From Clark RG: Clinical neuroanatomy and neurophysiology, ed 5, Philadelphia, 1975, FA Davis Co.

The evolution of the nervous system has allowed the more advanced reflexes to become superimposed on the more primitive. Therefore it is postulated that pathologic reflexes are manifestations of primitive reflexes that are normally supressed by supraspinal centers. This concept is now being challenged by proponents of the central control hypothesis, but it still provides a useful model for the therapists who use sensorimotor approaches. The concept is helpful in understanding the hierarchical organization of posture and motor control for testing and treatment. Table 17-3 summarizes and serves as a reference. The following is a brief summary of the segmental centers for motor control.*

Spinal Level

The spinal level regulates the more primitive, stereotypical movements. These are principally stretch reflexes arising from muscles. Because these reflexes are generated from muscles, they are often called *myotatic reflexes*. Spinal reflexes are "phasic" in that they occur rapidly and extinguish very fast. These reflexes are believed to be primitive responses to potentially harmful stimuli. Therefore a painful stimulus or quick stretch produces spinal level responses. The spinal level reflexes include (1) flexor withdrawal, (2) crossed extension, (3) extensor thrust, (4) positive supporting reaction, (5) negative supporting reaction, and (6) cutaneousfusimotor reflexes. These reflexes are fairly predictable when elicited in infants or persons with CNS lesions. They abide by the principles of reciprocal innervation and autogenic inhibition. They are evoked by primary and secondary endings in muscle spindles, Golgi tendon organs, and nonspecific cutaneous receptors.

Lower Brain Stem

The lower brain stem includes the nuclei in the medulla and the facilitory portion of the reticular formation. These centers have long-lasting effects on posture and therefore are called *tonic* reflexes. For example, the nuclei for the vestibular system are constantly discharging into motor neuron pools to sustain head and body alignment. The static labyrinthine reflex arises from the vestibule (utricle and saccule) and discharges during changes in head position and linear acceleration. The kinetic labyrinth includes the three semicircular canals and responds to head movement and rotatory motions. These reflexes regulate muscle tone (especially extensors) and balance reactions. The tonic neck reflexes are also exerting tonic influences on limbs and postural muscles in response to stretch

imposed on the neck muscles. The tonic lumbar reflex arises from joint and muscle proprioceptors in the lumbar segments. This reflex is divided into symmetric and asymmetric components. The symmetric response occurs when the trunk is ventroflexed, causing flexion of all four extremities, and dorsiflexed, causing extension of all four extremities. The asymmetric response is stimulated by rotation or lateral flexion of the trunk. Trunk rotation to one side results in flexion of the ipsilateral upper extremity and extension of the lower extremity. Simultaneously the contralateral upper extremity extends and the lower extremity flexes. These opposite effects contribute to the normal reciprocal movements of the limbs during gait pattern. Lateral flexion of the trunk results in ipsilateral upper extremity flexion and lower extremity extension. The contralateral response produces extension of the upper extremity and flexion of the lower. Lower brain stem reflexes include (1) tonic labyrinthine reflexes (static or kinetic), (2) tonic neck reflexes (asymmetric or symmetric), and (3) tonic lumbar reflexes. These reflexes arise from the proprioceptors in the neck muscles and trunk and the receptor organs in the vestibular apparatus.

Upper Brain Stem

The upper brain stem includes the midbrain and the diencephalon (hypothalamus and thalamus). This level includes "tonically" induced reflexes for more refined postural adjustments. Because these reflexes assist with the maintenance of the upright position, they are "righting" or "displacement reactions."[24]

The upper brain stem includes (1) labyrinthine righting reactions, (2) neck righting, (3) body-and-head righting, and (4) body-on-body righting.

Central Control Centers

The integrated circuits between the cerebral cortex, basal ganglia, and cerebellum supply an added dimension to posture and movement. Much research has been done to single out the functions of these structures. Although investigators are not in full agreement, they seem to work as feedback circuits to refine higher level motor functions. In general, skilled voluntary movement arises from the cerebral cortex. Descending impulses send collaterals to both the basal ganglia and the cerebellum. The basal ganglia are credited with the regulation of the more rhythmic automatic movement patterns.[25] The cerebellum tends to monitor the rate, range, force, and direction of movement. Therefore once the voluntary movement has been initated by the cortex, the subcortical structures refine and feed back information during the motor act.[21,25] Some reflexes or reactions associ-

---

*References 1, 15, 21, 24, 40, 41, 48, 91, 105.

Table 17-3 Hierarchical Organization of Postural Reflexes

Level	Reflex	Stimulus	Receptor	Motor response	Pathologic sign
Cerebral cortex (basal ganglia and cerebellum)	Optical righting	Visual cues	Eyes	Righting of head	Decorticate rigidity Spasticity Babinski's sign Hoffmann's sign Clasp-knife reflex
	Placing reaction Hopping reaction	Surface contact	Various proprioceptors*	Weight-bearing on palmar sole when placed on hard surface	
Upper brain stem (midbrain and diencephalon)	Labyrinthine righting	Tilt body	Vestibular apparatus	Face vertical and mouth horizontal	
	Neck righting	Stretch of neck muscles	Muscle spindles	Rights body in respect to neck	Romberg's sign Tremor
	Body on head righting	Pressure on side of body	Exteroceptors	Rights head in respect to gravity	Decerebrate rigidity
	Body on body reaction	Rotation of head or thorax	Exteroceptors	Rights head or thorax	
	Tonic lumbar reflex	Lateral flexion or rotation of trunk	Joint and muscle proprioceptors	Reciprocal movements of limbs, trunk, and pelvis for gait pattern	Ataxia Asynergies, weakness
Lower brain stem (medulla and reticular formation)	Tonic labyrinthine reflex (kinetic and static)	Head inversion (gravity)	Vestibular apparatus	Increased extensor tone	Vestibular shoot
	Tonic neck reflex	Rotation, flexion or extension of neck	Joint receptors Neck proprioceptors	Alterations in extensor or flexor tone of the limbs	Asynergistic movements; tonic changes in muscle tone
Spinal cord (reflex arc)	Flexor withdrawal	Nociceptive	Exteroceptive	Withdrawal of stimulated extremity	
	Crossed extension	Nociceptive	Exteroceptive	Flexion of stimulated limb and extension-abduction of contralateral limb	
	Extensor thrust	Nociceptive	Exteroceptive	Extension-abduction of contralateral limb	
	Positive supporting reaction	Contact with sole or palm	Proprioceptors and distal flexors	Leg extended to support body	Marie-Foix reflex
	Negative supporting reaction	Stretch	Proprioceptors in extensors	Release of positive supporting reaction	Flexion reflex and clonus
	Cutaneous-fusimotor reflex	Cutaneous stimuli	Exteroceptors and spindle afferents	Prolonged increase in muscle tone at segmental level	Hyperreflexia Hypertonia Romberg's sign Degrees of paralysis

*Pacinian corpuscles, Ruffini end organs, Golgi-Mazzoni muscle spindles, and several exteroceptors.

ated with the cerebral cortex are (1) optical righting reflexes, (2) placing reactions, and (3) hopping reactions.

Current interpretations of the nervous system do not subscribe to the linear or segmental function of the nervous system.[35] However, the segmental approach has merit for determining origins of pathological signs and symptoms. The new theories suggest that the nervous system functions more holistically through resonance rather than segmental connection. Another factor to consider are individual differences. No two nervous systems are entirely alike. Each brain has its own uniqueness and functional signature.

SPECIAL SENSE MECHANISMS
Olfactory

The special senses are often alluded to in sensorimotor techniques, but specific procedures are limited. The following discussion outlines some of the salient features of the special sense organs and how they might be used in therapy.

The physiologic components of the olfactory system are not well understood. There are many theories about how smell is transduced into neuronal messages, but the scientific facts are somewhat limited. Basically olfaction is a chemical process.[52] The receptors for smell are located in specialized epithelium in the roof of the nasal cavity. The olfactory epithelium contains three types of cells and small glands that secrete mucous substances for dissolving odorous materials. The receptor cells contain fine hairlike cilia, which are the most exposed nerve endings in the entire body. The olfactory epithelium is estimated to contain 100 million receptor cells, yet it only occupies an area the size of a dime.[34,48] The afferent fibers from these cells converge with the second order neurons in a ratio of 1000:1.[1]

The receptor cells for olfaction respond to a variety of stimuli. Some sources indicate that humans can distinguish between 2000 to 4000 different odors.[73] However, each of these odors may generate different impulses from the olfactory receptors and pass directly to many regions of the brain. The principal regions are the temporoal lobe of the cortex (area 28), structures in the limbic system, and subcortical nuclei and autonomic nuclei of the hypothalamus.[34,73] Furthermore, olfaction is the only sensory modality that bypasses the thalamus en route to the cortex.[44] So if the thalamus is damaged, olfactory stimulation can still reach certain portions of the CNS.

When using olfactory stimuli, the therapist should keep in mind that the receptors for smell adapt rather quickly. As many as 50% cease firing after the first few seconds of stimulation.[52] Therefore the strength of the odor has to be increased by about 30% to reactivate the adapted receptors. To allow for adaptation the therapist can use three vials of the same scent, each one containing a concentration 30% greater than the first. The therapist should start with a diluted scent first, then a solution of 60%, and last a solution of full strength. This process increases the times that the therapist can use a given scent for olfactory stimulation. Consequently, some noxious chemicals, such as ammonia and vinegar, cause irritation of the mucous linings in the nasal cavity. As a result, it causes more activity in the trigeminal nerve rather than the olfactory. These odors are more useful for stimulating avoidance reactions or facial expressions. It should also be noted that olfactory stimuli go directly into the amygdala of the limbic system.[15,48,87,106] Responses to olfactory stimuli may also elicit emotional responses or primal behaviors associated with survival.

Gustatory

Gustation or taste is also a chemical process. However, the act of eating is a multisensory experience that uses somatosensory receptors as well. The taste receptors are located in the tongue, soft palate, and upper regions of the throat.[73] The tongue contains three different types of taste buds that occupy specific locations. Basically there are four primary taste sensations: sweet, sour, salty, and bitter. Many flavors are combinations of the four taste sensations.[87] However, action potentials show the base of the tongue responds best to bitter, the outer edges to sour and salty, and the tip to sweet.[53]

The taste receptors transmit along the fibers of four cranial nerves: the glossopharyngeal (IX), trigeminal (V), facial (VII), and vagus (X). These cranial nerves transmit to nuclei in the brainstem, reticular formation, spinal and cranial reflex centers, thalamus, and regions of the parietal lobe of the cortex.[73,74]

Before beginning gustatory stimulation the therapist should evaluate swallowing and the gag reflexes to see if the glossopharyngeal (IX) and vagus (X) nerves are intact. Gustatory discrimination is similar to olfaction because it adapts readily and requires about a 30% change in concentration to distinguish differences.[45,87] Also, before a substance can be tasted, it must be somewhat water soluble. Therefore the therapist can use one of each primary flavor mixed in distilled water so the concentrations can be graded from weak to strong. Again the first solution should contain a 1:3 ratio, that is, one part flavor and three parts distilled water. Three vials can be mixed for each taste stimulus. The second vial can contain a solution 30% stronger than the first, and the last can be full strength. These solutions can be applied to the tongue with an eye dropper so they contact specific portions of the tongue. For example, the sweet flavor can be made with low calorie sweeteners and distilled water. In this case the drops would be applied to the tip of the tongue. The sour taste can be made with vinegar and distilled water and applied to the middle sides of the tongue. Salt flavor can be made with table salt or sodium fluoride and applied to the anterior edges of the tongue.[14,73] Because bitter tastes are detected in lower concentrations and can trigger avoidance reactions, they should be used last. In addition, sour and bitter tastes may also elicit *taste reflexes* that stimulate the parotid and submaxillary glands to secrete saliva. This is a natural way of promoting swallowing, but it may dilute the taste stimuli.

Auditory

The auditory system enables the perception of events that are taking place at a distance. This is a sophisticated sense that transduces sound waves into mechanical energy and ultimately neuronal impulses. The receptor cells for audition are housed in the cochlea in a structure called *Corti's organ.*[15,73] This structure contains hair cells similar in appearance to the cells in the vestibular system. The impulses from the receptor cells pass along nerve fibers of the spiral ganglion through the nerve root of cranial nerve VIII to special nuclei in the superior portion of the medulla. Second order neurons project to the contralateral side of the brain stem or ascend ipsilaterally to the olivary and accessory nuclei. Still other collaterals synapse on neurons in the reticular system or ascend by way of the lateral lemniscus to the inferior colliculus. Third-order neurons ascend to the medial geniculate body and then to the auditory cortex (Brodmann's area 41).[13]

The auditory system has its own set of reflexes that are related to protective behavior. It connects to the reticular formation and the evokes responses in the autonomic nervous system. In the midbrain the inferior colliculi feed into the tectospinal tract. This system is activated by sudden sounds, such as a car backfiring. Such a sound would transmit auditory input to centers believed to trigger reflexive movements of the head, neck, and upper extremities. The auditory system may be used with moderation in therapy. This does not imply that the therapist should use sudden sound stimuli to evoke reflex responses. However, it does imply that auditory stimuli feed into motor neuron pools that influence postural reflexes. It may also imply that the auditory stimuli going to the reticular formation can produce excitatory or inhibitory states, depending on the nature of the sound. For example, a novel sound stimulus tends to be excitatory. A constant sound stimulus, such as the waves of the ocean or city traffic, is suppressed by the reticular system. Soft melodic music is said to be restful, whereas "hard rock" music would have an excitatory effect. Some therapists use the sound of their voice as an inhibitory or excitatory stimulus. If the activity is designed to promote movement, the therapist should use simple, one-word commands, such as "reach," "pull," "stop," or "look." On the other hand, if the activity is designed to be inhibitory, the therapist should speak to the patient in a soft monotone. This is particularly helpful for elderly patients who have difficulty hearing sounds of high-pitched frequencies.

Background music can be very beneficial with certain patient populations. The key of A tends to be arousing, whereas the key of B can be emotionally depressing. High pitch has been shown to increase muscle tone whereas low pitch can lower muscle tone. A tempo of 70 to 80 beats per minute is physiologically soothing. A tempo greater than 70 to 80 beats per minutes can increase heart rate, blood pressure, and respiration.[2,27,38,64,90]

In therapy, a principle called vectoring is useful for agitated or hyperkinetic patients. The process involves selecting music to match the mood of the listeners; a concept called the isoprinciple.[107] The music is then gradually slowed down to a more tranquil rate. Studies show that motor activity also slows down in conjunction with the music.

There is some evidence that music releases endorphins.[28] In one study, music outperformed biofeedback as a means of relaxation for patients suffering from migraine headaches.[2] Studies also suggest that music creates specific emotional states because its input is more directed to the limbic brain than to the neocortex. The phenomenon of visualizing colors while listening to music indicates a fusion of senses occurring in the limbic system. This phenomenon, termed *synesthesia,* illustrates how one sensory modality can affect another.[6,10,35]

Visual

The visual system is one of the most relied-on senses for orientation in space. Vision is a remarkable biochemical process that transduces light stimuli into neuronal impulses. Basically light is an electromagnetic energy that passes through the lens of the eye to be cast on the retina. The retina is actually an extension of the brain. It is composed of specialized receptor cells (rods and cones) and photopigments that absorb the light stimulus. This causes an action potential, and impulses are conducted along visual pathways.[1,12] The visual pathway projects posteriorly to form the fiber tracts of cranial nerve II where it becomes the optic nerve. The visual pathway can be very confusing because the retina of each eye contains fibers from the nasal portion that cross at the optic chiasm. The fibers arising from the temporal portions of each retina do not cross at the optic chiasm but continue uninterrupted to the lateral geniculate bodies of the thalamus. From this juncture the fibers proceed posteriorly until they terminate on the occipital lobes of the cortex. The visual cortex is composed of Brodmann's area 17, which is the visual receptive area. Areas 18 and 19 are believed to be involved with visual reflexes and visual perception. Area 8 in the frontal lobe is associated with voluntary eye movements.[30]

The visual system mediates a number of protective and postural reflexes. For example, connections to the superior colliculus mediate reflexes for quick localization of potentially harmful stimuli. Connections to cranial nerves III, IV, VI and the vestibular apparatus provide a stabilizing influence on the eyes during head rotation. Other visual reflexes may include the light reflex, visual fixation, convergence, accommodation, pupillary constriction, blinking, and ciliospinal reflex.[1,15] Much evidence suggests that the visual motor system is linked to chains of motor neurons that modulate posture and movement.[73] In essence the extraocular muscles direct the eyes toward a stimulus in the periphery. If the eyes are turned laterally to converge on the object in the visual field, the head rotates in an effort to center the eyes. Rotation of the neck sets off a volley of postural responses (tonic neck and righting reactions) that attempt to realign the trunk with the neck. Therefore the eyes lead, the head follows, and the trunk and limbs adjust accordingly.

NEW FRONTIERS IN THERAPY

Although the nervous system is composed of many subdivisions, it functions as an integrated whole. Because the therapist cannot see the internal functions of the CNS, examination must be done through clinical observation. Sometimes the nervous system gives subtle clues about what is going on inside. The occupational therapist must be a skilled observer to interpret subtle signs such as body language, behaviors, and motor deficits that the patient exhibits.

Neurolinguistic Programming

A new approach to understanding the process of human communications offers some hints for understanding how a person perceives sensory input. This approach is called neurolinguistic programming.[8,56] Although neurolinguistic programming is in its infancy, it offers some interesting ways to observe and communicate with patients. As the name implies, the

nervous system is programmed to process information similar to a computer. Studies have shown that people process incoming information by channeling it through a dominant sensory modality. In our culture most people are biased to one of the three sensory-based categories: kinesthetic, visual, or auditory. Because the occupational therapist engages the patient in purposeful activities, it is important to ascertain which sensory modality the patient prefers to use. To do this, neurolinguistic programming provides some helpful hints. During the time the therapist is interviewing or evaluating the patient, some simple observations can be made. These findings may not be absolute but are true for many persons. First, the observer should focus on the patient's oculomotor system or the movement of the eyes. Interestingly, the direction in which a person is looking is in correlation with his or her thinking process. For example, when a person is speaking and the eyes are turned upward or defocused straight ahead, that person most likely is visualizing what is being described. If the patient looks upward frequently, it could mean the patient is a visual learner (Fig. 17-9A). Therefore functional activities may be more successful for this patient if introduced more visually or graphically. The therapist may reinforce this visualization process by looking upward and posing hypothetical questions. Often the patient follows the lead and answers the questions by looking upward to imagine the situation.

The person who is oriented to processing information auditorily usually oscillates the eyes from side to side. If the person is engaged in internal speech or talks to self while performing a task, the eyes usually turn in the direction of the nondominant hand (Fig. 17-9,B). The auditory person prefers sounds or words for learning. Thus the therapist may present functional activities more verbally and descriptively.

The kinesthetic person tends to be oriented toward emotions or physical action. The most common eye pattern is to look down toward the dominant hand while experiencing sensations or emotions (Fig. 17-9,C). This patient may profit from activities that are more physically oriented.

Hand gestures and breathing patterns also may reveal auditory, visual, or kinesthetic tendencies. People have been known to point toward or touch the sense organ that is associated with their thinking process. The auditory person gestures toward his ear; the visual gestures in the direction of the eyes; and the kinesthetic may point toward the heart, an organ equated with emotions. Kinesthetic persons exhibit deep abdominal respirations. Shallow thoracic breathing has been linked with visual perception, and even

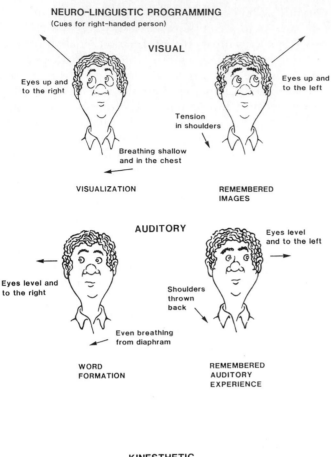

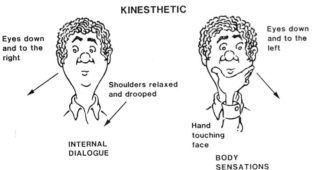

Fig. 17-9. Patterns of eye movements. Redrawn and modified from Dilts R, and Grinder J: Neuro-linguistic programming, Cupertino, CA, 1980, Meta Publications.

breathing with prolonged expiration is associated with auditory perception.

Touch Communication

Touch is another important aspect of interpersonal communication. It has been shown that touch is a form of primal communication, perhaps more powerful than the spoken word alone. Montagu has emphasized the importance of touch from an anthropologic standpoint.[68] More recently, Krieger has dem-

onstrated how the "laying on of hands" produces measurable physiological benefits.[57-59] *Therapeutic touch* is a process by which the therapist assesses or in a sense treats certain conditions by placing the hands within proximity of the patient. It is postulated that some form of energy is transmitted from the therapist to the patient.[57] Experimental research has produced some rather amazing results. Registered nurses, trained in therapeutic touch, treated 34 hospitalized patients and compared their blood samples to a control group of hospitalized patients who received only routine calls. Subjects exposed to therapeutic touch had many beneficial reactions. Blood studies show an increase in enzyme activity and hematocrit values. Hemoglobin levels are significant because hemoglobin carries oxygen molecules and oxygen promotes healing. Electroencephalographic studies show that subjects receiving therapeutic touch produce more alpha waves, indicating altered levels of consciousness and a relaxation response. Therapeutic touch when used with cotton to potentiate its effect has been found to relieve pain especially the discomfort associated with orthopedic injuries.*

The ancient practice of laying on of hands is not unique to occupational therapy. However, research shows that touch or cutaneous stimulation may have more implications than previously imagined. Some evidence suggests that touch changes the relationship of positive and negative ions, which in turn regulates "well-being" or "wellness."

In short, the body does not end at the skin. Some people evoke a state of mind in which the receiver really feels loved; this produces a measurable boost to their immune system.[23,26,50,60,102] Researchers have described this phenomenon as the *Mother Theresa* effect. It suggests that state of mind can give placebos a powerful therapeutic effect.

Psychoneuroimmunology

The recent discovery of neuropeptides has given rise to a new discipline called psychoneuroimmunology (PNI).[50,79,102] This exciting discipline brings much needed credence to therapeutic activities and holistic health practices. The neuropeptides connect the nervous system, the endocrine system and the immune system into a unified network.[102] They are the link between the mind and the body. In fact, neuropeptides are considered the neurotransmitters of emotions. Emotions generated in the limbic system are transmitted through the bloodstream in the form of neuropeptides. Among other things, neuropeptides

*References 19, 47, 54, 57-59, 83, 84, 103.

direct the movement of the monocytes (macrophages), which are critical for tissue repair, eliminating foreign bodies and communicating with T cells and B cells to fight disease.[27,28,50,60,102]

According to Pert, emotions are the key to health. The patient's state of mind affects the outcome of his recovery.[79] Neuropeptides not only are found in the brain but are strategically located throughout the body.* Peptides and receptor sites are found in the linings of the gastrointestinal tract and in brain stem nuclei as well. This may explain why some persons refer to "gut feelings" and why certain deep-breathing techniques affect levels of consciousness and pain thresholds. Even facial expression may influence the release of neuropeptides in the limbic system. Zajonic has theorized that facial expressions change emotional states.[20,108,109] Voluntary contraction of facial muscles may alter the blood flow to the brain, thereby changing its biochemistry. According to recent research, there may be feedback loop between facial expression and emotional states.[108] This raises some interesting therapeutic implications for occupational therapists. If emotions are indeed the key to health, occupational therapists are in a prime position to affect attitudes and emotions through purposeful activities. Banning and Nelson analyzed the therapeutic components of an activity eliciting humor and the effect of group structure. Their study found humor elicited laughter, altered affect, and the perceptions of the subjects. Humor was a significant component in group cohesion and therapeutic activity. From a psychoneuroimmunology perspective, humor elicited changes in facial expression, which released neuropeptides in the limbic system and thus biochemical changes in the immune, endocrine, and nervous systems. These biochemical changes generated feelings of well-being and confidence; thus producing another feedback loop.

Switchboards to the Brain

Concepts of neuronal transmission and brain mapping are changing. The earlier concept of tract systems and pathways being *hardwired* has given way to dynamic, nonlinear, and fluid concepts of neuronal transmission.[6,10,29,35,71] The fluids surrounding the brain are rich in peptides and neurotransmitter substances.[10,18] Neurotransmission may not be purely an

electrical and chemical process but also a glandular transmission through intracellular fluids. Certain types of therapeutic activities may produce more global effects than previously imagined. Prescribed movements combined with positive emotions and imagery may switch on many more neuronal circuits than an isolated movement directed toward one goal. It is possible that neuronal summation occurs where a variety of stimuli converge upon assemblies of neurons which act as "switchboards" to activate higher centers. For example, mental activity and movement exercises stimulate one hemisphere more than the other. A stimulus applied to one area of the body may influence a different part of the body.

In the past, the brain was mapped out by recording responses to primarily electrical stimulation. In 1954, Penfield and Jasper delineated the sensory-motor homunculus by showing topographic representation of brain cells to specific body parts.[78] More recently, Picard and Oliver analyzed the cortical representation of the tongue on 100 human subjects who underwent craniotomies.[82] Their findings suggest that the tongue has a much larger cortical representation than previously estimated. In fact, the tongue and the hand have the highest ratio of brain cell bodies proportional to their size. The cell bodies for the hand and the tongue are in close proximity to one another, and in some areas they overlap. Metabolic mapping studies record the distribution of blood flow to various regions of the brain and have revealed much overlap in functional brain cell activity.[46,71,80,81] Considering the closeness of the cell bodies representing the hand and the tongue on the homunculus, one might postulate that sensory stimulation applied to the hand can affect speech development. Conversely, sensory stimulation applied to the tongue might affect manual dexterity of the hand. In the past, this would have sounded preposterous; however the hand is an important vehicle for nonverbal communication and expression. Hand movements naturally accompany verbal expression and follow similar developmental patterns. Research shows that the physical body is innerconnected to the nerves in ways that are not yet understood. Thus, many questions are yet to be explored. Occupational therapists are beset with new challenges in the future to keep informed of new discoveries in the neurosciences. What seems to be speculation today may become new paradigms for therapeutic intervention tomorrow.

---

*References 13, 28, 33, 61, 76, 93.

REVIEW QUESTIONS

1. What are the two classifications of nerve fibers?
2. What is the primary function of gamma loop (fusimotor neuron)?
3. Differentiate between the functions of the sympathetic and the parasympathetic branches of the autonomic nervous system.
4. Why is the brain stem so important to sensorimotor integration?
5. Describe the two properties that

a neuron must possess to convey information.

6. Explain the terms *reverberating, excitation,* and *disinhibited.*
7. Describe the factors contributing to the rebound phenomenon.
8. List three factors associated with neuroplasticity.
9. Discuss how interoceptors are used in sensorimotor techniques.
10. Describe some of the therapeutic features associated with the pacinian corpuscle.
11. Contrast the basic functions of the Golgi tendon organ with the muscle spindle.
12. Describe the functions of the Ia afferent and secondary endings of the muscle spindle.
13. Describe the anatomic components of the static and kinetic labyrinthine systems.
14. List four functions of the vestibular system.
15. What are the functions of joint receptors?
16. Differentiate between the spinothalamic and the lemniscal tract systems.
17. Why is the trigeminal nerve considered to be an individual sensory tract system?
18. Describe how dermatomes relate to spinal cord segments and the topographic arrangement on the skin.
19. Describe the cutaneous reflex and its significance in sensorimotor therapy.
20. List the reflexes associated with each level of the nervous system.
21. Describe how the olfactory system can be used in sensorimotor therapy.
22. Discuss how gustation can be used in sensorimotor therapy.
23. How can auditory stimuli be used in sensorimotor therapy?
24. How can visual stimuli be used in sensorimotor therapy.?
25. Describe how neurolinguistic programming can be used in occupational therapy.
26. How does prolonged psychological stress contribute to dysfunction?
27. Name four therapeutic modalities for prolonged stress reactions.

28. How does the endocrine system contribute to the fight or flight response?
29. What have computerized tomography and metabolic mapping revealed about brain cell activity?
30. Describe how cutaneous stimulation might alleviate pain?
31. How might disturbances in fascia disrupt physical mobility?
32. What are three therapeutic benefits of acupressure?
33. Describe trigger points and how they may contribute to pain.
34. List three possible benefits of background music.
35. Define psychoneuroimmunology.

REFERENCES

1. Afifi A and Bergman R: Basic neuroscience, Baltimore, 1980. Urban & Schwarzenberg, Inc.
2. Andrasik F: Relaxation and biofeedback for chronic headaches. In Holzman A and Turk K, editors: Pain management: a handbook of psychological approaches, New York, 1986, Pergamon Press, pp. 213-239.
3. Appelberg B, Beson P, and LaPorte Y: Effects of dynamic and static fusimotor gamma fibers on the responses of primary and secondary endings, J Physiol 177:29, 1965.
4. Ayres J: The development of sensory integrative theory and practice, Dubuque, 1974, Kendall/Hunt Publishing Co.
5. Bach-y-Rita P, editor: Recovery of function: theoretical considerations for brain injury rehabilitation, Baltimore, 1980, University Park Press.
6. Bach-y-Rita P: Central nervous system lesions: sprouting and unmasking in rehabilitation Arch Phys Med Rehabil 62:413, 1981.
7. Balian R and Riggs H: Myelination of the brain in the newborn, Philadelphia, 1969, JB Lippincott Co.
8. Bandler R and Grinder J: The structure of magic, Palo Alto, 1975, Science & Behavior Books.
9. Banning MR and Nelson DL: The effects of activity elicited

humor and group structure on group cohesion and affective responses, J Occup Ther 41(8):510, 1987.
10. Barnes D: Brain architecture: beyond genes, Research News, 233:1 155-156, 1986.
11. Barnes J: Benefits of myofascial release. cranio-sacral therapy explained, Physical Therapy Forum 3(35):2, 1984.
12. Barr M: The human nervous system, ed 2, New York, 1974, Harper & Row Publishers, Inc.
13. Basbaum A, Clanton C and Fields H: Opiate and stimulus produced analgesia: functional anatomy of a medullospinal pathway, Proc Natl Acad Sci USA 73:4685, 1976.
14. Basbaum A and Fields H: Endogenous pain control mechanisms: review and hypothesis, Ann Neurol 4:451, 1978.
15. Basmajian J: Primary anatomy, ed 7, Baltimore, 1976, The Williams & Wilkins Co.
16. Battista J: The holistic paradigm and general systems theory, Gen Systems J, 22, 65, 1977.
17. Becker BO and Selden G: The body electric electromagnetism and the foundation of life, New York, 1985, William Morrow & Co.
18. Bergland R: Fabric of mind, New York, 1986, Viking Press.
19. Boguslawski M: Therapeutic touch: a facilitator of pain relief. Topics Clin Nurs 2(1):27, 1980.
20. Bower B: The face of emotion, Science News, 128:12, 1985.
21. Brown D: Neurosciences for allied health therapies, St. Louis, 1980, The CV Mosby Co.
22. Brudny J, et al: Helping hemiparetics to help themselves: sensory feedback therapy, JAMA 241:814, 1979.
23. Bry A: Visualization: directing the movies of the mind. New York, 1979, Barnes & Noble Books.
24. Chusid J: Correlative neuroanatomy and functional neurology, ed 18, Los Altos, CA, 1982, Lange Medical Publications.

25. Clark R: Clinical neuroanatomy and neurophysiology, ed 5, Philadelphia, 1975, FA Davis Co.

26. Cock J: The therapeutic use of music: a literature review. Nurs Forum, 20(3):252, 1981.

27. Colligan D: Wholemind, Omni 10(1):125, 1987.

28. Davis J: Endorphins, New York, 1983, Dial/Doubleday Books.

29. Diamond M: Brain research and its implication for education, California Infomedix Audiocassette, Physiology-Anatomy Department, University of California—Berkeley, 1987.

30. Downie P: Cash's textbook of neurology for physiotherapists, ed 4, Philadelphia, 1986, JB Lippincott Co.

31. Farber S: Neurorehabilitation: a multisensory approach, Philadelphia, 1982, WB Saunders Co.

32. Feigenson JS: Stroke rehabilitation: effectiveness, benefits and cost: some practical considerations, Stroke 10:1, 1979 (editorial).

33. Fox E and Melzack R: Comparison of transcutaneous electrical stimulation and acupuncture in the treatment of chronic pain, Adv Pain Research Ther 2:797, 1976.

34. Gardner E: Fundamentals of neurology, ed 6, Philadelphia, 1975, WB Saunders Co.

35. Garfinkel A: Nonlinear dynamics of movement patterns, Am J Physiol, 245:438, 1984.

36. Gartland J: Fundamentals of orthopaedics, ed 3, Philadelphia, 1979, WB Saunders Co.

37. Gellhorn E: Principles of autonomic-somatic integration, Minneapolis, 1967, University of Minnesota Press.

38. Gernandy B and Harlow A: Spinal motor responses to acoustic stimulation. Exp Neurol 10:52, 1964.

39. Gill A: Polarity therapy-integration of the senses through energy balancing and release. Physical Disabilities Special Interest Section Newsletter, American Occupational Therapy Association, vol 7:1, 1985.

40. Gilman S and Winans S: Manter and Gatz's essentials of clinical neuroanatomy and neurophysiology, ed 6, Philadelphia, 1982, FA Davis Co.

41. Gilroy J and Meyer JS: Medical neurology, ed 3, New York, 1979, Macmillan Publishing Co, Inc.

42. Golberg S: Clinical neuroanatomy made ridiculously simple, Miami, 1979, Medical Master, Inc.

43. Goodwin GM, McCloskey DI, and Matthews P: The contribution of muscle afferents to kinesthesia shown by vibration illusions of movement and by the effects of paralyzing joint afferents, Brain 95:705, 1972.

44. Goss CM: Gray's anatomy, ed 28, Philadelphia, 1970, Lea & Febiger.

45. Greenough W: Experimental modification of the developing brain, Am Sci 63:30, 1975.

46. Greenberg JH and Reivich M: Metabolic mapping of functional activity in human subjects with the fluorodeoxyglucose technique, Science, 212:678, 1981.

47. Grad B: Some biological effects of the laying on of hands: a review of experiments with animals and plants. J Am Soc Phys Research, 59:95, 1965.

48. Guyton A: Structure and function of the nervous system, Philadelphia, 1972, WB Saunders Co.

49. Hagbarth KE: Excitatory and inhibitory skin areas for flexor and extensor motoneurons, Acta Physiol Scand 26:1, 1952.

50. Hammer S: The mind as healer, Science Digest, 47-49, 1984.

51. Hughes J: Isolation of an endogenous compound from the brain with pharmacological properties similar to morphine, Brain Res 88:295, 1975.

52. Huss J: Sensorimotor treatment approaches. In Hopkins HL and Smith HD, editors: Willard and Spackman's occupational therapy, ed 6, Philadelphia, 1983, JB Lippincott Co.

53. Jacob S and Francone C: Structure and function in man, Philadelphia, 1974, WB Saunders Co.

54. Keller E and Bzdek V: Effects of therapeutic touch on tension headache pain, Nurs Research 4(35):101, 1986.

55. Kottke F, Stillwell K, and Lehmann J: Krusen's handbook of physical medicine and rehabilitation, ed 3, Philadelphia, 1982, WB Saunders Co.

56. Knowles R: Through neurolinguistic programming, Am J Nurs 83:1010, 1983.

57. Krieger D, Peper E, Ancoli S: Physiologic indices of therapeutic touch, Am J Nurs 79(4)660, 1979.

58. Krieger D: Healing by the laying-on of hands as a facilitator of bioenergetic change: the response of in-vivo human hemoglobin, Int J Psychoenergetic Systems 1:121, 1976.

59. Krieger D: Therapeutic touch: searching for evidence of physiological change, Am J Nurs 79:660, 1979.

60. Locke S and Colligan D: Mind cures, OMNI: 7(7)44, 1985.

61. Lundberg JM and Hokfelt T: Coexistence of peptides and classical neurotransmitters, Trends Neurosci 6(8):325, 1983.

62. Matthews PBC: Mammalian muscle receptors and their central actions, London, 1973, Edward Arnold (Publishers), Ltd.

63. McCloskey DI: Kinesthetic sensibility, Physiol Rev 58:763, 1978.

64. McGunigle-Reardon D and Bell G: Effects of sedative and stimulative music on activity levels. Am J Ment Defic 75(2):156, 1970.

65. Melzack R: Trigger points and acupuncture points for pain: correlation and implications, Pain, 3:3, 1977.

66. Melzack R: Myofascial trigger points: relationship to acupuncture and mechanisms of pain, Arch Phys Med Rehabil 82:47, 1981.

67. Merzennich M: The organization of neurotransmitters and receptors, Science 225:820, 1984.

68. Montagu A: Touching: the human significance of the skin, ed 2, San Francisco, 1978, Harper & Row, Publishers, Inc.

69. Moore J: A new look at the nervous system in relation to rehabilitation techniques, Am J Occup Ther 22:6, 1965.

70. Moore J: The Golgi tendon organ and the muscle spindle, Am J Occup Ther 28:7, 1974.

71. Moore J: Recovery potentials following CNS lesions: a brief historical perspective in relationship to modern research data on neuroplasticity. Am J Occup Ther 40(7):459, 1986.

72. Moore JC: Neuroanatomical considerations relating to recovery of function: theoretical considerations for brain injury rehabilitation. Baltimore, 1980, University Park Press.

73. Mountcastle VB: Medical physiology, ed 14, St Louis, 1980, The CV Mosby Co.

74. Noback C: The human nervous system, basic principles of neurophysiology, ed 2, New York, 1975, McGraw-Hill Book Co.

75. Nolte J: The human brain: an introduction to its functional anatomy, St Louis, 1981, The CV Mosby Co.

76. Ornstein R: The Amazing Brain, Boston, 1984, Houghton-Mifflin Co.

77. Pendleton B and Mehling B: Relax with self' therap/ease, New York, 1984, Prentice Hall Press.

78. Penfield W and Jasper H: Epilepsy and the functional anatomy of the human brain, Boston, 1954, Little, Brown & Co.

79. Pert C: Brain and biochemistry, Washington, 3-N256 NIMH Audiocassette, Soundworks Box 75890, Washington (Brain/Mind Bulletin), 1986.

80. Phelps ME, Keihl DE and Maggiotta JC: Metabolic mapping of the brain's response to visual stimulation: studies in humans, Science 211(27):1445, 1981.

81. Phelps M and Kuhl D: Sex and handedness differences in cerebral blood flow during rest and cognitive activity, Science 217:13, 1982.

82. Piccard C and Olivier A: Sensory cortical tongue representation in man, J Neurosurg 59:781, 1983.

83. Prudden B: Pain erasure, New York, 1977, Ballantine Books.

84. Randolph G: Therapeutic and physical touch: physiological response to stressful stimuli, Nurs Research 33(1):33, 1984.

85. Rausch P: A tactile and kinesthetic stimulation program for primative infants, In Brown C, editor: The many facets of touch. (special issue), 1984, Johnson & Johnson.

86. Rosner BS: Recovery of function and localization of function in historical perspective. In Stein DG, Rosen JJ, and Butlers N, editors: Plasticity and recovery of function in the central nervous system, New York, 1974, Academic Press, Inc.

87. Schmidt R: Sensory physiology, New York, 1977, Springer-Verlag New York, Inc.

88. Schmidt R: Fundamentals of neurophysiology, New York, 1978, Springer-Verlag New York, Inc.

89. Scholz J and Campbell S: Muscle spindles and the regulation of movement, Phys Ther 60:1416, 1980.

90. Scott T: The use of music to reduce hyperactivity in children. Am J Orthopsych 40(4):677, 1970.

91. Selkurt EE: Basic physiology for the health sciences, ed 2, Boston, 1982, Little, Brown & Co.

92. Smith F: Inner bridges: a guide to energy movement and body structure, Atlanta, Humanics, Limited, 26, 114, 1986.

93. Snyder S: Neurosciences: in integrated discipline, Science 225:4668, 1984.

94. Taubes G: An electrifying possibility. Discover, 7(4):22, 1986.

95. Teeguarden I: Acupressure way of health: Jin Shin Do. Tokyo, 1977, Japan Publications.

96. Thompson R: The neurobiology of learning and memory, Science, 233:941, 1986.

97. Travell J: Myofacial trigger points: clinical review In Bonica JJ and Alber-Fessard DG: Advances in pain therapy and research, vol I, New York, 1976, Raven Press.

98. Vallbo A, Hagbarth H, and Torebjard H: Somatosensory, proprioception sympathetic activity in human peripheral nerves, Physiol Rev 59:919, 1979.

99. Van Deusen J and Harlowe D: The efficacy of the ROM dance program for adults with rheumatoid arthritis, Am J Occup Ther 41(2)90:1987.

100. Van Leir P: Painful hemiplegic shoulder, Occup Ther Forum 2(38):3, 1987.

101. Vierck CJ: Alterations of spatiotactile discrimination after lesions of primate spinal cord, Brain Res 58:69, 1973.

102. Wechsler R: A new prescription: mind over malady, Discover 2(8):50, 1987.

103. Weiss S: Psychophysiological effects of caregiver touch on incidence of cardiac dysrhythmia. Heart Lung 15(5):495, 1986.

104. Wensel L: Acupuncture in medical practice, Reston, VA, 1980, Reston Publishing Co, Inc.

105. Werner JK: Neuroscience: a clinical perspective, Philadelphia, 1980, WB Saunders Co.

106. Williams P and Warwick R: Functional neuroanatomy of man, ed 35, Philadelphia, 1975, WB Saunders Co.

107. Wolf SL: EMG biofeedback applications in physical rehabilitation: an overview. Physiotherapy 31:65, 1979.

108. Zajonic R: The face of emotion. Science 128(4):1443, 1985.

109. Zajonic RB: Emotional and facial efference: a theory reclaimed, Science 228:15, 1985.

18 The Rood approach to the treatment of neuromuscular dysfunction

GUY L. McCORMACK

Margaret S. Rood was trained and registered in both occupational and physical therapy. Her theory originated in the 1940s and underwent many revisions before she died and it continues to do so today. She did not write extensively; she seemed to prefer clinical teaching to disseminate her ideas. Most of the literature that describes the Rood approach is based on interpretations by accomplished therapists. It is postulated that Rood may have been ahead of her time. She integrated neurophysiologic and developmental literature with clinical observations. At times her level of understanding was beyond the comprehension of the average clinician. Despite the controversy about the efficacy of Rood's techniques, current research in the neurosciences continues to support the importance of sensory stimulation.

Many knowledgeabe therapists, such as Shereen Farber, Jean Ayres, Joy Huss, Margot Heininger, and Shirley Randolph, have been greatly influenced by Rood's work. The purpose of this chapter is to summarize the major tenets of Rood's theory and to suggest new considerations for the use of sensory stimulation in occupational therapy.

Rood's basic hypothesis may be paraphrased as appropriate sensory stimulation can elicit specific motor responses. Rood combined controlled sensory stimulation with a sequence of positions and activities of normal ontogenetic motor development to achieve purposeful muscular responses.[54]

Thus, according to Rood, muscle action can be "activated, facilitated and inhibited through the sensory system."[85,86]

GOALS

The goals of Rood's theory are summarized in the following discussion.

Normalize Muscle Tone

Patients with neurologic dysfunction may have muscle tone ranging from hypertonic to hypotonic. Controlled muscle tone is a prerequisite to movement. Normal muscle tone flows smoothly and is constantly changing during a motor act. For example, to turn on the ignition of a car, one has to have fairly good eye-hand coordination, postural control of the trunk muscles, coinnervation of the proximal arm muscles, forearm pronation and supination, and moderately fine prehension and dexterity in the hands. Subsequently, the demands placed on the various muscle groups are different. Rood recognized this when she stated, "muscles have different duties," with some muscles predominantly used for heavy work and others for light work. The light work muscles (mobilizers) are primarily the flexors and adductors used for skilled movement patterns. The heavy work muscles (stabilizers) are principally the extensors and abductors used for postural support[41] (Table 18-1).

Rood also believed that a voluntary motor act is based on inherent reflexes and on modification of those reflexes at higher centers.[85] Therefore she began therapy by eliciting motor responses on a reflex level and incorporating developmental patterns to augment the motor response. The heavy work muscles are activated before the light work muscles except for the feeding and speech muscles.[84]

Treatment Begins at the Developmental Level of Functioning

The patient is evaluated developmentally and treated in a sequential manner. The patient does not proceed to the next level of sensorimotor development until some measure of voluntary (supraspinal) control is achieved. This principle follows the cephalocaudal rule. Treatment begins from the head and proceeds downward segment by segment from the proximal to the distal to the sacral area. The flexors are stimulated first, the extensors second, the adductors third, and the abductors last.[96]

Movement is Directed Toward a Purposeful Goal

Rood realized that the patient's motivation plays an important role in rehabilitation. The patient must first accept the activity as a meaningful event. Second, the patient must develop a subcortical program in his or her central nervous system (CNS) to perform a motor act in a coordinated manner.

Table 18-1 Characteristics of Heavy Work and Light Work Muscles

Characteristics	Heavy work (stabilizers)	Light work (mobilizers)
Function	Tonic position cocontraction (holding patterns and maintenance of posture)	Phasic movement (repetitive or rhythmic patterns of distal musculature and skilled movement)
Anatomy	Deep, close to bone and medial axis of body; fan-shaped with broad attachments	More superficial and lateral to midline axis; fusiform shaped, tendinous distal attachment
Fibers	Red fibers (aerobic); run obliquely, rich blood supply, low metabolic cost	White fibers (anaerobic), more energy; run parallel with long axis of muscle, high metabolic cost
Joints	Cross one major joint (uniarthrodial)	Cross two or more joints (multiarthrodial)
Specific muscles	Deep tonic extensors of neck and trunk, scapular adductors (rhomboid major and minor), downward rotators	Two joint extensors (longhead of the triceps brachii, gastrocnemius, flexors, and adductors)
Innervation	More reflexive (tonic) under extrapyramidal, vestibulospinal, reticulospinal, and medial motor system	More voluntary or willed under lateral corticospinal and rubrospinal tracts
Facilitation	Quick stretch, heavy joint compression and traction, pressure to skin surfaces bearing weight, static position of head in space; saccule and utricle of vestibular system	Quick stretch, nocioceptive stimuli light joint compression and traction, vibration, movement of head in space, e.g., semicircular canals of vestibular system
Exercise	Isometric resistance	Isometric or isotonic resistance
Testing	Inversion, joint compression of more than body weight	Quick stretch and light moving touch
Muscle innervation	Greater number of group II and fewer Golgi tendon organs	Greater number of Ia afferents

Modified from Farber S: Sensorimotor evaluation and treatment procedures for allied health personnel, Indianapolis, 1974, Indiana University and Purdue University at Indianapolis Medical Center; Rood M: Occupational therapy in the treatment of the cerebral palsied, Phys Ther Rev 32:220, 1952; Stockmeyer S: An interpretation of the approach of Rood to the treatment of neuromuscular dysfunction, NUSTEP proceedings, Am J Phys Med 46:900, 1967; Goff B: The Rood approach in Cash's textbook of neurology for physiotherapists, 4th ed, Philadelphia, 1986, JB Lippincott Co.

Neurologically, the pyramidal system (corticospinal) is used to control reflex activity and to perform isolated voluntary acts.[58] However, the coordination of the agonist muscle, antagonist muscle, and synergies is a function of the extrapyramidal system. Complex motor patterns rely on subcortical centers for modification and correction so that the cortex can concentrate on the purpose of the act.[22] In addition, when the patient performs a willed movement with an intended goal, more neurons throughout the nervous system must discharge to initiate the task.[88]

Repetition is Necessary for the Training of Muscular Responses

The importance of repetition to achieve coordination has been emphasized by Kottke.[58,59] Thousands of repetitions are required to formulate *engrams*. Engrams are interneuronal circuits involving specific neurons and muscles to perform a pattern of motor activity. Repetition, however, can be monotonous. Therefore activities that incorporate similar motor patterns add purpose and value to the exercise.

PRINCIPLES OF TREATMENT

In a journal article in 1956 Rood suggested four principles in the treatment of neuromuscular dysfunction.[85] Following is an interpretation of those principles.

Tonic Neck and Labyrinthine Reflexes Can Assist or Retard the Effects of Sensory Stimulation

The tonic neck receptors lie in the muscles and skin of the neck region and respond to changes in the relationship of the head to the neck. The tonic neck reflexes (TNR) are divided into symmetric and asymmetric.[49,52] According to Rood, the TNRs have a modifying influence on extensor tone, especially the "postural part." Fukuda studied postural reflexes in humans and offered the following summary.[35]

Dorsiflexion of the neck extends the upper extremities and flexes the lower extremities. Ventral flexion of the neck flexes the upper extremities and extends the lower extremities. Torsion or rotation of the neck toward one shoulder produces an increase in the extensor tone of the upper and lower extremities on the face side of that shoulder.

The labyrinthine receptors lie in the ampullae of the semicircular canals and in the vestibule.[22] These receptors are affected by the "position of the head in relation to gravity." Rood's description of labyrinthine influences on posture is not entirely clear.[84-86]

The following is a composite summary from several authors and is illustrated in Fig. 18-1 for clarification. In the normal upright bipedal stance (180°) (Fig. 18-1, A) TNR and tonic labyrinthine reflexes (TLR) cause slight flexion of the elbow joint and extension of the lower limbs.[82] As the face moves clockwise to the quadruped position, the head is slightly tilted, decreasing the influences of the TNR and TLR, [59] (Fig. 18-1, B).

In this position the vertebral column is almost horizontal, eliminating gravitational pressure on the intervertebral joints, and the face is looking downward, which reduces the activity of the TLR. In addition, weight-bearing is evenly distributed between the upper and lower extremities. If the subject assumes the quadruped position (Fig. 18-1, C) (−90°) in the horizontal plane and flexes or extends his neck, the TNRs prevail and the TLRs diminish.[77,82,98] If the subject assumes a position in which the head is lower than the shoulders (Fig. 18-1, D), extensor tone increases in selected muscles (extensor carpi ulnaris, extensor carpi radialis, and soleus).[95] A position of total inversion (Fig. 18-1, E) would elicit righting reactions,[82,95,98]

whereas a supine position with the head below the horizontal plane (Fig. 18-1, F and G) constitutes a combined TNR and TLR.[55] A patient in the supine-semireclining position (Fig. 18-1, H) at 60° above horizontal is in a position that maximizes the static TLR.[59] This position causes abduction, flexion, and external rotation of the arms and increased extensor tone in the trunk and lower extremities. Hellenbrant and his associates reported that this supine head-up position (45° to 60° above horizontal) suppresses the TNR.[49,50]

Rood suggested that if the subject is lying on the side with the ear toward the earth's surface, "the arm and leg of the down side will exhibit extensor tone while the up side will be predominated by flexor tone."[85] The side-lying position is also used for the neurologically impaired patient to reduce the influences of the TLR and TNR.[41]

Stimulation of Specific Receptors Can Produce Three Major Reactions

The three major reactions that can be produced by stimulation of specific receptors are homeostatic responses via the autonomic nervous system, reflexive-protective responses via spinal and brain stem circuits and adaptive responses that require greater integration of all regions of the nervous system.[3,43,100]

In 1970 Rood presented four rules of sensory input to clarify the procedure.[96] The first rule is "A fast

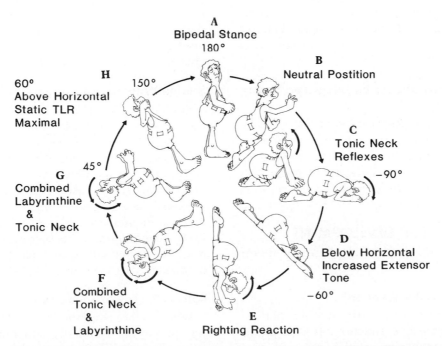

Fig. 18-1. Composite summary: tonic labyrinthine reflexes. **A,** Bipedal stance; **B,** neutral position; **C,** tonic neck reflexes (TNR); **D,** below horizontal increased extensor tone; **E,** righting reaction; **F,** combined TNR and TLR; **G,** combined TLR and TNR; **H,** sixty degrees above horizontal static TLR maximum.

brief stimulus produces a large synchronous motor output. This type of stimulus is used to confirm that the reflex arc is intact." The second rule is "A fast repetitive sensory input produces a maintained response." A stimulus, such as fast brushing with a battery-operated brush, activates nonspecific receptors that transmit impulses along the C fibers and probably the gamma fibers.[99] According to Rood, this stimulus feeds into the fusimotor system that can drive the alpha motor neuron of the muscle. The third rule is "A maintained sensory input produces a maintained response." The force of gravity is an example of a maintained sensory input. Gravity is an ever-present force that has a constant effect on the sensory system. Whether standing, sitting, or lying, the exteroceptors of the skin are in contact with a surface, thus discharging impulses into the nervous system to reinforce the presence of gravity.[97]

The fourth rule is "Slow, rhythmical, repetitive sensory input deactivates body and mind." Any constant low-frequency stimuli, such as slow rocking in an easy chair, soft music, or even firm pressure to the upper lip, abdomen, soles of the feet or palms of the hands, activates the parasympathetic system, causing a generalized calming effect.

Muscles Have Different Duties

Some muscles predominate as stabilizers, whereas other muscles undertake the duties of mobilization. According to Rood, both groups have distinct functions and characteristics. Table 18-1 is a summary of the characteristics of the heavy work and light work muscles.

Heavy Work Muscles Should be Integrated Before Light Work Muscles

The principle of integrating heavy work muscles before light work muscles primarily refers to the use of the upper extremities. For example, fine fingertip manipulation is not functional if the proximal muscles are not strong enough to lift or stabilize the position of the arms.

SEQUENCE OF MOTOR DEVELOPMENT

Rood proposed four sequential phases of motor control.[6,85,86]

Reciprocal Inhibition (Innervation)

Reciprocal inhibition is an early mobility pattern that subserves a protective function. It is a phasic (quick) type of movement that requires contraction of the agonist muscle as the antagonist muscle relaxes. This basic movement pattern is primarily a reflex governed by spinal and supraspinal centers.

Cocontraction (Coinnervation)

Cocontraction or coinnervation provides stability and is considered to be a tonic (static) pattern. This provides the ability to hold a position or an object for a longer duration. Cocontraction is defined as simultaneous contraction of the agonist muscle and antagonist muscle with the antagonist supreme.[34,48]

Heavy Work

Heavy work is described by Stockmeyer as "mobility superimposed on stability."[96] In this pattern the proximal muscles contract and move, and the distal segment is fixed. A good example is creeping. In the quadruped position the distal segments, wrist, and ankles are in a fixed position. The proximal joints, such as the neck and thorax, are stable whereas the shoulder and hip girdles are free to move.

Skill

Skill is the highest level of motor control and combines the effort of mobility and stability.[85] To execute a skilled pattern, the proximal segment is stabilized while the distal segment moves freely. The art of oil painting demonstrates this pattern as the artist stands back from the canvas, holds his or her arm at full length, and manipulates the brush freely in the hand.

ONTOGENETIC MOTOR PATTERNS

The sequence of motor development described previously occurs as the patient is put through the skeletal function sequence that Rood called ontogenetic motor patterns.[41] The eight ontogenetic motor patterns are briefly described and related to their neurologic benefits and are illustrated in Fig. 18-2.

Supine Withdrawal (Supine Flexion)

Supine withdrawal is a total flexion response toward the vertebral level of T10. This is a protective position because the flexion of the neck and the crossing of the arms and legs protects the anterior surface of the body. This is a mobility posture requiring reciprocal innervation. Yet it also requires heavy work of the proximal muscles and trunk.[85] Therapeutically, supine withdrawal aids in the integration of the TLR. Rood recommended this pattern for patients who do not have reciprocal flexion pattern and for patients dominated by extensor tone (Fig. 18-2, *A*).

Roll Over (Toward Side Lying)

When rolling over, the arm and leg flex on the same side of the body. This is a mobility pattern for the extremities and activates the lateral trunk musculature.[96] This pattern is encouraged for patients who are dominated by tonic reflex patterns in the supine position. The rolling action also stimulates the semi-

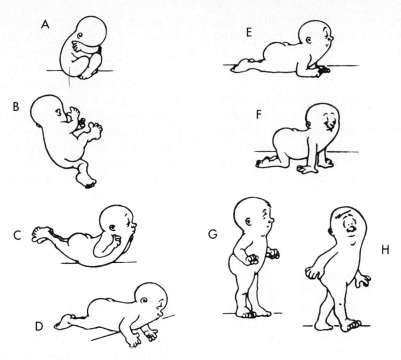

Fig. 18-2. Ontogenic motor patterns. **A,** Supine withdrawal; **B,** roll over toward side lying; **C,** pivot prone; **D,** neck cocontraction; **E,** prone on elbows; **F,** quadruped pattern; **G,** static standing; **H,** walking.

circular canals, which in turn activate the neck and extraocular muscles (Fig. 18-2, *B*).

Pivot Prone (Prone Extension)

The pivot-prone position demands a full range of extension of the neck, shoulders, trunk, and lower extremities. This pattern has been called both a mobility pattern and a stability pattern. The position is difficult to assume and hold. Therefore it plays an important role in preparation for stability of the extensor muscles in the upright position. The pivot-prone position has been associated with the labyrinthine righting reaction of the head. The ability to maintain the position indicates integration of the symmetric TNRs and the TLRs (Fig. 18-2, *C*).

Neck Cocontraction (Coinnervation)

Neck cocontraction is the first real stability pattern. In keeping with the cervicocaudal rule and cervicorostral rule, cocontraction of the neck precedes cocontraction of the trunk and extremities. As the head bobs up and down, the extensors and rotators are stretched. This action is said to activate both flexors and deep tonic extensors of the neck.[85] However, it is important to make sure the neck flexors are well established before the prone position is assumed. To raise the head against gravity, the patient needs to have good cocontraction of the flexors and extensors

of the neck.[33] Neurologically, this pattern elicits the tonic labyrinthine righting reaction when the face is perpendicular to the floor. As the head flexes, it stretches the proprioceptors in the neck and upper trapezius, causing them to contract against the forces of gravity.[77,82,83] This position also promotes neck stability and extraocular control (Fig. 18-2, *D*).

On Elbows (Prone on Elbows)

Following cocontraction of the neck and prone extension, weight bearing on the elbows is the next pattern to achieve. Bearing weight on the elbows stretches the upper trunk musculature to influence stability of the scapular and glenohumeral regions. This position gives the patient better visibility of the environment and an opportunity to shift weight from side to side. It is also inhibitory to the symmetric TNR[3] (Fig. 18-2, *E*).

All Fours (Quadruped Position)

The quadruped position follows stability of the neck and shoulders. The lower trunk and lower extremities are brought into a cocontraction pattern. Initially the position is static and the abdomen may sag at the T10 level, causing stretching of the trunk and limb girdles. This stretching develops cocontraction of the trunk flexors and extensors. Eventually weight shifting forward, backward, side to side, and diagonally provides a mobility superimposed on the stability phase. The weight shifting may be preparatory to equilibrium responses (Fig. 18-2, *F*).

Static Standing

Assuming the upright bipedal position, static standing is thought to be a skill of the upper trunk because it frees the upper extremities for prehension and manipulation.[96] At first, weight is equally distributed on both legs and then weight shifting begins. This position brings in higher level integration, such as righting reactions and equilibrium reactions (Fig. 18-2, *G*).

Walking

The gait pattern unites skill, mobility, and stability. According to Murray, normal locomotion entails the ability to support the body weight, maintain balance, and execute the stepping motion.[75] Walking includes a stance phase, push off, swing, heel strike, and stride length.[96] Walking is a sophisticated process requiring coordinated movement patterns of various parts of the body (Fig. 18-2, *H*).

SPECIFIC FACILITATION TECHNIQUES USED IN TREATMENT
Cutaneous Facilitation

Cutaneous facilitation can be used to stimulate the exteroceptors of the skin.[3,81,100] *Exteroceptors* are those end organs located immediately under the skin in subcutaneous tissues or in external mucous membranes.[102] Exteroceptors respond to stimuli arising from the external environment. In general, the exteroceptive system subserves protective withdrawal responses and produces states of alertness and rapid movements of the limbs.[6,16,31] The principal sensory modalities transmitted by the exteroceptive system are pain, temperature, and touch. These modalities are transmitted to the spinal cord along A delta (group III) and C fibers (group IV), which are thin, have little or no myelination, and are slow conductors. Nondiscriminative exteroceptive impulses travel to higher centers of the CNS by way of the spinothalamic and spinoreticular tracts. The more discriminative exteroceptive stimuli, vibration, stereognosis, and fine touch (conscious proprioception), ascend along the lemniscal (dorsal) columns.[2,31,34] Exteroceptive stimuli, such as icing and brushing, should be used judiciously because they have a profound effect on the reticular activating system and the autonomic nervous system.[48] Specific techniques of cutaneous facilitation are described later.

LIGHT MOVING TOUCH. Touch is important for normal growth and development.[72] Light touch stimuli send input to limbic structures and have been shown to increase corticosteroid levels in the bloodstream.[66,92] Corticosteroids aid in increasing resistance against disease, tissue repair, and fluid and electrolyte balance.[3,21] Rood used a light moving touch or stroking of the skin to activate the superficial mobilizing muscles. These muscles are classified as the light work group that perform skilled tasks.[83,84,96] Neurologically, the light stroke stimulus activates low threshold hair end organs and free nerve endings. The stimuli send impulses along A delta size sensory fibers, which synapse with the fusimotor system. As a result, light moving touch causes reciprocal innervation, which is clinically seen as a phasic withdrawal response.[77] Light moving touch is applied with the fingertip, camel hair brush, or cotton swab.

Originally, the frequency of the touch stimulus was done "two times per second and at least ten times, and then repeated three to five times."[85] The formula now suggested is to apply three to five strokes and allow 30 seconds to elapse between strokes.[34,48] The 30-second rest period is important because it prevents a presynaptic inhibitory response called *primary afferent depolarization*. This is a synaptic mechanism that prevents overstimulation.[34,88] Light moving touch is applied to the facial region after firm pressure is maintained on the upper lip.[33] This causes a generalized inhibitory response before the light moving stimulus is applied to the perioral region. The first area stimulated is the area from the nose to the chin (perioral midline). The stimulus may have to be applied several times before a response is elicited. In infants the response may cause a flexion pattern of the upper and perhaps the lower extremities.[34] A similar type of stimulus is to apply light stroking from the corner of the lip to the cheek (perioral lateral). This stimulus activates superficial musculature of the neck, and the head tilts laterally toward the side of the stimulus. In adults a unilateral flexion pattern can be facilitated by applying a light moving touch to the navel region or dermatome T10.[34,96] The stimulus is applied several times in a midline to lateral direction. Light moving touch can also be applied to the dorsal web spaces of the fingers and toes to elicit a withdrawal pattern of the extremities. More rapid results may be obtained if light moving touch is applied to the tips of the fingers or soles of the feet because it facilitates a "tickle withdrawal response" of greater magnitude.[84,100]

FAST BRUSHING. In 1964 Rood introduced a battery-operated brush to stimulate the C fibers, which send many collaterals to the reticular activating system.[88,92] The stimulation to this system was reported to have its maximal effect 30 minutes after stimulation.[84] Therefore fast brushing was used be-

Table 18-2 Dermatomes

Spinal segment	Dermatome location	Muscles facilitated	Function
CN V	Anterior facial region	Mastication	Ingestion
C3	Neck region	Sternocleidomastoid, upper trapezius	Head control
C4	Upper shoulder region	Trapezius (diaphragm)	Head control
C5	Lateral aspect of shoulder	Deltoid, biceps, rhomboid major and minor	Elbow flexion
C6	Thumb and radial forearm	Extensor carpi radialis, biceps	Shoulder abduction wrist extension
C7	Middle finger	Triceps, extensors of wrist and fingers	Wrist flexion, finger extension
C8	Little finger, ulnar forearm	Flexor of wrist and fingers	C8 finger flexion
T1	Axilla and proximal medial arm	Hand intrinsics	Abduction and adduction of fingers
T2-12	Thorax	Intercostals	Respiration
L1-2	Inside of thigh	Cremasteric reflex, accessory muscles	Elevation of scrotum
T4,T6	Nipple line	Intercostals	Respiration
T7-11	Midchest region Lower rib	Abdominal wall, abdominal muscles	T5-7 superficial abdominal reflex
T10	Umbilicus	Psoas, iliacus	Leg flexion
L2	Proximal anterior thigh	Iliopsoas, adductors of thigh	Reflex voiding
L3-4	Anterior knee	Quadriceps, tibialis anterior, detrusor urinae	Hip flexion, extensors of knee, abductors of thigh
L5	Great toe	Lateral hamstrings	Flexion at knee, toe extension
L5-S1	Foot region	Gastrocnemius, soleus, extensor digitorum longus	Flexor withdrawal, urinary retention
S2	Narrow band of posterior thigh	Small muscles of foot (flexor digitorum, flexor hallucis)	Bladder retention

fore all other forms of stimulation because of its prolonged latency effect. Spicer and Matyas compared brushing and icing as therapeutic modalities.[94] They found brushing to be a better stimulus than icing, but the greatest effect occurs during the time the stimulation is applied. Neurologically, fast brushing is a nonspecific, high-intensity stimulus that increases the fusimotor activity of selected muscles.[59,77] The key to fast brushing is to apply it over the dermatomes of the same segment that supplies the muscle (myotome) to be facilitated.[41,96] Fig. 18-3 shows the anterior and posterior distribution of the dermatomes. Table 18-2 shows the spinal segment, the location of the dermatome, the muscles facilitated at the spinal level, and the primary function. The stimulus is applied for 3 to 5 seconds and repeated after 30 seconds have elapsed.[86] Fast brushing can be applied adjacent to the vertebral column over the posterior primary rami to facilitate the deep tonic muscles of the back[96] (Figs. 18-4 and 18-5). Heininger and Randolph have sug-

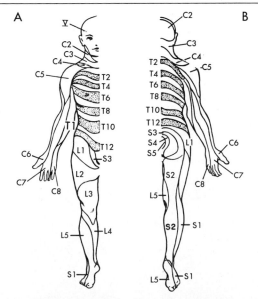

Fig. 18-3. A and **B,** Dermatomes. From Clark RG: Clinical neuroanatomy and neurophysiology, ed 5, Philadelphia, 1975, FA Davis Co.

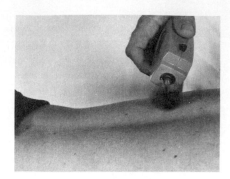

Fig. 18-4. Fast brushing to deep proximal muscles.

gested that the inverted position is more effective for this purpose.[48] The anterior primary rami can also be brushed to tonically facilitate the superficial muscles. Again the stimulus is applied to the dermatomal segment (T2 to T12) that corresponds to specific muscle groups.[85] Brushing appears to work best on isolated muscle groups where the dermatome lies over the muscle to be facilitated.[54]

Fast brushing is contraindicated for certain areas of the skin. The outer ring of the trigeminal nerve where C2 dermatome begins has a tremendous overlap of free nerve endings.[34,36] This area also has an extensive input to the reticular system. These fibers also transmit to the parasympathetic branch of the autonomic nervous system, causing a generalized inhibitory response.[34,100] Facial brushing should be avoided on patients with high cervical spinal cord or brain stem injuries because of autonomic dysreflexia and the possibility of inducing a coma.[11]

The pinna of the ear also has an abundant nerve supply. It receives sensory fibers from the trigeminal, facial, and vagus cranial nerves as well as the auricular and occipital nerves that surface from C2 and C3 spinal segments.[23,26,27] Dermatomal skin areas L1 and L2 connect with sympathetic fibers in the spinal cord and innervate the detrussor urinae. Fast brushing to this area can cause voiding. Stimulation to dermatomes S2 to S4 can improve bladder retention in in-

continent patients. This technique appears to work as an overflow mechanism similar to the referred pain phenomenon. The smooth muscle of the bladder responds to a stretch reflex controlled by the proprioceptors in its wall.[39] Fast brushing over dermatome S2 to S4 sends impulses to the proprioceptors of the sphincter muscle, thereby causing involuntary constriction of the sphincter muscles.[96]

Fast brushing also should be used with caution on infants and children with flaccid paralysis. These children have underdeveloped nervous systems, and autonomic nervous system responses are not yet well developed.[41]

ICING. Ice is an extreme in thermal facilitation and has been used for facilitation of muscle activity and autonomic nervous system responses.[84] Unfortunately, icing is a powerful stimulus and the results are not predictable. Rood has described three uses for icing.[84,85]

First, A icing or quick icing is used for patients with hypotonia and in a state of relaxation. A icing probably activates the more myelinated A delta fibers, causing a reflex withdrawal response in the superficial muscles.[96] The ice is applied to the skin in three quick swipes and the water blotted with a terry cloth towel between each swipe (Fig. 18-6). To elicit a withdrawal response of the limbs, the ice is applied to the dorsal web spaces or the palms and soles of the hands and feet[86] (Fig. 18-7). Ice also alerts the mental processes if applied to the palmar surfaces of the fingertips.[41] Second, C icing is a high-intensity nociceptive stimulus that affects the nonspecific C fibers.[86] This type of

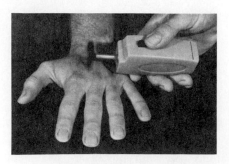

Fig. 18-5. Fast brushing to web spaces of fingers.

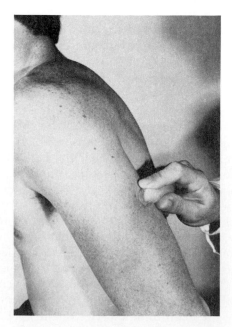

Fig. 18-6. "A" icing.

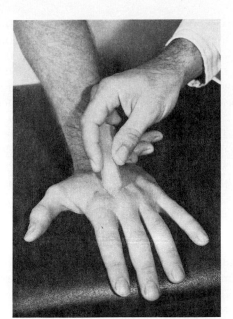

Fig. 18-7. "A" icing to dorsal web spaces of fingers.

icing is used to facilitate maintained postural responses. The ice cube is pressed to the skin of a dermatome serving the same spinal segment of the target muscles to be stimulated. The excess water is blotted away, and the response may take as long as 30 minutes because it must travel through spinal circuits and the reticular activating system.[86] Third, autonomic icing is a stimulus affecting the sympathetic nervous system and probably influences glandular output of the thyroid and adrenal glands[85] (Fig. 18-8). This area needs more research.

Rood has described the use of ice to promote the reciprocal pattern between the diaphragm and the abdominal muscles.[51] Ice is administered to the upper right quadrant of the abdomen (T7 through T9) along the angle of the lower rib. The stimulus is ap-

plied briefly two or three times from midline to the lateral direction. The melted water should be blotted instead of stroked.[85] This technique has been reported to increase breathing patterns, voice production, and general vitality.[84]

Ice chips have been used inside the mouth to stimulate the mucosa, to facilitate closure of the mouth, and to aid swallowing.[54] Ice can be used safely on the inner walls of the cheeks and the posterior of the tongue because fewer nerve endings are in this area.[24] In some patients ice applied to the lips can cause opening of the mouth.[34] Application of ice for 2 or 3 seconds to the upper sternal notch may induce swallowing in patients with dysphagia.[34]

Icing should be used more selectively than fast brushing. Aside from the mucosa of the mouth, ice should never be applied above the neck to the trigeminal nerve distribution or to the pinna of the ear. Furthermore, ice should not be applied along the midline axis of the body. The midline axis contains a greater concentration of free nerve endings and a greater capacity to feed into the sympathetic outflow of the autonomic nervous system.[24] In patients with spinal cord injury at the level of C4, C5, icing along midline may cause autonomic dysreflexia, which can bring on seizures, palpitations of the heart, and vasoconstriction.

Icing also should be avoided in patients with a history of cardiovascular problems. If ice is applied to the region of the left shoulder, angina or heart arrhythmia may occur. If applied behind the ear, ice can facilitate a sudden lowering of blood pressure.[41]

In general, the exteroceptive stimulation can be unpredictable. It is a divergent system that recruits other neurons and can cause discharge long after the stimulus is applied.[44] In the 1970s Rood began to abandon the use of exteroceptive stimuli and endorsed the use of proprioceptive input.[48]

Proprioceptive Facilitory Techniques

Proprioceptive stimulation refers to the facilitation of muscle spindles, Golgi tendon organs, joint receptors, and the vestibular apparatus.[69,102] In general, proprioceptive stimulation gives the therapist more control over the motor response. Proprioceptors adapt more slowly than exteroceptors and can produce sustained postural patterns.[16] There is little or no recruitment in the proprioceptive system. Therefore the motor response lasts as long as the stimulus is applied.[32,88]

HEAVY JOINT COMPRESSION. Heavy joint compression is defined as joint compression greater than body weight applied through the longitudinal axis of the bone.[6] The amount of force is more than that of

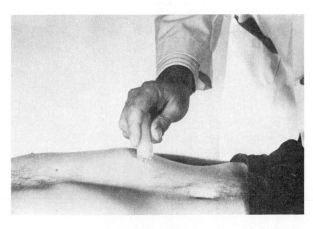

Fig. 18-8. "C" icing.

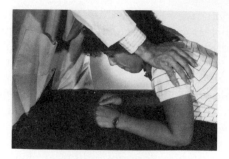

Fig. 18-9. Heavy joint compression.

the normal body weight above the supporting joint[34,48] (Fig. 18-9). Heavy joint compression is used to facilitate cocontraction at the joint undergoing compression. This can be combined with developmental patterns, such as prone on elbows, quadruped (Fig. 18-10), sitting, and standing positions. The joint compression may be done manually by the therapist or with weighted wrist cuffs or sandbags. Clinically, joint compression is most effective when applied through the longitudinal axis of long bones such as the humerus (glenohumeral joint) and the femur (acetabulum).

STRETCH. Stretch is a physiologic stimulus used to activate the proprioceptors in selected muscles of the body.[85] Quick stretch employs the principles of reciprocal innervation. The muscle undergoing stretch is facilitated through the Ia afferent of the muscle spindle and by alpha motor neurons. Quick stretch is applied by holding the proximal bony prominences of

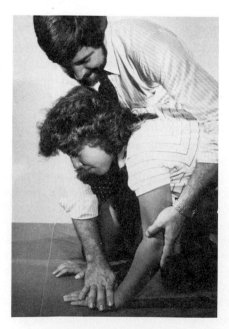

Fig. 18-10. Joint compression to elbow with stretch to wrist extensors in quadruped position.

the limb to be stretched while moving the distal joint in one direction. For example, the elbow joint is secured while the forearm is pushed into flexion to stretch the triceps. The response is immediate and short-lived. Quick stretch is used on light work muscle groups, such as physiologic flexors and adductors.[41,96]

INTRINSIC STRETCH. Intrinsic stretch pertains to Rood's use of the intrinsic muscles to promote stability of the scapulohumeral region.[96] For example, in the on-elbows position, shoulder stability can be enhanced if the patient engages in an activity requiring a resistive grasp. Resistance is a form of stretching because it increases fusimotor activity of the muscle spindle. Another variation of this principle can be used in the quadruped position if the patient bears more weight on the ulnar side of his or her hand.[96] Therapists have used cones, float trowels, and horizontal bars angled downward toward the lateral side of the forearm to distribute more weight on the ulnar side of the patient's wrist toward the pisiform bone.[34,41,96]

SECONDARY ENDING STRETCH. Rood combined resistance and maintained stretch to facilitate developmental muscle patterns. For instance, to promote the supine withdrawal pattern, the patient is placed supine on a mat with the knees flexed and feet flat on the supporting surface. A small book is placed under the head and a folded towel under the lumbosacral regions. The book and towel put the deep extensor muscles on full stretch. In principle, anytime a muscle is put on full stretch, it fires the secondary endings, which is always facilitory to the flexors and inhibitory to the extensors regardless of which muscle is being stretched.[48,54,96] Rood called this procedure "driving the flexors through the extensors." To reinforce the reciprocal action of this maneuver the patient is offered resistance to the flexors, adductors, and internal rotators of the shoulders by compressing a device, such as a bicycle pump. This is a very good technique for integrating the tonic labyrinthine reflex in the supine position.[6]

STRETCH PRESSURE. Stretch pressure affects both

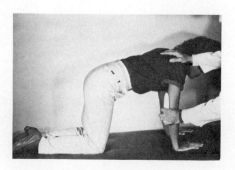

Fig. 18-11. Vibration combined with joint compression.

the exteroceptors and the Ia afferents of the muscle spindle. The stimulus is applied by placing the pads of the thumbs and index and middle fingers on the skin over a superficial muscle. Firm downward pressure and stretching motion is achieved as the thumb moves away from the fingers.[33,34] The degree of pressure and stretch should be sufficient to cause deformation of the skin and stretch the underlying muscle fibers. The stimulus should not exceed 3 seconds. This technique can be applied dermatomally or directly over the muscle belly. Because this stimulus is offensive to some patients, a lubricant can be used to reduce the friction on the skin.

RESISTANCE. Rood used heavy resistance to stimulate both primary and secondary endings of the muscle spindle. Resistance is used in an isotonic fashion in developmental patterns to influence the stabilizer muscles. According to Stockmeyer, resistance to contraction of muscles in the shortened range facilitates muscle spindle afferents in the deeper, tonic postural muscles.[96] Fast brushing is used over the stabilizers before resistance is applied to maximize the response. Farber uses quick stretch before resistance to increase the responsiveness of the muscle spindle.[34] In addition, when a muscle contracts against resistance, it assumes a shortened length that causes the muscle spindles to contract so they readjust to the shorter length. This is called "biasing" the muscle spindle so it is more sensitive to stretch. Intermittent resistance graded to the desired motion is better than manual stretching for alleviating tight muscles.[85]

TAPPING. The tapping technique is done by tapping over the belly of a muscle with the fingertips. The therapist percusses 3 to 5 times over the muscle to be facilitated. This may be done before or during the time a patient is voluntarily contracting the muscle. This stimulus acts on the afferents of the muscle spindle and increases the tone of the underlying skeletal muscle.

VESTIBULAR STIMULATION. Vestibular stimulation is a powerful type of proprioceptive input.[27] The static labyrinthine system can be used to promote extensor patterns of the neck, trunk, and extremities.[105] The kinetic labyrinth can be used to elicit phasic subcortical responses, such as protective extension.[35] Jones and Watt studied muscular responses to unexpected falls in human subjects.[55] Their findings demonstrate that the vestibular system activates the antigravity muscles and their antagonists before the stretch reflex of the muscle spindles.

The vestibular system is a divergent system that affects tone, balance, directionality, protective responses, cranial nerve function, bilateral integration, auditory-language development, and eye pur-

suits.[22,48,105] The vestibular system is stimulated during linear acceleration and deceleration in horizontal and vertical planes and angular acceleration and deceleration, such as spinning, rolling, and swinging. Vestibular stimulation can be either facilitory or inhibitory, depending on the rate of stimulation. Fast rocking tends to stimulate, whereas slow rhythmic rocking tends to relax.[5,6]

INVERSION. Rood encouraged the use of the inverted position to alter muscle tone in selected muscles. In the inverted position the static vestibular system produces increased tonicity of the muscles of the neck, midline trunk extensors, and selected extensors in the limbs.[48] Tokizane used human subjects to study the effects of head position on selected skeletal muscles. His findings indicate that extensor tone is maximized in certain muscles in the head-down position, whereas extensor tone is minimized in those muscles in the upright position. For best results, the head must be in normal alignment with the neck. If the neck is flexed or extended, the TNR interferes with the response.[82,98]

Inversion should be used with extreme care for patients with cardiovascular diseases. As the head approaches a point below the level of the shoulders, baroreceptors in the carotid sinus are stimulated by blood pressure changes. This produces a physiologic response through the parasympathetic nervous system and reduces blood pressure, decreases muscle tone, and promotes generalized relaxation. Inversion techniques can be combined with vibration or neck compression to change tone in selected muscles.[34,48]

THERAPEUTIC VIBRATION. Vibration may be defined as a series of rapid touch stimuli. Therapeutic vibration has been used for tactile stimulation, to desensitize hypersensitive skin, and to produce tonal changes in muscles.[34,48,54] Vibratory stimuli applied over a muscle belly activate the Ia afferent of muscle spindle, thereby causing contraction of that muscle, inhibition of its antagonist muscle, and suppression of the stretch reflex (Fig. 18-11). This response is called the tonic vibration reflex and is best elicited with a high-frequency vibrator that delivers 100 to 300 cycles per second. A low-frequency vibrator that delivers 50 to 60 cycles per second can be used to fire subcutaneous encapsulated receptors called pacinian corpuscles.[102] These receptors send impulses along the dorsal columns to higher centers of the nervous system in which the vibratory sense is consciously perceived.[1] Pacinian corpuscles do not elicit the tonic vibration reflex but may play a role in the suppression of pain perception at the cutaneous level.[8-12]

Because vibration is a proprioceptive therapeutic modality, it has a short latency period and lasts as long

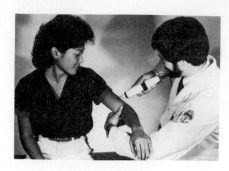

Fig. 18-12. Vibration with pressure to muscle insertion.

as the stimulus is applied.[8-12] To elicit the tonic vibration reflex, the vibrator should be applied over the muscle belly, parallel with the muscle fibers. If the vibrator is placed over the tendon, it may conduct along the bone and stimulate adjoining muscles. The muscle should be on stretch or contracting[45] (Fig. 18-12). The vibrator should be applied with light pressure because deep pressure is inhibitory and may interfere with the results. The duration of vibration should not exceed 1 to 2 minutes per application because heat friction will result.[11] The position of the patient may also be a factor. The prone position may be best while vibrating flexor muscle groups, and the supine position may enhance extensor muscle groups.[8-12] Temperature may also be a factor when using vibration. For example, ice compresses applied to painful joints may slow nerve conduction and have a dampening effect on the tonic vibration reflex. However, if the patient is in a cool environment, it may increase the activity of the sympathetic nervous system, increase muscle tone, and maximize the tonic vibration reflex. When using vibration for cutaneous stimulation, it is best to have the patient in a warm environment because the skin receptors are at a lower threshold for firing.[33]

The results of vibration are also influenced by the patient's response to the stimulus or his or her emotional state.[13] If the patient is depressed or angry, the tonic vibration reflex may be less effective than when the patient is calm. Certain medications such as muscle relaxants and barbiturates can block synaptic transmission at the myoneural junction or in the fusimotor system. These medications also decrease the tonic vibration reflex.[8-12] Vibration should not be used with children less than 3 years of age. Vibration is a powerful stimulus and the CNS is not well myelinated in children.[106] In addition, vibration should not be applied near joints in children, because it may interfere with bone cells in the growth (epiphyseal) plate.[45] In elderly persons over 65 years of age, the skin is thinner and the blood vessels, bones, and organs are more susceptible to vibratory stimuli. With extrapyramidal

or cerebellar lesions, vibration may increase tremors, promote irregular muscle tone, or impair the action of synergies.[8-12]

The electrical vibrator can be a useful tool when properly applied. More research needs to be done on vibration, and therapists should be properly trained before using vibration on patients with neurologic dysfunction.

OSTEOPRESSURE. Pressure on bony prominences has been used with some success to facilitate or inhibit voluntary muscles.[85] It is not clear whether the stimulus is affecting the nerve network in the periosteum of the bone or the subcutaneous pressure receptors (pacinian corpuscle) of the skin. According to Rood, osteopressure produces a slower reaction and needs to be preceded by a light moving touch stimulus. For example, if light moving touch is applied to dermatome C7 of the arm and pressure applied over the lateral epicondyle of the elbow, the arm extends.[85] Pressure on the medial aspect of the malleolus facilitates the lateral dorsiflexors, whereas pressure on the lateral malleolus facilitates the medial dorsiflexors and inhibits the calf muscles.[86]

The light moving touch is probably applied to dermatomes L3 and L4. This technique needs further research verification before it can be used as an effective treatment modality.

Pressure on or near bony prominences also may affect acupressure points. Traditional Chinese medicine recognizes two points located below the medial and lateral malleolus bones of the ankle joint, which are anatomically the same locations described by Rood. According to Chinese medicine, these points contribute to the promotion of deep sleep and correct insomnia.[53,67] Therefore, the mechanism that explains why osteopressure works remains obscure.

SPECIFIC INHIBITION TECHNIQUES USED IN TREATMENT
Neutral warmth

The neutral warmth technique most likely affects the temperature receptors of the hypothalamus and stimulates the parasympathetic nervous system.[88] Neutral warmth can be used for patients with hypertonia, particularly spasticity and rigidity. It may also be helpful for children with attention deficit disorders.[34]

The procedure entails having the patient assume a recumbent position while the entire body is wrapped in a cotton blanket or comforter for approximately 5 to 10 minutes. Neutral warmth provides a moderate amount of heat that is homeostatically compatible with the receptors of the hypothalamus. The patient usually feels relaxed and muscle tone is decreased.[33,54]

Table 18-3 Effects of Proprioceptive Facilitation

Stimulus	Light work (mobilizers) (flexors and adductors)	Heavy work (stabilizers) (extensors and abductors)
Quick stretch	Excitation of Ia afferents in muscles stretched and inhibition in antagonist (reciprocal innervation)	Not applicable
Full stretch in maximum range	Not applicable	Inhibition of group II or secondary ending of muscles on stretch and synergic muscles; excitation in antagonistic flexors of adductors
Joint compression (approximation)	Reduction of spasticity in flexor and adductor group	Promotes cocontraction especially facilitory to one joint extensors
Tendinous pressure over insertion of superficial muscles	Inhibition of tone in long flexors of elbow, fingers, and thumb	Not applicable
Vibration (musculotendinous insertion with the muscle on stretch or working)	Facilitation of underlying muscle via Ia afferents (tonic vibration reflex)	Facilitation via Ia afferents (prior positioning and cutaneous brushing enhances its effect.)
Firm pressure over palmar surface of metacarpals	Reduces tonicity in long flexors of fingers and thumb	Allows extensors to facilitate a more normal release pattern
Outside muscle resistance	Facilitation to muscle being resisted	Sustained contraction if applied proximally; cocontraction if applied distally
Active muscle setting; small range contractions with gravity eliminated (no resistance)	Inhibition via Golgi tendon organs (Ib); reduction of spasticity in flexor and adductor muscles	Facilitation; isotonic contraction of antagonistic extensor and abductor muscles
Input from semicircular canals, eg, movement of head in space	Facilitation; protective responses in limb muscles	Increased tone in postural muscles
Input from utricle and saccule, ie, static position of the head in space	Slight changes in tone depending on position of head	Facilitation predominantly to specific extensor muscles

Gentle shaking or rocking

Gentle shaking or rocking is a generalized inhibitory technique that uses light joint compression and traction of the cervical vertebrae and slow rhythmic circumduction of the head. The patient lies in the supine position, and the therapist places the palm of the right hand under the occiput of the head. The left hand is positioned on top of the patient's head. The neck is held in slight flexion and the head is slowly moved in a circumferential pattern (Fig. 18-13). The head is moved slowly and rhythmically, light joint compression is applied down through the cervical vertebrae with the left hand.[34] As the slow circumduction continues, the therapist uses the right hand to apply gentle traction. This is done by placing the fingertips under the ridge of the occipital bone and applying a slight pulling action after each light compression of the cervical vertebrae. The emphasis should be on a slow continuous motion to elicit a relaxation response.

This motion affects the proprioceptors of the neck and the vestibular apparatus because the joint receptors between the cervical vertebrae and the muscle spindles in the neck muscles are facilitated.[22,100] The slow circumduction of the neck causes the hair cells in the semicircular canals and in the vestibule to alter their rate of discharge. A similar technique can be applied to the shoulder and pelvic girdles to promote segmental relaxation of the upper extremities.

For the upper extremity, the patient lies in a supine position, and the therapist slides the left hand between the patient's left arm and chest (axilla) so that the hand is facing upward and supporting just beneath the scapula. The therapist places the right hand on the patient's left shoulder. With the left hand supporting below the scapula and the right hand firmly placed on top of the left shoulder, the therapist gently rotates the upper region of the shoulder backward (posteriorly). The shoulder may be rotated backward about 4 times, depending on the patient's shoulder mobility and the presence of pain in the shoulder. The immediate response is that the left shoulder will appear to be lower and fully resting on the supporting surface below. This technique should be used on the patient's

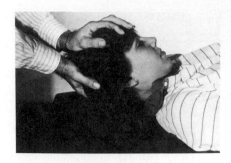

Fig. 18-13. Gentle shaking and rocking.

right shoulder to promote symmetry and also works well for patients with a spastic scapula. It slowly relaxes and mobilizes the scapula so it can glide along with the upper extremity. These procedures are continued until relaxation can be palpated in the muscles or observed in the patient's posture.

To apply gentle shaking and rocking to the pelvic girdle, the patient continues to lie in the supine position. The therapist stands over or straddles the patient so his or her hands can be placed around the lateral aspects of the pelvic girdle. The thumbs are placed on the pelvic crest and the fingertips under the gluteal muscles. Thus, the therapist can lift and gently rotate the pelvis from side to side.

The lower extremities can be relaxed in the following manner: The patient remains in the supine position, and the therapist moves to the bottom of the feet. The therapist places the palms of the hands under the patient's heels and slowly lifts the legs about 12 inches off the mat. At the same time, the therapist leans backward to put slight traction on the legs. As the therapist lowers the legs to the mat, they can be jiggled laterally in a scissoring fashion.

In addition, when the legs are slowly lowered to the mat, the therapist's hands remain under the heels (Achilles tendon) and carefully jiggle the patient's entire body toward the head and feet. This slow jiggling motion is very relaxing and allows the patient's body to become evenly distributed on the surface below.

Slow stroking

Slow stroking has been described as an inhibitory technique. The patient lies in the prone position while the therapist provides rhythmic, moving, deep pressure over the dorsal distribution of the primary posterior rami of the spine. The therapist applies fingertip pressure on both sides of the spinous process to affect the nerve endings and the sympathetic outflow of the autonomic nervous system. The stroking action is done slowly and continuously from the occiput to the coccyx. The hands are alternated so that as one hand reaches the bottom of the spine, the other is starting downward from the top.[34,48,54]

Several variations of slow stroking have been used by therapists. To achieve the best results, a lubricant such as hand cream can be used to prevent friction on the skin. Some therapists use the ends of the flexed proximal interphalangeal (PIP) joints of the index and long finger to provide firm and continuous downward pressure to both sides of the spinous process. Other therapists apply the ulnar side of the hands in a cascading motion with alternating pressure from the neck region to the lumbar area.

These inhibition techniques have been found to be clinically beneficial when accompanied by soft music. Music also has been used as a closure technique following sensory integrative therapy to calm children after vestibular and proprioceptive facilitation. This procedure should not exceed 3 minutes, because it may cause a rebound phenomenon, resulting in excitation of the sympathetic branch of the autonomic nervous system.[96]

Slow rolling

The patient is placed in a side-lying position. (The hemiplegic patient should first lie with the univolved side down.) The therapist kneels behind the patient and places one hand on the rib cage and the other hand on the lateral aspect of the patient's pelvis (Fig. 18-14, *A*). The patient is rolled slowly from a side-lying position to a prone position and back again in a rhythmic fashion[33,34] (Fig. 18-14, *B*). In addition to rolling the entire body from lying on the side toward a prone position, the therapist can incorporate some slow rotational movements between the hip and the trunk. This technique should be used on both sides of the body. With some patients it is necessary to place a pillow between the knees or under the head to prevent friction and malalignment of the body.

Light joint compression (approximation)

Joint compression of body weight or less than body weight can be used to inhibit spastic muscles around a joint.[86] This technique may be used with hemiplegic patients to alleviate pain and to temporarily offset the muscle imbalance around the shoulder joint.[34] The patient can be sitting or lying in the supine position. The therapist places one hand over the patient's shoulder and the other hand under the flexed elbow joint. The arm is abducted 35° to 45° and a compression force of body weight or less is applied through the longitudinal axis of the humerus.[6] This procedure compresses both the glenohumeral joint and the articulation between the humerus and ulna. Moreover, if applied properly, this technique compresses two joints but has the most dramatic effect on the shoulder. Once the muscles begin to relax, the therapist can slowly and gently circumduct the humerus in

A   B

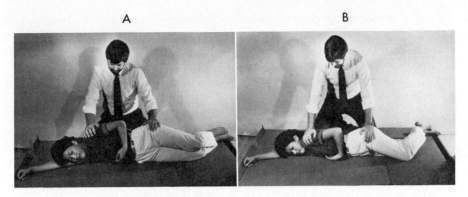

Fig. 18-14. A and **B,** Slow rolling.

small circles to reduce pain and stiffness in the shoulder joint.[34] Joint compression of the shoulder and elbow joints also can be achieved when the patient is in the on-elbows position.[96] Light joint compression is also beneficial when applied through the longitudinal axis of the wrist and elbow joints.[34] The therapist places one hand behind the elbow and places the patient's forearm in midposition; the wrist joint is extended, and compression is applied through the heel of the patient's hand. Joint compression has its greatest effect during the time that the stimulus is applied.[100]

Tendinous pressure

Manual pressure applied to the tendinous insertion of a muscle or across long tendons produces an inhibitory effect.[6,48] This pressure has a dramatic effect on spastic or tight muscle groups in which the tendons are accessible to the forces of pressure. Pressure provided by hard surfaces is preferable to that provided by soft surfaces.[26] Therefore many therapists use a hard cone in the hand with the tapered end toward the thumb side to inhibit the flexors.[33] A hard surface over the anterior aspect of the forearm is inhibitory to the extrinsic flexors of the hand.[86] This principle has been used in a number of orthotic devices to manage muscle imbalance and contractures provided by spasticity. It is postulated that the pacinian corpuscle is responsible for the inhibition of the muscle.[99] The Golgi tendon organ, however, may be also play a role in this response, because it is located in the musculotendinous insertions and monitors tendon tension.[73]

Maintained stretch

Rood recommended positioning hypertonic extremities in the elongated position for various periods to cause lengthening of the muscle spindles.[86] The rationale for this is to reset or "bias" the afferents of the muscle spindle to a longer position so that they are less sensitive to stretching. Rood did not advocate passive stretch for tight muscles. Instead, she recommended maintained stretch in the lengthened position for the stronger agonist muscle to increase the threshold of the muscle spindles. The antagonist muscle is then facilitated by cutaneous stimulation to offset the muscle imbalance.[85] Rood also used autogenic inhibition through the Golgi tendon organ to reciprocally facilitate the antagonist muscle.[84,86]

Goff suggests that spasticity is reduced if the patient is taught to practice very small range contractions of isolated muscles and their antagonists. If this is done repeatedly with no resistance and with gravity eliminated, spasticity can be reduced especially in extensor and abductor muscles.[41]

Rocking in developmental patterns

In keeping with the developmental sequence and the concept of mobility superimposed on stability, Rood encouraged movement as the patient gained mastery of the static position.[96] Developmentally, the patient first must assume and be able to achieve a static position and then integrate coordinated movements while maintaining the posture. Rood referred to this as the development of "skill." For example, in the quadruped position, the patient shifts weight to a three-point stance so that one hand is free to reach forward to grasp and explore. Movement may begin by shifting the weight forward and backward. The shifting may progress to side-to-side and diagonal patterns as the patient becomes comfortable with the rhythmic movements.[34] Hemiplegic patients are assisted in the quadruped position by achieving stability of the involved elbow (see Fig. 18-10) when the therapist applies pressure and stretch to the triceps brachii and anconeus. As the therapist applies compression that is greater than body weight to facilitate cocontraction, the pressure exerted on the extended wrist and heel of the hand inhibits the wrist flexors. Light moving touch over the dorsum of the hand is done to promote finger extension.[86] Rocking in the quadruped position should first be done with the neck in a straight normal relationship to the body so that the proprioceptors of the neck do not influence the tonicity of the limbs.[32] As the patient moves in an anteroposterior plane, the shoulder and pelvic girdles are being mobilized. Later in treatment, the therapist may want to incorporate flexion, extension, and rotation of the neck as a reflex inhibition measure.[77] See Table 18-3 for a summary of the effects of proprioceptive facilitation.

SPECIAL SENSES FOR FACILITATION OR INHIBITION

Rood suggested the use of olfactory and gustatory stimuli to facilitate cranial nerves and to influence the autonomic nervous system.[84,86] In principle, pleasant odors such as vanilla and banana oil may have a calming effect or evoke strong moods. Unpleasant odors such as sulfur and fresh horseradish can produce primitive protective responses such as sneezing and choking.[34] Rood used noxious substances such as ammonia and vinegar to affect the trigeminal nerve, which activates the muscles of mastication.[96]

Warm liquids may be calming to the oral musculature, whereas sweet foods or sour tastes can stimulate the salivary glands.[44] As with other stimuli, the intensity of warm liquids and sweet and sour tastes can be gauged to facilitate or inhibit the CNS. Rood did not provide specific guidelines for the stimulation of special senses.[84-86]

The importance of using many sensory modalities in the rehabilitation of neurologic dysfunction is emphasized by several therapists.[5,33,48] In theory, the CNS retains its capacity to produce adaptive changes to stimuli throughout life.[24,106] Bach-y-Rita has suggested that a process called "sensory substitution" can compensate for the loss of a particular sensory modality.[7] Sensory substitution is the process in which a blind person uses the tactile sense instead of vision in reading braille. Another example is the stroke patient who sees four objects on a table and with the eyes closed can identify the objects correctly by using the sense of touch alone. Farber refers to this phenomenon as "cross-modal" stimulation.[34] Regardless of what it is called, the ability to learn and relearn depends on the integration of sensory input. Rood's basic hypothesis, that sensory stimulation can elicit specific motor responses, continues to gain credence in the realm of physical medicine and rehabilitation.

APPLICATION OF THE ROOD APPROACH IN OCCUPATIONAL THERAPY

The occupational therapist uses the previously described techniques primarily to prepare the patient for purposeful activities. Patients who have undergone severe neurologic damage usually do not have voluntary control over their muscles. The motor responses exhibited by the patient may begin with primitive reflexive motions. Therefore the therapist may need to begin with the ontogenetic developmental patterns. During this phase of rehabilitation, the therapist must carefully select the pattern to be trained and control extraneous conditions. Next, the desired motor patterns should be done passively by the therapist and reinforced by sensory stimulation. The motor patterns should be repeated until the patient can actively perform the pattern in a slow, accurate manner. The speed of the movement should not be increased until precision is accomplished. The therapist should avoid fatiguing the patient and should not allow incorrect patterns to develop. Thousands of correct repetitions may be necessary before the speed and force of contraction are increased.[58,59] As the patient gains mastery of a motor pattern, the therapist should introduce purposeful activities into the repertoire. Hence, as mentioned earlier, a basic tenet of the Rood approach is that activity should be purposeful. The introduction of purposeful activities adds meaning and relevance to the endeavor. Routine exercises and neurophysiologic techniques alone can become redundant, and the patient may reach a plateua too early in therapeutic progression.

Ontogenetic motor patterns with activities

SUPINE WITHDRAWAL. The therapist may use an activity that promotes elbow flexion or shoulder adduction. The patient may squeeze an accordion or a large balloon to add resistance and to reinforce the pattern. An easel or macrame frame may be set up in such a way that the patient can lie supine, reach forward toward the midline, and paint an oil painting or tie cords for plant hangers. Certain leather craft projects and numerous minor crafts could be manipulated in this pattern. The incentive for the patient is an end product that can adorn his or her room or be given to a "significant other."

ROLL OVER. The roll-over pattern can be promoted by placing an object on either side of the patient so he or she has to visually fixate on the object and to roll reach for it. It is best to minimize extraneous demands and external stimuli in the room so that the patient can concentrate on the task at hand. The therapist may begin the roll-over pattern by having the patient lie on an equilibrium board tilted slightly to one side to remove some of the gravitational demands. Objects, such as cassette tape recorders and remote control for a television or video game, can provide an incentive to roll, reach, and manipulate an object.

PIVOT PRONE. The pivot-prone position is a stability pattern that places demands on the proximal extensor muscles. Scooter board activities are ideal for this pattern because the patient must lift the extremities against gravity. The scooter board may be equipped with a rope-and-pulley system so that the board can accelerate and decelerate forward and backward. This linear movement (forward and backward) stimulates the vestibular apparatus and enhances the tonicity of the extensor muscles. The prone-extension pattern (pivot prone) also can be reinforced with activities that provide light resistance. The patient can lie prone on a soft bolster (suspended or on a mat) and manipulate strings attached to bells or talking toys. The object of this activity is to entice the patient into looking up so that his or her neck extends and the arms pull backward away from the midline axis.

NECK COCONTRACTION. Neck cocontraction can be reinforced by positioning the patient in the prone position on a firm surface, such as a table. The head and neck should extend off the end of the table so the weight is distributed on the patient's chest region. In this position, the patient can suck through a straw to pick up objects and transfer them from one container to another. The object of the sucking action is to reinforce neck cocontraction. For an advanced activity, table tennis balls marked with numbers could be placed in a pan of water. The object would be to pick up these balls by sucking through the straw. The score board can be positioned on the wall in front of the patient so he or she has to extend the neck and look up to see the score.

ON ELBOWS. A patient on his or her elbows is in a position that is conducive to many activities. The patient may be positioned on a mat in front of a video game monitor. The control handle is placed near the midline so that the patient can use either hand to manipulate the controls. This activity provides concentration and fine eye-hand manipulation as the patient bears weight on the elbows. A number of minor crafts, games, and puzzles can be integrated into this pattern.

ALL FOURS (QUADRUPED). The quadruped position does not allow freedom of the hands for manipulation unless the patient can shift weight to a three-point stance. Thus if the patient can support his or her body weight on the knees and one hand, he or she can use one hand to draw or manipulate objects. In an effort to produce mobility in the quadruped position, the patient can support half of the body weight on a scooter board. For example, the hands and anterior part of the body can rest on the scooter board while the lower extremities provide forward propulsion. This activity does not provide coordina-

tion and reciprocal movements between the upper and lower extremities but does afford mobility and exploration of the environment. In addition, when the knees are resting on the scooter board and the upper limbs are used for propulsion, the patient is receiving some of the benefits of inversion.

STATIC STANDING. Standing provides the best position for activities of daily living (ADL) and purposeful activities. In this position, the arms are free to explore and manipulate while the task of weight-bearing is placed on the legs. The patient can begin with light resistive activities on a high bench and proceed to resistive crafts, such as woodworking, leather crafts, and ceramics. As the patient develops stability in standing and in activities that require weight shift and equilibrium, the responses can be integrated into the repertory of motor skills.

WALKING. Walking is the skilled level of mobility. The upright bipedal position requires an integration of many components of the CNS. The physical therapist usually undertakes the responsibility of gait training, whereas the occupational therapist provides purposeful activities to encourage walking for ADL, such as grocery shopping, visiting neighbors, and facilitating the cardiovascular system. The occupational and physical therapists should work together closely on walking skills so that the patient can receive a well-coordinated treatment plan.

NEW CONCEPTS FOR SENSORY STIMULATION

Margaret S. Rood was a pioneer in the field of sensory stimulation. She laid down the foundation for the use of sensory stimulation as it is known today and integrated neurophysiology with clinical techniques. However, current research warrants a new look at sensory stimulation and its implications as a therapeutic modality. The following are new concepts to consider.

First, sensory stimulation or touch has been found to be more complicated than simply facilitating receptors beneath the skin. A stimulus applied to the skin sets off a cascade of biochemical and neuroendocrinologic events, more pervasive and complex than previously imagined.[25,28,66,80] Up to this time, sensory stimulation in occupational therapy has focused on neuromuscular and possibly, psychosocial responses.[6,34,48] Today, growing evidence exists that touch or sensory stimulation has an integrating effect on many organ systems and homeostatic mechanisms throughout the body.[87,89,101] In the health care delivery context, five types of touch (sensory stimulation) have been identified.[87,101]

Social touch is skin-to-skin contact for the development of human relationships. Much has been written about the importance of touch in infancy and throughout life for human growth and development.[15,72,81] It is commonly agreed that social touch promotes social bonds, attachment, and emotional well-being.

Passive touch pertains to a sensory stimulus that is applied to the patient's skin to facilitate specific receptors and tract systems. For example, when fast brushing is applied dermatomally, a reflex arc is set off, which facilitates muscles of a myotome that serve the same spinal segment.[41]

Active touch provides the patient with the opportunity for manual exploration in which the receptors in the skin, joints, and muscles must function collaboratively to obtain information about the activity or the environment. Occupational therapy provides active touch experiences by engaging the patient in purposeful activities.[5,78]

Comforting touch is often used by care-givers for the purpose of assisting the patient to cope with dysfunction and its related stressors.[28] A touch on the shoulder for encouragement and holding the patient's hand are immeasurable therapeutic tools. Studies have shown that patients have a greater need for this type of touch during illness.[17-19]

Procedural touch is the result of science and technology in Western medicine. Health professionals are trained to use touch to evaluate, monitor, diagnose, and treat illnesses. According to Morse, the intent of this type of touch is to perform a procedure or activity that is important to the patient's physical health.[74] Procedural touch may be perceived by the patient as routine, directive, and controlling. Studies have shown that taking the pulse and measuring blood pressure in intensive care units has profound negative influences on the patient's heart rate and other physiologic responses.[19,66,71,101]

This brief overview of the types of sensory stimulation shows that touch is much more complicated than mastering the application of a technique. For instance, the patient's perception of touch can influence his or her response to the stimulus. Experimental evidence indicates that the precondition of the nervous system, that is the patient's emotional state prior to touch, affects the neurologic tract systems, and biochemical responses.[25,40,57,89] If the patient perceives the stimulus as being potentially harmful, the sympathetic branch of the autonomic nervous system is more likely to prevail and release catecholamines and various biogenic amines causing fight-or-flight responses.[40,71,93,101] Therefore, it is important for the therapist to set up the emotional climate that is conducive to the desired response before the stimulus is

applied. For example, if the patient is overly anxious about a noxious stimulus such as ice, the therapist should explain what will take place and should incorporate relaxation techniques such as deep breathing to induce relaxation responses.[25,47]

Scientific information is emerging about the skin that will have enormous influences on patient care in the future. Traditional concepts about the skin have suggested that it is the largest organ of the body, the first line of defense against infectious organisms, and a vehicle of communication.[38,57] New concepts of the human skin suggest even more profound characteristics. For example, the skin can be considered the organ of health. A study conducted at Ohio State University involved feeding rabbits a high-cholesterol diet.[76] After being fed the unhealthy diet for a period of time the rabbits were sacrificed and their coronary arteries examined for arteriosclerotic plaque. One subset of rabbits had 60% less fat build-up in their arteries than that of the others. The only variable in this subset was that the attendant made a practice of taking this group out of their cages and petting them. The researchers replicated the study 3 times, and the subgroup that was touched had significantly less arteriorsclerosis.[30,76] Similar results are reported on human subjects. Medalie and Goldboust conducted a study involving 10,000 males with arteriosclerotic heart disease.[70] The researchers found that the patients who had loving, supportive, and caring spouses reported an incidence of angina that was only half that of the group as a whole. Another study conducted at the University of Miami Medical School examined the effects of touch on premature infants.[14] The experimental group received gentle stroking and passive range of motion. The control group received the normal treatment and care. As a result, the experimental group showed a 47% greater weight gain per day with the same caloric intake. The infants who received gentle stroking required an average of 6 days less hospitalization at a savings of $3000 per child.

The literature also suggests that the skin influences internal homeostasis. It is well documented that the skin is the primary transducer of information to the nervous system. Rood's focus on neuromuscular dysfunction through sensory stimulation is still of major interest to occupational therapists. Research continues to suggest that certain types of sensory stimulation may be linked to facilitation of regional areas of the nervous system. Stimuli of long duration, high frequency, and strong intensity excite a greater number of neurons in the spinal thalamic system and limbic system. Sensory stimuli to areas of rich innervation, such as the face and hands, transmit to specific cell bodies in the cortex and association fibers.[19,90] Also evidence exists that the skin is connected to internal organs through complex reflex arcs.[20,29,67,80] In fact, many diseases of internal organs manifest on the surface of the skin like a mirror reflecting disturbances within. Liver deficiency results in a characteristic waxy yellow skin, whereas, heart disease causes cyanosis.[67]

This reflex arc phenomenon is best illustrated by referred pain. Dysfunction in an internal organ manifests as pain on the surface of the skin at a location that is some distance from the organ. For instance, pain arising from the stomach is transmitted to the skin of the upper abdomen and the adjacent part of the back. An explanation for this phenomenon is that the stomach and the skin areas are supplied by the same nerve segment (T7 and T8). An old remedy for stomach discomfort was a hot water bottle placed over the skin area where the pain was referred.[9] The reduction of pain indicates the presence of cutaneous-visceral reflexes transmitted by way of the nervous system.[38,67,88]

Rood's approaches were based on passive touch and sensory stimulation applied to specific dermatomal areas of the skin. The long-term effects on internal organs have not yet been fully determined. However, some research is showing positive effects of sensory stimulation due to the release of catecholamines, which are organic compounds known to stimulate the nervous and cardiovascular systems, metabolic rates, temperature, and smooth muscle.[63,71,89,104]

Researchers drawing on data from psychology, neurobiology and immunology are developing a new discipline called psychoneuroimmunology.[64,102] They are demonstrating that stimulation to the skin not only sends messages to the central nervous system but to the endocrine and immune systems as well. Studies conducted by Pertovaara have shown that *neuropeptides*, (small chains of amino acids including endorphins) play a prominent role throughout the body.[79] To date, neuropeptides have been associated with pain, anxiety, pleasure, appetite, learning, and a variety of moods. Movement and sensory stimulation have been found to trigger mechanisms in the brain to release neuropeptides into the bloodstream.[93] In the bloodstream, neuropeptides direct the movement of the key components of the immune systems, the *monocytes (macrophages)*. These specialized white blood cells are crucial to wound healing and elimination of foreign bodies, and they communicate with B cells and T cells to combat disease.[46,64,103] Neuropeptides are also the neurotransmitters of emotions and are greatly influenced by the patient's attitude. A positive attitude toward wellness increases the patient's chances for recovery from a catastrophic illness.[46,64] Blood tests show that patients who cope poorly with

illnesses have less active immune cells than those with a more positive attitude.[46,64] This explains why mental imagery has been beneficial to terminal cancer patients. The occupational therapist can use imagery and metaphors with sensory stimulation to potentiate these effects. Carl Simonton's book, *Getting Well Again*, and Norman Cousins' work, *Anatomy of an Illness*, offer many strategies for clinical practice. According to Pertovaara neuropeptides are strategically located throughout the body. For example, breathing techniques used in relaxation may release neuropeptides in the brain stem nuclei. This probably explains why deep breathing alters pain thresholds and levels of consciousness.[93] Breathing techniques were not suggested in Rood's original work. Yet clinical experience with children and adults has shown that inhibitory techniques such as slow stroking or gentle shaking and rocking are more effective when the patient uses deep breathing and visualization.[34,91]

The clinical signs of inhibition were not well outlined in Rood's work. Today, when using holistic and inhibitory techniques, the therapist can gauge the effectiveness of the techniques by observing the following:

1. If the eyes are open, the size of the pupils may constrict, indicating a parasympathetic response. In some patients the eyes remain partly open, and the pupils appear fixed or "glazed" when they are inhibited. The most important eye signs are the rapid eye movements (REM). This eye flutter is indicative of an altered state of consciousness. REMs are a natural occurrence during sleep and dreaming.[61,91]

2. The patient's respirations change because breathing is influenced by both the autonomic and the voluntary nervous systems. For some patients the respirations slow down and deepen. This may be preceded by large inspirations and expirations as if to "blow off" tension.[61,91,101]

3. A third manifestation to note is change in voice quality. Sometimes the therapist needs to elicit a verbal response by asking "how are you doing?" The patient's voice takes on a quality and vitality different than it was before the inhibition or relaxation techniques began.[61,91]

4. A fourth clinical sign often noticed is the presence of gurgling or rumbling sounds called borborygmus created by the gastrointestinal tract. This is a good sign because an increase in stomach motility indicates a parasympathetic response.

5. Changes in skin tone, due to dilation of the peripheral vascular system may be observed.

6. Muscle jerks unrelated to neurologic movement disorders also are observed. These muscle jerks

may appear as minor twitches, as seen in a person about to fall asleep.

It is important for the therapist to monitor these responses and not allow the patient to get too inhibited because it decreases purposeful neuromuscular responses.

The skin senses both pleasure or pain and a whole gamut of sensations in between. According to Smith, memories and emotions can be triggered during various forms of cutaneous stimulation.[91] The physiologic mechanism for this phenomenon is unknown at present, but possibly neuropeptides are involved.[46,57,64,93] As previously mentioned, neuropeptides have an influence on learning, moods, and emotions. Therefore, as the therapist is using sensory stimulation techniques, the patient may suddenly remember a past event or experience changes in emotions. The therapist should not brush aside these psychological responses. Although the therapist is working on a physical response the importance of the emotional response should not be underemphasized. If the patient wishes to express himself or herself, he or she should feel free to discuss psychosocial matters to a nonjudgmental therapist. Because the occupational therapist is trained to work with the whole person and because research indicates that the body is not biochemically separated from the mind, a holistic approach to treatment is feasible. Furthermore, the discussion of emotions or stressors related to the physical disability may help the patient to develop coping mechanisms and a better attitude about his or her disability.[17,46,57,74]

Another new concept is that the skin is incredibly dynamic. With the exception of the cornea and mucous membranes, the skin is one of the fastest growing tissues in the body.[29] A completely new skin is developed every 4 to 6 weeks. Radiographic studies have shown that 98% of the body's atoms are renewed each year, and the atoms of the skin are the first to be exchanged.[30] Some researchers are referring to the human body as a complex energy field.[20,53,56,62,80,91] Nordinstrom theorizes that the body is like a battery with electrical circuits containing positively and negatively charged ions. According to Nordinstrom, these ions regulate many systems of the body. Injury to tissues results in a buildup of positively charged ions in the affected area. In addition, macrophages or monocytes are attracted to these positively charged ions. Nordinstrom's preliminary research has shown that inserting electrodes into the skin can change the polarity of tissues and shrink benign tumors.

A less invasive approach to working with the skin's bioelectric energy has been developed by Doris Krieger in the field of nursing.[47,56,60,61,62] Since 1977, several studies have confirmed the efficacy of her technique called *therapeutic touch*. According to this theory, each person is composed of a complex energy field and forms of life energy. These fields of energy not only run through the skin, body, and bones but are in constant interaction and exchange with surrounding energy fields in the environment. Therapeutic touch is performed by directing the life energy through the hands of the therapist to the patient, who may then internalize it or use it to restore balance and promote self-regulation of healing.[56] At first, this concept was very controversial and regarded as little more than mysticism and nonscience. However, several well-controlled studies have revealed that subjects receiving therapeutic touch (TT) recorded increased hemoglobin levels, which bring more oxygen to tissues, increased relaxation responses verified by electroencephalograph readings, reduction of orthopedically related pain, and a balance of positive and negatively charged ions.[47,56,60,61,62] The practice of therapeutic touch goes beyond the scope of this chapter but it can be used effectively before touch and sensory stimulation. To date, one of the most important findings of this research is that touch is biochemically and psychologically more beneficial when the therapist performs it with unconditional kindness or with the intent to help or heal.[61,91]

Studies show that when the person performing therapeutic touch is mentally preoccupied, the physiologic benefits are significantly diminished.[56] In my opinion, the occupational therapy concept called *therapeutic use of self* is synonymous with the intent of therapeutic touch. It also appears that we are connected in ways that are not fully understood. Therefore, when applying any procedure in occupational therapy, the therapist should have clear intentions to help the person and keep in mind that the activity or modality is only a medium through which to communicate.

This brief review of the literature has revealed many new possibilities for sensory stimulation as a modality for treatment. The Rood approach to the use of sensory stimulation has opened the door to many possibilities. New avenues can be explored to expand the basic tenets of Rood's work. Occupational therapists should continue to use sensory stimulation with confidence while keeping an eye on new research literature for scientific verification of new techniques.

REVIEW QUESTIONS

1. List the four goals of the Rood approach.
2. Differentiate between the motor responses elicited by the TNR and TLR.
3. What are the three major reactions produced by sensory stimulation?
4. Describe the four rules for sensory stimulation.
5. List the four sequences of motor development.
6. Describe the eight ontogenetic motor patterns.
7. Differentiate between exteroceptive and proprioceptive stimulation.
8. Which size nerve fibers carry pain, temperature, and light touch?
9. Which nerve fibers carry conscious and subconscious proprioceptive messages?
10. Contrast the functions of the stabilizer and mobilizer muscles.
11. How often is the light touch stimulus applied and what happens if it is applied too often?
12. How long should fast brushing be applied to the skin?
13. Why should fast brushing be applied according to dermatomal segments?
14. List the skin areas in which fast brushing is contraindicated.
15. Describe the uses of C icing, A icing, and autonomic icing and the principal motor responses elicited by each.
16. Discuss the advantages of proprioceptive stimulation over cutaneous stimulation.
17. How is heavy joint compression differentiated from light joint compression?
18. Describe how inversion is used as a therapeutic modality.
19. Explain how therapeutic vibration can be used to activate muscles and cutaneous receptors.
20. Discuss three methods of reducing muscle tone.
21. List five types of touch and describe the benefits or adverse effects of each.
22. Discuss the potential benefits of therapeutic touch.
23. Under what conditions is therapeutic touch most beneficial to the patient?

REFERENCES

1. Abbruzzese G et al: Excitation from skin receptors contributing to the tonic vibration reflex in man, Brain Res 150:194, 1978.
2. Afifi A and Bergman R: Basic neuroscience, Munich, 1980, Verlag Urban und Schwarzenberg.
3. Alpern M, Lawrence N, and Wolsk D: Sensory processes, Belmont, Calif., 1976, Brooks/Cole Publishing Co.
4. Androsik F: Relaxation and biofeedback for chronic headaches. In Halzman A and Turk D, editors: Pain management—a handbook of psychological treatment approaches, New York, 1986, Pergamon Press.
5. Ayres J: Sensory integration and learning disorders, Los Angeles, 1972, Western Psychological Services.
6. Ayres J: The development of sensory integrative theory and practice, Dubuque, Iowa, 1974, Kendall/Hunt Publishing Co.
7. Bach-y-Rita P: Sensory substitution in rehabilitation of the neurological patient, Oxford, England, 1983, Basil Blackwell Publisher, Ltd.
8. Barr ML: The human nervous system, ed 2, New York, 1974, Harper & Row Publishers, Inc.
9. Beeson P and McDermott W: The textbook of medicine, Philadelphia, 1979, WB Saunders Co.
10. Bishop B: Vibratory stimulation. I, Phys Ther 54:1273, 1974.
11. Bishop B: Vibratory stimulation. II, Phys Ther 55:29, 1975.
12. Bishop B: Vibratory stimulation. III, Phys Ther 55:139, 1975.
13. Bishop B: Spasticity: its physiology and management, Parts I, II, and III, Phys Ther 57:4, 1977.
14. Bower B: Different strokes. Science News 128:301, 1985.
15. Bowlby J: The nature of the child's tie to his mother, Int J Psychoanal 39:350, 1958.
16. Buchwald J: Exteroceptive reflexes and movement, Am J Phys Med 46:121, 1967.
17. Burnside IM: Caring for the aged: touching is talking, Am J Nurs 73:2060, 1973.
18. Burton A and Heller L: The touching of the body, Psychoanal Rev 51:122, 1964.
19. Buschsbaum M and Pfefferbaum A: Individual differences in stimulus intensity response, Psychophysiology 8:600, 1971.
20. Capra F: The Tao of physics, Boulder, Colorado, 1975, Shambhala Publications.
21. Chusid JG: Correlative neuroanatomy and functional neurology, ed 18, Los Altos, Calif., 1982, Lange Medical Publications.
22. Clark B: The vestibular system. In Mussen PH, and Rosenzweig MR, editors: Annual review of psychology, New York, 1970, Harper & Row Publishers, Inc.
23. Clark R: Clinical neuroanatomy and neurophysiology, ed 5, Philadelphia, 1975, FA Davis Co.
24. Colavila F: Sensory changes in the elderly, Springfield, Ill., 1978, Charles C Thomas, Publisher.
25. Day F: The patients' perception of touch. In Anderson D, Bergersen M, Duffey M, Lohr R, and Rose M, editors: Current concepts in clinical nursing, St Louis, 1973, The CV Mosby Co.
26. Dayhoof N: Re-thinking stroke: soft or hard devices to position hands? Am J Nurs 7:1142, 1975.
27. DeQuiros JB: Diagnosis of vestibular disorders in the learning disabled, J Learning Disabilities 9:50, 1974.
28. Dominion J: The psychological significance of touch, Nurs Times 67:896, 1971.
29. Dossey L: The biodance in space, time, and medicine, Boulder, Colorado, 1982, Shambhala Publications.
30. Dossey L: The skin: what is it? Topics Clin Nurs 5:1, 1983.
31. Eldred E: The dual sensory role of muscle spindles, Phys Ther 45:290, 1965.
32. Eldred E: Peripheral receptors: their excitation and relation to

reflex patterns, Am J Phys Med 46:69, 1967.

33. Farber S: Sensorimotor evaluation and treatment procedures for allied health personnel, Indianapolis, 1974, Indiana University and Purdue University Medical Center.

34. Farber S: Neurorehabilitation: a multisensory approach, Philadelphia, 1982, WB Saunders Co.

35. Fukuda T: Studies on human dynamic postures from the viewpoint of postural reflexes, Acta Otolaryngol 161(suppl):8, 1961.

36. Fulton JF: Physiology of the nervous system, vol 179, ed 3, New York, 1949, Oxford University Press, Inc.

37. Gardner E: Fundamentals of neurology, ed 6, Philadelphia, 1975, WB Saunders Co.

38. Geldard F: The human senses, New York, 1972, John Wiley & Sons, Inc.

39. Gilman S and Winans S: Essentials of clinical neuroanatomy and neurophysiology, ed 6, Philadelphia, 1982, FA Davis Co.

40. Glick G and Brauwald E: Relative roles of the sympathetic and parasympathetic system in the reflex control of heart rate, Circ Res 16:363, 1965.

41. Goff B: The Rood approach. In Cash's textbook of neurology for physiotherapists, ed 4, Philadelphia, 1986, JB Lippincott Co.

42. Goldberg S: Clinical neuroanatomy made ridiculously simple, Miami, 1979, Medical Master, Inc.

43. Greenberg JH, Reivich A, Alavi A, and Hand P: Metabolic mapping of functional activity in human subjects with the fluorodeoxyglucose technique, Science 212:678, 1981.

44. Guyton A: Structure and function of the nervous system, Philadelphia, 1972, WB Saunders Co.

45. Hagbarth KE and Edlund G: The muscle vibrator: a useful tool in neurological therapeutic work, Scand J Rehabil Med 1:26, 1969.

46. Hammer S: The mind as healer, Science Digest, 47, April 1984.

47. Heidt P: Effect of therapeutic touch on anxiety level in hospitalized patients, Nurs Res, 30(1):32, 1981.

48. Heininger M and Randolph S: Neurophysiological concepts in human behavior, St Louis, 1981, The CV Mosby Co.

49. Hellebrandt F, Schade M, and Carns M: Methods of evoking the tonic neck reflexes in normal human subjects, Am J Phys Med 41:89, 1962.

50. Hellebrandt F et al: Tonic neck reflexes in exercise of stress in man, Am J Phys Med 35:144, 1956.

51. Henderson A and Coryell J: The body senses and perceptual deficit. Proceedings of the Occupational Therapy Symposium, Boston, 1973.

52. Hirt S: The tonic neck reflex mechanism in the normal human adult, Am J Phys Med 46:362, 1967.

53. Holbrook B: The stone monkey: an alternative Chinese-scientific reality, New York, 1981, William, Morrow and Company.

54. Huss AJ: Sensorimotor approaches. In Hopkins H and Smith H, editors: Willard and Spackman's occupational therapy, ed 5, Philadelphia, 1978, JB Lippincott Co.

55. Jones GM and Watt D: Muscular control of landing from unexpected falls in man, J Physiol (Lond.) 219:729, 1971.

56. Keller E and Bzdek V: Effects of therapeutic touch on tension headache pain, Nurs Res 35(2):101, 1986.

57. Kenshalo D: Sensory functions of the skin of humans, New York, 1977, Plenum Press.

58. Kottke F: From reflex to skill: the training of coordination, Arch Phys Med Rehabil 61:551, 1980.

59. Kottke F, Stillwell K, and Lehmann J: Krusen's handbook of physical medicine and rehabilitation, ed 3, Philadelphia, 1982, WB Saunders Co.

60. Krieger D: Healing by the laying on of hands as a facilitator of bioenergetic change. The response of in vivo hemoglobin, Psychenergetic Systems 1:121, 1976.

61. Krieger D: The therapeutic touch: how to help your hands to help or heal, Englewood Cliffs, NJ, 1979, Prentice-Hall Books.

62. Krieger D, Peper E, and Ancoli S: Therapeutic touch: searching for evidence of physiological change, Am J Nurs 79:660, 1979.

63. Lagercrantz H and Slotkin T: The stress of being born, Scientific American p. 100 1986.

64. Locke S and Colligan D: Mind cures, OMNI 7:(7)44, 1986.

65. Loeb GE and Hoffer JA: Muscle spindle function: in muscle receptors in movement control, London, 1981, Macmillan Publishing Co.

66. Lynch JJ, Thomas SA, Mills ME, Matinow K, and Kotcher A: The effects of human contact on cardiac arrhythmia in coronary care patients, J Neurol Ment Dis 158:88, 1974.

67. Mann F: Acupuncture: the ancient Chinese art of healing, New York, 1972, Vintage Books—Random House, Inc.

68. Matthews PBC: Muscle spindles and their motor control, Physiol Rev 44:219, 1964.

69. McCloskey DI: Kinesthetic sensibility, Physiol Rev 58:763, 1978.

70. Medalie JH and Goldbourt U: Angina pectoris among 10,000 men with psychosocial and other risk factors as evidenced by a multivariate analysis of a five year incidence study, Am J Med 60(6):920, 1978.

71. Mills ME, Thomas SA, Lynch JJ, Katcher AH: Effect of pulse palpation on cardiac arrhythmia in coronary care patients, Nurs Res 25:378, 1976.

72. Montague A: Touching: the significance of the skin, ed 2, San

Francisco, 1978, Harper & Row Publishers, Inc.

73. Moore J: The Golgi tendon organ and the muscle spindle, Am J Occup Ther 28:415, 1974.

74. Morse JM: An ethnoscientific analysis of comfort: a preliminary investigation, Nursing Papers 15:6, 1983.

75. Murray MP: Gait as a total pattern of movement, Am J Phys Med 46:290, 1967.

76. Nerem RM, Levesque MJ, and Cornhill JF: Social environment as a factor in diet-induced atherosclerosis. Science 208(4451):1475, 1980.

77. Payton R, Hirt E, and Newtown G, editors: Scientific basis for neurophysiologic approaches to therapeutic exercise: an anthology, ed 2, Philadelphia, 1978, FA Davis Co.

78. Pedretti LW: Occupational therapy: practice skills for dysfunction, St Louis, 1981, The CV Mosby Co.

79. Pertovaara M: Modification of human pain threshold by specific tactile receptors, Acta Physiol Scand 107:339, 1979.

80. Randolph G: Therapeutic and physical touch: physiological response to stressful stimuli, Nurs Res 33(1):33, 1984.

81. Rausch P: A tactile and kinesthetic stimulation program for premature infants. In Brown C, editor: The many facets of touch. Special issue, Skillman, NJ, 1984, Johnson & Johnson Companies, Inc.

82. Roberts T: Neurophysiology of postural mechanisms, New York, 1976, Plenum Publishing Co.

83. Rood M: Occupational therapy in the treatment of the cerebral palsied, Phys Ther Rev 32:220, 1952.

84. Rood M: Neurophysiological reactions as a basis for physical therapy, Phys Ther Rev 34:444, 1954.

85. Rood M: Neurophysiological mechanisms utilized in the treatment of neuromuscular dysfunction, Am J Occup Ther 10:4, 1956.

86. Rood M: The use of sensory receptors to activate, facilitate and inhibit motor response, automatic and somatic, in developmental sequence. In Sattely C, editor: Approaches to the treatment of patients with neuromuscular dysfunction, Dubuque, Iowa, 1962, Wm C Brown Book Co, Publishers.

87. Rose S: Preterm responses of passive, active and social touch. In Brown C, editor: The many facets of touch. Special Issue, Skillman, NJ, 1984, Johnson & Johnson Companies, Inc.

88. Schmidt R: Fundamentals of sensory physiology, New York, 1978, Springer-Verlag, Inc.

89. Schwartz P, Malliani A: Electrical alteration of the T wave: clinical and experimental evidence of its relationship with the sympathetic nervous system and with the long Q-T syndrome, Am Heart J 89:45, 1976.

90. Sinclair D: Cutaneous sensation, New York, 1967, Oxford University Press.

91. Smith F: Inner bridges: a guide to energy movement and body structure, Atlanta, Georgia, 1986, Humanic, New Age.

92. Smythies JR: Brain mechanisms and behavior, ed 2, New York, 1970, Academic Press, Inc.

93. Synder S: Neurosciences: an integrative discipline, Science 225(4468):1255, 1984.

94. Spicer SD and Matyas TA: Facilitation of the tonic vibration reflex (TVR) by cutaneous stimulation, Am J Phys Med 59:223, 1980.

95. Stejskal L: Postural reflexes in man, Am J Phys Med 58:1, 1979.

96. Stockmeyer S: An interpretation of the approach of Rood to the treatment of neuromuscular dysfunction, NUSTEP proceedings, Am J Phys Med 46:900, 1967.

97. Taubes G: An electrifying possibility, Discover 7(4):22, 1986.

98. Tokizane T et al: Electromyographic studies on tonic neck, lumbar and labyrinthine reflexes in normal persons, Jpn J Physiol 2:30, 1951.

99. Trombly CA and Scott AD: Occupational therapy for physical dysfunction, Baltimore, 1977, Williams & Wilkins Co.

100. Vallbo A et al: Somatosensory proprioceptive and sympathetic activity in human peripheral nerves, Physiol Rev 4:59, 1979.

101. Weiss S: Psychophysiological effects of caregiver touch on incidence of cardiac dysrhythmia, Heart and Lung, 15(5):495, 1986.

102. Werner J: Neuroscience: a clinical perspective, Philadelphia, 1980, WB Saunders Co.

103. Weschsler R: A new prescription: mind over malady, Discover 2(8): 50, 1987.

104. Williams P and Warwick R: Functional neuroanatomy of man, Philadelphia, 1975, WB Saunders Co.

105. Wilson VJ and Paterson BW: The role of the vestibular system in posture and movement. In Mountcastle V, editor: Medical physiology, ed 14, St Louis, 1979, The CV Mosby Co.

106. Yakovlev P and Lecours A: Regional development of the brain in early life, vol 3, Oxford, 1967, Minkowski Blackwell Scientific Publications.

Chapter

19 Movement therapy

THE BRUNNSTROM APPROACH TO TREATMENT OF HEMIPLEGIA

LORRAINE WILLIAMS PEDRETTI

PROFILE

Signe Brunnstrom was a physical therapist from Sweden. Her practice, teaching, and theory development in the United States extended from the World War II years through the 1970s. Her clinical observation and research at major treatment and educational institutions were done in the Northeast and led to the development of the treatment approach that she called *movement therapy*. Brunnstrom published three major works in the United States, co-authored a book with Donald Kerr, *Training the Lower Extremity Amputee,* and later published the well-known *Clinical Kinesiology.* Her third book was *Movement Therapy in Hemiplegia,* published in 1970 in which she described movement therapy, also known as the *Brunnstrom approach* to the treatment of hemiplegia. Signe Brunnstrom died in February, 1988.[8] The material presented in this chapter is summarized primarily from *Movement Therapy in Hemiplegia.*[3]

The theoretical foundations, treatment goals, and methods are intended as an overview and introduction to some of the procedures that the new practitioner may find helpful. To learn the details of the treatment approach and additional procedures the reader is referred to the original source for further study.

THEORETICAL FOUNDATIONS

Brunnstrom evolved her treatment approach on the basis of an extensive review of the literature in neurophysiology, central nervous system (CNS) mechanisms, effects of CNS damage, sensory systems and related topics, and clinical observation and application of training procedures.[3]

The work of several major theorists, such as Gellhorn, Denny-Brown, Hagbarth, Jackson, Magnus, and Sherrington, served as a foundation for the treatment approach. A few of the important concepts are summarized briefly here. Sherrington, whose work dates to the late 1800s, stated that afferent-efferent (sensory-motor) mechanisms in phylogenesis are re-

tained in man. These mechanisms served as the basis for the evolutionary process that resulted in man's movements being more voluntary than automatic, as seen in lower animals. Sherrington also discovered that sensory denervation abolished all voluntary movement that revealed the necessity of sensation for effective movement.[3]

In the early 1900s Magnus stated that peripheral influences continuously affect the CNS and may work together to facilitate a movement or exert opposite influences that compete with each other. Magnus demonstrated in experimental animals that the same stimulus may evoke opposite motor responses, depending on the position of the responding part.[3] The studies of Magnus support the hypothesis that sensory stimuli and positioning can be used to influence motor function.

In the late 1800s Hughlings Jackson described the successive levels of CNS integration. He postulated that the spinal cord and cranial nerve nuclei are located at the *lowest motor centers* and that muscles in all parts of the body are represented at this level, but few movement combinations are possible. Movements are simple and more automatic than voluntary at this level. He described the *middle motor centers* in the Rolandic region of the brain. All the muscles represented at the lowest motor centers also are represented here. However, more complex movements are possible, but movement is still more automatic than voluntary at the middle motor centers. Jackson stated that the frontal lobes contain the *highest motor centers,* along with corresponding sensory centers. The body parts represented at the middle and lowest motor centers are represented here in a still more complex manner than before. This level subserves complex voluntary movement.[9] Jackson hypothesized that the damaged CNS has undergone an "evolution in reverse." The same reflexes present in earlier phylogenesis and ontogenesis are present once again after CNS damage. Therefore, these reflexes are considered normal for the regressed CNS. Jackson also stated that reflexes are precursors of purposeful movement and that they support purposeful movement.[3] Brunnstrom's treatment approach is based on Jackson's hypotheses.

The successive levels of CNS integration and the reflexes and reactions integrated at each level are summarized as follows:

Spinal level (apedal). Flexor withdrawal, extensor thrust, crossed extension

Brain stem level (apedal). TNR, TLR, associated reactions, positive and negative supporting reactions

Midbrain level (quadrupedal). Neck righting, body righting, labyrinthine righting, optical righting, amphibian reaction, Moro reflex

Cortical level (bipedal). Equilibrium reactions[5]

Twitchell described a sequence of motor recovery after cerebrovascular accident (CVA). He hypothesized that recovery after CVA constitutes a reversal of the regression of CNS function. He stated that primitive responses are the bases for the evolution of more elaborate motor responses. Twitchell also noted that all proprioceptive responses are influenced by neck and body righting reactions, reflexes, and tactile stimulation. He replicated Sherrington's study and proved that (1) sensation is critical to movement, (2) without sensation a limb is essentially useless, (3) preservation of cutaneous sensation in the hand is indispensable for motor function of the upper limb, and (4) movements of the upper limb, particularly grasp function, are directed by contactual stimuli. The recovery process after CVA described by Twitchell is summarized sequentially by the presence of the following:

1. Flaccidity
2. Stretch reflexes
3. Complex proprioceptive reactions such as the proximal traction response
4. Limb synergies with ability to use these movement patterns
5. Decline in spasticity
6. Improvement of willed movement and ability to be influenced by tactile stimuli[10]

Brunnstrom subscribed to the concept that the damaged CNS has undergone an evolution in reverse and regresses to phylogenetically older patterns of movement. These include the *limb synergies,* gross patterns of limb flexion and extension that are primitive spinal cord patterns, and primitive reflexes.[2,3] These primitive movement patterns are modified in man through the influence of higher centers of nervous system control during development. After CVA, they return to their primitive, stereotyped character. When the influence of higher centers is disturbed or destroyed, primitive and pathologic reflexes, such as the tonic neck reflex (TNR), tonic lumbar reflex, and tonic

labyrinthine reflex (TLR), reappear, and normal reflexes, such as the deep tendon reflexes (DTR), become exaggerated. These reflexes were present at an earlier phylogenetic period and therefore may be considered normal when, as in hemiplegia, the central nervous system (CNS) has regressed to an earlier developmental stage.[3]

The Brunnstrom approach to the treatment of hemiplegia is based on the use of motor patterns available to the patient at any point in the recovery process. It enhances progress through the stages of recovery toward more normal and complex movement patterns, and thus reintegration of the CNS.

Brunnstrom saw synergies, reflexes, and other abnormal movement patterns as a normal part of the process that the patient must go through before normal voluntary movement can occur. Synergistic movements are used by normal persons all of the time, but they are controlled, occur in a wide variety of patterns, and can be modified or stopped at will. Brunnstrom maintained that the synergies appear to constitute a necessary intermediate stage for further recovery. Gross movement synergies of flexion and extension always precede the restoration of advanced motor functioning following hemiplegia.[3] Therefore during the early stages of recovery (stages 1 to 3), Brunnstrom maintained that the patient should be aided to gain control of the limb synergies and that selected afferent stimuli (TNR, TLR, cutaneous and stretch stimuli, and positioning and associated reactions) can be advantageous in helping the patient to initiate and gain control of movement. Once the synergies can be performed voluntarily with some ease, they are modified, and simple to complex movement combinations can be performed (stages 4 and 5), which deviate from the stereotypical synergy patterns of flexion and extension.[3]

The advisability of using pathologic and primitive reflexes and movement patterns to affect motion is challenged by Bobath.[1] It is argued that no pathologic responses should be used in training for fear that by repeated use the efferent pathways will become too readily available for use at the expense of normal pathways.[2,3] However, Brunnstrom concluded that the opposite was true. She maintained that during the early stages of recovery, the development of the synergies should be facilitated. The use of selected exteroceptive and proprioceptive stimuli is justified for this purpose.[2,3] Both Bobath and Brunnstrom based their hypotheses on neurophysiology. Brunnstrom proposes that the approaches may not be as opposed as they appear. She stated that at an early recovery stage, only reflex movement is available and is considered normal, whereas at later stages, reflex activity is inhibited and more normal movement is possible. Brunnstrom proposed that both approaches can be useful if applied to a specific patient at a specific time.[3]

The Limb Synergies

A *limb synergy* of flexion or extension, seen in hemiplegia, is a group of muscles acting as a bound unit in a primitive and stereotypical manner.[3] The muscles are neurophysiologically linked and cannot act alone or perform all of their functions. If one muscle in the synergy is activated, each muscle in the synergy responds partially or completely. The patient then cannot perform isolated movements when bound by these synergies.

The flexor synergy of the upper limb consists of scapular adduction and elevation, shoulder abduction and external rotation, elbow flexion, forearm supination, wrist flexion, and finger flexion. Spasticity is usually greatest in the elbow flexion component, and least in shoulder abduction and external rotation (Fig. 19-1). The extensor synergy consists of scapula abduction and depression, shoulder adduction and internal rotation, elbow extension, forearm pronation, and wrist and finger flexion or extension. Shoulder adduction and internal rotation are usually the most spastic components of the extensor synergy, and elbow extension is usually the least spastic component (Fig. 19-2).

In the lower limb the flexor synergy consists of hip flexion and abduction and external rotation, knee flexion, ankle dorsiflexion and inversion, and toe extension. Hip flexion is usually the component with the greatest spasticity, and hip abduction and external rotation are the components with the least spasticity. The extensor synergy is composed of hip adduction, extension, and internal rotation; knee extension; ankle plantar flexion and inversion; and toe flexion. Hip adduction, knee extension, and ankle plantar flexion are usually the most spastic components, whereas hip extension and internal rotation are usually less spastic.

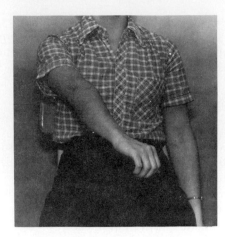

Fig. 19-2. Extensor synergy of upper limb in hemiplegia.

Characteristics of Synergistic Movement

The flexor synergy dominates in the arm, and the extensor synergy dominates in the leg. Performance of synergistic movement, either reflexively or voluntarily, may be influenced by the primitive postural reflex mechanisms. When the patient performs the synergy, the components with the greatest degree of spasticity are often most apparent, rather than the entire classic patterns described above. By the same token the resting posture of the limb, particularly the arm, is usually characterized by a position that represents the most spastic components of both flexor and extensor synergies, that is, shoulder adduction, elbow flexion, forearm pronation, and wrist and finger flexion. However, with facilitation or voluntary effort the more classic synergy pattern can usually be evoked.[3]

Motor Recovery Process

Following CVA resulting in hemiplegia, the patient progresses through a series of recovery steps or stages in fairly stereotypical fashion (Table 19-1). The progress through these stages may be rapid or slow.

The recovery follows an ontogenetic process, usually proximal to distal so that shoulder movement can be expected before hand movement. Flexion patterns occur before extension patterns in the upper limb. Reflex motion occurs before controlled, volitional movement, and gross movement patterns can be performed before isolated, selective movement.[3]

Recovery may cease at any stage, and is influenced by factors such as sensation, perception, cognition, motivation, affective states, and concomitant medical problems. Few patients make a very good recovery of arm function, and the greatest loss is usually in the wrist and hand.

It should be noted that no two patients are exactly alike. There is much individual variation in the char-

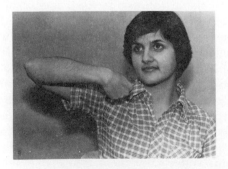

Fig. 19-1. Flexor synergy of upper limb in hemiplegia.

Table 19-1 Motor Recovery Following Cerebrovascular Accident

Stage	Characteristics		
	Leg	*Arm*	*Hand**
1	Flaccidity	Flaccidity; inability to perform any movements	No hand function
2	Spasticity develops; minimal voluntary movements	Beginning development of spasticity; limb synergies or some of their components begin to appear as associated reactions	Gross grasp beginning; minimal finger flexion possible
3	Spasticity peaks; flexion and extension synergy present; hip-knee-ankle flexion in sitting and standing	Spasticity increasing; synergy patterns or some of their components can be performed voluntarily	Gross grasp, hook grasp possible; no release
4	Knee flexion past 90° in sitting, with foot sliding backward on floor; dorsiflexion with heel on floor and knee flexed to 90°	Spasticity declining; movement combinations deviating from synergies are now possible	Gross grasp present; lateral prehension developing; small amount of finger extension and some thumb movement possible
5	Knee flexion with hip extended in standing; ankle dorsiflexion with hip and knee extended	Synergies no longer dominant; more movement combinations deviating from synergies performed with greater ease	Palmar prehension, spherical and cylindrical grasp, and release possible
6	Hip abduction in sitting or standing; reciprocal internal and external rotation of hip combined with inversion and eversion of ankle in sitting	Spasticity absent except when performing rapid movements; isolated joint movements performed with ease	All types of prehension, individual finger motion, and full range of voluntary extension possible

*NOTE: Recovery of hand function is variable and may not parallel the six recovery stages of the arm.
From Brunnstrom S: Movement therapy in hemiplegia, New York, 1970, Harper & Row Publishers, Inc.

acteristic motor disturbances and the recovery process among patients. The motor behavior and recovery process described represent common characteristics that may be observed in most persons after CVA occurs.[3]

DEFINITIONS OF TERMS

Some definitions of terms are necessary to comprehend the discussion of treatment principles that follows.

Associated reactions are movements seen on the affected side in response to voluntary forceful movements in other parts of the body.[3] Resistance to flexion movements of the normal upper extremity usually evokes a flexion synergy or some of its components in the affected upper extremity. By the same token resistance to extension on the sound side evokes extension on the affected side. In the lower extremities the responses are reversed. Resisted flexion of the normal limb evokes extension of the affected limb and vice versa.[7]

Homolateral limb synkinesis is a mutual dependency between the synergies of the affected upper and lower limbs. The same or similar motion occurs in the limb on the same side of the body. For example, efforts at

flexion of the affected upper extremity evoke flexion of the lower extremity.[3,7]

The mirroring of movements attempted or performed on the affected side by the unaffected side, perhaps in an effort to facilitate the movement, is called *imitation synkinesis*.[3]

Several specialized reactions can be noted in the hemiplegic hand. These are the proximal traction response, grasp reflex, instinctive grasp reaction, instinctive avoiding reaction, and Souques' finger phenomenon. The *proximal traction response* is elicited by a stretch to the flexor muscles of one joint of the upper limb, which evokes contraction of all flexors of that limb, including the fingers. It may therefore be used to elicit the flexion synergy. To elicit the *grasp reflex* deep pressure is applied to the palm and moved distally over the hand and fingers, mostly on the radial side. The responses are complex but in general adduction and flexion of the digits are present. The *instinctive grasp reaction* is differentiated by Brunnstrom from the grasp reflex. It is a closure of the hand in response to contact of a stationary object with the palm of the hand. The person is unable to release the object-stimulus once the fist has been closed.

A hyperextension reaction of the fingers and thumb

in response to forward-upward elevation of the arm is the *instinctive avoiding reaction*. Brunnstrom reported that, with the arm in this position, stroking distally over the palm and attempting to reach out and grasp an object resulted in an exaggeration of the reaction. The automatic extension of the fingers when the shoulder is flexed is known as *Souques' finger phenomenon* and can be observed in some but not all hemiplegic patients. Brunnstrom found that although this phenomenon may not be exhibited, the elevated position of the affected arm is favorable for the facilitation of finger extension.[3]

MOTOR EVALUATION OF HEMIPLEGIC PATIENT

Brunnstrom in *Movement Therapy in Hemiplegia* described an evaluation procedure that assesses muscle tone, stage of recovery, movement patterns, motor speed, and prehension patterns of the upper extremity.[3]

The evaluation is based on the recovery stages after the onset of hemiplegia. The test requires the patient to perform motor acts that are graduated in complexity and require increasingly finer neuromuscular control. Thus the degree of recovery of the CNS can be evaluated.

Progress through the recovery stages is gradual, and signs of two stages may be apparent at any given time in the patient's recovery. Because it is not possible to establish an absolute demarcation between one recovery stage and the next, the patient may be classified as stages 2 and 3 or 3 and 4, for example. This indicates progression from one stage to the next. The Hemiplegia Classification and Progress Record is presented in Fig. 19-3. The reader should refer to this while reading the directions for test administration, which have been summarized from *Movement Therapy in Hemiplegia*.

Gross Sensory Testing

Sensory evaluation precedes motor evaluation and includes assessment of passive motion sense and touch localization in the hand. Tests of passive motion sense of the shoulder, elbow, forearm, wrist, and fingers are carried out by procedures similar to those described in Chapter 11. Results are recorded on the first and second pages of the form (shown in Fig. 19-3, *A* and *B*).

Fingertip recognition is evaluated by asking the subject to localize touch stimuli to specific fingers. The subject is seated with forearms pronated and resting on a pillow in the lap. The test is given with the vision occluded after a rehearsal in full view. The palmar surface of the fingertips is lightly touched with a pencil eraser in a random sequence. The subject must indicate which finger is being touched. Results are recorded on the second page of the form (Fig. 19-3, *B*).

Motor Tests, Upper Extremity

The subject is classified as being in recovery stage 1 when no voluntary movement of the affected arm can be initiated.[3] The examiner should move the limb passively through the synergy patterns and assess the degree of resistance to passive movement. The subject should be asked to attempt movement during these maneuvers. During recovery stage 1 the limb is predominantly flaccid and will feel heavy, there will be little or no resistance to passive movement, and the subject is unable to initiate or effect any movement voluntarily. At this time the subject is likely to be confined to bed and to be too weak for extensive evaluation.

During recovery stage 2 spasticity begins to increase, and the limb synergies or some of their components may be evoked on voluntary effort or as associated reactions. The flexor synergy usually appears first.[3] The examiner may again move the limb passively, alternating between flexor and extensor synergy patterns. The examiner should ask the subject to "help" in the movements. Thus it is possible to assess the degree of spasticity and to assess whether the subject's voluntary efforts are evoking any movement responses.

During recovery stage 3, spasticity is increased and may be marked. The limb synergies or some of their components are performed voluntarily. The subject may remain at this stage for a long period of time. Severely involved hemiplegics may never progress beyond it. The pectoralis major, pronators, and wrist and finger flexors may be very spastic, causing limited performance of their antagonists.

The subject is seated, and the complete flexor synergy is demonstrated by the examiner. The subject is asked to perform the movement pattern with the unaffected side to demonstrate that the directions are understood. The subject is then asked to perform the movement pattern with the affected side after a command, such as "touch your ear" or "touch your mouth," which gives purpose and direction to the effort.

A similar procedure is used to evaluate performance of the extensor synergy. The subject is asked to reach forward and downward to touch the examiner's hand, which is held between the subject's knees.

The responses may be influenced by the predominant spasticity seen in components of each of the synergies. For instance, the very spastic pectoralis major and elbow flexors may predominate during the subject's efforts and result in the subject reaching across the thorax to touch the opposite shoulder.

The status of the synergies is recorded on the evaluation form in terms of the active joint range achieved for each motion in the pattern. The joint ranges are estimated and recorded as 0, ¼, ½, ¾, or full range.

When the subject has reached recovery stage 4, there is a decrease in spasticity, and the subject is capable of performing gross movement combinations that deviate from the limb synergies. Brunnstrom

chose three movements to represent stage 4. These are (1) placing the hand behind the body to touch the sacral region, (2) raising the arm forward to 90° of shoulder flexion with elbow extended, and (3) pronating and supinating the forearm with the elbow flexed to 90° and stabilized close to the side of the body. The subject performs all of the movements while seated, and as in all test items, no facilitation is allowed. During the test for pronation-supination, bilateral performance is allowed so that the examiner can make a comparison of the two sides.

```
HEMIPLEGIA  CLASSIFICATION AND PROGRESS RECORD

              Upper limb-test sitting

Name _____ Age ____ Date of onset ____ Side affected _____

Date _____

____ Passive motion sense:  Shoulder _____ Elbow _____

____ Pronation-supination _____ Wrist flexion-extension_____

____ 1. NO MOVEMENT INITIATED OR ELICITED _____

____ 2. SYNERGIES OR COMPONENTS FIRST APPEARING.  Spasticity developing ____
____    Flexor synergy_____
____    Extensor synergy_____

____ 3. SYNERGIES OR COMPONENTS INITIATED VOLUNTARILY.  Spasticity marked ____
```

FLEXOR SYNERGY		ACTIVE JOINT RANGE		REMARKS
Shoulder girdle	Elevation			
	Retraction			
Shoulder joint	Hyperextension			
	Abduction			
	External rotation			
Elbow	Flexion			
Forearm	Supination			
EXTENSOR SYNERGY				
Shoulder	Pectoralis major			
Elbow	Extension			
Forearm	Pronation			
4. MOVEMENTS DEVIATING FROM BASIC SYNERGIES. Spasticity decreasing	Hand to sacral region			
	Raise arm forward-horizontally			
	Pronate-supinate elbow at 90 degrees			
5. RELATIVE IN-DEPENDENCE OF BASIC SYNERGIES. Spasticity waning	Raise arm sideways -horizontally			
	Raise arm over head			
	Pronate-supinate elbow extended			
6. MOVEMENT COORDINATION NEAR NORMAL. Spasticity minimal				

Continued.

Fig. 19-3. A, Hemiplegia classification and progress record. From Brunnstrom S: Movement therapy in hemiplegia, New York, 1970, Harper & Row Publishers, Inc.

```
┌─────────────────────────────────────────────────────────────────────────┐
│              HEMIPLEGIA  CLASSIFICATION AND PROGRESS RECORD                │
│                                                                           │
│                    Upper limb-test sitting  cont'd                        │
│                                                                           │
│     Name _____                                      │
│                                                                           │
│     Date _____                                      │
│                                                                           │
│                                                                           │
│         SPEED TESTS FOR Classes 4, 5, 6      Strokes per 5 second         │
│                                                                           │
│         Hand from          Normal        ┌──────────┬──────────┐          │
│    ___  lap to chin        Affected      │          │          │          │
│                                          ├──────────┼──────────┤          │
│         Hand from lap      Normal        │          │          │          │
│    ___  to opposite knee   Affected      │          │          │          │
│                                          └──────────┴──────────┘          │
│    ___  Passive motion sense, digits_____ │
│                                                                           │
│    ___  Fingertip recognition _____ │
│                                                                           │
│         Wrist stabilization   1.  Elbow extended_____ │
│    ___  for grasp                                                         │
│                               2.  Elbow flexed_____  │
│         Wrist flexion         1.  Elbow extended_____  │
│         and extension                                                     │
│    ___  Fist closed           2.  Elbow flexed_____  │
│    ___  Wrist circumduction _____  │
│                                                                           │
│         DIGITS                                                            │
│                                                                           │
│    ___  Mass grasp_____ Dynamometer test  Normal_____lb.     │
│                                                       Affected_____lb.    │
│                                                                           │
│    ___  Mass extension _____ │
│                                                                           │
│    ___  Hook grasp (handbag, 2 lb.)_____ │
│                                                                           │
│    ___  Lateral prehension (card)_____ │
│                                                                           │
│    ___  Palmar prehension (pencil)_____ │
│                                                                           │
│    ___  Cylindrical grasp (small jar)_____ │
│                                                                           │
│    ___  Spherical grasp (ball)_____ Catch_____ Throw_____  │
│                                                                           │
│         Indiv. thumb movements                                           │
│    ___  hands in lap          1.  Vertical movements _____  │
│         Ulnar side down       2.  Horizontal movements_____   │
│                                                                           │
│    ___  Individual finger movements_____  │
│                                                                           │
│    ___  Button and unbutton shirt     Using both hands_____   │
│    ___                                 Using affected hand only_____    │
│                                                                           │
│    ___  Other skilled activities _____  │
└─────────────────────────────────────────────────────────────────────────┘
```

Continued.

Fig. 19-3, cont'd. B, Hemiplegia classification and progress record. From Brunnstrom S: Movement therapy in hemiplegia, New York, 1970, Harper & Row Publishers, Inc.

Further decrease of spasticity and ability to perform more complex combinations of movement characterize recovery stage 5. The subject is relatively free of the influence of the limb synergies and performs the stage 4 movements with greater ease. Three movements chosen to represent stage 5 are (1) raising the arm to 90° of shoulder abduction with the elbow extended and forearm pronated, (2) raising the arm forward, as in stage 4, but above 90° of shoulder flexion, and (3) pronating and supinating the forearm with the elbow extended. The third movement is performed with the arm in the forward or side horizontal position and is not isolated from shoulder internal and external rotation.

Hemiplegics who progess to recovery stage 6 are able to perform isolated joint motions and demonstrate coordination that is comparable or nearly comparable to that of the unaffected side. On close observation the trained observer may detect some awkwardness of movement, and there may be some incoordination when rapid movement is attempted. The subject may be evaluated while performing a va-

HEMIPLEGIA   CLASSIFICATION AND PROGRESS RECORD

Trunk and lower limb

Name_____ Evaluation date_____

SUPINE

Passive   Hip_____ Knee_____
motion
sense   Ankle_____ Big toe _____

Flexor synergy_____

Extensor synergy_____

Hip: Abduction_____ Adduction_____

SITTING ON CHAIR   STANDING

Trunk balance   With_____ Without_____ support
(no back support)   Balance, normal limb   sec.

Sole sensation   Correct _____   Double scale   (a) _____   (b)_____
(no. of answers)   Incorrect   reading†

Hip-knee-ankle flexion   Hip-knee-ankle flexion

Knee flexion-extension small range   Knee flexion-extension small range

Knee flexion beyond 90 degrees   Knee flexion hip extended

Ankle, isolated dorsiflexion   Ankle, isolated dorsiflexion

Reciprocal hamstring action*   Hip abduction knee extended

AMBULATION   Evaluation date _____

Brace?_____ Cane?_____ In parallel bars_____

Supported_____ Escorted_____ Alone_____

Arm in sling_____ Arm swings loosely_____ Elbow held flexed_____

Arm swings near normal _____

GAIT ANALYSIS   Evaluation date_____

STANCE PHASE   SWING PHASE

Ankle_____ _____   _____

Knee_____ _____   _____

Hip_____ _____   _____

Walking cadence: Steps per min.   Speed: Feet per min.

*Inward and outward rotation at knee with inversion-eversion at ankle.
†Recorded as normal/affected; (a) preferred stance, (b) weight shift on affected limb.

Fig. 19-3, cont'd. C, Hemiplegia classification and progress record. From Brunnstrom S: Movement therapy in hemiplegia, New York, 1970, Harper & Row Publishers, Inc.

riety of daily living tasks, provided that recovery of hand function has kept pace with recovery of arm function.

The tests of motor speed on the second page of the evaluation form (Fig. 19-3, B) may be used to assess spasticity during any recovery stage, provided that the subject has enough range of active motion to perform the necessary movement. The tests are especially useful in stages 4, 5, and 6. The normal side is tested first for comparison; then the affected side is tested. The two movements that are tested are (1) hand to chin and (2) hand to opposite knee. The subject is seated in a sturdy chair without armrests. The trunk should be stabilized against the back of the chair, and the head should be erect. The hand is closed, but not tightly, and rests in the lap. For the hand-to-chin test the forearm is at 0° neutral between pronation and supination. The examiner asks the patient to bring the hand from lap to chin as rapidly as possible, first with the unaffected side and then with the affected side, and records the number of full back-and-forth movements accomplished in 5 seconds. If speed is slow because of marked spasticity, half movements may be counted. The same procedure is followed for the hand-to-opposite knee test, except that the forearm is positioned in full pronation on the lap. The hand is moved from the lap to the opposite knee, using full range of elbow extension. These two tests measure the spasticity of elbow flexors and extensors.

Wrist stabilization, which is automatic during normal grasp, is often lacking after a stroke. Therefore it is important to evaluate wrist stabilization during fist closure. This is done with the elbow both flexed and extended. During the recovery stages when the synergies are dominant, the wrist tends to flex when the elbow flexes. The subject is asked to make a fist while the elbow is extended across the front of the body. The subject is then asked to make a fist while the elbow is flexed at the side of the body. Whether the wrist remains stabilized in the neutral position or extends slightly is observed. This test is followed by a request for wrist flexion and extension with the fist closed. The subject holds an object such as a wide (1¾ inches, or 4.5 cm) dowel, and extends and flexes the wrist. This is done in the elbow-extended and elbow-flexed positions as on the previous test.

Circumduction of the wrist indicates significant recovery to the advanced stages. When evaluating the ability to perform this movement, the examiner should stabilize the forearm in pronation. The upper arm should be stabilized against the trunk.

Mass grasp is tested with a dynamometer, which measures pounds of pressure of grasp strength. The normal side is tested first; then the affected side is

tested, and the results are recorded for comparison. Mass extension is evaluated by asking the subject to release and actively extend the fingers to the degree possible. Whether active extension was accomplished and the approximate amount of range achieved should be noted on the form. Active release to full range of extension is very difficult for many persons with CVA.

All types of prehension are evaluated in order of their difficulty. Everyday tasks that require the particular prehension pattern should be used. Hook grasp may be assessed by asking the subject to hold a handbag. Holding a card demands lateral prehension. Palmar prehension is required for grasping a pencil. Cylindrical grasp may be assessed by asking the subject to hold a small, narrow jar. Grasping a ball requires spherical grasp. The subject's ability to catch and throw the ball may be observed. These are difficult activities for hemiplegics, because they require rapid grasp and release, coordination of the entire limb, and time-space judgment. In all the prehension tests the normal side should be observed first for purposes of comparison.

Individual thumb movements are evaluated with the subject's hand resting in the lap, ulnar side down. The normal side is observed first; then the affected side is observed. The subject is asked to move the thumb up and down (flexion-extension) and side to side (adduction-abduction).

Individual finger movements are evaluated by asking the subject to tap the index and middle fingers on the tabletop or on a pillow held in the lap. Isolated control of metacarpophalangeal (MP) flexion and extension is assessed and noted on the evaluation form.

Fine, coordinated use of the affected hand/arm and of both hands together usually is indicative of advanced recovery. Subjects who have succeeded well at the prehension tests may be asked to button and unbutton a shirt, first using both hands, then using the affected hand only. Other skilled activities, such as writing, threading a needle, removing a small bottle cap, and picking up and placing ¼-inch (0.6 cm) mosaic tiles, may be used to further test skilled hand use.

Motor Tests, Trunk and Lower Extremity

To evaluate trunk and lower extremity function the patient is tested first in the supine position, then in the sitting position, and then in the standing position. If the patient is ambulatory, a gait analysis is made (Fig. 19-3, C). Tests in the supine position include tests of passive motion sense, flexor and extensor synergies, and hip abduction and adduction. In the sitting position trunk balance, sole sensation, and specific movements of the lower limb are tested. These include hip-knee-ankle flexion, knee flexion and extension in small range, knee flexion beyond 90°, isolated ankle dorsiflexion, and reciprocal hamstring action (which is inward and outward rotation at the knee with inversion-eversion at the ankle). In the standing position balance and selected movements are evaluated. These are hip-knee-ankle flexion, knee flexion-extension in small range, knee flexion with the hip extended, isolated ankle dorsiflexion, and hip abduction with the knee extended. The lower extremity evaluation concludes with a gait analysis, including timed walking cadence.[3]

In facilities where evaluation is coordinated between physical therapy and occupational therapy the physical therapist is primarily responsible for the trunk and lower limb testing, and the occupational therapist may test for upper extremity function. However, each therapist working with the patient must be aware of the test results and use an integrated approach in treatment. An integrated approach incorporates upper limb, trunk and lower limb function, according to prescribed treatment goals.

GENERAL PRINCIPLES OF FACILITATING MOTOR FUNCTION

The goal of Brunnstrom's movement therapy is to facilitate the patient's progress through the recovery stages that occur after onset of hemiplegia (see Table 19-1). Use of the available afferent-efferent mechanisms of control is the means for attainment of this goal. Some of these mechanisms are summarized here.

Postural and attitudinal reflexes are used as means to increase or decrease tone in specific muscles.[7] For instance, changes in head and body position can influence muscle tone by evoking the tonic reflexes, such as the TNR, tonic lumbar reflex, TLR, and equilibrium and protective reactions. Associated reactions may be used to initiate or elicit synergies in the early stages of recovery by giving resistance to the contralateral muscle group on the normal side. Efforts at flexion synergy of the affected leg may be used to elicit a flexion synergy of the arm through homolateral limb synkinesis.

Stimulating the skin over a muscle by rubbing with the fingertips produces contraction of that muscle and facilitation of the synergy to which the muscle belongs. An example is briskly stimulating the triceps muscle during other efforts at performance of the extension synergy, which enhances elbow extension and amplifies the synergy pattern. Muscle contraction is facilitated when muscles are placed in their lengthened position, and the quick stretch of a muscle facilitates its contraction and inhibits its antagonist. Resistance

facilitates the contraction of muscles resisted. Synergistic movement may be augmented by the voluntary effort of the patient. Visual stimulation through the use of mirrors, videotape of self, and movement of parts can facilitate motion in some patients as can auditory stimuli in the forms of loud and repetitive commands to perform the desired movement.

The strongest component of one synergy inhibits its antagonist through reciprocal innervation. It follows that if relaxation of the stronger or spastic muscle can be effected, it may be possible to evoke some activity in the weaker antagonist, which may appear to be functionless because of its inability to overcome the very spastic agonist.[2,7]

GENERAL TREATMENT GOALS AND METHODS

Before the initiation of any intervention strategies the occupational and physical therapists must make a thorough evaluation of the motor, sensory, perceptual, and cognitive functions of the adult hemiplegic. The motor evaluation yields information about stage of recovery, muscle tone, passive motion sense, hand function, sitting and standing balance, leg function, and ambulation. The treatment goals and methods summarized are directed primarily to the rehabilitation of the hemiplegic upper extremity. The point at which the therapist initiates treatment depends on the stage of recovery and muscle tone of the individual patient.

Bed Positioning

Proper bed positioning begins immediately after the onset of the stroke when the patient is in the flaccid stage.[3] During this period the limbs can be placed in the most favorable positions without interference from spastic muscles. Correct bed positioning is often the responsibility of the nurse; therefore it is essential that the physical therapist or occupational therapist provide information about the influence of the limb synergies on bed postures.

If left unsupervised, the lower limb tends to assume a position of hip external rotation and abduction and knee flexion. This posture is partly a result of mechanical influences on the flaccid limb, that is, the weight of the part tends to pull the hip into external rotation. Neurologically, this position mimics the flexor synergy of the lower extremity. The advent of muscular tension in the flexor and abductor muscle groups of the hip and the flexor group of the knee contributes to the posture of the lower extremity as described above.

If the extensor synergy is developed in the lower extremity, a different position may be present. Spasticity of the extensor muscles usually exceeds that of the flexor muscles in the lower limb. In this case the posture of the lower extremity is characterized by extension and adduction at the hip, knee extension, and ankle plantar flexion. If adductor spasticity is severe, the patient may habitually place the unaffected leg under the affected leg, which allows the affected limb to adduct even more and results in a crossed-limb posture.

If the extensor synergy dominates in the lower limb, the recommended bed position in the supine position is slight flexion of the hip and knee maintained by a small pillow under the knee. Lateral support of the leg at the knee with pillows or a rolled blanket or bolster should be provided to prevent abduction and external rotation. The bed clothes should be supported to prevent them from resting on the foot. This helps to prevent excessive ankle plantar flexion. The position of slight flexion at the hip and knee is beneficial because it has an inhibitory effect on the extensor muscles of the knee and ankle, counteracting the development of severe spasticity in these muscles, which hinders ambulation.

If the flexor synergy dominates in the lower limb, the knee must be maintained in extension. Hip external rotation can be prevented with supports as described above. The choice of bed position is determined on an individual basis. The position selected should be opposite the pattern of the greatest amount of muscle tone to effect the inhibition of excessive spasticity.

The affected upper extremity is supported on a pillow in a position comfortable for the patient. Abduction of the humerus in relation to the scapula should be avoided, because in this position the stabilizing action of the lower portion of the glenoid fossa on the humeral head is reduced and the superior portion of the joint capsule is slackened. This position can predispose the humeral head to downward subluxation. In handling the patient, traction on the affected upper extremity is to be avoided. The patient is instructed to use the unaffected hand to support the affected arm when moving about in bed.

Bed Mobility

Turning toward the affected side is easier for patients than turning toward the unaffected side, because it requires little activity of the affected limb(s). The affected arm is placed close to the body and the patient rolls over the affected arm when turning. Turning toward the unaffected side requires muscular effort of the affected limbs. The unaffected arm can be used to elevate the affected arm to a vertical position over the face, with the shoulder in 80° or 90° of flexion and the elbow fully extended. The affected lower extremity is positioned in partial flexion at the knee and hip and can be stabilized in this position momentarily by the therapist. The patient turns by swinging the arms and the affected knee across the body toward the unaffected side. The movements of the limbs assist in the turn of the upper body and pelvis. When control improves, the patient can carry out the maneuver independently in one smooth, continuous movement to turn from the supine position to the side-lying position on the unaffected side.

Trunk Movement and Balance

One of the early goals in treatment is for the patient to achieve good trunk or sitting balance. Most hemiplegic persons demonstrate "listing" to the affected side, which may result in a fall if the appropriate equilibrium responses do not occur. To evoke balance responses the therapist deliberately disturbs the patient's erect sitting posture in forward-backward and side-to-side direction. This may be done while the patient sits on a chair, edge of a bed, or mat table. The patient is prepared for the procedure with an explanation and is pushed, at first, gently, then more vigorously. The patient may support the affected arm by cradling it to protect the shoulder. This prevents the patient from grasping the supporting surface during the procedure. Later the therapist initiates and assists the patient with bending the trunk directly forward and obliquely forward. The patient sits and supports the affected arm as previously described. The therapist's hands are held under the patient's elbows. The therapist may use the knees to stabilize the patient's knees if balance is poor. In this position the therapist guides the patient while inclining the trunk forward and obliquely and attains some passive glenohumeral and scapular motion at the same time.

Trunk rotation is encouraged in a similar manner, with the therapist sitting in front of the patient or standing behind and supporting the patient's arms as before. Trunk rotation is first performed through a limited range and is gently guided by the therapist. The range is gradually increased. Some neck mobilization may be attained almost automatically during these maneuvers. As the trunk rotates, the patient cradles the affected arm and swings the arms rhythmically from side to side to achieve shoulder abduction and adduction alternately as the trunk rotates. The shoulder components of the flexor and extensor synergies might be evoked during these procedures through the TNR and tonic lumbar reflexes.[3]

Shoulder Range of Motion

A second important early goal in treatment is to maintain or achieve pain-free range of motion (ROM) at the glenohumeral joint. There appears to be a relationship between the shoulder pain, so common in adult hemiplegics, and the stretching of spastic muscles around the shoulder joint. Traditional forced passive exercise procedures may actually produce this stretching and contribute to the development of pain. Such exercise is harmful and contraindicated. Once the patient has experienced the pain, the anticipation of it increases the muscular tension that in turn decreases the joint mobility and increases the pain experienced on passive motion. Therefore the shoulder joint should be mobilized without forceful stretching of hypertonic musculature about the shoulder and shoulder girdle.

This is accomplished through guided trunk motion. The patient sits erect, cradling the affected arm. The therapist supports the arms under the elbows while the patient leans forward. The more the patient leans, the greater the range of shoulder flexion that can be obtained. The therapist guides the arms gently and passively into shoulder flexion while the patient's attention is focused on the trunk motion. In a similar fashion the therapist can guide the arms into abduction and adduction while the patient rotates the trunk from side to side. The TNR and tonic lumbar reflex facilitate relaxation of muscles during this maneuver. When the patient is confident that the shoulder can be moved painlessly, active-assisted movements of the arm in relation to the trunk can begin.

First, the patient moves both shoulders into elevation and depression and scapula adduction and abduction. These are then combined with glenohumeral movements. The arm is supported by the therapist from behind, with the shoulder between forward flexion and abduction, the elbow flexed less than 90°, and the wrist supported in slight extension. The therapist may ask the patient to elevate the shoulders while tapping the upper trapezius with the fingertips. At the same time the therapist is assisting the patient to elevate the arm as well. Active shoulder elevation tends to elicit other components of the flexor synergy that in turn tends to inhibit the very spastic adduction component of the extensor synergy (pectoralis major), allowing the therapist to elevate the arm into abduction by small degrees each time the patient repeats the active shoulder girdle elevation. The procedure is repeated, and the therapist gives the appropriate verbal commands "pull up, let go." The abduction movement is at an oblique angle between forward flexion and full abduction. Sideward abduction with the arm in the same plane as the trunk is likely to be painful and should be avoided. Alternate pronation and supination of the forearm by the therapist should accompany the elevation and lowering of the arm throughout the procedure. The forearm should be supinated when the shoulder is elevated and pronated when the arm is lowered. Head rotation to the normal side inhibits activity in the pectoralis major muscle through the TNR. When abduction movement above the horizontal has been accomplished without pain, the patient can be directed to reach overhead and straighten out the elbow if there has been sufficient recovery to do so. The patient is directed to rotate the head to the affected side to facilitate the elbow extension while observing the movement of the arm.

These techniques result in increased ROM at the shoulder and also help the development of the flexor synergy. A small ROM in the path of the extensor synergy should be performed between the patient's efforts at flexion so that both synergies are developed. As training progresses, greater emphasis is placed on the development of the extensor synergy.

Shoulder Subluxation

Glenohumeral subluxation appears to be a result of dysfunction of the rotator cuff muscles: supraspinatus, infraspinatus, teres minor, and subscapularis. Activation of these muscles in treatment is necessary if subluxation is to be minimized or prevented. Function of the supraspinatus muscle is particularly important for the prevention of subluxation. Slings have been used in an effort to hold the humeral head in the glenoid fossa, but they do not in any way activate the muscles needed to protect the integrity of the shoulder joint.[3] Recently, the use of slings has been found to be of little value and may actually be harmful.[4] A more complete discussion of shoulder problems and slings appears in Chapter 20.

METHODS OF TREATMENT
Upper Limb Training

The training procedures for improving arm function are geared to the patient's recovery stage. During stages 1 and 2 when the arm is essentially flaccid or some components of the synergy patterns are beginning to appear, the aim is to elicit muscle tone and the synergy patterns on a reflex basis. This is accomplished through a variety of facilitation procedures. Associated reactions and tonic reflexes may be employed to influence tone and evoke reflexive movement. The proximal traction response may be used to activate the flexor synergy. Tapping over the upper and middle trapezius, rhomboids, and biceps may elicit components of the flexor synergy. Tapping over the triceps and stretching of the serratus anterior may activate components of the extensor synergy. Passive movement alternately through each of the synergy patterns is not only an excellent means for maintaining ROM of several joints but provides the patient with proprioceptive and visual feedback for the desired patterns of early movement. Quick stretch and surface stroking of the skin over them are also used to activate muscles.

These methods are not employed in any set order or routine but are selected to suit the particular responses of each individual patient. Because the flexor synergy usually appears first, it may be useful to begin trying to elicit the flexor patterns. This should be followed immediately with facilitation of the extensor synergy components, because these tend to be weaker and more difficult to perform in later stages of recovery.[3,6]

When the patient has recovered to stages 2 and 3, the synergies or their components are present and may be performed voluntarily. Spasticity is developing and reaches its peak in stage 3. During this period the aim is for the patient to achieve voluntary control of the synergy patterns. This is accomplished by repetitious alternating performance of the synergy patterns, first with the assistance and facilitation of the therapist. Facilitation is provided through resistance to voluntary motion, verbal commands, tapping, and cutaneous stimulation. This is followed by voluntary repetition of the synergy patterns without the facilitation and, finally, concentration on the components of the synergies from proximal to distal with, then without, facilitation. Bilateral rowing movements with the therapist holding the patient's hands are a useful activity for reciprocal motion of the synergies that should be started during this time.[3,6]

The treatment aim during stages 4 and 5 is to break away from the synergies by mixing components from antagonistic synergies to perform new and increasingly complex patterns of movement. One means for accomplishing this goal is to use skateboard or powder board exercises in arcs of movement to get elbow flexion, combined with shoulder horizontal adduction and forearm pronation, and alternating with shoulder horizontal abduction and elbow extension with forearm supination (Fig. 19-4). These same movement patterns may be used to perform the therapeutic activities just mentioned. Later the patient may be able to perform the more complex figure eight pattern on the skateboard or powder board.

In the final recovery stages 5 and 6 increasingly complex movement combinations and isolated motions are possible. The aims in treatment are to achieve ease in performance of movement combina-

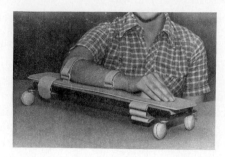

Fig. 19-4. Skateboard exercises for synergy or combined movement patterns in gravity-eliminated plane.

tions and isolated motion and to increase speed of movement.

It should be noted that the hemiplegic upper extremity seldom makes a full recovery. If voluntary and spontaneous movement is possible, the patient should be trained to use the limb as an assist to the sound arm to the extent possible in bilateral activities.

Hand Training

Methods for retraining hand function are treated separately, because recovery of hand function does not always coincide with arm recovery. Hand retraining commensurate with the recovery status of the patient should be carried out continuously.

The first goal of hand retraining is to achieve mass grasp. The proximal traction response and grasp reflex may be used to elicit early grasp movement on a reflex level. During the proximal traction response maneuver the therapist should maintain the patient's wrist in extension and give the command "squeeze."

Because the normal association between wrist extension and grasp is disturbed, another important aim is to achieve wrist fixation for grasp. Wrist extension often accompanies the extensor synergy. Wrist extension can be evoked if the therapist applies resistance to the proximal palm or fist while supporting the arm in the position described earlier for elevation of the arm into abduction. Percussion of the wrist extensors with the elbow in extension and arm elevated and supported by the therapist can activate wrist extension. The proximal portion of the extensors are tapped, and the therapist directs the patient to "squeeze" simultaneously. The commands to "squeeze" and "stop squeezing" are given at appropriate points in the facilitation procedures. During the wrist extension and fist closure the therapist carries the elbow forward into extension. During the wrist and finger relaxation the therapist carries the elbow back into flexion. While the patient is maintaining fist closure, the therapist may withdraw the wrist support and give the command "hold." The therapist may continue tapping the wrist extensors while the patient attempts to hold the posture. The goal is to synchronize the muscles for fist closure with wrist extension.

This procedure should be alternated with a command to "stop squeezing," and the wrist should be allowed to drop and fingers opened while the elbow is moved into flexion. These steps are alternated and the wrist extension-fist closure is performed gradually with increasing amounts of elbow flexion so that the patient can learn to grasp with wrist stabilization when the arm is in a variety of positions.

A third objective in hand retraining is to achieve active release of grasp. This is difficult, because there is usually a considerable degree of spasticity in the flexor muscles of the hand. A release of tension in the finger flexors, then, is primary to the achievement of any active finger extension. Active grasp should be alternated with manipulations to release tension in the flexors. The therapist sits facing the patient and pulls the thumb out of the palm by gripping the thenar eminence. The forearm is supinated. The wrist is allowed to remain in slight flexion. The therapist maintains the grasp around the thumb and alternately pronates and supinates the forearm with emphasis on supination. Pressure on the thumb is decreased during pronation and increased during supination. Cutaneous stimulation is given to the dorsum of the hand and wrist when the forearm is supinated. This manipulation is likely to develop some tension in the finger extensors, and the fingers extend. The patient may actually participate in opening the hand when the forearm is supinated. However, strong efforts on the part of the patient may evoke flexion instead and should be avoided.

If this manipulation is inadequate, stretch of the finger extensors may be used. With the therapist and patient positioned and the hand manipulated as just described, the therapist uses the free hand for distally directed, rapid stroking movements over the proximal phalanges of the affected hand. This causes momentary flexion of the metacarpophalangeal joints (MP), which then bounce back into partial extension. The stroking movement is performed so that the proximal, then distal interphalangeal (IP) joints are included. The movement is performed rapidly and continuously, causing rapid flexion and then bounce back of MP and IP joints. The fingers become extended, and the finger flexors are relaxed because they are reciprocally inhibited by the stretch reflex response in the extensors. If the flexors are stretched or stroking is performed over the palmar surface of the fingers, the spasticity returns to the finger flexors, and they act to close the hand.[3] For this reason the fingers should not be pulled into extension.

Active finger extension may be further facilitated by the use of a finger extension exercise glove with rubber bands, which the patient uses while the hand is manipulated into supination with the thumb pulled out of the palm as described earlier (Fig. 19-5).

Elevation above the horizontal position evokes the extensor reflexes of the fingers. After flexor spasticity has been decreased by the maneuvers just described, the therapist stands on the affected side and maintains the thumb in abduction and extension and the forearm in pronation. The fingers are kept in extension by pressure over the IP joints and stabilization of the fingertips. The grip on the thumb is released, and the arm is raised above the horizontal position. The therapist strokes distally over the IP joints with the heel of her hand. The fingers extend or hyperextend, and the therapist gradually discontinues contact with the patient's hand. If the patient is ready, slight voluntary mental effort can be superimposed on the reflex extension which may bring about additional extension of the fingers.

If the forearm is supinated while the arm is elevated, thumb extension is enhanced. The hand should be positioned overhead for this maneuver. To facilitate extension of the fourth and fifth fingers the forearm should be pronated as the arm is elevated and friction should be applied over the ulnar side of the dorsum of the forearm.

When reflex extension of the fingers is well established, alternate fist opening and closing can begin. The arm is lowered passively, and the elbow is flexed. The forearm and wrist are supported, and the patient is asked to "squeeze" then "stop squeezing." As soon as the fingers relax, the manipulations to facilitate finger extension are carried out. These two steps are alternated, and the patient's voluntary efforts are superimposed on the reflex activity so that the movements begin to assume a semivoluntary character. Semivoluntary finger extension is influenced by the position of the limb and appears to be linked to gross movements other than the synergy patterns.

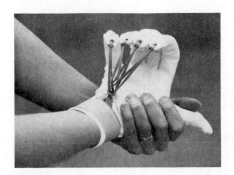

Fig. 19-5. Finger extension exercise glove.

Voluntary movements of the thumb appear when semivoluntary mass extension becomes possible. Once the flexor muscles have been relaxed, the hand can be placed in the patient's lap, ulnar side down, and the patient can attempt to move the thumb away from the first finger, a preliminary for lateral prehension. The therapist may stimulate the tendons of the abductor pollicis and the extensor pollicis brevis by tapping or friction at the point where they pass over the wrist to enhance the patient's effort. The patient can learn to "twiddle" the thumbs to attain further control of thumb motion. The patient folds hands, wrists slightly flexed, and moves the thumbs around each other. Initially the normal thumb may push the other around, but the involved thumb may begin to participate actively. The willed effort, visual input, and sensory feedback from affected and unaffected sides contribute to the development of this movement. During treatment sessions the patient must be comfortable and relaxed. The patient's willed efforts must be slight because too much effort may evoke a flexor rather than an extensor response that is desired. Excessive muscle tension in the limb and entire body must be avoided or finger extension will not occur.

Many adult hemiplegics never achieve good voluntary extension or coordinated, fine hand motions. However, if semivoluntary extension can be well established, voluntary extension usually follows, so that the patient can open the hand in all positions.[3]

The accomplishment of palmar prehension and fine hand movements requires the achievement of voluntary opening of the hand, opposition of the thumb to the fingers, and ability to release objects in contact with the palm of the hand.

Lower Limb Training

Lower limb training is directed toward restoring safe standing and the development of a gait pattern that is as nearly normal as possible. The goal is to modify the gross movement synergies and facilitate movement combinations that are more nearly like those used during normal ambulation. Lower limb training includes trunk balance and activation of specific muscle groups followed by gait training.

Training procedures for the lower extremity are primarily the domain of the physical therapist. However, when training the patient in functional activities, the occupational therapist can use procedures that are in concert with the work of the physical therapist. To name a few examples, transfer training, dressing, toileting, and ambulating about in the occupational therapy clinic involve motor activity of the lower limb. Therefore it is important for the occupational therapist to know which training procedures are in prog-

ress, which movement patterns are to be encouraged or inhibited, and which methods facilitate the desired gait pattern when assisting or accompanying the patient during functional tasks.

OCCUPATIONAL THERAPY APPLICATIONS

Controlled movements achieved in upper limb training have more significance if the patient can use them for functional activities. Even with limited control, the affected limb can be used in many ways to assist with function. Encouraging the use of the affected arm in everyday activities decreases the possibility of the patient functioning strictly as a one-handed person.

During stages 3 and 4 when the patient has voluntary control of the synergies and may begin to be able to use movement combinations that deviate from the synergies, the occupational therapist should help the patient to use the newly learned movement for functional and purposeful activities. Some of the activities that can be adapted to use the synergy patterns or gross combined movement patterns are skateboard or powder board exercises (see Fig. 19-4), sanding, leather lacing, braid weaving, finger painting, sponging off tabletops, and using a push-broom or carpet sweeper. Activities that demand too much cortical control and conscious effort on the part of the patient tend to increase fatigue and muscle tension and should be avoided.

Brunnstrom described several possible uses for the flexor and extensor synergies in stage 3.[3] The extensor synergy may be used to stabilize an object on a table while the unaffected arm is performing a task. Examples are stabilizing stationery while writing letters or stabilizing fabric for sewing. The extensor synergy may also be used to stabilize a jar against the body while unscrewing the lid or to hold a handbag or newspaper under the arm. When pushing the affected arm through the sleeve of a garment, the garment can be positioned so that the arm follows the path of the extensor synergy. (However, this requires the forearm to be pronated first to facilitate elbow extension.) The flexor synergy or its components may be used to carry a coat or handbag over the forearm and to hold a toothbrush while the unaffected hand squeezes the toothpaste, for example. Bilateral pushing and pulling activities that alternate the paths of both synergies may be helpful for some patients. Examples of these are sweeping, vacuuming, and dusting. Such activities may be performed with the unaffected hand stabilizing the affected one. The affected hand may be more a hindrance than a help until greater control is gained. Strongly motivated patients will try to use available movements under the guidance and encouragement of the occupational therapist.

To promote transition from stage 3 to stage 4 movement combinations are facilitated and practiced in upper limb training. These movements are hand to chin, hand to ear on the same side and opposite side, hand to opposite elbow, hand to opposite shoulder, hand to forehead, hand to top of head, hand to back of head, and stroking movements from top to back of head and from dorsum of the forearm to the shoulder and toward the neck on the normal side. As soon as possible, these movement patterns should be translated to functional activities. Success at functional tasks increases motivation and establishes a purpose for the training. Also contact with body parts where sensation is intact is instrumental in guiding the hand to its goal. Examples of application of these movements to function are hand-to-mouth motions used in eating finger foods, combing hair, washing the face, washing the unaffected arm, and reaching the opposite axilla for washing or application of deodorant.[3] The therapist's role is to analyze activities for movement patterns that are possible for the patient to per-form, and to select activities with the patient that have meaning and are interesting.

At this time the occupational therapist should stress the use of any voluntary movement of the affected limb in performance of activities of daily living. Using the arm for dressing and hygiene skills translates the movements to purposeful use. It should be borne in mind that the degree to which purposeful, spontaneous use of the arm is possible depends on the sensory status of the limb and not only on the motor recovery achieved.

If the patient surpasses stage 4, the number of activities that can be performed increases, and more movement combinations are possible. The involvement of the affected limbs in activities of daily living should be encouraged. The activities mentioned earlier can be performed now in their usual manner and can be graded to demand finer and more complex movement patterns. Loom weaving, block printing, gardening, furniture refinishing, leather tooling, rolling out dough, sweeping, dusting, and washing dishes are a few of the activities that may enlist the use of the affected arm purposefully if hand recovery is adequate.

REVIEW QUESTIONS

1. List the stages of recovery of arm function after CVA, as described by Brunnstrom.
2. List the motions in the flexor and extensor synergies of the arm, and draw stick figures to illustrate the positions.
3. What is the most spastic component of the flexor synergy of the arm?
4. What is the least spastic component of the extensor synergy of the arm?
5. What is the basis of the Brunnstrom approach to the treatment of hemiplegia?
6. For what purposes does Brunnstrom recommend the use of primitive reflexes and associated reactions in the early recovery stages after onset of hemiplegia?
7. Define or describe the following terms: limb synergy, associated reactions, imitation synkinesis, proximal traction response, grasp reflex, and Souques' finger phenomenon.
8. Describe or demonstrate the procedure that Brunnstrom recommended to maintain or achieve pain-free ROM at the glenohumeral joint.
9. What is the aim of treatment for functional recovery of the arm during stages 1 and 2? Stages 2 and 3? Stages 3 and 4?
10. List two treatment methods that could be used to achieve each of these aims.
11. Describe three activities other than those listed in the text that may be used in occupational therapy to enhance voluntary control of the flexor and extensor synergies.
12. What is the effect of the proximal traction response on muscle function?
13. Describe or demonstrate the procedure that Brunnstrom recommends to establish wrist fixation in association with grasp.
14. Describe the procedure that may be used to relax spastic finger flexion and facilitate finger extension.
15. Which muscle group is thought to play a significant role in maintaining glenohumeral joint stability?
16. Describe proper bed positioning for the patient with a dominant extensor synergy of the leg. What is the rationale for this position?

REFERENCES

1. Bobath B: Adult hemiplegia: evaluation and treatment, London, 1978, Wm. Heinemann Medical Books, Ltd.
2. Brunnstrom S: Motor behavior in adult hemiplegic patients, Am J Occup Ther 15:6, 1961.
3. Brunnstrom S: Movement therapy in hemiplegia, New York, 1970, Harper & Row Publishers, Inc.
4. Cailliet R: The shoulder in hemiplegia, Philadelphia, 1980, FA Davis Co.
5. Fiorentino MR: Reflex testing methods for evaluating CNS development, Springfield, IL, 1973, Charles C Thomas.
6. Perry C: Principles and techniques of the Brunnstrom approach to the treatment of hemiplegia, Am J Phys Med 46:789, 1967.

7. Sawner K: Brunnstrom approach to treatment of adult patients with hemiplegia: rationale for facilitation procedures, Buffalo, 1969, State University of New York. Unpublished.

8. Schleichkorn J: Signe Brunnstrom remembered for contributions as therapist, OT Week, Rockville, MD, American Occupational Therapy Association, 2:2, 1988.

9. Taylor J, editor: Selected writings of Hughlings Jackson (Abstract), New York, 1958, Basic Books. Cited in Brunnstrom S: Movement therapy in hemiplegia, New York, 1970, Harper & Row Publishers, Inc.

10. Twitchell TE: The restoration of motor function following hemiplegia in man (Abstract), Brain, 74:443-480, 1951. Cited in Brunnstrom S: Movement therapy in hemiplegia, New York, 1970, Harper & Row Publishers, Inc.

Chapter

20 Neurodevelopmental treatment

THE BOBATH APPROACH TO THE TREATMENT OF ADULT HEMIPLEGIA

JAN ZARET DAVIS

This chapter introduces and orients the reader to the Bobath approach in the treatment of adult hemiplegia: neurodevelopmental treatment (NDT). It is designed to provide a basic foundation in the principles of treatment, to describe treatment techniques, to identify problems with the hemiplegic shoulder, and to provide specific management of the painful shoulder. Those interested in expanding their knowledge in this area are directed to readings from the references, particularly *Adult Hemiplegia: Evaluation and Treatment* by Berta Bobath and *Steps to Follow* by Patricia Davies.[2,6]

Berta Bobath, a physical therapist, and her physician husband, Dr. Karel Bobath, have been developing a special method of treatment in London since the 1940s. This method, referred to as NDT in the USA, is commonly used in the treatment of cerebral palsy and acquired adult hemiplegia. It is most effective when used by the entire health care team in the 24-hour per day care of the patient. The principles of treatment can be followed by all those concerned with the patient's care. These include the nursing staff, occupational therapists, physical therapists, speech therapists, and family. It is ideal to begin treatment immediately during the acute stages of illness, but effective treatment can be started at any time. The information and principles described in this chapter are meant to be used specifically in the treatment of adult hemiplegia.

Rationale for Use of Neurodevelopmental Treatment Techniques with Adult Hemiplegics

The primary goal of NDT is to relearn normal movements. The techniques used are intended for more than just the movements of an arm or leg; they treat the person as a whole, encouraging the use of both sides. The patient uses less adaptive equipment (for example, slings, braces, and canes) and is more able to move about freely with normal muscle tone.[2] This creates a better atmosphere for the psychosocial adjustment to family and everyday living. The more

normal a person appears to others, with less deformity from spasticity, the better he or she is accepted.

The Bobaths use specific treatment principles to inhibit abnormal patterns of movement. This suppression or inhibition of abnormal patterns (synergies) must be accomplished before normal, selective isolated movement can take place. It is impossible to superimpose normal movement on a person with abnormal tone.[2]

The following terms often are used in describing the NDT techniques of Bobath. These are defined as they are used throughout this chapter.

Positioning
Rotation of trunk
"Placing"
Spasticity
Inhibition
Weight bearing
Scapular mobility
Normalization of tone
Postural reactions
    Righting reactions
    Equilibrium reactions
Protective extension

Additional terms associated with this approach and their definitions are:

ASSOCIATED MOVEMENTS. Extraneous movements that occur normally and are seen in children and adults when new and difficult tasks are learned. For example, a child displays associated movements when cutting with scissors when he or she sticks the tongue in and out. The movements can also be the same types of movements of both limbs, and the activity of the limb not involved in the motor task reinforces that of the limb on the opposite side of the body involved in the motor task.[2]

ASSOCIATED REACTIONS. In the hemiplegic patient, activity that requires excessive effort of the unaffected limbs can result in apparent limb movement, usually in a synergy pattern with a palpable increase in tone, of the affected limbs. Associated reactions are

351

abnormal and occur as a result of tonic reflexes or released postural reactions in muscles deprived of voluntary control. These reactions must be prevented in treatment and therefore the patient should be careful when using any part of his or her body with excessive effort.[2]

KEY POINTS OF CONTROL. Points on the body, usually proximal (for example, shoulder and pelvic girdles), when handled by the therapist in a specific manner can be used to change part of an abnormal pattern to increase normal movement throughout the body and to guide the patient's active movements. Spasticity of the limbs can be influenced and reduced from these key points of control.[2]

POSTURAL TONE. Postural tone, as defined by the Bobaths, is normal central nervous system (CNS) activation of large groups of muscles in patterns for the maintenance of posture. Normal postural tone is high enough to resist gravity and low enough to give way to movement.[2]

REFLEX INHIBITING PATTERNS. Patterns of movement, which are opposite to spastic patterns and guided by the therapist from key points of control, are used to inhibit abnormal motor activity and facilitate more normal motor activity.[2]

For more complete definitions and discussion, consult the original source.[2]

EVALUATION

The initial phase in treatment is the evaluation. To do an accurate evaluation, the therapist should not only have a good understanding of normal development and normal movement but also extremely good observation skills. Therapists must observe patients' movements, contrast them with what is normal and identify discrepancies in order to list specific problem areas. "Normal postural reflex activity forms the necessary background for normal movements and functional skills. The *normal postural reflex mechanism* consists of a great number and variety of automatic movements that gradually develop along with the maturation of the infantile brain. For the purpose of assessment and treatment, three large groups of automatic reactions can be differentiated as follows:"

1. Righting reactions: "The righting reactions are automatic reactions which serve to maintain and restore the normal position of the head in space and its normal relationship with the trunk, together with the normal alignment of trunk and limbs."

2. Equilibrium reactions: "Equilibrium reactions are automatic reactions which serve to maintain and restore balance during all our activities, especially when we are in danger of falling. Another important automatic reaction which is closely associated

with the development of equilibrium reactions is the protective extension of the arms."

3. Automatic adaptation of muscles to changes of posture: "In a normal person, the postural reflex mechanism controls the weight of a limb during movements both into and against gravity." It allows for smooth and well-controlled mobility against the forces of gravity. "The normal person does not relax when being moved—relaxation, unless fully supported, being a voluntary learnt ability. The limb can be 'placed.' It feels light to the examiner, follows the movement actively and is controlled throughout its whole range by adequate contraction of the antigravity muscles."[2]

An NDT evaluation includes the assessment of the previously mentioned reactions as well as sensation and postural tone. Refer to the original source for a more complete discussion of the evaluation.[2] The occupational therapist must also include an activities of daily living (ADL) and a perceptual evaluation in the assessment. The patient is evaluated by the therapist to see what he or she can or cannot do. Emphasis is placed on the *quality of movement,* that is, the ways in which the patient moves, his or her coordination, tonus changes, and postural reactions rather than on muscles and joints.[2] It is important to understand what is "normal" and "abnormal" in the posture and movement of the body. Most patients display at least one abnormal reaction following a cerebrovascular accident (CVA). Normal and abnormal movements are listed here for comparison.

Normal	Abnormal
Muscle tone at rest	Flaccidity, spasticity or mixed tone
Voluntary selective movement	Abnormal postural tone
Isolated control	Synergistic movement
Associated movements	Associated reactions
Postural reactions	Lack of or reduced equilibrium reactions

TYPICAL PROBLEMS OF ADULT HEMIPLEGIA

The adult hemiplegic patient often has many problems that can be debilitating either alone or in combination. The following are some of the most common problems seen in adult hemiplegia:

1. Asymmetry. Asymmetry is the most obvious problem seen in hemiplegia. This is seen in the trunk, extremities, and face. Asymmetry may also be influenced by any of the following listed problems.

2. Non-weight-bearing. Most patients are afraid to bear weight on the affected side of their body.

Instead of the weight being evenly distributed, it is usuallly shifted to the nonhemiplegic side.

3. Fear. Fear may be the most debilitating factor for many patients. Fear magnifies other problems that cause the patient to be dependent rather than independent. Fear can be caused by loss of sensation, poor balance reactions, lack of protective extension (fear of falling), perceptual or cognitive problems and is a major factor influencing spasticity.[5]

4. Sensory loss. Sensory loss may include loss of stereognosis, kinesthetic awareness, light touch, and pressure. The functional potential of an extremity can be dependent on the sensation. Often a patient's extremity remains useless because of sensory loss even though he or she has good motor control.[2,5]

5. Neglect. Unilateral neglect can be a combination of one or more of the following: sensory, perceptual, cognitive, or visual field cut (homonymous hemianopsia). The patient may have good motor recovery but be unable to use it functionally because of the neglect.[1,5]

Many other problems related to CVA, such as aphasia, apraxia, and a variety of perceptual motor problems occur. These are discussed in Chapter 34.

MOTOR PROBLEMS

The major motor problem in hemiplegia is the lack of postural control affecting voluntary movement. Flaccidity is most common at the onset of a CVA. During this time the patient is often passive, displaying low endurance and low tolerance to activity. This may last a few days or as long as several months. Although the patient displays no movement in the affected extremities at this time, a proper treatment program can have a strong impact on the eventual functional outcome.[2]

Following the flaccid stage, patients enter a stage of mixed tone; displaying a combination of flaccidity and spasticity. For example, the upper extremity might have an increase in tone proximally but a decrease in tone distally.

Spasticity is the most common and most difficult motor problem to treat following a CVA. If not treated correctly, spasticity can progress to the point at which independent living is nearly impossible. Spasticity interferes with the patient's ability to move by interfering with selective motor function. It produces abnormal sensory feedback and contributes to weakness of the antagonist muscles. It can cause contractures, pain, and an all-consuming fear in many patients. Fear, pain, and spasticity are often so intertwined that a vicious cycle appears. The spasticity can cause an increase in pain, which can cause an increase in fear,

which in turn increases the amount of spasticity.[5]

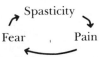

If measures are taken to reduce pain and fear, the therapist has a much better chance for success with the methods used to reduce spasticity. Other factors that can influence the amount of spasticity are stress (either emotional or physical), temperature, effort, and the rate at which an activity is done.

The typical posture of the adult hemiplegic patient (Fig. 20-1) is a combination of the strongest components of the flexion and extension synergies and can be described as follows:

• Head. Lateral flexion toward the involved side with rotation away from the involved side
• Upper extremity
  1. Scapula—depression, retraction
  2. Shoulder—adduction, internal rotation
  3. Elbow—flexion
  4. Forearm—pronation
  5. Wrist—flexion, ulnar deviation
  6. Fingers—flexion
• Trunk. Lateral flexion toward the involved side (trunk shortening)
• Lower extremity
  1. Pelvis—posterior elevation, retraction
  2. Hip—internal rotation, adduction, extension
  3. Knee—extension
  4. Ankle—plantar flexion, supination, inversion
  5. Toes—flexion

The one fortunate characteristic about spasticity is the fact that *it can be influenced*. This means that therapists can reduce or inhibit the effects of spasticity to some degree. Normalization of muscle tone may be

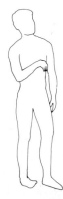

Fig. 20-1. Typical posture of hemiplegic adult in standing position. Courtesy of Graphic Arts Department, Harmarville Rehabilitation Center, Pittsburgh

accomplished by using one or more of the following techniques:[2,5,7]
1. Proper positioning
2. Weight-bearing over the affected side
3. Trunk rotation
4. Elongation of the affected side
5. Shoulder protraction
6. Careful gradation of stimulation

These six points provide the foundation for treatment of the adult hemiplegic using the Bobath approach. As previously stated, the techniques are most effective and provide the best potential in rehabilitation when they are started in the acute phase at the time of admittance to the hospital. These techniques, however, can be used in any phase throughout the treatment program.

TREATMENT

In each medical setting the roles of occupational therapy and physical therapy may differ slightly. Yet the techniques described are imperative for proper patient treatment, and all persons in professional services should be aware of them and be able to apply them appropriately. The Bobaths strongly emphasize that this is not a series of exercises and the upper and lower extremities must not be separated.[2] The occupational therapist must be constantly aware of the tonus, motor patterns, positions, and reflex mechanisms of both the upper and lower extremities.

Tips for Nursing, Family, and Staff

The following tips help the patient to become more aware of the hemiplegic side, to better integrate both sides of the body, and to increase sensory stimulation to the hemiplegic side. By following these tips, some problems that are characteristic of hemiplegia can be prevented or minimized.
1. Room position. The hemiplegic side of the patient should face the source of stimulation. The patient's hemiplegic side should face the door and be positioned so that the telephone, the nightstand, and the television, encourage the patient to turn toward that side, thus increasing integration of both sides of the body (Fig. 20-2). The one exception being the call light for the nurse.[4]
2. Approach. Always approach the patient from the hemiplegic side to encourage eye contact. Sometimes the patient has difficulty turning the head and may need assistance. The therapist should simply assist the patient by gently but firmly turning the head until he or she is able to establish eye contact. Family members can be encouraged to give tactile input to the patient by holding his or her hand or stroking his or her arm.

3. Naming. During nursing tasks, such as washing, name each body part to increase awareness of it.
4. Encouraging independence. The patient should begin to assist in simple ADL. If the patient is unable to complete a task independently, the therapist can guide the patient's hands, in order to get the feel of the movement pattern necessary to complete an activity. This encourages the patient to learn to carry out the task sooner.[1]
5. Bed position. The patient should be properly positioned (see Figs. 20-3 to 20-6). The reasons that patients should be positioned in this manner are (1) weight-bearing inhibits spasticity; (2) weight-bearing increases awareness of the hemiplegic side; and (3) lengthening of the hemiplegic side inhibits spasticity.

The three basic positions are listed in order of their therapeutic value: lying on the affected side, lying on the unaffected side, and lying supine. Patients should be repositioned as often as nursing procedures require (usually every 2 hours) for the prevention of decubiti. For the best therapeutic results, position the patient on the hemiplegic side[2,7] (Fig. 20-3). The back of the patient should be parallel with the edge of the bed. The head is placed on the pillow symmetrically but not in extreme flexion. The shoulder is fully protracted with at least 90° of shoulder flexion (less than 90° encourages a flexion synergy). The forearm is supinated and the wrist is supported on the bed or can be slightly off the bed, which encourages wrist extension. The nonaffected leg is placed on a pillow. The affected leg is slightly flexed at the knee. A pillow can be placed behind the patient to keep him or her from rolling onto the back. For a slight variation of this position, have the patient place the affected hand under the pillow under the head. This does, however, require a significant amount of shoulder external rotation.

To position the patient on the nonhemiplegic side (Fig. 20-4), the back should be parallel with the edge

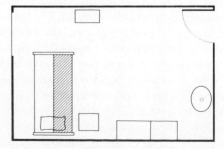

Fig. 20-2. Room arranged so that patient must turn to affected side. Shaded area represents affected side of body.

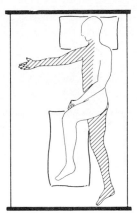

Fig. 20-3. Bed position when lying on affected side.

of the bed.[2,5] The head is placed symmetrically on the pillow. The shoulder is in full protraction with the shoulder in at least 90° of flexion. The arm and hand are fully supported on a pillow. The wrist should not be allowed to drop off the pillow into flexion. The affected lower extremity is in hip flexion and knee flexion, and fully supported on a pillow. The foot and ankle must be supported to keep the foot from inverting.

To position the patient in a supine position (Fig. 20-5), the head is symmetric on the pillow.[2,5] The body and trunk are also symmetric (to prevent the shortening of the hemiplegic side of the trunk). A pillow is placed under the affected shoulder, supporting the shoulder so it is at least level with the nonhemiplegic shoulder (it is common for the affected shoulder to be pulled back into retraction). The affected arm is fully supported, with the elbow extended and forearm in supination and entirely supported on a pillow in elevation. A small pillow can be placed under the hip to reduce retraction of the pelvis. *Do not place a pillow under the knees or a foot board at the end of the bed,* because

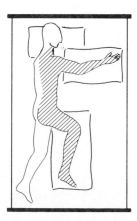

Fig. 20-4. Bed position when lying on unaffected side.

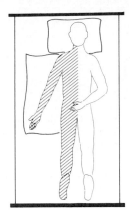

Fig. 20-5. Bed position when lying supine.

this encourages knee flexion contractures and extension synergy of the lower extremity.

To position the patient in a sitting position, the trunk should be supported symmetrically in extension (Fig. 20-6). The hips are flexed and knees extended. The arms are forward, not allowing the scapulae to pull into retraction. The hands can be clasped together with the hemiplegic thumb on top (see Fig. 20-18) or the hand can lay flat on the table, and the entire forearm is supported on a bed table. This position of the arms inhibits the flexion synergy.

THE OCCUPATIONAL THERAPY PROGRAM
Application of Bobath Principles

The basic principles of the Bobath approach in the treatment of adult hemiplegia can be applied in all areas of the occupational therapy program. These include ADL, therapeutic activities, and home exercise programs. Following the initial evaluation of the patient, the therapist begins to formulate the treatment program. It is important that meaningful activities are selected that best meet the patient's needs and goals as well as therapeutic goals. Throughout the treatment session, the therapist must continually observe not only what the patient is doing, but also *how* he or she is doing it. The therapist is constantly aware of both the involved and uninvolved sides as well as the position of the patient's trunk and upper and lower extremities. For example, if the therapist is working on reducing the tone in the upper extremity and if the patient's lower extremity goes into an extension synergy, the lower extremity must be corrected before full inhibition of the upper extremity is obtained.

As stated previously, specific handling methods are used to prevent or to reduce spasticity.

1. Proper position. In lying, the proper position has already been discussed (see Figs. 20-3 to 20-5). In sitting (Figs. 20-6 and 20-7), the patient should

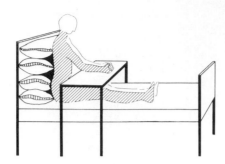

Fig. 20-6. Bed position when sitting upright.

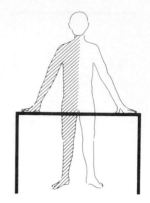

Fig. 20-8. Symmetry when standing with weight-bearing on upper limbs.

have the feet flat on the floor, ankles, knees, and hips in 90° of flexion, and trunk extended (no thoracic flexion). The head should be in midline and the arm fully supported when working at the table. In standing the head should be in midline, trunk symmetric, and weight equally distributed on both lower extremities (Fig. 20-8).

2. Weight-bearing. Whether in lying (see Fig. 20-3), sitting (Fig. 20-9), or standing (see Fig. 20-8), the most effective method of normalizing tone is through weight-bearing over the hemiplegic side. The effects are quite amazing. Patients typically bear weight only on the nonhemiplegic side, encouraging abnormal postural tone. In all activities the therapist must constantly check to see whether or not the patient has weight over the affected side. However, a patient should never bear weight over a painful extremity or swollen hand.

3. Trunk rotation (Fig. 20-10). Several things occur as a patient rotates the trunk. Rotation encourages weight-bearing and elongation of the hemiplegic side, and provides vestibular input. Through trunk rotation, the patient not only helps to normalize tone but also learns to better integrate both sides of the body.

4. Elongation of the trunk on the affected side. Be-

cause a hemiplegic patient typically exhibits an asymmetric trunk with possible shortening (lateral flexion) on the affected side of the trunk, it is important that the therapist work toward symmetry of the trunk. This can be accomplished in lying, sitting, or standing position through proper positioning and the use of reflex inhibiting patterns as explained by Bobath.[2] A prolonged stretch not only reduces tone in the proximal regions but has an effect distally as well.

5. Shoulder protraction (Fig. 20-11). Shoulder protraction accomplishes two goals. First, it helps to normalize tone, and second, it helps to maintain scapular mobility. When the patient pulls back into scapular retraction, an increase in tone in the flexor pattern can be detected throughout the extremity. Shoulder protraction is an effective method that is easily incorporated into the occupational therapy program.

6. Careful gradation of stimulation. Stimulation can refer to a number of things. Auditory stimulation affects muscle tone. The therapist's voice, background noise, or any loud noise can produce an increase in muscle tone.[1] Tactile stimulation (in-

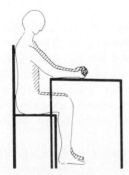

Fig. 20-7. Position when sitting in chair at table. Hands clasped in front, elbows extended, and entire forearm supported.

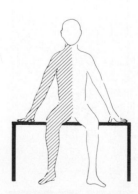

Fig. 20-9. Weight-bearing position of upper limbs when in sitting position.

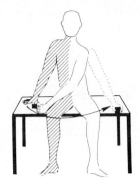

Fig. 20-10. Trunk rotation is practiced while patient bears weight on affected arm and transfers objects from one side of bench to other.

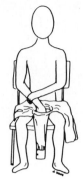

Fig. 20-12. Dressing training. Shirt positioned across patient's knees, arm hole visible, and sleeve dropped between knees.

cluding vibration and temperature) can also increase or decrease muscle tone depending on how and the length of time it is applied. Stimulation can also be the rate (how fast) an activity or facilitation technique is performed.

Practical Application in Occupational Therapy Activities

DRESSING ACTIVITIES

Purpose. The patient learns to inhibit his or her own spasticity. The procedure breaks up typical hemiplegic patterns of lower extremity extension synergy and upper extremity flexion synergy. Using the NDT approach, dressing is learned faster than traditional, one-handed methods, especially for patients with perceptual problems. The patient learns to carry over techniques of inhibition into daily living skills.

Tips. The patient should not attempt to get dressed in bed. Instead, the patient should be seated on a chair (preferably a straight chair next to the bed. The therapist should *always* assist from the affected side. Always begin dressing with the hemiplegic side. The same sequence in dressing is maintained to increase learning.

PROCEDURE
Donning shirt (Figs. 20-12 and 20-13)

1. Position shirt across patient's knees with arm hole visible and sleeve between knees.
2. Bend forward at hips (inhibiting extension synergy of the lower extremity), placing affected hand in sleeve.
3. Arm drops into sleeve; shoulder protraction and gravity inhibit upper extremity flexion synergy.
4. Bring collar to neck.
5. Sit upright, dress nonhemiplegic side.
6. Button shirt from bottom to top.

Donning underclothes and pants (Fig. 20-14)

1. Clasp hands and cross affected leg over nonhemiplegic leg. (Therapist helps when needed).
2. Release hands. Hemiplegic arm can "dangle" and should not be trapped in lap.
3. Pull pant leg over hemiplegic foot.
4. Clasp hands to uncross leg.
5. Place nonhemiplegic foot in pant leg (no need to cross legs). This is difficult, because the patient must bear weight on hemiplegic side.
6. Pull pants to knees.
7. While holding onto waistband, patient stands with therapist's facilitation.
8. Zip and snap pants.
9. Therapist facilitates patient returning to sitting position.

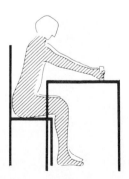

Fig. 20-11. Shoulder protraction demonstrated during bilateral activity of upper limbs.

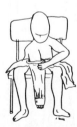

Fig. 20-13. Patient bends forward at hips (inhibiting extension synergy of lower extremity) and places affected hand into sleeve.

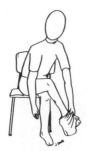

Fig. 20-14. Proper position while putting on pants and underclothes.

Donning shoes and socks (Fig. 20-15)

1. Clasp hands and cross legs (as before).
2. Put sock and shoe on hemiplegic foot.
3. Cross nonhemiplegic leg, put on sock and shoe.

THERAPEUTIC ACTIVITIES. There are three ways to incorporate the involved upper extremity into functional activities. First, weight-bearing through the involved upper extremity. Therapeutic activities that encourage weight-bearing on the hemiplegic side (see Figs. 20-8 and 20-9) in sitting and standing positions must be included in the treatment program. The purposes of weight-bearing are to provide proprioceptive input to the hemiplegic side, encourage more normal postural tone and balance reactions, decrease fear, reduce spasticity, and prevent contractures of the wrist and fingers.

Second, bilateral activities (Figs. 20-16 and 20-17) with hands clasped together (Fig. 20-18) are used to increase awareness of the hemiplegic side, increase sensory input to the hemiplegic side, bring the affected arm into the visual field, begin "purposeful" movement of the hemiplegic arm, discourage flexion synergy by protraction of the scapula and extension of the elbow and wrist, develop abduction of fingers and thumb that discourages spasticity of the hand, and teach the patient reflex inhibiting patterns that he or she can perform without any help.

Third, the therapist can guide the patient's hand through normal patterns of movement during func-

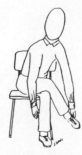

Fig. 20-15. Proper position while putting on shoes and socks.

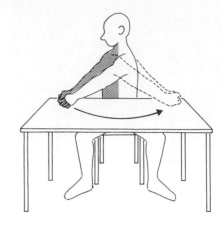

Fig. 20-16. Bilateral activity incorporating trunk rotation.

tional activities. This can be done by placing his or her hand over the patient's hand with firm but not forceful movements.

Each therapeutic activity can be done sitting or standing, depending on the level of the patient's progress. At every possible opportunity the patient should be treated in a straight chair (or standing) rather than the wheelchair to obtain maximal benefit.

The activity plans (box on p. 359) demonstrate how the Bobath principles can be applied to activities. Positioning of the patient, goals, therapist facilitation, common errors, correction, and variations are included. This format can be used to design many other activities.

THE SHOULDER IN HEMIPLEGIA

The variety of problems relating to the hemiplegic shoulder are often frustrating and confusing to the occupational therapist. Pain can hinder the entire rehabilitation program. The responsiblity of the therapist is to learn how to evaluate these problems and

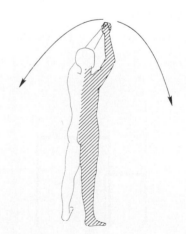

Fig. 20-17. Proper position in standing for activities incorporating bilateral use of upper extremities.

Occupational therapy application: activities

"BOWLING" WITH LIGHT-WEIGHT BALL

Positioning of patient
Sitting on chair or bench
Trunk and hips forward
Shoulders forward
Arm hanging down
Knees 90°

Common errors	*Correction*
Patient "braces with unaffected arm, causing associated reactions.	Bring both arms forward.
Patient tries to swing arm too hard, increasing flexor spasticity.	Encourage light movements.
Patient uses back by sitting up rather than arm.	Keep patient forward.
Patient slides hemiplegic foot under instead of flat on floor.	Bring weight over hemiplegic side.

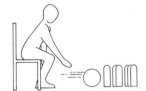

Goals
Symmetry of body
Bringing weight forward
Isolated control of shoulder flexion and wrist extension
Facilitation of finger extension
Shoulder protraction
What therapist does
Stands on hemiplegic side (one hand on hemiplegic shoulder, especially for patients with poor balance)
Guides patient through movement until moving independently
Stops patient if spasticity increases; repositions
Checks position throughout activity
Variations
Pins placed to left or right (encourages head rotation and compensation for neglect)
Both hands clasped together to bowl
Size of ball
Box or crate as goal instead of pins
Number or color pins (makes game more challenging)

LINOLEUM BLOCK PRINTING

Positioning of patient
Standing with table directly in front
Weight evenly distributed on both feet
Feet comfortably apart
Hands clasped around grip
Ink or paint on hemiplegic side

Common errors	*Correction*
Patient puts weight only on unaffected leg.	Stand closer to patient; use firmer contact.
Patient leans against table too much.	Help patient to find balance point.
Patient buckles knee.	Position therapist's leg to control patient's leg.
Patient presses unevenly or printing block pulls back.	Keep shoulder forward; support under elbow.

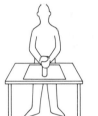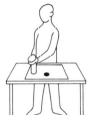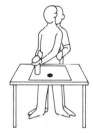

Goals
Trunk rotation
Increased standing (or sitting) tolerance
Increased awarenes of hemiplegic side (good compensation training for hemianopsia)
Bilateral use of upper extremities
Increased shoulder protraction, elbow extension
What therapist does
Stands on patient's hemiplegic side
Places hands on patient's hips to facilitate weight bearing onto hemiplegic leg
Checks hands
Checks elbows for good extension
Variations
Shape and size of grip
Sitting instead of standing
Size of paper
Complexity of design
Placement of paint to increase truck rotation
Stencil used to reduce complexity

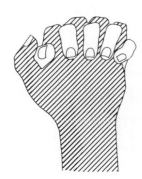

Fig. 20-18. During bilateral activity and in sitting position, hands are clasped as shown. Affected hand is shaded. Note that hemiplegic thumb is always on top.

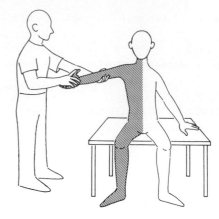

Fig. 20-20. Therapist assists patient to obtain reflex-inhibiting pattern for arm.

prepare a treatment program that is effective in dealing with them. It is important to understand the basic anatomy and functional mechanism of the shoulder girdle. Those interested in expanding their knowledge in this area are directed to readings from the references, particularly *The Shoulder in Hemiplegia* by Rene Cailliet.[3]

The shoulder girdle is made up of seven joints (Fig. 20-19): (1) glenohumeral, (2) suprahumeral, (3) acromioclavicular, (4) scapulocostal, (5) sternoclavicular, (6) costosternal, and (7) costovertebral.

To have full pain-free range of motion (ROM), all seven joints need to be working synchronously. The glenohumeral joint allows for considerable mobility but is unfortunately an unstable joint. It is dependent on the proper alignment of the scapula and humerus (for mechanical support) as well as the supraspinatus.

It is important to understand the relationship of the scapula to the humerus and its significance in pain-free shoulder flexion and abduction. When the arm is raised in forward flexion or abduction, the scapula must glide and rotate upward. The humerus and the

scapula work in unison; more specifically, they work in a 2:1 ratio pattern. In other words, if the shoulder moves 90° of abduction, the humerus moves 60° and the scapula moves 30°. Another example might be 180° of shoulder flexion in which the humerus moves 120° and the scapula 60° (again, a 2:1 ratio).[3]

If for any reason the arm is raised in shoulder flexion or abduction without the scapula gliding along, joint trauma and pain can occur. The therapist must be aware of this and take it into consideration during ROM, ADL, transfers, and all other activities.

In the hemiplegic shoulder, the scapula can fall into downward rotation because of a heavy, flaccid upper extremity or the muscles that move the scapula in downward rotation (rhomboids, latissimus dorsi, and levator scapulae) are spastic. This makes it difficult for the scapula to glide upward, which is necessary for pain-free movement. The scapula must first be mobilized and the spasticity reduced to regain the ROM and allow for selective movement. The arm must never be fully raised before the scapula has been mobilized and the therapist can feel its gliding movements. Even in a seemingly flaccid arm, the scapula can be influenced by spasticity of the rhomboids, trapezius, and latissimus dorsi. The techniques previously described assist the therapist.

Because the hemiplegic shoulder can often be pulled back into retraction, the emphasis of treatment is placed on forward gliding of the scapula. By protracting the scapula, the patient is able to reduce the hypertonicity of the upper extremity, allowing for more isolated movement and selective control. When the spasticity is too strong for the patient to obtain protraction of the shoulder, the therapist must assist. The therapist should use reflex inhibiting patterns to control and reduce spasticity. As Bobath stated, "The

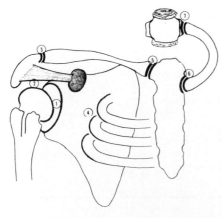

Fig. 20-19. Composite drawing of shoulder girdle. From Cailliet R: The shoulder in hemiplegia, Philadelphia, 1980, FA Davis Co.

main reflex inhibiting pattern counteracting spasticity in the trunk and arm is the extension of neck and spine and external rotation of the arm at the shoulder with elbow extended. Further reduction of flexor spasticity can be obtained by adding extension of the wrist with supination and abduction of the thumb."[2] (Fig. 20-20).

Subluxation

Many professionals are particularly concerned about the subluxed shoulder. Numerous efforts are made to protect it and "prevent" it. Subluxation cannot be prevented. If the muscles around the shoulder girdle, which are attached to the humerus and scapula, are weak enough, the shoulder will be subluxed. Slings do not help subluxation. They keep the arm in a poor position and may contribute to pain and swelling. Subluxation itself does not cause pain. The pain is caused by improper *handling* of a subluxed arm. Forcing the head of the humerus back into place can cause trauma and pain. Doing standard ROM procedures on an arm without a gliding scapula can also cause pain. Treatment of the subluxed arm should include proper sitting (see Figs. 20-6 and 20-7), weight-bearing (see Figs. 20-8 and 20-9), and mobilization of the scapula and proper positioning in bed (see Figs. 20-3 to 20-6).

Slings

The application of a sling to the hemiplegic arm is a source of considerable controversy. It has been demonstrated over the past several years that "the commonly used hemiplegic sling has no appreciable effect on ultimate ROM, subluxation, pain, or peripheral nerve traction injury."[9] It has also been stated that "there is no need to support a pain free shoulder in order to prevent or correct subluxation since the sling does not prevent, improve, cure or reduce such a deformity."[8] The use of a sling on the hemiplegic arm can actually contribute to subluxation and lead to a painful, disabling condition called shoulder-hand syndrome. It is important to realize that when a patient wears a sling, the arm is supported in a position that is compatible with the typical hemiplegic posture and discourages the patient from using the arm either bilaterally or unilaterally. Even the sling previously described by the Bobaths is *no longer being used.*[2] This sling was found to hinder the the circulation of the arm and push the head of the humerus into lateral subluxation as well.

If the patient has a painful shoulder or swollen hand, a thorough evaluation should be done to determine the cause and appropriate treatment instituted.

PREPARING THE PATIENT FOR HOME

The benefits of the treatment program are lost if the patient is not adequately prepared for returning home. This preparation should include prescribing a home exercise program, family education, and communication with the follow-up therapist when applicable. The hospital or clinic is a very secure setting, and it is very important that both the patient and family feel comfortable and confident on their return home. The home exercise program is important to maintain mobilization and movement. The therapist should select exercises that can be done easily and correctly without assistance. If stress or excessive effort is used to complete the exercises, the patient is likely to form bad habits, and spasticity will increase.

After the selection of exercises the therapist must train the patient in each of them. To encourage consistency, the patient should follow the same sequence of exercises each day. This should begin long before discharge from occupational therapy so that it is a well-established part of the daily routine.

Each exercise should be written down in the proper sequence, including how often the exercises should be done (for example, twice a day), the number of repetitions (for example, 10 times each), and diagrams if necessary.

Next, the family should be trained so that they are also well acquainted with each exercise. Thus they can guide the home program properly. For best results in family teaching the occupational therapist should demonstrate and explain the importance of tasks; emphasize each major point (for example, position of arm and placement of hands), have the family work with the patient under the therapist's guidance, and repeat instructions as often as needed until the family and patient are confident enough to do the exercises at home alone. Family education should include a home exercise program and ADL training in areas of dressing, eating, grooming, hygiene, bathing, transfers, and cooking. This program should also include instruction in proper positioning (lying, sitting, and standing) and proper use of equipment. Before discharge from the treatment center the therapist should give the family his or her name and telephone number at work, set up a date for a reevaluation if necessary, and contact the therapist treating the patient following discharge from the treatment facility to ensure proper carry-over.

General treatment principles

1. Never exercise—*retrain!* The brain knows patterns and movements, not muscles and bones.
2. Start and finish a treatment session with something positive, something the patient can do well.
3. Use slow, controlled movements; fast movements can increase spasticity.

4. The patient must find the treatment useful, purposeful, and meaningful.
5. Do not magnify pain by dwelling on it.
6. If the patient thinks there has been no progress, it may be caused by memory loss.
7. Proper sequence of activities leads to success.
8. After spasticity is inhibited, follow with a purposeful movement—put it to use! Do not inhibit spasticity unless you plan to use the limb.
9. Do not ask a patient who is influenced by spasticity to relax; he or she cannot.
10. Encourage the patient to look at his or her arm.
11. Tell the patient when a movement has been done correctly so that the patient can *feel* it.
12. It is of great importance to train proprioceptive, tactile, and spatial sensation.
13. Discourage stressful or excessive efforts of the sound arm, which increase associated reactions of the affected arm.
14. Ask for "automatic movements" to reduce stress. The patient then thinks about the activity rather than the arm.
15. If spasticity starts, *stop!*
16. The patient often has to relearn movements, even on his "good" side.[5]

Popular misconceptions about adult hemiplegia

1. Shoulder subluxation causes pain.
2. A person with hemiplegia has a normal side.
3. Slings prevent shoulder subluxation.
4. The harder the patient tries, the better the patient gets.
5. Strength is more important than control.
6. Hemianopsia is the primary reason for neglect of the hemiplegic side.

7. Hemiplegia of long standing cannot be changed.
8. Return of sensation is totally dependent on the lesion.
9. Walking is enough of a rehabilitation goal.
10. If the affected arm has no functional use, forget it.
11. An arm with an intravenous drain in place is an immobilized arm.[5]

SUMMARY

The NDT approach was developed by Karel and Berta Bobath. It may be effectively used with a wide variety of CNS dysfunctions but is most widely known for its application in treatment of cerebral palsy and adult hemiplegia.

The NDT approach is based on normal neuromotor development and function. Its primary goal is to enhance the relearning of normal movement patterns. Special techniques of positioning and motion are used to inhibit spasticity, abnormal patterns of movement, and abnormal reflex activity.

Emphasis is on treating the client as a whole rather than using an isolated approach to treatment of the arm, leg, or trunk. Quality of movement, control, and coordination is developed through the treatment techniques rather than through muscle strength and joint motion per se.

Sensory reeducation and involvement of the family in the rehabilitation program are important elements in this approach to treatment.

REVIEW QUESTIONS

1. What is the fundamental or primary goal of the NDT approach?
2. List three advantages of the NDT approach stated in the text.
3. What are the elements of an NDT evaluation?
4. List four factors that can cause or increase spasticity.
5. Describe the vicious cycle that may contribute to the maintenance of spasticity.
6. What are some of the factors that contribute to the neglect of the hemiplegic side?
7. Describe the positions that Bobath recommends to reduce this neglect in sitting and standing.
8. What are the purposes of trunk rotation? Bilateral activities?
9. Describe recommended positioning and mobilization procedures used to prevent shoulder pain and severe spasticity around the shoulder and shoulder girdle.
10. How is subluxation treated in the

NDT approach?
11. What is the role of the occupational therapist in preparing the patient to go home?
12. Why does Bobath stress scapula protraction in positioning and movement of the hemiplegic arm?
13. According to the NDT approach, how should the hemiplegic arm be positioned when the patient is seated? What is the rationale for this position?
14. Describe and assume the typical posture of the adult hemiplegic.
15. What is meant by "trunk shortening?" What is its cause?
16. Why is the common hemiplegic sling contraindicated?

REFERENCES

1. Affolter F: Perceptual processes as requisites for complex human behavior, Bern, Switzerland, 1980, Hans Huber.
2. Bobath B: Adult hemiplegia: evaluation and treatment, London, 1978, William Heinemann Medical Books Ltd.
3. Cailliet R: The shoulder in hemiplegia, Philadelphia, 1980, FA Davis Co.
4. Cash J: Neurology for physiotherapists, London, 1977, Faber & Faber, Ltd.
5. Davies P: Treatment techniques for adult hemiplegia. Study course, Klinik Valens, Valens, Switzerland, 1979.
6. Davies P: Steps to follow. Berlin, 1985, Springer-Verlag.
7. Eggers O: Occupational therapy in the treatment of adult hemiplegia, Rockville, MD, 1984, Aspen Systems Corp.
8. Friedland F: Physical therapy. In Licht S editor: Stroke and its rehabilitation. Baltimore, Williams & Williams Co., 1975.
9. Hurd MM, Farrell KH, and Waylonis FW: Shoulder sling for hemiplegia: friend or foe? Arch Phys Med Rehab 55:519, 1974.

Chapter

21 The proprioceptive neuromuscular facilitation approach*

SARA A. POPE-DAVIS

The purpose of this chapter is to introduce the reader to proprioceptive neuromuscular facilitation (PNF) and its application to evaluation and treatment in occupational therapy (OT). The basic principles, diagonal patterns, and a few of the more commonly used facilitation techniques are presented here. A case study is used to apply the concepts discussed. To use PNF effectively, it is necessary to understand the concepts, learn the motor skills to use the techniques, and apply the concepts and techniques to OT activities. This chapter should form the basis for further reading and training under the supervision of a therapist experienced in PNF.

Proprioceptive neuromuscular facilitation is based on normal movement and motor development. In normal motor activity the brain registers total movement and not individual muscle action.[12] Encompassed in the PNF approach are mass movement patterns that are spiral and diagonal in nature and that resemble movement seen in functional activities. In this multisensory approach, facilitation techniques are superimposed on movement patterns and postures through the therapist's manual contacts, verbal commands, and visual cues. PNF is effective in the treatment of numerous conditions, including Parkinson's disease, spinal cord injury, arthritis, stroke, head injury, and hand injuries.

HISTORY

Proprioceptive neuromuscular facilitation originated with Dr. Herman Kabat, physician and neurophysiologist, in the 1940s. He applied neurophysiologic principles, based on the work of Sherrington, to the treatment of paralysis secondary to poliomyelitis and multiple sclerosis. In 1948 Kabat and Henry Kaiser founded the Kabat-Kaiser Institute in Vallejo, California. Here he worked with physical therapist Margaret Knott to develop the PNF method of treatment. By 1951 the diagonal patterns and several techniques were established. Essentially no new techniques have been developed since 1951, although new methods of application have been advanced. PNF is now used to treat numerous neurologic and orthopedic conditions.

In 1952 Dorothy Voss, a physical therapist, joined the staff at Kaiser-Kabat Institute. She and Knott undertook the teaching and supervision of staff therapists. In 1954 Knott and Voss presented the first two-week course in Vallejo. Two years later, the first edition of *Proprioceptive Neuromuscular Facilitation* by Margaret Knott and Dorothy Voss was published by Harper & Row.

During this same period there were several reports in the *American Journal of Occupational Therapy* that described PNF and its application to OT treatment.* It was not until 1974 that the first PNF course for occupational therapists taught by Dorothy Voss, was offered at Northwestern University. Since then Beverly Myers, an occupational therapist, and others have been offering courses for occupational therapists throughout the United States. In 1984, PNF was first taught *concurrently* to both physical and occupational therapists at the Rehabilitation Institute in Chicago, and has since been offered annually.[15,22]

PRINCIPLES OF TREATMENT

Voss presented 11 principles of treatment at the Northwestern University Special Therapeutic Exercise Project in 1966. These principles were developed from concepts in the fields of neurophysiology, motor learning, and motor behavior.[20]

1. *All human beings have potentials that have not been fully developed.* This is the underlying philosophy of PNF. Therefore, in evaluation and treatment

*Nancy D. Thompson, RPT, is gratefully acknowledged for introducing the subject of this chapter in the second edition. This material was rewritten from the original draft.

I want to thank Beverly Myers, OTR, and Diane Harsch, MS, OTR, for their assistance in reviewing and editing this chapter. I also want to thank Barbara Gale, MS, OTR, for using her technical skills to take photographs for the illustrations and Diane Harsch for her patience in posing for them.

*References 3, 5, 6, 13, 19, 23.

planning, the patient's abilities and potentials are emphasized. For example, the patient who has weakness on one side of his body can use the intact side to assist the weaker part. Likewise, the hemiplegic patient who has a flaccid arm can use the intact head, neck, and trunk musculature to begin reinforcement of the weak arm in weight-bearing activities.

2. *Normal motor development proceeds in a cervicocaudal and proximodistal direction.* In evaluation and treatment the cervicocaudal and proximodistal direction is followed. When severe disability is present, attention is given to the head and neck region, with its visual, auditory, and vestibular receptors, and to the upper trunk and extremities. If the superior region is intact, an effective source of reinforcement for the inferior region is available.[22] The proximodistal direction is followed by developing adequate function in the head, neck, and trunk prior to developing function in the extremities. This is of particular importance in treatment that often facilitates fine motor coordination in the upper extremities. Unless there is adequate control in the head, neck, and trunk region, fine motor skills cannot be developed effectively.

3. *Early motor behavior is dominated by reflex activity. Mature motor behavior is supported or reinforced by postural reflexes.* As the human being matures, primitive reflexes are integrated to allow for progressive development such as rolling, crawling, and sitting. Reflexes also have been noted to have an effect on tone changes in the extremities. Hellebrandt and coworkers studied the effect of the tonic neck reflex (TNR) and the asymmetric tonic neck reflex (ATNR) on changes in tone and movement in the extremities of normal adults. She found that head and neck movement significantly affected arm and leg movement.[10] In applying this to treatment, weak elbow extensors can be reinforced with the ATNR by having the patient look toward the side of weakness. Likewise, the patient can be assisted in assuming postures with the influence of reflex support. For example, the body-on-body righting reflex supports assuming side-sitting from side-lying position.

4. *Early motor behavior is characterized by spontaneous movement which oscillates between extremes of flexion and extension. These movements are rhythmic and reversing in character.* In treatment it is important to attend to both directions of movement. When working with the patient on getting up from a chair, attention also must be given to sitting back down. Often with an injury the eccentric con-

traction (sitting down) is readily lost and becomes very difficult for the patient to regain. If not properly treated, the patient may be left with inadequate motor control to sit down smoothly and thus may "drop" into a chair. Similarly, in activities of daily living (ADL) training, the patient must learn how to get undressed as well as dressed.

5. *Developing motor behavior is expressed in an orderly sequence of total patterns of movement and posture.* In the normal infant the sequence of total patterns is demonstrated through the progresion of locomotion. The infant learns to roll, to crawl, to creep, and finally to stand and walk. Throughout these stages of locomotion the infant also learns to use his or her extremities in different patterns and within different postures. Initially the hands are used for reaching and grasping within the most supported postures such as supine and prone. As postural control develops, the infant begins to use the hands in side-lying, sitting, and standing.

The use of extremities in total patterns requires interaction with component patterns of the head, neck, and trunk. For example, in swinging a tennis racquet in a forehand stroke, the arm and the head, neck, and trunk move in the direction of the swing. Without the interaction of the distal and proximal components, movement becomes less powerful and less coordinated.

6. *The growth of motor behavior has cyclic trends as evidenced by shifts between flexor and extensor dominance.* The shifts between antagonists help to develop muscle balance and control. One of the main goals of the PNF treatment approach is to establish a balance between antagonists. Developmentally the infant does this prior to creeping, that is, when rocking forward (extensor dominant) and backward (flexor dominant) on hands and knees. Postural control and balance must be achieved before movement can begin in this position. In treatment it is important to establish a balance between antagonistic muscles by first observing where imbalance exists and then facilitating the weaker component. For example, if the stroke patient demonstrates a flexor synergy (flexor dominant), extension should be facilitated.

7. *Normal motor development has an orderly sequence but lacks a step by step quality. Overlapping occurs. The child does not perfect performance of one activity before beginning another more advanced activity.* In trying to ascertain in which total pattern to position the patient, normal motor development should be

heeded. If one technique or developmental posture is not effective in obtaining the desired result, it may be necessary to try the activity in another developmental posture. For example, if an ataxic patient is unable to write while sitting, it may be necessary to practice writing in a more supported posture, such as prone on elbows. Just as the infant reverts to a more secure posture when attempting a complex fine motor task, so must the patient. The cognitive demands of the task in relation to the developmental posture also must be considered. When the patient's position is varied, either by changing the base of support or shifting weight on different extremities, the quality of visual and cognitive processing is influenced.[1]

8. *Locomotion depends upon reciprocal contraction of flexors and extensors, and the maintenance of posture requires continual adjustment for nuances of imbalance. Antagonistic pairs of movements, reflexes, muscles, and joint motion interact as necessary to the movement or posture.* This principle restates one of the main objectives of PNF—to achieve a balance between antagonists. An example of imbalance is the head-injured patient who is unable to maintain adequate sitting balance for a table-top cognitive activity because of a dominance of trunk extensor tone. Another example is the hemiplegic patient with tight finger flexors secondary to flexor dominant tone in the hand. In treatment, emphasis would be placed on correcting the imbalances. In the presence of spasticity this may have to be done first by inhibiting the spasticity and then by facilitating the antagonistic muscles, reflexes, and postures.

9. *Improvement in motor ability is dependent upon motor learning.* Multisensory input from the therapist facilitates the patient's motor learning and is an integral part of the PNF approach. For example, the therapist may work with a patient on a shoulder flexion activity such as reaching into the cabinet for a cup. The therapist may say, "reach for the cup," to add verbal input. This also encourages the patient to look in the direction of the movement to allow vision to enhance the motor response. Thus, tactile, auditory, and visual input are used. Motor learning has occurred when these external cues are no longer needed for adequate performance.

10. *Frequency of stimulation and repetitive activity are used to promote and for retention of motor learning, and for the development of strength and endurance.* Just as the therapist who is learning PNF needs the opportunity to practice the techniques, the patient needs the opportunity to practice new motor skills. In the process of development the infant constantly repeats a motor skill until it is mastered. This becomes apparent to anyone who has watched a child learning to walk. Numerous attempts fail, but efforts are repeated until the skill is mastered. After the activity is learned, it becomes part of the child. He or she is able to use it automatically and deliberately as the occasion demands.[22] The same is true for the person learning to play the piano or to play tennis. Without the opportunity to practice, motor learning cannot successfully occur.

11. *Goal directed activities coupled with techniques of facilitation are used to hasten learning of total patterns of walking and self care activities.* When applying facilitation techniques to self-care the objective is improved functional ability, but improvement is obtained by more than instruction and practice alone. Correction of deficiencies is accomplished by directly applying manual contacts and techniques to facilitate a desired response.[11] In treatment this may mean applying stretch to finger extensors to facilitate release of an object or providing joint approximation through the shoulders and pelvis of an ataxic patient to provide stability while standing to wash dishes.

MOTOR LEARNING

As discussed previously, motor learning requires a multisensory approach. Auditory, visual, and tactile systems are all used to achieve the desired response. The correct combination of sensory input with each patient should be ascertained, implemented, and altered as the patient progresses. The developmental level of the patient and the ability to cooperate also should be taken into consideration.[22] The approach used with an aphasic patient differs from the approach used with a hand-injured patient. Similarly the approach with a child varies greatly from that with an adult.

Auditory

Verbal commands should be brief and clear. Timing of the command is important so that it does not come too early or too late in relation to the motor act. Tone of voice may influence the quality of the patient's response. Buchwald states that tones of moderate intensity evoke gamma motor neuron activity and that louder tones can alter alpha motor neuron activity.[4] Strong sharp commands simulate a stress situation and are used when maximal stimulation of motor response is desired. A soft tone of voice is used to offer reassurance and to encourage a smooth movement, as in the presence of pain. When the patient is giving his best effort, a moderate tone can be used.[22]

Another effect of auditory feedback on motor performance was studied by Loomis and Boersma.[14] They used a "verbal mediation" strategy to teach patients with right CVA wheelchair safety prior to transferring out of the chair. They taught patients to say aloud the steps required to leave the wheelchair safely and independently. They found that only patients who used verbal mediation learned the wheelchair drill sufficiently to perform safe and independent transfers. Their retention of the sequence also was better, suggesting that verbal mediation is beneficial in reaching independence with better sequencing and fewer errors.

Visual

Visual stimuli assist in initiation and coordination of movement. Visual input should be monitored to ensure that the patient is tracking in the direction of movement. For example, the therapist's position is important because the patient often uses the therapist's movement or position as a visual cue. If the desired direction of movement is forward, the therapist should be positioned diagonally in front of the patient. In addition to the therapist's position, placement of the OT activity also should be considered. If the treatment goal is to increase head, neck, and trunk rotation to the left, the activity is placed in front and to the left of the patient. Because OT is activity-oriented, an abundance of visual stimuli is offered to the patient.

Tactile

Developmentally, the tactile system matures before the auditory and visual systems.[7] Furthermore, the tactile system is more efficient because it has both temporal and spatial discrimination abilities as opposed to the visual system, which can make only spatial discriminations, and the auditory system, which can make only temporal discriminations.[8] Affolter states that during development, processing of tactile-kinesthetic information can be considered fundamental for building cognitive and emotional experience.[2] Looking at and listening to the world does not result in change. However, the world cannot be touched without some change. A Chinese proverb often cited at PNF courses reinforces this viewpoint: I listen—I forget, I see—I remember, I do—I understand.

It is important for the patient to *feel* movement patterns that are coordinated and balanced. With the PNF approach, tactile input is supplied through the therapist's manual contacts to guide and reinforce the desired response. This may mean gently touching the patient to guide movement, using stretch to initiate movement, and providing resistance to enhance movement. The type and extent of manual contacts depend on the patient's clinical status, which is established through evaluation and reevaluation.

To increase speed and accuracy in motor performance, the patient needs the opportunity to practice. Through repetition, habit patterns that occur automatically without voluntary effort are established. The PNF approach uses the concepts of part-task and whole-task practice. In other words, to learn the whole task, emphasis is placed on the parts of the task that the patient is unable to perform independently. The term *stepwise procedures* is descriptive of the emphasis on a part of the task during performance of the whole.[22] Performance of each part of the task is improved by practice, combined with appropriate sensory cues and techniques of facilitation. For example, the patient learning to transfer from a wheelchair to a tub bench may have difficulty lifting his leg over the tub rim. This part of the task should be practiced, with repetition and facilitation techniques to the hip flexors, during performance of the transfer. When the transfer becomes smooth and coordinated, it is no longer necessary to practice each part individually.

In summation, several components are necessary for motor learning to occur. In the PNF treatment approach, these components include multisensory input from the therapist's verbal commands, visual cues, and manual contacts. Touch is the most efficient form of stimulation and provides the opportunity for the patient to feel normal movement. The patient must practice motor activities in varying situations with immediate and constant feedback given.

EVALUATION

Assessment requires astute observational skills and knowledge of normal movement. An initial evaluation is completed to determine the patient's abilities, deficiencies, and potential. After the treatment plan is established, ongoing assessment of the patient is necessary to ascertain the effectiveness of treatment and to make modifications as the patient changes.

The PNF evaluation follows a sequence from proximal to distal. First vital and related functions are considered, such as breathing, swallowing, voice production, facial and oral musculature, and visual/ocular control. Any impairment or weakness in these functions is noted.

The head and neck region is observed next. Deficiencies in this area directly affect the upper trunk and extremities. Head and neck positions are observed in varying postures and total patterns during functional activities. It is important to note (1) dominance of tone (flexor or extensor), (2) alignment (midline or shift to one side), and (3) stability/mobility (more or less needed).[15]

After observation of the head and neck region, the evaluation proceeds to the following parts of the body: upper trunk, upper extremities, lower trunk, lower extremities. Each segment is evaluated individually in specific movement patterns, as well as in developmental activities in which interaction of body segments occurs. For example, shoulder flexion can be observed in an individual upper extremity movement pattern as well as during a total developmental pattern such as rolling.

During assessment of developmental activities and postures, the following issues should be addressed:
1. Is there a need for more stability or mobility?
2. Is there a balance between flexors and extensors, or is one more dominant?
3. Is the patient able to move in all directions?
4. What are the major limitations (weakness, incoordination, spasticity, contractures)?
5. Is the patient able to assume a posture and to maintain it? If not, which total pattern or postures are inadequate?
6. Are the inadequacies more proximal or distal?
7. Which sensory input does the patient respond to most effectively (auditory, visual, tactile)?
8. Which techniques of facilitation does the patient respond to best?

Finally, the patient is observed during self-care and other ADL to determine whether performance of individual and total patterns is adequate within the context of a functional activity. The patient's performance may vary from one setting to another. After the patient leaves the structural setting of the OT or PT (physical therapy) clinic, for the less structured home or community environment, deterioration of motor performance is not unusual. Thus the treatment plan must accommodate for practice of motor performance in a variety of settings in locations appropriate to the specific activity.

TREATMENT IMPLEMENTATION

After the previously mentioned factors are determined, a treatment plan is developed, which includes goals that the patient hopes to accomplish. The techniques and procedures that have the most favorable influence on movement and posture are used. Similarly, appropriate total patterns and patterns of facilitation are selected to enhance performance.

Diagonal Patterns

The diagonal patterns used in the PNF approach are mass movement patterns observed in most functional activities. Part of the challenge in OT evaluation and treatment is recognizing the diagonal patterns in activities of daily living. Knowledge of the diagonals is necessary to identify areas of deficiency. Two diagonal motions are present for each major part of the body: head and neck, upper and lower trunk, and extremities. Each diagonal pattern has a flexion and extension component together with rotation and movement away from or toward the midline.

The head, neck, and trunk patterns are referred to as (a) flexion with rotation to the right or left and (b) extension with rotation to the right or left. These proximal patterns combine with the extremity diagonals. The upper and lower extremity diagonals are described according to the three movement components at the shoulder and hip: (1) flexion/extension, (2) abduction/adduction, and (3) external/internal rotation. Voss introduced shorter descriptions for the extremity patterns in 1967 and referred to them as diagonal 1 (D_1) flexion/extension and diagonal 2 (D_2) flexion/extension.[20] The reference points for flexion and extension are the shoulder and hip joints of the upper and lower extremities, respectively.

The movements associated with each diagonal and examples of these patterns seen in self-care and other ADL follow. Note that in functional activities, not all components of the pattern or full range of motion are necessarily seen. Furthermore, the diagonals interact during functional movement, changing from one pattern or combination to another, when they cross the transverse and sagittal planes of the body.[16]

UNILATERAL PATTERNS
1. UE (upper extremity) D_1 flexion (antagonist of D_1 extension). Scapula elevation, abduction, and rotation; shoulder flexion, adduction, and external rotation; elbow in flexion or extension; forearm supination; wrist flexion to the radial side; finger flexion and adduction; thumb adduction (Fig. 21-1, A). Examples in functional activity: hand-to-mouth motion in feeding, tennis forehand, combing hair on left side of head with right hand (Fig. 21-2, A), rolling from supine to prone.

2. UE D_1 extension (antagonist of D_1 flexion). Scapula depression, adduction, and rotation; shoulder extension, abduction, and internal rotation; elbow in flexion or extension; forearm pronation; wrist extension to the ulnar side; finger extension and abduction; thumb in palmar abduction (Fig. 21-1, B). Examples in functional activity: pushing a car door open from the inside (Fig. 21-2, B), tennis backhand stroke, and rolling from prone to supine.

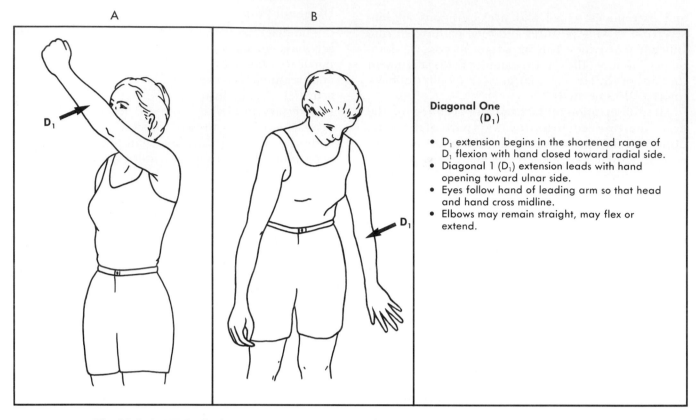

Fig. 21-1. **A,** UE D₁ flexion pattern. **B,** UE D₁ extension pattern. From Meyers BJ: Unit I: PNF diagonal patterns and their application to functional activities, videotape study guide, Rehabilitation Institute of Chicago, 1982.

3. UE D₂ flexion (antagonist of D₂ extension). Scapula elevation, adduction, and rotation; shoulder flexion, abduction, and external rotation; elbow in flexion or extension; forearm supination; wrist extension to the radial side; finger extension and abduction; thumb extension (Fig. 21-3, *A*). Examples in functional activity: combing hair on right side of head with right hand (Fig. 21-4, *A*), lifting racquet in tennis serve, back stroke in swimming.

4. UE D₂ extension (antagonist of D₂ flexion). Scapula depression, abduction, and rotation; shoulder extension, adduction, and internal rotation; elbow

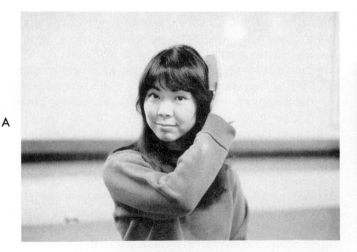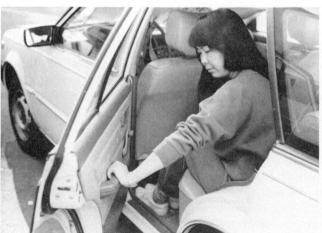

Fig. 21-2. **A,** UE D₁ flexion pattern is used in combing hair, opposite side. **B,** UE D₁ extension pattern is used in pushing a car door open.

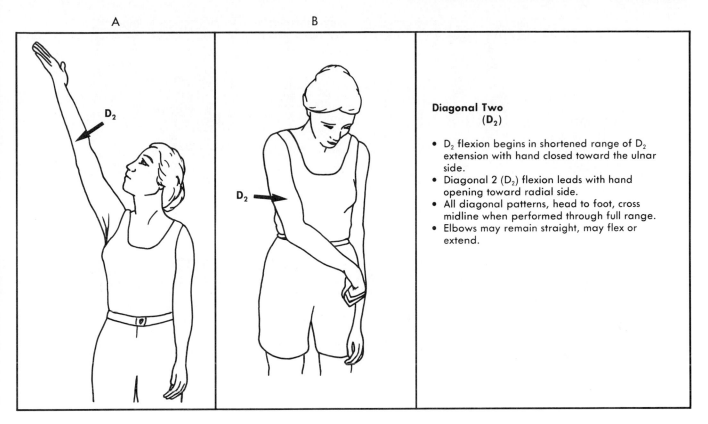

**Diagonal Two
(D₂)**

- D₂ flexion begins in shortened range of D₂ extension with hand closed toward the ulnar side.
- Diagonal 2 (D₂) flexion leads with hand opening toward radial side.
- All diagonal patterns, head to foot, cross midline when performed through full range.
- Elbows may remain straight, may flex or extend.

Fig. 21-3. A, UE D₂ flexion pattern. **B,** UE D₂ extension pattern. From Meyers BJ: Unit I: PNF diagonal patterns and their application to functional activities, videotape study guide, Rehabilitation Institute of Chicago, 1982.

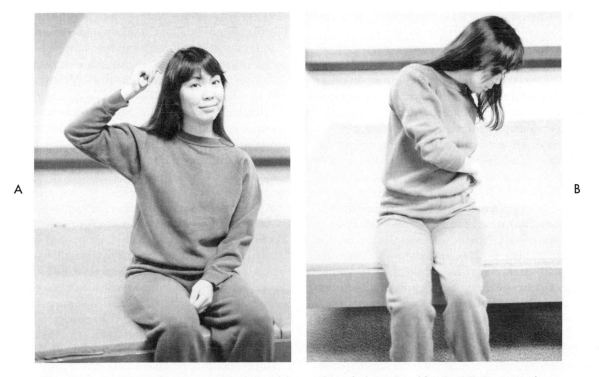

Fig. 21-4. A, UE D₂ flexion pattern is used in combing hair, same side. **B,** UE D₂ extension pattern is used in buttoning trousers, opposite side.

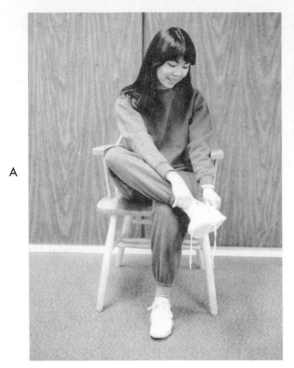
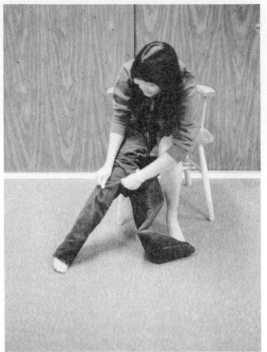

Fig. 21-5. A, LE D₁ flexion pattern is demonstrated in the crossed leg when putting on a shoe.
B, LE D₁ extension pattern is used when pulling on trousers.

in flexion or extension; forearm pronation; wrist flexion to the ulnar side; finger flexion and adduction; thumb opposition (Fig. 21-3, *B*). Examples in functional activity: pitching a baseball, hitting ball in tennis serve, buttoning pants on left side with right hand (Fig. 21-4, *B*).

The rotational component in lower extremity D₁ flexion and extension parallel the upper extremity patterns.

5. LE (lower extremity) D₁ flexion (antagonist of D₁ extension). Hip flexion, adduction, and external rotation; knee in flexion or extension; ankle and foot dorsiflexion with inversion and toe extension. Examples in functional activity: kicking a soccer ball, rolling from supine to prone, putting on a shoe with leg crossed (Fig. 21-5, *A*).

6. LE D₁ extension (antagonist of D₁ flexion). Hip extension, abduction, and internal rotation; knee in flexion or extension; ankle and foot plantar flexion with eversion and toe flexion. Examples in functional activity: putting leg into pants (Fig. 21-5, *B*), rolling from prone to supine.

The rotational component of lower extremity D₂ flexion and extension is opposite to the upper extremity patterns.

7. LE D₂ flexion (antagonist to D₂ extension). Hip flexion, abduction, and internal rotation; knee in flexion or extension; ankle and foot dorsiflexion with eversion and toe extension. Examples in functional activity: karate kick (Fig. 21-6, *A*), drawing the heels up during the breaststroke in swimming.

8. LE D₂ extension (antagonist of D₂ flexion). Hip extension, adduction and external rotation, knee in flexion or extension; ankle and foot plantar flexion with inversion and toe flexion. Examples of functional activity: push-off in gait, the kick during the breaststroke in swimming, long sitting with legs crossed (Fig. 21-6, *B*).

BILATERAL PATTERNS. Movements in the extremities may be reinforced by combining diagonals in bilateral patterns as follows:

1. Symmetric patterns. Paired extremities perform like movements at the same time (Fig. 21-7, *A*). Examples: bilateral symmetric D₁ extension, such as pushing off a chair to stand (Fig. 21-8, *A*); bilateral symmetric D₂ extension, such as starting to take off a pullover sweater (Fig. 21-8, *B*); bilateral symmetric D₂ flexion, such as reaching to lift a large item off a high shelf (Fig. 21-8, *C*).

2. Asymmetric patterns. Paired extremities perform movements toward one side of the body at the same time (Fig. 21-7, *B*). The asymmetric patterns can be performed with the arms in contact such as in the chopping and lifting patterns in which greater trunk rotation is seen (Figs. 21-9 and 21-10). Furthermore, with the arms in contact, self-touching oc-

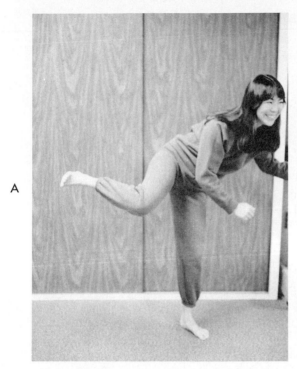
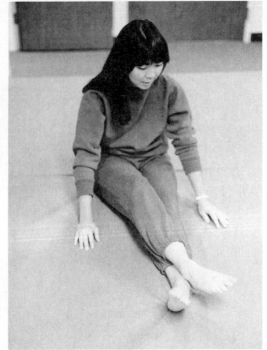

Fig. 21-6. A, LE D₂ flexion pattern is shown in this karate kick. **B,** LE D₂ extension pattern is used in long sitting with legs crossed.

curs, which is frequently observed in the presence of pain or in reinforcement of a motion when greater control or power is needed.[22] This phenomenon is observed in the baseball player at bat and in the tennis player who uses a two-handed backhand to increase control and power. Examples: bilateral asymmetric flexion to the left, with the left arm in D₂ flexion and the right arm in D₁ flexion, such as putting on a left earring (Fig. 21-11); bilateral asymmetric extension to the left, with the right arm in D₂ extension and the left arm in D₁ extension, such as zipping a left side zipper.

3. Reciprocal patterns. Paired extermities perform movements in opposite directions at the same time (see Fig. 21-7, *C*). Reciprocal patterns have a stabilizing effect on the head, neck, and trunk, because movement of the extremities is in the opposite direction from that of the head and neck remaining in midline. During activities requiring high-level balance, the reciprocal patterns come into play with one extremity in D₁ extension and the other extremity in D₂ flexion. Examples: pitching in baseball, walking, sidestroke in swimming, and walking a balance beam with one extremity in a diagonal flexion pattern and the other in a diagonal extension pattern (Fig. 21-12).

COMBINED MOVEMENTS OF UPPER AND LOWER EXTREMITIES. Interaction of the upper and lower

extremities results in (1) ipsilateral patterns with extremities of the same side moving in the same direction at the same time, (2) contralateral patterns with extremities of the opposite sides moving in the same direction at the same time, and (3) diagonal reciprocal patterns with contralateral extremities moving in the same direction at the same time while opposite contralateral extremities move in the opposite direction (Fig. 21-7, *D–F*).

The combined movements of the upper and lower extremities are observed in activities such as crawling and walking. Awareness of these patterns is important in the evaluation of the patient's motor skills. The ipsilateral patterns are more primitive developmentally and indicate lack of bilateral integration. Less rotation also is observed in ipsilateral patterns. Therefore, the goal in treatment is to progress from ipsilateral to contralateral to diagonal reciprocal patterns.

There are several advantages to using the diagonal patterns in treatment. First, crossing of midline occurs. This is of particular importance in the remediation of perceptual motor deficits such as unilateral neglect, in which integration of both sides of the body and awareness of the neglected side are treatment goals. Second, each muscle has an optimal pattern in which it functions. For example, the patient who has weak thumb opposition benefits from active movement in D₂ extension. Similarly, D₁ extension is the

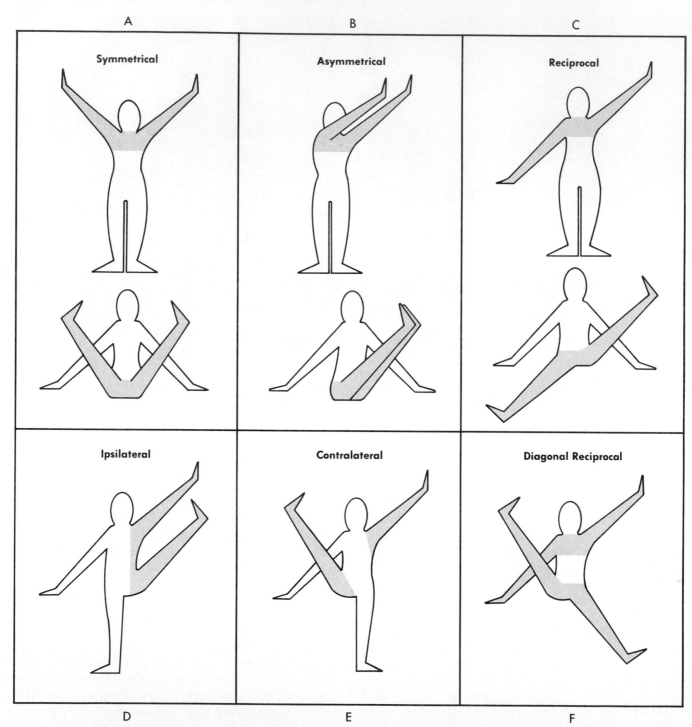

A, Symmetrical   B, Asymmetrical   C, Reciprocal

D, Ipsilateral   E, Contralateral   F, Diagonal Reciprocal

Fig. 21-7. A, Symmetric patterns; **B,** asymmetric patterns; **C,** reciprocal patterns; **D,** ipsilateral pattern; **E,** contralateral pattern; **F,** diagonal reciprocal pattern. From Meyers BJ: Unit I: PNF diagonal patterns and their application to functional activities, videotape study guide, Rehabilitation Institute of Chicago, 1982.

optimal pattern for ulnar wrist extension. Third, the diagonal patterns use groups of muscles, which is typical of movement seen in functional activities. For example, in eating, the hand-to-mouth action is accomplished in one mass movement pattern (D₁ flexion)

that uses several muscles simultaneously. Therefore, movement in the diagonals is more efficient than movement performed at each joint separately. Finally, rotation is always a component in the diagonals (trunk rotation to the left or right and forearm pronation/

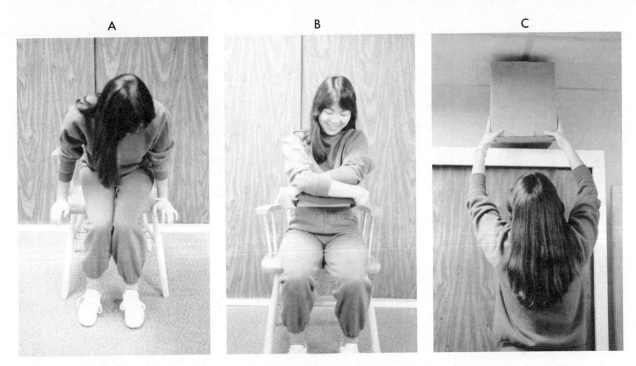

Fig. 21-8. A, UE bilateral symmetric D_1 extension pattern is shown in pushing off from a chair. **B,** UE bilateral symmetric D_2 extension pattern is used when starting to take off a pullover shirt. **C,** UE bilateral symmetric D_2 flexion pattern is used when reaching to lift a box off a high shelf.

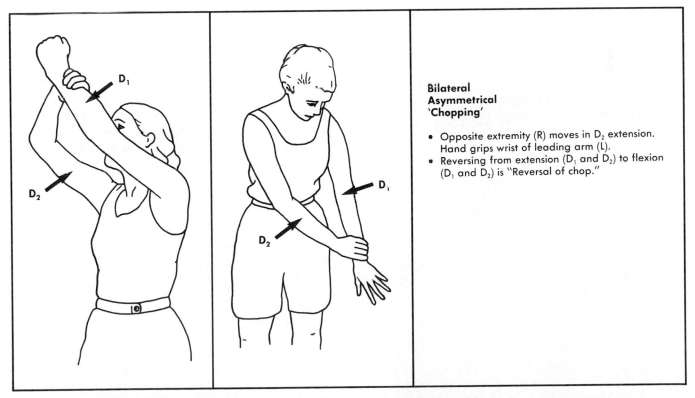

Fig. 21-9. Bilateral asymmetric chopping. From Meyers BJ: Unit I: PNF diagonal patterns and their application to functional activities, videotape study guide, Rehabilitation Institute of Chicago, 1982.

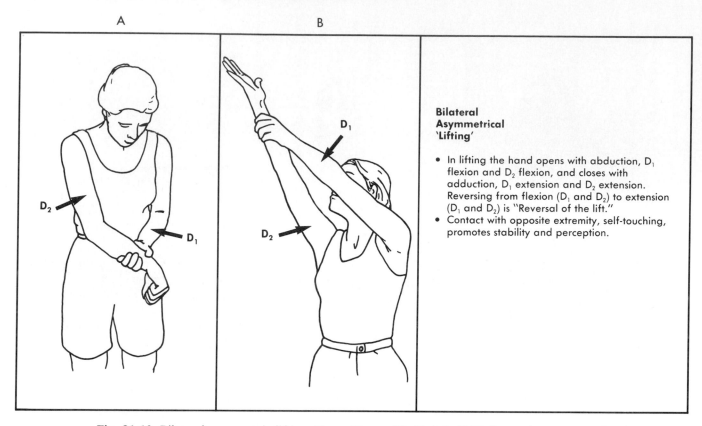

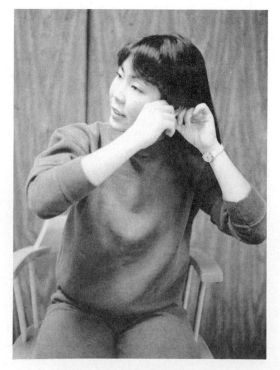

A   B

Bilateral Asymmetrical 'Lifting'

- In lifting the hand opens with abduction, D_1 flexion and D_2 flexion, and closes with adduction, D_1 extension and D_2 extension. Reversing from flexion (D_1 and D_2) to extension (D_1 and D_2) is "Reversal of the lift."
- Contact with opposite extremity, self-touching, promotes stability and perception.

Fig. 21-10. Bilateral asymmetric lifting. From Meyers BJ: Unit I: PNF diagonal patterns and their application to functional activities, videotape study guide, Rehabilitation Institute of Chicago, 1982.

Fig. 21-11. Putting on an earring requires the use of the UE bilateral asymmetric flexion pattern.

supination). With an injury or the aging process, rotation frequently is impaired and can be facilitated with movement in the diagonals. In treatment, attention should be given to placement of activities so that movement occurs in the diagonal. For example, if the patient is working on a wood-sanding project, trunk rotation with extension can be facilitated by placing the project on an inclined plane in a diagonal.

Total Patterns

In PNF, developmental postures also are called total patterns of movement and posture.[17] Total patterns require interaction between proximal (head, neck, and trunk) and distal (extremity) components. The assumption as well as the maintenance of postures is important. When posture is unable to be sustained, emphasis should be placed on the *assumption* of posture.[21] In other words, before the patient can be expected to sustain a sitting posture, he or she must have ability in lower developmental total patterns of movement, such as rolling and moving from sidelying to side-sitting. Active assumption of postures can be included in OT activities. For example, a reaching and placing activity could be set up so that the patient must reach for the object in supine posture and place

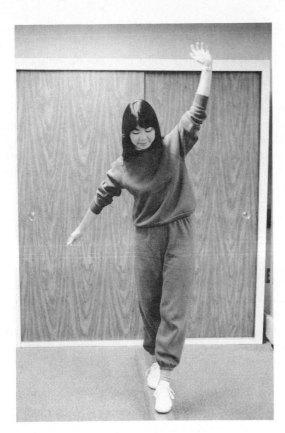

Fig. 21-12. A bilateral reciprocal pattern of the upper extremities is used to walk the balance beam.

the object in side-lying posture. The use of total patterns also can reinforce individual extremity movements. For example, in an activity such as wiping a table top, wrist extension is reinforced while the patient leans forward over the supporting arm.

Several facts support the use of total patterns in the PNF treatment approach.[17] First, total patterns of movement and posture are experienced as part of the normal developmental process in all human beings. Therefore, recapitulation of these postures is meaningful to the patient and acquired with less difficulty. Second, movement in and out of total patterns and the ability to sustain postures enhance components of normal development, such as reflex integration and support, balance between antagonists, and development of motor control in a cephalocaudal, proximodistal direction. Third, use of total patterns improves the ability to assume and maintain postures, which is important in all functional activities.

The sequence and procedures for assisting patients to the developmental postures were developed by Voss. In 1981 Myers developed a videotape for use of the sequence and procedures in OT.[17] Refer to this video for further information on application of the total patterns and postures to OT.

Procedures

Proprioceptive neuromuscular facilitation techniques of facilitation and inhibition are superimposed on movement and posture. Among these techniques are basic procedures considered essential to the PNF approach. Two procedures, verbal commands and visual cues, have been discussed previously. Other procedures are described in the following sections.

Manual contacts refer to the placement of the therapist's hands on the patient. Pressure from the therapist's touch is used as a facilitating mechanism and serves as a sensory cue to help the patient understand the direction of the anticipated movement.[22] The amount of pressure applied depends on the specific technique being used and the desired response. Location of manual contacts is chosen according to the groups of muscles, tendons, and joints responsible for the desired movement patterns. If the patient is having difficulty reaching to comb the back of his or her hair because of scapular weakness, the desired movement pattern would be D_2 flexion. Manual contacts would be on the posterior surface of the scapula to reinforce the muscles that elevate, adduct, and rotate the scapula.

Stretch is used to initiate voluntary movement and enhance speed of response and strength in weak muscles. This procedure is based on Sherrington's neurophysiologic principle of reciprocal innervation.[18] When a muscle is stretched, the Ia and II fibers in the muscle spindle send excitatory messages to the alpha motor neurons, which innervate the stretched muscle. Inhibitory messages are sent to the antagonistic muscle simultaneously.[7]

When stretch is used in the PNF approach, the part to be facilitated is placed in the extreme lengthened range of the desired pattern (or where tension is felt on all muscle components of a given pattern). This is the completely shortened range of the antagonistic pattern. Special attention is given to the rotatory component of the pattern because it is responsible for elongation of the fibers of the muscles in a given pattern. After the correct position for the stretch stimulus has been achieved, stretch is superimposed on the pattern. The patient should attempt the movement at the exact time that the stretch reflex is elicited. The use of verbal commands also should coincide with the application of stretch to reinforce the movement. Discrimination should be exercised when using stretch to prevent increasing pain or muscle imbalances.

Traction facilitates the joint receptors by creating a separation of the joint surfaces. It is thought that traction promotes movement and is used for pulling motion.[22] In activities such as carrying a heavy suitcase or pulling open a jammed door, traction can be felt on joint surfaces. Although traction may be contraindicated in patients with acute symptoms, such as after surgery or a fracture, it can sometimes provide relief of pain and promote greater range of motion in painful joints.

Approximation facilitates joint receptors by creating a compression of joint surfaces. It promotes stability and postural control and is used for pushing motion.[22] Approximation is usually superimposed on a weight-bearing posture. For example, to enhance postural control in prone on elbow, approximation may be given through the shoulders in a downward direction.

Maximal resistance is a procedure that applies Sherrington's principle of irradiation, namely, that stronger muscles and patterns reinforce weaker components.[18] This procedure is frequently misunderstood and applied incorrectly. It is defined as the greatest amount of resistance that can be applied to an active contraction allowing full range of motion to occur or to an isometric contraction without defeating or breaking the patient's hold.[22] It is *not* the greatest amount of resistance that the therapist can apply. The objective is to obtain maximal effort on the part of the patient, because strength is increased by movement against resistance that requires maximal effort.[9]

If the resistance applied by the therapist results in uncoordinated or jerky movement or if it breaks the patient's hold, too much resistance has been given. Movement against maximal resistance should be slow and smooth. In order to use this technique effectively, the therapist must sense the appropriate amount of resistance. For patients with neurologic impairment or pain, the resistance may be very light, and is probably maximal for the patient's needs. In the presence of spasticity, resistance may increase existing muscle imbalance and needs to be monitored. For example, if an increase in finger flexor spasticity is noted with resisted rocking in the hands-knees position, resistance should be decreased or eliminated, or an alternate position used.

Techniques

Specific techniques are used in conjunction with these basic procedures. A few have been selected for discussion. These techniques are divided into three categories: those directed to the agonist, those that are reversal of the antagonists, and those that promote relaxation.[22]

TECHNIQUES DIRECTED TO THE AGONIST

Repeated contractions is a technique based on the assumption that repetition of an activity is necessary for motor learning and helps develop strength, range of motion, and endurance. The patient's voluntary movement is facilitated with stretch and resistance using isometric and isotonic contractions. Repeated contractions could be used to increase trunk flexion with rotation in the patient who has difficulty reaching to put on a pair of shoes from the sitting position. The patient bends forward as far as he or she can go. At the point when active motion weakens, he or she is asked to "hold" with an isometric contraction. This is followed by isotonic contractions, facilitated by stretch, as the patient is asked to "reach toward his feet." This sequence is repeated until fatigue is evident or the patient is able to reach his or her feet. The pattern can be reinforced further by asking the patient to hold with another isometric contraction at the end of the sequence.

Rhythmic initiation is used to improve the ability to initiate movement, a problem that may be seen with Parkinson's disease or apraxia. This technique involves voluntary relaxation, passive movement, and repeated isotonic contractions of the agonistic pattern. The verbal command is, "Relax and let me move you." As relaxation is felt, the command is, "Now you do it with me." After several repetitions of active movement, resistance can be given to reinforce the movement. Rhythmic initiation allows the patient to *feel* the pattern prior to active movement. Thus the proprioceptive and kinesthetic senses are enhanced.

REVERSAL OF ANTAGONIST'S TECHNIQUES.
Reversal of antagonist's techniques employs a characteristic of normal development, namely, that movement is reversing and changes direction. These techniques are based on Sherrington's principle of successive induction in which the stronger antagonist facilitates the weaker agonist.[18] The agonist is facilitated through resistance to the antagonist. The contraction of the antagonist can be isotonic, isometric, or a combination of both. In patients in whom resistance of antagonists increases symptoms such as pain and spasticity, these techniques may be contraindicated. For example, the facilitation of finger extension (agonist) would not be effectively achieved through resistance applied to spastic finger flexors (antagonist). In this situation, finger extension may be better facilitated through the use of repeated contractions, in which the emphasis is only on the extensor surface.

Slow reversal is an isotonic contraction (against resistance) of the antagonist followed by an isotonic contraction (against resistance) of the agonist. **Slow reversal-hold** is the same sequence, with an isometric contraction at the end of the range. For the patient who has difficulty reaching his mouth for oral hygiene because of weakness in the D_1 flexion pattern, the slow reversal procedure is as follows: An isotonic contraction against resistance in D_1 extension with verbal command "push down and out" followed by an isotonic contraction of D_1 flexion against resistance with verbal command "pull up and across." An increase or buildup of power in the agonist should be felt with each successive isotonic contraction.

Rhythmic stabilization is used to increase stability by eliciting simultaneous isometric contractions of antagonistic muscle groups. Cocontraction results if the patient is not allowed to relax. Because this technique requires repeated isometric contractions, increased circulation or the tendency to hold one's breath or both occurs. Therefore, rhythmic stabilization may be contraindicated for patients with cardiac involvement, and no more than three or four repetitions should be done at a time.

Manual contacts are applied on both agonist and antagonist muscles with resistance given simultaneously. The patient is asked to "hold" the contraction against graded resistance. Without allowing the patient to relax, manual contacts are switched to opposite surfaces. Rhythmic stabilization is useful with patients lacking postural control due to ataxia or proximal weakness. Used intermittently during an activity requiring postural stability, such as meal preparation in standing posture, this technique enhances muscle balance, endurance, and control of movement.

RELAXATION TECHNIQUES. Relaxation techniques are an effective means of increasing range of motion, particularly in the presence of pain or spasticity, which may be increased by passive stretch.

Contract-relax involves an isotonic contraction of the antagonistic pattern against maximal resistance, followed by relaxation, then passive movement into the agonistic pattern. This procedure is repeated at each point in the range of motion in which limitation is felt to occur.[22] Contact-relax is used when no active range in the agonistic pattern is present.

Hold-relax is performed in the same sequence as contract-relax but involves an isometric contraction of the antagonist, followed by relaxation, then active movement into the agonistic pattern. Because this technique involves an isometric contraction against resistance, it is particularly beneficial in the presence of pain or acute orthopedic conditions. For the reflex sympathetic dystrophy (RSD) patient who has pain with shoulder flexion, abduction, and external rotation, the therapist asks the patient to "hold" against resistance in the D_2 extension pattern, followed by active movement into the D_2 flexion pattern. This technique is beneficial for the RSD patient during self-care activities such as shampooing hair and zipping a shirt in back.

Slow reversal-hold-relax begins with an isotonic contraction, followed by an isometric contraction,

then by relaxation of the antagonistic pattern, and then by active movement of the agonistic pattern. When the patient has the ability to actively move the agonist, this technique is preferred. For example, to increase active elbow extension in the presence of tight elbow flexors, the therapist asks the patient to perform D_1 flexion with elbow flexion as resistance is applied to the elbow flexors. When the range of motion is complete, the patient is asked to hold with an isometric contraction followed immediately by relaxation. When relaxation is felt, the patient moves actively into D_1 extension with elbow extension. This technique helps to increase elbow extension for such activities as reaching to lock the wheelchair brakes or picking up an object off the floor.

Rhythmic rotation is effective in decreasing spasticity and increasing range of motion. The therapist passively moves the body part in the desired pattern. When tightness or restriction of movement is felt, the therapist rotates the body part slowly and rhythmically in both directions. After relaxation is felt, the therapist continues to move the body part into the newly available range. This technique is effective in preparing the paraplegic patient with lower extremity spasticity or clonus to put on a pair of pants and also in preparing for splint fabrication on a spastic extremity.

SUMMARY

Emphasis in the PNF approach is on the patient's abilities and potential so that strengths assist weaker components. Strengths and deficiencies are evaluated and addressed in treatment within total patterns of movement and posture. A battery of techniques are superimposed on these total patterns to enhance motor response and facilitate motor learning.

Proprioceptive neuromuscular facilitation uses multisensory input. Coordination and timing of sensory input are important in eliciting the desired response from the patient. The patient's performance should be monitored and sensory input adjusted accordingly.

To use PNF effectively, an understanding of the developmental sequence and the components of normal movement is necessary. Second, it is necessary to learn the diagonal patterns and how they are used in ADL. Third, the therapist must know when and how to use the techniques of facilitation and relaxation. This requires observation and practice under the supervision of an experienced PNF therapist. Finally, the therapist applies patterns and techniques of facilitation to OT evaluation and treatment.

CASE STUDY

A 50-year-old woman was referred to OT with a right cerebral vascular accident (CVA) resulting in left hemiplegia. Before the CVA, she had a history of hypertension but otherwise good health. Referral to OT was made 10 days after onset for evaluation and treatment in ADL, visual perceptual skills, and left upper extremity function.

Evaluation

Initial evaluation revealed intact vital and related functions, such as oral/facial musculature and swallowing. Voice production was good. Patient had a tendency to hold her breath during activities, and subsequent decreased endurance was noted. Visual tracking was impaired with inability to scan past midline and apparent left side neglect.

Head and neck were observed to be frequently rotated to the right and slightly flexed due to weak extensors. Trunk was noted to be asymmetric in sitting posture with most of the weight supported on the right side. Posture was flexed because of weak extensors. Static sitting balance was fair and dynamic sitting balance was poor, with patient listing forward and left.

Right arm was normal in sensation and strength, although motor planning was impaired. Left arm was essentially flaccid with impaired sensation of light touch, pain, and proprioception. Patient complained of mild glenohumeral pain during passive movement at end ranges of shoulder abduction and flexion. Scapular instability was noted. No active movement could be elicited in left arm.

Perceptual evaluation showed apraxia (especially during activities requiring crossing of midline), and left side neglect. Patient was alert and oriented with good attention span and memory. Carryover in tasks was adequate.

Patient needed moderate assistance in ADL and moderate to maximum assistance with transfers. Impaired balance and apraxia were most limiting factors in performance of ADL.

Treatment Implementation

Following cervicocaudal direction of development, alignment of head and neck was appropriate starting point for treatment. Left side awareness, sitting posture, and trunk balance were directly influenced by position of head and neck. Before the start of self-care activities patient performed head and neck patterns of flexion and extension with rotation. To reinforce rotation to left, therapist was positioned to left of patient. Clothing and hygiene articles also were placed to left of patient.

Lack of trunk control was another problem. During bending activities patient reported fear of falling and was unsure of her ability to return to upright position. Consequently, she had difficulty leaning forward to transfer from wheelchair. Slow reversal-hold technique was used to reinforce trunk patterns during ADL. For example, as patient prepared to don her left pant leg, therapist was positioned in front and to left of patient. Manual contacts were on anterior aspect of either scapula. Therapist moved with patient and applied resistance as she leaned forward to don her pants. At end of the range, patient was instructed to hold with isometric contraction. After pants were donned, manual contacts switched to posterior surface of either scapula. Resistance was applied as patient returned to upright position. Verbal command was, "look up and over your right shoulder." When patient was upright she was again instructed to hold with isometric contraction. In addition to reinforcing trunk control, this technique alleviated patient's fear of leaning forward, because therapist was in continual contact with patient.

An indirect benefit of the flexion and extension patterns of the head, neck, and trunk was reinforcement of respiration. Patient was encouraged to inhale during extension and exhale during flexion. This eliminated the patient's tendency to hold her breath.

Treatment consisted of total patterns and techniques to facilitate proximal stability in left upper extremity and provide proprioceptive input. Weight-bearing activities were selected because no active movement was available in the left arm. Patient performed perceptual tasks in diagonal patterns with right upper extremity, such as a mosaic tile design, paper and pencil activities and board games. These activities were performed to include side-lying posture on left elbow, prone posture on elbows, side-sitting posture with weight on left arm, and all fours. To reinforce stability at the shoulder girdle, approximation and rhythmic stabilization were used with manual contacts at both shoulders and then shoulder and pelvis. Performance of perceptual tasks in diagonals improved patient's motor planning, left-side awareness, and trunk rotation.

Patient was instructed in bilateral asymmetric chopping and lifting patterns to support scapula and left upper extremity in rolling and other activities. These also enhanced left-side awareness and trunk rotation. To facilitate scapular movement during chop and lift patterns, therapist applied stretch to initiate movement followed by slow reversal technique. In preparation for lift pattern, manual contacts were placed on posterior surface of scapula. Stretch was applied in lengthened range. As patient initiated lifting pattern, resistance was given and maintained throughout range. This was repeated for antagonistic or reverse of lift pattern with manual contacts switching to anterior surface of scapula.

About 3 to 4 weeks after injury, patient was able to initiate left upper extremity movement in synergy with predominance of flexor tone. Weight-bearing activities and rhythmic rotation were helpful in normalizing tone, and both techniques were used with ADL such as dressing and bathing. Wrist and finger extensions were facilitated in the D_1 extension and D_2 flexion patterns using repeated contractions.

Results

Reevaluation after 5 weeks of OT revealed increased endurance and ability to coordinate breathing with activity, and consistency in crossing midline during visual scanning activities. Patient was able to turn head and neck to the left without cues from therapist. Fear of falling forward with bending had diminished, and patient automatically turned her head to look up and over her shoulder to reinforce assumption of upright position. As trunk strength continued to improve, reinforcement with head and neck rotation was no longer necessary. Visual tracking alone, in direction of movement, was sufficient to reinforce assumption of upright position. Eventually, patient was able to obtain an upright position without apparent visual or head and neck reinforcement. Sitting balance improved with bilateral weight bearing through both hips. Shoulder pain decreased, as well as improved scapular stabilty during weight-bearing activities. Patient initiated left upper extremity movement out of flexor synergy pattern. Right upper extremity motor planning was within functional limits for ADL. Transfers and self-care required only minimal assistance, and cues were no longer needed for left upper extremity awareness.

REVIEW QUESTIONS

1. Give examples of how the TNR and the ATNR reinforce motor performance.
2. Is rolling from prone to supine a flexor or extensor dominant activity?
3. In the presence of pain, what tone of voice should be used when giving verbal commands?
4. Discuss the significance of auditory, visual, and tactile input in motor learning.
5. Which upper extremity diagonal pattern is used for the hand-to-mouth phase of eating? For zipping front-opening pants?
6. Discuss the advantages of using the chop and lift patterns.
7. Which trunk pattern is used when donning a left sock?
8. List three advantages of using the diagonal patterns.
9. What is the developmental sequence of total patterns?
10. If a patient needs more stability, which of the following total patterns should be chosen: sidelying or prone posture on elbows?
11. Which PNF technique facilitates postural control and cocontraction?
12. Discuss the neurophysiologic

principles of Sherrington upon which the PNF techniques of facilitation are based.
13. What would be an effective technique to prepare the patient with upper extremity flexor spasticity to don a shirt?
14. Define maximal resistance.
15. Name two PNF techniques that facilitate initiation of movement.

REFERENCES

1. Abreu BF and Toglia JP: Cognitive rehabilitation: a model for occupational therapy, Am J Occup Ther 41(7):439, 1987.
2. Affolter F: Perceptual processes as prerequisites for complex human behavior, Int Rehabil Med 3(1):3, 1981.
3. Ayres JA: Proprioceptive neuromuscular facilitation elicited through the upper extremities. Part I. Background 9(1):1, Part II. Application 9(2):57, Part III. Specific application to occupational therapy, Am J Occup Ther 9(3):121, 1955.
4. Buchwald JS: Exteroceptive reflexes and movement, Am J Phys Med 46(1):121, 1967.
5. Carroll J: The utilization of reinforcement techniques in the program for the hemiplegic, Am J Occup Ther 4(5):211, 1950.
6. Cooke DM: The effects of resistance on multiple sclerosis patients with intention tremor, Am J Occup Ther 12(2):89, 1958.
7. Farber SD: Neurorehabilitation: a multisensory approach, Philadelphia, 1982, WB Saunders Co.
8. Hagbarth KE: Excitatory and inhibitory skin areas for flexor and extensor mononeurons, Acta Physiol Scand 26(suppl 94):1, 1952.
9. Hellebrandt FA: Physiology. In Delorme TL and Watkins AL: Progressive resistance exercise, New York, 1951, Appleton, Century, & Crofts.
10. Hellebrandt FA, Schade M, and Carns ML: Methods of evoking the tonic neck reflexes in normal human subjects, Am J Phys Med 4(90):139, 1962.
11. Humphrey TL, Huddleston OL: Applying facilitation techniques to self care training, Phys Ther Rev 38(9):605, 1958.
12. Jackson JH: Selected writings, vol 1, London, 1931, Hodder and Staughton (edited by J Taylor).
13. Kabat H and Rosenberg D: Concepts and techniques of occupational therapy neuromuscular disorders, Am J Occup Ther 4(1):6, 1950.
14. Loomis JE and Boersma FJ: Training right brain damaged patients in a wheelchair task: case studies using verbal mediation, Physiother Can 34(4):204, 1982.
15. Myers BJ: Proprioceptive neuromuscular facilitation: concepts and application in occupational therapy as taught by Voss, Notes from Course at Rehabilitation Institute of Chicago, September 8–12, 1980.
16. Myers BJ: PNF: patterns and application in occupational therapy, Chicago, Rehabilitation Institute of Chicago, 1981 (videotape).
17. Myers BJ: Assisting to postures and application in occupational therapy activities, Chicago, Rehabilitation Institute of Chicago, 1981 (videotape).
18. Sherrington C: The integrative action of the nervous system, New Haven, 1961, Yale University Press.
19. Voss DE: Application of patterns and techniques in occupational therapy, Am J Occup Ther 8(4):191, 1959.
20. Voss DE: Proprioceptive neuromuscular facilitation, Am J Phys Med 46(1):838, 1967.
21. Voss DE: Proprioceptive neuromuscular facilitation: the PNF method. In Pearson PH and Williams CE, editors: Physical therapy services in the developmental disabilities, Springfield, Ill, 1972, Charles C Thomas, Publisher.
22. Voss DE, Ionta MK, and Myers BJ: Proprioceptive neuromuscular facilitation, ed 3, Philadelphia, 1985, Harper & Row Publishers, Inc.
23. Whitaker EW: A suggested treatment in occupational therapy for patients with multiple sclerosis, Am J Occup Ther 4(6):247, 1950.

22 Wheelchairs and wheelchair transfers

LORRAINE WILLIAMS PEDRETTI
GREGORY STONE

WHEELCHAIRS

The wheelchair provides a comfortable and efficient mode of ambulation for those persons whose physical dysfunction makes walking impossible or impracticable (Figs. 22-1 and 22-2). Others who ordinarily walk with supportive devices such as canes or crutches may find a wheelchair helpful when daily activities require speed or physical endurance that would be overtaxing. A wheelchair for such persons can enrich life experiences by making possible activities such as trips to shopping centers, theaters, and amusement parks, and sight-seeing vacations.

In a sense the wheelchair becomes an extension of the self or the body.[13] The user must learn to manage the wheelchair skillfully, safely, and efficiently, learn to measure space and judge speed and distance with the wheelchair, adapt to viewing the world from a different eye level, and cope with the symbolic meaning of the device to self and society.

The folding wheelchair makes possible a normal life pattern.[10] Wheelchair accessibility in the community and in public buildings has improved significantly in recent years. Curbs, building entrances, restrooms, buses, airports, airplanes, restaurants, and concert halls have been adapted to accommodate the wheelchair user. Consequently, there are many more wheelchair users visible in the community, and their presence is no longer unusual.[10]

The wheelchair is an aid to recreation and socialization. Skillful wheelchair users can participate in sports, dance, and dramatic productions.[10]

Occupational and physical therapists are usually responsible for evaluating, measuring, and selecting a wheelchair for the patient, and for teaching wheelchair safety and mobility. An individualized wheelchair prescribed for the unique needs of the patient is essential for maximal physical independence.

The unprescribed wheelchair is potentially hazardous. Yet "it has been estimated that 80-95 percent of the wheelchairs sold are obtained without professional guidance or prescription."[10] The possible hazards of the unprescribed wheelchair include undue fatigue, potential trauma, secondary deformity, and failure to achieve optimal function.[10]

Wheelchair Evaluation

When evaluating the patient for a wheelchair, the therapist must consider the patient's clinical, mobility, and environmental needs. The therapist must make careful observation of the patient's physical status and functional abilities, overall psychological state, and attitude about the wheelchair. The financial arrangements also are an important consideration. Careful documentation and justification of need by the therapist are essential to enable the patient to receive reimbursement for durable medical equipment.[1] The therapist(s) should make a home evaluation to ascertain wheelchair accessibility and maneuverability. Deep pile carpets, doorsills, stairs, arrangement of furniture and appliances, floor plan, and entrance can influence wheelchair use in the living place. Modifications to the home, as well as to the wheelchair, may need to be considered. In some instances a change of living place is necessary to accommodate the wheelchair.

If a ramp needs to be installed to allow the wheelchair user to enter and exit, it should be 1 foot in length for every inch of stair height of the home entrance. At this incline the wheelchair user can usually manage the ramp safely and independently.

WHEELCHAIR MEASUREMENT

For best comfort and use efficiency the wheelchair should fit the person who is going to use it. Therefore the occupational or physical therapist should measure the patient, as a preparatory step to completing a wheelchair prescription. When properly fitted the

Carole Adler, OTR, Clinical Supervisor, Occupational Therapy Department, Santa Clara Valley Medical Center, is gratefully acknowledged for her assistance with this chapter.

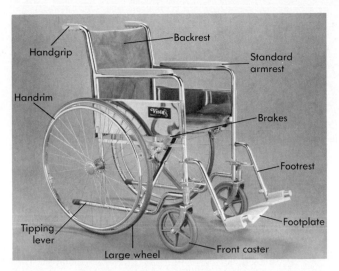

Fig. 22-1. Standard adult wheelchair with standard armrests and detachable swing-away footrests. Reproduced by permission, Everest and Jennings, Inc, Camarillo, Calif.

wheelchair should conform to the following specifications:[1,13]

1. The seat width should be 2 inches (5 cm) wider than the widest point across the patient's hips or thighs. This is to prevent pressure of the body against the sides of the chair. If braces are worn, the measurement across the hips should include the braces.

2. The seat depth should be 2 or 3 inches (5 to 7 cm)

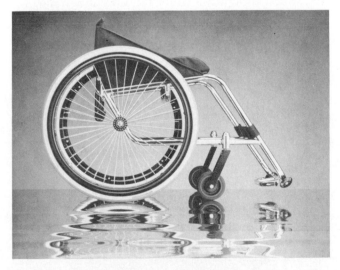

Fig. 22-2. A low-back, high mobility wheelchair. Reproduced by permission, Everest and Jennings, Inc, Camarillo, Calif.

less than the distance from the rear of the buttocks to the inside of the bent knee. This is to distribute weight evenly along the thighs, relieving pressure on the buttocks, and to prevent pressure in the popliteal area.

3. To obtain the correct footrest and seat height adjustment, these must be evaluated together. Leg length measurement is taken from the heel of the shoe or from the heel of the foot, if shoes are not to be worn, to under the thigh, just behind the bent knee. Seat height is determined by adding 2 inches (5 cm) to this measurement.[13] The correct adjustments result in a clearance of 1 inch (2.5 cm) of height and 1½ inches (3.8 cm) of depth under the thighs, whereas the foot plates clear the floor by at least 2 inches (5 cm) for safety. If a wheelchair cushion is to be used, this must be considered when measuring for seat height and footrest adjustments. Special seat heights are available for unusually tall persons.

4. The wheelchair armrest helps in maintenance of posture and balance and provides a comfortable support for the arms. The armrest height should be approximately 1 inch (2.5 cm) more than the distance from the seat level to the bottom of the elbow when flexed to 90°. When the armrest is properly fitted, the patient's shoulders should not be elevated nor should the patient lean to meet the armrests. If a cushion is to be used, this must be considered when measuring for arm height. Adjustable height arms are available and could be more economical than ordering special custom arms, in some cases.[13]

5. The current trend is toward low back rest, high mobility wheelchairs (see Fig. 22-2). The backrest height required depends on the extent of the disability and the amount of back support required. It should provide support that is adequate for physical needs and activity requirements.[13] The height of the standard seat back is 4 inches (10 cm) less than the distance from the seat level to the posterior aspect of the axilla when the shoulder is flexed to 90°. The seat back should provide support to the patient's back, help to maintain posture, and permit free arm movement without irritation. If full trunk support is required, semi-reclining or reclining seat backs or a headrest extension is available.

It is possible to fit most wheelchair users with a manufacturer's standard sizes. However, custom modifications are possible at some additional cost to accommodate individual needs.[13] Such modifications include changes in seat width, depth, and height, back height, armrest height, and footrest height.[1]

Wheelchair Selection

After wheelchair evaluation, the therapist and patient must decide on the following:

1. Wheelchair size
2. Frame style and weight
3. Mode of propulsion
4. Rental or purchase of wheelchair
5. Special accessories and modifications
6. Type of wheelchair cushion[1]

Wheelchair Size

Wheelchairs are available in three major sizes: (1) standard or adult size, (2) intermediate or junior size, and (3) children's size. The standard adult size is suitable for most adults. It can be obtained with a wider (20 inches or 50.8 cm) or narrower (16 inches or 40.6 cm) than standard seat width (18 inches or 45.7 cm) to accommodate wide and narrow adults. The intermediate or junior size is suitable for small adults and older children. The children's size is suitable for children less than age 6 years.[4]

FRAME STYLE AND WEIGHT. Wheelchair frames are rigid or folding, light-weight or standard folding styles.[1]

The outdoor frame with the large wheels in the rear and 8-inch front casters in the most frequently recommended frame for wheelchair users. It is designed for indoor and outdoor use and is easily modified.[15]

The patient with a bilateral lower extremity amputation may benefit from the amputee frame. On this type the large wheels are set further back than on the outdoor frame to improve balance. Because the patient's weight is concentrated toward the rear of the chair, the amputee frame prevents the patient from tipping backward.[15]

The indoor frame has the large wheel in front and the casters in the rear. It is primarily for indoor use and has many disadvantages in maneuverability, compared with the outdoor frame. It may be more useful for persons with limited range of motion (ROM), however.[8,15]

Five factors for selecting frame style are summarized from Adler as follows[1]:

Clinical picture. What is the specific disability? Is ROM limited? Are strength and endurance limited? How old is the patient? What is the prognosis of the condition? How long is the patient expected to use the wheelchair?

Activities of daily living (ADL). What is the patient's life-style? Is the patient active or sedentary? Which type or types of transfers does the patient use? What is the maneuverability of the wheelchair in the patient's home: entrance, door width, turning radius in bathroom and hallways, floor surfaces, ratio of indoor to outdoor activities?

Environment. Where will the wheelchair be used: at school, at work, and in the community? What mode of transportation will be used? What special needs exist in each of the environment, for example, work heights, available assistance, accessibility of toilet facilities, parking facilities?

Leisure skills. Does the patient participate in sports activities? Indoor or outdoor sports? Special types of casters and tires are available for sports, as well as special track and road racing wheelchairs.

Financial considerations. Who will pay for the wheelchair? Can accessories and special modifications be justified or are they luxury items? What are the patient's resources for equipment maintenance?

MODE OF PROPULSION

Propelling a wheelchair may be accomplished in a variety of ways, depending on the physical capacities of the user. In the standard drive wheelchair (see Fig. 22-1) the hand rims are attached directly to the large wheels. These are operated by pushing and pulling motions of the arms and by grasp. Standard drive is the most common type of propulsion and assumes sufficient grasp, arm strength, and physical endurance to propel the chair and body weight for daily living.[15]

When grasp strength is inadequate but arm strength and motion are sufficient, a hand rim with projections may be ordered (Fig. 22-3). The chair is operated by pushing the heel of the hand against the hand rim projections to push the large wheels. This type of operation is often used by quadriplegics with good arm function but inadequate grasp strength.

The one-arm drive wheelchair has both hand rims on the same side of the chair (Fig 22-4). The outer rim, which is slightly smaller than the inner rim, operates the opposite wheel. The inner rim is attached directly to the wheel on the same side.[15] This propulsion system is used by persons with only one functional upper extremity and with lower extremity involvement as in triplegia. One-arm drive may be used

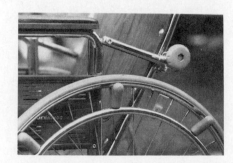

Fig. 22-3. Hand rim projections on wheelchair hand rim.

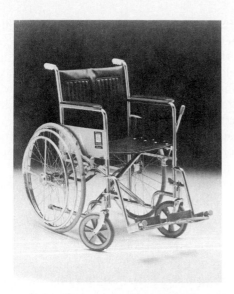

Fig. 22-4. One-arm drive wheelchair. Reproduced by permission, Everest and Jennings, Camarillo, Calif.

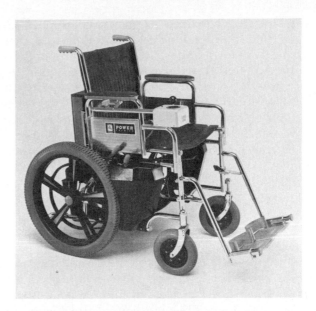

Fig. 22-6. Electric or power-driven wheelchair. Reproduced by permission, Everest and Jennings, Inc, Camarillo, Calif.

by persons with hemiplegia in some instances. However, they can benefit from a hand and foot method of wheelchair propulsion using a standard wheelchair (Fig 22-5).

For those with severe disability and minimal use of the arms the power drive or electric wheelchair is the choice if some independence is to be achieved (Fig. 22-6). The typical system has a control box that can

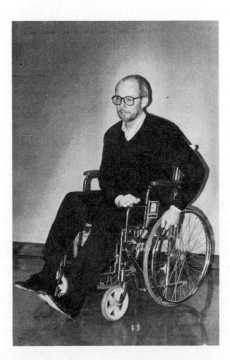

Fig. 22-5. Persons with hemiplegia can propel standard wheelchair by using unaffected arm and leg.

be located near either hand, with a single stick lever projecting from it. The wheelchair is operated by pushing the lever in different directions to effect the desired movement. If upper extremity function is insufficient for this control system, the controls can be adapted for operation by head, chin, mouth, elbow, foot, or toe.[15]

RENTAL OR PURCHASE OF WHEELCHAIR

The question of whether a patient should rent or purchase the wheelchair should be considered. This decision depends on several functional, psychological, and disability factors. The rental chair is appropriate for short-term or temporary use, such as when the patient's clinical picture, functional status, or body size are changing. Rental chairs may be necessary when the permanent wheelchair is being repaired. A rental wheelchair also may be useful when the patient cannot accept a wheelchair and needs to experience it as a temporary piece of equipment, initially.[1]

A permanent wheelchair is indicated for the full-time user and for the patient with limited need for a wheelchair over a long period of time. The patient who has a permanent or nearly permanent clinical status, who requires custom features, who has a permanent disability, and who has demonstrated acceptance of the disability is a good candidate for a permanent wheelchair.[1]

SPECIAL ACCESSORIES AND MODIFICATIONS. Many wheelchair accessories are available. Some of the major accessories and their benefits are discussed here.

Armrests come in fixed, fixed offset, desk, and detachable styles. The fixed armrest is a continuous part of the frame and is not detachable. It limits proximity to table, counter, and desk surfaces and prohibits side transfers. Fixed offset armrests give extra width for those wearing casts or braces without increasing the overall width of the chair. Desk armrests have a "step" in the front to permit fitting under desk or table surfaces. Detachable armrests permit side transfers.[15]

Footrests may be standard, swinging detachable, or swinging detachable and elevating. The standard footrests are fixed to the wheelchair frame and do not move. They prevent the person from getting close to counters and may make some types of transfers more difficult. The swinging detachable footrests can be moved to the side of the chair or removed entirely from the chair. They allow a closer approach to bed, bathtub, and counters and, when removed, reduce the overall wheelchair length and weight for easy loading into a car. They lock into place when on the chair with a locking device. Swinging detachable footrests are recommended for most wheelchair users. The foot plates may have heel loops, heel loops with ankle straps, or toe loops. The heel loops prevent the foot from slipping backward off the foot plate. The toe loops or ankle straps help to control involuntary motion and maintain the position of the foot on the foot plate.[15]

Use of elevating legrests is recommended to aid circulation and when disability necessitates periodic rest. They may be appropriate when knee flexion is limited or lower extremity edema is a problem.[4] Elevating legrests usually are used when the wheelchair has a reclining backrest.[15]

Backrests are standard or reclining—fully reclining or semireclining. A headrest extension can be added to any backrest to give greater trunk support. The backrest may be obtained in detachable or zip-open styles that allow for a rear transfer.

A reclining or semireclining backrest might be a feature selected for patients who have postural hypotension, as in a spinal cord injury.[4]

Wheelchair tires are usually solid. Pneumatic tires are available as well, primarily for rough and uneven surfaces.[15] They are more difficult to use indoors than the solid tires. Some wheelchair users who are active in the outdoors choose to have two wheelchairs to meet their needs.

Contact wheelchair manufacturers for a description of all the possible wheelchair modifications and accessories with their uses and advantages.

TYPES OF WHEELCHAIR CUSHIONS
A cushion is usually used on the wheelchair seat. Sensory loss necessitates the use of a cushion 4 inches (10 cm) thick to help prevent pressure sores.[4] Some types of wheelchair cushions are foam, air-filled, gel, and gel/foam combination types. Air-filled cushions, such as the ROHO,* consist of many balloonlike, air-filled cells that are attached to a common base, each with an inflation valve. The cushions come with cells that are either 2 or 4 inches (5–10 cm) high. Air is displaced freely between the cells until it fits the natural shape of the body. The combination foam/gel cushion has a deeply contoured foam base with a gel-filled pad for pressure relief at the rear to cushion the ischial area. It conforms to the body without pushing back. Foam cushions are made of compressible foam with a memory and come in three thicknesses and three densities.[1]

Seat boards under the cushions can improve lower extremity posture. A horseshoe-shaped cushion with the opening positioned at the back of the wheelchair seat can provide an area of noncontact between the cushion and the sacral-coccygeal area, which is so vulnerable to pressure sores.[4]

When the type, size, and features of the wheelchair have been selected, it is most desirable for the patient to try a wheelchair of similar size and features before his or her own chair is ordered. Many rehabilitation facilities have a sample group of wheelchairs available for trial use. These should include chairs of various sizes with special features, such as detachable armrests, reclining backrests, desk arms, and swing-away detachable footrests. If the patient is allowed to use a wheelchair most similar to the one prescribed, the staff can best evaluate the selection and make any necessary adjustments in the prescription before the actual purchase. If sample chairs are not available, it may be possible to rent a wheelchair from a local rehabilitation equipment company for a trial period.[4] The process of wheelchair selection and prescription should be carefully guided by the professionals working with the patient and the family to obtain a wheelchair that fits properly, provides comfort and increases mobility, and is adequate for the patient's lifestyle.

Psychology of the Wheelchair
The wheelchair evokes feelings and attitudes in its user and in observers. It has a functional and symbolic meaning to the user and a symbolic meaning to the observer.[10] These feelings, attitudes, and meanings may be negative (evoke fear, threat, and concepts of total disablement) or positive (evoke feelings of special status and greater mobility and environment control). The therapist who is responsible for wheelchair train-

---

*ROHO, Inc, Belleville, IL.

ing needs to understand the meaning of the wheelchair to the patient. He or she may have to facilitate a change of attitude from negative to positive in some patients and their families. The understanding therapist can facilitate the patient's physical and psychological adjustment to life in a wheelchair.

Some patients readily accept and tolerate the wheelchair. They see it as a necessity that meets specific physical and functional needs and improves their functioning. Others become attached to the wheelchair because it is easier and less taxing than ambulation, and they may cling to the use of the wheelchair when it is no longer necessary or desirable. Still others regard the wheelchair as a punishment, following the disability, which is the primary punishment.[10]

It is difficult for some patients to accept the wheelchair as a necessary part of their rehabilitation. They may regard it as a sign of complete disability and total surrender. This attitude can be related to the symbolic meaning of the wheelchair to the patient, to nonacceptance of the disability, and to an unrealistic assessment of physical capacities. Such patients require support and encouragement and can benefit from extended trials with the wheelchair to learn the benefits of decreased fatigue, increased safety, mobility, and function, and they should have realistic confrontations with the reactions of family, friends, and the public.

Often patients consider the wheelchair a status symbol and may value it as a car is valued. The possibility of shiny chrome, special upholstery colors, and extra gadgets makes a given wheelchair special and affords its user status in some social groups.[10]

Wheelchair Safety

Elements of safety for the wheelchair user and an assistant are as follows:
1. Brakes should be locked during all transfers.
2. Foot plates should never be stood on and should be up during transfers.
3. In most transfers it is an advantage to have footrests swung away if possible.
4. If an assistant is pushing the chair, he or she should be sure that the patient's elbows are not protruding from the armrests and the hands are *not* on the hand rims. If approaching from behind to assist in moving the wheelchair, the assistant should inform the patient of this intent and check the position of the feet and arms before proceeding.
5. If the assistant wishes to push the patient up a ramp, he or she should move in a normal, forward direction. If the ramp is negotiated independently, the patient should lean slightly forward while propelling the wheelchair up the incline.[14]

6. If the assistant wishes to push the patient down a ramp, he or she should tilt the wheelchair backward by pushing the foot down on the tipping levers to its balance position, which is a tilt of approximately 30°. Then the assistant should ease the wheelchair down the ramp in a forward direction, while maintaining the chair in its balance position. The assistant should keep his or her knees slightly bent and the back straight.[14] The assistant may also move down the ramp backward while the patient maintains some control of the large wheels to prevent rapid backward motion. This approach is useful if the grade is relatively steep. Ramps with only a slight grade can also be managed in a forward direction if the assistant maintains grasp and pull on the hand grips, and the patient again maintains some control of the big wheels to prevent rapid forward motion. If the ramp is negotiated independently, the patient should move down the ramp facing forward while leaning backward slightly and maintaining control of speed by grasping the hand rims. Gloves are recommended to reduce the effect of friction.[14]
7. An assistant can manage ascending curbs by approaching them forward, tipping the wheelchair back, and pushing the foot down on the tipping levers, thus lifting the front casters onto the curb and pushing forward. The large wheels then are in contact with the curb and roll on with ease as the chair is lifted slightly onto the curb.
8. To descend the curb using a forward approach the wheelchair is tilted backward, and the large wheels are rolled off the curb in a controlled manner, while the front casters are tilted up. When the large wheels are off the curb, the assistant can slowly reduce the tilt of the wheelchair until the casters are once again on the street surface. The curb may be descended using a backward approach. The assistant can move him or herself and the chair around as the curb is approached and pull the wheelchair to the edge of the curb. Standing below the curb, the assistant can guide the large wheels off the curb by slowly pulling the wheelchair backward until it begins to descend. After the large wheels are safely on the street surface, the assistant can tilt the chair back to clear the casters, move backward, lower the casters to the street surface, and then turn around.[14]

With good strength and coordination, many patients can be trained to manage curbs independently. To mount and descend a curb, the patient must have a normal grip, good arm strength, and good balance. Quadriplegic patients with lesions at T1 and below may achieve this skill. To mount the curb, the patient tilts the chair onto the rear wheels and pushes forward until the front wheels hang over the curb, then lowers them gently. The patient then leans forward and forcefully pushes forward on the hand rims to bring the rear wheels up on the pavement. To descend a curb, the patient should lean forward and push slowly backward until the rear and then the front wheels roll down the curb.[3]

The ability to lift the front casters off the ground and balance on the rear wheels is a useful skill and expands the patient's independence in the community for curb management and in rural settings for movement over grassy, sandy, or rough terrain. Patients who have good grip, arm strength, and balance usually can master this skill and perform safely. The technique involves being able to tilt the chair on the rear wheels, balance the chair on the rear wheels, and move and turn the chair on the rear wheels. The patient should not attempt to perform these maneuvers without instruction and training in the proper techniques, which are beyond the scope of this chapter. Refer to the references for specific instructions on teaching these skills.[3]

TRANSFER TECHNIQUES

The major and most obvious purpose of transfers is to move a patient from one surface to another. Transfer techniques for moving the patient specifically from wheelchair to bed, chair, toilet, or bathtub are included in this section. Assuming that a patient has some physical incapacity, it will be necessary for the therapist to assist in or supervise a transfer. Many therapists question which transfer to employ or feel perplexed when a particular one does not succeed with the patient. It is important to remember that each patient, therapist, and situation is different. The techniques outlined here are not all-inclusive but are basic ones. Each must be adapted for the particular patient and his or her needs.

Preliminary Concepts

It is important for the therapist to be aware of the following concepts when selecting and carrying out transfer techniques:

1. The therapist should be aware of the patient's assets and deficits, especially his or her physical and cognitive abilities.
2. The therapist should know his or her own assets and limitations and whether he or she can communicate clear, sequential instructions to the patient.
3. The therapist should be aware of and employ correct moving and lifting techniques. The following are adapted from the guidelines of the Sister Kenny Institute.[16]

   a. Maintain broad base of support by standing with feet apart (shoulder's width), hips flexed, knees flexed, and one foot slightly forward. Head and trunk should remain upright.
   b. Maintain center of gravity by carrying, supporting, and lifting others as close to the body as possible.
   c. Lift with the legs, not the back.
   d. Avoid spine rotation; move the feet to turn.
   e. Know personal limitations: do *not* lift alone if in doubt.
4. The therapist should be acutely aware of the safety aspects of transfers.
   a. Maintain all equipment in proper order and state of repair.
   b. Stabilize or lock all surfaces, including wheelchairs, beds, and chairs.
   c. Employ a transfer belt securely fastened around the patient's waist.
   d. Clear the work area by removing wheelchair footrests when possible and armrests when appropriate.
5. The therapist should employ the following basic principles applicable to most trnasfers:
   a. Stabilize surfaces (for *safety*).
   b. Equalize heights of surfaces as much as possible.
   c. Unless otherwise necessary, position wheelchair to bed, chair, or toilet at optimal angle of approximately 60°.
   d. Support the patient by using a transfer belt or by grasping the waistband of the trousers. If a transfer belt is used, apply it securely enough that it can't come undone or slide up the trunk. If necessary to hold onto the patient, support the patient around his or her back with an open hand.
   e. Avoid grasping the patient's arm, because, in general, this offers poor support.
   f. Always briefly explain the transfer procedure to the patient so that both patient and therapist are working toward the same goal.

It is important for the therapist to be familiar with as many types of transfers as possible so that he or she can resolve each situation as it arises. Some excellent resources regarding transfers, which go beyond the scope of this text, are included in the references.*

Directions for some transfer techniques that are most commonly employed in practice are outlined later. The standing-pivot transfers and the seated-sliding transfers to bed, chair, toilet, and bathtub are included.

---

*References 3, 5-7, 11, 14, 16.

Many classifications of transfers exist, based on the amount of therapist participation. Classifications can range from dependent, in which the patient is unable to participate and the therapist moves the patient, to independent, in which the patient moves himself or herself while the therapist merely supervises or observes. In general, progression of therapist participation should begin with active assistance; then gradually the assistance is withdrawn if and when the patient's abilities and performance improve.

Standing-Pivot Transfers

The standing-pivot transfer requires the patient to be able to come to standing and pivot on one or both feet. It is most commonly used with those patients who have hemiplegia, hemiparesis, or general loss of strength or balance.

WHEELCHAIR-TO-BED ASSISTED TRANSFER (Fig. 22-7). The procedure for accomplishing the wheelchair-to-bed assisted transfer with patient and therapist is as follows:

1. The therapist positions the wheelchair at an approximately 60° angle next to the bed, which should be on the patient's stronger side.
2. The therapist sets the brakes and removes the footrests.
3. The therapist positions the patient's feet (with shoes on) securely on the floor 6 to 10 inches (15.2 to 25.4 cm) apart, directly below and slightly behind the knees.
4. The therapist applies a transfer belt, if one is used.
5. The therapist should be sure the patient knows the transfer procedure.
6. The therapist positions him or herself in front of the patient on the affected side, stabilizing the patient's foot and knee with his or her own. NOTE: Some therapists prefer assisting by standing at a slightly oblique angle to the patient.
7. The therapist asks the patient to lean forward so that the shoulders are above the knees.
8. The therapist grasps the transfer belt or waistband of the trousers at the patient's back and lifts by extending his or her knees and hips, *not* the back!
9. At the same time the patient pushes on the armrest(s) and straightens the lower extremity or extremities.
10. The patient comes to a complete standing position.
11. The patient pivots on the unaffected foot, as the therapist pivots and repositions his or her rear foot.
12. The patient reaches for the bed and sits as the

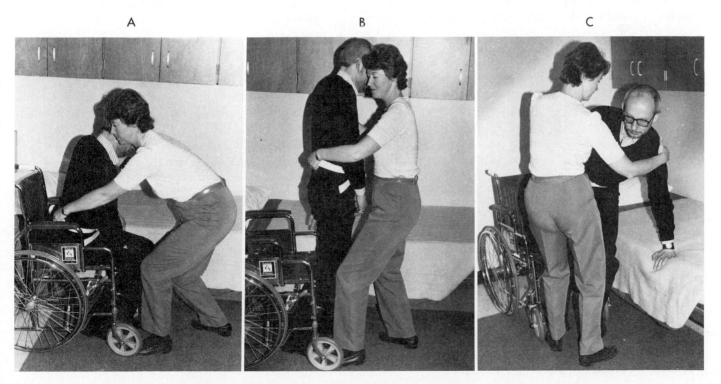

| A | B | C |

Fig. 22-7. The standing pivot transfer—wheelchair-to-bed assisted. **A,** Wheelchair and patient are prepared for transfer, and therapist is positioned to assist patient to stand. **B,** Patient is standing and therapist assists patient to pivot to prepare to sit down on bed. **C,** Patient pivots, reaches bed, and sits as therapist assists.

therapist flexes his or her knees and hips to lower the patient, avoiding the use of his or her back for this maneuver.

13. The therapist then ensures that the patient is firmly and safely seated on the bed and assists the patient to recline.

14. The therapist removes the transfer belt, if one was used.

BED-TO-WHEELCHAIR TRANSFER (Fig. 22-8). The bed-to-wheelchair transfer procedure is essentially the same as the wheelchair-to-bed assisted transfer, except for the following points:

1. The patient is positioned on the edge of the bed, sitting with feet securely on the floor. The therapist should be aware of the bed's instability and the possibility of the patient slipping from its edge.

2. It is more difficult for the patient to come to a standing position, because there is no armrest, and it is difficult to push off from the soft bed.

3. After coming to a standing position and pivoting, the patient reaches for the armrest to assist in sitting.

4. After the patient is sitting, the therapist removes the transfer belt, fastens the seat belt (if used), and repositions the footrests.

WHEELCHAIR-TO-CHAIR AND RETURN TRANSFER (Fig. 22-9). The wheelchair-to-chair and return transfer is similar to the transfer to bed, as described earlier, except for the following differences:

1. The therapist and the patient should be aware that the chair may be light and less stable than a bed.

2. When lowering to the chair, the patient reaches for the *seat* of the chair. The patient avoids reaching for the armrest or back of the chair, because this may cause the chair to tip over.

3. When moving from the chair to the wheelchair, the patient pushes with arm(s) from the seat of the chair as he or she comes to standing.

4. Standing from a chair is often more difficult if the chair is low or the seat cushions are soft. It is wise to select a chair that is as near as possible to the height of the wheelchair. Secure and firm cushions may be added to chairs that are lower.

WHEELCHAIR-TO-TOILET AND RETURN TRANSFER (Fig. 22-10). In general, the wheelchair-to-toilet and return transfer is a very difficult transfer for both the therapist and the patient because of the confined space of most bathrooms, compounded by the patient's usual and justified fear of transferring to the slick and small surface area of a toilet seat. Problems that may arise include the following:

1. It may be necessary, due to lack of space, to position the wheelchair at a angle greater than 60°, often even facing the toilet, requiring up to a 180° pivot.

2. It may not be possible to position the wheelchair so that a hemiplegic patient moves *toward* the strong side.

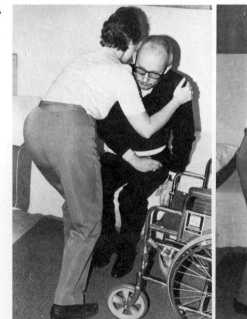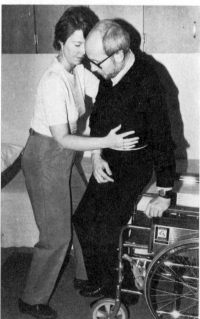

Fig. 22-8. Standing pivot transfer—bed-to-wheelchair assisted. **A,** Patient is seated on bed ready to move toward wheelchair. The therapist is positioned to assist. **B,** Patient has stood and pivoted, reaches for wheelchair armrest, and lowers body into wheelchair.

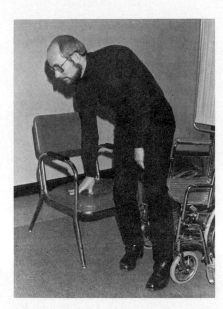

Fig. 22-9. Patient in midtransfer, reaches for seat and chair, pivots, and lowers body to sitting.

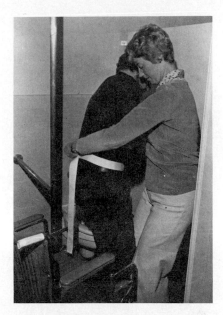

Fig. 22-10. Standing pivot transfer—wheelchair to toilet.

3. The confined quarters may force both the therapist and the patient to assume foot positions of less than optimal stability.
4. The patient may have to reach for and sit on the toilet seat, but therapist and patient should be aware of the instability of the hinged seat.

Some important points should be made concerning removal of lower clothing for toilet use. There are advantages and disadvantages in removing clothing before the transfer or after being seated on the toilet. *Before* the transfer, waist closures may be loosened so that trousers and underwear can be lowered when coming to standing. Skirts or dresses may be rolled up and tucked into the belt. This can present problems, because it is often difficult to lower clothing when standing and because clothing dropped to knees-ankles may encumber the pivot. *After* the transfer, clothes may be removed when the patient is seated on the toilet. This, however, requires leaning and hip-hiking (often difficult for the patient), and the clothes may get wet in the bowl. No simple solutions are available, except for therapist and patient to discover the best and safest method.

INDEPENDENT PIVOT TRANSFER (Fig. 22-11). All of the transfers just discussed may be accomplished by the patient independently; the obvious difference here is that the patient does *all* of the tasks. An independent transfer from one surface to another requires the patient to perform the following steps:
1. Position wheelchair and set brakes.
2. Flip up footplates and remove footrests, if possible.
3. Scoot forward in chair.
4. Position feet directly below and slightly behind

knees at 6 to 10 inches (15.2 to 25.4 cm) apart.
5. Lean forward so that shoulders are over the knees, and look up.
6. Push down with the arm(s) on the armrest(s) while extending the knees and hips.
7. Come to a complete standing position and pivot.
8. Reach for the stable area of a bed, chair, or toilet, and sit.
9. Unlock the wheelchair and reposition (if necessary) to be ready for the return transfer.

Seated-Sliding Transfers

Seated-sliding transfers are best suited for those who cannot bear weight on the lower extremities or who are too unstable to accomplish a standing transfer. The transfers require the ability to use the upper extremities and are most often employed with persons who have lower extremity amputations or paraplegia or those who have quadriplegia with adequate upper extremity function.

In the previous section on standing-pivot transfers, each was first discussed as a therapist assisted the transfer. Subsequently the independent transfer was outlined. In this section the techniques are discussed from the point of view of the therapist *supervising* the transfer. Active assistance is assumed to be minimal. Initial assistance might include helping the patient to move his or her body by lifting on the transfer belt or waistband or ensuring that the patient does not fall or injure himself or herself.

It is assumed that all proper lifting, moving, and *safety* techniques are employed. In general, use of additional equipment is discouraged so that the patient

A   B   C

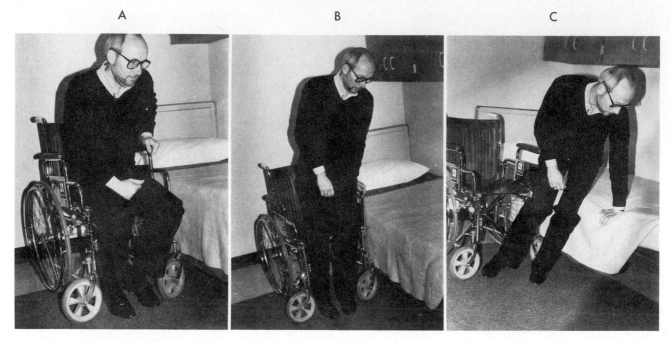

Fig. 22-11. Independent pivot transfer. **A,** Patient is properly positioned and leaning on armrest, ready to stand. **B,** Patient comes to standing position and begins to pivot. **C,** Patient reaches for bed and lowers body to sitting position.

may learn to perform as independently as possible. With these transfers, however, instruction often begins with the use of a sliding board that is eventually eliminated if and when the patient has become stronger and more stable and confident in his or her transfer abilities. NOTE: The patient may initially manifest poor balance and decreased strength, which requires

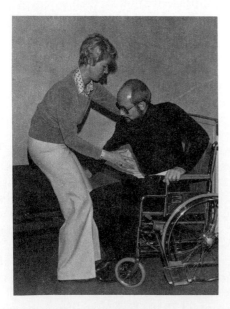

Fig. 22-12. Seated-sliding transfer. Patient and wheelchair are positioned, and transfer board has been placed under buttocks and on edge of bed.

more assistance from the therapist. In general, the therapist should position himself or herself in front of the patient to offer both physical and psychological support (Fig. 22-12).

WHEELCHAIR-TO-BED AND RETURN TRANSFER WITH SLIDING BOARD (Fig. 22-13). The wheelchair-to-bed transfer with a sliding board can be accomplished by using the following procedure:

1. The patient positions the locked wheelchair next to the bed at approximately a 60° to 90° angle.
2. The patient removes the armrest of the wheelchair that is nearest the bed.
3. The patient slips the transfer board under buttocks, as shown, and bridges the board securely across to the bed.
4. The patient then elevates his or her body by pushing down with one hand on the sliding board and the other hand on the seat or arm of the wheelchair.
5. Then by lifting the buttocks from the surface, the patient moves on the board toward the bed in a series of small shoves or moves.
6. When secure on the bed surface, the patient removes the sliding board and lifts his or her legs onto the bed.

To return, the following procedure is used:

1. The patient sits on the edge of the bed with the feet on the floor for stability (if the bed is low enough).

A   B   C

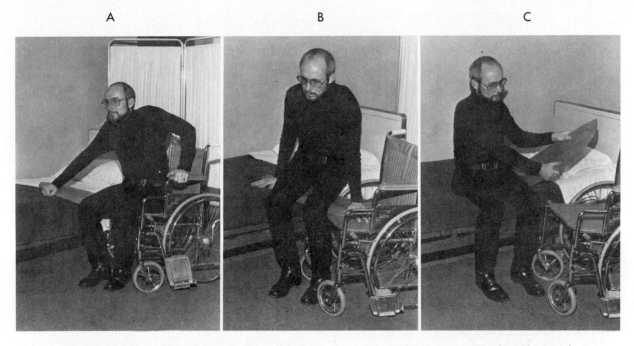

Fig. 22-13. Wheelchair-to-bed transfer with sliding board. **A,** Patient moves across board toward bed. **B,** Patient is on middle of transfer board, lifting weight from surface. **C,** Patient reaches bed and removes transfer board.

2. The sliding board is positioned under the buttocks and bridged to the wheelchair.
3. Again, in a series of small moves, the patient lifts his or her body weight and edges to the wheelchair seat.

NOTE: In moving from the wheelchair to the bed or return, there is a tendency for the weaker, less stable patient to pitch forward or backward. Also, this transfer is made more difficult if surfaces are of unequal heights.

WHEELCHAIR-TO-BED AND RETURN TRANSFER WITHOUT SLIDING BOARD (Fig. 22-14). Two techniques are recommended if the patient is stronger and more stable and does not require the use of a sliding board.

The first technique, similar to the transfer just discussed, is as follows:
1. The patient positions the locked wheelchair at a 60° to 90° angle next to the bed with the armrest nearest the bed removed.
2. The patient positions himself or herself in the wheelchair as close to the bed as possible.
3. The patient places one hand on the seat or armrest of the chair (seat preferred for stability) and the other hand approximately 12 to 18 inches (30.5 to 45.7 cm) onto the bed surface.
4. The patient pushes his or her body weight up from the seat and swings the buttocks onto the bed.
5. The process is reversed to return to the wheelchair.

The second technique is a forward-backward approach, whereby the locked wheelchair is positioned directly facing and touching the edge of the bed. This technique, more easily used to move from the bed to the wheelchair, is as follows (Fig. 22-15):

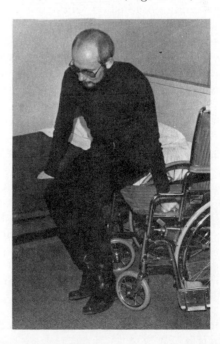

Fig. 22-14. Wheelchair-to-bed transfer without sliding board. Patient has pushed up and is shifting from wheelchair to bed without transfer board.

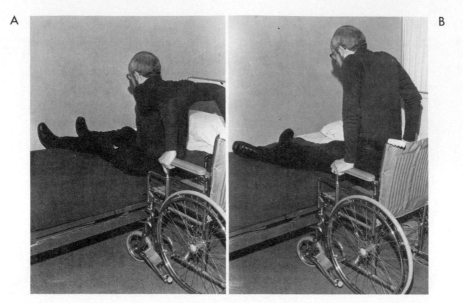

Fig. 22-15. A, Patient is positioned and ready to move backward into wheelchair. **B,** Patient pushes up and pulls body back into wheelchair.

1. The patient sits on the bed with the back toward the wheelchair.
2. The patient places a hand on each armrest.
3. The patient pushes his or her body up and over into the seat of the wheelchair.

WHEELCHAIR-TO-CHAIR AND RETURN TRANSER. The wheelchair-to-chair and return process is very similar to the wheelchair-to-bed transfer. In general, it is best accomplished when the patient can transfer without using a sliding board, because a chair allows less room for maneuverability. This transfer is further complicated because a chair is less stable or secure than a bed. The steps are as in the first seated-sliding transfer described earlier. This transfer is easier than a bed transfer if the chair used is a hard, straight-back type and is of equal height to the wheel-chair.

WHEELCHAIR-TO-TOILET TRANSFER (Fig. 22-16). The wheelchair-to-toilet transfer is also like the first wheelchair-to-bed transfer described earlier if the wheelchair can be positioned next to or at an acute angle to the toilet. In some instances a second method is employed, whereby the wheelchair is positioned facing the toilet as closely as possible. Then by performing a forward-backward transfer the patient slides directly on and off the toilet, facing the rear or tank end of the bowl.

Wheelchair-to-Bathtub, Standing or Seated, Transfers (Fig. 22-17)

The bathtub transfer is more dangerous than others because the bathtub is considered one of the most hazardous areas of the home. It is *not* recommended that a patient transfer directly from the wheelchair to the floor of the bathtub but rather from the wheelchair to either a commercially produced bathtub chair or a well-secured straight back chair placed in the bathtub. Therefore whether a standing or sliding transfer is employed, the technique is basically similar to a wheelchair-to-chair transfer. However, the transfer is further complicated by the confined space, the slick bathtub surfaces, and the bathtub wall between the wheelchair and the bathtub seat.

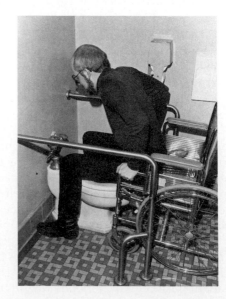

Fig. 22-16. Forward-backward transfer—wheelchair to toilet.

If a standing pivot transfer is employed, it is recommended that the locked wheelchair be placed at a 60° angle to the bathtub if possible. The patient should stand, pivot, sit on the bathtub chair, and *then* place the lower extremities into the bathtub.

If a seated transfer is used, the wheelchair is placed next to the bathtub with the armrest removed. The patient should then slide to the bathtub chair (with or without a sliding board). In some instances more capable patients may transfer to the edge of the bathtub and then to the bathtub chair or even the bathtub floor. This obviously requires greater strength and balance and good judgment on the part of the patient.

In general, the patient may exit by first placing his or her feet securely outside the bathtub on a nonskid floor surface and *then* performing a standing or seated transfer back to the wheelchair.

Dependent Transfers

The dependent transfer is designed for use with the patient who has little functional ability. If this transfer is performed incorrectly, it is potentially hazardous for both therapist and patient. This transfer should be practiced with able-bodied persons and used initially with the patient only when standby assistants are available.

The purpose of the dependent transfer is to move the patient from surface to surface. The requirements are that the patient be cooperative and willing to follow instructions. The therapist should be keenly aware of correct body mechanics as well as his or her own physical limitations.

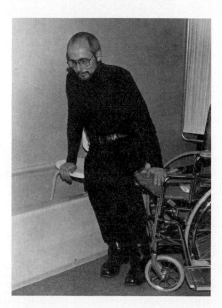

Fig. 22-17. Seated transfer from wheelchair to bathtub chair. Legs are lifted into bathtub following transfer.

WHEELCHAIR-TO-BED DEPENDENT TRANSFER (Fig. 22-18). The procedure for transferring the patient from wheelchair to bed is as follows[2]:

1. The therapist removes the wheelchair footrest closest to the bed (inside footrest) and positions the patient's inside foot over the outside foot on the remaining footrest. The therapist positions the wheelchair close to the bed at a slight angle (30° to 60°), locks the brakes, and turns the front casters backward so that they are aligned with the big wheels.

2. The therapist removes the inside armrest and unfastens trunk or hip restraints, if any.

3. The therapist positions the patient's feet together on the floor directly under the knees and swings the outside footrest away.

4. The therapist grasps the patient's legs from behind the knees and pulls the patient slightly forward in the wheelchair so that the buttocks clear the big wheel when the transfer is made (Fig. 22-18A).

5. A sliding board should be placed under the patient's inside thigh, midway between the buttocks and the knee, to form a bridge from bed to wheelchair. The sliding board is angled toward the patient's outside hip.

6. The therapist then stabilizes the patient's feet by placing his or her own feet laterally to each of the patient's feet.

7. The therapist stabilizes the patient's knees by placing his or her knees firmly against the anterolateral aspect of the patient's knees (Fig. 22-18B).

8. The therapist assists the patient to lean over the knees by pulling him or her forward from the shoulders. The patient's head and trunk should lean opposite the direction of the transfer. The patient's hands can rest on the lap.

9. The therapist reaches under the patient's outside arm and grasps the waistband of the trousers or under the buttock. On the other side, the therapist reaches over the patient's back and grasps the waistband or under the buttock (Fig. 22-18C).

10. After the therapist's arms are correctly positioned, they are locked to stabilize the patient's trunk. The therapist keeps the knees slightly bent and braces them firmly against the patient's knees.

11. The therapist then gently rocks with the patient to gain some momentum and prepare to move after the count of three. Both therapist and patient count to three aloud. On "three," with his or her knees held tightly against the patient's knees, the patient's weight is transferred over his

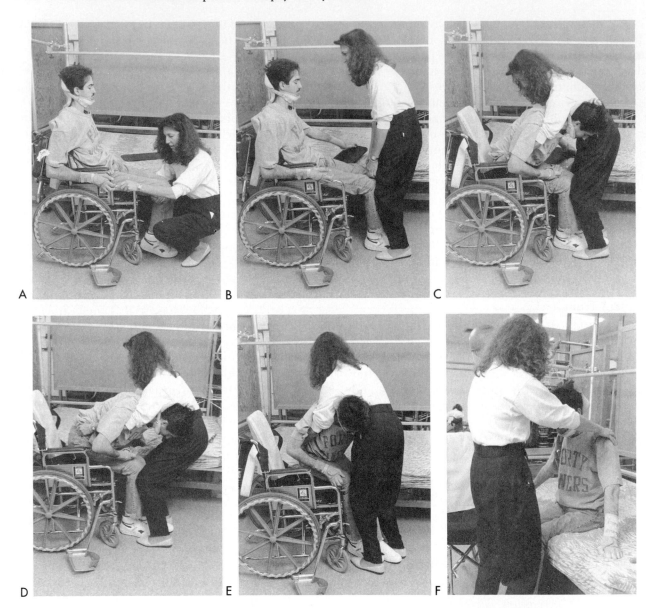

Fig. 22-18. The dependent transfer. **A,** Therapist positions wheelchair and patient and pulls patient forward in chair. **B,** Therapist stabilizes patient's knees and feet after placing sliding board. **C,** Therapist grasps waistband of patient's trousers. **D,** Therapist rocks with patient and shifts his weight over his feet. **E,** Therapist pivots with patient and moves him onto the sliding board. **F,** Patient is stabilized on the edge of the bed.

or her feet. The therapist's back must be kept straight to maintain good body mechanics (Fig. 22-18*D*).

12. The therapist pivots with the patient and moves him or her onto the sliding board (Fig. 22-18*E*). The therapist repositions himself or herself and the patient's feet and repeats the pivot until the patient is firmly seated on the bed surface, perpendicular to the edge of the mattress and as far back as possible. This usually can be achieved in two or three stages (Fig. 22-18*F*).

13. The therapist can secure the patient on the bed by easing him or her against the back of an elevated bed or on the mattress in side-lying posture, then by lifting the legs onto the bed.

This transfer can be adapted to move the patient to other surfaces. It should be attempted only when therapist and patient feel secure with the wheelchair-to-bed transfer.

LIFT TRANSFER. Some patients are completely dependent during transfers. The *cervical lift* or *through arm lift* method requires two assistants and can be used to transfer the patient to and from the mat, bed, or chair.[3,11]

To transfer the patient from bed to wheelchair, use the following steps[3,11]:

1. Position the chair at an angle about 30 degrees to the bed.
2. Position the patient in long sitting with the head and trunk flexed and the arms folded across the lower chest.
3. The first assistant stands behind the patient with one leg on each side of the rear wheel that is closest to the bed. The therapist reaches under the patient's arms and around the chest, grips the patient's lower thorax with his or her forearms, and grasps the patient's forearms, which are crossed over the lower thorax.
4. The second assistant stands facing the side of the lower end of the bed and grasps the patient's legs, using one arm under the upper thighs and the other under the lower legs. The arm that supports the thighs must be placed higher for heavier patients.
5. The assistants agree on a prearranged signal to coordinate the lift. For example, "On the count of three—lift"; "One, two, three—lift." As they lift, the first assistant, holding the trunk, takes a step sideways and the second assistant, holding the legs, takes a step backward. They must lift the patient high enough to clear the rear wheel and also avoid bumping the patient's spine against the wheelchair handle or backrest support.[3,11]

MECHANICAL LIFT TRANSFER. A hydraulic mechanical lifting device (such as the Hoyer Patient Lifter) can be used to transfer patients who are totally dependent and require excessive lifting or who are too heavy or require extensive assistance to transfer. A properly trained assistant, even one who is considerably smaller than the patient, can learn to use the lifter safely and independently. Family members, attendants, and other care givers should be trained in the use of the patient lifter.[4,11,14] Various models of lifters are available. There are mobile lifts and fixed models that attach directly to the floor or overhead.[9,11] The patient's physical size, disability status, and the uses to which the lift will be put must be considered when ordering the appropriate hydraulic lift.

SUMMARY

A wheelchair that fits well and can be managed safely and easily by its user and an attendant is the most significant factor in the patient's ability to perform activites of daily living with maximal independence.[13] Each wheelchair user must learn the capabilities and limitations of the wheelchair and safe methods of performing ADL. If there is an assistant, he or she needs to be thoroughly familiar with safe and correct techniques of handling the wheelchair and the patient.

Transfer skills are among the most important activities that must be mastered by the physically disabled person. The ability to transfer increases the possibility of mobility and travel. Yet transfers can be hazardous. Safe methods must be learned and followed.[14] Several basic transfer techniques are outlined in this chapter. Additional methods and more detailed training and instructions are available, as cited previously.

It should be recognized that many wheelchair users with exceptional abilities have developed unique methods of wheelchair management. Although such innovative approaches may work well for the person who has devised and mastered them, they cannot be considered basic procedures that can be learned by everyone.[14]

REVIEW QUESTIONS

1. If the wheelchair is properly fitted, what is the correct seat width?
2. What is the danger of having a wheelchair seat that is too deep?
3. What is the minimal distance for safety from the floor to the bottom of the wheelchair step plate?
4. List three types of wheelchair frames and the general uses of each.
5. Describe three types of wheelchair propulsion systems and when each would be used.
6. What are the advantages of detachable desk arms and swing-away footrests?
7. Discuss the factors for consideration before wheelchair selection.
8. Name and discuss the rationale for at least three general wheelchair safety principles.
9. Describe or demonstrate how descend a curb in a wheelchair with the help of an assistant.
10. Describe or demonstrate how to descend a ramp in a wheelchair with the help of an assistant.
11. List four safety principles for correct moving and lifting technique during wheelchair transfers.
12. Describe or demonstrate the basic standing-pivot transfer from wheelchair to bed and wheelchair to toilet.
13. Describe or demonstrate the wheelchair-to-bed transfer, using a sliding board.
14. What is meant by the "balance position" of the wheelchair?
15. List and discuss three possible attitudes of patient's toward their wheelchairs as outlined in this chapter.
16. List the requirements for patient and therapist to perform the dependent transfer safely and correctly.
17. Describe the lift transfer. Under what circumstances would this transfer be used?
18. When is the mechanical lift transfer most appropriate?

REFERENCES

1. Adler C: Wheelchairs and seat cushions: a comprehensive guide for evaluation and ordering, San Jose, 1987, Santa Clara County, Santa Clara Valley Medical Center, Occupational Therapy Department.
2. Adler C: Personal communication, May 26, 1988.
3. Bromley I: Tetraplegia and paraplegia: a guide for physiotherapists, ed 3, London, 1985, Churchill Livingstone.
4. Ellwood P Jr: Prescription of wheelchairs. In Kottke FJ, Stillwell GK, and Lehmann JF: Krusen's handbook of physical medicine and rehabilitation, ed 3, Philadelphia, 1982, WB Saunders Co.
5. Ford JR and Duckworth B: Physical management for the quadriplegic patient, Philadelphia, 1974, FA Davis Co.
6. Hale G, editor: The source book for the disabled, London, 1979, Paddington Press, Ltd.
7. Kamenetz HL: The wheelchair book, Springfield, Ill, 1969, Charles C Thomas, Publisher.
8. Modification and accessory analysis (form), Camarillo, Calif, 1979, Everest and Jennings, Inc.
9. Pernichief, JM et al: Rehabilitation. In Ruskin AP, editor: Current therapy in physiatry, Philadelphia, 1984, WB Saunders Co.
10. Pezenik D, Itoh M, and Lee M: Wheelchair prescription. In Ruskin AP: Current therapy in physiatry, Philadelphia, 1984, WB Saunders Co.
11. Turner A, editor: The practice of occupational therapy, ed 2, New York, 1987, Churchill Livingstone.
12. Wheelchair prescription (form), Camarillo, Calif, 1978, Everest and Jennings, Inc.
13. Wheelchair prescriptions: measuring the patient (Booklet no 1), Camarillo, Calif, 1979, Everest and Jennings, Inc.
14. Wheelchair prescriptions: safety and handling (Booklet no 3), Camarillo, Calif, 1983, Everest and Jennings, Inc.
15. Wheelchair prescriptions: wheelchair selection, (Booklet no 2), Camarillo, Calif, 1979, Everest and Jennings, Inc.
16. Yates J and Lundberg A: Moving and lifting patients: principles and techniques, Minneapolis, 1970, Sister Kenny Institute.

23 Mobile arm support and suspension slings

LORRAINE WILLIAMS PEDRETTI
CAROLE ADLER

The mobile arm support and the suspension sling are both devices that support the upper extremity in a plane parallel to the floor. They are devices that facilitate useful upper extremity motion in the presence of significant muscle weakness.

MOBILE ARM SUPPORTS

The mobile arm support (MAS) may also be called a balanced forearm orthosis or a ball-bearing feeder.[6] It is usually mounted on the wheelchair, but it can be mounted on a table or working surface. It consists of a trough that supports the user's forearm and a pivot and linkage system under the trough. This system can be preset and adjusted so that the user can produce elbow and shoulder motion with slight motions of the trunk or shoulder girdle[1] (Fig. 23-1).

The MAS is adjusted so that gravity is used to assist weak muscles. Various adjustments are possible, and these are individualized to suit the needs of the particular patient. The MAS provides assistance for shoulder and elbow movement by using gravity to aid lost muscle power. It provides a large, usable range of arm motion that would otherwise not be available to the patient. It helps support, assist, and strengthen weakened musculature and enables patients to perform simple activities of daily living (ADL) and leisure activities that they could not perform without them.[6]

Candidates for Use of the MAS

Generally those patients with disabilities that result in muscle weakness, such as poliomyelitis, cervical spinal cord injuries, Guillain-Barré syndrome, muscular dystrophy, and amyotrophic lateral sclerosis, are candidates for MAS. When there is moderate to severe muscle weakness in the upper extremities [muscle grades Trace(1) to fair (3) at the elbow and grades Trace(1) to 3 at the shoulder] and limited endurance for sustained movement, the MAS could increase function.[6]

The patient must have a source of muscle power to initiate movement of the MAS. This may be at the neck, trunk, shoulder, or leg. There should be adequate, pain-free range of motion (ROM) as follows: (1) shoulder flexion to 90°, abduction to 90°, external rotation to 30°, and internal rotation to 80°; (2) elbow flexion from 0° to 140°; (3) full forearm pronation from midposition and supination to midposition; and (4) hip flexion from 0° to 95°, required for the upright sitting position.[7]

The patient must have sufficient coordination to cope with and control movement of the freely swinging arms of the MAS. Involuntary movement precludes effective use.[6] There must be adequate trunk and neck stability provided by the patient's own muscle power or by outside support. A consistently stable sitting posture and good body alignment are key factors in the successful use of the MAS. The MAS works best when the user is sitting in an upright position. Successful use decreases as the user reclines. A recline of 30° is about maximum, and in this position there are some limitations in use.[6] Sitting tolerance and balance and gadget tolerance[5] must be adequate to engage in the training program and later, make use of the MAS worthwhile.[2]

There must be sufficient motivation to use the MAS and adequate frustration tolerance to persevere at the training program until use is mastered.[2] It is important that the patient know the purpose in using the MAS. The patient should be aware that the motion provided will strengthen muscles and that the device may not necessarily be for permanent use.[7] Motivation to take care of personal needs, eat independently, or enjoy avocational activities that would otherwise be impossible can be a determining factor in acceptance and mastery of the MAS. Successful experience with the MAS can be a motivating factor.[5,6]

Parts of the MAS and Their Functions[5,6]

The parts of a standard MAS are shown in Fig. 23-2. There are several types of MAS. Additional attachments and assisting devices are available to suit individual needs.[5,6] The semireclining, adjustable *bracket assembly* holds the MAS to the wheelchair. It supports the proximal arm and controls the height of

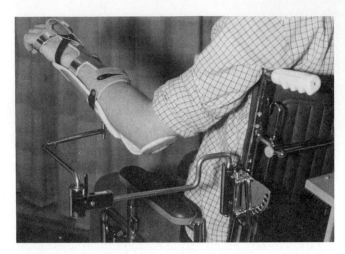

Fig. 23-1. Mobile arm support, mounted on wheelchair with patient's arm positioned in the forearm trough.

the MAS. It can be adjusted to assist horizontal movement at the shoulder and elbow. It may be adapted for use in the reclining position, but the upright position is most desirable.[2,6] The standard *proximal swivel arm* permits horizontal abduction and horizontal adduction at the shoulder and contains the distal ball bearings. Both the bracket assembly and the proximal ball-bearing housing have stops that can be set at any position on the circumference of the housing unit to limit horizontal motion. The proximal ball-bearing housing on the proximal swivel arm can also be tilted so that gravity assists elbow flexion or extension.[6]

The *distal swivel arm* permits forearm motion in the horizontal plane. It supports the rocker arm assembly and forearm trough. Attached to the forearm trough

is the *rocker arm assembly*. It is positioned in the distal swivel arm and permits vertical (hand-to-mouth) motions. It swivels to produce added horizontal motion. The *forearm trough* supports the forearm. It offers stable elbow support but may limit elbow extension. The elbow dial can be bent to produce adjustments for comfort and vertical motion.[6] The assembled mobile arm support is shown in Fig. 23-3.

How the MAS Works

The patient must have adequate muscle power to activate the mobile arm support. Some source of power at the neck, trunk, shoulder girdle, shoulder, and elbow may serve alone or in combination to operate the mobile arm support. Some controlling muscle in both elbow and shoulder is necessary if the user is to have control of motions in the horizontal plane over the lapboard.[6]

The mobile arm support allows horizontal and vertical motions. The device assists horizontal motions across the tabletop. Vertical movement allows tabletop-to-face activity. To assist horizontal motion the bracket assembly and the proximal ball-bearing housing on the proximal swivel arm can be adjusted to produce an inclined plane in the direction of horizontal abduction or horizontal adduction, as the need may be. Gravity then assists motion to the low point in the plane, and muscular effort must be exerted to return the arm to the high point of the plane.[6]

Adjustments for vertical motions are somewhat more complex. The rocker arm assembly is fastened to the underside of the forearm trough and acts as the fulcrum of this lever. There are several holes in the length of the forearm trough so that the fulcrum can be moved toward or away from the elbow (force end). Any force applied by the user proximal to the fulcrum lifts the weight of the hand and anything in the hand toward the face. Shoulder elevation and depression are used to effect the vertical motions of the forearm trough. The distance of the fulcrum from the elbow will determine whether the mechanical advantage is on the load side (hand) or force side (elbow) of the lever.[6]

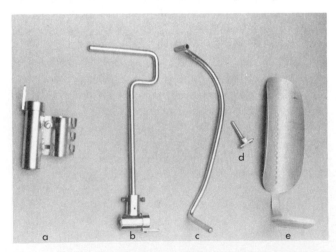

Fig. 23-2. Parts of the MAS. **A,** Bracket assembly with stop. **B,** Proximal swivel arm and proximal ball bearing housing with stop. **C,** Distal swivel arm. **D,** Rocker arm assembly. **E,** Forearm trough.

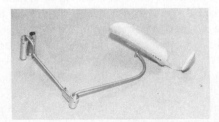

Fig. 23-3. The assembled mobile arm support.

Adjustment and Checkout of the MAS[3,6]

To adjust the MAS the therapist must find the best position for the patient in the wheelchair, choose the correct bracket assembly for the arm being fitted, since the right and left are not interchangeable, and set the height of the bracket to position the whole MAS at the proper height. The forearm trough is then fitted to the patient. It is balanced for maximal range and force in vertical motion. The bracket is adjusted for maximal range and force in horizontal motion at the glenohumeral joint. The therapist must then tilt the distal bearing, if necessary, to produce the maximal range and force in horizontal motion at the elbow joint. The therapist should then reevaluate range and force of combined horizontal motions of the glenohumeral and elbow joints and reevaluate the vertical motion of the trough. Some patients may require special attachments, such as straps, to stabilize the forearm in the trough.[6]

The following questions can serve as a guide for the therapist to determine the correctness of fit and adjustments of the MAS.[3]

1. Are the hips set back in the chair?
2. Is the spine in good vertical alignment?
3. Is there good lateral trunk stability?
4. Is the chair seat adequate for comfort and stability?
5. Is the patient able to sit upright?
6. If the patient wears hand splints, are they on?
7. Does the patient have adequate passive ROM?
8. Is the bracket tight on the wheelchair?
9. Are all arms and joints freely movable?
10. Is the proximal arm all the way down in the bracket?
11. Is the bracket at the proper height so that the shoulders are not forced into elevation?
12. Does the elbow dial clear the lap surface when the trough is in the "up" position?
13. When the trough is in the "up" position, is the patient's hand as close to the mouth as possible?
14. Can the patient obtain maximal active reach?
15. Is the trough short enough to allow active wrist flexion, if present?
16. Are the trough edges rolled so that they do not contact the forearm?
17. Is the elbow secure and comfortable in the elbow support?
18. Is the trough balanced correctly?
19. In vertical motion is the dial free of the distal arm?
20. Can the patient control motion of the proximal arm from either extreme?
21. Can the patient control motion of the distal arm from either extreme?
22. Can the patient control vertical motion of the trough from either extreme?
23. Have stops been applied to limit range, if necessary?
24. Can the patient lift a sufficient amount of weight to perform appropriate functional tasks?

Training in Use of the MAS

The therapist should be sure that supports are fitting well and correctly adjusted before attempting to instruct the patient in their use. If two MASs are used, the patient should practice with one at a time until each is mastered. Bilateral use of MASs requires considerable practice. Early use includes training in vertical motions (external and internal rotation of the shoulder). External rotation is accomplished by depressing the shoulder to elevate the hand, shifting the body weight to the side of the MAS, rolling the shoulder back, tilting or turning the head toward the side of the device, or leaning backward. Internal rotation is accomplished by gravity, elevating the shoulder on the same side as the mobile arm support, shifting the body weight to the opposite side from the device, rolling the shoulder forward, tilting and turning the head to the opposite side from the MAS, or leaning forward. Work is started on horizontal adduction and abduction with the trough balanced at midposition. Then the patient can proceed to practice these motions with the trough at various heights between wheelchair tray and head. Practice progresses to include elbow flexion and extension with the trough at various heights. Activities that are designed to offer practice in the use of MASs are typing or computer work, turning book pages, using the phone, grooming, hygiene at sink, and playing games such as checkers, cards, and puzzles.

The MAS offers the patient who demonstrates upper extremity weakness the necessary assistance to make maximal use of minimal muscle power. Once assembled, fitted, and adjusted it enables the patient to perform a variety of self-care and leisure activities that promote self-esteem, and independence. The reader is referred to the references for more comprehensive discussion of MASs and their use.[2,5,6]

SUSPENSION SLINGS

The suspension sling supports the upper extremity in a plane parallel to the floor. The suspension sling is used to facilitate horizontal movement during activity or exercise in which the force of gravity on the movement of the upper extremity needs to be minimized (Fig. 23-4).[4]

Parts of the Suspension Sling

A bracket holds the suspension rod to the back of the wheelchair. The bracket can be adjusted to keep the top of the suspension rod parallel to the floor. It

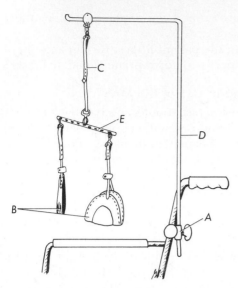

Fig. 23-4. Suspension sling. **A,** bracket. **B,** Arm cuff. **C,** Suspension strap. **D,** Suspension rod. **E,** Horizontal supporting device for cuffs. Modified with permission from Occupational Therapy Department, Rancho Los Amigos Hospital, Downey, CA.

also allows for adjustments in height. The suspension sling is hung from the suspension rod with a spring or a strap. The length of the suspension device de-

termines the height of the sling in relation to the user's body. The suspension device also swivels to eliminate friction or twisting and to allow maximal mobility. If a spring suspension is used, it adds to the amount of motion that the user can produce in the sling but may decrease coordination.

The cuffs of the suspension sling are fastened to a horizontal bar that has holes along its entire length. These allow the cuffs of the sling to be placed for optimal balance to assist vertical or horizontal motions of the arm. A forearm trough, as used on the mobile arm support, is sometimes substituted for the arm cuffs shown in Fig. 23-4, and the assembly is referred to as a suspension feeder.[4]

Use of the Suspension Sling

In many instances the suspension sling can be used with patients who have the same diagnoses as previously cited, although somewhat greater muscle power is required for effective use. Use of the suspension sling may be initiated with enabling exercise to establish patterns of horizontal abduction and adduction, hand-to-body movements, and hand-to-face movements. Use may then progress to activities, such as eating, hygiene at sink, table top communication skills, and leisure activities.

REVIEW QUESTIONS

1. Which patients are good candidates for use of the MAS (in terms of disability or muscle grades)?
2. Which patients are poor candidates for use of the MAS? Why?
3. List the five criteria a patient must meet to use the MAS successfully.
4. Describe how the MAS works (refer to parts and their functions, how the device is activated, and how it is adjusted so that gravity assists movement).
5. What activities can be performed with the MAS which could not be performed without it?
6. List the three major steps in training the patient to use MAS.
7. List two ways external rotation motion can be accomplished.
8. List two ways internal rotation motion can be accomplished.
9. What are some activities that are good for practicing use of the MAS?
10. What is the primary purpose of

the suspension sling?
11. List three purposeful activities that may be performed by patients with significant upper extremity dysfunction while using a suspension sling. Can you think of some that were not listed in the text?

REFERENCES

1. Bender LF: Upper extremity orthotics. In Kottke FJ, Stillwell GK, and Lehmann JF: Krusen's handbook of physical medicine and rehabilitation, ed 3, Philadelphia, 1982, WB Saunders Co.
2. Dicus RG: Mobile arm supports, part 1, (film), Downey, CA, 1970, Rancho Los Amigos Hospital, SRS Service Dept. (Available at the Instructional Resources Center, San Jose State University.)
3. Rancho Los Amigos Hospital: Check-out sheet for feeders. In Marshall E: Occupational therapy management of physical dysfunction, Loma Linda, CA, 1976, De-

partment of Occupational Therapy, School of Allied Health Professions, Loma Linda University. (Distributed by Fred Sammons, Inc., Box 32, Brookfield, IL, 60513.)
4. Rancho Los Amigos Hospital: Suspension feeders and slings: parts and their functions. In Marshall E: Occupational therapy management of physical dysfunction, Loma Linda, CA, 1976, Department of Occupational Therapy, School of Allied Health Professions, Loma Linda University. (Distributed by Fred Sammons, Inc., Box 32, Brookfield IL, 60513).
5. Thenn JE: Mobile arm support: installation and use, San Jose, CA, 1975. (Self-published.) (Distributed by Fred Sammons, Inc., Box 32, Brookfield, IL, 60513.)
6. Wilson DJ, McKenzie MW, and Barber LM: Spinal cord injury: a treatment guide for occupational therapists, Thorofare, NJ, 1974, Charles B Slack, Inc.

24 Hand splinting

LORRAINE WILLIAMS PEDRETTI

The hand is a very specialized organ that functions to obtain information and to execute motor acts essential to human interaction with the environment.[11] The ability to use the hand normally requires sensation, mobility, and stability. The highly developed, well coordinated sensorimotor function of the hand is dependent upon intact neuromuscular, skeletal, articular, vascular, and soft tissue structures. A dysfunction in any of these elements will have an effect on hand function and appearance.[2,4]

The proximal joints of the upper limb are essential to normal hand function. The wrist, elbow, and shoulder joints must be capable of stability and mobility for maximum hand function. The upper limb enables the hand to move away from the body and to be positioned exactly for the performance of any given activity. Especially important are the movements of the wrist and forearm which make fine adjustments of hand position possible. The vascular and nervous systems of the hand are continuous with that of the arm, and some of its muscles originate in the forearm. Therefore the hand must be evaluated in relation to total upper extremity functioning.[11]

The hand functions to obtain information about the environment through its exquisite sensory abilities. It is the organ of accomplishment of almost all daily activities, work, and creative tasks. The hand is essential to the nutrition of the organism, functioning to prepare food and present it to the mouth. The hand is an organ of expression, since through its gestures it supplements speech and conveys emotions. For many hearing impaired persons it is the primary organ of communication. The hand functions to touch, caress, convey feelings of warmth, caring, and love. It plays an important role in sexual functioning. Conversely, the hand functions as an organ of offense or defense. The fist or ulnar border of the hand can be used to strike another, and the open hand to slap.[11]

The cosmetic value of the hand is significant. The use of skin-softening agents, manicures, nail lacquers and decorations, and jewelry on the hands are all testimony to the importance of its attractiveness in interpersonal relationships.

Because of its primary role in daily interaction with the human and physical world, psychosocial problems are often associated with injuries and dysfunction of the hands.[11] Splinting is one of several therapeutic modalities that has as its aim the maximum restoration of hand function and appearance.

The purposes of this chapter are (1) to briefly review the structure and function of the hand, (2) to introduce the reader to the basic principles of hand splinting, and (3) to provide direction for construction and evaluation of two basic hand splints through the use of a self-instruction program.

ROLE OF THE OCCUPATIONAL THERAPIST

The occupational therapist is frequently called upon to fabricate splints. Hand splints are most commonly made by occupational therapists, but splints for knees, ankles, and feet, as well as contour splints, are also made by occupational therapists. Therefore it is important for the occupational therapist to understand the principles of hand splinting and to be able to construct some types of hand splints. The occupational therapist is usually the professional who works most closely with hand rehabilitation. The therapist is depended on to analyze hand dysfunction, make suggestions for splinting needs, evaluate splint performance, and train the patient in the use of the splint.[6,9] The occupational therapist may determine when the goals of splinting have been achieved, recommend changes in the splint, or see that its use is discontinued.[6]

Splints made of high- and low-temperature thermoplastic materials are often constructed by the occupational therapist. These splints are usually used in treating temporary conditions of muscle weakness and joint limitation. They may be used to prevent or correct deformity, substitute for lost muscle power, and assist weak muscles in normal patterns of motion.

Splints required for long-term use to treat permanent conditions are often made by a certified orthotist.[1,10]

STRUCTURE OF THE HAND

This is a brief review of some hand structures that are important for consideration in splinting. It is assumed that the reader has studied hand anatomy and kinesiology. A detailed review is beyond the scope of this chapter. The references 2, 5-8, and 11 and kinesiology texts are recommended for further study.

Bones

The hand and wrist are composed of 27 bones. Of these, 19 are metacarpals and phalanges. The remaining 8 are the carpals of the wrist. The metacarpals articulate with the distal row of carpals, and the radius and ulna of the forearm articulate with the proximal row of carpals. The combined wrist and forearm movements provide the versatility of position and movement needed for grasp and prehension in any activity.[2,7,11]

Alignment of the Digits

There is a precise relationship between the length, mobility, and position of each digit or finger and between the thumb and the fingers. The relative lengths of the fingers vary with hand movements. The fingertips converge toward the pulp of the thumb during palmar prehension.[11] When flexed individually, the fingers converge to touch a small area at the base of the thenar eminence.[2,7,11] When flexed simultaneously, however, contact of the fingertips to the palm is more parallel, from the middle of the first metacarpal to the hypothenar eminence.[2]

Arches of the Hand[5,6] (Fig. 24-1)

The bones of the hand are arranged in three arches. There are two transverse arches and one longitudinal arch. The first transverse arch is the carpal arch. It has a deep palmar concavity,[11] is located at the wrist, and is formed by the annular ligaments and carpal bones.[6] The flexor tendons and neurovascular structures traverse through this arch so that the concavity is not apparent externally.[2] The carpal arch provides

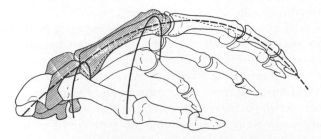

Fig. 24-1. Longitudinal and transverse arches of the hand. Reprinted by permission from Tubiana, R. et al.: Examination of the hand and upper limb, Philadelphia 1984, W.B. Saunders Co.

the mechanical advantage to the finger flexor tendons by acting as the fulcrum.[6]

The second transverse arch is the metacarpal arch, which lies across the distal metacarpal heads at a slightly oblique angle. The second and third metacarpal bones are relatively stable elements in the arch, whereas the fourth and fifth metacarpal bones are the more mobile elements. The normal arch increases as the hand is used functionally. The dexterity and function of the fingers are dependent on the mobility and flexibility of this arch. Grasp function will be impaired if the mobility of the metacarpal bones is limited and if the metacarpal transverse arch is flattened or prevented from increasing during functional use. These conditions can be caused by poor positioning of the hand in the splint, poorly constructed or ill-fitting splints, intrinsic muscle paralysis, edema, and scarring and contracture of the dorsal skin of the hand.[6]

The longitudinal arch follows the long lines of the carpal and metacarpal bones at a slightly oblique angle and primarily involves the third finger. The carpal and metacarpal bones are the fixed units, and the fingers through their flexion and extension abilities are the mobile units. This flexibility allows for a wide range of prehension patterns. The function of the longitudinal arch can be disturbed by intrinsic muscle paralysis, poor hand positioning, edema, scarring of the dorsal skin, and adhesions of extensor tendons or bony obstructions.[6]

Dual Obliquity of the Hand

The transverse axis of the palm corresponds to the metacarpalphalangeal (MP) joints and lies approximately across the distal palmar crease. The longitudinal axis is described through the middle metacarpal and finger. The transverse axis is not perpendicular to the longitudinal axis. Rather, it lies at an oblique angle because of the decreasing length of the metacarpals from the radial to the ulnar side of the hand.[2,11]

Because of the successive decrease in length of the metacarpals from the radial to the ulnar side of the hand, objects grasped in the hand are held at two oblique angles. The first is an oblique angle formed by the decreasing length of the metacarpals. An object held using cylindrical grasp with the hand in full pronation will be parallel to the metacarpal heads and *not* parallel to the axis of the wrist joint (Fig. 24-2, *A*). The second oblique angle is formed by the transverse metacarpal arch and the mobility of the fourth and fifth metacarpals when the hand is used. Because of the arch and the metacarpal mobility, an object grasped with a cylindrical grasp will be higher on the radial side than on the ulnar side of the hand and

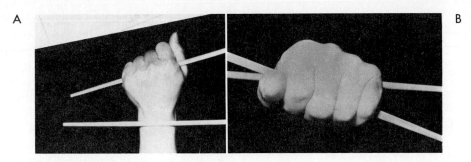

Fig. 24-2. Dual obliquity of the hand. **A,** Oblique angle of metacarpal heads in relation to axis of wrist joint. **B,** Oblique angle of metacarpal heads from radial to ulnar side of hand. Reproduced by permission, George Wu, MD, San Francisco.

thus *not* parallel to the floor when the hand is in full pronation[2,5] (Fig. 24-2, *B*).

Fixed and Mobile Elements

The structure of the hand is composed of stable and mobile elements. The more stable or fixed elements are the distal row of carpal bones and the second and third metacarpals. These two metacarpals are relatively fixed and act as stable posts. The mobile elements are the phalanges and the fourth and fifth metacarpals. The latter are more mobile than the second and third metacarpals and give the metacarpal transverse arch its flexibility.[2,11]

Collateral Ligaments

Because of their eccentric insertions and the shape of the metacarpal heads, the collateral ligaments of the MP joints are somewhat lax or in their shortened position when the MPs are extended. This allows for the lateral mobility of these joints when the fingers are in extension. The MP collateral ligaments are taut or lengthened when in the flexed position, and lateral mobility of the joints is limited in flexion.[2,11] The proximal interphalangeal (PIP) and distal interphalangeal (DIP) joints have strong ligamentous support. This support and the nature of the hinge joint prohibit lateral flexibility. Unlike the MP joint ligaments, these become lax on flexion and are tightest during extension.[2]

Fibrous Structure

The fibrous structure of the hand is composed of aponeuroses, ligamentous structures, and fibrous sheaths that are attached to the bones and skin. This structure reinforces the bony skeleton and allows considerable adaptability. The fibrous structure has several functions: It unites bone segments and stabilizes the arches of the hand. It provides fixation for the palmar skin. It contains the structures of the hand and separates the hand into compartments. It pro-

vides protection and padding of the fingers. It connects the volar plates and the extensor tendons and provides guidance for the tendons.[11]

Blood Supply

Blood is conveyed to the hand by the radial and ulnar arteries. The ulnar artery lies lateral to the flexor carpi ulnaris tendon and divides at the wrist into large and small branches. The large branch forms the superficial arterial arch, and the smaller branch forms the lesser part of the deep palmar arch. The radial artery divides into a superficial branch that completes the superficial arterial arch. The deep radial branch forms the deep palmar arch. Exiting the superficial arterial arch are the digital branches that in turn bifurcate into phalangeal branches.[2]

Venous drainage of the hand is accomplished by two sets of veins: a superficial and a deep group. The superficial venous system forms a large network of vessels over the dorsum of the hand. Injuries to the dorsum of the hand which disrupt venous drainage can result in severe edema.[2]

The rich vascular network of the hand gives it an important role in thermal regulation. Thermal regulation is mediated by the large exposed surface of the hand and its abundance of sweat glands.[11]

Creases and Skin of the Hand

The dorsal skin of the hand is fine, supple, and mobile. These characteristics allow it to move freely during flexion and extension of the fingers. Scar formation or dorsal edema disrupts the normal mobility of the dorsal skin and will limit hand function.[11]

The palmar skin is thick and inelastic.[11] It is tough and not very pliable or mobile. It functions for protection and support. It is firmly attached to underlying structures to prevent slippage between the skeleton and the object grasped[11] and allows for stability and fixation of the palmar skin during motion. The palm has several skin creases (Fig. 24-3) that can act as

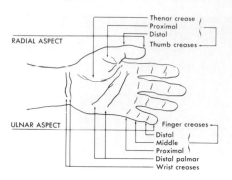

Fig. 24-3. Palmar creases of hand. From Malick MH: Manual on static hand splinting, Pittsburgh, Harmarville Rehabilitation Center.

guides in individual design and fitting of splints. These include the wrist creases; the thenar crease; the proximal and distal palmar creases; and the proximal, middle, and distal finger creases.[6,7]

Muscles of the Hand

Movements of the hand and wrist are effected by 20 extrinsic muscles and 19 intrinsic muscles. Each movement of the hand and wrist is the result of many muscular actions.[11] The long flexors and extensors of the wrist and fingers, pronators and supinators, are extrinsic and lie in the forearm. The intrinsic muscles are those of the thenar and hypothenar eminences, the lumbricals, and interossei.[2]

Nerve Supply

The hand is supplied by three peripheral nerves. In general the radial nerve supplies the extensor/supinator group of muscles. Its sensory fibers supply the dorsal surface of the radial side of the hand. The median nerve supplies the flexor/pronator muscles, the thenar group, and the first and second lumbricals. It conveys sensation from the radial side of the palmar surface of the hand and thumb and plays a critical role in grasp, prehension, and tactile discriminative functions. The ulnar nerve supplies the intrinsic muscles of the hand except for the first and second lumbricals. Its sensory fibers supply both the dorsal and volar surfaces of the ulnar fingers and ulnar side of the hand. The reader is referred to Chapters 11, 28, and 32 for a more detailed discussion of the sensory and motor supply to the hand.

NORMAL HAND FUNCTION

The occupational therapist must understand normal hand function and hand-to-upper extremity relationships to perform splint design and construction accurately and effectively.

The joints of the upper extremity must have adequate range of motion (ROM) to ensure normal hand function. This will allow the hand to reach the object or perform the activity. Joints of the hand and arm must have stability and the ability to be fixed or to cocontract at any point in their ROM. The hand and arm must have enough muscle power for the reaching, placing, performing, or holding that is required by the task to be done.[6]

Wide ranges of shoulder motions are critical to placing the hand at some distance from the body, such as extending over the head and reaching behind and out to the side of the body. A lesser degree of shoulder motion is essential for hand-to-mouth and hand-to-body activities such as toileting and combing hair.[6]

To perform hand-to-face activities the elbow must have full range of flexion. Full extension is required if activities at some distance from the body are to be accomplished, such as putting on socks or reaching to high shelves. Pronation and supination are essential for placing the hand at the correct angle for holding or activity performance. Full pronation is required if the hand is to perform adequately. Supination to midposition is sufficient for adequate function.

Lesser ROM at the wrist is required for basic hand function. More important is the wrist's stability. For the hand to function maximally it should be possible to stabilize the wrist at any point in its ROM and make fine adjustments in the degree of wrist motion. This ability to stabilize and make fine adjustments in the wrist contributes to the fine coordination possible in the hand. Wrist extension is most important, since finger flexion and grasp are best performed with the wrist in extension. If the wrist is flexed, grasp will be limited and the arches of the hand will tend to flatten. When the wrist is flexed because of pain, paralysis, or deformity, the long extensor tendons stretch, the metacarpal transverse arch flattens, and the thumb drifts into the plane of the palm of the hand.

The MP joints are the key joints of the fingers. Their ability to flex and be stabilized at any point in their range of flexion is critical to grasp and prehension. When the MP joints are hyperextended, the interphalangeal (IP) joints flex as a result of the pull on the long flexor tendons of the fingers.

The carpal and metacarpal transverse arches are critical to hand function. Motion and opposition of the thumb and little finger, ability to grasp round or large objects, convergence of the fingers during flexion, and strength or pressing with the palm are dependent on these arches.[9]

The thumb is the most valuable element of the hand. One or two other fingers and the thumb will make a more functional hand than four fingers and no thumb. Thumb opposition is critical to all of the prehension patterns. It acts as a flexible force in strong grasp patterns. It must be possible for the thumb to rotate at the carpometacarpal (CMC) joint if true opposition of thumb pad to finger pads is to take place. Hand splints are often used to stabilize and position the thumb properly for some grasp and prehension patterns.[9] In some instances splints may be used to assist thumb extension, abduction, or opposition.[7]

Sensation is a major asset of the normal hand. The normal hand has the ability to sense pain and temperature and to interpret the qualities of objects, such as size, weight, and texture. Splinting can do nothing to aid sensation and actually limits sensation during wear.[2,9]

The normal hand has many assets, several of which cannot be replaced or helped with splints. The normal hand is capable of mobility and stability at all joints. Splinting can provide one or the other but usually not both.[5,9] The normal hand has considerable dexterity and can move in a quick, accurate manner. The use of a splint may aid in the ultimate recovery of dexterity, but while the splint is being worn, dexterity is hindered or limited.

The cosmetic appearance of the hand can be improved by splinting. However, during splint wear or use the hand may be less cosmetically appealing. This may influence the patient's acceptance and use of the device.[9]

The normal hand can perform a wide variety of prehension and grasp patterns. The finer prehension patterns require minimal strength and flexibility in the hand, whereas grasp patterns require more strength and flexibility in the hand.[9] Splinting may assist in only one or two patterns, such as palmar prehension or grasp.[5] The grasp and prehension patterns that may be provided by hand splinting are determined by the muscles that are functioning, potential and present deformities, and how the hand is to be used.[9]

Prehension and grasp are the primary functions of the hand. Hand movements are complex and occur in smooth sequence and combinations. However, it is possible to reduce these movements to several basic types of prehension and grasp.[6]

Types of Prehension and Grasp[5,6,9] (Fig. 24-4)

FINGERTIP PREHENSION (Fig. 24-4, *A*). Fingertip prehension, contact of the thumb pad with that of the index or middle fingers, is used to pick up small objects, such as pins, nails, and buttons, and to fasten buttons and snaps and hold a needle for sewing. It requires very fine coordination.

PALMAR PREHENSION (Fig. 24-4, *B*). Palmar prehension, also called "three-jaw chuck grip" or "palmar tripod pinch,"[6] is the contact of the thumb pad with

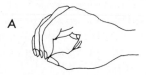

A

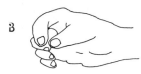

B

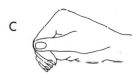

C

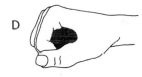

D

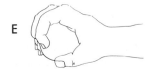

E

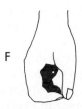

F

Fig. 24-4. Basic types of prehension and grasp. **A,** Fingertip prehension. **B,** Palmar prehension. **C,** Lateral prehension. **D,** Cylindrical grasp. **E,** Spherical grasp. **F,** Hook grasp.

the middle and index fingers. It is the most common type of prehension and requires a high level of coordination. It is used to pick up and hold small square, cylindrical, or spherical objects, such as a marble, pen, or small cube, and is the prehension pattern used for holding a pen or eating utensil.

LATERAL PREHENSION (Fig. 24-4, *C*). During lateral prehension the thumb pad is in contact with the lateral surface of the index finger at the middle or distal phalanx. For this to be a functional prehension pattern the thumb and index finger must have good stability and the first dorsal interosseous muscle must have good to normal strength. The fourth and fifth fingers must act as a support to the index and middle fingers. Lateral prehension is used for turning a key or thumbscrew, carrying a plate or teacup, and winding a watch. It is a stronger type of prehension than fingertip or palmar prehension and requires less coordination to perform.

CYLINDRICAL GRASP (Fig. 24-4, *D*). The cylindrical grasp is the position the normal hand assumes when holding objects such as a tumbler, rail, hammer, or pot handle. The object is stabilized against the palm by the fingers, which close or flex around it. Intrinsic and thenar muscle strength are essential to the power of this grasp. It is one of the earliest grasp patterns, occurring reflexly in infants and developing later into voluntary gross grasp.[6]

SPHERICAL GRASP (Fig. 24-4, *E*). The spherical grasp, also called "ball grasp," is the position the normal hand assumes when grasping a small rubber ball, such as a tennis ball. The five fingers are flexed around the object and hold it against the palm, which is in an arched position. It is used to hold balls, apples, oranges, and round doorknobs. Its power depends on the stability of the wrist and finger joints and the strength of the intrinsic and extrinsic muscles of the hand.

HOOK GRASP (Fig. 24-4, *F*). The hook grasp is the position the normal hand assumes when carrying a briefcase or similar bag handle. The grip can be accomplished entirely by the fingers. The thumb remains outside the fingers and is relatively passive. It acts simply to close the hook, but its presence and power are not essential to hook function. The hook grasp requires strength and stability of the IP joints, primarily. The MP joints and the wrist remain in the neutral position and need not be completely stabilized. This type of grasp is used to carry heavy objects, such as pails, suitcases, and shopping bags, and may also be used to pull open drawers and cabinets with hardware that require four fingers to hook to pull them.

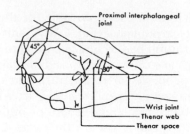

Fig. 24-5. Functional position, lateral view, right hand. From Malick MH: Manual on static hand splinting, Pittsburgh, Harmarville Rehabilitation Center.

Positions of the Hand and Tendon Action

FUNCTIONAL POSITION (Fig. 24-5). The functional position of the hand is a position similar to that which the hand assumes when grasping a ball. The wrist is in 20° to 30° of extension. The transverse metacarpal arch is rounded. The thumb is in abduction and is in opposition to the pads of the four fingers. The metacarpal joints are flexed to about 30° and the PIP joints are flexed to about 45°.[6,8]

The functional position of the hand may be described as the midposition of the ROM of every joint. In this position there is equal tension of all musculature, and the muscles are in the best mechanical position for efficient function.

The functional position is an important concept, since it is usually desirable to splint the hand in a position as near the functional position as possible.[5,9] Placing the hand in the functional position alone will improve its performance and decrease the possibility of developing deformity in many instances.

RESTING POSITION (Fig. 24-6). The resting position is slightly more relaxed than the functional position. It is similar to the position the normal hand assumes when resting passively on a tabletop. The wrist is in 10° to 20° of extension. All finger joints are slightly flexed. The thumb is in partial opposition and abduction, and the thumb pad faces the pad of the index finger. The metacarpal, carpal, and longitudinal arches are maintained when the hand is in the resting position.[6] The hand is often splinted in this position in a static resting splint if joint rest or pre-

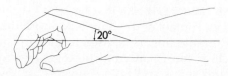

Fig. 24-6. Resting position. From Malick MH: Manual on static hand splinting, Pittsburgh, Harmarville Rehabilitation Center.

vention of deformity is desirable in conditions such as peripheral nerve injuries and rheumatoid arthritis.

NONFUNCTIONAL POSITION. The normal hand naturally falls into a nonfunctional position when the wrist is dropped passively as when hanging over the end of a table, mattress, or arm chair. In this position the transverse metacarpal arch is flattened, the fingers are extended, and the thumb is adducted and extended (Fig. 24-7). This is a position of potential deformity for the injured or paralyzed hand. If left untreated this position could contribute to the development of a claw hand or intrinsic minus deformity. Positioning the wrist in slight-to-moderate extension with a splint or positioning device will do much to obviate this problem.

TENDON ACTION. The tendon or tenodesis action of the long finger flexors and extensors can be an important consideration when evaluating hand function and for splinting. In the normal hand when the wrist is flexed, the fingers are passively pulled into extension by tendon action. This is because the length of the finger extensors is insufficient for flexion at all of the joints that they cross. The reverse is also true. When the wrist is extended, the fingers tend to pull into flexion. The length of the finger flexors is inadequate for extension at all of the joints that they cross. This tenodesis action results in a passive prehension pattern. This may be used to gain some functional prehension with the aid of a dynamic splint in the hand with some wrist function but absent finger function.[2]

PRINCIPLES OF HAND SPLINTING
Types of Splints

STATIC SPLINTS. *Static splints* have no moving parts. It is usually desirable to hold the involved part

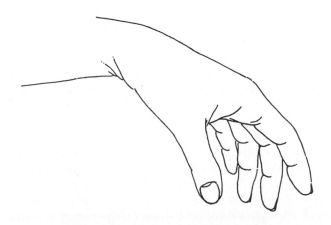

Fig. 24-7. Non-functioning position.

in a functional position or as close to a functional position as is physically possible. The antideformity splint for the burned hand (see Fig. 26-5) and the postoperative flexor tendon splint (see Fig. 28-10) are two examples of exceptions to this rule. To the extent possible, the patient should be able to perform daily living tasks while wearing the splint. This of course depends on the type of splint and its purpose. Some splints necessarily eliminate most or all functioning. The use of the functional position in splinting will help to ensure the ability to perform activities of daily living (ADL) when the splint is removed even if function is not possible when the splint is being worn. However, the physician's requirements regarding the position of the hand for splinting may vary with the diagnosis and purposes of the splint. These requirements must be considered when designing splints, and the therapist with the physician must plan for facilitating the regaining of maximal function following the splinting period.[5]

All splints should be designed to meet the patient's physiological and functional needs. The splint must achieve the desired purposes while not creating dysfunction. All static splints must be removed periodically for exercise of the affected part, and the patient should be encouraged to use the part as frequently as possible while wearing the splint.[6]

Static splints may be used for three major purposes. The first purpose is for protection of weak muscles. A static splint can protect weak muscles from overstretching and therefore prevent their antagonists from contracture. Prevention of overstretching muscles weak because of temporary paralysis is important to ensure good function when nerve and muscle recovery occurs.

The second major purpose of static splints is for support. A joint may be supported or immobilized for resting purposes, as in rheumatoid arthritis, or for healing purposes, as in tendon lacerations and skin grafting. The function of the hand can often be improved if the wrist is supported in extension. Therefore a simple static wrist cock-up splint can improve finger function for grasp and prehension.

The third major purpose of static splinting is for prevention or correction of deformity. The splint may be designed to force the involved joint into correct or near-correct alignment, such as the protective ulnar drift splint used in rheumatoid arthritis.[8]

DYNAMIC SPLINTS. The *dynamic hand splint* has a static base and one or more moving parts. Thus the same splint may incorporate both static and dynamic elements. Some parts may be supported in their best anatomical position for function, whereas other parts

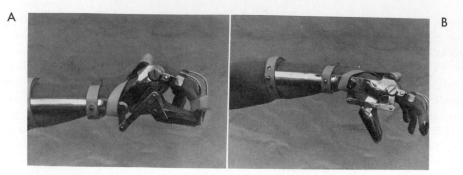

Fig. 24-8. Wrist-hand orthosis. **A,** Prehension affected by wrist extension. **B,** Release of prehension affected by relaxation of wrist extension.

are assisted in movement by the dynamic features of the splint. The splint is designed to apply a relatively constant force on a part as it moves. It provides mobility to the joints with control on the direction and degree of motion. This splint is designed to assist weak muscles or substitute for lost muscle power.[7]

Movement in dynamic splints may be effected by another part of the body or available muscle group, as in the wrist-driven flexor hinge splint, also called the "wrist-hand orthosis" (Fig. 24-8); or by springs, pulleys, and rubber bands, as in the long opponens splint with MP stop and extensor assist (Fig. 24-9); or by an external power source, such as an electronic or pneumatic unit.[2,5,7] Dynamic splints also use traction through rubberbands, springs, cords, or Velcro, to increase joint ROM.[2]

CONTOUR SPLINTS. Contour splints are molded to fit the contour of a part very closely. They are used in burn rehabilitation to prevent hypertrophic scarring through the application of pressure. Thus they minimize skin contracture and deformity. Examples of contour splints include the neck conformer, transparent face mask, and airplane splint. These are illustrated in Chapter 26.

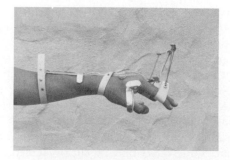

Fig. 24-9. Long opponens splint with MP stop and extensor assist.

Principles of Splinting

BONE. When the therapist is molding and fitting splints, bony prominences must be considered. Soft tissue is thin over these areas, and there is potential for pressure and resultant skin breakdown from a poorly fitted splint. The most vulnerable areas are the ulnar and radial styloids, the pisiform, the metacarpal heads, and the base of the thumb metacarpal. When splinting, bony prominences should be avoided or the area of application over them should be widened.[2]

ALIGNMENT OF THE DIGITS. The normal alignment of the fingers should be maintained by the splint. For example, a traction device used to maintain or increase finger flexion should not originate from a single point at the wrist but from four points that coincide with the normal alignment of the fingers when they are flexed simultaneously.[2]

ARCHES OF THE HAND. The metacarpal transverse arch and the longitudinal arch must be preserved when splinting. The metacarpal transverse arch should be apparent in any splint that includes the metacarpals and any splint parts that extend beyond the metacarpals, such as a lumbricals bar.[2,5] The splint should be designed to maintain the normal arch of the hand and allow the arch to increase during hand use. If the metacarpal transverse arch is flattened, the thumb will be unable to oppose the fingers and thus hand function will be seriously impaired.[5,6]

The longitudinal arch permits flexion of the MPs and IPs. Any splint covering these joints should have some curvature to support the longitudinal arch in part or in its entire length, depending on the length and type of splint being used.[2,5]

DUAL OBLIQUITY. When making hand splints, the dual obliquity of the hand, described earlier, must be considered. The radial side of the splint must be longer or more distal than the ulnar side (Fig. 24-10, *A*), and the splint must be higher on the radial side than on the ulnar side[2,5] (Fig. 24-10, *B*).

JOINTS. To prevent the nonfunctional position of

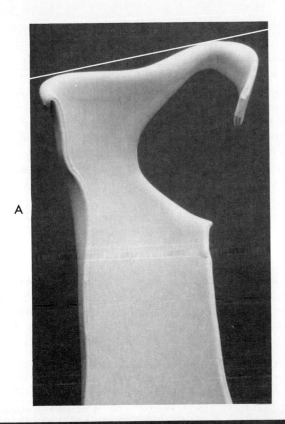

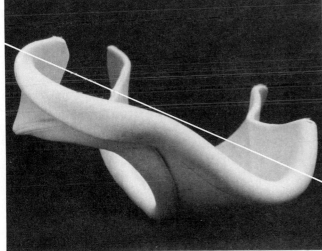

Fig. 24-10. Distal end of cock-up splint demonstrates dual obliquity.

the wrist and subsequent potential deformity from developing, the wrist should be splinted in slight extension. There are exceptions, of course, depending on the particular dysfunction, limitations already present at the wrist, degree of paralysis, and goals of hand splinting. Individual variations in wrist positioning will depend on these factors and should be determined by the therapist in concert with the supervising physician.

Dynamic traction should be applied at 90° angle of pull to the splinted part. In this position the rotational element of the force is maximized.[3] This is accomplished by positioning the distal end of the outrigger at a point that allows the dynamic assist (such as a finger sling suspended by a rubber band) to pull at a 90° angle on the bone to be mobilized. As the ROM increases, the length of the outrigger must be changed to maintain the pull at 90°.[2,7] The pull should also be perpendicular to the rotational axis of the joint. The location of the joint axis is determined by observation of joint movement in the plane in which it is to be splinted.[2]

Of greatest importance is the prevention of the adverse effects of immobilization. Prolonged immobility from splinting or positioning can produce limitations in joint ROM and ultimately joint stiffness and immobility. All static splints must be removed periodically for active or passive exercise, unless contraindicated by surgery, infection, or trauma.

Joints that do not require splinting should not be limited or immobilized by the splint. All joints proximal and distal to the splinted joint(s) should be used actively or exercised passively if active motion is not possible.[6,9]

A splint cannot provide both mobility and stability of a joint, as in the normal hand, at the same time. Therefore a choice for one or the other must be made in relation to the dysfunction, purposes of splinting, potential deformities, and use of the hand.

COLLATERAL LIGAMENTS. The length of the collateral ligaments should be maintained in a splint. Therefore in a splint that requires IP joint immobilization the IP joints should be splinted in nearly full extension. Conversely, the length of the MP ligaments can be preserved by splinting these joints in nearly full flexion. If the MP collateral ligaments are allowed to shorten, there will be a loss of MP flexion and possibility of contracture.[2]

FIBROUS STRUCTURE AND BLOOD SUPPLY. The normal hand has unique padding on the palm and fingertips which contributes to the effectiveness of grasp and pinch. Splinting may limit or hinder the function of this unique padding. The hand is supplied with complex blood-vascular and lymphatic systems. Effective splinting and splint use can aid good circulation, whereas poor splinting can limit circulation.[9]

To ensure that proper fit and comfort have been achieved, the splint should be removed after short periods of wear (½ hour to 1 hour) and the part should be checked for indentations of the skin, redness, edema, pain, and changes in the degree of joint mobility.

CREASES AND SKIN OF THE HAND. The skin creases correspond to the underlying joints and are good landmarks for splint boundaries. If motion of a particular joint is to be allowed, the general rule is that the distal end of the splint should terminate just proximal to the specific crease.[2] For example, splints should not obstruct the distal palmar crease if full MP flexion is to be allowed. The thenar crease must not be obstructed if opposition is to occur or if the hand is to be in the position of function.[6] Conversely, if the joint is to be immobilized, then the splint should extend almost to the creases of the next segment, both proximally and distally, to provide the best support.[2]

To avoid skin pressure the area of splint application should be wide enough to disperse the pressure. The splint material should be contoured for the full length of the segment being splinted. The distal end of the splint should be rolled, and the proximal end rolled or flared. Padding must be used judiciously. It is easily contaminated and should not be used to compensate for poor fitting.[2] If the splint is to be padded, this must be allowed for when first molding the splint by padding the patient's arm or applying the padding to the thermoplastic *before* the splint is molded. Any padding added to the splint after it is molded will increase the pressure. The use of padding is generally undesirable. The discomfort of perspiration can be alleviated by wearing an absorbent "sock," such as stockinette tubing, over the part or over the splint.[5]

SENSORIMOTOR FUNCTION. Motion and sensation are intimately related in hand and upper extremity function. Sensory information and feedback from the parts are essential to normal motion. A person with severely limited sensation will have limited motor function even if muscles are normal or near normal. Splinting cannot aid in the restoration of sensation. Splints reduce the amount of sensory information being received from the part. The possibility of the development of pressure points and the resultant skin breakdown from splints is greater in the person with sensory deficits. Such patients must be taught how to compensate for and guard the affected part by using their vision. The therapist and the patient must be responsible for vigilant precautions against the adverse effects of splinting.[9]

Purposes of Splints[9]

A hand splint may be prescribed and fitted for more than one purpose. If there is limited joint motion, the splint may be a positioning or corrective device, and more function may not be achieved until the ROM is improved. In such instances performance of hand skills may be greater without the splint, although not necessarily in the most desirable patterns of motion.

A splint may be a positioning device to enhance function during the day and a corrective device at night.

The ultimate and idealistic goal of hand splinting is to assist in the development of as near a normal hand as possible. The following are some specific goals of hand splinting:

1. Prevent deformity caused by joint tightness or muscle contracture. Contracture of muscles whose antagonists are weak or paralyzed can be prevented by placing the muscle at its resting length in the functional position and facilitating motion through the splint or passively.
2. Protect weak muscles from overstretching so that maximal efficiency will be obtained when the muscle regains its function. This goal is related to number 1.
3. Prevent increased muscle imbalance by providing assistance to the weaker muscle group, for example using rubber bands, to pull the part through the full ROM. This will enable weak muscles to work and allows active ROM.
4. Strengthen weak muscles by providing assistive motion first. Assistance is gradually decreased as muscle function improves. This goal is related to number 3. The MP extensor assist or opponens assist are examples of splints with these purposes.
5. Correct or prevent deformity by maintaining the ROM gained in forced stretching exercise or maintaining corrected alignment of joints.
6. Provide temporary support for a painful part while permitting motion of uninvolved segments. An example is the wrist cock-up splint to support an arthritic wrist while allowing some hand function.
7. Prepare the hand for future surgery by approximating the position or motions to be gained by surgery and provide the needed ROM and strength, if possible.
8. Place the hand in the correct or appropriate position after burn, surgery, trauma, or skin grafting.
9. Aid in the development of a useful tenodesis tightness in the long finger flexors for the wrist-hand orthosis.
10. Transfer power from one joint to another for increased function. An example is the wrist-hand orthosis where wrist extension effects palmar prehension and wrist flexion effects release through the splint. Later with the controlled development of some finger flexor tightness many patients can discard this splint and use the tenodesis action of the hand for some prehensile function.
11. Substitute for permanently paralyzed muscles through the use of external power such as elec-

tricity. Examples of this type of splint are the battery-driven wrist-hand orthosis and the Rancho electric arm.

12. Encourage use of normal movement patterns, prevent substitutions, and facilitate muscle reeducation. These purposes may be achieved by placing the part in a functional position and providing as near a normal range as possible. Return of function will be facilitated by use of the hand in coordinated movement patterns. Proper position and motion will aid returning muscles to work to their maximal potential but will have no effect on reinnervation of the muscle itself.[9]

Criteria for Assessing Splints

The splint should be evaluated periodically for fit and function. The frequency of evaluation will depend on the disability and the purposes of the splint. For example, a splint for the burned hand should be evaluated at least daily, whereas one that is used during regeneration of a radial nerve could be evaluated weekly or at each patient visit. The therapist must determine if the splint is achieving the desired goals, making no difference, or possibly increasing dysfunction or deformity.[6,9]

Static splints should be fitted soon after injury, surgery, or disease. They should be simple in design, easily adjustable, lightweight, cosmetically pleasing, and comfortable and should offer adequate support to achieve the objectives of the splint. It should be possible to fabricate the splint in a reasonable period. The splint should be inexpensive when materials and the therapist's time for construction are considered.[6] The splint should be neat, durable, and easy to clean.

The splint should follow the natural contours of the hand and arm as closely as possible without causing pressure areas. The arches of the hand must be maintained, and the normal padding of the fingers and the hypothenar and thenar eminences must not be flattened. Joints should be positioned in correct anatomical alignment, and the hand should be positioned in or as nearly as possible to the position of function unless contraindicated.[9] The therapist should be aware of and check the splints for shifts in position, which therefore change their function and support of the part. If the splint is used for progressive increase of joint motion, three points of pressure should be used[9,13] (Fig. 24-11).

INDEPENDENT SPLINT CONSTRUCTION: A SELF-INSTRUCTION PROGRAM

The following self-instruction program was designed to enable the reader to construct two simple static splints frequently fabricated by occupational therapists. These are the volar radial bar wrist cock-up splint and the resting splint. The wrist cock-up splint may be used to immobilize the wrist in a functional position while allowing finger function. It is used for rheumatoid arthritis, if rest or stabilization of the wrist is desirable, and also to protect the wrist and finger extensors from overstretching when there is muscle weakness producing the wrist-drop position.

The resting splint is worn for similar purposes but immobilizes the thumb and fingers as well as the wrist in the position of rest or function. It may be modified to the antideformity position required for splinting the hand with dorsal burns. In this position the wrist is at neutral, the MP joints are flexed to approximately 80°, and the IP joints are in full extension. The thumb is midway between radial and palmar abduction to maintain full stretch on the thumb web space.

The resting splint is sometimes used to prevent contractures of the hand with flexor spasticity. When the patient wears the splint, no hand function is possible. Therefore it is often worn when the patient is at rest or asleep or is worn on one side at a time if bilateral splinting is required.

Steps in Making a Hand Splint Independently

Study the preceding sections of this chapter and review the illustrations of grasp, prehension, hand creases, position of function, and position of rest. Then with a partner, begin construction of a splint.

THE RADIAL BAR WRIST COCK-UP SPLINT

MAKING A SPLINT PATTERN

Supplies
A pencil or felt-tip pen, a piece of paper towel 18 to 20 inches (45.7 to 50.8 cm) long, scissors, and a ruler.

Make a tracing of the hand[10]

The pattern will be drawn over a tracing of the hand to be splinted. To trace the hand follow these steps:

1. Position the hand and forearm to be splinted palm down on the piece of paper towel. The fingers should be slightly abducted, and the wrist should be in neutral deviation with the thumb slightly abducted.

2. Draw around the hand and forearm, keeping the pen perpendicular at all times. It is not necessary to trace around each finger.

3. With the hand still in place, mark the wrist joint and the MP joints of the fingers on the radial and ulnar sides and the MP joint of the thumb.

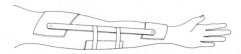

Fig. 24-11. Three-point elbow extension splint illustrates points of pressure proximal and distal to elbow joint and over it to increase or maintain extension.

4. Take a measurement on the volar surface of the forearm from the distal wrist crease to the elbow crease. Make a mark on the tracing of the forearm equal to ⅔ of this distance plus ½ inch (1.3 cm). Use the marks for the wrist joint as the point of reference.

Marking the splint pattern on the tracing

1. On the tracing of the hand, draw a line connecting the MP joint marks across the palm. Extend this line 1½ inches (3.8 cm) out on the radial side and ¾ inch (1.9 cm) on the ulnar side of the hand.

2. Draw a line 1 inch (2.5 cm) down from the radial side of this line. This forms the radial bar. On the ulnar side draw a line parallel to the side of the hand and extend it to the wrist. Follow the general contour of the hand.

3. At the level of the MP joint of the thumb, make a mark in the palm of the hand about ¼ inch (0.6 cm) off center, toward the radial side of the hand. This mark designates the thenar crease.

4. Draw a curved line from the radial bar to the wrist. Arch this line through the mark in the palm. If this is drawn correctly, the line will have a C shape.

5. Draw a line across the mark on the forearm tracing for the length of the forearm trough. Extend this line on either side of the forearm tracing a distance equal to one half the thickness of the forearm at this level. The thickness of the arm may be estimated by eye, or a ruler or a pen can be used to measure half the height of the upper forearm. Make a mark at each end of the line across the upper forearm.

6. On the radial side of the wrist, make a mark beyond the width of the tracing, which is about one half the thickness of the forearm at wrist level.

7. From the marks at the wrist, draw two lines extending proximally to meet the line at the upper end of the forearm. Taper these lines outward to accommodate for the increasing thickness of the forearm. Be sure not to make the lines concave or convex (Fig. 24-12).

8. Cut the pattern out and place it over your partner's forearm. With the pattern in place and wrist slightly extended, flex the MP joints. there should be no more than a ¼-inch (0.6-cm) fold-over when this is done. Then, oppose the thumb. There should be no more than a ¼-inch (0.6-cm) fold-over at the thenar eminence when this is done. Check to see that the sides of forearm trough extend about half way around the forearm. Trim the pattern to fit, if necessary.

CUTTING THE SPLINT OUT OF THE THERMOPLASTIC[5,12]

Supplies

The pattern, a piece of low-temperature thermoplastic material such as Polyform, Polyflex, or Kay-splint, about 8 by 12 inches (20.3 × 30.5), and a ball-point pen or an awl. To heat the thermoplastic use a shallow pan such as an electric frying pan, with water about 1-inch (2.5-cm) deep and heated to the correct temperature for the specific thermoplastic. A thermometer to monitor the water temperature, a heat gun, a folded towel, large scissors, and a wooden tongue blade will also be needed. Place a folded towel on the work surface next to the heating pan. Keep the scissors and tongue blades in the work area.

Practicing

Before you mold the splint, take some scrap thermoplastic material and soften it in the pan. Remove it from the pan

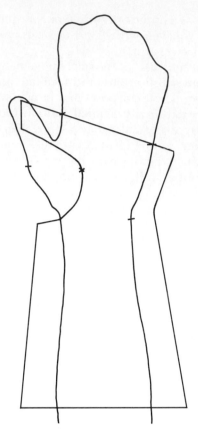

Fig. 24-12. Cock-up splint pattern.

and blot it gently on the towel. Check the temperature by holding the material against your own cheek or forearm. If it is too hot, let it rest for a minute or so. Mold it over your MP joints with smoothing motions. The purpose of this is to get the feel of the material before making the splint.

Cutting the pattern out of the thermoplastic

1. Place the splint pattern on the thermoplastic material and trace around it with the awl or ball-point pen. If a ball-point pen is used, be careful not to let it slip under the paper pattern since ball-point ink cannot be easily removed.

2. To cut the pattern out, take the large piece of thermoplastic material and cut off any excess length. Do this by heating the scrap end first and cutting it off.

3. Then heat the thermoplastic to the correct temperature for the specified time until it is uniformly flexible. Test for flexibility by lifting a corner with a tongue blade.

4. When it is flexible, remove the thermoplastic from the heating pan. Be careful not to suspend it vertically since it can stretch. Gently pat it on the folded towel. Be sure it is cool enough to handle. Touch it to your forearm to test the temperature.

5. Supporting the material with one hand, cut out the splint pattern on the marking. Round all of the corners. When cutting out the pattern, hold the material near the work surface and be careful not to suspend it vertically to prevent stretching (Fig. 24-13).

MOLDING THE SPLINT

When the pattern is cut out of the thermoplastic material, it may be setting a little. Reheat it very briefly to soften it

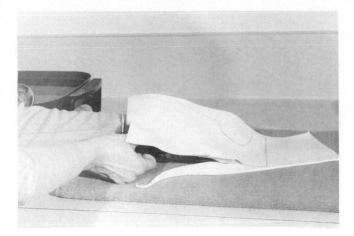

Fig. 24-13. Cutting the splint out of the thermoplastic.

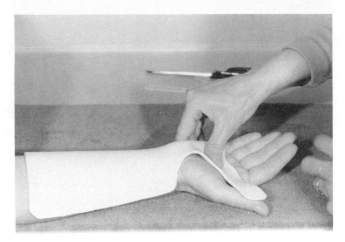

Fig. 24-14. Thermoplastic draped on forearm and thumb pressed into palm to attain metacarpal transverse arch.

enough for molding. Once the thermoplastic is softened, you have about 3 to 5 minutes to mold the splint. It can be reheated to make adjustments, but it is best not to reheat more than once or twice.

1. Remove the material from the heating pan and pat it dry on a towel. Cool it until it is comfortable to the touch. Test it for temperature before applying it to the forearm to be splinted. Position the forearm in supination and about 30° of wrist extension.

2. Drape the material over the forearm without squeezing it. Smooth proximally over the forearm trough and be careful not to twist the trough to either side.

3. Next, place your thumb into the palm of the hand to get the contour of the arch molded into the splint (Fig. 24-14).

4. Have your partner oppose the thumb to the little finger. This will cause a fold at the border of the thenar eminence.

5. Then with your partner's thumb back out of the way, roll this edge over at the fold. This should be rolled back far enough to allow full opposition of the thumb to the little ringer. Roll over the edge almost to the full length of the radial bar. This rolled edge adds comfort and strength to the splint (Fig. 24-15).

6. Bring the radial bar through the thumb web space and mold it flat against the dorsum of the hand.

7. Next have your partner flex the MP joints that will cause a fold at the distal edge of the splint. Then open the hand and fold over this edge. Be sure to fold it at an oblique angle to follow the oblique line of the proximal and distal palmar creases. It should be rolled back far enough so that full flexion of the MP joints is possible with the splint in place.

8. Allow the splint to set until it is somewhat rigid and then remove it from your partner's forearm. (Setting may be hastened by using Cold Spray or by immersion in cold water.)

Finishing

When the basic molding is completed, make some finishing touches on the splint.

1. First, hold the splint vertically and heat the proximal end in the heat pan. When slightly softened, gently flare this end out. This will prevent the proximal end of the splint from irritating the forearm.

2. If there are any jagged edges, they may be smoothed by heating the edge in water or by using the heat gun and smoothing carefully with your finger.

APPLYING STRAPS TO THE SPLINT

Supplies

Two pieces of self-adhesive Velcro hook, 3 inches (7.6 cm) each, and two peices 1 inch (2.5 cm) each; a piece of Dura Val or Velfoam strapping material about 18 inches (45.7 cm) long; a heat gun; and thermoplastic solvent.

1. The Velcro is attached to the outside of the splint. One 3-inch (7.6 cm) piece is attached at the proximal end of the splint, and another just proximal to the ulna styloid at the wrist. A 1-inch (2.5-cm) piece is attached at the distal end of the splint on the ulnar side, and the other is attached to the end of the radial bar.

2. Abrade the finish of the thermoplastic by applying some solvent to the spots where the pieces of Velcro are to be applied or by scraping the finish off the material with the blade of a scissors.

3. Then heat each spot until slightly sticky, before the Velcro is applied. Before removing the backing from the Velcro, briefly warm the adhesive side over the heat gun.

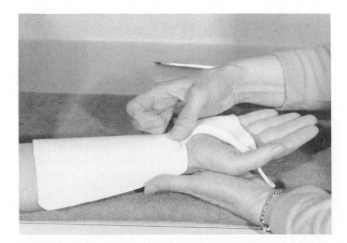

Fig. 24-15. Therapist rolls over the thenar edge of the splint.

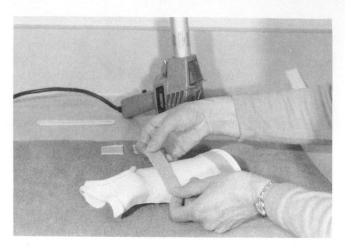

Fig. 24-16. Velcro closures are applied to the splint for the straps.

Then remove the paper backing and apply the Velcro to the prepared area on the splint. Do this to all four pieces. The piece that is applied to the radial bar may need to be trimmed to shape (Fig. 24-16).

4. The straps should be long enough to cover the arm and completely cover the Velcro. Cut one strap to go across the forearm, one for the wrist, and one for the hand. Round the corners of the strap end that covers the radial bar.

Evaluation of the Splint (Fig. 24-17)

Evaluate the splint for function, fit, and appearance, measuring it against the following criteria.

For function

1. Are the arches of the hand maintained? Look at the hand from the front with the MPs flexed and see if the metacarpal transverse arch is preserved. Look at the palmar side of the splint and see if it has a concave contour.

2. Is there full ROM at the MP joints with the splint in place? Place one hand over your partner's wrist and

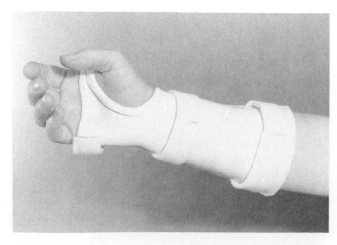

Fig. 24-17. Completed radial bar wrist cock-up splint.

have your partner flex the MP joints fully. If the splint is too long, there will be some wrist flexion to compensate and the wrist will rise in the splint. If the splint is the correct length, the wrist should remain comfortably in the splint.

3. Is there full opposition to the fifth finger? Ask your partner to oppose the thumb to the fifth finger and observe for obstruction of the thenar eminence as it rotates toward the palm. Watch for compensatory flexion of the thumb MP joint to reach the little finger. Have your partner oppose with both hands and compare the amount of thumb MP flexion which is used on the splinted hand as opposed to the normal hand. The splinted hand should not have any more MP flexion than the unsplinted hand if the thenar eminence is not obstructed.

4. Is the wrist extended at least 10 to 30 degrees? Take your goniometer and measure wrist extension on the radial side of the hand. The measurement should be 10° to 30° of extension.

For fit

1. Are the straps correctly placed for stability and to avoid pressure points?
2. Do the sides of the forearm trough extend half way around the forearm at all points or is the trough twisted? Check to see if it is higher on one side than on the other when the splint is on the arm.
3. Does the splint fit loosely enough to prevent pressure areas along the edges and over bony prominences? Have your partner wear the splint for 30 minutes and check for reddened areas on the skin!

For appearance

1. Is the splint smooth and free of marks, dents, cuts, and jagged edges?
2. Are all of the corners rounded and the edges smoothed?
3. Are the straps clean and attached in correct alignment?
4. If this splint were prescribed for you, would the appearance be acceptable?

RESTING SPLINT

MAKING A SPLINT PATTERN

Supplies

A pencil or felt-tip pen, a piece of paper towel 18-20 inches (45.7 to 50.8 cm) long, and a ruler.

Making a tracing of the hand[10]

Draw the pattern over a tracing of the hand to be splinted. To make the tracing follow these steps:

1. Position the hand and forearm palm down on the piece of paper towel. The fingers and the thumb should be slightly abducted, and the wrist in neutral deviation.
2. Draw around the hand, forearm, and thumb, keeping

the pencil perpendicular at all times. It is not necessary to trace around each finger.

3. With the hand still in place, mark the wrist joint on the radial and ulnar sides, the CMC joint of the thumb, the MP joint of the index finger and the MP joint of the thumb. Make a dot at the apex of the thumb web space and between the index and middle finger.

4. Take a measurement on the volar surface of your partner's forearm from the distal wrist crease to the elbow crease. Make a line on the tracing of the forearm equal to ⅔ of this distance plus ½ inch (1.3 cm). Use the marks at the wrist joint as the point of reference.

Marking the splint pattern on the tracing

1. On the tracing of the hand, beginning at the MP joint of the index finger, draw a line ½ inch (1.3 cm) away around the hand tracing, ending at the wrist on the ulnar side. Extend the line on the radial side straight down to the CMC joint of the thumb and then another ½ inch (1.3 cm).

2. Draw a horizontal line from the dot at the thumb web space and a vertical line from the dot between the index and middle fingers. Make a dot where the two lines intersect.

3. Now, draw a line from this dot toward the wrist. This line is parallel to the outer edge of the tracing next to the thumb and equal to the length of the thumb from the thumb MP joint plus ½ inch (1.3 cm). Taper this line in slightly and round the bottom.

4. Go back to the dot at the intersecting lines and draw another line down, slightly away from the first, and curve it around so that it comes out at the wrist mark.

5. Extend the line across the forearm tracing a distance equal to one half the thickness of the forearm on each side. The thickness of the arm may be estimated by eye, or measure half the height of the upper forearm with a ruler or a pencil.

6. On the radial side of the wrist make a mark beyond the width of the tracing, which is about one half the thickness of the forearm at wrist level.

7. From the marks at the wrist draw two lines extending proximally to meet the line at the upper end of the forearm. Taper these lines outward. Be sure not to make the lines concave or convex (Fig. 24-18).

8. Cut the pattern out and place it over your partner's hand. With the pattern in place and the wrist slightly extended, have your partner assume the resting position with the hand. Look at the contour of the pattern over the palm and place the thumb piece backward to form a trough around the thumb.

The pattern should extend about ½ inch (1.3 cm) beyond the width of the hand all the way around. The thumb piece should be about ½ inch (1.3 cm) wider than the thumb and should extend about ½ inch beyond the length of the thumb. Check to see that the forearm trough extends about half way around the arm at all points. Trim the pattern to fit.

CUTTING THE SPLINT OUT OF THE THERMOPLASTIC[5,12]

Supplies

The pattern, a piece of low-temperature thermoplastic material such as Polyform, Polyflex, or Kay-splint, about 8 by 18 inches (20.3 cm by 45.7 cm), a leather punch, and an awl or a ball-point pen. A shallow pan such as an electric frying pan, with water about 1-inch (2.5-cm) deep, a ther-

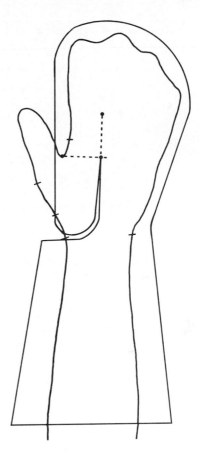

Fig. 24-18. Resting splint pattern.

mometer to monitor the water temperature, a heat gun, a folded towel, large scissors, and a wooden tongue blade will also be needed. Place the thermometer in the pan. Place a folded towel on the work surface next to your heating pan. Keep the scissors and tongue blade in the work area.

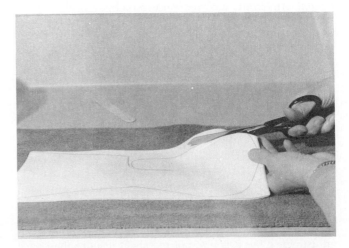

Fig. 24-19. Cutting the splint out of the thermoplastic.

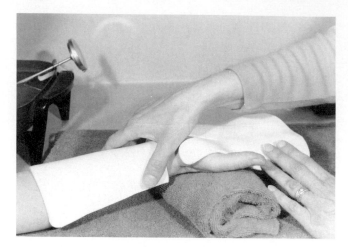

Fig. 24-20. Therapist smoothes thermoplastic over the patient's forearm.

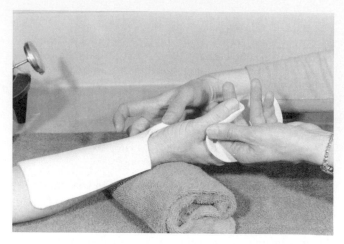

Fig. 24-21. Thumb trough is molded and thenar edge is rolled back.

Practicing

1. The water should be heated to the correct temperature for the specific thermoplastic. The temperature and timing will depend on which thermoplastic is being used. Follow the manufacturer's instructions.

2. Before you mold the splint, take some scrap thermoplastic material and soften it in the pan for a minute or so. Remove it from the pan and blot it gently on the towel. Check the temperature by holding the material against your cheek or forearm. If it is too hot, let it rest for a minute or so. Mold it over your MP joints with smoothing motions. The purpose of this is to get the feel of the material before making the splint.

3. Place the splint pattern on the thermoplastic material and trace around it with the awl. If a pen is used, be careful not to let the pen slip under the paper pattern since ball-point ink cannot be easily removed.

Cutting the pattern out of the thermoplastic

1. To cut the pattern out of the material take the large piece of thermoplastic, and if it is too long to fit in the pan, heat the scrap end first and cut it off.

2. Then heat the thermoplastic to the correct temperature and time until it is uniformly flexible. You can test for flexibility by lifting a corner with the tongue blade.

3. When it is flexible, remove the thermoplastic from the heating pan. Be careful not to suspend it vertically since it can stretch. Gently pat it on the folded towel. Be sure it is cool enough to handle.

4. Supporting the material with one hand, cut out the splint pattern on the marking. Hold the material near the work surface and be careful not to suspend it vertically. Punch a hole at the top end of the cut between the thumb piece and the palm. This reduces stress at this point. Round all the corners. Be very careful not to stretch it in the wrist area where it is narrowest (Fig. 24-19).

MOLDING THE SPLINT

When the pattern is cut out, the material may be setting a little. Reheat it very briefly to soften it enough for molding. Once the thermoplastic is softened, you have about 3 to 5 minutes to mold the splint. It can be reheated to make adjustments, but it is best not to reheat it more than once or twice. Remove the thermoplastic from the heating pan and pat it on the towel. Cool it for a minute or so. Test it for temperature before applying it to your partner's arm.

1. Position the forearm in supination with the hand in the resting position. It is difficult to maintain this position when the forearm is supinated, so while molding the splint, watch that your partner's wrist does not deviate or flex and that the thumb does not drift laterally.

2. Drape the material over your partner's forearm without squeezing it. Smooth proximally over the forearm trough and be careful not to twist it to either side (Fig. 24-20).

3. Place your thumb into the palm of the hand to get the contour of the arch of the hand molded into the splint.

4. Move the thumb into place for the resting position. The pad of the thumb should oppose the pads of the index and middle fingers. The thumb MP and IP joints should be extended, and the CMC in a moderate amount of palmar abduction.

5. When the thumb is in the correct position, you can gently mold the thumb trough around it and hold it lightly with one hand while with the other, you roll back the material around the thenar eminence (Fig. 24-21).

6. Around the hand, flare the sides of the splint material upward to create a little fence around the hand section.

7. Check to see that the wrist is not deviated and that it has remained extended 20° or 30°.

8. Allow the splint to set before removing it from your partner's arm.

Finishing

When the basic molding is completed, put some finishing touches on the splint.

1. First try the splint on and check the length of the forearm trough. Have your partner flex the elbow while wearing the splint. If the trough is too long, the skin will be pinched when the elbow flexes. If this happens, hold the proximal end of the splint vertically in the hot water until it softens, and trim off some length.

2. Then gently flare this end out. This will prevent the proximal end from irritating the forearm.

3. If there are any jagged edges, they may be smoothed by heating the edge in water or by using the heat gun and smoothing the edge carefully with your finger.

APPLYING STRAPS TO THE SPLINT

Supplies

Two pieces of self-adhesive Velcro hook 3 inches (7.6 cm) long, and 3 pieces 1 inch (2.5 cm) long; a piece of Dura Val or Velfoam strapping material about 22 inches (55.8 cm) long; a heat gun; and some thermoplastic solvent.

1. The Velcro is attached to the outside of the splint. One 3-inch (7.6 cm) piece is attached to the proximal end of the splint, and the other just proximal to the wrist. The 1-inch (2.5-cm) pieces are attached on either side of the hand at the level of the proximal phalanges, and one is attached on the under side of the thumb piece (Fig. 24-22).

2. Abrade the finish of the thermoplastic by applying some solvent to the spots where the pieces of Velcro are to be applied, or by scraping the finish off with the scissors blade.

3. Then heat each spot slightly just before applying the Velcro. Before removing the paper backing from the Velcro, briefly warm the adhesive side over the heat gun. Then remove the paper backing and apply the Velcro to the prepared area on the splint. Do this to all four pieces.

4. The straps should be long enough to go over the arm or hand and completely cover the Velcro. Cut one strap to go across the forearm, one for the wrist, one for the hand, and one to go around the thumb. Be sure to position the strap at the wrist so that it does not go directly over the ulna styloid, and on the hand and thumb so that they are not directly over the IP joints.

Evaluation of the Splint (Fig. 24-23)

A goniometer is needed to evaluate the splint. It should be analyzed for fit, function, and appearance. Examine the splint and measure it against the following criteria:

For function

1. Are the arches of the hand maintained? Look at the splinted hand from the front and see if the metacarpal heads are arched. Look at the palmar surface of the splint and see if it has a concave contour. Look at the splinted hand from the side. Is the longitudinal arch preserved?

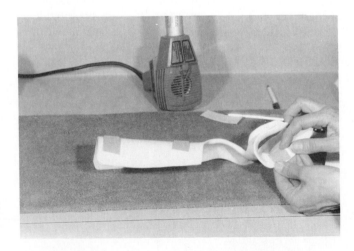

Fig. 24-22. Velcro closures are applied to splint.

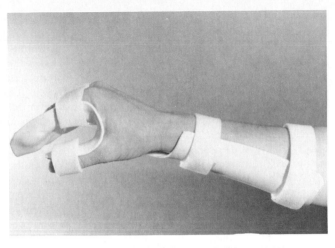

Fig. 24-23. The completed resting splint.

2. Is the hand splinted in the resting position? Is the wrist extended 10° to 30°? Are the MP joints in 20° to 30° of flexion?—and are all of the IP joints slightly flexed? Check to see that the little finger is flexed as much as the others. Is the thumb in palmar abduction?—and is the thumb pad opposed to the pad of the index finger?

For fit

1. Are the straps correctly placed for stability and to avoid pressure points?

2. Do the sides of the forearm trough extend half way around the forearm at all points?

3. Is the thumb trough deep enough and long enough to support the thumb?

4. Does the splint fit loosely enough to prevent pressure areas along the edges and over bony prominences such as the radial styloid? Have your partner wear the splint for 30 minutes and check for reddened areas on the skin!

For appearance

1. Is the splint smooth and free of marks, dents, cuts, and jagged edges?

2. Are all of the corners rounded and the edges smoothed?

3. Are the straps clean and attached in correct alignment?

4. If this splint were prescribed for you, would the appearance be acceptable?

SUMMARY

This chapter presents an overview of normal hand function and basic principles of hand splinting. Instructions for the construction of two hand splints are outlined. This information is intended as an introduction to splinting for the novice, and the reader is referred to the references 2,5-7 for further study of the subject.

REVIEW QUESTIONS

1. What is the role of the occupational therapist in hand splinting?
2. List five assets of the normal hand.
3. Describe the relationship of shoulder, elbow, and wrist function to hand use.
4. Which type of prehension is used to pick up a straight pin?
5. Which type of prehension is used to turn a key in a lock?
6. Which type of grasp is used to hold a tumbler?
7. What is the role and importance of the metacarpal transverse arch in hand function?
8. What happens to hand function if the metacarpal transverse arch is flattened?
9. Describe the nonfunctional position of the hand. Why should this posture be avoided in the paralyzed or injured hand?
10. In which position are the muscles of the hand at the best mechanical advantage to function efficiently?
11. Describe and demonstrate the dual obliquity of the hand. Why is it an important consideration in hand splinting?
12. Compare the tension in flexion and extension between the collateral ligaments of the MP and the IP joints.
13. Name the three nerves that supply sensation and motion to the hand. Which one is most critical to tactile discriminative function? Why?
14. Name three major classifications of splints. Give one example of each.
15. How are the adverse effects of immobilization by splinting best prevented?
16. What is the optimal position for splinting the wrist?
17. What effect does wrist flexion have on hand function?
18. Why is it important to splint the MP joints in some flexion if these joints are to be splinted?
19. What is the optimal position for splinting the thumb?
20. Describe six purposes of splinting.
21. List and describe three limitations of splints.
22. What are the factors that influence the practicability of splint construction by the occupational therapist?
23. Lit six general rules for achieving optimal fit and function of the splint.
24. Describe the purposes of the resting and wrist cock-up splints.

REFERENCES

1. Bender LF: Upper extremity orthotics. In Kottke FJ, Stillwell GK, and Lehmann JF: Krusen's handbook of physical medicine and rehabilitation, ed 3, Philadelphia, 1982, WB Saunders Co.
2. Fess EE, Gettle KS, and Strickland JW: Hand splinting: principles and methods, St Louis, 1987, Times Mirror/Mosby College Publishing.
3. Gribben M: Splinting principles for hand injuries. In Moran CA: Hand rehabilitation, New York, 1986, Churchill Livingstone.
4. Hardy MA: Preserving function in the inflamed and acutely injured hand. In Moran CA, editor: Hand rehabilitation, New York, 1986, Churchill Livingstone.
5. Kiel JH: Basic hand splinting: a pattern designing approach, Boston, 1983, Little, Brown & Co.
6. Malick M: Manual on static hand splinting, vol 1, rev ed, Pittsburgh, 1972, The Harmarville Rehabilitation Center.
7. Malick M: Manual on dynamic hand splinting with thermoplastic materials, Pittsburgh, 1982, The Harmarville Rehabilitation Center.
8. Melvin JL: Rheumatic disease: occupational therapy and rehabilitation, Philadelphia, 1977, FA Davis Co.
9. Principles of hand splinting, Downey, CA, 1962, Occupational Therapy Department, Rancho Los Amigos Hospital. (Unpublished.)
10. Splinting manual, Jamaica Plain, MA, 1972, Occupation Therapy Department, Lemuel Shattuck Hospital. (Unpublished.)
11. Tubiana R: Architecture and functions of the hand. In Tubiana R, Thomine J, and Mackin E: Examination of the hand and upper limb, Philadelphia, 1984, WB Saunders Co.
12. Von Prince K: Orthoplast splint construction, San Jose, CA, 1971, special study, Department of Occupational Therapy, San Jose State College. (Unpublished.)
13. Willis B: The use of orthoplast isoprene splints in the treatment of the acutely burned child: preliminary report, Am J Occup Ther 23:57, 1969.

PART THREE

TREATMENT APPLICATIONS

Chapter

25 Amputations and prosthetics

LORRAINE WILLIAMS PEDRETTI
SHARON PASQUINELLI

Limb loss can result from disease, injury, or congenital causes. Congenital amputees or those whose amputations occurred very early in life grow and develop sensorimotor skills and self-images without the amputated part. The individual who incurs amputation of a part in adolescence or adulthood is confronted with the task of adjusting to the loss of a part that was well-integrated into the body scheme and self-image.

These two types of amputees present somewhat different problems for the rehabilitation worker.[22] This chapter will be limited to discussion of the adult with acquired upper or lower extremity amputations. The preprosthetic and prosthetic training of the upper extremity (UE) amputee is the primary responsibility of the occupational therapist. Controls and use training, and wearing tolerance are important aspects of the occupational therapy program.[22]

Occupational therapy intervention for the lower extremity (LE) amputee includes positioning, basic and advanced activities of daily living (ADL) training, UE exercise, and discharge planning. Psychosocial adjustment, prevocational, and avocational training are integral components of the occupational therapy program.

Physical therapy is usually responsible for the preprosthetic preparation and prosthetic training of the LE amputee. Additional physical therapy management for LE amputees may include exercise, stump and wound care, and the application of physical modalities to promote healing or minimize pain.

Mr. Lawrence L Mott, Director, Central Fabrication and Education Program, OTTO BOCK Orthopedic Industries, Inc, Minneapolis, MN, is gratefully acknowledged for his assistance with this chapter.

ETIOLOGY/INCIDENCE

Amputations may result from trauma, peripheral vascular disease (PVD); peripheral vasospastic diseases such as Buerger's and Raynaud's diseases; chronic infections such as gas gangrene and osteomyelitis; chemical, thermal, or electrical injuries; and malignant tumors. The most common cause of UE amputations in adults is trauma. LE amputations are most frequently the result of peripheral vascular disease, including diabetes.[2]

It is estimated that 1 American in every 300 to 400 has had a major amputation.[4,19] LE amputations occur three times as frequently as those of the UE.[2,19] The incidence of amputation remains fairly constant between the ages of 1 and 15. However, from 15 to 54 years of age there is a gradual increase in incidence due to work related injuries and highway accidents. Over 55 years of age there is a sharp increase in the incidence of LE amputation, which is indicative of the large number of patients with PVD.[2]

SURGICAL MANAGEMENT

The surgeon attempts to preserve as much tissue as possible during the amputation procedure. During and after surgery it is a primary goal to form the stump in a way to maintain maximal function of the remaining tissue and obtain a result that will allow maximal use of the prosthesis.[22] Blood vessels and nerves are severed and allowed to retract so that stump pain is minimized during prosthetic use. Bone beveling is a surgical procedure that smoothes the rough edges and prevents spur development of the remaining bone. Muscles are sutured to the bones distally by a surgical process called "myodesis."[16] In any amputation the muscles involved in the function of the amputated part are affected by the loss.

A closed or open surgical procedure may be performed. The open method allows drainage and minimizes the possibility of infection. The closed method reduces the period of hospitalization but also reduces free drainage and increases the risk of infection. In either case the stump that results must be strong and resilient. It must be possible to fit the prosthesis socket to the stump snugly and comfortably, since the amputee will be exerting much pressure on the stump when using the prosthesis.[22]

SPECIAL CONSIDERATIONS AND PROBLEMS

Several factors and potential problems can affect the outcome of the amputee's rehabilitation. Stump length, skin coverage, stump edema, hypersensitivity, rate of healing, infections, and allergic reactions to the prosthesis are some of the physical problems that can affect the fitting and use of the prosthesis.

Skin

Skin complications account for the major portion of postsurgical problems among amputees. These complications occur in either the preprosthetic or the postprosthetic phase. Delayed healing and extensive skin grafting are complications that occur during the preprosthetic phase. Skin breakdown, ulcers, stump "corns," and infected sebaceous cysts occur in the postprosthetic phase. Stump edema can occur in either phase.

PREPROSTHETIC PHASE. *Delayed healing* of the incision site is one of the earliest preprosthetic complications. This complication is most common among LE amputees who have PVD resulting in compromised circulation. As a result prosthetic fitting is postponed and necrotic areas may develop. If the necrotic area is less than ½ inch (1.3 cm) wide, surgical intervention is not usually necessary. However, when the necrotic area is greater than ½ inch (1.3 cm) wide, surgical closure is indicated.[2]

Immediately following surgery the stump is normally *edematous* as a result of the fluid that has collected within the soft tissues. Swelling is usually most prominent in the distal portion of the stump.[7]

In order to achieve a stump length suitable for prosthetic use the surgeon may perform *extensive skin grafting*. The grafted area can pose a problem in prosthetic use, as adherent grafted skin will not withstand the pressure exerted by the prosthesis. If the skin graft adheres to a bone in the weight-bearing area the grafted area may ulcerate and require a stump revision.[2] Daily massages by the patient and therapist will decrease the adherence of grafts to underlying bones.

POSTPROSTHETIC PHASE. During the postprosthetic phase *skin breakdown* may be caused by an ill-fitting socket or by wrinkles in the stump sock.[8] *Ul-*

ceration of the stump is associated with ischemia and pressure exerted by the prosthesis on the stump.[16] The ulcer is treated by rest, elevation, and hot compresses.[21] If these problems persist, surgical revision of the amputation to a more viable tissue level is needed before further rehabilitation can occur.[16]

Some patients may develop stump "*corns*" similar to those that appear on the foot. The cornified areas may be resected or pared down to minimize discomfort.

Above-knee amputees (AKAs) are predisposed to the development of *sebaceous skin cysts*. These cysts are caused by the torqueing forces between the socket and the stump. When the cyst becomes infected, drainage ensues and enucleation of the cyst wall may be required.

The development of stump *edema* during the postprosthetic phase is usually indicative of an ill-fitting socket. Proximal tightness of the socket may result in distal stump edema. A new, well-fitted socket is the solution.[2]

Sensory Problems

The loss of sensory feedback from the amputated part is one of the major problems that confronts the amputee. The amputee must rely on visual and proprioceptive sensory feedback to control the use and function of the prosthesis. Sensation in the stump is functionally lost when the prosthesis is applied. An ill-fitting socket or a stump that is not well formed at the distal end can cause pain and discomfort when the prosthesis is worn. Besides the loss of normal sensation the amputee must become accustomed to new sensations as well. The pressure of the stump inside the socket and the feeling of the harnessing system must be accommodated.[22] Stump hyperesthesia, neuromas, and phantom sensation or pain are problems that may interfere with use of the prosthesis.

Hyperesthesia of the stump limits functional use. The stump is desensitized by tapping and gentle massage.[8] Sympathetic nerve blocks are sometimes used to medically manage stump hypersensitivity.[21]

A *neuroma* is a small ball of nerve tissue occurring in a stump following amputation. It is caused by excessive growth of axons attempting to reach the distal portion of the stump. As these axons grow into the soft tissue, they turn back on themselves thus producing a ball of nerve tissue. Most neuromas occur 1 to 2 inches (2.5 cm to 5.0 cm) proximal to the stump end and therefore are not troublesome. However, subcutaneous neuromas cause pain when they are pressed or moved.[2] Treatment includes surgical excision or ultrasound. Additionally, the stump socket may be fabricated to accommodate the neuroma.[25]

Phantom sensation is a common experience among amputees. It is the sensation of the presence of the amputated part or a distal portion of it. The phantom sensation may be present for life or may eventually disappear. Phantom sensation does not usually interfere with good prosthetic usage. A much less common phenomenon that can prohibit good use of the prosthesis is phantom pain. In this condition the amputated limb is not only perceived as present but is painful as well.[25]

Surgical revision of the stump is sometimes necessary to alleviate the discomfort. Phantom sensations occur most frequently in crush injuries and are usually felt as distal parts, that is, a hand or foot, rather than the entire extremity. Supportive counseling and early use of the stump with a temporary or permanent prosthesis are effective measures for dealing with phantom sensations.[22] The therapist can allay the patient's fears about these phenomena by offering information, support, and reassurance. Unless the therapist considers these fears an indication of some mental imbalance it is best not to dwell on discussion of phantom sensation but rather to focus on prosthetic training and the advantages of using a prosthesis. The appearance of phantom pain or overconcern with phantom sensation may require the intervention of a psychiatric specialist who may work with the patient or provide advice to the occupational therapist.[25]

Bone and Joint Problems

Joint contractures are common preprosthetic problems among LE amputees.[2] The AKA typically develops an external rotation and abduction contracture of the affected hip. The below-knee amputee (BKA) develops an external rotation and flexion contracture of the hip and a flexion deformity of the knee.[16]

The formation of *bone spurs* is another complication that may occur during the preprosthetic phase. Since most bone spurs are not palpable, an x-ray is needed to confirm their presence or absence. Large bone spurs that cause pain or result in persistent stump drainage require surgical excision.

PSYCHOLOGICAL ADJUSTMENT
Reactions to Amputation

Amputation is likely to be accompanied by a profound psychological shock. Reactions are less severe in patients who have been well-prepared for amputation surgery and more severe in persons who have experienced sudden traumatic injury that causes or necessitates amputation.[5,12]

The reaction to amputation is determined by the amputee's personality, age, cultural background, training, and psychological, social, economic, and vo-

cational resources. Ultimately, the amputee must come to terms with the facts of limb loss, less physical wholeness, and decreased attractiveness. The amputee is confronted with discomfort, inconvenience, expenses, loss of function, increased energy expenditure, and possible curtailment of favored activities. It may be necessary for the amputee to change occupations, deal with social discrimination, and cope with resultant medical problems.[5]

Cultural factors are significant in the reaction to amputation. If the society in which the individual lives tends to have aversive reactions to amputation, the amputee is likely to hold these same feelings. Such attitudes can result in self-hatred and self-deprecation. In some social, cultural, or religious groups, the amputation may be considered a means of punishment or atonement for sin. Such beliefs will affect the patient's reactions and adjustment to the disability.[5]

It is not uncommon for the amputee to feel self-pity, anxiety, shock, grief, depression, anger, frustration, and feelings of futility in response to amputation.[5,12] Older persons may demonstrate postoperative confusion, whereas younger persons may have a sense of mutilation, emasculation, or castration.[5,12]

Shock may be significant when the amputee views the stump for the first time. Later reactions may include fear for the future, panic, and compensatory rage and anger. Grief, self-pity, despair, and suicidal impulses can also occur.

Depression is considered a normal part of the adjustment process after amputation unless it is severe and prolonged. The preexisting personality of the patient determines the severity and duration of the reactions and ultimately the adjustment to the amputation and to prosthetic use.[5]

Facilitating Adjustment

The amputee will need a lot of reassurance during the preoperative, postoperative, and rehabilitative phases of care.[12] In the acute postoperative phase the amputee may have hostile reactions that can be directed to self and the medical team. Caregivers should not respond with counterhostility. The patient's hostility may be masked by oversolicitousness and overfriendliness to the medical team. Involvement in the rehabilitation process and with other amputees enhances the patient's movement toward solving the problems of returning to former life roles. Depression can be reduced with an activity program and medication if necessary.[5]

Adjustment to the prosthesis depends upon the adjustment to the amputation. Loss of a body part necessitates a revision of the body image. The amputee must accept the new body image.[22] The prosthesis can assist with reintegration of the body image, since its presence replaces the missing part in the patient's body image.[5] Such adjustment will have a beneficial effect on prosthetic training, since the amputee must integrate the prosthesis into the body scheme. The prosthesis must become part of the self before it can be used most effectively.[22] The prosthesis is a way to conceal the amputation. This is advantageous, since the prosthesis enhances a more normal appearance and helps the amputee avoid reactions of pity and identify with able-bodied individuals.[5] Difficulties with acceptance of body image change may cause difficulties in prosthetic training.[22]

The amputee experiences many fears about returning to family, social, vocational, and sexual roles. Frequent discussion of fears and possible solutions to real or imagined problems is important to facilitate adjustment. The availability of a similar, successfully rehabilitated amputee to talk to the patient may be very helpful. This may help to decrease fear and encourage emotional expression.[5]

Following a mourning period the amputee may minimize the significance of the amputation and actually joke about it. When this phase of adjustment has subsided, the amputee begins to seriously consider the future. At this point social, vocational, and educational planning should be stressed.[5]

LEVELS OF AMPUTATION AND FUNCTIONAL LOSSES IN THE UPPER EXTREMITY (Fig. 25-1)

The higher the level of amputation the greater the functional loss of the part, and the more the amputee must depend on the prosthesis for function and cosmesis. The higher level amputations require more complex and extensive prostheses and prosthetic training. The more complex prostheses can be more difficult to operate and use effectively.[22]

The shoulder forequarter and shoulder disarticulation (SD) amputations will result in the loss of all arm and hand functions. The short above-elbow (AE) amputation will result in the loss of all hand, wrist, and elbow functions and rotation of the shoulder. The long AE and elbow disarticulation amputations will result in loss of hand, wrist, and elbow functions, but good shoulder function will remain. The short below-elbow (BE) amputation will result in loss of hand and wrist function, forearm pronation and supination, and reduction in the force of elbow flexion. Shoulder function will be intact and good. The long BE amputation will result in loss of hand and wrist function and most of the forearm pronation and supination. Elbow function and force of elbow flexion will be good. The wrist disarticulation will result in complete loss of hand and wrist function and about 50% loss

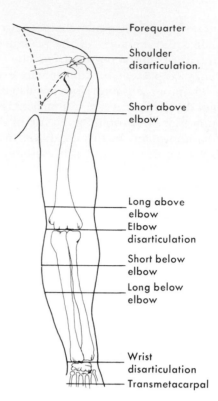

Fig. 25-1. Levels of UE amputation.

of pronation and supination. Amputations below the wrist across the metacarpal bones are called transmetacarpal or partial hand amputations. Functions of all the joints of the arm are intact, and there may be some hand function available, depending on whether the thumb was amputated or left intact.

ACCESSORIES AND COMPONENT PARTS OF THE UE PROSTHESIS (Fig. 25-2)

Many types of prostheses are available for each level of amputation. Each prosthesis is individually prescribed according to the patient's needs and lifestyle and is individually fitted and custom-made.[22]

Terminal Device

Two types of terminal devices (TDs) that are available are the hook and the cosmetic hand. These may be either voluntary-opening or voluntary-closing in design.

The voluntary-opening TD opens when the amputee exerts tension on the control cable, which connects to the "thumb" of the TD. When tension is released, rubber bands, springs, or coils close the fingers of the TD. The voluntary-opening type is the most frequently prescribed.[1,25]

The voluntary-closing TD is also activated when tension is applied to the control cable. The tension

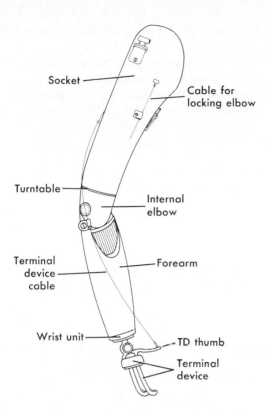

Fig. 25-2. Component parts of standard above-elbow (AE) prosthesis. Adapted from Santschi W, editor: Manual for upper extremity prosthetics, ed 2, Los Angeles, 1958, University of California Press.

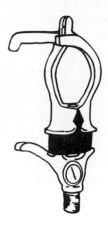

Fig. 25-3. "Farmer's hook," Dorrance model 7, heavy-duty stainless steel.

effects locking and maintaining the grasp forces on the object in the desired position.

The hook TD may be made of aluminum or steel. It may have canted or lyre-shaped fingers and usually has a neoprene lining for the protection of the objects grasped and for the prevention of slippage. It is the most functional and most frequently prescribed and used TD. Several types of hooks are available to meet the individual needs of the amputee. The farmer's and carpenter's hooks allow for ease in handling tools, and narrow-opening hooks may be used for handling fine objects (Fig. 25-3). On the hook TD, the number of rubber bands controls the amount of grasp pressure. Training usually begins with one rubber band, and the number increases to three to four rubber bands as training progresses.

The cosmetic TD, designed to duplicate the amputee's hand as nearly as possible, is available in addition to the hook. One type of cosmetic hand that is used primarily for its appearance is the flesh-colored glove, which covers a partial hand. It may be used to hold light objects or to position objects by pushing or pulling. Another type of cosmetic hand is the functional hand, which may be attached to the wrist unit and activated by the same control cable that operates

the hook. It comes in voluntary-opening and voluntary-closing types. The thumb of the functional hand is prepositioned manually in either of two positions to accommodate small or large objects. The fingers are controlled at the metacarpophalangeal (MP) joints by the prosthesis control cable, and palmar prehension between the thumb and these two fingers is possible through the control system. A natural-looking plastic glove fits over the mechanical hand.[22]

Wrist Unit

The wrist unit joins the TD to the forearm socket. There are three basic types of wrist units. These are the friction, locking, and oval types. The wrist unit allows prepositioning of the TD to accommodate the task to be performed. It serves as a disconnecting unit so that TDs may be interchanged. The locking unit allows wrist flexion by manual operation or with the aid of another object, such as the edge of a table. It is usually used by the bilateral amputee for facilitating activities close to the body. The friction unit requires prepositioning of the TD manually or with the aid of another object. There is a rubber washer in the unit which creates the friction sufficient to hold the TD, as it was prepositioned, against moderate loads.[1,22,25,28]

The oval unit is used with the wrist disarticulation prosthesis. It minimizes the length of the components so that the prosthesis will match the length of the sound arm more closely.

The wrist unit is usually selected for its ability to meet the use needs of the amputee in daily living and vocational activities.[22]

Elbow Unit

The elbow unit on the AE prosthesis allows the maximal range of motion (ROM) possible, locking of the elbow in various degrees of motion, and prepositioning of the prosthesis for arm rotation by a manual control friction turntable unit.

A spring-loading device is available for the elbow unit. This device allows the amputee to preset the spring by winding the device so that the amount of effort needed to flex the elbow is reduced by the assistance of the spring mechanism. The spring tension can be set to different levels by the degree to which the device is wound. The tension is reduced by releasing a small pin. The spring-loading device is helpful for lifting heavy loads and for accommodating a short AE stump.[28]

The BE prosthesis has flexible metal or leather hinges that allow amputees with longer stumps to use the available normal pronation and supination.

A rigid metal hinge with a step-up mechanism is available for the short BE stump. It allows the amputee to achieve a range of elbow flexion which would otherwise not be possible. The forearm socket and TD flex 2° for every 1° of flexion of the stump through this mechanism.

The forearm socket on the AE prosthesis provides the connection between the wrist and elbow units. It contains the wrist unit and TD and is fabricated to fit the arm length requirements of the individual amputee. The forearm lift loop, which allows the amputee to flex the prosthesis forearm, is fastened to this forearm socket.[25]

Upper-arm Cuff

The upper-arm cuff is used on the BE prosthesis to increase stability and control of the prosthesis and to provide an anchor point through which the cable passes to the TD. It prevents the control cable from floating freely and incorporates the elbow hinges to hold the forearm socket to the harness.

Socket

The forearm socket for the BE amputee is made of plastic resins and may have a single or double wall. The socket must be anchored stably on the stump to allow the wearer full power and control of the prosthesis. The BE stump socket may be constructed to allow any remaining pronation and supination to be used. The single wall socket is used when the outside diameter of the distal end of the stump is sufficient to permit tapering to the wrist unit. The double wall socket is used when the stump is too short or slender to achieve the desired contour or tapering. The inner wall conforms to the stump, and the outer wall gives the required length and contour for the forearm replacement. A rotation unit that fastens to the inner socket and rotates inside the outer shell may be used to increase the remaining pronation and supination.

This unit is driven by the forearm stump and has a step-up ratio of 2:1.[22,25]

The AE stump socket is a double wall unit. There is a locking elbow unit laminated onto the socket. The elbow unit provides elbow flexion, extension, and locking at various points on the ROM by the control cable system. The socket must fit snugly and firmly but allow full ROM at the shoulder.[22,25]

Cable and Components

The cable is made of stainless steel and is contained in a flexible stainless steel housing. It is fastened to the prosthesis by a retainer unit made of a base plate and a retainer butterfly or a housing crossbar and a leather loop. A ball or ball swivel fitting at one end of the cable attaches it to the TD while a T bar or hanger fittings at the other end attach it to the harness.[1,20,25]

Harness

The purposes of the harness are to suspend the prosthesis and to provide the anchor point for the control cables. The figure eight Dacron harness is a commonly used design, although others are available. Extra straps may be added to the figure eight as needed.[20,22,25] The higher the level of amputation the more complex the harnessing system. The amount of muscle power and ROM loss may necessitate variations in the harness design. Fig. 25-4 illustrates the lateral and medial aspect of an AE prosthesis.

Stump Sock

A stump sock of knit wool, cotton, or Orlon-Lycra is usually worn by the amputee. It absorbs perspiration and protects from potential discomfort or irritation that could result from direct contact of the skin with the socket of the prosthesis. It accommodates volume change in the stump and aids with fit and comfort of the stump in the socket.[22,38]

THE UE PROSTHETIC TRAINING PROGRAM
Preprosthetic Training

During the period between the amputation and the fitting of the prosthesis the amputee is engaged in a training program designed to promote stump shrinkage, desensitize the stump, maintain ROM of proximal joints, and increase the strength of the stump and proximal muscles. In addition, aiding in adjustment to the loss and achieving independence in self-care are important aspects of the training program.[15,25]

During the preprosthetic period the amputee should be encouraged to use the sound arm to perform activities of daily living (ADL). If the dominant arm was amputated, special training may be required

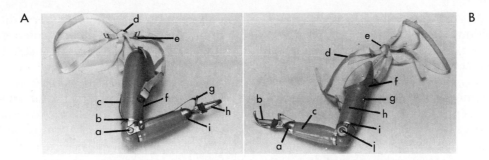

Fig. 25-4. A, Lateral side of AE prosthesis. *a,* Elbow unit. *b,* Turntable. *c,* Control cable. *d,* Harness ring. *e,* Figure harness. *f,* Elbow lock cable. *g,* TD thumb. *h,* Hook TD. *i,* Wrist flexion unit. **B,** Medial side of AE prosthesis. *a,* Wrist unit. *b,* Hook TD. *c,* Forearm. *d,* Harness. *e,* Harness ring. *f,* Control cable. *g,* Baseplate and retainer. *h,* Socket. *i,* Turntable. *j,* Spring-loading device.

for the nondominant limb to assume the dominant role. Practice in writing and activities requiring dexterity and coordination may be helpful in the retraining process.[22,25] Most amputees change dominance to the sound extremity automatically.

During the preprosthetic period the patient may be counseled about the acceptance of the amputation and about the prosthesis and its benefits. It is important for the therapist to be aware of what the amputation and the prosthesis may mean to the patient. It is also important to consider whether the amputee's primary need is function or cosmesis, in selecting the prosthesis and presenting it to the amputee.

With medical approval stump exercises may be commenced. These are designed to encourage use of the stump, maintain ROM of joints proximal to the amputation site, and strengthen muscles of the arm and shoulder. Many of these muscles will ultimately be used to operate the prosthesis, so strength and endurance are the desired results of training.

The loss of weight of the amputated part will cause a shift in the body's center of gravity. Early exercise programs geared toward correcting faulty body mechanics can help to prevent muscular atrophy, scoliosis, and compensatory curves, which can result from this shift in the center of gravity.

The patient is encouraged to move and use the stump as much as possible during the healing period. After complete healing the stump is massaged. This increases circulation, aids with desensitization, reduces swelling, and discourages adhesions from scar tissue. It helps the patient overcome fear of handling the stump.

Stump shrinkage and shaping are effected with Ace bandaging or an elastic stump shrinker sock. The bandage is applied to the stump several times a day, from the distal to the proximal end of the stump. The bandage must be applied smoothly, evenly, and not too tightly[22,25] (Fig. 25-5).

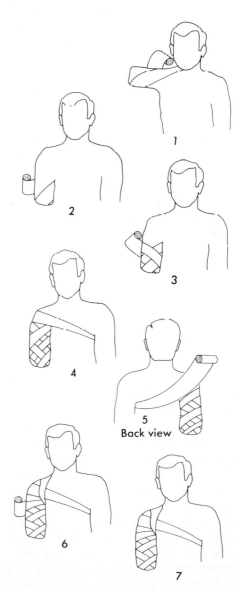

Fig. 25-5. Steps in stump bandaging for AE amputee.

Small utensils may be strapped to the stump to encourage its functional use. A temporary prosthesis fashioned of plaster or leather may be applied to the stump. This enhances early use of the stump for function and helps to accustom the amputee to prosthesis wear and use. Bilateral activities should be encouraged during the preprosthetic period. The early use of a temporary prosthesis may aid in psychological adjustment and increase the possibility of the acceptance and use of the prosthesis by the amputee.

Checkout of the Prosthesis

When the prosthesis is received, it is checked by the members of the rehabilitation team to ensure that it is functioning efficiently, is mechanically sound, and meets prescription requirements. The prosthesis is checked for fit and function against specific mechanical standards that were developed from actual tests on prostheses worn by amputees. Ranges of motion with the prosthesis on and off are compared. Control system function and efficiency, TD opening in various positions, degree of slippage of the socket on the stump under various degrees of load or tension, compression fit and comfort, and force required to flex the forearm are several of the factors that are measured against prescribed standards during the initial checkout.[1,25] The following methods and standards for the prosthesis checkout were adapted primarly from Wellerson.[25]

To perform a prosthetic checkout the therapist needs a spring scale (50 pound, 23 kg); ruler; goniometer; tape measure; masking tape; small woodblock (½ inch by ¾ inch by ½ inch or 1.3 cm by 1.9 cm by 3.8 cm); and three special, short adapter cables to connect the scale to the hook or hand TD and harnessing system; a pencil; and a looped, leather strap.

Checkout of BE Prosthesis

ROM. The therapist checks for range of elbow flexion with the prosthesis off and then when the amputee is wearing the prosthesis. The ROM of elbow flexion should be the same in each case or lacking no less than 10° except if there are joint or muscle limitations.

Pronation and supination of the BE stump are measured by positioning the stump in neutral rotation and marking a vertical line on the end with the skin pencil. The line is used as a point of reference for goniometer placement and reading of ROM. The measurement is repeated while the prosthesis is worn. The TD is positioned in neutral rotation, and the TD thumb can be used as a point of reference for goniometer placement. Forearm rotation with the prosthesis on should be no less than 50% of the rotation possible without the prosthesis. This is true for long BE and wrist

disarticulation amputations. Very short BE stumps will have little usable forearm rotation.

CONTROL SYSTEM EFFICIENCY. The amputee is positioned with the arm at the side and the elbow flexed to 90°. The TD should be in neutral rotation, and the small woodblock is placed between its fingers. The TD should have no less than 3 pounds (1.4 kg) of pressure (three rubber bands on the voluntary-opening type). The cable is then disconnected from the TD, and the spring scale is attached to the terminal device with a special adapter cable. The therapist stands behind the amputee and applies force to the scale in the same direction as force is applied by the regular control cable. The force on the scale is read at the moment that the finger of the TD begins to move away from the woodblock. Three readings are taken, and the cable of the prosthesis is then reconnected to the TD. This cable is then disconnected from the harness at the back, and the spring scale is connected to the proximal end of the control cable by use of a special adapter cable. Once again force is applied to the control cable in its direction of pull, and three readings are taken. If the procedure was done correctly and the mechanism is not faulty, the readings should not deviate from one another by more than ½ pound (0.2 kg). One reading is selected. The control system efficiency is calculated by dividing the force at the cable into the force at the TD. The efficiency should be 70% or better.

$$E = \frac{\text{Force at TD}}{\text{Force at control cable}}$$

TD OPENING AT 90° ELBOW FLEXION. With elbow flexed to 90° the amputee is asked to open the TD fully. The opening is measured with the ruler. The TD should have full opening in this position.

TD OPENING AT MOUTH AND FLY. The TD opening is measured as just described with the TD near the mouth (elbow fully flexed) and again near the fly of the trousers (elbow extended). The amputee should be able to achieve 70% to 100% of TD opening in these two positions.

TENSION STABILITY. The prosthesis is straightened to the side of the body. The scale is hooked over the TD, or the scale is hooked to the leather strap used around the wrist of the cosmetic hand. The stump or stump sock is marked with the skin pencil at the level of the upper rim of the socket. Force is then applied straight down on the scale until it reads 50 pounds (23 kg). The top of the socket pulls away from the pencil mark, and the distance from the pencil mark to the top of the socket is measured. A 50-pound (23-kg) force should not displace the socket more than 1 inch (2.5 cm), nor should it cause failure of any part of the prosthesis or harness. An alternative method is to measure the distance from the medial or lateral epicondyle to a specific point at the top edge of the socket before and during the application of the force.

COMPRESSION FIT AND COMFORT. The amputee flexes the elbow to 90° and places the back of the elbow against a firm support, such as a wall. The therapist holds the TD, pushes the prosthesis toward the wall, and also pushes down on the TD. These forces should cause no discomfort or pain to the amputee. When the prosthesis is removed, there should be no irritation, blisters, abrasions, or signs of pressure.

Checkout of AE Prosthesis

STUMP ROM WITH PROSTHESIS. With the prosthesis on and the elbow locked the amputee is instructed to move the stump (humerus) into shoulder flexion, extension, abduction, and internal and external rotation. The ROM of each of these is measured with a goniometer. Minimal standards for shoulder ROM with the prosthesis on are: flexion, 90°; extension, 30°; abduction, 90°; and rotations, 45°.

FLEXION OF MECHANICAL ELBOW. While the amputee is not wearing the prosthesis, the therapist flexes the mechanical elbow and measures the ROM with the goniometer. The ROM should be at least 135°. The forearm should not be flexed more than 10° when the mechanical elbow is resting in extension.

The amputee is then instructed to put the prosthesis on and actively flex the mechanical elbow. The range of active flexion is measured with the goniometer and should not be less than 135°.

SHOULDER FLEXION REQUIRED TO FLEX THE MECHANICAL ELBOW. While wearing the prosthesis the amputee is instructed to slowly flex the shoulder, flexing the mechanical elbow. With the goniometer the therapist measures the amount of shoulder flexion which is required to fully flex the mechanical elbow. This measurement should not exceed 45°.

FORCE REQUIRED TO FLEX THE ELBOW. While the amputee wears the prosthesis, the therapist tapes the TD closed and makes sure the elbow is unlocked. The therapist than attaches the special cable adapter and the spring scale to the control cable at the point where it attaches to the harness. The therapist supports the forearm in 90° flexion, and the upper arm is stabilized in adduction. The therapist then pulls the scale along the normal line of the cable, slowly releasing the forearm so that it remains at 90°. The therapist continues pulling the spring scale until some further elbow flexion is apparent. The force at the moment of this additional flexion should be noted. The force required to flex the mechanical elbow

should not be more than 10 pounds (4.5 kg).

LIVE LIFT. The therapist tapes the TD closed, and the amputee flexes the forearm to 90° without locking the elbow. The scale is hooked over the prosthesis a distance of 12 inches (30.5 cm) from the axis of the elbow joint. It may be necessary to use the leather loop strap over the prosthesis at the correct distance. The therapist pulls straight down on the scale while the amputee resists the pull. The scale is read when the forearm slips below 90° flexion. It should be possible for the amputee to resist a force of at least 3 pounds (1.4 kg) at 12 inches (30.5 cm) from the elbow axis.

CONTROL SYSTEM EFFICIENCY. The prosthetic elbow is locked, and the control cable should be disconnected from the TD. The spring scale is attached to the hook thumb or the cosmetic hand by the adapter cable. The small woodblock is placed between the fingers of the TD. The therapist stands behind the amputee and pulls on the scale in the same direction as the pull normally exerted by the control cable. The force required to just move the TD away from the woodblock is recorded after three trials. If the procedure was done correctly and the mechanics of the prosthesis are not faulty, the readings on the three trials should not deviate more than ½ pound (0.227 kg) from one another. The cable is then reconnected to the TD.

With the elbow flexed to 90° and locked the control cable is disconnected from the harness at the back. The small woodblock is placed between the fingers of the TD. The scale is attached to the T bar of the control cable by use of a special adapter cable. The humerus is stabilized in adduction at the side of the trunk. The therapist exerts force on the spring scale, pulling in the same direction as the regular control cable. There should be three trials and three readings taken. One reading is selected to designate the force required to open the TD. The control system efficiency should be greater than 50%. This is calculated by dividing the force measured at the cable into the force measured at the TD.

$$E = \frac{\text{Force at TD}}{\text{Force at control cable}}$$

TD OPERATION AT 90° ELBOW FLEXION. The amputee flexes the TD to 90°, locks the elbow, and then actively operates the TD. The therapist measures the TD opening with the ruler. The amputee should obtain full TD opening in this position.

TD OPERATION AT MOUTH AND FLY. The same procedure just described for elbow flexion at 90° is used, except the measurements are taken in full elbow flexion with elbow locked (TD at mouth) and an elbow extension with elbow locked (TD at fly of trousers). The TD opening is measured in both positions, and at least 50% of full opening should be obtained.

INVOLUNTARY ELBOW LOCKING. With the elbow unlocked the amputee is asked to walk a short distance, swinging the prosthesis as in normal arm swing during gait. The therapist faces the amputee and asks him or her to abduct the prosthesis to 60°. There should be normal arm swing during ambulation without elbow locking, and with the arm abducted to 60° the elbow should not lock involuntarily.

MOVEMENT OF THE TD DURING ELBOW LOCKING. The therapist stands directly in front of the amputee and holds the end of a ruler at the lateral aspect of the waist and horizontal to the floor. The amputee is asked to flex the elbow to 90° without locking it and is instructed to hold the TD on top of the ruler, touching the therapist's waist and then actively locking the elbow. The TD should not move more then 6 inches (15.2 cm) from the original position. An alternative method would be to measure with a goniometer the amount of shoulder extension required to lock the TD.

TENSION STABILITY. With the prosthesis extended at the side of the body the elbow is locked. The scale is hooked over the TD, or the leather loop strap may be used around the wrist of the cosmetic hand with the scale hooked to the strap. The stump or stump sock is marked with the skin pencil at the level of the top edge of the socket. The therapist pulls straight down on the scale until it reads 50 pounds (23 kg). The socket should not pull more than 1 inch (2.5 cm) away from the pencil mark, and there should be no failure of any part of the prosthesis or harness. An alternative method is to measure the distance from the acromion to a specific point on the top edge of the socket before and during the application of the force.

FIT AND COMFORT. The amputee flexes the elbow to 90° and locks the elbow, and then is instructed to abduct the stump to 60° and then rotate the humerus. The amputee should be able to control the prosthesis during this motion. The socket should not slip around the stump.

With the forearm flexed to 90° and the elbow locked the scale is hooked over the prosthesis at a distance of 12 inches (30.5 cm) from the axis of the elbow joint. The amputee is instructed to resist the pull of the scale as force is applied from the lateral direction. The procedure is then repeated with the scale positioned on the medial side of the TD and the force applied from a medial direction. It should be possible for the amputee to withstand 2 pounds (0.9 kg) of pull at 12 inches (30.5 cm) in both medial and lateral positions. If the prosthesis has a turntable, it should be adjusted to withstand at least 2 pounds (0.9 kg) of pull.

With elbow flexed to 90° and locked the amputee rests the forearm on a table, and is then instructed to force the stump down into the socket. The elbow is then moved off the table, and the therapist pushes down on the TD and instructs the amputee to resist the push. There should be no pain or discomfort during these maneuvers. When the prosthesis is removed, the stump should not appear discolored or irritated.

The prosthesis checkout also includes a technical inspection of the prosthesis to determine correct length, fit, and mechanical function of all of its parts. Various forms have been devised to record all of the information for the complete checkout of the prosthesis. The initial checkout is done before prosthetic training is started, and the final checkout is done following all revisions and adjustments of the prosthesis and during or following prosthetic training.

Common Considerations in Training

The amputee should be instructed in stump hygiene and care of the stump sock in the early phase of the prosthetic training program. The stump and armpits should be washed daily and blotted dry. Underarm deodorant or deodorant powder should be applied every day. At least six stump socks of cotton, wool, or Orlon-Lycra should be obtained. A clean stump sock should be worn every day. The socks should be washed daily and squeezed out—not wrung—gently. The sock is placed on a flat surface to dry and spread out gently to its original dimension and contours. A T shirt for men and an underblouse for women are recommended for wear under the harness. These will absorb perspiration and protect the skin from irritation in the axillae and across the back. Stump socks and undergarments may need to be changed twice a day in very warm weather.[25,28]

The amputee should learn the names and functions of the parts of the prosthesis. This is important so that the amputee can communicate with the therapist, physician, or prosthetist, using terminology understood by all. It is especially important if the amputee is having difficulties with the prosthesis or if it is in need of repairs. The amputee then is trained in donning and removing the prosthesis with ease.[25,28]

Training the Unilateral BE Amputee

DONNING AND REMOVING THE PROSTHESIS. The amputee dons the stump sock with the sound arm. To apply the prosthesis the amputee places it on a table or bed and pushes the stump between the control cable and Y strap from the medial side into the socket. The harness is placed across the shoulder on the amputated side, and the opposite axilla loop is allowed to dangle down the back. The sound hand reaches around the back and slips into the axilla loop. The amputee then slips into the harness as if putting on a coat. The shoulders are shrugged to shift the harness forward and into the correct position.[1,20,25]

To remove the prosthesis the amputee slips the axilla shoulder strap off on the sound side with the TD and then slips the shoulder strap off on the amputated side. The harness is then slipped off like a coat.[20,25]

CONTROLS TRAINING, TD CONTROL. Scapula abduction and glenohumeral flexion on the amputated side are the motions necessary to operate the TD. The therapist takes the movable finger on the TD and opens it, holding it to show the amputee that the control cable in back is slack. The therapist then pulls the prosthesis forward so that the amputee's shoulder is in a flexed position and releases the TD, asking the amputee to maintain the tension on the control cable (Fig. 25-6). This will hold the TD open. The amputee is then asked to gradually move the shoulder back into extension, releasing the tension on the control cable and allowing the TD to close. The therapist will then hold one hand at the back of the amputee's stump and passively move the humerus into flexion (Fig. 25-7).[1,28] The therapist returns the stump to the neutral position at the amputee's side. During this procedure the amputee watches the TD operate and gains a sense of the tension on the prosthesis control cable. The amputee then repeats the motions without the therapist's assistance and verbalizes the actions that occurred during operation.

This same procedure is repeated, except that scapula abduction is used as the control motion. The therapist stands in front of the amputee and passively draws the shoulders together, rounding the back. The amputee feels and observes the effect of the motion

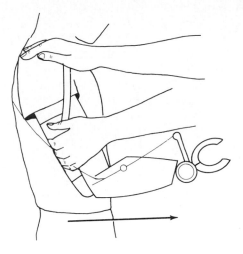

Fig. 25-7. Therapist moves stump forward to attain cable tension and TD opening.

on the TD and repeats the motion actively. This procedure is again repeated, using scapula depression as the control motion. The therapist instructs the amputee to hold the humerus at the side with the elbow extended. The therapist places one hand directly under the TD and asks the amputee to push down and push the hand away. The amputee again feels and observes the effect on the TD and repeats the movements, verbalizing the actions that are occurring.

If the forearm stump is more than 50% of the normal forearm length, pronation and supination should be practiced. The therapist stands behind the amputee and asks him or her to flex the elbow to 90°. The therapist holds the amputee's elbow adducted to the side of the body, and the amputee pronates and supinates the forearm stump, observing the effect on the TD. The amputee then repeats the motion without assistance. The therapist then instructs the amputee to repeat all of these motions in one continuous sequence in both sitting and standing positions until they are smooth and natural.[25]

The amputee will then be instructed to open and close the TD in a variety of ranges of elbow and shoulder motion. TD opening and closing should be accomplished easily with the elbow extended, and at 30°, 45°, 90°, and full elbow flexion, as well as with the arm overhead, down at the side, out to the side, and leaning over to the floor level.[28]

Training the Unilateral AE Amputee

CONTROLS TRAINING, ELBOW FLEXION. After learning to don and remove the prosthesis as just described, the AE amputee is instructed in elbow controls. Learning to flex the mechanical elbow is the first step in the training process. The therapist should protect the amputee's face when teaching elbow flexion

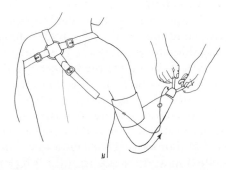

Fig. 25-6. Therapist pulls prosthesis forward, to open TD, asks amputee to maintain tension on control cable, and then releases hands.

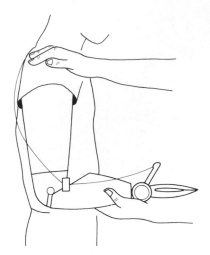

Fig. 25-8. Therapist passively flexes elbow to cause slackening of control cable.

control. The therapist can place a hand in front of the amputee's face or have the amputee place the sound hand in front of the face. This is important because initially the amputee may have poor control over elbow flexion, which could result in the TD hitting the face.[1]

The therapist places one hand on the amputee's shoulder and the other on the forearm. The therapist passively flexes the prosthesis into full elbow flexion for the amputee, noting that the control cable is slackened by this maneuver (Fig. 25-8). The therapist then flexes the amputee's shoulder forward and asks the amputee to hold this position while the therapist releases his or her hands (Fig. 25-9). The amputee gains a sense of the control cable tension across the scapula from this maneuver. The amputee is then asked to relax the stump to the side of the body once again, slowly allowing the forearm to extend (Fig. 25-10). This procedure is repeated by asking the amputee to

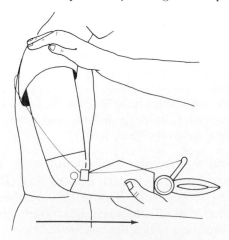

Fig. 25-9. Forearm is moved forward, which causes tension on control cable, to maintain elbow flexion.

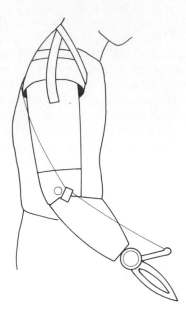

Fig. 25-10. Amputee relaxes stump to allow controlled extension of forearm.

flex the humerus and abduct the scapula to accomplish elbow flexion and relax the stump back slowly into shoulder extension to achieve elbow extension. This is repeated until the amputee gains enough control of cable tension to accomplish elbow flexion and extension smoothly and with ease.[1,28] The therapist should be aware of the possible need for adjustment of the prosthesis and should consult with the prosthetist if this need becomes apparent.

CONTROLS TRAINING, ELBOW LOCKING. The therapist then teaches elbow locking by placing one hand on the amputee's shoulder and the other hand on the TD. The therapist passively pushes the humerus into hyperextension with the elbow flexed thus locking the elbow (Fig. 25-11). The therapist brings the arm back to the neutral position and removes his or her hands from the prosthesis, demonstrating that the elbow mechanism is locked. The therapist repeats this maneuver, demonstrating that the elbow is now unlocked. The amputee is then asked to lock the elbow by moving the humerus into hyperextension and rolling the shoulder forward, using scapular depression and abduction at the same time to lock the elbow. This control motion may be difficult to master. It requires practice and the development of a "proprioceptive memory." The same motions are used to unlock the elbow mechanism. The amputee is then asked to practice locking and unlocking the elbow in various ranges of elbow flexion and extension until full flexion and extension are obtained[1,28] (Fig. 25-12).

TD CONTROL. Once elbow controls have been mastered, TD control training can begin. With the elbow

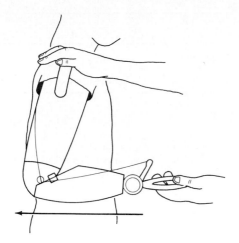

Fig. 25-11. Therapist pushes humerus into hyperextension to lock elbow.

locked the same motions of shoulder flexion and scapula abduction which were used to flex the forearm can now be used to control the TD. The amputee is instructed to lock the elbow, first at 90°, and perform the control motions to open the TD. The sequence of elbow flexion, elbow locking, TD operation, elbow unlocking, and elbow extension is repeated at various points in the range of elbow motion from full extension to full flexion.[1,28]

Once elbow controls are achieved, the therapist should show the amputee how to position the forearm in internal or external rotation. The elbow is flexed to 90°; then the amputee is instructed to rotate the

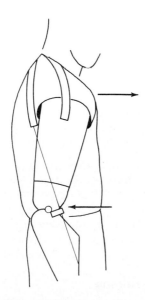

Fig. 25-12. Shoulder is rolled forward, scapula abducted, and humerus hyperextended to lock or unlock elbow at various points in ROM.

forearm to the desired degree of internal or external rotation by passively moving the forearm medially (toward the body) or laterally (away from the body).

Use Training for AE and BE Amputees

PREPOSITIONING. Once controls of the prosthesis are mastered, use training is commenced. The first stage in use training is prepositioning the TD. This involves rotating the TD to the best position to grasp an object or perform a given activity. The BE amputee is instructed to rotate the TD into the desired degree of pronation or supination to accomplish the activity. For the AE amputee this involves flexing and locking the elbow and rotating the turntable to the desired degree of rotation before prepositioning the TD. The goal of prepositioning the TD should be to allow the amputee to approach the object or activity with as near normal a movement as one would with a normal hand and to avoid awkward body movements used to compensate for poor prepositioning.[20]

PREHENSION TRAINING. Along with prepositioning, prehension training should begin, first using large, hard objects such as blocks, cans, and jars, and progressing to soft, then to crushable objects, such as rubber balls, sponges, paper boxes, cones, and paper cups. These objects should be placed at various heights and positions that demand prepositioning and opening and closing the TD, elbow flexion, and locking and unlocking, at various heights.[25,28]

A training board with common household hardware attached or actual hardware found in the training facility may be used as the next step in use training. Items such as a pencil sharpener, door lock, padlock and key, jar and lid, and bottle opener should be used to challenge the amputee.[1,25] The amputee should be encouraged to use a problem-solving approach to these and other tasks to determine the best position for the TD and an appropriate use of the sound arm and the prosthesis in bilateral activities (Table 25-1). The prosthesis should be regarded as an assistive device and not as a primary member.[25]

ADL

Use training should progress to performance of necessary ADL. The amputee is encouraged to analyze and perform the activities of personal hygiene and grooming, dressing, feeding, home management, communication and environmental hardware, avocation, and vocation as independently as possible. The therapist may help the amputee analyze and accomplish a task when needed or aid in task achievement through the use of a special method or gadget or repetitive practice to achieve the desired level of speed and skill.[25]

Table 25-1 Use Training Suggestions for Unilateral UE amputees[20,22,25]

Activity	Suggestion	
	Sound arm	**Prosthesis**
Dressing		
Tie shoes	Use one-handed methods or elastic shoelaces	
	Tie double knot, complete bow	Hold one loop of bow
Tie necktie	Manipulate knot	Hold and stabilize short end of necktie
Don shirt, blouse	Insert in sleeve second, adjust shirt	Insert in sleeve first
Button and unbutton shirt or blouse	Manipulate buttons	Hold fabric taut
Button shirt cuff on sound arm	Hold cuff fabric taut	Button, using amputee buttonhook, if necessary
Don trousers	Tuck in shirt; fasten waist; zip zipper	Hold trousers up; hold bottom of zipper
Hang clothes on hanger	Place hanger in garment and hang in closet	Hold garment
Feeding		
Cut meat	Cut with knife (procedure may be reversed)	Hold fork with handle resting on TD thumb
Butter bread	Hold bread (procedure may be reversed)	Spread butter (TD at neutral, knife stabilized between TD fingers and over thumb)
Fill glass	Hold glass	Turn faucet handle
Open bottle	Open, remove, or unscrew cap	Stabilize carton or bottle
Carry tray	Hold one side of tray	Hold other side of tray, TD in neutral position
Sharpen pencil	Hold pencil	Operate crank
Read book	Turn pages	Hold book
Open envelope	Tear or cut open	Hold envelope
Home management		
Open jar	Unscrew lid	Hold jar
Wash dishes	Hold dish	Hold dish mop or sponge
Dry dishes	Hold dish	Hold towel
Iron	Maneuver iron	Stabilize and adjust garment
Use egg beater	Turn handle	Stabilize beater
Use mop or broom	Guide or push implement	Hold implement
Hammer nail	Use hammer	Hold nail
Hygiene and grooming		
Shave (safety razor)	Insert blade; shave	Hold razor
Apply toothpaste	Hold tube and turn (procedure may be reversed)	Hold cap
Communication and environmental hardware		
Use phone	Dial phone; write message	Hold receiver
Write	Hold pen (if dominant arm); hold paper (if nondominant arm)	Hold pen with TD in 90° pronation (if dominant arm); hold paper (if nondominant arm)
Type	Use one-handed method	Hold typing stick with TD in 90° pronation to operate keys, space bar, and shift key

WORK-RELATED ACTIVITIES. Prevocational evaluation may be included in the use training phase of the rehabilitation of the amputee. The therapist will need to assess the amputee's potential for returning to a former occupation or consider a change of occupation. Work tolerance may need to be improved through the use of increasingly long periods at job samples. Alternate but related occupations may be considered, or training or education for new jobs may

be necessary. Home management skills and child care should be included as part of the amputee's assessment when appropriate to life roles.[22]

Duration of Training

The average adult unilateral BE amputee who is otherwise healthy and well-adjusted will require approximately 5 to 10 hours of training to master control and use of the prosthesis for daily living. The unilateral AE amputee under the same conditions will require approximately 8 to 13 hours of training.[25]

The initial training session should be about 1 hour long, and subsequent sessions should steadily increase in time duration in accordance with the increasing tolerance for the prosthesis, capabilities in use of the prosthesis, and physical endurance for activity until a full day of wear can be tolerated.[25]

When controls training and initial use training are mastered, the amputee is allowed to take the prosthesis home for an overnight trial so that the therapist can check for problems and correct faulty use habits before they become well-established. Use of the prosthesis over the weekend should follow before the amputee makes the prosthesis a part of his regular daily life.[25]

The Myoelectric Prosthesis

The myoelectric prosthesis (Fig. 25-13) uses signals from muscle contraction within the stump to activate a battery-driven motor that operates specific component functions of the prosthesis.[13,23] It is possible to operate the cosmetic hand, wrist rotation, and elbow flexion and extension with myoelectrical controls. Both conventional and myoelectrical controls may be used within the same prosthesis in some instances.[23] This type of prosthesis is cosmetically and functionally superior to a conventional prosthesis and has no harnessing system.[13,14]

Control is based on a philosophy of mimicking natural body motion or function. Contraction of the wrist extensors is used to open the TD, and contraction of the wrist flexors to close it. Pronation and supination are activated by the natural rotation used before amputation. The myoelectric prosthesis allows more accurate control with less energy expenditure as compared with the conventional prosthesis. A greater range of operation around the body allows function over the head and behind the back and neck. The stump does not remain inactive and is healthier because of increased circulation and muscle tone, which results from the muscle contraction. The availability of natural-appearing hands with gloves enhances cosmesis. This prosthesis is more likely to become an integral part of the wearer than the conventional prosthesis.[14]

The first myoelectric prosthesis dates back to 1948 before the era of transistors.[13] Although research was in progress, the first functional myoelectric prosthesis was not shown until 1958 at the Brussels exhibit by the USSR.[14] Early models were controlled by a relatively large external control unit. The device underwent further evolution with the advent of transistors, which enabled the control unit to be integrated into the prosthesis.[13] There are five manufacturers that currently offer components for external-powered or myoelectric systems in the United States. They are: OTTO BOCK Orthopedic Industries, Inc, Hosmer-Dorrance, Liberty Mutual Insurance Co, The University of New Brunswick, and Motion Control, Inc (Utah Artificial Arm). Their systems allow fittings for patients from 2 years old to adults with amputations from below-elbow up to shoulder disarticulation amputation.[14]

The components of the below-elbow myoelectric prosthesis are (1) an intimately fitted forearm socket; (2) surface contact electrodes placed in the proximal end of the socket, lying over the muscles that have been selected to activate the terminal device; (3) a wrist connection unit that can be controlled manually or electrically; (4) a motor located in the terminal device; (5) a battery charger and rechargeable battery; and (6) a terminal device.[13] In some cases the electric hand may be interchangeable with an electric hook style device.[14]

PATIENT SELECTION. Not every amputee is a candidate for a myoelectric prosthesis. Before the prosthesis is prescribed, the level of amputation, limb condition, amount of muscle power, and control of the remaining limb and body are evaluated by a prosthetist to determine the appropriateness of the candidate.[23]

Candidates for myoelectrical prostheses are selected for potential success in mastering control and use of the device. Extrinsic factors essential to success with the myoelectrical prosthesis are the proximity of prosthetist, adequate funding sources, available prosthetic training, and appropriateness of the device to the amputee's vocation.[23]

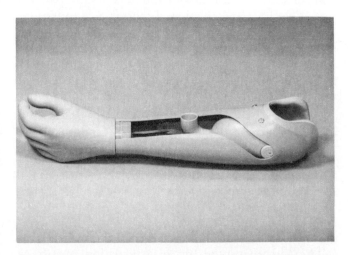

Fig. 25-13. The myoelectric prosthesis. The MYOBOCK prosthesis for long to short amputation level. Closed forearm shell with supracondylar inner socket. Quick disconnect wrist with manual pronation and supination. Reproduced with permission, Otto Bock, Minneapolis, MN.

Intrinsic factors include good intelligence and high motivation. In addition, it must be possible for the amputee to learn to isolate the muscle contractions that are to activate the prosthesis. The amputee must understand that the myoelectric prosthesis will not closely simulate the motor and sensory function of a normal arm and hand. Its capabilities and limitations must be appreciated realistically.[13]

Training

The amputee is initially trained with a myotester that is an electromyographic (EMG) device that measures muscle contraction. Prior to use of the myotester the prosthetist shows the patient the motions necessary to control the prosthesis such as tensing the wrist extensors to activate hand opening and tensing wrist flexors for hand closing. These muscle contractions are practiced with the sound arm and duplicated on the amputated side. After adequate practice, the prosthetist selects the optimal site for electrode placement.[13,14]

The training program is similar to that used with the conventional prosthesis. The amputee is taught the component parts of the prosthesis and stump care. Stump socks are not worn over the area where the surface contact electrodes are placed. The elbow is flexed to 90° to don the prosthesis. It is necessary for the battery to be recharged every night when the prosthesis is not being worn. The socket must be cleaned with a cloth that has been dampened with alcohol every day.[13,14]

Initial training involves repetitive practice of the control motions. When these are mastered, grasp and release of various sized objects are practiced, graded from large to small and from hard to soft. Bilateral ADL are introduced next, followed by work and/or leisure tasks that are among the patient's life roles.[13]

LEVELS OF AMPUTATION AND FUNCTIONAL LOSSES IN THE LE

Hemipelvectomy and hip disarticulation amputations result in loss of the entire lower extremity; thus hip, knee, ankle, and foot functions are lost.[2] AKA and knee disarticulation amputations result in loss of knee, ankle, and foot motion. The stump of the AKA may vary in length from 10 to 12 inches (25.4 cm to 30.5 cm) below the greater trochanter.[16,21] The stump of the BKA is approximately 4 to 6 inches (10.1 cm to 15.2 cm) in length from the tibial plateau.[16,21] Some classification systems further delineate between upper 1/3, middle 1/3, and lower 1/3 above-knee (AK) and below-knee (BK) amputation respectively[16] (Fig. 25-14). The Symes amputation is equivalent to an ankle disarticulation[2] with removal of the medial and lateral

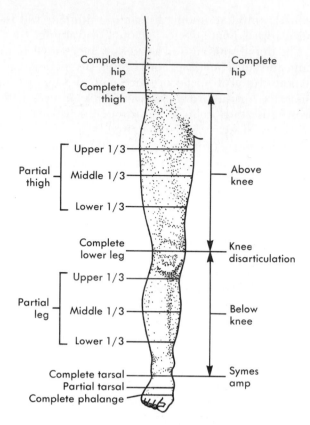

Fig. 25-14. Levels of lower extremity amputation. Comparison of systems for classifying acquired amputations of the lower limb and functional loss at each level. *Left,* System established by the Task Force on Standardization of Prosthetic-Orthotic Terminology. *Right,* Older system. From O'Sullivan SB, Cullen K, and Schmitz T: Physical rehabilitation: evaluation and treatment procedures, Philadelphia, 1981, FA Davis Co.

malleoli and the last inch of the tibia. These patients lose ankle and foot function. Transtarsal amputations are avoided.[2] In a transmetatarsal amputation the foot is severed through the metatarsal bones and ankle function remains intact.[2] Loss of the small toes does not result in functional impairment. Loss of the great toe, however, prevents "toe-off" during ambulation.[24]

ACCESSORIES AND COMPONENT PARTS OF THE LE PROSTHESIS

The major components of the LE prosthesis include a suspension device, a socket, an artificial knee joint, a shin, an ankle joint, and an articulated foot.[19] The type of prosthesis selected depends on the level of amputation and on the individual's needs. Some of the commonly used prostheses are described briefly below.

The Canadian-type hip disarticulation prosthesis meets the needs of the hemipelvectomy and hip disarticulation patient. This prosthesis is suspended from the pelvis and is equipped with hip and knee joints, a shaft, and solid ankle cushioned heel (SACH) foot. Pelvic movements provide energy for limb use.[24]

The AKA benefits from either a suction socket or a conventional above-knee prosthesis. The conventional socket prosthesis is held in place by a silesian bandage or a pelvic belt.[8,17,21] The suction socket is held in place by negative air pressure. Both these prostheses have a quadrilateral-shaped socket, a knee joint that permits flexion and extension, a shank, and a SACH foot.

BKAs use either the patella tendon-bearing (PTB) prosthesis or the standard BK prosthesis. The PTB below-knee prosthesis has a soft socket for the BK stump. It is composed of a strap around the thigh just above the patella[8,17] for suspension, a shank, and the ankle foot assembly.[9] The standard BK prosthesis consists of a thigh corset, lateral hinges for a knee joint, a shin piece, and the ankle foot assembly.

The Symes amputee utilizes the Canadian-type Syme prosthesis or "Plastic Syme." This prosthesis consists of a total contact plastic socket and SACH foot; there is no ankle joint.[24]

Transmetatarsal and toe amputations do not require prostheses. These amputees need a shoe- or toe-filler.[2] Lamb's wool is sometimes used.[24]

MANAGEMENT OF THE LE AMPUTEE
The Rehabilitation Team

Rehabilitation of the LE amputee is best accomplished by a multidisciplinary team.[4,6,17] Following surgery, the patient may be transferred to an amputee center or a rehabilitation facility. The basic rehabilitation team includes the physician, nurse, physical and occupational therapists, prosthetist, and social worker. In some facilities the health care team also includes a vocational counselor, psychologist,[21] discharge planner, dietitian, and recreation therapist.

The physician is responsible for overseeing the patient's medical management. This includes reviewing the patient's past medical history; performing a physical examination; making a complete diagnosis of the patient's present medical problems; providing an account of the surgical procedure; and ordering medications, laboratory studies, and therapies.

In general the nursing staff is responsible for administering medication, monitoring vital signs, caring for the patient during hospitalization, and offering psychological support. The nursing staff is also responsible for wound care, such as daily dressing changes, inspection of the surgical site, and prevention of contractures and bed sores. As the patient progresses, the nursing staff permits the patient to perform self-care skills that have been learned in therapy.

The physical therapist is responsible for evaluating

ROM, strength, sensation, coordination, balance, pain, stump condition, and gait. Depending on the evaluation results a treatment program may include therapeutic exercise, stump and wound care, pain management, and gait training. The physical therapist assists in prosthetic selection and determines the appropriate device for use during ambulation. As the patient's ambulation status progresses, instruction in stair climbing, outdoor ambulation, and floor transfers is provided.

The prosthetist specializes in fabricating artificial limbs. Based on the individual's needs, the prosthetist advises on the selection of the prosthesis and its component parts. "The prosthetist should be able to design innovative prosthetic systems for difficult and unusual cases."[2]

The social worker interviews the patient and the patient's family members to assess the patient's social environment and the patient's psychological functioning since the onset of the disability. Recommendations regarding family problems, housing, and finances are provided. The social worker may be involved with third-party payers and other sources of financing the patient's care.

Occupational therapy may be initiated in the preoperative or postsurgical phases of amputee care. The preoperative visit(s) provides a means of introducing the patient to the proposed postoperative regimen and rehabilitation care plan.[4,16,24] Preoperative training may include a baseline evaluation, exercises to improve cardiovascular endurance and muscle strength, and instruction in postoperative positioning techniques. An explanation of phantom sensation and the methods employed to minimize these sensations should be discussed.[4,24]

OT Evaluation

The first step in the postoperative phase is evaluation. The reader is referred to Part 2 of this text for a detailed description of evaluation principles and procedures.

Knowledge of the patient's medical condition assists the therapist in establishing a treatment plan and in determining the patient's rehabilitation potential. Significant information includes: (1) date and level of amputation, (2) reasons for amputation, (3) whether amputation is associated with disease such as PVD or diabetes, (4) presence of amputation-associated symptoms, and (5) past medical history.[2]

The occupational therapy assessment can be categorized into five major areas: physical, basic ADL, advanced ADL, vocational status, and leisure skills. Components of the physical status evaluation include manual muscle test, range of motion, sensation, pain, edema, stump and skin condition, condition of the remaining leg, and endurance. A basic ADL evaluation assesses bed mobility, wheelchair mobility and parts management, hygiene, dressing, transfers, and balance. Most amputees are dependent in advanced ADL and vocational activities postoperatively. Sedentary leisure interests, however, may be easily performed. When indicated the occupational therapy assessment also includes cognitive, psychological, visual, and perceptual components.

OT Treatment Plan

Basic ADL

Positioning. Prevention of muscle contractures is an immediate postoperative concern.[4] The purpose of positioning is to prevent abduction, flexion, external rotation of the hip, and flexion deformity at the knee.[8,16,24] To prevent hip flexion contractures the patient is encouraged to sleep and rest in the prone position. When prone the patient turns the head toward the unaffected side to avoid flexing the affected hip. Positions that encourage knee and hip flexion, such as prolonged sitting in a bed or chair, are avoided. In supine or sitting positions pillows should not be placed beneath the knee in a BKA, under the stump in an AKA, or between the legs.

BKAs benefit from the use of a stumpboard (Fig. 25-15) or knee extension splint. The stumpboard and knee extension splint keep the knee of the affected extremity passively extended while the amputee is sitting in a regular chair or wheelchair. (The calf pad of an elevated wheelchair legrest may be used temporarily).

Both the BKA and the AKA need a firm sitting surface for pelvic support. As a result of prolonged use wheelchairs develop a hammock-type seat that causes poor sitting and posterior pelvic tilt postures and spinal scoliotic complications. A solid seat insert remediates these problems and prevents secondary low back pain. Hemipelvectomy and hip disarticulation amputees may benefit from the use of a hemipelvectomy wheelchair cushion.

Because the amputee's center of gravity in a sitting position is shifted posteriorly, an amputee wheelchair is needed. The amputee wheelchair is constructed so that the axis of the rear wheels is set back 1⅞ inches (4.7 cm) from that of a standard wheelchair. This axis compensates for the transfer of weight due to limb loss, maintains proper chair balance, and prevents the chair from tipping backward. Antitipping devices for wheelchairs are available. If an amputee wheelchair is not available, an amputee adapter offsets the rear wheels by 2 inches (5.0 cm). A semireclining or reclining wheelchair may temporarily be substituted, as

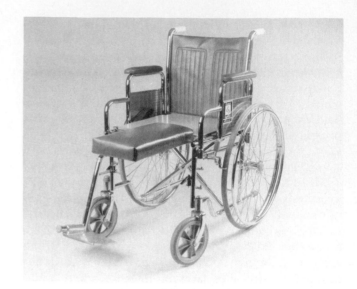

Fig.25-15. The stump board maintains knee extension and prevents flexion deformity. It is fastened to the wheelchair at the back with a Velcro strap, which goes under the seat.

the axes on these wheelchairs are also set back 2 inches (5.0 cm) from a standard wheelchair.[26] For amputee use, the primary disadvantage of reclining wheelchairs is the added weight [approximately 6 to 10 pounds (2.7 to 4.5 kg)] and back height which make wheelchair self-propulsion more difficult.

Stump hygiene. After the wound is healed and the sutures are removed, stump hygiene is initiated. The purpose of stump hygiene is to prevent irritation, injury, and infection. The following basic principles of hygiene are taught until the amputee incorporates them into the daily routine independently.

1. The stump is washed daily with warm water and mild soap. Thorough cleansing prevents a buildup of salt deposits, skin flakes and debris. Use of a medicated soap, such as Phisohex, decreases bacteria count.

2. Rinsing with clean water and thorough towel drying are essential. Soap residue and dampness irritate the skin and facilitate bacterial growth.

3. Skin folds are cleansed with a cotton swab.

4. The patient is instructed in skin inspection techniques. Using a long-handled mirror the patient checks the stump for skin breakdown, blisters, sores, reddened areas, and skin separations or ulcerations. If any of these conditions are observed, the doctor is notified immediately.

5. Application of oils, creams, or alcohol is not recommended. Oils and creams soften the skin, making it difficult to tolerate the prosthesis. Alcohol dries the skin and may cause skin sloughing and breakdown.

Because of the increased demand placed on the unaffected leg, skin inspection techniques and hygiene principles are equally important in maintaining skin integrity of the remaining leg. To prevent skin breakdown and absorb perspiration, a well-fitted shoe and wool sock are recommended. Since geriatric and diabetic patients may have impaired vision, poor eye-hand coordination, and reduced sensation in the foot, callous removal and toenail trimming should be performed by a podiatrist. Thick toenails should be soaked and then cut straight across.

These hygiene principles must be performed indefinitely and on a daily basis for both lower extremities. When the patient is independent in these activities, stump bathing should be carried out in the evening. Evening care is preferred so that the stump is not softened prior to daily prosthetic use. The stump shrinker or Ace wrap is applied after hygiene.

Dressing training. Most LE amputees are independent in all areas of dressing except for hiking pants, donning shoes and socks, tying shoelaces, and donning and doffing the prosthesis. Impaired dynamic standing balance initially interferes with the amputee's ability to stand independently and pull up the pants. LE dressing training may be graded from donning pants in bed to sitting and standing positions. When dressing in bed the patient either rolls from side to side to pull up the garment or bridges while pulling up the pants. LE dressing in sitting and standing positions provides an opportunity to treat impaired dynamic sitting and standing balance.

The diabetic or geriatric amputee may have problems with donning and doffing shoes and socks, as well as tying shoelaces as a result of the impaired sitting balance, vision, or eye-hand coordination which often accompany these conditions. For these deficits, the reader is referred to the dressing techniques described in Chapter 15.

AKAs don the prosthesis in a standing position. The stump is pushed into the socket while steadying the prosthesis against a firm object. The adductor longus tendon fits into the adductor longus tendon groove, and the ischial tuberosity rests on the ischial shelf. The amputee must exert weight into the prosthesis while fastening the suspension apparatus to prevent hip internal rotation and the concomitant gait deviation.[2] If the patient has difficulty with sock wrinkling, the sock is placed in the socket prior to donning the prosthesis.

The BKA dons the prosthesis in a sitting position. Initially the stump is flexed. After the stump enters the socket, the knee is extended. To properly align the stump and socket, the amputee stands and bears weight on the prosthesis.

Bed mobility. The amputee is taught bed mobility activities so that it is possible to move independently in bed without the assistance of an overhead trapeze bar, bed rails, or an electric hospital bed. Rolling from side to side, scooting up and down, and bridging activities are achieved by flexing the hip and knee of the unaffected leg and pushing the foot down into the bed. The upper extremities naturally assist in rolling, scooting, and bridging activities. To sit at the edge of the bed the patient rolls to sidelying; slides the LEs off the bed; and using upper extremity strength, pushes to an upright sitting position.

Wheelchair mobility and parts management. Following surgery the amputee's primary mode of mobility is the wheelchair. Wheelchair propulsion is practiced on level and uneven surfaces, indoors and outdoors, and eventually on ramps and curbs. To propel straight forward the patient places both hands on the hand rims and pushes forward with equal force. If one arm exerts more effort than the other, the wheelchair will not roll straight forward. To make a right turn the patient pulls backward with the right arm and pushes forward with the left. To make a left turn the opposite actions are performed. The unaffected LE uses a walking action to provide control and to guide the wheelchair direction.[27]

An amputee with good bilateral UE strength and endurance can be instructed to manage ramps with inclines less than 10°. As the patient propels up a ramp, the upper body leans slightly forward to accommodate for the gravitational forces that pull backward on the patient and wheelchair. During instruction the occupational therapist stands behind the patient to prevent loss of steering control and/or tipping over backward. If the patient must regularly negotiate ramps a "grade-aid" may be used. The grade-aid prevents backward rolling on an incline. To descend a ramp the patient leans slightly backward. Speed is controlled by gripping the handrims. The wheel brakes are *not* used to slow the descent. Attempting to use the brake for slowing may result in accidental locking. Such an abrupt stop could pitch the wheelchair forward or cause it to veer to one side and tip over sideways.[27] The reader is referred to Chapter 22 for details on curb management.

In order to use a wheelchair safely the amputee is instructed in wheelchair parts management. This may include locking and unlocking the brakes, removing and replacing armrests and legrests, elevating and lowering legrests, and folding the wheelchair for transport.

Transfer training. Unilateral LE amputees use the stand-pivot transfer technique described in Chapter 22. Ninety-degree stand-pivot transfers to the uninvolved side are the safest and easiest to perform. One hundred-eighty degree stand-pivot transfers and ninety-degree stand-pivot transfers to the amputated side are practiced for restrictive environments. When transferring to the toilet and bathtub, the amputee may benefit from adaptive equipment such as toilet rails and tub seats.

Bilateral LE amputees use the sliding board transfers shown in Chapter 22. Another option for transfers is available for those amputees who have a zippered-back or detachable back wheelchair. These accessories allow for transfers to and from the rear of the wheelchair. The patient reverses in, locks the brakes, detaches or unzips the back, and slides backward onto the surface. The patient slides forward to return to the wheelchair.

As the amputee progresses in the gait training program, the occupational therapist supervises practice of ambulating transfers. The ambulation aid and techniques used are recommended by the physical therapist. From sitting to standing the amputee is instructed to use the arms to push up to a standing position before reaching for or using the ambulation aid. From standing to sitting, the amputee is taught to feel the chair with the back of the legs, reach backward with both hands to the arms of the chair or sitting surface, and then sit down.

Bathing. Bathing is a self-care activity that includes dressing and undressing, transferring to and from the shower or tub, and balance activities to reach the faucets and body parts. A survey of 130 amputees found that 55% of the respondents had difficulty bathing and 25% used adaptive bathing equipment.[10] These patients had not received occupational therapy intervention.

Adjunctive Methods and Enabling Activities

EDEMA REDUCTION. Although edema is a normal part of the postsurgical process, an early rehabilitation goal is to reduce edema. If edema persists, it can cause secondary complications such as pain, contractures, and soft tissue adhesions. Edema reduction techniques include Ace wrapping, stump shrinkers or socks, intermittent compression pump therapy, elevation with precautions against increasing hip flexion contractures, and the use of a temporary prosthesis or pylon.

The occupational therapist incorporates Ace wrapping techniques or the use of stump shrinkers into the patient's dressing training program. There are several methods of wrapping stumps; most methods are based on similar principles. These include application of firm pressure distally which decreases as the bandage is applied proximally; application of turns in a slightly oblique angle; and reapplication of the bandage 3 to 4 times a day. "The patient is instructed to bandage himself and instructed to wear the bandage at all times except when the prosthesis is worn."[2] The advantages of Ace wrapping are that it allows for individual contouring and frequent checking of the wound. The disadvantages are that improper wrapping may result in a poorly shaped stump and impairment of blood supply to the distal portion of the stump.[19] Additionally, some individuals have difficulty managing this technique independently. Because of these disadvantages clinicians may choose to use stump shrinkers or shrinker socks.[19] The primary advantage of shrinker socks is that they are easily applied and removed. The shrinker sock is donned as follows: (1) the sock is turned so that the bulky seam at the end is on the outside; (2) the top is turned so that it is folded back on itself about two thirds of the way; (3) the end of the sock is stretched so that it fits smoothly on the end of the stump; and (4) the sock is gently pulled up over the stump.[3] The therapist must instruct the patient to check the fit of the shrinker sock so that wrinkles do not occur and so that the top rim of the sock does not roll over into an elastic band. This would impair circulation and cause distal stump edema. The major disadvantage of the shrinker sock is that it is available in only three sizes.

In addition to controlling edema both of these techniques prevent hemorrhage, promote stump shaping, provide a sense of security, assist in desensitizing the stump, and aid in venous return. Ace bandages and shrinker socks should be washed frequently, rinsed thoroughly, and dried on a flat surface. "A bandage or stump sock that has lost its elasticity should be discarded."[17]

UE EXERCISE AND ENDURANCE ACTIVITIES. On initial evaluation the amputee's strength may well be within the good to normal range. Because of the deconditioning effects of bedrest and surgery, however, amputees require an exercise program to regain the strength and endurance needed for independent basic and advanced ADL. Therapeutic exercise programs serve the multiple goals of strengthening specific muscle groups, conditioning the cardiovascular system, and increasing endurance. Scapular depressors, elbow extensors, and wrist extensors are specifically exercised as these muscles are needed for sit-to-stand activities during transfers and ambulation. Trunk exercises are incorporated into the program for these same reasons. Patients with peripheral vascular disease require close monitoring while exercising to avoid undue fatigue.

Some examples of grading activities for endurance include increasing the number of repetitions of an exercise or activity within the same time allotment, increasing the total time the patient performs the activity, or increasing the distance the patient propels a wheelchair. Wheelchair mobility activities can be graded from level to uneven surfaces as a means of simultaneously providing UE exercise, endurance, and wheelchair mobility training.

BALANCE ACTIVITIES. Good dynamic sitting and standing balance is a basic need of the amputee and a prerequisite to ADL performance. The amputee who lacks good balance will have difficulty with activities such as bending over to bathe the LEs, pulling up pants, reaching into a cupboard, and retrieving an object from the floor. These activities tax the patient's ability by demanding that postural adjustments be made to regain equilibrium. Balance activities that involve reaching in all directions are graded by increasing the reaching radius.

PAIN MANAGEMENT. Successful pain management begins with a thorough physical and psychosocial evaluation. The physical examination includes inspecting the stump for poorly healed areas, neuromas, bone fragments, and abcesses or infection. The psychosocial assessment includes questions regarding the patient's family background, level of education, cooperation, pending lawsuits, description of pain, attitude toward health care, and the family's attitude toward the patient's problem.[2]

There is no strict treatment protocol for patients with phantom limb pain.[2] The physician may treat the pain by injecting anesthetics into the tender area or by using sympathetic nerve blocks. Biofeedback, transcutaneous electrical nerve stimulation (TENS), ultrasound, progressive relaxation exercises, and controlled breathing exercises may assist in reducing chronic stump pain. Many patients find that activities such as rubbing, tapping, and/or applying pressure and heat or cold to the stump provide relief.

Advanced ADL

ENERGY CONSERVATION AND WORK SIMPLIFICATION. Amputees expend more energy during ADL than nonamputees of the same sex, age, and stature.[2] Energy expenditure increases with age and obesity.[19] Several studies suggest that there is a statistically significant correlation between stump length and energy demands.[2] Below-knee amputees average a 10% increase in energy expenditure, whereas AKAs average a 40% increase. For these reasons amputees benefit from instruction in work simplification and energy conservation techniques. The reader is referred to Chapters 27 and 29 for more detail on these techniques.

HOME MANAGEMENT. To live alone at home the amputee must be independent in all basic ADL and in some advanced ADL. Minimally, the amputee must be able to prepare a simple meal and request emergency help if needed. Activities of home management are discussed in Chapter 15.

DRIVING. The ability to drive increases independence and may enhance vocational opportunities. Hand controls and assistive devices are commercially available for UE and LE amputees. They are mounted near the steering wheel in such a manner that they do not impede use of the car by other drivers. Hand control systems are classified into three types: pull-push, right angle-push, and twist-push.

Safe driving requires that the appropriate adaptive equipment be used. An UE amputee benefits from the use of a spinner knob that allows for steering with one hand. Directional signal levers mounted on the steering column may require extensions so that they are accessible to the unaffected UE. Some BKAs have enough kinesthetic awareness to use a gas pedal, clutch, and floor-mounted parking brake. If the sensory feedback is not adequate, the left BKA will need a left-hand-operated clutch and a hand parking brake. The right BKA will require a left foot accelerator. AKAs use the same types of adaptive equipment as below knee amputees since kinesthetic feedback is usually not adequate for driving without assistive devices.

Although the occupaitonal therapist may not be responsible for conducting an on-the-road driving test, the therapist does assess predriving skills. a predriving evaluation may include an assessment of visual acuity, traffic signal recognition, color vision, glare recovery, night vision, peripheral vision, depth perception, reaction time, UE function, trasferring to and from the car, and wheelchair management. When necessary, additional cognitive, visual, and perceptual skills are evaluated.

Upon completion of the predriving evaluation the therapist is responsible for making driving recommendations. These may include treatment for remediation of deficits, referral to a driver education center for driving training and installation of assistive devices, and a statement regarding the patient's potential for safe driving. If the patient is unble to resume driving, the ability to use public transportation should be evaluated by the occupational therapist.

In some states, patients are required to report the amputation to the motor vehicle department and to their insurance company. Failure to do so may result in a noninsured driver.

PREVOCATIONAL AND VOCATIONAL ACTIVITIES. Given a well-fitted prosthesis and a multidisciplinary rehabilitation program, unilateral BKAs usually have a minimal disability and can return to their former jobs. A unilateral AKA may have difficulty performing a job that requires carrying heavy objects and/or standing and walking for extended periods of time. Bilateral LE amputees, on the other hand, need to be employed in a wheelchair-accessible environment and where they can be seated most of the day.[24]

Prevocational and vocational evaluations assist in determining whether the amputee will be able to return to the former job or whether job retraining is needed. Prevocational and vocational assessments may include evaluation of physical capacities, work habits and behaviors, and intellectual abilities needed to perform the job. Performance of real or simulated job tasks may be included. Prevocational training may include job site modification and occupational therapy intervention to remediate the deficits noted upon evaluation. Work evaluation and work hardening are discussed in Chapter 16.

LEISURE ACTIVITIES. Two different surveys of the recreational activities of amputees revealed that approximately 60% of the respondents were active in sports. Fishing and swimming were the most common leisure activities. Sports requiring running, jumping, and walking long distances caused the greatest discomfort and were least frequently enjoyed. Factors limiting recreational activities included excessive perspiration of the residual LE, pain, fatigue, sores, cramping, and swelling.[10,11]

Recreational LE prostheses are available for golfing, swimming, and skiing. Golfers may consider installing a rotator inside the prosthesis. Swimmers often use a waterproof prosthesis. Unilateral LE amputees participate in cross-country skiing without the use of a special prosthesis, as the gliding action of the skis allows them to cover a greater distance than they can negotiate when walking. Unilateral BKAs who do downhill skiing may use a specially designed prosthesis that permits knee flexion. Unilateral AKAs ski downhill on their unaffected leg and attach outrigger miniature skis to their ski poles. This is called the "track three method."[2,11]

SEXUAL ADJUSTMENT. There is a lack of literature regarding sexual adjustment following LE amputation. One study found a statistically significant decrease in frequency of sexual intercourse following amputation. The decreased frequency was greater for males than for females. Men cited less interest as the reason for decreased frequency, and women reported fear of injury. None of the respondents cited "uncomfortable position" as a reason for the decline in frequency. Of the 60 respondents, only 15 discussed sexuality with a health care professional following amputation. The authors concluded that there is a risk of sexual dysfunction following amputation and that sexual counseling should be included in the rehabilitation process.[18]

Discharge Planning

Discharge planning includes family training and provision of a home exercise program and necessary equipment. A home evaluation may be completed in anticipaiton of discharge.

FAMILY TRAINING. Depending on the level of independence achieved by the amputee, the family may need training in some or all aspects of ADL. Frequently family members require training in transfer techniques, wheelchair mobility, and wheelchair parts management. Following instruction and demonstration, family members and the patient should be given the opportunity to perform transfer techniques with the occupational therapist's guidance. If the patient is nonambulatory, instruction in community wheelchair mobility skills such as up and down stairs, ramps, curbs, and on and off elevators is included. Wheelchair parts management and loading the wheelchair into the car are necessary components of family training for the nonambulatory or partially ambulatory patient.

HOME PROGRAM. A home exercise program is developed to maintain the skills acquired during rehabilitation, to prevent regression, and to facilitate further progress. Prior to discharge the patient receives a written copy of the home program and instruction in performing the activities listed. The amputee's home program may include exercises, proper positioning techniques, ADL techniques, energy conservation principles, safety measures, instructions in LE care and wheelchair parts management and maintenance information.

ORDERING EQUIPMENT. The occupational therapist is responsible for ordering all discharge equipment with the exception of ambulation aids. Wheelchairs are ordered for the nonambulatory patient, for assistance with long-distance community mobility, or as a back up for conventional walking aids. In selecting a wheelchair consideration is given to the patient's size, weight, age, prognosis, and proposed wheelchair use. Lightweight and standard weight amputee wheelchairs are available. If a standard wheelchair is used, amputee adapters are needed to maintain proper chair balance. Wraparound armrests, detachable desk armrests, swingaway elevating legrests, pneumatic tires, zipper backs, detachable backs, grade-aid, and reduce-a-width are some of the available options.[27]

Patients whose unilateral LE amputation is a result of PVD have a 33% chance of becoming a bilateral LE amputee within 5 years.[6] If these individuals choose to purchase a wheelchair, detachable armrests may be ordered to allow for the potential consequences of PVD, which will necessitate a sliding board transfer. Wheelchair cushions are available for those individuals who spend prolonged time sitting in the wheelchair. The cushions are designed to minimize presure on bony prominences. Several varieties are available including foam, gel, or air-filled interiors. A wheelchair cushion pressure evaluation may be indicated prior to ordering the cushion.

Most LE amputees find that the use of bathroom equipment provides safety in bathing and toileting. Bath and shower benches permit the patient to bathe independently. Without a bath bench, the amputee has to either transfer to the bottom of the tub or stand while bathing. Grab bars may be affixed to walls or clasped on the side of the tub to aid with transfers and with dynamic balance activities performed while bathing. Soap dishes and towel racks cannot be substituted for grab bars as they are not designed to hold body weight and are easily detached from the wall. A raised toilet seat and/or a toilet versa frame facilitate independent toilet transfers. If the bathroom is inaccessible, a commode chair and alternate bathing arrangement are indicated.

HOME VISIT. The home evaluation or an extensive verbal environmental assessment assists the occupational therapist in determining whether or not structural modifications are required. When stairs render the home inaccessible, a ramp is needed. The preferred gradient is 1 foot (30 cm) of length for each inch (2.5 cm) of rise. The ramp width needs to allow for unobstructed wheelchair maneuvering. Ramp landings approximately 2 feet × 5 feet (6.0 cm × 150 cm) are needed to accommodate the wheelchair and swing doors.[2]

The home environment will influence wheelchair width and the type of transfer used at home. To pass through a doorway a wheelchair needs a minimal clearance of 2 feet and 6 inches (75 cm). To self-propel a wheelchair in a hallway, a minimum of 3 feet and 2 inches (95 cm) is needed. Minor home modifications can be made to improve safety. These include removing scatter rugs and electrical cords and removing casters on furniture to improve stability during transfers. Wooden bed or chair blocks can be made to increase height and ease transfers.[2]

SUMMARY

Acquired UE and LE amputations can occur as a result of trauma, infection, neoplasms, electrical or thermal injuries, and vascular diseases. Occupational therapists play an important role in the rehabilitation of the amputee.

In the rehabilitation of the UE amputee, the occupational therapist addresses stump conditioning and care, preprosthetic exercise, and prosthetic training. Independent management of ADL and resumption of work and leisure roles are the desired outcomes of occupational therapy intervention for the UE amputee.

Occupational therapy for the LE amputee includes stump positioning, ADL training, UE strengthening, and functional use of the prosthesis in daily activities. Evaluation and training for resumption of work and leisure roles are also part of the occupational therapy program for the LE amputee. Facilitating psychosocial adjustment to limb loss is an integral part of occupational therapy for both UE and LE amputees.

REVIEW QUESTIONS
1. What do the following abbreviations mean?
   a. AE
   b. TD
   c. BE
2. Which arm function is lost and which functions are maintained in a long BE amputation?
3. Name two common problems of amputees can interfere with prosthetic training. How is each solved?
4. What are the purposes of preprosthetic training?
5. Describe activities and exercises suitable for the preprosthetic period.
6. List the five major steps in prosthetic training.
7. What is the sequence of training in learning controls of the AE prosthesis?
8. What is the sequence of training in learning use of the prosthesis?
9. What motion of the arm accomplishes elbow lockig on the AE prosthesis?
10. Before an AE amputee can operate the TD, what must he do?
11. What motions accomplish TD opening?
12. How is the TD prepositioned by the amputee?
13. Name two types of TDs. Which is more frequently prescribed and used?
14. How is use training graded?
15. When is the proper time for the amputee in a prosthetic training program to take his prosthesis home?
16. The best position for the TD when holding a coffee cup is at _____ ° _____.
17. When using an eggbeater the ____ holds the top of the beater while the _____ cranks the handle.
18. What is the most common cause of LE amputation?
19. Describe the desired positioning for the LE stump following amputation surgery.
20. List three methods for reducing edema in the LE stump.
21. What method can be used to teach the LE amputee to don pants in bed?

22. How is the LE amputee evaluated for driving? What role can the occupational therapist play in this evaluation?
23. Describe some of the home adaptations that can be made to increase safety and independence for the LE amputee?

REFERENCES

1. Anderson MH, Bechtol CO, and Sollars RE: Clinical prosthetics for physicians and therapists, Springfield, IL, 1959, Charles C Thomas.
2. Banerjee SJ: Rehabilitation management of amputees, Baltimore, 1982, Williams and Wilkins.
3. Borcich D, Beukma L, and Olves T: Amputee care: a handout for patients with below knee amputations, Stanford, CA, 1986, Department of Physical and Occupational Therapy, Stanford University Hospital. (Unpublished.)
4. Engstrand JL: Rehabilitation of the patient with a lower extremity amputation, Nurs Clin North Am 11:4, 1976.
5. Friedman LW: The psychological rehabilitation of the amputee, Springfield, IL, 1978, Charles C Thomas.
6. Goldberg RT: New trends in the rehabilitation of lower extremity amputees, Rehabil Lit 45:2, 1984.
7. Hill SL: Interventions for the elderly amputee, Rehabil Nurs 10:23, 1985.
8. Hirschberg G, Lewis L, and Thomas D: Rehabilitation, Philadelphia, 1964, JB Lippincott Co.
9. Kathrins RJ: Lower extremity amputations.In Logigian MK, editor: Adult rehabilitation: a team approach for therapists, Boston, 1982, Little, Brown & Co.
10. Kegel B, Carpenter ML, and Burgess EM: Functional capabilities of lower extremity amputees, Arch Phys Med Rehabil 59:109, March 1978.
11. Kegel B, Webster J and Burgess EM: Recreational activities of lower extremity amputees: a survey, Arch Phys Med Rehabil 61:258, June 1980.
12. Larson CB and Gould M: Orthopedic nursing, ed 8, St Louis, 1974, CV Mosby Co.
13. Maiorano LM and Hunter JM: Myoelectric prosthesis: prescription and training. In Hunter JM, et al editors: Rehabilitation of the hand, St Louis, 1984, CV Mosby Co.
14. Mott LL: Personal communication, July 6, 1988.
15. Olivett BL: Management and prosthetic training of the adult amputee. In Hunter JM, et al, editors: Rehabilitation of the hand, St Louis, 1984, CV Mosby Co.
16. O'Sullivan S, Cullen K, and Schmitz T: Physical rehabilitation: evaluation and treatment procedures, Philadelphia, 1981, FA Davis Co.
17. Palmer ML and Toms JE: Manual for functional training, ed 3, Philadelphia, 1982, FA Davis Co.
18. Reinstein L, Ashley J, and Miller KH: Sexual adjustment after lower extremity amputation, Arch Phys Med Rehabil 59:501, November 1978.
19. Rusk H and Taylor E: Rehabilitation medicine: a textbook of physical medicine and rehabilitation, ed 2, St Louis, 1964, CV Mosby Co.
20. Santschi WR editor: Manual of upper extremity prosthetics, ed 2, Los Angeles, 1958, University of California Press.
21. Shands A, Raney R, and Brashear H: Handbook of orthopaedic surgery, ed 2, St Louis, 1963, CV Mosby Co.
22. Spencer EA: Amputations. In Hopkins HL and Smith HD, editors: Willard and Spackman's occupational therapy, ed 5, Philadelphia, 1978, JB Lippincott Co.
23. Spencer EA: Functional restoration: amputations and prosthetic replacement. In Hopkins HL and Smith HD, editors: Willard and Spackman's occupational therapy, ed 7, Philadelphia, 1988, JB Lippincott Co.
24. Stoner EK: Management of the lower extremity amputee. In Kottke FJ, Stillwell GK, and Lehmann JF: Krusen's handbook of physical medicine and rehabilitation, ed 3, Philadelphia, 1982, WB Saunders Co.
25. Wellerson TL: A manual for occupational therapists on the rehabilitation of upper extremity amputees, Dubuque, IA, 1958, Wm C Brown Co, Publishers.
26. Wheelchair prescription booklet no. 3: Safety and handling, Camarillo, CA, 1983, Everest & Jennings, Inc.
27. Wheelchair catalog, Camarillo, CA, 1980, Everest & Jennings, Inc.
28. Wright G: Controls training for the upper extremity amputee (film), San Jose, CA, Instructional Resources Center, San Jose State University.

Sample treatment plan

CASE STUDY

Mr. K is 41 years old. He is a member of a minority group and has lived in poverty all of his life. He is intellectually limited, although some of this may be a result of a poor educational advantage. Mr. K recently sustained a left AE amputation because of a traumatic injury. The stump is well healed, and there is good stump shrinkage. There are no medical complications.

Mr. K is receiving state aid, and a prosthesis and vocational training have been authorized for him. He has done janitorial work and tobacco picking in the past. He reads the basic vocabulary necessary for everyday life at home and in the street (for example, signs and simple newspaper headlines). When employed Mr K is a steady and hard worker. He is married and has four children, all living at home. His interests are watching television, playing cards, and light gardening.

The client is accepting the prosthesis and is no longer depressed about the loss of his arm. Strength in the stump musculature is good to normal. He was referred to occupational therapy as an outpatient for prosthetic training and vocational evaluation. He will be scheduled for daily treatment sessions.

Personal data

Name: Mr. K
Age: 41
Diagnosis: Traumatic injury to left arm
Disability: Left AE amputation
Treatment aims as stated in referral:
Prosthetic training
Vocational evaluation

OTHER SERVICES

Medical
Social service
Vocational counseling
Sheltered employment and community social groups
(possibly)

EVALUATION SUMMARY

Frame of reference/treatment approaches
Occupational performance
Biomechanical and rehabilitative approaches

OT EVALUATION

Performance components

Motor
    Strength: Manual muscle test to muscles of stump
    Active and Passive ROM: Left shoulder, test
    Physical endurance: Observe
    Manual dexterity, unilateral: Observe
    Speed of movement and motor planning skill: Observe
Sensory integrative
    Sensation (touch, pain, temperature) of end of stump: Test
    Pain: Observe
Cognitive/psychological
    Judgment: Observe

Problem-solving skills: Observe
    Language skills: Observe
Adjustment to disability: Observe
Social
    Dyadic and group interaction skills: Observe

Performance skills

Potential work skills: Observe, test
Work habits and attitudes: Observe
Self-care independence: Test, observe
Independent travel: Observe or test
Leisure interests/activities: Interview

EVALUATION SUMMARY

Muscle test of Mr. K's stump musculature revealed grades of N(5) in shoulder flexors, extensors, and abductors. Grades of G(4) were noted for shoulder rotators and adductors. Active and passive ROM for all shoulder motions are within normal limits. Sensory modalities of touch, pain, and temperature are intact in the stump. There is no stump pain. Physical endurance for light to moderate activity is adequate for a full day's work. Mr. K will need some additional practice in one-handed skills to improve right-handed manual dexterity.

Mr. K's reading skills are limited, and he cannot follow written directions. He needs assistance with problem solving but succeeds with some verbal guidance. The patient tends to be quiet, cooperative, and compliant. He socializes when drawn into group interaction but is somewhat hesitant and shy in interactions with the therapist. He appears to be well-motivated for the prosthesis and for return to employment.

Mr. K is performing most self-care activities independently, using the sound right arm, except for bilateral activities, such as cutting meat, buttoning the shirt, applying deodorant, carrying large objects, and tying shoes. He needs some assistance in analyzing methods for one-handed performance.

There is good potential for performance of unskilled work similar to that done in the past. Janitorial or assembly work and simple use of tools will be part of the last phases of the prosthetic use training program.

ASSETS

Good use of right arm
Motivated to use prosthesis
Motivated to return to work
Cooperative
Family support
Positive adjustment to limb loss

PROBLEM LIST

1. Muscle weakness
2. Limited literacy and problem-solving skills
3. ADL dependence
4. Loss of role as family provider
5. Inability to use AE prosthesis

Continued.

Sample treatment plan—cont'd

TREATMENT PLAN

PROBLEM 1

Muscle weakness

Objective

Strength of shoulder rotators and adductors will increase from good to normal

Method

Progressive resistive exercise (PRE) to shoulder adductors, using wall pulleys; PRE to shoulder rotators, using weighted cuffs on stump; client holds stump in 90° shoulder flexion, then 90° shoulder abduction and rotates shoulder internally and externally

Gradation

Increase resistance by adding weight; increase number of repetitions from 10 to 30 per day

PROBLEM 3

ADL dependence

Objective

Achieve proficiency in stump care within the first week of the treatment program, so that stump care is carried out independently on a daily basis at home

Method

Washing and drying stump; application and removal of stump socks; washing out stump socks; daily change of stump socks

Gradation

Decrease amount of direction and assistance as proficiency is achieved

PROBLEM 5

Inability to use AE prosthesis

Objective

To know the names and functions of all the parts of the prosthesis by the end of the first week of training

To put on and remove the prosthesis smoothly and efficiently within 5 minutes

Achieve proficiency in controls of elbow flexion, elbow locking, and TD opening and closing, so that each control motion is performed when needed with little or no hesitation

Method

Review names and functions of parts of prosthesis; review repetitively

Repetitive application and removal of prothesis for practice.

Practice in elbow flexion control, elbow locking, and TD opening and closing; practice in performing these tasks in sequence

Gradation

Decrease repetitions

Decrease amount of supervision and assistance

Decrease assistance and direction; increase time spent in training sessions and wearing

PROBLEMS 5,2

Inability to use prosthesis, limited problem-solving skill

Objective

To preposition the TD when using practice objects, so that he can preposition the TD and pick up 75% of the objects with little or no hesitation

Method

Grasp and release of objects of various weights, textures, sizes, and shapes in a variety of positions, for example, cans, jars, wood cylinders, blocks, pencils, door knob, and cabinet handles

Gradation

Hard to soft objects; large to small objects; progress from table surface to grasp and release at side, overhead, and on floor

PROBLEMS 3,2

ADL dependence, limited problem-solving skill

Objective

Achieve moderate skill in performance of bilateral ADL, so that he is performing 75% of these activities independently at home

Method

Fasten trousers; handle wallet; tie shoes; clean fingernails; apply deodorant; tie necktie; button shirt; use phone; cut food. Cue patient to analyze best use for prosthesis and best role for sound arm in each activity.

Gradation

Simple to complex activities client is expected to perform; decrease amount of supervision and assistance

PROBLEMS 4,2

Loss of vocational role, limited problem-solving skill

Objective

Evaluate potential for employment so that specific information about potential work skills, work habits and attitudes, and work tolerance can be conveyed to the vocational counselor

Method

Janitorial work—floor cleaning, emptying trash

Assembly jobs—electronic parts assembly

Use of hand tools in light woodwork, such as sawing, hammering, drilling, using a screwdriver, planing, and sanding. Cue patient to analyze best use for prosthesis and sound arm in bilateral work activities.

Gradation

Increase complexity, speed, and duration at work tasks; and amount of manipulation required of prosthesis; decrease amount of instruction and supervision

26 Burns

SHIRLEY W. CHAN
LORRAINE WILLIAMS PEDRETTI

The skin is the largest organ of the body and primarily functions as an environmental barrier. It prevents foreign organisms from invading the body, reduces loss of essential body fluids, assists in control of body temperature, regulates heat loss, and serves as a sensory organ. Anatomically the skin consists of two layers: the epidermis, a nonvascular layer made up of epidermal cells, and the dermis, a network of capillaries, sweat glands, sebaceous glands, nerve endings, and hair follicles.[4]

In a burn injury the skin and possibly the underlying structures are damaged, causing a destruction of the environmental barrier. It is one of the most severe forms of trauma to the body, and it can be a life-threatening injury in severe cases.

Burns are categorized as thermal, chemical, and electrical. Thermal injuries can be caused by flame, steam, hot liquid, hot metals, and extreme cold.[4] The extent and severity of the injury depend on the amount of skin surface area involved and the depth of the burn. Although burns are often accidental, it is known that children, the elderly, the physically handicapped, and the mentally unstable are high-risk groups.

Possible disabilities that can result from a burn injury include (1) loss of joint motion because of contractures of scar tissue or heterotopic ossification; (2) loss of muscle strength caused by disuse or nerve involvement; (3) loss of sensation resulting from destruction of the sense receptors in the skin or concomitant nerve damage; (4) loss of body parts, especially common to fingers; (5) disfigurement; and (6) associated injuries, such as loss of vision, neurovascular damage, and fractures.

MEDICAL MANAGEMENT

Following the burn injury the extent and depth of the burn must be medically evaluated to determine

Treatment procedures described in this chapter are modeled after those used at the Bothin Burn Center of Saint Francis Memorial Hospital, San Francisco.

its severity. The patient's age, general health, past medical history, part of the body involved, and other associated injuries are important factors in determining the severity of the burn injury.[8]

The percentage of the burn surface area is usually measured by the rule of nines in persons over 16 years of age. The measurements are modified for children to accommodate the difference in proportion of limbs to trunk to head. The rule of nines is used to estimate the total body surface area (TBSA) that has been injured. It divides the body surface into areas of 9% or multiples of 9%[8] (Fig. 26-1).

The depth of the burn is measured by degrees or thickness of the skin injured. This is determined primarily by appearance of the wound and the presence of sensation, such as pain.[4] With a first-degree burn, such as a sunburn, only the epidermis is involved and damage is minimal. The wound is quite painful, characteristically erythematous and dry but without vesicles. It usually heals by itself in 1 week without scarring. Treatment usually consists of minor measures to relieve discomfort and prevent infection.[1]

With a second-degree burn, also referred to as "partial thickness burn,"[8] the epidermis and some portion of the dermis is injured. These burns may be superficial or deep depending on the thickness of the dermis involved. The wound is painful, erythematous, possibly exudative with vesicles, and there is subcutaneous edema.[1,8] Healing occurs as a result of regeneration from epithelium-lined skin appendages, which are the hair follicles and sebaceous and sweat glands. A superficial second-degree wound will epithelialize in about 10 to 14 days without scarring. A deep second-degree wound requires 3 to 4 weeks to epithelialize and may require skin grafting. Scarring will occur, and if the burn is over a joint, contracture may also develop. Infection can convert the second-degree burn to a third-degree burn.[1]

The third-degree burn, or full thickness burn, destroys the entire epidermis and dermis down to the subcutaneous tissue.[1] There may be muscle, tendon, or bone damage as well,[8] which is sometimes referred

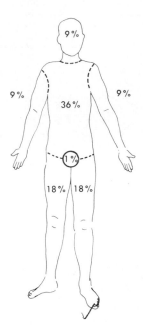

Fig. 26-1. Rules of nines.

to as a "fourth-degree burn." The burn is not painful, since all nerve endings have been destroyed. The wound is leathery and can be pearly white or charred with considerable subcutaneous edema.[4] Spontaneous healing is not possible, and regeneration of the epidermis is only at the margins of the wound. Skin grafting is required to promote wound healing and minimize scarring and contracture.[1]

Psychosocial Factors

The burn injury can result in serious psychosocial problems that the rehabilitation team should be aware of and deal with in their treatment of the patient. These include depression and withdrawal; adverse reactions to disfigurement; anxiety and uncertainty about the ability to resume work, family, community, and leisure roles; financial difficulties; and concern about being accepted by family and friends.

A major burn and its associated treatment is extremely stressful to the patient, the family, and the treatment staff. During the period of hospitalization the patient is confronted with isolation, dependency, pain, monotony, and threatened identity.[12] Anger, fear of deformity, and depression can influence the recovery of the burn patient.[6]

Members of the treatment team must subject the patient to activities and procedures that produce discomfort and pain. Consequently, they may be subject to hostility and abuse by the patient and/or the family members. This is stressful to the staff, and they often need support to continue with work in this specialty area. Following hospitalization the patient is subject

to curiosity and perhaps even hostility and aversive responses from other persons.[12]

The adjustment of the burn patient can be facilitated by providing emotional support, supplying patient education, confronting problems, and helping the patient to develop coping mechanisms and self-directedness. Self-esteem can be maintained or improved by involving the patient in setting goals and planning treatment.[6]

A comprehensive patient education program that incorporates information about the physical, psychological, and social components of burn injury can facilitate patient cooperation and adjustment to the injury. Occupational therapists are well-qualified to present patient education programs because of their holistic training and approach. Educational methods must be geared to the patient's needs and level of understanding.[6]

COURSE OF RECOVERY

The course of recovery from a burn injury can be divided into three phases: (1) shock or emergent phase; (2) acute or infection phase; and (3) rehabilitation phase.[1,4]

Shock Phase

The shock phase is the first 2 to 3 days immediately after the injury. During this period there is increased permeability of blood vessels, causing rapid leakage of protein-rich fluid to extravascular tissue thus resulting in intravascular hypovolemia.[1,8,9] The lymphatic system, which would normally carry away the excess fluid in the tissues, becomes overloaded,[8] causing subcutaneous edema. Fluid resuscitation, using intravenous fluid, such as Ringer's lactate solution, is extremely essential in this phase to replace venous fluid and electrolytes.[9]

The fluid volume required is determined by various formulas, such as Parkland and modified Brook formulas and is based on the extent of the burn and the weight of the patient.[1,8] The rate of fluid infusion is monitored by pulse rate, urinary output, central venous pressure, hematocrit, and state of consciousness.

In the case of circumferential full thickness burns, the edema can produce a rise in interstitial pressure sufficient to impair capillary filling of the distal portion of the extremity, causing limb ischemia.[4] Escharotomy, or incision of the eschar (necrotic tissue), is performed to relieve such pressure and is usually painless because of the destroyed nerve endings. In deep wounds a fasciotomy or an incision down to the fascia is occasionally needed for adequate pressure relief.

Inhalation injury is a common secondary diagnosis

with thermal injury, especially in facial burns, and is a major cause of mortality in burn patients. When there is objective evidence of inhalation injury, bronchoscopy, arterial blood gas, and chest x-ray examinations are used to confirm the diagnosis. Treatment usually includes giving the patient high flow oxygen and intravenous steroids. Nasotracheal intubation and ventilatory support may be required along with vigorous respiratory therapy and nasotracheal suctioning. A tracheostomy is generally not performed unless absolutely necessary.[17]

Daily hydrotherapy is carried out in the Hubbard tank or tub to allow thorough cleansing of the wound as well as the uninvolved areas and to allow a total assessment of the wound and enable exercising without restriction of dressings.[4] Debridement may be initiated to remove debris and loose epidermis. Topical and systemic antibiotic therapy may also be initiated.[1]

Acute Phase

The acute phase follows immediately after the shock phase and continues until the burn wounds are nearly healed. During this period vulnerability to wound infection, sepsis, and septic shock is especially great, and treatment is focused on promoting healing and minimizing infection. Burn wound colonization begins at the moment of injury, and by the fourth day the normal bacterial flora can be replaced by gram-negative organisms, such as *Pseudomonus aeruginosa*, which lives on dead tissue.[1,16] Wound cultures and biopsies are routinely performed to monitor the severity of the infection, since it can convert into sepsis when there is systemic bacterial penetration.[9] Septic shock is a state of circulatory collapse, a cardiovascular response to bacteria and their by-products (endotoxins), and the result can be fatal. The syndrome is characterized by ischemia, diminished urine output, tachycardia, hypotension, tachypnea, hypothermia, disorientation, or coma.[1]

Infection is treated with topical and systemic antibiotics. Some of the commonly used topical antibiotics are silver sulfadiazine cream, povidone-iodine, polymyxin B sulfate, Neosporin, and mafenide acetate (Sulfamylon cream).

Debridement is also carried out to remove eschar and can be done chemically using topical ointments, such as proteolytic enzymes (Travase and Collagenase), which act enzymatically to digest dead tissue, or mechanically with forceps, scissors, and dressings, or surgically.

Eschar must be completely removed to allow healing and for skin grafting to be successful. There are three types of skin grafts: (1) xenograft, (2) homograft, and (3) autograft. A xenograft or heterograft is processed pigskin, and a homograft or allograft is processed human skin from another person. These are used as biological dressings to provide temporary wound coverage and pain relief. Autograft is a surgical procedure in which skin is harvested from an unburned area of the patient (donor site) and applied to the clean granulating tissues of the burn wound (graft site). With proper care, the donor site will re-epithelialize by itself and the skin graft is permanent once it "takes."

Adequate nutrition is absolutely essential during this phase, since the metabolic rate of the burn patient is greatly increased and the protein, vitamin, mineral, and calorie needs are correspondingly increased. Protein is essential for wound healing and must be provided in substantial amounts. Nutritional requirements are calculated based on the TBSA and patient's admission weight. Calorie and protein counts and the patient's weight are monitored daily to ensure proper intake. If the patient is unable to meet individual requirements through diet, high protein and calorie supplements are given either orally or through a nasogastric tube. Intravenous hyperalimentation is occasionally necessary.

Since burn injuries and treatment procedures are often painful, narcotic analgesia is often liberally used.[9] Relaxation and imagery techniques are also employed to reduce stress and anxiety. The amount of narcotic analgesia given will be gradually decreased as the wound heals, and patients usually require minimal pain medications on discharge.

During the shock and acute phases positioning, splinting, and exercising are an integral part of the total treatment program and are carried out consistently to prevent contracture and deformity and to maintain range of motion (ROM).

Rehabilitation Phase

The third phase of recovery is the rehabilitation phase. This is the postgrafting period when the patient is medically stable. The goals of treatment are maximal self-care independence; prevention of deformity, contracture, and hypertrophic scarring; recovery of strength and ROM; preparation for discharge from the hospital; vocational exploration; and psychosocial adjustment.

The rehabilitation team is composed of the physician, psychiatrist or psychologist, physical and occupational therapists, nurse, dietitian, social workers, art and play therapists, recreational therapist, vocational counselor, patient, and family. The team works closely together to help the patient achieve individual rehabilitation goals.

During this phase patient and family education is

especially important so that the patient can be familiar with his or her care in preparation for discharge. Patient education is done by the entire team, and the family is asked to observe and practice assisting the patient with his or her care. Visiting nurses are particularly helpful in assisting the patient and the family through the initial period following discharge to readjust to the home environment. Reassessment on an outpatient basis is routinely carried out by the team to ensure progressive recovery. If reconstructive surgery is necessary to correct excessive scarring and joint contracture, the patient will need to return for a short hospital stay.

THE ROLE OF OCCUPATIONAL THERAPY
Pregrafting Stage

During the initial stage following a burn injury medical management is of utmost importance for the survival of the patient, and the goal of occupational therapy is primarily prophylactic in nature, such as preventing contractures, deformities, and loss of ROM and strength. As the patient recovers and progresses toward the rehabilitation phase, he or she will require less medical intervention and occupational and physical therapy become the main focus of the treatment program to assist the patient in returning to the previous level of function. Although the role delineation between occupational and physical therapy differs in each facility, it is essential that the two disciplines work closely together and communicate frequently in a team approach so that the patient benefits from the skills and viewpoints of both disciplines.

The occupational therapy evaluation should be completed soon after admission, and a treatment program should be established early. This is so that a baseline of the patient's level of functioning can be obtained, rapport can be established, and the patient can get accustomed to the therapy procedures as part of the daily routine. Pertinent information such as type, percentage, depth, and location of the thermal injury; other secondary diagnoses; past medical history; functional ability before the injury; and psychosocial status can be obtained from the medical history and through a patient interview.[8] Active and passive ROM of affected and unaffected extremities should be measured or estimated without dressings if possible. Any preexisting contractures or deformities should be noted. Muscle strength can be estimated through observation of functional activities. Initially manual muscle testing is not indicated in the involved extremities, since it could cause excessive bleeding and increased pain.

In cooperation with the aims of the other members of the rehabilitation team, the treatment aims of oc-

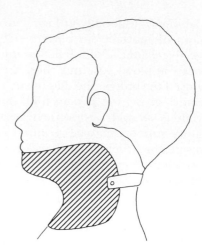

Fig. 26-2. Neck conformer splint to prevent flexion contracture of neck skin.

cupational therapy are to prevent deformity and joint contractures, prevent loss of ROM and strength in affected and unaffected parts, achieve the maximal self-care independence possible at this stage, and provide psychological support.

Treatment is conducted in a sterile environment, using aseptic techniques, so the therapist must be familiar with infection control procedures.

To prevent contractures and deformity a splinting and positioning regimen is indicated when there is a burn over a joint, especially over a flexor surface.[3,8,12] This should be established soon after admission. The principle of positioning is to maintain the affected extremities in antideformity positions or keep them extended and abducted, since the position of comfort is the position of contracture. Elevating the extremities at the same time will also decrease dependent edema. Positioning techniques are listed in Table 26-1.

Some of the commonly used positioning devices are (1) foam head donut for patients with anterior neck burns to prevent neck flexion contracture and excessive pressure on the occiput, since pillows are not allowed, (2) foam ear protector to prevent pressure on a burned ear, (3) arm trough to keep shoulders abducted, (4) bed extension for prone positioning, and (5) foot board to keep ankles at a neutral position when supine. Pillows are often used to elevate the extremities.

Splinting plays an important role in maintaining antideformity positions.[12] Splints are usually not fabricated until approximately 12 hours after the injury to allow edema to occur, and they are made of low-temperature thermoplastics molded on the patient over the dressings. Splints should be thoroughly cleaned and dried before each application, and their

Table 26-1 Antideformity Positioning and Splinting[8,16]

Body part and splint	Position		
	Supine	Prone	Side lying
Neck Neck conformer, soft cervical collar	Slight extension; no pillow, except small roll behind neck and/or foam head donut may be used	Extension; small role under forehead or head turned to side	Extension; pillows can be used to maintain position as needed
Shoulders Axillary or airplane splints	Abducted at least 90° with slight internal rotation	Same as for supine position	Position free shoulder at or near 90° flexion
Elbows Elbow conformer, three-point extension splint	Position in 5° to 10° flexion and forearm in supination when anterior surface is involved	Alternate between 5° to 40° flexion	5° to 10° flexion; splints may be used to maintain extended position
Wrist and hand Antideformity splint Cock-up splint	Splint to maintain antideformity position or maintain wrist extension by placing roll between thumb and fingers, elevate above heart level	Same as for supine position	Splint to maintain antideformity position
Hips Abductor wedge	Extension with approximately 15° of abduction to separate thighs	Same as for supine position	Alternate extension of hips
Knees Three-point extension splint or knee conformer	Extension; splinting if knee, posterior thigh, or leg are burned	Extension; same as for supine position	Alternate extension of knees
Ankles and feet Footboard, foot drop splints	Ankles at neutral position with no pressure at heel and the plantar surface supported; foot drop splint to maintain position; elevate part	Hang feet over edge of mattress to maintain the position	Maintain neutral position; splint if necessary; keep pressure off malleoli

fit should be reevaluated at least daily. Revisions are made as often as needed.[8] The splint should be labeled with the patient's name and body part to ensure proper application and to prevent cross-contamination.

Depending on the area involved some splints that may be used to maintain antideformity positions are the neck conformer (Fig. 26-2), axillary or airplane splint (Fig. 26-3), elbow or knee conformer (Fig. 26-4), antideformity hand splint (Fig. 26-5), cock-up splint, three-point extension splint for the elbow or knee, and ankle or foot drop splint. All splints should be removed at least two to three times daily to allow wound cleansing, dressing changes, and exercising the involved joints.

In addition to splinting and positioning the occupational therapy program should include active ROM exercises.[12] Exercising during dressing changes or hydrotherapy is also beneficial, since friction from dressings and bandages is eliminated, thus allowing more joint excursion.[8] Several short sessions of active or gentle passive ROM exercise with five to seven repetitions of each motion are often more effective than a single long session, especially for patients with major burns. Slow, complete motions are encouraged rather than short, jerky movements.

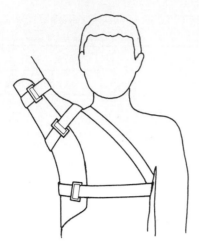

Fig. 26-3. Axillary or airplane splint to prevent adduction contracture of shoulder.

If there are deep second- or third-degree dorsal burns of the hands and fingers, fist making and passive proximal interphalangeal (PIP) flexion should not be performed to protect the extensor mechanism.[10] Progressive resistive exercises may be used for unaffected areas to maintain strength and ROM but are generally avoided for burned areas until good skin coverage is evident. This is to prevent capillary trauma and bleeding during a crucial and tenuous period of healing.

Although physical therapists are generally responsible for gait training, it is important that occupational therapists be aware of the precautions for lower extremity burns as well. When there is lower extremity involvement, elastic bandage wraps must be applied to support the capillary bed in the new granulating tissue and to prevent edema before the patient is allowed to dangle the feet or to ambulate. Elastic bandage wraps should be applied from the metatarsal heads, including the heel, to the groin in figure eight or spiral patterns. Static standing or dangling the feet should be avoided, but if it is necessary, such as when shaving at the sink, the patient should be instructed to take steps in place to improve circulation. The lower extremities should be elevated as soon as the patient returns to bed or sits down. Should there be burns

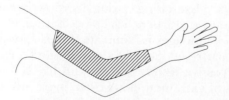

Fig. 26-4. Elbow conformer splint to prevent elbow flexion contracture.

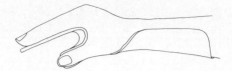

Fig. 26-5. Antideformity splint for dorsal burn of hand to prevent clawhand deformity.

on the soles of the feet, weight bearing on the feet should be eliminated entirely, which includes bridging in bed, standing, and ambulating, until the soles of the feet are healed.

Simple craft activities and self-care activities that are within the patient's ability may be used to encourage purposeful use of affected parts, promote independence, enhance self-esteem, and divert attention from the dysfunction to functional capacities.[3] For patients with hand burns adaptive equipment, such as built-up utensils, may be necessary. Patients who are intubated will need an alphabet board, since they cannot communicate verbally.

The occupational therapist needs to offer the patient reassurance and psychological support. Physical proximity to other people and facilitation of the relationship between the patient and important others in his or her life can help to overcome feelings of revulsion and aversion to self.

Grafting Stage

Since it is essential to immobilize and minimize pressure to the new graft after an autograft procedure, additional splints and positioning devices may be needed. It is important that the occupational therapist discuss postoperative positioning needs with the physician and nurses before surgery so that splints and positioning devices are readily available immediately after the surgical procedure. The joints proximal and distal to the graft site are generally immobilized for 5 to 7 days to allow the graft to "take."[7] Gentle active ROM exercise can then commence with the physician's consent and should be done without dressings to avoid shearing on the new graft. At 7 to 10 days, the patient is allowed to exercise with the dressings on, and active assisted exercises can be started. As the graft heals, the treatment can progress to include resistive exercises and use of exercise equipment, such as reciprocal pulleys. Active exercise to donor sites is generally permitted after 2 to 3 days if there is no excessive bleeding. Lower extremity donor sites are treated similarly to lower extremity burns, and therefore elevation and wrapping with elastic bandage are used. In lower extremity autografts the patient is not allowed to ambulate for 7 to 10 days. With the physician's consent the patient is then encouraged and assisted to ambulate for short distances and thus slowly increase his or her endurance. Wrapping with an elastic bandage, elevation, and avoidance of static stance are particularly important to protect the graft.

Throughout the grafting stage, active and resistive exercise to the uninvolved extremities should be continued if possible to maintain ROM and strength. Environmental stimulation, self-care, and avocational activities should be continued and increased if possible, commensurately with the patient's physical abilities and tolerance level.

Depending on the parts involved, activities that can be used include leather lacing, ceramic tile work, peg games, painting, knitting, and puzzles.[3,7] The condition of the skin must be considered when selecting activities. Unless skin is well-healed, hazardous tools, irritating materials, and those activities or tools that would apply shearing forces to the skin should be avoided.

Initially activities should be relatively simple with assured success. They can be graded in difficulty to challenge the patient to improve performance.[3]

Postgrafting Stage

When the grafts heal and activity level increases, the patient is in the rehabilitation phase.

During this phase a more thorough occupational therapy evaluation can be carried out with greater emphasis on assessment of performance skills.

Active and passive ROM measurements should be taken. Muscle strength can be measured by the manual muscle test, although this should be done only if the graft has taken well and with extreme caution when applying resistance on skin surface. Endurance and performance of self-care and home management activities should be evaluated, including the need for assistive devices. As the patient is being discharged from the hospital, home visits may be needed, depending on the patient's independence, social situation, and home environment. Psychological adjustment should be assessed by observation, interview, and consultation with other members of the rehabilitation team, especially the psychologist or psychiatrist and the social worker. Some patients may require driving evaluation. Evaluation of vocational potential should be undertaken in the later stages of rehabilitation if residual dysfunction necessitates a change in former vocational role.

During the rehabilitation phase the treatment aims are to (1) familiarize the patient with necessary care in preparation for discharge from the hospital, (2) increase ROM of affected joints, (3) improve strength and physical endurance for return to community and employment, (4) prevent hypertrophic scarring, (5) achieve independence in activities of daily living (ADL), (6) explore vocational potential, and (7) aid psychological adjustment, including the restoration of self-confidence, social adjustment, and community reentry.

Because of the damaged or destroyed sebaceous glands, artificial lubrication to the healed area is necessary. A lubricant is applied 3 to 4 times daily while massaging the scars in a circular fashion. This will assist in softening the scars and is especially beneficial when done before exercising. It is also a form of desensitization. Sunlight exposure to the involved area should be avoided, since the new skin is more prone to sunburn and hyperpigmentation. The patient should be encouraged to use the involved extremities during functional activities. An active resistive exercise and therapeutic activity program should be established so that they can be carried out after discharge from the hospital.

Training in self-care and home management activities and the use of assistive devices as needed are carried out. Training in mobility, transfers, and ambulation is appropriate with lower extremity burns and especially if wheelchair or other ambulation aids are required.

Hypersensitivity of burned areas may be decreased through the self-application of handling, touch, and pressure stimuli, and activities using tools and materials may be graded from soft to hard. This must be done with extreme caution to avoid blistering and breakdown of the newly healed skin.

Pressure splints, bandages, and pressure garments are used to prevent hypertrophic scarring.[2,12] The occupational therapist is often responsible for the measurement, ordering, and fitting of the pressure garments[7] and for patient instruction regarding their application and care.[6] These are designed to conform to the burned part with the desired amount of pressure at different points in the garment.[2] They are used from approximately 2 weeks after grafting and have proved to be effective in reducing hypertrophic scars and contractures.

The occupational therapist should maintain a supportive and reassuring approach, yet not give excessive or false praise or demonstrate pity. Activities that require gradually increasing amounts of decision making, responsibility, and initiative can increase self-determination and self-confidence.

Splinting at this stage is used to correct deformities, increase ROM, and apply extra pressure to problem areas. Static and dynamic splints may be used, depending on the need. Nighttime splinting allows functional use of the extremity during the day and prevents contractures at rest.

Outpatient follow-up visits are important to assess the patient's progress and monitor for new problems that may arise. Reassessment of ROM, scars, effectiveness of the pressure garments, splints, home program, activity level, ADL independence, and psychosocial readjustment should be carried out every 6 to 8 weeks for 1 year or sometimes longer. Driving evaluation and prevocational assessment using simulated work activities or work sample testing may also be needed. More frequent outpatient occupational therapy may be necessary to provide a more structured treatment program for complications and special needs. Physical tolerance assessment and workhardening may be indicated for patients preparing for work return or vocational rehabilitation. These decisions are made by the physician and the occupational therapist on an individual basis.

COMPLICATIONS OF BURN INJURY
Heterotopic Ossification

Heterotopic ossification is a calcium deposit in a joint, frequently at the elbow, that causes progressively limited joint excursion with a stiff endpoint and considerable joint pain. It occurs more commonly in circumferential burns of the extremities, and the therapist should be aware of its early signs. If they appear, the physician should be notified. It has been found that positioning the elbow in 5° to 10° of flexion instead of full extension can help decrease potential disability. Once it has developed, frequent active ROM exercise to the joint should be carried out within the pain-free range to maintain joint motion. Use of splints and forceful passive stretching to the involved joint should be discontinued. The condition may resolve itself with time or surgical intervention may be required.

Peripheral Nerve Injury

Peripheral nerve injury can result from improper splinting, awkward positioning, and prolonged immobilization. Frequent reassessment of the patient's neurological status is advisable, and notice should be taken of any signs, such as decreased muscle strength or sensation. Common injury sites are at the brachial plexus and peroneal nerve.

Decubitus Ulcer

Decubitus ulcers are caused by excessive pressure, usually over a bony prominence, for a prolonged period of time. They can be prevented by proper positioning; frequent change of position; and devices, such as foam donuts and water bags, placed under areas where excessive pressure is anticipated.

Hypertrophic Scarring, Contracture Formation, and Pressure Therapy

Most burn wounds have a satisfactory flat appearance on healing. It can worsen with time, however, because the healed burn wound does not become elevated until 1 to 2 months after basic wound coverage. The process of healing of burn wounds is conducive to the formation of hypertrophic scars and concomitant contractures. The following are characteristics of a hypertrophic scar:

1. *Marked increase in vascularity.* A scar that remains hyperemic at the end of 2 months following healing and becomes progressively firmer will become hypertrophic.
2. *Marked increase in fibroblasts, myofibroblasts, collagen, and interstitial material.* The contractile properties of fibroblasts, myofibroblasts, collagen, and interstitial material may exert sufficient force to cause contractures, and the burn wound will shorten until it meets an opposing force.
3. *Voluntary muscle contraction.* Most patients prefer to assume a flexed, adducted position for comfort. This permits the new collagen fibers in the wound to fuse together. The collagen becomes compact and piled up in whorls and nodules, which results in scar contracture. New hypertrophic scar contracture, which is made of collagen, is easily influenced by mechanical forces. Because collagen linkage is less stable in new scars, it will readily respond to pressure and splinting. Early and consistent intervention using pressure garments and splinting to prevent hypertrophic scarring and contracture formation is the treatment of choice.[11]

Because scar formation begins the first few weeks after burn injury, pressure dressings should be introduced as soon as the graft has taken or epithelialization begins.[12] In the early stages, however, fragile skin is not able to tolerate commercial pressure garments.[2] Bruster and Pulliam[2] described a program of four stages of gradient pressure which begins with Ace bandaging, progresses to commercial tubular elastic bandaging, then to fabricated garments, and finally to commercial pressure garments. Gradation of pressure is determined by the ability of the skin to tolerate shearing and the location of the burn.

Pressure garments are indicated for all donor sites, graft sites, and burn wounds that need more than 2 to 3 weeks to heal spontaneously. Pressure can be applied when the open area is smaller than 1 inch (2.5 cm) in diameter. Pressure garments should provide approximately 35 mm Hg pressure to the involved area and must be worn continuously and consistently for 23 hours a day to be effective. They should be removed only for bathing and changing into a clean set. Both custom-made garments and

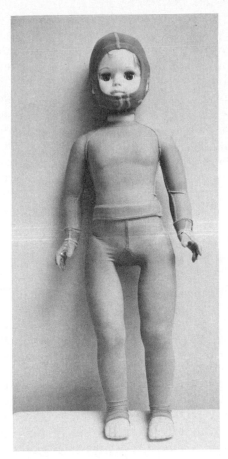

Fig. 26-6. Pressure garments.

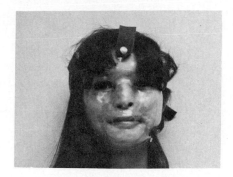

Fig. 26-7. Transparent face mask.

ready-made garments are available commercially.* Ready-made garments are often used temporarily while waiting for custom-made garments to be fabricated. All custom-made garments need to be measured and ordered following the special instructions of each company. The companies will provide order forms and instructions on request.

Some of the most commonly used garments are the face mask, chin strap, vest, sleeve, glove, gauntlet, panty brief, waist height support, knee height support, and anklet (Fig. 26-6). Willis[18] described and illustrated a variety of Jobst garments. Generally two of each garment are ordered to allow for laundering. Because of the resilient construction of the fabric, it is essential that the garments be hand washed with pure soap and air dried in the shade. Use of washing machines, dryers, and direct heat should be avoided

to prolong the life of the garments. If they are properly cared for, the garments will last approximately 3 months before a new set is needed. Children will need replacements more frequently resulting from their growth and active life-style.

Pressure should be applied to the burned area for approximately 6 to 12 months or until the scarring process is complete. Donor sites and sites of reconstructive surgery can also benefit from pressure therapy for 2 to 3 months. When the scar matures, there is resolution of the hyperemia, the area is flat and soft to the touch, and wrinkles appear when gently squeezed. When scar maturation occurs, the patient is instructed to remove the pressure garments or to reduce the time spent wearing them until they are no longer needed.

For facial hypertrophic scars, the standard treatment used to be the elastic face mask. However, because of the multiple openings for the eyes, nose, and mouth and the contours of the face, it was found that the ordinary face mask does not provide adequate pressure in the central area of the face. In recent years the transparent face mask (Fig. 26-7) made with a high-temperature material, Uvex, has been used. This provides more adequate pressure than the elastic face mask and is more cosmetically acceptable, since it is transparent and the patient's face and expression can be seen.[13] Transparent face masks are custom-made by therapists and orthotists at many burn centers throughout the country. Burns around the oral area can lead to microstomia, or "small mouth," caused by tight scars around the mouth. Mouth stretching exercises are essential and a microstomia device (Fig. 26-8) that acts as a mouth splint is commercially available.[5]*

---

*Custom-made garments are available from the Jobst Institute, Inc in Toledo, OH and Bio-Concepts, Inc in Phoenix, AZ. Ready-made garments are available from Genetic Laboratories, Inc in St Paul, MN and from Tubigrip, which is distributed by Mark One Health Care Products, Inc in West Point, PA.

---

*One type, the microstomia prevention appliance, can be obtained from the Microstomia Prevention Appliance, Inc, in Iowa City, IA, and is available in several sizes.

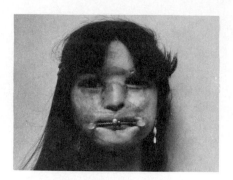

Fig. 26-8. Microstomia device.

THE BURNED HAND

A burn injury of the hand requires special consideration, since it is a common injury. It can result in serious dysfunction if not treated appropriately. These injuries are primary concerns of the occupational therapist.[8]

Dorsal burns are more common than those on the palmar surface. A dorsal burn can result in a clawhand deformity. A contracture of the skin on the dorsal surface of the hand will tend to flatten the metacarpal transverse arch and pull the metacarpophalangeal (MP) joints into hyperextension and the thumb will assume the adducted and extended position. The extensor tendons, which lie superficially on the dorsum of the hand, are especially vulnerable to injury as they cross the proximal interphalangeal (PIP) joint. The central slip of the extensor tendon, inserting at the PIP joint, may rupture. If this occurs, a boutonnière deformity can result.[8,14]

Serious palmar burns are uncommon because of the thickness of the palmar skin and because the hands are used instinctively to protect the face or body.[16] Palmar burns usually result from direct contact with a hot object, electricity, or chemical substance. The deformity that could result from the palmar burn is severe flexion and adduction contractures of the fingers and thumb.[16]

Treatment of the Dorsal Burn

The elements of treatment of a dorsal burn of the hand consist of active exercise; or active-assisted exercise if the patient is incapable of active motion; splinting; and elevation of the hand above heart level from the first day after the injury occurs. Elevation can be done by securing a tube stockinette over the arm to a position above the elbow and attaching the other end as high as possible to an intravenous stand. Another method, less effective when there is severe edema, is to rest the hand on pillows. When the dorsum of the fingers are burned, the hand is splinted in the antideformity position,[8] which is 0° to 30° of wrist extension, 45° to 70° of MP flexion, complete PIP and distal interphalangeal (DIP) extension, and extension and palmar abduction of the thumb.[14] This position prevents contracture of the collateral ligaments and protects the central slip of the extensor tendon over the PIP joint from rupture, and maintains the dorsal skin and thumb web space fully stretched. The splint is applied over the dressing with a bias-cut stockinette or rolled gauze. The splint should be wrapped securely, particularly across the PIP joints, but not so tightly as to inhibit circulation. This will prevent the hand from slipping on the splint, which could cause the hand to assume a clawhand position.[8] Hand position should be checked at least daily, and the splint should be remolded when necessary. If the fingers are spared, a cock-up splint with 0° to 30° of wrist extension is adequate.

In first-degree or superficial second-degree burns splinting may not be necessary unless there is edema and resulting tendency to revert to the claw position. Active exercise is initiated on the first day with no restrictions of motion. Fist making is allowed, and the patient is encouraged to use the hand functionally.

In moderate to deep second- to third-degree burns continuous splinting is necessary during the edema phase except during exercise periods and dressing changes. When edema has subsided, the splint is removed for periods of supervised functional activities and exercise during the day to encourage motion. To protect the extensor mechanism, passive PIP flexion and fist making are contraindicated, and the patient should be made aware of this. ROM exercise is modified so that active PIP and DIP flexion exercises are allowed if the MP joints are stabilized in extension, and MP flexion exercise is done with the IP joints extended. Full finger extension and abduction and wrist and thumb motions are allowed. The patient is encouraged to perform ADL, such as self-feeding, brushing teeth, and marking hospital menus. Adaptive equipment, such as built-up utensils and pen, is needed to avoid excessive stretching of the extensor tendons. Continuous splinting is maintained until full coverage of dry skin over the MP and PIP joints is visible. At this time, fist making is allowed and encouraged. Other hand activities, such as squeezing a foam ball, manipulating therapy putty, simple hand crafts, writing, and muscle strengthening exercises are performed.[14] A pressure glove is necessary, and should be ordered as soon as the hand has good dry skin coverage. A thorough hand evaluation should be administered to obtain baseline data. The hand evaluation should include passive and active ROM, strength, sensation, coordination, and functional testing.

Treatment of the Palmar Burn

The treatment of the full thickness palmar burn also involves splinting, positioning, and exercise. The antideformity position is 0° to 20° of wrist extension, full extension and abduction of the fingers, and extension and radial abduction of the thumb.[8,14] A volar pancake splint can be used to maintain the hand in this position, and a bulky dressing is used to keep the fingers abducted. An alternative is the banjo splint applied to the dorsum of the hand. Dressmaker's hooks, glued to each fingernail with a polymer adhesive, allow the fingers to be held in gentle traction by fastening rubber bands from each of them to the distal end of the splint.[15] There is no contraindication to fist making or to ordinary ROM exercise. Functional use of the hand should be encouraged as tolerated. Guidelines for applying pressure garments are the same as for the dorsal burn of the hand.

When there is a circumferential burn of the hand, the dorsal and palmar antideformity splints can be used alternately.

Some of the common complications of hand burns are web space contracture, tendon adhesion, finger flexion contracture, and boutonnière deformity, which is sometimes accompanied by a sharp abduction and rotation contracture usually seen in the fifth digit. Splinting, exercise, and pressure devices are needed. Finger web spacers can be ordered from companies that make custom-made pressure garments* or can be inexpensively made by using foam inserts between fingers under the pressure glove to provide extra pressure to each web space involved. A dynamic finger extension splint with a lumbricals bar is often used to increase PIP and DIP extension while preventing hyperextension of the MP joint. A dynamic MP flexion splint, which is made by attaching rubber bands and finger cuffs at the volar surface of a cock-up splint, is also commonly used to increase ROM. Surgical intervention is often needed to acquire maximal functional or cosmetic results. After surgery splinting, exercise, and pressure may be indicated to achieve the best outcome.

*These can be ordered from Jobst Institute, Inc in Toledo, OH, or Bio-Concepts, Inc in Phoenix, AZ.

REVIEW QUESTIONS

1. What is the role of the occupational therapist in the pregrafting stage of treatment of the burn patient?
2. What is the purpose of splinting after burn injury?
3. Describe or demonstrate the antideformity position for bedrest in the supine position.
4. What types of exercise are commenced 7 days after grafting?
5. What is the precaution for exercising a hand with a dorsal burn? Why is this so?
6. What is the purpose of pressure garments?
7. In which position is the hand with palmar burn splinted?
8. Which important tendon can be ruptured when there is a dorsal burn? How can this be prevented?
9. How can the occupational therapist help the patient accept him or herself and prepare the patient for return to the community?
10. What are some of the social and psychological problems that the burn-injured patient may experience? Discuss how occupational therapy can help to prevent or minimize these problems during early phases of treatment and later during the extended rehabilitation program.
11. What are the precautions for lower extremity burns?
12. What are the indications to use pressure garments, and when are they discontinued?

REFERENCES

1. American Burn Association: Aims of the American Burn Association: prevention, care, teaching, research, New Orleans, American Burn Association. Unpublished.
2. Bruster JM and Pullium G: Gradient pressure, Am J Occup Ther 37:485, 1983.
3. Curreri PW and Pruitt BA: Evaluation and treatment of the burned patient, Am J Occup Ther, 24:475, 1970.
4. Dyer C: Burn care in the emergent period, J Emerg Nurs 6:9, 1980.
5. Gorham JA: A mouth splint for burn microstomia, Am J Occup Ther 31:2, 1977.
6. Kaplan SH: Patient education techniques used at burn centers, Am J Occup Ther 39:655, 1985.
7. Krocker C, Denor B, and Nicoud B: Occupational therapy in the rehabilitation of burn patients, Milwaukee, 1977, St Mary's Hospital.
8. Malick MH: Burns. In Hopkins HL and Smith HD, editors: Willard and Spackman's occupational therapy, ed 7, Philadelphia, 1988, JB Lippincott Co.
9. Nolan WB: Acute management of thermal injury, Ann Plast Surg 7:3, 1981.
10. O'Donnell LK: Hand protocol: Bothin Burn Center rehabilitation therapy procedure manual, Saint Francis Memorial Hospital, San Francisco, (Unpublished.)
11. O'Donnell LK: Hypertrophic scarring and contracture formation: Bothin Burn Center rehabilitation therapy procedure manual, Saint Francis Memorial Hospital, San Francisco. (Unpublished.)
12. O'Shaughnessy EJ and Heimbach D: Management and rehabilitation of burns. In Kottke FJ, Stillwell KG, and Lehmann JF: Krusen's handbook of physical medicine and rehabilitation, ed 3, Philadelphia, 1982, WB Saunders Co.
13. Rivers EA, Strate RG, and Solem

LD: The transparent face mask, Am J Occup Ther 33:2, 1979.

14. Tanigawa MC, O'Donnell LK, and Graham PL: The burned hand: a physical therapy protocol, J Phys Ther 54:9, 1974.
15. Von Prince K, Curreri W, and

Pruitt BA: Application of fingernail hooks in splinting burned hands, Am J Occup Ther 24:556, 1970.
16. Von Prince K and Yaekel M: The splinting of burn patients, Springfield, IL, 1974, Charles

Thomas, Publisher.
17. Weil R et al: Smoke inhalation injury, Ann Plast Surg 4:2, 1980.
18. Willis BA: Burn scar hypertrophy: a treatment method, Galveston, TX, 1973, Shriners Burn Institute.

Sample treatment plan

CASE STUDY

Mr. B is a right-handed, 45-year-old automobile assembly worker who was burned in an automobile accident. He sustained deep second- and third-degree burns in the region of the left shoulder, left axilla, anterior surface of the left arm, and dorsum of the hand.

Mr B is considered a well-adjusted family man. He lives with his wife and two teenaged children in their own home. He is the sole support of his family. His leisure activities include spectator sports, card playing, gardening, golf, and home repairs.

He has been admitted to the burn unit of a rehabilitation center. Occupational therapy has been called on to treat Mr. B through all phases of rehabilitation. The objectives are to maintain ROM; prevent contractures, deformity, and hypertrophic scars; restore maximal functional independence; and aid with adjustment to disability.

Personal data

Name: Mr B
Age: 45
Diagnosis: 10% TBSA of deep second- and third-degree flame burns to the left upper extremity
Disability: Potential axillary contracture, elbow flexion contracture, and clawhand deformity, and hypertrophic scars
Surgery: Debridement and split thickness skin graft to left upper extremity
Donor site: Left thigh
Treatment aims as stated in referral:
Prevent contractures and deformity
Maintain or increase ROM and strength
Prevent hypertrophic scars
Restore to maximal functional independence
Aid with adjustment to disability
Precautions:
Contraindications until dorsum of fingers are healed
—No fist making
—No passive PIP flexion
—MP and IP joints are exercised separately
Elastic bandages wrap lower left extremity when up after surgery

OTHER SERVICES

Physician: Wound and medical assessment; prescribe medication; perform debridement or escharotomy as needed; supervise rehabilitation therapies; grafting
Nursing: Nursing care; positioning; administer medications; change dressings; carry out ADL
Physical therapy: Prevent contractures through ROM and strengthening exercises; hydrotherapy procedures
Psychologist: Evaluate psychological status; counsel; consultant to staff
Social worker: Explore financial problems; counsel patient and family
Family: Provide support, acceptance, encouragement, and assistance
Vocational counseling: Explore feasibility of return to same or similar job; explore job alternatives, if needed
Recreational therapy: Mental stimulation; activities for enjoyment and diversion; function of affected and nonaffected parts
Dietitian: Assess and monitor calorie and protein requirements and intake; provide supplemental diet as needed

FRAME OF REFERENCE:

Occupational performance

TREATMENT APPROACHES:

Biomechanical and rehabilitative

OT EVALUATION

Pregrafting.
Active and passive ROM: Observe
Muscle strength: Observe for function
ADL: Observe
Need for splints and positioning: Observe
Psychological status: Observe, interview, and consult with psychologist
Postgrafting.
Active and passive ROM: Measure
Muscle strength: Functional muscle test with precautions
Hand function: Test
ADL: Evaluate performance
Pressure garments: Assess need, measure, order, fit, and monitor
Psychological adjustment: Observe
Vocational exploration: Evaluate simulated work skills
Assistive devices: Observe need

EVALUATION SUMMARY

Pregrafting

Active ROM limited to 0° to 145° of shoulder flexion and abduction; full active flexion and extension of elbow and wrist; full finger extension; finger flexion limited by edema and pain as follows: MP joints (0° to 45°), PIP joints (0° to 30°), and DIP joints (0° to 5°); all remaining extremities are within normal limits

Patient able to do most hygiene and grooming, feeding, and dressing activities with uninvolved hand, using one-handed techniques, except for washing hair. Patient is depressed and withdrawn as a result of pain and fear of potential disability

Postgrafting

Shoulder flexion and abduction ROM increased to 0° to 150°, full motion possible at elbow and wrist and full finger extension; finger flexion increased as follows: MP (0° to 60°), PIP (0° to 45°), and DIP (0° to 10°); opposition only possible to tip of fourth finger; in fist making fingertips are 1 inch (2.5 cm) away from palm; strength in left arm rated good in all muscle groups; all remaining extremities are within normal limits

Patient is independent in all self-care activities and light home management activities using mostly his right hand. Patient is protective of his left hand and tends to use it in a guarded manner

Right hand function is normal; left hand is unable to perform gross grasp; maximal lateral pinch 3 pounds (1.4 kg) (below 10th percentile); maximal palmar prehension 2 pounds (0.9 kg) (below 10th percentile); performed below 10th percentile on all subtests of Jebsen-Taylor Hand Function Test

This initial depression and withdrawal is gradually being replaced by increasing motivation to recover and resume former life roles; active involvement and participation in the rehabilitation program increasing; patient realistic about injury, medical status, and future potential

ASSETS

Normal right arm and lower extremities
Good coping skills
Supportive family
Good potential for reemployment
Severe deformity prevented in pregrafting and grafting stages of treatment
Intelligent, realistic outlook
Good motivation and cooperation with medical and rehabilitation efforts

PROBLEM LIST

Pregrafting
1. Potential contracture and deformity of left shoulder, elbow, wrist, and hand
2. Depression and withdrawal initially
3. Anxiety about hospitalization and potential disability
Grafting
4. Joint movement inpedes graft take
Postgrafting
5. Decreased physical endurance
6. Limitation of strength in left arm and hand
7. Limited ROM in left shoulder and hand
8. Limited left hand function and coordination
9. Potential hypertrophic scarring

PROBLEM 1

Potential joint contracture and deformity of left upper extremity

Objective

Contracture and deformity will be prevented at shoulder, elbow, wrist, and fingers

Method

Positioning and splinting the shoulder in 90° of abduction, elbow in 5° of flexion and hand with wrist extended, MPs flexed to 45°, PIP and DIP in complete extension, thumb abducted and extended

Elevate arm above heart to reduce edema

Frequent active ROM exercise, if possible for all joints, for short periods of time following precautions outlined on p. 456.

Gradation

Revise splints as edema decreases to maintain maximal deformity positions

Passive to active assisted exercise if active ROM is not possible initially

PROBLEM 4

Joint movement impedes graft take during grafting phase

Objective

Grafted areas will be prevented from moving to promote healing

Method

Axillary splint with shoulder abducted to 110°, hand elevated

Elbow conformer splint to maintain full extension

Antideformity splint for hand

Splints worn 24 hours per day for 5 to 7 days

Gradation

Assess and revise splints as needed. Reduce splint wear on nighttime only after skin grafts are taken

PROBLEM 6

Muscle weakness in uninvolved extremities during grafting stage resulting from inactivity

Objective

Muscle strength will be maintained at good grade in uninvolved areas

Method

Active and resistive exercise to right upper extremity and both lower extremities

Gradation

Increase resistance and number of repetitions of exercises

PROBLEM 7

Limited range of motion in left shoulder and hand, postgrafting

Objective

Shoulder flexion and abduction to increase from 150° to 160°. Distance of fingertips to palm in fist making to decrease from 1 inch to 0 inch (2.5 cm to 0 cm)

Method

Left shoulder abducted at 90° at all times

Left axillary and hand splints at night

Passive stretching and active ROM exercise program to shoulder and hand

Functional hand activities with shoulder in flexion

Gradation

Decrease assistance in exercise program until patient carries it out independently

Discontinue splinting when full ROM is gained

PROBLEM 9

Potential hypertrophic scars

Objective

Hypertrophic scarring will be minimized or prevented over grafted areas and donor site

Method

Measure, order, and fit Jobst vest with long left sleeve, left glove, and panty brief to be worn 23 hours per day for 9 to 12 months

Instruct patient rationale, use and care of garments

Gradation

Discontinue pressure garments when scars are no longer active

Chapter

27 Rheumatoid arthritis

LORRAINE WILLIAMS PEDRETTI
JOCELYN M. HITTLE
MARY C. KASCH

Rheumatoid arthritis is a chronic systemic disease that can affect the lungs, cardiovascular system, and eyes in some patients. However, joint involvement resulting from inflammatory disease of the synovium is the primary clinical feature.[8,16,19] The disease may range from mild to severe and can result in joint deformity and destruction of varying degrees.[16]

Although rheumatoid arthritis occurs most frequently between the ages of 20 and 40[8] and about three times more frequently in women than in men, it can occur from infancy to old age.[8,16,19]

The cause of the disease is unknown; however, it now appears that there are genetic factors that precipitate a continued immune reaction in the synovium. It has been documented that rheumatoid factor complex binding with synovial fluid complement precipitates the inflammatory reaction in a rheumatoid joint which results in its inflammation and pannus formation.[8,36] This can progress to erode the joint capsule, tendons, ligaments, and eventually cartilage and bone.[8,19]

DIAGNOSIS

The diagnosis is usually made by an analysis of the initial symptoms, the presence of rheumatoid nodules usually over bony prominences, radiological evidence of cartilage destruction or bony erosions, and presence of the rheumatoid factor in the blood serum.[19] Certain macroglobulins or antiglobulins constitute the rheumatoid factor.[8,36]

The number of clinical features present determines the classification of the disease. It can be designated as *possible*, *probable*, *definite*, or *classic* rheumatoid arthritis.[1,19]

COURSE

The onset of rheumatoid arthritis is usually gradual or insidious, although it may be abrupt. It is characterized by bilateral, symmetrical involvement of the small joints of the hands and feet.[1,19] The joints are typically painful, stiff, tender, hot, and occasionally, red.

Muscles that act on the involved joints may decrease in strength and size fairly early in the course of disease because of disuse. Range of motion (ROM) is limited because of edema and pain in the early stages and later may be due to destructive changes in the joint.[1]

The systemic manifestations should not be overlooked. Signs, which may be present in varying degrees, include fever, weight loss, weakness, fatigue, and generalized stiffness.[1] There may be an apparent depression and lack of motivation that may be related to the fatigue and organic symptoms and should be differentiated from the same symptoms that can be psychogenic.[19]

The course of the disease is unpredictable. Some individuals experience a single, brief episode, and others experience multiple episodes of varying severity. A small percentage of patients experience a gradual and continuous progression to severe joint deformity and dysfunction.[1]

The course is usually characterized by exacerbations and remissions. The patient's level of function and independence can fluctuate from independent to completely dependent, varying with the stage and severity of the disease process.[16,19]

DRUG THERAPY

Drugs used include aspirin and other nonsteroidal anti-inflammatory drugs (NSAIDs), intraarticular and oral steroids, gold salts, antimalarials, and cytotoxic agents. Aspirin is often the drug of choice because of the low cost, but often other NSAIDs are selected because administration is easier and improved compliance may result.[14]

There are several classifications of NSAIDs, and trials from the different groups of these drugs may be used either individually[14] or in conjunction with others such as steroids or the remission–inducing drugs. NSAIDs relieve inflammation but do not alter the course of the disease, and although some have potentially serious side effects, their occurrence is rare.

Steroids are used as anti-inflammatory agents, which usually are very effective. However, because of the multiplicity and potential seriousness of their side effects, they are reserved for patients who would become severely disabled without them. They may be used in low dosage, however, with relatively few side effects and as such, when used as an adjunct to other drug therapy, may make a significant difference in those patients whose disease is not adequately controlled on other medications alone.[21]

Gold salts and penicillamine suppress inflammation and unlike NSAIDs can alter the course of the disease.[29] The mechanism of their action is unknown. Because of the close monitoring of the patient, which is required to identify potential toxicity, and the seriousness of the possible side effects, the use of gold salts is reserved for patients who are dependable, will comply with frequent visits for urinalysis and blood testing, are alert to side effects that must be reported immediately, and have failed to respond to more conservative forms of treatment.

Antimalarial drugs such as hydroxycloroquine may also be effective but require close medical supervision. Cytotoxic agents can benefit selected patients but again require careful monitoring because of potentially serious side effects. Imuran has been FDA approved for the treatment of rheumatoid arthritis, and Methotrexate is currently being evaluated. The latter is rapidly gaining acceptance because of its effectiveness and the ease of controlling the side effects.[12]

Remission-inducing drugs and cytotoxic agents are slow acting, with 2 to 3 months of drug therapy required before their full benefit is realized. During this time, steroids may improve the patient's functional status and it is important that supportive measures such as joint protection, energy conservation, and splinting be employed until synovitis is controlled.

PSYCHOLOGICAL FACTORS

The so called "rheumatoid personality" is undoubtedly a myth arising from research done in the 1950s and 1960s. Its validity has since been questioned. These reports suggested that persons with rheumatoid arthritis show characteristics of rigidity, hostility, and a variety of other personality variables. These have since been shown to be conclusions drawn from inadequate data.[26]

Personality factors seen in patients with rheumatoid arthritis are found in persons with other chronic diseases and in the healthy population. The psychological factors are probably a response to chronic disease

rather than a predisposing cause.[19] The patient may have suffered a serious change in physical function and life roles, and even appearance may be altered by deformity and drug side effects. These changes evoke an adjustment process akin to the grief process after a death. The patient may respond to the disability with depression, denial, a need to control the environment, and dependency.[19]

Some aspects of the illness which may contribute to the psychological state include constant pain and fear of pain; changed body image and perception of self as a sick person; continuous uncertainty about the course and prognosis of the disease because of remissions and flares; sexual dysfunction because of pain or deformity; and altered social, family, vocational, and leisure roles.

Rehabilitation workers need to be aware of the patient's response to disability and the adjustment that is in progress. All the factors and behaviors just cited will have an influence on rehabilitation. The interaction of personnel with the patient can facilitate the development of healthy coping mechanisms and acceptance of disability. The reader is referred to Melvin[19] for a more detailed discussion of this subject.

JOINT PROBLEMS AND DEFORMITIES*
Pathogenesis of Joint Destruction

The initial event and prime cause of joint destruction is proliferation of the synovial membrane. The synovial membrane becomes so proliferated that it grows over and into cartilage, bone, and tendons and secretes enzymes that destroy them. The major microscopic fibers that hold the tissues of bone, cartilage, and tendons together are called collagen. The destruction of collagen is a major event, causing joint damage. This destruction is caused by the abnormal secretion of the enzymes collagenase and elastase by the abnormal synovium. The abnormal synovium also produces a thin, watery synovial fluid that is a poor lubricant and nutrient.

Polymorphonuclear white blood cells produced by the inflamed synovium bathe the joint by the millions, and when they break down, they release lysosomal enzymes and other enzymes that further alter the synovial fluid viscosity, cartilage, bone, and tendons to create a vicious cycle.

This destruction process can result in tendon, muscle, and nerve dysfunction and a variety of joint deformities. Tests for specific deformities or potential

---

*Adapted from Lages W, MD: Pathogenesis of joint destruction; and from Specific joint problems in rheumatoid arthritis, San Jose, CA, 1976 and 1980, Santa Clara Valley Medical Center. (Unpublished).

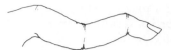

Fig. 27-1. Swan-neck deformity results in PIP hyperextension and DIP flexion.

deformities of the hand should be administered as appropriate. The therapist might evalute for possible carpal tunnel syndrome, swan-neck deformities, boutonnière deformities, flexor tendon nodules, ulnar drift, metacarpophalangeal (MP) and wrist subluxation, intrinsic and extrinsic muscle tightness, ruptured tendons, extensor tendon displacement, and laxity of the MP collateral ligaments[5] (Figs. 27-1; 27-2; 27-3; 27-4).

Specific Problems

EXTRINSIC MUSCLE TIGHTNESS. To test for tightness (contracture) or adherence of the extensor digitorum communis (EDC) tendon, the wrist is positioned at neutral. Then the MP joint is passively flexed to different positions, and simultaneously the proximal interphalangeal (PIP) and distal interphalangeal (DIP) joints are flexed. The test is positive if the position of the proximal joint (MP) influences the degree of flexion possible at the distal joints (IPs). For example, when the MP joint is fully flexed, the PIP joint will lack full active or passive flexion. When the PIP joint is fully flexed, it will not be possible to fully flex the MP joint because the tendon does not have sufficient length to go over all the joints it crosses when they are all flexed.[9,19]

When performing this test, forceful flexion of the wrist and fingers should be avoided and all joint movements should be done gently. If there is any attrition of the extensor tendons, forceful flexion of these joints could cause tendon rupture.[32]

DIP AND PIP JOINTS OF SECOND TO FIFTH FINGERS

Swan-neck deformity. Swan-neck deformity results in hyperextension of the PIP joint and incomplete extension or slight flexion of the DIP joint. There are several causes of swan-neck deformity. Three types are discussed here. It is important for the therapist

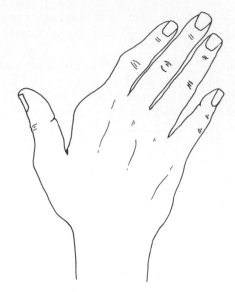

Fig. 27-3. MP joint ulnar drift.

and physician to know the underlying cause if appropriate treatment is to be instituted.

One type of swan-neck deformity is caused by initial involvement at the MP joint[19] and results in intrinsic muscle tightness. To test for this type the test for extrinsic muscle tightness is applied first to prove that the extensor tendons do not have adhesions.[9,25] Then the MP joint is passively moved into full extension, and the PIP joint is flexed. Resistance to PIP flexion indicates intrinsic tightness. The PIP joint will not flex fully in this position if the intrinsic muscles are shortened. The reason for this is that the lumbricales act to extend the IP joints during MP flexion. By extending MP joints and flexing PIP joints these muscles are fully stretched. If they have become shortened, there will be insufficient elasticity or length to achieve the test position. Intrinsic muscles become weak, scarred, and shortened when they are invaded by pannus during the rheumatoid disease process.[5,19] This can create an excessive pull on the PIP joint, causing hyperextension.[20] Whenever intrinsic muscle tightness is found, patients should be taught intrinsic muscle stretching exercise.

Another type of swan-neck deformity is a result of initial involvement at the DIP joints[19] and rupture of the lateral slips of the extensor tendons (Fig. 27-5). To test for this type the test for extrinsic tightness is

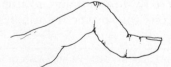

Fig. 27-2. Boutonnière deformity results in DIP hyperextension and PIP flexion.

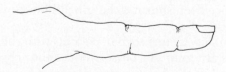

Fig. 27-4. MP palmar subluxation.

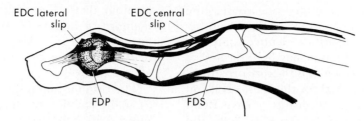

Fig. 27-5. Swan-neck deformity resulting from rupture of lateral slips of EDC tendon.

applied first to prove that there is no adherence of the extensor tendon.[19] Then the MP joint is moved into extension, and the PIP joint is flexed to prove that there is no intrinsic tightness. Then the patient should extend the finger actively. If there is a rupture of the lateral slips of the extensor tendon, the DIP joint will drop into flexion because ruptured lateral slips of the EDC cannot function to extend the joint. The middle slip of the EDC, acting on the PIP joint, pulls too hard and hyperextends the joint when active extension is attempted, resulting in the swan-neck appearance.

A swan-neck deformity with initial involvement at the PIP joint[19] is caused by rupture of the flexor digitorum superficialis (FDS) tendon (Fig. 27-6). To test for this the test for extrinsic tightness is applied as before. The MP joint is moved into hyperextension, and the PIP joint is flexed to rule out intrinsic tightness. The patient is then asked to flex the finger into the palm actively. If the FDS tendon is ruptured, it will not be possible to flex the PIP joint. The tendon rupture is a result of synovitis of the PIP joint with infiltration of the FDS tendon. Bony spurs producing tendon erosion may also cause the tendon to rupture.[19]

Intervention. Direct surgery involving the lateral slips of the extensor tendons is rarely done because of poor technical results. Sometimes synovectomy is indicated early to remove the invading synovium at the MP joints. Daily passive ROM and gentle stretching are indicated for the DIPs. Active ROM should be done daily to the MPs, PIPs, and DIPs to prevent contractures. A small, short *dynamic* splint may be applied to the PIPs during daily activity to prevent pro-

gressive hyperextension. A three-point finger splint is sometimes used to maintain range of PIP flexion and relieve stress to the volar aspect of the PIP joint resulting from severe hyperextension.[19] Flexion contractures of the MPs, PIPs, and DIPs should be treated by active muscle contraction with stretch and not with passive or device stretch.

Isotonic and isometric resistive exercise to the finger extensors will not strengthen damaged tendons and may damage them further.

Boutonnière deformity. Boutonnière deformity can occur when synovitis at the wrist, MP, or PIP joints weakens or destroys the central slip of the extensor tendon which inserts into the base of the middle phalanx. There is often associated PIP joint arthritis. The result is incomplete and weak-to-absent extension at the PIP joint with overbalanced contraction of the lateral slips of the extensor tendon which insert into the base of the distal phalanx with hyperextension at the DIP joint (Fig. 27-7). The central slip of the extensor tendon is the major extensor of the finger, and if this problem is recent (days) and if *the physician does not know of it,* he or she should be informed immediately. Invariably a flexion contracture of the PIP joint and hyperextension of the DIP joint with loss of flexion range will ensue. Function of the finger will be seriously compromised.

Intervention. Direct surgery of the central slips is often done if caught early enough, but there may be severe damage to the extensor tendon by the synovium, which may require a tendon graft from another site or may be irreparable. Because of this the fourth

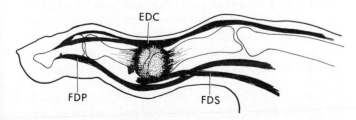

Fig. 27-6. Swan-neck deformity as a result of rupture of FDS tendon.

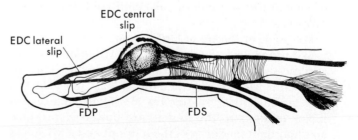

Fig. 27-7. Boutonnière deformity caused by rupture or lengthening of central slip of EDC tendon.

and fifth fingers are rarely operated on, whereas the second and third fingers often are operated on because of hand function priorities. Synovectomy will not restore tendon integrity but may be indicated to prevent the invasion of other tendons in proximity. Daily passive ROM is indicated for the MPs, PIPs, and DIPs to correct or prevent deformity. Active ROM exercises should be done daily to the MPs, PIPs, and DIPs to preserve joint ROM and muscle tone. *Dynamic* extension splints of the second and third fingers may be indicated to improve function and opposition.

Isotonic and isometric exercise or resistive exercise to the extensors will not help this deformity and may further damage tendons.

Trigger finger. Trigger finger deformity is caused by a nodule or thickening of the FDS tendon at the entrance to the flexor tunnel (tendon sheath). This is caused by a rheumatoid nodule on the FDS tendon which blocks or makes difficult the slipping of the tendon through its sheath, preventing full extension of the PIP joint.[5,19] To test for this problem the examiner should ask the patient if the fingers ever catch or stay closed when attempts are made to open the hand. If the patient reports that this is the case, the examiner should determine if it occurs rarely, occasionally, or consistently; if there is any pain associated with it; and if it inhibits function. The therapist should palpate for a nodule over the flexor pulleys.[19] A click or crepitation may be palpated at the point where the nodule is pulled through the sheath. The palpation point is in the palm distal to the palmar creases at the base of the involved finger. The deformity is described as mild if there is inconsistent, painless triggering during active motion; as moderate if there is constant triggering during active motion or if it is intermittent but painful; and as severe if it prevents full active motion and is severely painful.[19]

INTERVENTION. If persistent triggering occurs, it may result in lost range of motion or tendon rupture. Treatment includes hydrocortisone injection, tendon protection techniques, splinting and the use of heat to improve tissue mobility and cold to decrease inflammation.[5] ADL evaluation and training as well as instruction in the use of heat and cold may be appropriate.

MP Joints of Second to Fifth Fingers

MP ulnar drift. Synovitis of the MP joints leads to weakness or destruction of the MP ligaments. The MP ligaments, particularly when the MPs are flexed at 45°, give medial and lateral stability. Both the extensor and flexor tendons to the fingers are bowed to produce an ulnar drift tendency of the tendons at the MP joints during normal contraction. Forced contractions and especially forceful hand grip accentuate this tendency. With MP ligaments weakened the normal forces result

in ulnar drift. The fifth MP joint buttresses the remainder of fingers from static, postural ulnar drift, but when the fifth MP ligament loses stability, ulnar drift can occur with gravity and posture even at rest (Fig. 27-3).

The result is that if the MP ligament damage is mild or if the stability of the fifth joint is preserved, the ulnar drift may occur only dynamically with finger extension-flexion. This gives weak pinch, which may result in thumb adduction and lateral pinch being substituted for true opposition. If the MP ligament damage is severe or if the stability of the fifth MP joint is lost, there will be ulnar drift even at rest, posturally, and the problem of opposition will be severe.

The dynamic and static ulnar drift plus lifting of the extensor hood by MP synovitis will result in dislocation of the extensor tendons from the extensor hood over the metacarpal heads into the space between the heads, leading to possible tendon injury and loss of ability to completely extend the MP joints. The lateral pinching of the thumb will result in radial subluxation and deformity of the IP joint of the thumb.

The therapist may test for the deformity by measuring the angle between the proximal phalanx and the MP joints during active extension. This measurement should be compared with the normal ROM. The index finger normally has 10° to 20° of ulnar deviation during active extension. The severity of the ulnar drift is described as follows:

Severity	Index finger	Fingers 3 to 5
Mild	20° to 30°	0° to 10°
Moderate	30° to 50°	10° to 30°
Severe	50° or more	30° or more[19]

Intervention. Treatment consists of early synovectomy, which may prevent progressive MP ligament damage. Extensor tendons dislocated ulnarly may be able to be replaced surgically with excision of MP synovial tissue. Severe problems may require replacement of the MP joints, since the MP ligaments cannot be successfully repaired surgically. Daily passive ROM exercises of the MP joints are indicated only if daily active ROM does not produce full flexion and extension. A joint protection program is strongly indicated to prevent forceful flexion and extension in activities of daily living (ADL). *Dynamic* ulnar deviation splints during the day coupled with *static* splints with the MPs in neutral deviation and 45° of flexion at night may halt progression of deformity and improve opposition.

Isotonic and isometric exercise or resistive exercise of the fingers will not help this deformity and may produce further MP ligament damage.

MP palmar subluxation-dislocation. Synovitis of the MPs results in MP ligament damage. Since finger flexors are much stronger and much more used than extensors, palmar dislocation will result. Palmar dislocation is often associated with ulnar drift but may occur by itself. Loss of effective MP extension and shortening and weakening of the intrinsic muscles are the usual isolated problems. Complete dislocation can occur (Fig. 27-4).

The therapist can test for this deformity by palpating over the dorsum of the joint when it is at the 0° neutral position. If there is subluxation, a "step" can be felt between the metacarpal and the first phalanx. The deformity is described as mild if the step is palpable, but full extension is possible; as moderate if the step is visible, palpable, and there is a slight limitation of extension; and as severe if there is gross malalignment and definite limitation of ROM.[19]

Intervention. Early, complete surgical replacement or repair of the MP joints is the only effective treatment. Passive and active ROM exercises of the MPs to prevent loss of ROM are indicated. No exercises or splints are effective in correcting or treating this problem. A joint protection program is strongly indicated to prevent further progressive damage during ADL.

THUMB

Flexion of MP joint with hyperextension of the IP joint (Type I deformity). Chronic MP synovitis causes attenuation of the joint capsule, MP collateral ligaments, and the overlying extensor mechanism. Pain and distention of the joint capsule cause damage of the intrinsic muscles of the thumb. This may progress to MP palmar subluxation and ulnar-volar displacement of the extensor pollicis longus tendon. Once displaced this tendon acts as an MP flexor and with intrinsic muscle damage, causes hyperextension of the IP joint. The result is MP flexion and IP hyperextension.[19]

Flexion of MP joint with IP hyperextension and carpometacarpal CMC involvement (Type II deformity). Type II deformity appears similar to type I deformity, but CMC joint damage and subluxation, a result of chronic synovitis of this joint, are the major factors. Once there is subluxation of the CMC joint, the adductor pollicis muscle pulls on the first metacarpal, which can result in a fixed adduction contracture with hyperextension of the *distal* phalanx.[19]

MP hyperextension, IP flexion, and CMC joint involvement (Type III deformity). The dynamics of type III deformity are initially the same as those described for type II deformity. However, type III deformity will result if there is a natural or pathological laxity of the MP joint with hyperextension of the proximal phalanx.[19]

Intervention. These problems may be treated surgically by extensor tendon repair, synovectomy, ar-

throdesis, or joint replacement. A joint protection program is indicated, and a CMC stabilization splint may be helpful to relieve pain and increase hand function.

WRIST JOINT

Wrist subluxation. Subluxation of the wrist (Fig. 27-8) is a volar slippage of the carpal bones on the radius. It is caused by weakness of the supporting ligaments caused by chronic synovitis. To test for wrist subluxation, the therapist should palpate from the distal radius to the carpals on the dorsal side of the forearm. If there is subluxation, there will be a step. It may be merely palpable if mild, visible if moderate, and grossly malaligned if severe.[19]

INTERVENTION. Wrist splinting adds stability (1) to improve function, (2) to relieve pain, and (3) to prevent tendon rupture of digital extensor tendons. A flexible splint during the day with rigid splinting at night may be the most appropriate approach. The patient who does not wear splints all the time should be taught to use his or her splint during those activities that will be particularly stressful to the structures of the wrist.[20]

Carpal tunnel syndrome. The carpal tunnel under the transverse flexor carpal ligament is a tightly closed space, and inflammation can lead to high pressure on the median nerve, which runs in the carpal tunnel. This produces pain and sensory disturbances over the median nerve distribution in the hand and median nerve motor weakness and atrophy of the opponens pollicis, abductor pollicis brevis, and thenar atrophy. *If not already known by the physician, this should be promptly brought to his or her attention for treatment.* Sensory and motor deficits over the median nerve distribution and severe pain in the hand can result and can progress to permanent loss of feeling in the hand and weak-to-lost thumb opposition, which are serious impairments to hand use.

Intervention. Until medically treated, heat and any exercises of the wrist other than active ROM are contraindicated. A cock-up splint with a neutral wrist position is worn at night and in some cases during the day as well. Techniques to reduce edema may be used,

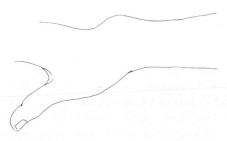

Fig. 27-8. Flexion subluxation of wrist.

such as use of cold packs, contrast baths, and elevation. ADL training to prevent aggravation of the problem is important, and some job tasks or household activities may need to be modified.[25] Corticosteroid injection may be beneficial, but if none of these measures is effective, surgical release of the transverse carpal ligament is indicated.

Synovial invasion of extensor tendons. Dorsal swelling can be seen and felt in cases of invasion of the extensor tendon sheaths. This can lead to their weakness or rupture, resulting in weak to lost extension of the fingers at the MP, PIP, and DIP joints, flexion contractures, and loss of hand function, which is serious.

Intervention. As soon as discovered, surgical synovectomy can correct and prevent further problems. Tendon repair may be done if caught promptly. Active ROM exercises at the wrist and night splints for the wrist can preserve function before surgery but are not substitutes for surgery. Passive and active ROM of the MP, PIP, and DIP are indicated to prevent flexion contracture.

Isotonic and isometric exercise or resistive exercise of the wrist extensors is of no value and may produce further damage.

Synovial invasion of the carpal bones. Synovial invasion of the carpal bone results in erosion and destruction of the intercarpal ligaments and joints. It can result in progressive loss of wrist motion, contracture of the wrist in a nonfunctional position, or in flexion subluxation-dislocation of the wrist (Fig. 27-8).

Intervention. Loss of ROM can be minimized by active ROM exercise. Passive ROM should be gentle to avoid damaging ligaments. Using volar resting splints at night with the wrist in the position of function (neutral radioulnar position and slight wrist extension) can prevent contracture in nonfunctional positions. Surgery is not feasible except to fuse in more functional positions. Since surgery can only offer wrist fusion in the position of function, *static* wrist splints in the position of function produce the same end result. Splints causing loss of pronation-supination are contraindicated. Active pronation-supination ROM exercise and gentle passive ROM are indicated several times a day with the wrist out of the splint to prevent this. Joint protection against forceful flexion is strongly indicated. Isometric strengthening of wrist extensors is indicated.

Isotonic and isotonic resistive exercise may lead to subluxation-dislocation.

Synovial invasion of radioulnar joint. Synovitis of the radioulnar joint, causing erosion of joint cartilage, usually results in progressive loss of pronation and supination at the wrist, particularly if there is associated elbow disease. It can result in partial-to-complete loss of pronation and supination of the wrist with severe functional impairment.

Intervention. Surgical resection of the distal ulna can be done to restore lost pronation-supination. Active pronation-supination ROM exercises and passive ROM are indicated daily to prevent loss. Pronation-supination in ADL is encouraged.

Isotonic or resistive exercises are contraindicated.

ELBOW JOINT

Elbow synovitis. The humeroulnar joint is a hinge joint, and synovitis results in loss of ROM. Disease of the radiohumeral joint can result in loss of pronation-supination at the elbow. Loss of flexion can result in contracture that prevents feeding and many other ADL. Loss of extension can result in contracture that makes ADL and crutch use difficult and some tasks impossible. Loss of pronation-supination severely compromises the use of the hands and wrists in ADL. A dominant arm with severe loss of extension and pronation makes writing and other activities extremely difficult. Both elbows with severely limited flexion seriously impair ADL and functional activities; both elbows with severely limited extension make transfers and crutch use extremely difficult.

Intervention. Flexion and extension contractures of the elbows are extremely difficult to improve surgically. The radial head can be resected to improve pronation-supination. With disease in the elbows splints and slings limiting movement are contraindicated unless daily ROM is preserved by a therapist or nurse. Active and passive ROM exercises are strongly indicated daily for the elbow. Isometric exercise is indicated for strengthening only if isotonic exercise is too painful. Isotonic exercise is best given through proper ADL instruction. Pain that may limit exercise can be reduced by corticosteroid injection. Loss of ROM is a greater concern than is joint damage, since the only surgical corrections for contractures are destructive of joints. Sometimes surgery is aimed toward improving extension at the expense of flexion in the dominant arm, to permit crutch use and writing and improving flexion at the expense of extension in the nondominant extremity for feeding and personal grooming.

SHOULDER JOINT

Shoulder Synovitis. The shoulder is a ball-and-socket joint that has some susceptibility to loss of motion.

The main result of synovitis is loss of some planes of ROM. A complication of shoulder synovitis is "frozen shoulder," which means very restricted ROM, and unfortunately is common. This results in major prob-

lems in ADL and in crutch ambulation. With shoulder contracture there is extremely severe restriction of ADL and other functions.

Intervention. Surgery is of little value in treating this problem. Corticosteroid injection early is very effective in reducing pain and restricted motion. Aggressive active and passive ROM and isotonic exercise are imperative, especially preceded by hot packs. A joint protection program is strongly indicated. Slings are a hazard and should be avoided.

SURGICAL INTERVENTION

Treatment of the patient with long-term rheumatoid arthritis will often include operative procedures to repair soft tissue or replace joints destroyed by the rheumatoid process.

Surgical procedures that may be of benefit to patients with rheumatoid arthritis include synovectomy, tendon repair and transplant, soft tissue reconstruction, joint replacement, bone resection, and joint fusion.[1,19]

Synovectomy, which is a surgical process of removing excessive synovium in an effort to control its proliferation, may be performed when the inflammation cannot be controlled by more conservative methods. It is most often delayed until soft tissue, such as finger extensors, appear to be jeopardized by the synovitis.

Resection implant arthroplasty is performed more successfully and more often since the development of high-grade Silastic spacers and joints. Early models of joints made out of metal and Silastic failed because of breakage of the implants from shearing forces applied during daily use. Current implant spacers are reinforced with Dacron and withstand normal hand usage more reliably than earlier models. Metal implants are generally no longer used in the fingers.

MP Joint Arthroplasty

Although implants exist to replace almost any joint affected by arthritis, resection arthroplasty of the MP joints is the most common rheumatoid surgery in the hand. Guidelines given for timing of treatment vary with the surgeon, the patient, and the expertise of the treating therapist. The program described was developed for the Swanson-type Silastic implant, but the general principles would apply to other types of spacers as well.

Some joint replacements, such as in the total hip replacement, are designed to work like the joint they replace. However, the MP joint arthroplasty uses a joint spacer that is not a joint but acts as an interface between the metacarpal bone and the proximal phalanx. The stems of the Swanson spacer are not fixed

within the intermedullary canal but move with a piston action within the bone. This allows adequate excursion of the implant for finger flexion and extension and reduces stress on the implant.

During the healing phase following the MP arthroplasty the implants go through an encapsulation period. During this time the tissue surrounding the Silastic forms a capsule that supports the stems of the spacer. Collagen fibers are present microscopically on the fourth or fifth day and gradually change from the cellular formation into collagen fibers.[18] This process appears to be complete by the end of the sixth week. During the encapsulation period it is extremely important that the joints be held in the desired position of extension and slight radial deviation.

During surgery the head of the metacarpal is resected and cleaned. The proximal phalanx is prepared but usually not resected. The bone canals are also prepared, and the spacer carefully inserted. Soft tissue release of the ulnar intrinsic muscles, reconstruction of the radial intrinsic muscles, and reconstruction and alignment of the extensor hood may be performed during surgery.

The patient's hand is placed in a bulky dressing and immobilized for 3 to 6 days postoperatively. At that time a dynamic splint is applied, which places the fingers in slight radial deviation at the MP joints while lightly supporting the fingers into full extension and allowing active flexion to 70°[35] (Fig. 27-9). A splint is worn 24 hours a day for the next 6 weeks. Some surgeons prefer a static splint, which maintains the fingers in the proper position while sleeping, and a dynamic splint during all waking hours. Frequent splint adjustments and goniometric measurements are necessary during this postoperative period to monitor joint position and excursion.

Starting with the application of the dynamic splint, passive ROM may be performed by the therapist on a daily basis to maintain 70° of pain-free passive flexion and full extension. Passive motion is applied gently with consideration to tissue reaction. Increased pain or edema would indicate that the treatment was too aggressive. The patient is instructed to perform active ROM and light ADL only in the splint for the first 6 weeks. This ensures that the fingers will not be used in an ulnarly deviated position. Heavy activities are restricted. During the 4- to 6-week period the patient may begin active flexion while wearing the splint under the supervision of the therapist. Care is taken that flexion occurs at the MP joints and not primarily at the IP joints. Individual finger splints may be placed on the fingers to prevent IP flexion during active MP flexion.[35] Also during this period flexion splinting may be begun if the patient has not regained

Treatment applications

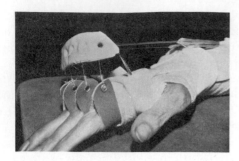

Fig. 27-9. Low profile dynamic splint is used to assist MP joints into extension while maintaining about 15° of radial deviation following implant arthroplasty of MP joints. MP joints should not be pulled into hyperextension by splint.

a full 70° of flexion. The flexion cuff should allow for slight radial pull and should not be painful or cause swelling of the fingers.

Other exercises that should be stressed are "radial walking" of the fingers individually toward the thumb and active exercise of the extensors by placing the fingers in the intrinsic minus position (IP joints slightly flexed) while extending the MP joints.

Extension and flexion splints are adjusted for fit and wearing time based on goniometric measurements. Strength usually returns as the patient is allowed to use the hand for normal activities. Heavy resistive exercise is contraindicated.

Night splinting is continued for 12 to 14 weeks, although the patient may go without the splint during the day following the sixth week.

The principles of wound healing and encapsulation may be applied to joint implant arthroplasty of other joints. A balance of controlled splinting and active motion should be achieved following any joint arthroplasty.

PRINCIPLES OF REHABILITATION

Rehabilitation of the rheumatoid patient is somewhat different than that of a patient with an acute or traumatic condition.[13] Because of the chronic and progressive nature of the disease, rehabilitation intervention may be required periodically for months or even years depending on the course of the disease and the individual patient.

The goals of the basic treatment regime are to decrease inflammation and pain, preserve function, and prevent deformity. The treatment methods used include systemic, emotional, and joint rest; drug therapy; and appropriate exercise[8] and activity. In some instances surgery is required.[13]

Joint rest in non-weight-bearing positions and prone lying to prevent hip and knee flexion contractures are part of the program of rest. Splints to pro-

vide temporary rest of individual joints are used.[13]

The amount of rest required varies with the individual patient. In some instances complete bed rest will be necessary, whereas in others the patient may continue with normal daily living, incorporating 2 hours of rest into the daily schedule.[8]

It is of primary importance in the treatment program to preserve function of the hips, knees, elbows, and MP joints. Therefore exercise to other joints must not interfere with functions of these joints or be done at their expense. Complete joint rest is applicable to acutely involved joints only. Self-care activities are permitted to pain tolerance, even in acute athritis.

Indications for Exercise

The concomitant use of the appropriate therapeutic exercise along with rest in proper balance is basic to the management of rheumatoid arthritis. The objectives of the exercise program are to preserve joint integrity, muscle strength, and endurance. Active-assisted exercises are useful and can be performed within limits of pain tolerance from the outset in the treatment program. As disease activity subsides and tolerance for exercise increases, gradation of the program may be increased to include active and resistive exercises.[8]

ACUTE STAGE. During the acute stage involved joints are inflamed and swollen. There may be systemic signs and symptoms, and rest may be required. Splints, braces, and positioning are used to provide joint rest and prevent deformity.

Active or passive ROM is done only to the point of pain in the acute stage with no stretching at the end of the range. Usually 1 to 2 repetitions of full joint ROM per day is enough to preserve ROM, although because of stiffness it may take several repetitions before maximum joint range is achieved.[19]

Isometric exercise without added resistance (muscle setting) may be used to maintain muscle tone. During the acute stage 1 isometric contraction per day is probably sufficient to preserve muscle strength.[19,33] Active exercises should be performed in a manner to prevent active stretching and joint stress. Pain or discomfort that results from exercise and lasts more than 1 hour indicates that the exercise was too stressful and should be decreased.[19]

Active resistive exercise, isometric exercise against added resistance, and stretching exercise are contraindicated during the acute stage of the disease.[38]

SUBACUTE STAGE. During the subacute stage of the disease a few joints are actively involved and there may be mild systemic symptoms. Short periods of rest and splints for corrective or preventive purposes are used.

Gentle passive stretch and active isotonic exercise

with minimal joint stress may be added to the passive or active ROM exercise program. Their purpose is to regain lost ROM in those joints that have become limited. A graded isometric strengthening program may be used to maintain or increase muscle strength and endurance.[38]

CHRONIC-ACTIVE AND CHRONIC-INACTIVE STAGES. During the chronic-active and chronic-inactive stages, stretch at the end of the ROM during exercise is recommended to increase ROM.[19] Active ROM, isometric, and isometric resistive exercises may also be continued.

Isotonic resistive exercise has traditionally been thought to produce excessive and undesirable joint stress.[19,38] This is undoubtedly true for joints in the acute stage of the disease, when synovitis is present, or when there is instability of the joint from stretching or deformity. However, in some postsurgical cases or when weakness is present in a chronic patient with a stable inactive joint, an individually prescribed isotonic resistive exercise program may be appropriate.[19,22,33]

HOME PROGRAM. A home exercise program that is designed for the particular patient should be carried out. It is best for the therapist to write out the directions for exercises for the patient to follow. The exercises should be done when the patient is feeling best, often after a warm shower or bath or in the afternoon when joint stiffness is at a minimum. Patients should be advised that taking pain medication in preparation for exercise or other physical activity is rarely recommended because of the need to use pain as a guideline for monitoring duration or intensity of the activity. Application of heat or cold for muscle relaxation and analgesic effect may benefit some patients.[8,20]

There is some conflict in the literature about the appropriateness of having arthritic patients adhere to a prescribed exercise program over the long term versus incorporating the therapeutic activities and goals into the patient's normal ADL routine. This may best be decided on an individual basis with "exercise to tolerance"[13] as a guideline and keeping principles of joint protection and energy conservation in mind. For a patient recovering from an acute flare an exercise program should be as efficient as possible so as not to take away valuable energy from one who may be barely able to cope with self-care.[23] For most patients, however, there comes a time when ADL will not be sufficient to enhance improved muscle tone, which aids in joint protection,[22] or to maximize general physical fitness.

In addition to well-accepted therapeutic exercise such as ROM and strengthening, there is recent evidence that arthritic patients may benefit from general conditioning exercise and recreational exercise with appropriate modifications to protect involved joints.[2,3] Particularly low-intensity aerobic activities such as walking, swimming, and bicycle riding, or a well-designed low-impact aerobics class have been shown to not only improve exercise tolerance and aerobic capacity but to decrease fatigue and improve functional status as well.[11]

Indications for Splinting

Splints may be used to rest inflamed joints; to improve function; or in the case of dynamic splints, to correct position or deformity. Splints are frequently used for the wrist and fingers but may also be used for the cervical spine, elbows, knees, and ankles. All splinting must be preceded by careful evaluation and be applied with skill, as inappropriate application may be not only ineffective but damaging as well.[30]

It is important to remember that splinting one joint may increase stress to the joints proximal and distal to it. This is particularly true of wrist splints that may increase stress to MP joints.[19]

Some of the splints commonly used in treatment of the arthritic hand are summarized from Melvin.[19] These include the volar resting, wrist stabilization, protective MP, combined, and ulnar drift positioning splints.

VOLAR RESTING SPLINT. The volar resting splint is indicated when there is acute synovitis of the wrist, fingers, and thumb. Its purpose is to rest involved joints and thus decrease inflammation and pain. It is also used when multiple joint contractures are beginning to develop for the purpose of maintaining proper positioning during sleep.

WRIST STABILIZATION SPLINT. A wrist stabilization splint immobilizes the wrist but allows motion of the MP joints. It is used when hand function is limited by wrist pain, to improve hand function and grip strength. It may be helpful when there is severe chronic wrist pain or inflammation to provide joint rest, and protect extensor tendons from attenuation and rupture.

PROTECTIVE MP SPLINT. The protective MP splint maintains the MP joints in normal alignment, allowing 0° to 25° of MP flexion. It is used to protect the MP joints from ulnar deviation and the forces of volar subluxation.

COMBINED WRIST STABILIZATION AND PROTECTIVE MP SPLINT. A combined wrist stabilization and protective MP splint is used when both the wrist and MP joints are involved for the purposes just described.

ULNAR DRIFT POSITIONING SPLINT. An ulnar drift positioning splint prevents ulnar drift and maintains normal alignment of MP joints during pinch and grasp activities.

Splints and other orthoses must be removed regularly for ROM exercises to the involved joints.

The reader is referred to *Rheumatic Disease: Occupational Therapy and Rehabilitation* by JL Melvin for a full dicussion and description of a wide variety of hand splints and their uses in the treatment of rheumatoid arthritis.

Indications for Activity

Treatment principles that apply to therapeutic exercise also apply to therapeutic activities. The activities that are selected should be nonresistive and provide opportunities for the maintenance or increase of ROM and strength. They should be meaningful and interesting to the patient. Joint protection principles, to be discussed subsequently, should be employed during leisure and work activities and ADL.

Crafts and games as therapeutic modalities are not as frequently or effectively used as therapeutic exercise regimes. However, they can be of value and interest to some patients and should not be overlooked as a purposeful application of therapeutic exercise procedures. Activities that can be useful in the treatment of rheumatoid arthritis include weaving, Turkish knotting, macrame, and peg games.[19]

The use of crocheting, knitting, and similar traditional needlecrafts is controversial. In principle they are to be avoided because they involve the use of prolonged static contraction of hand muscles in the intrinsic-plus position for holding tools and material. They also facilitate MP ulnar drift and MP volar subluxation through the forces in the hand during the performance of the activity. Melvin points out that in general the only conditions in which knitting and crocheting can be harmful are when there are active MP synovitis, beginning swan-neck deformity caused in part by intrinsic tightness, and degenerative joint disease of the CMC joint of the thumb.[19]

Adverse effects can be prevented by using an MP extension splint, performing intrinsic stretching exercises, and using a thumb CMC stabilization splint, depending on the specific potential problem. Frequent rest breaks during the activity or performing the activity for short, intermittent periods may also be helpful in preventing adverse effects. These are important considerations for those patients who would derive much pleasure and psychological benefit from these traditional and readily available leisure activities.[19]

ADL, including self-care and home management skills, is an important part of the rehabilitation program for the patient with rheumatoid arthritis. Self-care activities to pain and fatigue tolerance should be performed even during early acute stages of the disease episode. The number and types of activities are gradually increased as the patient's endurance and strength improve and pain and discomfort subside.[19]

These activities can be used to maintain or improve joint ROM, muscle strength, and physical endurance. Joint protection, work simplification, and energy conservation principles should be applied during the performance of these activities. The patient, with the aid and direction of the therapist, needs to work out a daily schedule of intermittent rest and activity which is suitable for the stage of the disease, activity tolerance, and any special systemic or joint problems that affect performance.

These principles apply to work activities. Since there are more women than men affected by arthritis, there has been an emphasis in the literature on home management activities, and joint protection principles related to these focused on the traditional role of woman as homemaker. The therapist must not lose sight of the facts that men also perform homemaking tasks and that a substantial percentage of women are employed outside of their homes. Therefore job analysis and application of joint protection and energy conservation principles may be an important part of the rehabilitation program for both men and women. Prevocational evaluation may be necessary if a job change is necessitated by the disability.

For juvenile rheumatoid arthritis school and leisure activities need to be considered and appropriate pacing of activities employed.

Assistive Equipment

Assistive devices and equipment are used to reduce pain, decrease joint stress, and increase independence.[19]

In general the purposes of various devices are to (1) facilitate grasp (built-up soft handles on tools); (2) compensate for lost ROM (dressing sticks or reachers); (3) facilitate ease of performance (lightweight equipment or electrical appliances); (4) stabilize materials or equipment (nonskid mats or suction brushes); (5) prevent deforming stresses (extended faucet handles or adapted key holder); (6) prevent prolonged static contraction (book stand or bowl holder); (7) compensate for weak or absent motor function (universal cuffs or stocking devices); and (8) prevent accidents (bathtub grab bars and nonskid mats for shower or bathtub).

Principles of Joint Protection

The purpose of joint protection training is to instruct the patient in methods of reducing joint stress, decreasing pain, preserving joint structures, and conserving energy.[19]

The arthritic joint is predisposed to deterioration from abuse that can lead to reduced performance abilities.[7] Patients with rheumatoid arthritis need to employ joint protection principles in all of their daily activities when in an active phase of the disease or where joint instability is present, in order to maintain maximal function and prevent joint damage and deformity.

MAINTAIN MUSCLE STRENGTH AND JOINT ROM. During daily activities each joint should be used at its maximal ROM and strength consistent with the disease process. For example, long, sweeping, flowing strokes to maintain and increase ROM can be employed when ironing. The arms should be straightened as far as possible, especially on flat work (Fig. 27-10). When vacuuming or mopping the floor a long, forward stroke of the implement, then pulling it in close to the body so the arm is first fully straightened, then fully bent, will achieve full or nearly full range of elbow flexion and extension and shoulder motion. The use of dust mitts on both hands keeps fingers straight and prevents the static contraction and potentially deforming forces of holding a dust cloth. Light objects, such as cereal, oats, or sugar, can be kept on high shelves so that full ROM in the shoulder can be used with reaching.[17]

AVOID POSITIONS OF DEFORMITY AND DEFORMING STRESSES. Positions that place internal forces (such as tight grasp) and external forces (such as propping the chin on the side or back of the fingers) may contribute to deformity and should be avoided during daily activity. Some applications of this principle include always turning the fingers toward the thumb side, such as turning a doorknob toward the thumb or opening the door with the right hand and closing it with the left. Jars should be opened with the right hand and closed with the left (Fig. 27-11). Dishcloths or hand laundry can be placed over the faucet

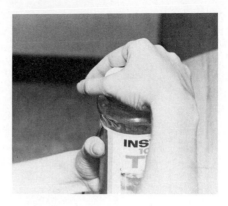

Fig. 27-11. Jar cap is twisted off, using palm of hand, and opened with right hand to prevent ulnar drift.

and squeezed between the palms or rolled in a towel to absorb water.[17]

Pressures along the thumb side of fingers should be avoided. These pressures contribute to ulnar deviation. This position of ulnar deviation decreases the use of the hands. Pressure can be prevented by (1) avoiding leaning chin on fingers or palm of hand; (2) picking up coffee cup with two hands instead of with index, middle finger, and thumb; (3) twisting a jar cap off and on with the palm of the hand and not with the fingers (Fig. 27-11); (4) installing level extensions on faucet handles to avoid use of fingers to turn on and off; and (5) using electric can opener instead of hand-operated type, since this device requires sustained grasp of one hand and forced motion of the thumb and fingers of the other hand for operation.

Tight grasp should be avoided. This position increases the strength of the muscles that allow grasp and therefore, contributes to ulnar deviation and dislocation of joints. This happens in activities such as carrying pails and baskets; using pliers, scissors, and screwdrivers; and holding spoons to stir or mix foods.

When standing up, the patient should be instructed to take the body weight through the wrist with fingers straight rather than on the fingers (Fig. 27-12). The palm of the hand, rather than the fingers, should be used when taking down or hanging clothes in the closet. The palm can be used to lift the hanger at the exposed area in its apex. This method is most useful in heavy coats and jackets.

Excessive and constant pressure against the pad of the thumb should be avoided. For example, pressure against the pad of the thumb to open a car door, sew through thick fabric, and rise to a standing position all contribute to dislocation of the thumb joints.[17]

USE EACH JOINT IN ITS MOST STABLE ANATOMICAL AND FUNCTIONAL PLANE. The patient should

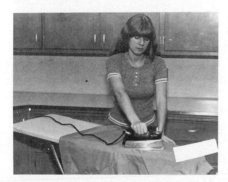

Fig. 27-10. During ironing, full extension at elbow can be practiced.

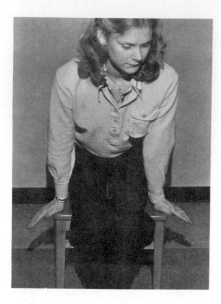

Fig. 27-12. Use of palms to push off chair helps to prevent dislocation of finger joints.

be instructed to stand up straight from any sitting position. The patient should stand or position self directly in front of a drawer to open it and not pull while standing to one side. In reaching for objects on a shelf the patient should stand or position self directly in front of or under the shelf, not at the side. The wrist and fingers should always be used in good alignment.[19]

USE THE STRONGEST JOINTS AVAILABLE FOR THE ACTIVITY. Applications of using the strongest joints include using the hips and knees, not the back, when lifting and using the entire body to move heavy things. Carts and chairs should be pushed from behind; use straps for opening and closing heavy doors and drawers; and roll objects on counters and floors rather than lifting them. If any objects must be lifted, they should be scooped up in both hands, palms upward. This technique can be used when handling baking pans and casseroles if long oven mitts are used and in handling dishes, packages, books, and laundry.[17]

AVOID USING MUSCLES OR HOLDING JOINTS IN ONE POSITION FOR ANY UNDUE LENGTH OF TIME. Sustained muscle contraction is fatiguing and can contribute to joint subluxation and dislocation. Applications of this principle include (1) using a book stand instead of holding the book while reading; (2) when mixing, stabilizing the bowl with the palm of the hand and fingers against the body or a wall or in an open drawer to avoid holding the bowl with the fingers and thumb; (3) holding the mixing spoon with the thumb side pointing upward, not with the thumb pointing

downward, and using a built-up handle to decrease the force of grasp (Fig. 27-13); (4) using a brush to scour pans, not the fingertips; (5) using the palm of the hand or the bend in the elbow instead of fingers in carrying handbags and coats; (6) holding objects, such as a vegetable peeler or knife, parallel to MP joints and not across the palms.[17,19]

NEVER BEGIN AN ACTIVITY THAT CANNOT BE STOPPED IMMEDIATELY IF IT PROVES TO BE TOO TAXING. In climbing up and down stairs, standing balance should be adequate to allow stopping and resting. In transferring from bed to wheelchair a sliding board should be used for less stress and to allow for stopping if necessary. In getting in and out of a bathtub graded platforms to ascend and descend gradually at individual speed and tolerance can be used.

RESPECT PAIN. Some discomfort during treatment and activity may be tolerable and acceptable. If rest produces rapid relief, the level of activity need not necessarily be considered excessive.[7] However, pain lasting 1 or more hours after activity is a sign that the activity needs to be stopped or modified.[7,19] Pain can evoke protective muscle spasm and inhibit muscle contraction.[7]

Energy Conservation and Work Simplification

Since prevention of fatigue is an important consideration in the management of rheumatoid arthritis, methods of simplifying work to save energy should be employed. One of the most important means to the end is to determine and carry out an appropriate balance between rest and play. The recommended

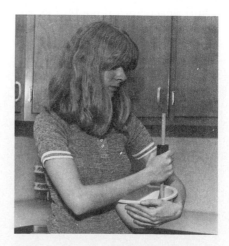

Fig. 27-13. Mixing bowl is stabilized with forearm. Spoon with soft, built-up handle is held so that pressure is toward radial side of hand.

amount of rest is 10 to 12 hours of rest per day, including a 1- to 2-hour nap in the afternoon.[19]

Short rest breaks of 5 to 10 minutes during daily activities can be very helpful in increasing overall endurance. In general, 5 to 10 minutes of rest to 20 minutes of activity is adequate. It may be difficult for the patient to accept the notion of these short rest breaks, since it is often the desire to get work or housekeeping over with as quickly as possible. However, intermittent rest can actually save energy for more enjoyable tasks.[19] Work can be planned for an entire week and month. Light and heavy tasks can be alternated and work paced throughout the week, instead of doing a lot of work in one day. Work should be planned so that it is efficient, that is, not requiring getting up and down and moving to and fro repeatedly.

Time management needs to be explored if rushing is a tendency of the patient. Rushing increases tension and fatigue. Most importantly the patient should learn an energy-saving program and work schedule that prevent pushing to exhaustion.[17]

Other suggestions for conserving energy include (1) avoid bending and stooping by using long-handle reachers and flexible-handle dust mops; (2) avoid long periods of standing during activities such as ironing and food preparation; rather, use a high stool; (3) avoid extra trips by using a utility cart to convey as many items as needed at once; and (4) relax homemaking standards by using prepackaged foods and by air drying dishes, for example.

Work may be simplified by adjusting the work height for maximal comfort. The elbows should be flexed to 90°, and shoulders should be in a relaxed position. This can be accomplished without expensive home modification by using an adjustable ironing board as a work surface, placing a board over an open drawer, or using a high stool with a backrest to work at counters. A rack may be placed in the sink bottom to elevate the dishpan and thus prevent stooping during dish washing.

Work areas can be rearranged so that frequently used tools, equipment, and supplies are stored nearby and at easily reached levels. Counter tops may be used for convenient storage of small appliances. Commercial organizers, such as step shelves and revolving turntables, can make work easier.[17]

OCCUPATIONAL THERAPY FOR RHEUMATOID ARTHRITIS

The patient with rheumatoid arthritis should be seen for occupational therapy services shortly after the diagnosis of arthritis is made. However, it is often the case that occupational therapy may not be initiated until many joints are involved, after surgery, or when the disease is severe enough to cause hospitalization or moderate-to-severe performance limitations.

Evaluation

OBSERVATION. The occupational therapist should observe the appearance of the hand for heat, redness, edema, deformity, deforming tendencies on motion, skin quality, and joint enlargement. In the early stages of the disease joints may appear puffy and soft. If the disease is active, joints may be red and hot.

ROM. The occupational therapy evaluation includes active and passive ROM measurements. These may take a considerable amount of time if there is discomfort or pain in the joints. It may be necessary to perform the measurements gradually over two or three treatment sessions. The therapist should be aware of how the joints feel, that is, stiff, unstable, or crepitant. A major discrepancy between active and passive ROM may be caused by pain secondary to inflammation in the joint or soft tissue, as well as from weakness[25] or tendon involvement.[5]

STRENGTH. Testing of muscle strength may be done by group or individual muscle testing. The usual procedures for manual muscle testing need to be adapted for the patient who has arthritis. Resistance should be applied within the patient's pain-free ROM rather than at the end of the ROM, as is usual in manual muscle testing. It is not unusual for patients with arthritis to have pain in the last 30° to 40° of joint motion. Therefore if resistance is applied within the pain-free range, the inhibition of muscle strength by pain will be avoided.[19]

The use of the manual muscle test is controversial, since some physicians prohibit any resistance that can cause harm to diseased tissue and joints and place deforming forces on the joint.[37] Functional muscle or motion testing may be used if resistance is prohibited.

In both the ROM assessment and the muscle strength test the therapist should make note of the time of day and the amount of anti-inflammatory or analgesic medication taken. These medications can affect results of the evaluation.[19]

HAND FUNCTION. Hand function testing is important. Pinch and grip strength testing with instruments is controversial for the reasons just stated.[37] Grip and pinch can be tested with an adapted blood pressure cuff and measured in millimeters of mercury.[19,25] A test of hand function that evaluates grasp and prehension patterns, such as the Jebsen Test of Hand Function[15] or the Quantitative Test of Upper Extremity Function,[4] should be administered.

SENSATION. Sensory evaluation is indicated if there is potential nerve compression caused by swelling. Modalities that should be tested are senses of touch, pain, temperature, and position. Paresthesias should be noted.

ENDURANCE. The patient's physical endurance should be evaluated by observation and an assessment of the daily or weekly schedule. Specific lower extremity evaluation may be carried out by the occupational or physical therapist. The occupational therapist should observe the gait pattern and mode of rising and sitting and the patient's posture during ambulation and when sitting. The therapist should observe for any obvious joint limitations and weakness in the lower extremities and have data from specific evaluation of ROM, strength, and deforming tendencies in the legs. These factors are important considerations in planning treatment, presenting joint protection and energy-conservation techniques, and positioning to prevent loss of ROM in the lower extremities.

PERFORMANCE. Assessment of performance is a very important part of the occupational therapy program. Evaluation of ADL, including self-care, child care, home management, and work activities, should be carried out by interview and observation. A home evaluation should be carried out to assist the client in learning new methods and in making modifications to simplify work, save energy, and protect joints from undue stress. Job performance may be evaluated by observation in a real or simulated situation. The job tasks can be analyzed, and joint protection principles can be applied, if possible. Pacing of work responsibilities may be a consideration to incorporate the required rest periods into the working day.

Treatment Objectives

The general objectives of treatment for patients with rheumatoid arthritis are to (1) maintain or increase joint mobility; (2) maintain or increase muscle strength; (3) increase physical endurance; (4) prevent or correct deformities, if feasible; (5) minimize the effect of deformities; (6) maintain or increase ability to perform daily life tasks; (7) increase knowledge about the disease and the best methods of dealing with physical, performance and psychosocial effects; and (8) aid with stress management and adjustment to physical disabilty.

Treatment Methods

Methods used by occupational therapists to minimize the dysfunction that can result from rheumatoid arthritis include a variety of exercises, just described, tailored to the patient's needs and stage of the disease.

Training in ADL is an important aspect of the occupational therapy program for many patients. This includes training in joint protection, energy-conservation techniques, and use of assistive devices and special equipment. Self-care, child care, home management, and work activities may be included in the ADL training program. Joint protection principles and energy-saving techniques should be introduced gradually, and the number and complexity of procedures should be increased as the patient incorporates previously learned skills into daily life. For some patients arts and crafts or games, as described earlier, can be a meaningful part of the treatment program. This will depend on the patient's needs, interests, and life-style and should be explored with the patient and not overlooked.

Splints to protect joints and prevent or retard the development of deformity are usually made by the occupational therapist. The therapist may recognize the need for splints and recommend them to the physician in some instances. Some splints that may be of benefit in the treatment of rheumatoid arthritis include the resting, cock-up, ulnar drift, MP extensor assist, flexor assist, CMC stabilization, and three-point finger extension splints.[19]

Psychosocial factors may be treated by exploring the patient's attitude toward the disability, the patient's goals, how the patient deals with pain and fear, and performance priorities and objectives. Activity groups, such as movement or exercise classes, home management classes, or arthritis education classes, can serve as mutual support and problem-solving groups. Occupational therapists may lead or participate with other rehabilitation specialists in such activity groups. Sexual counseling may be necessary to teach joint protection techniques during sexual activity and explore attitudes about body image, self-acceptance, and acceptance by the partner as a sexual being. Several excellent treatments of this subject are available.[6,28,31]

Education of the patient and family about the disease, potential disability, treatment, and home program to achieve maximal function is essential. Such education can be provided through classes and literature available from the Arthritis Foundation. Family roles may need to be changed or modified as a result of one member's physical dysfunction. Therefore it is important for families to understand and support the disabled member and lend aid for tasks the patient cannot or should not do.[24,26]

The occupational therapist should assist in designing a home program for the patient. This should include a suitable work and rest schedule, activities, and exercises that will maximize function and minimize deformity and dysfunction. The home program should be outlined for the patient in writing.

Treatment Precautions

Fatigue should be avoided, and pain should be respected. It may be difficult for the patient to do things in the morning because of stiffness of joints. A warm shower may be helpful to begin moving. Static, stressful, or resistive activities should be avoided. The use of a ball, putty, or clay for squeezing should be avoided, since these involve forceful flexion of the fingers, which can produce ulnar deviation, MP subluxation, and extensor tendon displacement.[10,19] If warmth is used to relax muscles and increase mobility, it should be limited to 20 minutes. Longer periods of warmth can increase inflammation and, later, produce increased swelling and pain. Resistive exercises for strengthening muscles do *not* improve joint stability and should not be used with this as an objective. Joint instability is usually caused by ligamentous laxity, and resistive exercises can make this worse.[38]

If sensation is impaired, the patient may not be aware of it, as the onset may be insidious and manifest itself subtly as gradual weakness and loss of hand function.[34] This may be attributed to other disease factors or hand deformity.[5] Because of possible involvement of the cervical spine in RA, it should be determined if any peripheral neuropathy is due to a cervical myelopathy or to a more distal lesion.[34] Appropriate protective mechanisms should be taught.

REVIEW QUESTIONS

1. What is the outstanding clinical feature that produces joint limitation and deformity in arthritis?
2. What sex and age groups are most frequently affected by arthritis?
3. What is meant by "rheumatoid factor"?
4. List four systemic signs of rheumatoid arthritis.
5. What is the characteristic course of the disease?
6. Describe the appearance and mechanics of two common finger deformities that may affect the DIP and PIP jonts in rheumatoid arthritis.
7. What are the deformities that can result at the MP joints? How are they treated or prevented?
8. What are the major problems at the elbow and shoulder in arthritis? How can they be prevented?
9. What kinds of exercises are appropriate for arthritis patients in the acute stage of disease?
10. When is stretching exercise indicated?
11. When is joint rest indicated in treatment of arthritis?
12. Which joints should not be splinted in treatment of arthritis?
13. Which joints are frequently splinted in treatment of arthritis?
14. What is the role of the occupational therapist in splinting for arthritis?
15. List appropriate occupational therapy evaluation procedures for rheumatoid arthritis.
16. What are the general objectives of occupational therapy in treatment of arthritis?
17. What kinds of activities are contraindicated for the arthritis patient during the acute stage of disease?
18. What kinds of activities are appropriate during the acute stage?
19. When the acute stage of the disease has abated, how can the patient's activity be graded?
20. Discuss some of the ways work can be simplified for the arthritis patient.
21. List some of the principles of joint protection directed toward maintaining ROM of the elbow and shoulder joints. Give some practical examples of methods of application of the principles to household tasks.
22. List five assistive devices for self-care or home management which could be useful to an arthritis patient, and give the rationale for each.

REFERENCES

1. Arthritis Foundation: Arthritis manual for allied health professionals, The Professional Manual Subcommittee of the Education Committee, Allied Health Professions Section, New York, 1973, The Arthritis Foundation.
2. Banwell B: Exercise behaviors. Presentation at The Arthritis Health Professions Association Annual Conference State of the Art Exercise and Arthritis, Washington, DC, June 1987.
3. Banwell B: Physical therapy in arthritis management. In Ehrlich

G, editor: Rehabilitation management of rheumatic conditions, ed 2, Baltimore, 1986, Williams & Wilkins.

4. Carroll D: A quantitative test for upper extremity function, J Chronic Dis 18:479, 1965.

5. Colditz J: Arthritis. In Malick M and Kasch M, editors: Manual on management of specific hand problems, Pittsburgh, 1984, AREN Publications.

6. Comfort A: Sexual consequences of disability, Philadelphia, 1978, George F Stickley Co.

7. Cordery JC: Joint protection: a responsibility of the occupational therapist, Am J Occup Ther 19:285, 1965.

8. Engleman E, and Shearn M: Arthritis and allied rheumatic disorders. In Krupp M and Chatton M, editors: Current medical diagnosis and treatment, Los Altos, CA, 1980, Lange Medical Publications.

9. Flatt A: The care of the arthritic hand, ed 4, St Louis, 1983, CV Mosby Co.

10. Fries JF: Arthritis: a comprehensive guide to understanding your arthritis, Reading, MA, 1986, Addison-Wesley Publishing Co, Inc.

11. Harcom TM et al: Therapeutic value of graded aerobic exercise training in rheumatoid arthritis, Arthritis and rheumatism 28:32, Jan 1985.

12. Healey L: The current status of methotrexate use in rheumatic diseases. Bull on the rheum dis 36(4), Atlanta, 1986, The Arthritis Foundation.

13. Hollander J: Rheumatoid arthritis. In Riggs G. and Gall E, editors: Rheumatic diseases: rehabilitation and management, Boston, 1984, Butterworth Publishers.

14. Huskisson E: Routine drug treatment of rheumatoid arthritis and other rheumatic diseases. In Huskisson E, editor: Clin rheum dis 5:697, Aug 1979.

15. Jebsen RH et al: An objective and standardized test of hand function, Arch Phys Med Rehabil 50:311, 1969.

16. Larson CB and Gould M: Orthopedic Nursing, ed 8, St Louis, 1974, CV Mosby Co.

17. Lorig K and Fries JF: The arthritis helpbook, ed 2, Reading, MA, 1986, Addison-Wesley Publishing Co, Inc.

18. Madden JW, DeVore G, and Arem AJ: A rational postoperative management program of metacarpal joint implant arthroplasty, J Hand Surg 2:26, 1977.

19. Melvin JL: Rheumatic disease: occupational therapy and rehabilitation, ed 3, Philadelphia, 1989, FA Davis Co.

20. Melvin JL: Hand dysfunction associated with arthritis. In Riggs G and Gall E, editors: Rheumatic diseases: rehabilitation and management, Boston, 1984, Butterworth Publishers.

21. Million R et al: Long term study of management of rheumatoid arthritis, Lancet, 1:812, April 1984.

22. Minor M: Aerobics. Presentation at The Arthritis Health Professions Association Annual Conference State of the Art Exercise and Arthritis, Washington, DC, June 1987.

23. Moncur C: Attacking the sacred cows. Presentation at The Arthritis Health Professions Association Annual Conference State of the Art Exercise and Arthritis, Washington, DC, June 1987.

24. Navarro A: Rheumatic conditions causing hip pain. In Rigg G and Gall E, editors: Rheumatic diseases: rehabilitation and management, Boston, 1984, Butterworth Publishers.

25. Polley H and Hunder G: Rheumatologic interviewing and physical examination of the joints, ed 2, Philadelphia, 1978, WB Saunders Co.

26. Potts MG: Psychosocial aspects of rheumatic disease. In Riggs G and Gall E, editors: Rheumatic diseases: rehabilitation and management, Boston, 1984, Butterworth Publishers.

27. RL Petzoldt Memorial Center for Hand Rehabilitation: Carpal tunnel syndrome protocol, RL Petzoldt Memorial Center for Hand Rehabilitation, 1987, San Jose, CA. (Unpublished.)

28. Richards JS: Sex and arthritis, Sexuality and dis 3:97, 1980.

29. Rodnan G and Schumacher HR, editors: Primer on the rheumatic diseases, ed 9, Atlanta, 1988, The Arthritis Foundation.

30. Seeger M: Splints, braces and casts. In Riggs G and Gall E, editors: Rheumatic diseases: rehabilitation and management, Boston, 1984, Butterworth Publishers.

31. Sidman JM: Sexual functioning and the physically disabled adult, Am J Occup Ther 31:81, 1977.

32. Simpson C: Exercise and arthritis. Presentation at the Northern California Chapter of The Arthritis Health Professionals, Arthritis Foundation, San Francisco, June 1987.

33. Sliwa J: Occupational therapy assessment and management. In Ehrlich G, editor: Rehabilitation management of rheumatic conditions, ed 2, Baltimore, 1986, Williams & Wilkins.

34. Sturge RA: The remote effects of rheumatic diseases on the hand and their management. In Wynn-Parry CB, editor: Clinics in rheumatic diseases, vol 10, London, 1984, WB Saunders Co.

35. Swanson A, Swanson G, and Leonard J: Postoperative rehabilitation in flexible implant arthroplasty of the digits. In Hunter JM et al: Rehabilitation of the hand, St Louis, 1984, CV Mosby Company.

36. Swezey RL: Rehabilitation in arthritis and related conditions. In Kottke FJ, Stillwell GK, and Lehmann JF, editors: Krusen's handbook of physical medicine and rehabilitation, Philadelphia, 1982, WB Saunders Co.

37. Trombly CA and Scott AD: Occupational therapy for physical dysfunction, Baltimore, 1977, Williams & Wilkins.

38. Wickersham B: The exercise program. In Riggs G and Gall E, editors: Rheumatic Diseases: rehabilitation and management, Boston, 1984, Butterworth Publishers.

Sample treatment plan

The treatment plan is not comprehensive. It deals with three of eight problems identified and two stages of the disease process. The reader is encouraged to add objectives and methods to the plan to make it more complete.

CASE STUDY

Mrs. J is a 36-year-old woman with a diagnosis of rheumatoid arthritis. The onset was 3 years ago. She is a wife and the mother of an 8-year-old girl. She lives with her husband and daughter in a three-bedroom, single-level tract home. Mrs J's primary role is that of homemaker. However, she has held a part-time job at a florist shop doing wreath design and construction and flower arranging. She both enjoys this work and sees her salary as a necessary adjunct to the family income.

Mrs. J experiences intermittent acute disease episodes that have primarily involved the elbows, wrists, MP, and PIP joints bilaterally. There are slight losses of ROM and strength at all involved joints.

To date there is no permanent deformity, but ulnar deviation, MP subluxation, boutonnière deformity, wrist subluxation, and further limitation of ROM at all involved joints are possible deformities.

Medical management has been through rest and salicylates. Medical precautions are no strenuous activity, no resistive exercise or activity, and avoidance of fatigue.

She was referred to occupational therapy during the acute phase of her most recent episode for prevention of deformity and loss of ROM and maintenance of maximal function. She continued with occupational therapy services during the subacute period with the same goals.

Personal Data

Name: Mrs. J

Age: 36

Diagnosis: Rheumatoid arthritis

Disability: Limited ROM, decreased strength, potential deformity of elbows, wrists, MP and PIP joints bilaterally.

Treatment aims stated in the referral: Prevent deformity, prevent loss of ROM, maintain maximal function

OTHER SERVICES

Physician: Supervise medical management and rehabilitation therapies

Physical therapy: May be used for specific exercise program

Social services: Patient and family counseling, if needed; financial arrangements, if appropriate

Vocational counseling: Explore feasibility of return to same or modified occupation in floral work.

FRAME OF REFERENCE/TREATMENT APPROACH

Occupational Performance

Biomechanical and Rehabilitation Approaches

OT EVALUATION

Performance components

Motor functioning
  Active and passive ROM: Test
  Muscle strength: Observe, test
  Hand deformities: Observe, test MP stability
    Ulnar drift: (Measure if present)
    Wrist subluxation
    MP subluxation
    Boutonnière deformity
    Swan-neck deformity
    Thumb deformities
  Hand function: Test
Sensory integrative functioning
  Sensation: Test
  Carpal tunnel syndrome: Test
Cognitive functioning
  Memory: Observe, interview
  Motivation: Observe, interview
  Functional language skills: Observe, interview comprehension of written/spoken
Psychological functioning
  Adjustment to disability: Observe, interview
  Interpersonal and coping skills: Observe

Performance skills

Social functioning

Family and community support: Interview

Self-care: Observe, interview

Home management: Observe, interview

Prevocational: Observe, interview

Endurance: Observe, interview

Play/Leisure: Observe, interview

EVALUATION SUMMARY

Weakness is noted particularly in wrist and finger extensors (F +) and to a lesser degree in flexor groups (G). Mild ROM limitations are present in elbows, wrists, and fingers with some MP instability noted (10° ulnar drift). No subluxation or other deformities were noted. Hand function testing revealed difficulty with fingertip prehension, and pinch and grip are good but not normal in strength. Forceful use of the thumb in opposition enhances ulnar drift and produces MP discomfort.

Continued.

Sample treatment plan—cont'd

Sensation is intact, and cognitive state appears to be within normal limits.

The patient's family has noted that the patient demonstrates withdrawal from social situations during flares and has limited patience when fatigued and in pain. Her family appears to be supportive, and her daughter helps with household tasks. During inactive periods she is independent for light housekeeping, self-care, and work. She fatigues after 2 hours of light to moderate activity and requires a 20-minute rest period. During flares she is severely limited in ADL, leaves home management tasks to her family, and is unable to work. She manages to do only light self-care activities independently.

Observation of the job by another worker and Mrs. J in simulated tasks revealed that some aspects of her job would contribute to development of deformity. Cutting and twisting floral wire, forcing stems and stem supports into Styrofoam, and binding wreaths were thought to be likely to enhance ulnar drift and MP subluxation because of the resistance and direction of joint forces. However, wreath design and layout and fresh flower arrangement are possible alternatives. Ms. J's employer is willing to retain her on a part-time basis to perform these duties.

ASSETS

No lower extremity involvement
Good preservation of function
Supportive and intact family unit
Potential job skills, flexible employer
Intelligence, motivation

PROBLEM LIST

1. Muscle weakness
2. Limited ROM
3. Potential deformity
4. Fluctuating vocational role
5. Limited ADL independence
6. Fluctuating role as wife and mother
7. Tendency to social withdrawal
8. Limited endurance

ACUTE STAGE

PROBLEM 1

Muscle weakness
Objective
Muscle strength will be maintained
Method
Isometric exercise without added resistance to biceps, triceps, flexor and extensor carpi radialis and ulnaris, 1 to 3 repetitions once a day. Active ROM exercise to elbows and wrists, 2 to 3 repetitions once a day; and self-care to tolerance.
Gradation
Increase number of exercise sessions or repetitions as synovitis and pain subside

PROBLEM 2

Limited ROM
Objective
ROM of affected joints will be maintained
Method
Active or active-assisted ROM exercises to elbow, MP and PIP flexion and extension, wrist flexion, extension, radial and ulnar deviation. Active ROM exercises may be carried out in a warm bath or shower or immediately following bathing
Gradation
Grade to active exercise and add gentle active and passive stretching during subacute stage

PROBLEM 5

Limitied ADL independence
Objective
With adaptive aids and use of joint protection techniques the patient will perform self-care activities independently
Method
Therapist will provide instruction in joint protection and make specific recommendations for modifications to existing equipment (building up handles on toothbrush, hairbrush, eating utensils, etc). Patient will be provided with necessary self-care adaptive equipment (button hook, washing mitt, etc) and instruction in their use. Treatment sessions within the clinic will include dressing and grooming tasks to facilitate problem solving and permit patient to demonstrate competence in the use of adaptive equipment and techniques
Gradation
As synovitis subsides patient will gradually be able to taper the use of adaptive equipment and to increase her activity level

SUBACUTE STAGE

PROBLEM 1

Muscle weakness
Objective
Strength of weakened muscles will increase by ½ grade as compared with the initial evaluation
Method
Patient's activity level in the home will increase to include light housekeeping activities (ironing, dust mopping, dish washing). Patient will be given isometric exercise with resistance to elbow and wrist flexors and extensors, MP and PIP extensors, 3 to 10 repetitions 3 times daily.
Gradation
Increase the amount of physical activity as tolerated. Increase the number exercise repetitions as tolerated

PROBLEM 2

Limited ROM
Objective
ROM of affected joints will be increased or maintained
Method
Active ROM exercise to elbow, wrist, MP and PIP joints, gentle passive stretching to elbow flexion, and extension and PIP extension. Patient will be instructed to use full ROM for light resistance ADL such as dust mopping, folding linen, and ironing
Gradation
Increase resistance for stretching exercise as tolerated

Chapter

28

Acute hand injuries

MARY C. KASCH

Treatment of the upper extremity is important to all occupational therapists who work with physically disabled persons. The incidence of upper extremity injuries is significant and accounts for about one third of all injuries. The nearly 16 million upper extremity injuries that occur annually in the United States result in 90 million days of restricted activity and 12 million visits to physicians. The upper extremities are involved in about one third of work-related farm injuries and one third of disabling industrial injuries. In addition, disease and congenital anomalies contribute to upper extremity dysfunction, and it is estimated that only about 15% of those suffering from severe cerebral vascular accident recover hand function.[56]

The hand is vital to human function and appearance. It flexes, extends, opposes, and grasps thousands of times daily, allowing the performance of necessary daily activities. The hand's sensibility allows feeling without looking and provides protection from injury. The hand touches, gives comfort, and expresses emotions. Loss of hand function through injury or disease thus affects much more than the mechanical tasks that the hand performs. Hand injury may jeopardize a family's livelihood and at the least affects every daily activity. The occupational therapist with training in physical and psychological assessment, prosthetic evaluation, fabrication of orthoses, and assessment and training in the activities of daily living (ADL), and in functional restoration is uniquely qualified to treat upper extremity disorders.

Hand rehabilitation, or hand therapy, has grown as a specialty area of both physical and occupational therapy, and some of the treatment techniques used with hand patients have emerged from both specialties to be used by the hand therapist. It is not the purpose of this chapter to instruct the occupational therapy student in physical modalities. Rather, treatment techniques that have been found to be beneficial to hand injury patients are presented. It is assumed that these techniques will be provided by the therapist best trained to provide them. Hand rehabilitation requires advanced and specialized training by both physical and occupational therapists. A role delineation study of hand therapy which includes definition and scope of practice has been reported.[22]

Treatment techniques, whether thermal modalities or specifically designed exercises, are used as a bridge to reach a further goal of returning to functional performance. Thus some modalities may be used as "enabling modalities" in preparation for functional use. It is within this context that treatment techniques will be presented in this chapter.

Treatment of the injured hand is a matter of timing and judgment. Following trauma or surgery a healing phase must occur in which the body performs its physiological function of wound healing. Following the initial healing phase when cellular restoration has been accomplished, the wound enters its restorative phase. It is in this phase that hand therapy is most beneficial. Early treatment that occurs in this restorative phase is ideal and in some cases essential for optimal results. Although sample timetables may be presented, the therapist should always coordinate the application of any treatment with the referring physician. Surgical techniques may vary, and inappropriate treatment of the hand patient can result in failure of a surgical procedure.

Communication between the surgeon, therapist, and patient is especially vital in this setting. A comfortable environment in which group interaction is possible may increase patient motivation and cooperation. The presence of the therapist as an instructor and evaluator is essential, but without the patient's cooperation limited gains will be achieved. Treating the psychological loss suffered by the patient with a hand injury is an integral part of the rehabilitative therapy as well.

The author gratefully acknowledges the staff of the Hand Rehabilitation Center of Sacramento: Lynne Hester Finney, OTR; Susan Chapman Williams, OTR; and Anne Greensfelder, OTR, for their assistance in reviewing and making recommendations for revision of the material in this chapter.—MCK

EXAMINATION AND EVALUATION

When approaching a patient who has a hand injury, the therapist must be able to evaluate the nature of the injury and the limitations it has produced. First the injured structures must be identified by consulting with the hand surgeon, reviewing operative reports and x-ray films, and discussing the injury with the patient. Evaluation of bone, tendon, and nerve function must be ascertained using standardized evaluation techniques whenever possible.

The patient's age, occupation, and hand dominance should be taken into account in the initial evaluation. The type and extent of medical and surgical treatment that has been received and the length of time since such treatment are important in determining a treatment plan. Any further surgery or conservative treatment that is planned should also be noted. The treatment plan should have the written approval of the referring physician.

The purposes of hand evaluation are to identify (1) physical limitations, such as loss of range of motion (ROM) (2) functional limitations, such as inability to perform daily tasks (3) substitution patterns to compensate for loss of sensibility or motor function and (4) established deformities, such as joint contracture.

The movement of the arm and hand must be coordinated for maximum function. Shoulder motion is essential for positioning the hand and elbow for daily activities.[20]

The wrist is the key joint in the position of function.[15] Skilled hand performance depends on wrist stability, mobility, and ability to make fine adjustments in position. It also depends on arm and shoulder stability and mobility for fixing or positioning the hand for functional use. The thumb is of greater importance than any other finger. Effective pinch is almost impossible without a thumb, and attempts will always be made to salvage or reconstruct an injured thumb.

Within the hand, the proximal interphalangeal (PIP) joint is critical for grasp and is considered to be the most important small joint.[15] Limitations in flexion or extension will result in significant functional impairment.

Observation and Topographical Evaluation

The occupational therapist should observe the appearance of the hand and arm. The position of the hand and arm at rest and the carrying posture can yield valuable information about the dysfunction. How the patient "treats" the disease or injury should be observed. Is it overprotected and carefully guarded or ignored? The skin condition of the hand and arm should be noted. Are there lacerations, sutures, or evidence of recent surgery? Is the skin dry or moist? Are there scales or crusts? Does the hand appear swollen? Does the hand have an odor? Palmar skin is less mobile than dorsal skin normally. The degree of mobility and elasticity and the adherence of scars is determined. Trophic changes in the skin should be observed. The vascular system is assessed by observing the skin color and temperature of the hand and evaluating for presence of edema. Are these contractures of the web spaces? The therapist should observe the relationship between hand and arm function as the patient moves about and performs test items or tasks.

The therapist should ask the patient to perform some simple bilateral ADL, such as buttoning a button, putting on a shirt, opening a jar, and threading a needle, and observe the amount of spontaneous movement and use of the affected hand and arm.

Physical Evaluation

The effect of trauma or dysfunction on anatomical structures is the first consideration in evaluating hand function. The joints must be assessed for active and passive mobility, fixed deformities, and any tendency to assume a position of deformity. The ligaments must be evaluated for laxity or contracture and their ability to maintain joint stability. Tendons must be examined for integrity, contracture, or overstretching; muscles are tested for strength and function.

SOFT TISSUE TIGHTNESS. Joints may develop dysfunction following trauma, immobilization, or disuse. Mennell emphasizes the importance of the small, involuntary motions of the joint which he refers to as "joint play."[77] Others[67] describe these as "accessory motions." Joint play or accessory motions are those movements that are nonvoluntary, physiologic, and can be performed only by someone else.[54] Examples of accessory motions are joint rotation and joint distraction. If accessory motions are limited and painful, the active motions of that joint cannot be normal. Therefore it is necessary to restore joint play through the use of joint mobilization techniques before attempting passive or active range of motion.[78]

Joint mobilization may date back to the fourth century BC, when Hippocrates first described the use of spinal traction.[54] In the 1930s an English physician, James Mennell, encouraged physicians to perform manipulation without anesthesia, a practice that is advocated today by James Cyriax, who explored the use of manipulation of the intervertebral discs. Current theorists include Cyriax, Robert Maigne, FM Kaltenborn, GD Maitland, Stanley Paris, and John Mennell, son of the late James Mennell. While physicians originally practiced manipulation, therapists have adapted the techniques, which are now called "joint mobilization."

The techniques used to assess joint play are also

used in the treatment of joint dysfunction. During assessment the evaluator determines the range of accessory motion and the presence of pain by taking up the slack only in the joint. During treatment a high-velocity, low-amplitude thrust or graded oscillation is applied to regain motion and relieve pain.[67]

Guidelines must be followed in applying joint mobilization techniques, and they should not be attempted by the untrained or inexperienced practitioner. Postgraduate courses are offered in joint mobilization of the extremities, and the therapist must be familiar with the orthokinematics of each joint as well as with the techniques used.

Joint mobilization is generally indicated with restriction of accessory motions or the presence of pain due to tightness of the joint capsule, meniscus displacement, muscle guarding, ligamentous tightness, or adherence. It is contraindicated in the presence of infection, recent fracture, neoplasm, joint inflammation, rheumatoid arthritis, osteoporosis, degenerative joint disease, or many chronic diseases.[54]

Limitations in joint motion may also be caused by tightness of the extrinsic or intrinsic muscles and tendons. If the joint capsule is not tight and accessory motions are normal, the therapist should test for extrinsic and intrinsic tightness.

To test for extrinsic extensor tightness the metacarpophalangeal (MP) joint is passively held in extension and the PIP joint is moved passively into flexion. Then the MP joint is flexed, and the PIP joint is again passively flexed. If the PIP joint can be flexed easily when the MP joint is extended but not when the MP joint is flexed, the extrinsic extensors are adherent.[2]

If there is extrinsic flexor tightness, the PIP and DIP joints will be positioned in flexion with the MP joints held in extension. It will not be possible to pull the fingers into complete extension. If the wrist is then held in flexion, the IP joints will extend more easily as a result of slack being placed on the flexor tendons.

Tightness of the intrinsic musculature is tested by passively holding the MP joint in extension and applying pressure just distal to the PIP joint. This is repeated with the MP joint in flexion. If there is more resistance when the MP joint is extended, intrinsic tightness is indicated.[2]

If there is no difference in passive motion of the PIP joint when the MP joint is held in extension or flexion and there is limitation of PIP joint flexion in any position, tightness of the joint capsule is indicated. The therapist should assess the joint for capsular tightness if this has not already been done.

EDEMA ASSESSMENT. Hand volume is measured to assess the presence of extra- or intracellular edema. It is generally used to determine the effect of treatment and activities. By measuring volume at different times of the day the effects of rest versus activity may be measured as well as the effects of splinting or treatment designed to reduce edema.

A commercially available volumeter[27] may be used to assess hand edema. The volumeter has been shown to be accurate to 10 ml[105] when used in the prescribed manner. Variables that have been shown to decrease the accuracy of the volumeter include (1) the use of a faucet or hose that introduces air into the tank during filling, (2) movement of the arm within the tank, (3) inconsistent pressure on the stop rod, and (4) the use of a volumeter in a variety of places. The same level surface should always be used.[43] The evaluation is performed as follows (Fig. 28-1):

1. A plastic volumeter is filled and allowed to empty into a large beaker until the water reaches spout level. The beaker is then emptied and dried thoroughly.
2. The patient is instructed to immerse the hand in the plastic volumeter, being careful to keep the hand in the midposition.
3. The hand is lowered until it rests gently between the middle and ring fingers on the dowel rod. It is important that the hand does not press onto the rod.

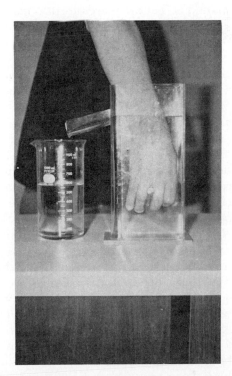

Fig. 28-1. Volumeter is used to measure volume of both hands for comparison. Increased volume indicates presence of edema.

4. The hand remains still until no more water drips into the beaker.
5. The water is poured into a graduated cylinder. The cylinder is placed on a level surface, and a reading is made.

A method of assessing edema of an individual finger or joint is circumferential measurement using either a circumference tape[60] or jeweler's ring-size standards. Measurements should be made before and after treatment and especially following the application of thermal modalities or splinting. While patients often will have subjective complaints relating to swelling, objective data of circumference or volume will help the therapist to assess the response of the tissues to treatment and activity. Edema control techniques will be discussed later in this chapter.

SENSIBILITY

Mapping. Sensibility testing can begin with sensory mapping of the entire volar surface of the hand.[17] The hand must be supported by the examiner's hand or be resting in a medium such as putty. Either the examiner or the patient can draw a probe, usually the eraser end of a pencil, lightly over the skin from the area of normal sensibility to the area of abnormal sensibility. The patient must immediately report the exact location where the sensation changes. This is done from proximal to distal and radial and ulnar to medial directions. The areas are carefully marked and transferred to a permanent record. Mapping should be repeated at monthly intervals during nerve regeneration.

Categories of tests. A variety of evaluations may be required to adequately assess sensibility. These tests can be divided into three categories: (1) Modality tests for pain, heat, cold, and touch-pressure; (2) functional tests to assess the quality of sensibility, or what Moberg described as "tactile gnosis." Examples of functional tests are stationary and moving two-point discrimination and the Moberg Pick-up Test; (3) objective tests that do not require active participation by the patient. These include the wrinkle test, the Ninhydrin sweat test, and nerve-conduction studies.[17]

Sympathetic function. Recovery of sympathetic response (sweating, pain, and temperature discrimination) may occur early but does not correlate with functional recovery.[30] O'Rain[83] observed that denervated skin does not wrinkle. Therefore nerve function may be tested by immersing the hand in water for 5 minutes and noting the presence or absence of skin wrinkling. This test may be especially helpful in diagnosing a nerve lesion in young children. The ability to sweat is also lost with a nerve lesion. A ninhydrin test[81] evaluates sweating of the finger.

The wrinkle test and the ninhydrin test are objective tests of sympathetic function. Recovery of sweating has not been shown to correlate with the recovery of sensation, but the absence of sweating correlates with the lack of discrimatory sensation. Other signs of sympathetic dysfunction are smooth, shiny skin; nail changes; and "pencil-pointing" or tapering of the fingers.[106]

Nerve compression and nerve regeneration. Sensibility testing is done to assess the recovery of a nerve following laceration and repair, as well as to determine the presence of a nerve compression syndrome and the return of nerve function following surgical decompression, or the efficacy of conservative treatment to reduce compression. Therefore tests such as vibratory tests may be interpreted differently depending on the mechanism of nerve dysfunction. In the following section tests will be described and differences drawn as appropriate to assist the therapist in selecting the correct evaluation technique as well as in planning treatment based on the evaluative measures.

Tinel's sign and Phalen's test. While these tests are not considered to be tests of sensibility, they are used to assess the rate of nerve recovery (Tinel's) and are considered "provocative" tests in nerve compression syndromes because they will elicit the pathological response of the nerve when employed.

During the first 2 to 4 months following nerve suture, axons will regenerate and travel through the hand at a rate of about 1 mm per day or 1 inch (2.54 cm) per month. Tinel's sign may be used to follow this regeneration.[59] The test is performed by tapping gently along the course of the nerve, starting distally and moving toward the nerve suture to elicit a tingling sensation in the fingertip. The point at which tapping begins to elicit a tingling sensation is noted and indicates the extent of sensory axon growth. As regeneration occurs, hypesthesias will develop. Although this hypersensitivity may be uncomfortable to the patient, it is a positive sign of nerve growth. A treatment program for desensitization of hypersensitive areas can be initiated as soon as the skin is healed and can tolerate gentle rubbing and immersion in textures. Desensitization is discussed further in the treatment section.

The examiner can also attempt to elicit Tinel's sign in nerve compression by percussing the median nerve at the level of the wrist carpal tunnel.[94] Tinel's sign is positive if there is tingling along the course of the nerve distally when percussed. Phalen's test will also produce the nerve paresthesias present in compression of the median nerve. The patient is asked to hold the wrist in a fully flexed position for 60 seconds. It is considered positive if tingling occurs within this time.[94]

Vibration. Dellon advocated the use of 30-cps and 256-cps tuning forks for assessing the return of vibratory sensation following nerve repair as regeneration occurs and as a guideline for initiating a sensory reeducation program.[31] He found that an orderly progression of sensory return occurred: pain, perception of 30-cps stimuli, moving touch, constant touch, and 256-cps stimuli. When using a tuning fork for testing the hand should be supported by resting on a table. The examiner hits the tuning fork briskly and places the prong on the fingertip, moving it proximally until the vibration is perceived by the patient. The corresponding contralateral finger is then tested, and the patient asked if the vibration is more, less, or the same. Vibration is considered altered if it is not the same on both digits.[32]

Two vibrometers are now available to test vibratory threshold: the Bio-Thesiometer[33,96] and the Bruel and Kjaer Vibrometer.[63] They have been found to be highly sensitive in detecting nerve compression when two-point discrimination is still normal. Gelberman[45] found that vibration and touch perception as measured by the Semmes-Weinstein monofilaments are altered before two-point because they measure a single nerve fiber innervating a group of receptor cells. Two-point discrimination is a test of innervation-density which requires overlapping sensory units and cortical integration. Thus it will be altered following nerve laceration and repair but will remain normal if the nerve is compressed as long as there are links to the cortex. Bell[9] has also found normal two-point values in the presence of decreased sensory function. Vibration and the Semmes-Weinstein test are more sensitive in picking up a gradual decrease in nerve function in the presence of nerve compression where the nerve circuitry is intact. They also correlate with decreases in sensory nerve action-potential amplitude as measured by nerve conduction studies.[96] Therefore vibration, Semmes-Weinstein, and electrical testing are reliable and sensitive tests for early detection of carpal tunnel syndrome. Vibration and Semmes-Weinstein can be performed in the clinic with no discomfort to the patient and are excellent screening tools when nerve compression is suspected.

Touch pressure. Moving touch is tested using the eraser end of a pencil. The eraser is placed in an area of normal sensibility and, pressing lightly, is moved to the distal fingertip. The patient notes when the perception of the stimulus changes. Light and heavy stimuli may be applied and noted.[30]

Constant touch is tested by pressing with the eraser end of a pencil, first in an area with normal sensibility and then moving distally. The patient responds when the stimulus is altered again; light and heavy stimuli may be applied.[30]

The Semmes-Weinstein monofilaments are the most accurate instrument for assessing cutaneous pressure thresholds.[10] The test is composed of 20 nylon monofilaments housed in plastic hand-held rods. The diameter of the monofilaments increases and when applied correctly exert a force ranging from 4.5 mg to 447 g. Markings on the probes range from 1.65 to 6.65 but do not correspond to the grams of force of each rod. Normal fingertip sensibility has been found to correspond to the 2.44 and 2.83 probes.

The monofilaments must be applied perpendicularly to the skin and are applied just until the monofilament bends. The skin should not blanch when the monofilament is applied. Probes 1.65 through 2.83 are bounced three times. Probes marked 3.22 to 4.08 are applied three times with a bend in the filament, and probes marked 4.17 to 6.65 are applied once. The larger monofilaments do not bend, and therefore skin color most be observed to determine how firmly to apply the probe.

The examiner should begin with a probe in the "normal" range and progress through the rods in increasing diameters to find the patient's threshold for touch throughout the volar surface.[10] A grid should be used to record the responses so that varying areas of touch perception can be demonstrated. Two out of three correct responses are necessary for an area to be considered as having intact sensibility. It is preferable to place the monofilaments randomly rather than to concentrate on an area, in order to allow the nerves recovery time. When a filament is placed three times, it should be held for a second, rested for a second, and reapplied.

Results can be graded from normal light touch (probes 2.83 and above) to loss of protective sensation (probes 4.56 and below). Diminished light touch and diminished protective sensation are in the range reflected by the central probes.[10]

Two-point and moving two-point discrimination. Discrimination, the second level of sensibility assessment, requires the subject to distinguish between two direct stimuli. Static or stationary two-point discrimination measures the slowly adapting fibers. The two-point discrimination test, first described by Weber in 1853, was modified and popularized by Moberg,[80] who was interested in a tool that would assess the functional level of sensation. A variety of devices have been proposed to use in measuring two-point discrimination. The bent paper clip is inexpensive but often has burrs on the metal tip. Other devices include industrial calipers,[21] and the Disk-Criminator.[35] A device with parallel prongs of variable distance and blunted ends should produce replicable results.

The test is performed as follows:[59]
1. The patient's vision is occluded.
2. An area of normal sensation is tested as a reference, using a blunt caliper or bent paper clip.
3. The calipers are set 10 mm apart and are randomly applied starting at the fingertip and moving proximally and longitudinally in line with the digital nerves, with one or two points touching. The skin should not be blanched by the caliper. The distance is decreased until the patient no longer feels two distinct points, and that distance is measured. Three to four seconds should be allowed between applications, and the patient should have four out of five correct responses.[9] Because this test indicates sensory function, it is usually administered at the tips of the fingers. It may be used proximally to test nerve regeneration. Normal two-point discrimination at the fingertip is 6 mm or less.[2]

Moving two-point discrimination measures the innervation density of the quickly adapting nerve fibers for touch. It is slightly more sensitive than stationary two-point discrimination.[61] The test is performed as follows:[30]
1. The patient's vision is occluded.
2. An area of normal sensation is tested as a reference, using a blunt caliper or bent paper clip.
3. The fingertip is supported by the examining table or the examiner's hand.
4. The caliper, separated 5 mm to 8 mm, is moved longitudinally from proximal to distal in a linear fashion along the surface of the fingertip. One and two points are randomly alternated. The patient must correctly identify the stimulus in seven out of eight responses before proceeding to a smaller value. The test is repeated down to a separation of 2 mm.

Two-point values increase with age in both sexes, with the smallest values occurring between the ages of 10 and 30. Females tend to have smaller values than men, and there is no significant difference between dominant and nondominant hands.[61]

Modified Moberg pick-up test. Recognition of common objects is the final level of sensory function. Moberg used the phrase "tactile gnosis" to describe the ability of the hand to perform complex functions by feel. Moberg described the Picking-Up Test in 1958,[80]

and it was later modified by Dellon.[30] This test is used with either a median nerve injury or a combination of median and ulnar nerves. Clinically it has been observed that it takes twice as long to perform the tests with vision occluded than with vision. The test is performed as follows:

1. Nine or ten small objects (coins, paper clip, etc) are placed on a table, and the patient is asked to place them one at a time in a small container as quickly as possible while looking at them. The patient is timed.

2. The test is repeated for the opposite hand with vision.

3. The test is repeated for each hand with vision occluded.

4. The patient is asked to identify each object one at a time with and then without vision.

It is important to observe any substitution patterns that may be used when the patient cannot see the objects.

Grip and Pinch Strength

Upper extremity strength evaluation is usually performed following the healing phase of trauma. Strength testing is *not* indicated following recent trauma or surgery. Testing should not be performed until the patient has been cleared for full-resistive activities, usually 8 to 12 weeks following injury.

A standard adjustable handle dynamometer is recommended for assessing grip strength (Fig. 28-2).

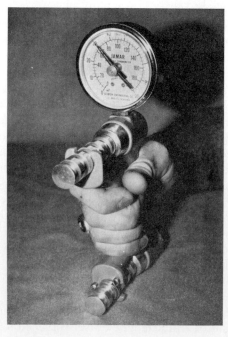

Fig. 28-2. Jamar dynamometer is used to evaluate grip strength in both hands.

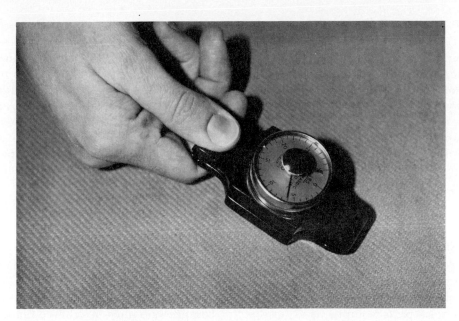

Fig. 28-3. Pinch gauge is used to evaluate pinch strength to variety of prehension patterns of pinch.

The subject should be seated with the shoulder adducted and neutrally rotated, the elbow flexed at 90°,[75] forearm in the neutral position, and the wrist between 0° and 30° extension and between 0° and 15° of ulnar deviation. Three trials are taken of each hand with the dynamometer handle set at the second position.[73] The dynamometer should be lightly held by the examiner to prevent accidental dropping of the instrument. A mean of the three trials should be reported. The noninjured hand is used for comparison. Normative data may be used to compare strength scores.[55,74] Variables, such as age, will affect the strength measurements.

Pinch strength should also be tested using a pinch gauge. The pinch gauge by B & L Engineering has been found to be the most accurate.[73] Two-point pinch (thumb tip to index fingertip), lateral or key pinch (thumb pulp to lateral aspect of the middle phalanx of the index finger), and three-point pinch (thumb tip to tips of index and long fingers) should be evaluated. As with the grip dynamometer, three successive trials should be obtained and compared bilaterally[43] (Fig. 28-3).

Manual muscle testing is also used to evaluate upper extremity strength. Accurate asessment is especially important when preparing the patient for tendon transfers or other reconstructive surgery. The student who wishes to study muscle testing of the hand is referred especially to JV Basmajians's work.[5]

Maximum voluntary effort during grip, pinch, or muscle testing will be affected by pain in the hand or extremity and it should be noted if the patient's ability to exert full force is limited by subjective complaints. Localization of the pain symptoms and consistency in noting pain will help the therapist to evaluate the role that pain is playing in the recovery from injury. Pain problems will be discussed in more detail later in this chapter.

Functional Evaluation

Evaluation of hand function or performance is important because the physical evaluation does not measure the patient's ingenuity and ability to compensate for loss of strength, ROM sensation, or presence of deformities.[20]

The physical evaluation should precede the functional evaluation because awareness of physical dysfunction can result in a critical analysis of functional impairment and an understanding of why the patient functions as he or she does.[76]

The effect of the hand dysfunction on the use of the hand in activities of daily living (ADL) should be observed by the occupational therapist. In addition, some type of a standardized performance evaluation, such as the Jebsen Test of Hand Function[49] or the Carroll Quantitative Test of Upper Extremity Function,[20] should be administered.

The Jebsen Test of Hand Function[49] was developed to provide objective measurements of standardized tasks with norms for patient comparison. It is a short test that is assembled by the administrator. It is easy to administer, and inexpensive. The test consists of seven subtests, comprising (1) writing a short sentence, (2) turning over 3 × 5-inch cards, (3) picking

up small objects and placing them in a container, (4)
stacking checkers, (5) eating (simulated), (6) moving
empty large cans, and (7) moving weighted large cans.
Norms are provided for dominant and nondominant
hands for each subtest and also are divided by sex
and age. Instructions for assembling the test, as well
as specific instructions for administering it, are provided by the authors.[49] This has been found to be a
good test for overall hand function.

The Quantitative Test of Upper Extremity Function described by Carroll[20] was designed to measure
ability to perform general arm and hand activities
used in daily living. It is based on the assumption that
complex upper extremity movements used to perform ordinary ADL can be reduced to specific patterns of grasp and prehension of the hand, supination
and pronation of the forearm, flexion and extension
of the elbow, and elevation of the arm.

The test consists of six parts, comprising (1) grasping and lifting four blocks of graduated sizes to assess
grasp; (2) grasping and lifting two pipes of graduated
sizes from a peg to test cylindrical grip; (3) grasping
and placing a ball to test spherical grasp; (4) picking
up and placing four marbles of graduated sizes to test
fingertip prehension or pinch; (5) putting a small
washer over a nail and putting an iron on a shelf to
test placing; and (6) pouring water from pitcher to
glass and glass to glass; placing hand on top of head,
behind head, and to mouth; and writing the name to
assess pronation, supination, and elevation of the arm.
The test uses simple, inexpensive, and easily acquired
materials. Details of materials and their arrangement,
test procedures, and scoring can be found in the original source.

Other tests that have been found to be useful in the
evaluation of hand dexterity are the Crawford Small
Parts Dexterity Test,[26] the Bennett Hand Tool Dexterity Test,[12] the Purdue Pegboard Test,[98] and the
Minnesota Manual Dexterity Test.[79] All of these tests
include comparison with normal subjects working in
a variety of industrial settings. These tests are especially useful when administering a work capacity evaluation. Tests may be purchased and come with instructions for administering the test and the standardized norms. Melvin lists a variety of additional
hand function tests.[76]

Clinical Tests for Specific Dysfunction

PERIPHERAL NEUROPATHY. Several quick clinical observations to detect dysfunction of peripheral
nerves are available, based on the sensory and motor
function of the individual nerve.

The ulnar nerve may be tested by asking the patient
to pinch with the thumb and index finger and palpate

the first dorsal inteosseous muscle. The radial nerve
may be tested by asking the patient to extend the wrist
and fingers. Median nerve function is tested by asking
the patient to oppose the thumb to the fingers and
flex the fingers.[23] The median nerve may be affected
by carpal tunnel compression in conditions such as
rheumatoid arthritis. Early signs of median nerve
compression are sensory in nature and may be tested
by performing Phalen's test and percussing over the
median nerve at the wrist to elicit Tinel's sign as described earlier in this chapter.

Patients may also develop compression syndromes
of the ulnar and radial nerves which will be indicated
by paresthesias along the course of those nerves. Tinel's sign may also be present. In patients with rheumatoid arthritis, it is important to test for nerve
compression periodically, since synovial proliferation
can cause compression in closed areas. Nerve
compression must be relieved before motor fibers are
damaged.

TREATMENT
Fractures

In treating a hand or wrist fracture the surgeon will
attempt to achieve good anatomical position through
either a closed (nonoperative) or open (operative) reduction. Internal fixation with Kirschner wires, metallic plates, and/or screws may be used to maintain
the desired position. External fixation may also be
used with internal fixation. The hand is usually immobilized in wrist extension and MP joint flexion with
extension of the distal joints whenever the injury allows this position[110] Trauma to bone may also involve
trauma to tendons and nerves in the adjacent area.
Treatment must be geared toward the recovery of all
injured structures, and this fact may influence treatment of the fracture.

Occupational therapy may be initiated during the
period of immobilization, which is usually 3 to 5
weeks. Uninvolved fingers of the hand must be kept
mobile through the use of active motion. Edema
should be carefully monitored, and elevation is required whenever edema is present.

As soon as there is sufficient bone stability, the surgeon will allow mobilization of the injured part. The
surgeon should provide guidelines for the amount of
resistance or force that may be applied to the fracture
site. Activities that correct poor motor patterns and
encourage use of the injured hand should be started
as soon as the hand is pain free. Early motion will
prevent the adherence of tendons and reduce edema
through stimulation of the lymphatic and blood vessels.

Closed functional treatment of fractures, or fracture bracing, is a technique described by Sarmiento[89] in which the fracture is treated with rigid immobilization for a brief period of time until the pain subsides. Immobilization is then discontinued, and the fracture is placed in a fracture brace that stabilizes the fracture while allowing function.

Fracture bracing is predicated on the belief that bone contact, end to end or otherwise, is not required for bony union; and that rigid immobilization of joints above and below a fracture, as well as prolonged rest, are detrimental to fracture healing. Closed functional bracing of fractures calls for functional activity in order to obtain greater osteogenesis.[89]

Occupational therapists may participate in the fabrication of fracture braces and may supervise a program of progressive functional activity for the patient who is treated with closed functional bracing. Ferraro[42] documented the success of closed functional bracing of metacarpal fractures with minimal interference in the ADL and work activities of the patients.

As soon as the brace or cast is removed, the patient's hand must be evaluated. If edema remains present, edema control techniques can be initiated using techniques described later in this chapter. A baseline ROM should be established, and the application of appropriate splints may begin. A splint may be used to correct a deformity that has resulted from immobilization, or it may be used to protect the finger from additional trauma to the fracture site. An example of this type of splinting would be the application of a Velcro "buddy" splint (Fig. 28-4) or a Bedford finger stall[69] (Fig. 28-5). A dorsal block splint that limits full extension of the finger may be used following a fracture or dislocation of the PIP joint. A dynamic splint may be used to achieve full ROM or prevent the development of further deformity at 6 to 8 weeks following fracture.

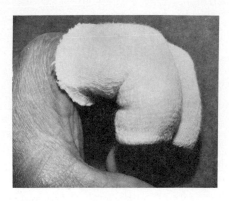

Fig. 28-5. Bedford finger stall may be used as "fellow traveler" to protect injured finger. Slight compression applied by stretch gauze may reduce edema, and pressure may alleviate pain. Finger stall can be worn for prolonged periods of time.

Intraarticular fractures may result in injury to the cartilage of the joint, resulting in additional pain and stiffness. An x-ray examination will indicate if there has been damage to the joint surface which might limit the treatment of the joint. Joint pain and stiffness following fracture without the presence of joint damage should be alleviated by a combination of thermal modalities, restoration of joint play, or joint mobilization and corrective and dynamic splinting followed by active use. Resistive exercise can be started when bony healing has been achieved.

Wrist fractures are common and may present special problems for the surgeon and therapist. Colles' fractures of the distal radius are the most common injury to the wrist[15] and may result in limitations in wrist flexion and extension, as well as pronation and supination resulting from the involvement of the radioulnar joint. Use of splints, active motion that emphasizes wrist movement, and joint mobilization may be beneficial. The weight well (Fig. 28-6) may be used to provide resistance to wrist motions.

The carpal scaphoid is the second most commonly injured bone in the wrist[15] and is often fractured when the hand is dorsiflexed at the time of injury. Fractures to the proximal portion of the scaphoid may result in nonunion because of poor blood supply to this area. Scaphoid fractures will require a prolonged period of immobilization, sometimes up to several months in a cast, with resulting stiffness and pain. Care should be taken to mobilize noninvolved joints early.

Trauma to the carpal lunate may result in avascular necrosis of the lunate or Kienböck's disease.[15] This may result from a one-time accident or may be caused by repetitive trauma. Lunate fractures are usually immobilized for 6 weeks. Kienböck's disease may be treated with a bone graft, Silastic implant, or partial wrist fusion.

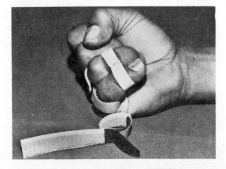

Fig. 28-4. Velcro "buddy" splint may be used to protect finger following fracture or to encourage movement of stiff finger. Smalley and Bates, Inc, 85 Park Avenue, Nutley, NJ.

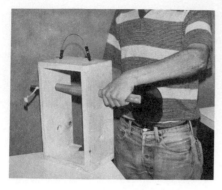

Fig. 28-6. Weight well is used for strengthening upper extremity with progressive resistance applied to weakened musculature and is also useful in retaining prehension of pinch and grip.

Stiffness and pain are common complications of fractures, but the control of edema coupled with early motion and good patient instruction and support will minimize these complications.

Nerve Injuries

Nerve injury may be classified into the following three categories:
1. Neurapraxia is contusion of the nerve without wallerian degeneration. The nerve recovers function without treatment within a few days or weeks.
2. Axonotmesis is an injury in which nerve fibers distal to the site of injury degenerate but the internal organization of the nerve remains intact. No surgical treatment is necessary, and recovery usually occurs within 6 months. The length of time may vary, depending on the level of injury.
3. Neurotmesis is a complete laceration of both nerve and fibrous tissues. Surgical treatment is required. Microsurgical repair of the fascicles is common. Nerve grafting may be necessary in situations where there is a gap between nerve endings.[14]

Peripheral nerve injuries may occur as a result of disruption of the nerve by a fractured bone, laceration, or crush injury. Symptoms of nerve injuries will include weakness or paralysis of muscles that are innervated by motor branches of the injured nerve and sensory loss to areas that are innervated by sensory branches of the injured nerve. Before evaluating the patient for nerve loss the therapist must be familiar with the muscles and areas that are innervated by the three major forearm nerves.

MEDIAN NERVE. The median nerve innervates the flexors of the forearm and hand and is often called the "eyes" of the hands because of its importance in sensory innervation of the volar surface of the hands. Median nerve loss may result from lacerations as well as from compression syndromes of the wrist, such as the carpal tunnel syndrome.

Motor distribution of the median nerve is to the pronator teres, palmaris longus, flexor carpi radialis, flexor digitorum profundus to the index and long fingers, flexor digitorum superficialis, flexor pollicis longus, pronator quadratus, abductor pollicis brevis, opponens pollicis, superficial head of the flexor pollicis brevis, and first and second lumbricals.

Sensory distribution of the median nerve is to the volar surface of the thumb, index, and middle fingers; radial half of the ring finger and dorsal surface of the index and middle fingers; and radial half of the ring finger distal to the PIP joints.

Clinical signs of a high-level median nerve injury are ulnar flexion of the wrist caused by loss of the flexor carpi radialis, loss of palmar abduction, and opposition of the thumb. Active pronation will be absent, but the patient may appear to pronate with the assistance of gravity. In a wrist-level median nerve injury the thenar eminence will appear flat and there will be a loss of thumb flexion, palmar abduction, and opposition.[87]

The sensory loss associated with median nerve injury is particularly disabling because there will be no sensation to the volar aspects of the thumb and index and long fingers and the radial side of the ring finger. The patient when blindfolded will substitute pinch to the ring and small fingers to compensate for this loss. An injury in the forearm that involves the anterior interosseous nerve will not result in sensory loss. Motor loss will include paralysis of the flexor pollicis longus, the flexor digitorum profundus of the index and long fingers, and the pronator quadratus. The pronator teres is not affected. Pinch will be affected.

Splints that position the thumb in palmar abduction and slight opposition will increase functional use of the hand (Fig. 28-7). If clawing of the index and long fingers is present, a splint should be fabricated to prevent hyperextension of the MP joints. Patients report that they avoid use of the hand with a median nerve injury because of lack of sensation rather than because of muscle paralysis. Despite this, the weakened or paralyzed muscles should be protected.

ULNAR NERVE. The ulnar nerve in the forearm innervates only the flexor carpi ulnaris and the median half of the flexor digitorum profundus. It travels down the volar forearm through the canal of Guyon, innervating the intrinsic muscles of the hand, including the palmaris brevis, abductor digiti minimi, opponens digiti minimi, flexor digiti minimi, dorsal and volar interossei, third and fourth lumbricals, and medial head of the flexor pollicis brevis.

The sensory distribution of the ulnar nerve is the

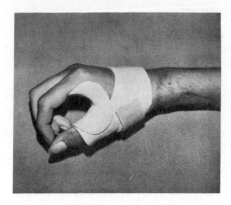

Fig. 28-7. Thumb stabilization splint may be used with median nerve injury to protect thumb and to improve functioning by placing the thumb in position of pinch. Normal pinch cannot be achieved with median nerve injury because of paralysis of thumb musculature.

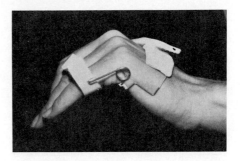

Fig. 28-8. Dynamic ulnar nerve splint blocks hyperextension of MP joints that occurs with paralysis of ulnar intrinsic muscles and allows MP flexion, which maintains normal ROM of MP joints. Splint, courtesy of Mary Dimick, OTR, University of California–San Diego Hand Rehabilitation Center.

dorsal and volar surfaces of the little finger ray and the ulnar half of the dorsal and volar surface of the ring finger ray.

A high-level ulnar nerve injury results in hyperextension of the MP joints of the ring and small fingers (also called "clawing") resulting from overaction of the extensor digitorum communis that is not held in check by the third and fourth lumbricals.[87] The IP joints of the ring and small fingers will not demonstrate a great flexion deformity because of the paralysis of the flexor digitorum profundus. The hypothenar muscles and interossei will be absent. The wrist will assume a position of radial extension caused by the loss of the flexor carpi ulnaris. In a low-level ulnar nerve injury the ring and small fingers will claw at the MP joints and the IP joints will exhibit a greater tendency toward flexion because the flexor digitorum profundus will be present. Wrist extension will be normal.

Clinical signs of a high-level ulnar nerve injury may include clawhand with a loss of the hypothenar and the interosseous muscles. In a low-level ulnar nerve injury the flexor digitorum profundus and flexor carpi ulnaris will be present and unopposed by the intrinsic muscles. When attempting lateral or key pinch the IP joint of the thumb will flex instead of extend because of paralysis of the intrinsic muscles. This is also known as "Froment's sign." Longstanding compression of the ulnar nerve in the canal of Guyon will result in a flattening of the hypothenar area and conspicuous atrophy of the first dorsal interosseous muscle.[15]

With a low-level ulnar nerve injury a small splint may be provided to prevent hyperextension of the small and ring fingers without limiting full flexion at the MP joints. Stabilization of the MP joints will allow

the extensor digitorum communis to fully extend the IP joints (Fig. 28-8).

Sensory loss of the ulnar nerve results in frequent injury to the ulnar side of the hand, especially burns. Patients must be instructed in visual protection of the anesthetic area.

RADIAL NERVE. The radial nerve innervates the extensor-supinator group of muscles of the forearm, including the brachioradialis, extensor carpi radialis longus, extensor carpi radialis brevis, extensor digitorum communis, extensor digiti minimi, extensor indicis, extensor carpi ulnaris, supinator, abductor pollicis longus, extensor pollicis brevis, and extensor pollicis longus. The sensory distribution of the radial nerve is a strip of the posterior upper arm and the forearm; dorsum of the thumb; and index and middle fingers and radial half of the ring finger to the PIP joints. Sensory loss of the radial nerve does not usually result in dysfunction.

Clinical signs of a high-level radial nerve injury (above the supinator) are pronation of the forearm, wrist flexion, and the thumb held in palmar abduction resulting from the unopposed action of the flexor pollicis brevis and the abductor pollicis brevis.[87] Injury to the posterior interosseous nerve will spare the extensor carpi radialis longus and brevis. Posterior Interosseus Nerve Syndrome will include normal sensation and wrist extension with loss of finger and thumb extension. Clinical signs of a low-level radial nerve injury include incomplete extension of the MP joints of the fingers and thumb. The interossei will extend the interphalangeal (IP) joints of the fingers, but the MP joints will rest in about 30° of flexion.

A dorsal splint that provides wrist extension, MP extension, and thumb extension should be provided to protect the extensor tendons from overstretching during the healing phase and to position the hand for

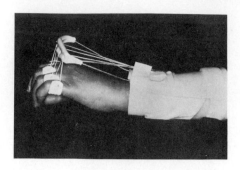

Fig. 28-9. Low-profile radial nerve splint is carefully balanced to pull MP joints into extension when wrist is flexed and allows the MP joints to fall into slight flexion when wrist is extended, thus preserving normal balance between two joints and preserving joint contracture. Splint, courtesy of Judy C Colditz, OTR, Raleigh Hand Rehabilitation Center.

functional use (Fig. 28-9). A dynamic splint is commonly provided.

POSTOPERATIVE MANAGEMENT FOLLOWING NERVE REPAIR. Following nerve repair the hand is placed in a position that will minimize tension on the nerve. For example, following repair of the median nerve, the wrist will be immobilized in a flexed position. Immobilization usually lasts for 2 to 3 weeks, after which protective stretching of the joints may begin. The therapist must exercise great care not to put excessive traction on the newly repaired nerve.

Correction of a contracture may take 4 to 6 weeks. Active exercise is the preferred method of gaining full extension, although a light dynamic splint may be applied with the surgeon's supervision. Splinting to assist or substitute for weakened musculature may be necessary for an extended period during nerve regeneration. Splints should be removed as soon as possible to allow for active exercise of the weakened muscles. However, it is important to instruct the patient in correct patterns of motion so that substitution is minimized.

Initially treatment is directed toward the prevention of deformity and correction of poor positioning during the acute and regenerative stages. Patients must be instructed in visual protection of the anesthetic area. ADL should be evaluated, and new methods or devices may be needed for independence. Use of the hand in the patient's work should be evaluated, and the patient should be returned to employment with any necessary modifications of his or her job or adaptations of equipment as soon as possible.

Careful muscle, sensory, and functional testing should be done frequently. As the nerve regenerates, splints may be changed or eliminated. Exercises and activities should be revised to reflect the patient's new

gains, and adapted equipment should be discarded as soon as possible.

As motor function begins to return to the paralyzed muscles, a careful program of specific exercises should be devised to facilitate the return. Proprioceptive neuromuscular facilitation techniques, such as hold-relax, contract-relax, quick stretch, and icing may assist a fair strength muscle and increase ROM. Neuromuscular electrical stimulation (NMES)[11] will also provide an external stimulus to help strengthen the newly innervated muscle. When the muscle has reached a good rating, functional activities should be used to complete the return to normal strength.

Sensory reeducation. Evaluation of sensibility has been described in some detail earlier in this chapter. This information should be used to prepare a program of sensory reeducation following nerve repair.

When a nerve is repaired, regeneration is not perfect and results in fewer and smaller nerve fibers and receptors distal to the repair. The goal of sensory reeducation is to maximize the functional level of sensation or tactile gnosis. Parry first described sensory reeducation in 1966,[87] and Dellon reported a highly structured sensory reeducation program in 1974.[31] Dellon divided his program into early and late phase training, based on vibratory sensation for early phase and perception of moving and constant touch sensation for late phase reeducation. Localization of stimuli and recognition of objects was used by both Parry and Dellon. Higher cortical integration was achieved by focusing attention on the stimuli through visual clues and by employing memory when vision was occluded. The patients were taught to compensate for sensory deficits by improving specific skills and generalizing them to other sensory stimuli. Daily repetition appears to be a necessary component of reeducation.

Callahan[17] has outlined a program of protective sensory reeducation and discriminative sensory reeducation if protective sensation is present and there has been a return of touch sensation to the fingertips. Waylett-Rendall[106] has also described a sensory reeducation program utilizing crafts and functional activities as well as desensitization techniques. All programs emphasize a variety of stimuli used in a repetitive manner to bombard the sensory receptors. A sequence of eyes-closed, eyes-open, eyes-closed is used to provide feedback during the training process. Sessions are limited in length to avoid fatigue and frustration. Objects must not be potentially harmful to the insensate areas, in order to avoid further trauma. A home program should be provided to reinforce learning that occurs in the clinical setting.

The authors[17,30,106] have found that sensory reeducation can result in improved functional sensibility in motivated patients. Objective measurement of sensation following reeducation must be performed and then compared with initial testing to accurately assess the success of the program.

Tendon transfers. If, following a minimal period of 1 year after nerve repair, a motor nerve has not reinnervated its muscle, the surgeon may consider tendon transfers to restore a needed motion. The rules of tendon transfer are to evaluate (1) what is absent, (2) what is needed for function and (3) what is available to transfer.[44] Some muscles, such as the extensor carpi radialis longus and the sublimis to the ring finger, are commonly used for transfers because their motions are easily substituted by the extensor carpi radialis brevis and flexor digitorum profundus to the ring finger, respectively. The surgeon may request assistance in evaluating motor status from the therapist to determine the best motor transfer.

Therapy before tendon transfer is essential if the motor being used is not of normal strength. A muscle will lose a grade of strength when transferred, and a strengthening program of progressive resistive exercises, NMES, and isolated motion will help ensure success of the transfer.

Following transfer, many patients require instruction to perceive the correct muscle during active use of the transfer. Use of biofeedback, careful instruction, and supervised activity to note any substitution patterns during active use will usually help the patient to use the transfer correctly. Therapy must be initiated before the patient has time to develop incorrect use patterns. NMES may be used to isolate the muscle and to strengthen it postoperatively.

Tendon Injuries

FLEXOR TENDONS. Injuries to tendons may be isolated or may occur in conjunction with other injuries, especially fractures or crushes. Flexor tendons injured in the area between the distal palmar crease and the insertion of the flexor digitorum superficialis are considered to be the most difficult to treat, because the tendons lie in their sheaths in this area beneath the fibrous pulley system and any scarring will cause adhesions. This area is often referred to as zone 2 or "no-man's-land."

Primary repair of the flexor tendons within zone 2 is most frequently attempted following a clean laceration. Several methods of postoperative management have been proposed with the common goal to promote gliding of the tendons and to minimize the formation of scar adhesions.

Controlled mobilization of acute flexor tendon in- **juries: Louisville technique.** Dr. Harold Kleinert of the University of Louisville School of Medicine was an early advocate of rubberband traction following repair of flexor tendons in zone 2. This technique is often referred to as the "Kleinert technique." The doctor and therapist do not actively participate in moving the tendon or finger when this protocol is followed as outlined by Kutz.[57]

Following surgical repair, rubberbands are attached to the nails of the involved fingers using a suture through the nail or with a hook held in place with cyanoacrylate glue. A dorsal blocking splint is fabricated out of low-temperture thermoplastic material, with the MP joints held in about 60° of flexion. The splint is constructed so that the IP joints are able to fully extend to the splint. The rubberbands are passed through a safety pin in the palm and are attached to the distal strap of the splint. The rubberbands should be placed in sufficient tension to hold the PIP joints in 40° to 60° of flexion without tension on the rubberbands. The patient must be able to fully extend the IP joints actively within the splint, or joint contractures will develop (Fig. 28-10).

The patient wears this splint 24 hours a day for 3 weeks and is instructed to actively extend the fingers several times a day in the splint, allowing the rubberbands to pull the fingers into flexion. This movement of the tendon through the tendon sheath and pulley system minimizes scar adhesions while enhancing tendon nutrition and blood flow.

The dorsal blocking splint is removed at 3 weeks and the rubberband is attached to a wristband, which

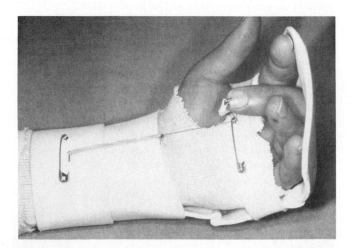

Fig. 28-10. Following flexor tendon repair, the wrist is placed in 30° flexion with traction applied from the nail through a safety pin pulley in the palm and attached to the proximal strap of the splint. The MP joints should be maintained in about 70° flexion, allowing full passive IP joint flexion and active extension.

is worn for 1 to 5 additional weeks, depending on the judgment of the surgeon.

The primary disadvantage of this technique is that contractures of the PIP joints frequently occur as a result of too much tension on the rubberband or incomplete IP extension within the splint. Dynamic extension splinting of the PIP joint can be started at 5 to 6 weeks if a flexion contracture is present. This technique requires a motivated patient who thoroughly understands the program in order to be successful.

Controlled passive motion: Duran and Houser technique. Duran and Houser[37] suggested the use of controlled passive motion to achieve optimal results following primary repair, allowing 3 mm to 5 mm of tendon excursion. They found this to be sufficient to prevent adherence of the repaired tendons. On the third postoperative day the patient begins a twice daily exercise regimen of passive flexion and extension of 6 to 8 motions for each tendon. Care is taken to keep the wrist flexed and the MPs in 70° of flexion during passive exercise. Between exercise periods the hand is wrapped in a stockinette. At 4½ weeks the protective dorsal splint is removed and the rubberband traction is attached to a wristband. Active extension and passive flexion are done for 1 additional week and gradually increased over the next several weeks.

Immobilization technique. A third postoperative program is complete immobilization for 3½ weeks following tendon repair. Immobilization has not resulted in consistently good results and may lead to a great incidence of tendon rupture following repair because a tendon gains tensile strength when submitted to gentle tension at the repair site.[95]

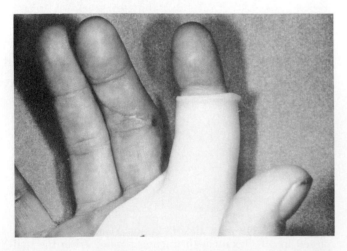

Fig. 28-11. A blocking splint can be used to isolate tendon pull-through and joint range of motion by blocking out the proximal joints. This splint is being used to facilitate motion at the DIP joint following repair of the FDP tendon.

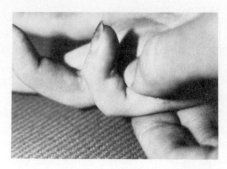

Fig. 28-12. Manual blocking of MP joint during flexion of PIP joint.

Postacute Flexor Tendon Rehabilitation. When active flexion is begun out of the splint following any of the postoperative management techniques described above, the patient should be instructed in exercises to facilitate differential tendon gliding.[107] Wehbe[108] recommends three positions, hook, straight fist, and fist, to maximize isolated gliding of the flexor digitorum superficialis and the flexor digitorum profundus tendons, as well as stretching of the intrinsic musculature and gliding of the extensor mechanism. Tendon gliding exercises should be done for 10 repetitions of each position, 2 to 3 times a day.

Isolated exercises to assist tendon gliding may also be performed using a blocking splint (Fig. 28-11) or the opposite hand (Fig. 28-12).

The MP joints should be held in extension during blocking so the intrinsic muscles that act on it cannot overcome the power of the repaired flexor tendons. Care should be taken not to hyperextend the PIP joint and overstretch the repaired tendons.

After 6 to 8 weeks passive extension may be started and splinting may be necessary to correct a flexion contracture at the PIP joint. A cylindrical plaster splint may be fabricated to apply constant static pressure on the contracture as described by Bell (Fig. 28-13). Static splinting may be especially effective with a flexion contracture greater than 25°. A finger gutter splint may be made using ⅟₁₆-inch (0.16-cm) thermoplastic material for static extension at night. This will help maintain extension gains made during the day. Gentle dynamic traction may be applied using a commercial splint such as an LMB finger extension splint[60] (Fig. 28-14) or one that is fabricated by the therapist (Fig. 28-15). Dynamic flexion splinting may be necessary if the patient has difficulty regaining passive flexion.

At about 8 weeks the patient may begin light resistive exercises and activities. The hand can now be used for light ADL, but the patient should continue to avoid heavy lifting with or excessive resistance to the affected hand. Sports activities should be discouraged.

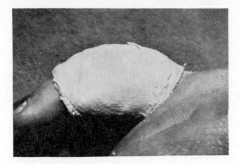

Fig. 28-13. Plaster cylindrical splint is used to apply static stretch of PIP joint contracture. It is not removed by patient and must be replaced frequently by therapist with careful monitoring of skin condition.

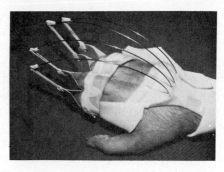

Fig. 28-15. Dynamic outrigger splint using spring steel outriggers with a lumbrical block can be used to assist PIP joint extension, stretch against scar adhesions of extrinsic flexors, or reduce PIP joint contractures. Proper fit and tension of rubber bands must be assessed frequently by therapist.

However, activities such as clay work, woodworking, and macrame are excellent. Full resistance and normal work activities can be started at 3 months following surgery.

When evaluating a hand that has sustained a tendon injury, passive versus active limitations of joint motion must be evaluated. Limitations in active motion may indicate joint stiffness, muscle weakness, or scar adhesions. If passive motion is greater than active motion, the therapist should consider that tendons may be caught in the scar tissue. The therapist should be able to determine if a tendon is adhering and causing a flexion contracture or if the tendon is free but the joint itself is stiff. Treatment should be based on this type of evaluation.

ROM, strength, function, and sensibility testing (if digital nerves were also injured) should be performed frequently with splints and activities geared to prog-

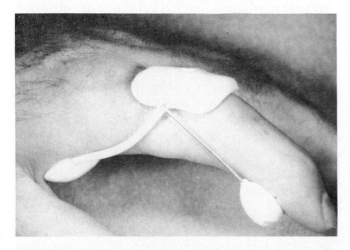

Fig. 28-14. This commercially available finger splint is used to increase extension of the PIP joint. Available from LMB Hand Rehabilitation Products, Inc, PO Box 1181, San Luis Obispo, CA 93406.

ress. Although performance of ADL is generally not a problem, the therapist should ask the patient about any problems he or she may have or anticipate. Disuse and neglect of a finger, especially the index finger, are common and should be prevented.

Gains in flexion and extension may continue to be recorded for 6 months postoperatively. A finger with limber joints and minimal scarring preoperatively will function better after repair than one that is stiff and scarred and has trophic skin changes.[16] It is important therefore that all joints, skin, and scars be supple and movable before reconstructive surgery is attempted. A "functional" to "excellent" result is obtained if the combined loss of extension is less than 40° in the PIP and distal interphalangeal (DIP) joints of the index and middle fingers and is less than 60° in the ring and little fingers[80] and if the finger can flex to the palm.[16]

If the tendon is damaged as a result of a crush injury or the laceration cannot be cleaned up enough to allow for a primary repair, staged flexor tendon reconstruction may be done. At the first operation a Silastic rod is inserted beneath the pulley system and attached to the distal phalanx. Other reconstructive procedures, such as pulley reconstruction, are performed at the same time. A mesothelial cell-lined pseudosheath is formed about the rod and a fluid similar to synovial fluid is formed in the postoperative recovery phase.[58] The second stage is performed about 4 months later when the digit can be moved passively to the palm. A tendon graft is inserted and the Silastic rod removed. The postoperative program is carried out in the same manner as for a primary tendon repair.

Following a two-stage tendon reconstruction or primary repair, a tenolysis may be performed if there is a significant difference between the active and passive motion. Tenolysis is usually not performed for 6 months to 1 year after tendon repair. At the time of tenolysis surgery scar adhesions are removed from the tendon and gliding of the tendons is assessed. Patients are often asked to move their fingers in the operating room at the time of lysis to determine the extent of scar removal. Active motion is begun within the first 24 hours using bipuvacaine hydrochloride (Marcaine) blocks[90] or transcutaneous electrical nerve stimulation (TENS)[18] to control pain.

LaSalle and Strickland[58] have recommended a system for evaluating the results of tenolysis surgery by comparing the preoperative passive IP joint motion with the postoperative IP joint motion. Based on this LaSalle and Strickland found that in one group of patients undergoing tenolysis, 40% had an improvement in motion of 50% or better compared with their preoperative status.

EXTENSOR TENDONS. Dorsal scar adherence is the most difficult problem following injury to the extensor tendons, because of the tendency of the dorsal extensor hood to become adherent to the underlying structures and thus limit its normal excursion during flexion and extension.

Extensor tendons in zones V, VI, and VII (proximal to the MP joints) become adherent because they are encased in paratenon and synovial sheaths and respond to injury in a way similar to flexor tendons, resulting in either incomplete extension, also known as "extensor lag," or incomplete flexion resulting from loss of gliding of the extensor tendon. Evans[40,41] studied the normal excursion of the extensor digitorum communis in zones V, VI, and VII in order to suggest guidelines for early passive motion of extensor tendons. She concluded that 5 mm of tendon glide following repair was safe and effective in limiting tendon adhesions and designed a postoperative splint that allows slight active flexion while providing passive extension.[40] The splint is worn for 3 weeks, with the initiation of active motion between the third and fourth weeks. A removeable volar splint is used between exercise periods to protect the tendon for 2 additional weeks. Dynamic flexion splinting may be started at 6 weeks postoperative to regain flexion if needed.

Injuries to extensor tendons proximal to the MP joint may be immobilized for 3 weeks. After this the finger may be placed in a removable volar splint that is worn between exercise periods for an additional 2 weeks. Progressive ROM is begun at 3 weeks, and if full flexion is not regained rapidly, dynamic flexion may be started at 6 weeks.

Extensor tendon injuries that occur distal to the MP joint require a longer period of immobilization, usually 6 weeks. A progressive exercise program is then initiated with dynamic splinting during the day and a static night splint to maintain extension.

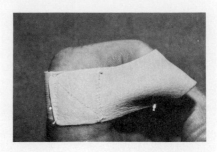

Fig. 28-16. PIP-DIP splint may be used to increase flexion of both PIP and DIP joints. Tension can be adjusted with Velcro closure. Wearing time should be determined by therapist.

Dynamic splints may include a PIP-DIP splint first described by Hollis and now available commercially[60] (Fig. 28-16), a web strap made of lamp wick or elastic, a fingernail hook with rubber band traction, a traction glove, or another splint.

If a lysis of scar tissue is required because of persistent scar adhesion, the surgeon may place a thin sheet of Silastic between the tendon and bone at the time of surgery to reduce further scar adherence. The patient begins exercising within the first 24 hours, and splints are applied as needed. Active exercise is essential, and the patient must be carefully instructed in a home program. The patient is encouraged to use the hand for all activities except those requiring heavy resistance. After 4 to 6 weeks the Silastic sheet is removed and ROM should be maintained.

TOTAL ACTIVE MOTION AND TOTAL PASSIVE MOTION. Total active motion (TAM) and total passive motion (TPM) is a method of recording joint ROM which is used to compare tendon excursion (active) and joint mobility (passive). It is the measure of flexion minus extensor lag of three joints. TAM and TPM have been recommended for use in reporting joint motion by The American Society for Surgery of the Hand.[2]

TAM is computed by adding the sum of the angles formed by the MP, PIP, and DIP joints in flexion minus incomplete active extension at each of the three joints. For example, MP joint flexion is 85° with full extension; PIP is 100° and lacks 15° extension, and DIP is 65° with full extension; therefore

$$TAM = 85 + 100 + 65 - 15 = 235°$$

TAM should be measured while making a fist. It is used for a single digit and should be compared with the same digit of the opposite hand or subsequent measurements of the same digit. It should not be used to compute a percentage of loss of impairment.

TPM is calculated in the same manner but measures only passive motion.

Edema

Edema is a normal consequence of trauma but must be quickly and aggressively treated to prevent permanent stiffness and disability. Within hours of trauma vasodilation and local edema occur with an increase in white blood cells to the damaged area.[66] The inflammatory response to the injury results in a decrease in bacteria to control infection.

Early control of edema should be achieved through elevation, massage, compression, and active ROM. The patient is instructed at the time of injury to keep the hand elevated, and a compressive dressing is used to reduce early swelling. Pitting edema is present early and can be recognized as a bloated swelling that "pits" when pressed. This may be more pronounced on the dorsal surface where the venous and lymphatic systems provide return of fluid to the heart. Active motion is especially important to produce retrograde venous and lymphatic flow.

If the swelling continues, a serofibrinous exudate invades the area. Fibrin is deposited in the spaces surrounding the joints, tendons, and ligaments, resulting in reduced mobility, flattening of the arches of the hand, tissue atrophy, and further disuse.[66] Normal gliding of the tissues is eliminated, and a stiff, often painful hand will be the result. Scar adhesions will form and further limit tissue mobility. If untreated, these losses may become permanent.

Early recognition of persistent edema through volume and circumference measurement is important. It may be necessary to use several of the suggested edema control techniques.

ELEVATION. Early elevation with the hand above the heart is essential. Slings tend to reduce blood flow and should be avoided. Resting the hand on pillows while seated or lying down is effective. Resting the hand on top of the head or using devices that elevate the hand with the elbow in extension have been suggested. Suspension slings may be purchased or fabricated.

The patient should use the hand for ADL within the limitations of resistance prescribed by the physician. Light ADL that can be accomplished while the hand is in the dressing are permitted.

CONTRAST BATHS. Alternating soaks of cold and warm water that is 66° and 96° F (18.9° and 35.6° C) have been recommended as a method preferred over warm water soaks or whirlpool baths. The contrast baths can be done for 20 minutes, alternating the hand between cool water for 1 minute and warm water for 1 minute. Start and end with cool water. A sponge can be placed in each tub so that the hand is moved during the soaking period. The tubs should be placed as high as possible to provide elevation of the extremity. The alternating warm and cool water will cause vasodilation and vasoconstriction, resulting in a pumping action on the edema. Combined with elevation and active motion edema may be reduced and pain is often alleviated by this technique.

RETROGRADE MASSAGE. A retrograde massage may be done by the therapist, but it should be taught to the patient so that is can be done frequently through the day. The massage assists in blood and lymph flow. It should be started distally and stroked proximally with the extremity in elevation.[29] Active motion should follow the massage but muscle fatigue should be avoided.

PRESSURE WRAPS. Wrapping with Coban elastic wrap[36] may be employed to reduce edema (Fig. 28-17). Starting distally, the finger is wrapped snugly with Coban. Each involved finger should be wrapped distally to proximally until the wrap is proximal to the edema. The wrap remains in place for 5 minutes and then is removed. Active exercise may be done while the finger is wrapped or immediately following. Measurements should be taken before and after treatment to document an increase in ROM and a decrease in edema. The wrapping may be repeated 3 times a day.

Light compression may be applied throughout the day with a light Coban wrap, an Isotoner glove,[48] or a custom-made garment by Jobst or Bio-Concepts (Fig. 28-18). The compression should not be constricting and should be discontinued if ischemia results.

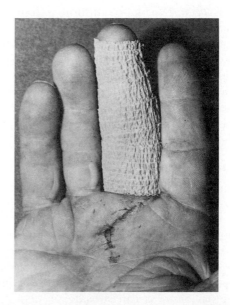

Fig. 28-17. One-inch Coban is wrapped with minimal pressure from distal end to proximal crease of digit. Patient is instructed to be aware of vascular compression or "tingling." Coban may be worn several hours a day to reduce edema. Available from Medical Products Division/3M, St. Paul, Minn.

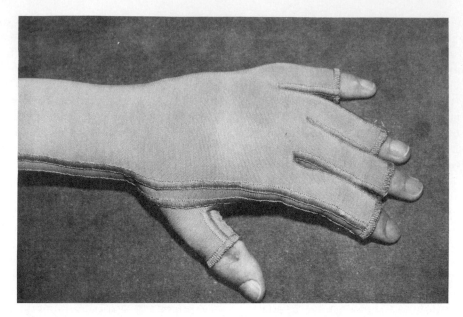

Fig. 28-18. Custom-fit Jobst garment may be used to reduce edema and to reduce and prevent hypertrophic scar formation following burns or trauma. Inserts may be used in conjunction with garment to increase pressure over natural curves, such as dorsum of wrist.

A variety of pressure wraps are used by hand centers. Tubular gauze, Digi-sleeves,[2,34] and Bedford finger stalls provide compression to a specific finger. No one method is superior to the other. A combination of techniques may be used at different stages of healing and according to patient comfort and may be the most effective.

ACTIVE ROM. Normal blood flow is dependent on muscle activity. Active motion does not mean wiggling the fingers but rather maximum available ROM done firmly. Casts and splints must allow mobility of uninjured parts while protecting newly injured structures. The shoulder and elbow should be moved several times a day. The importance of active ROM for edema control, tendon gliding, and tissue nutrition cannot be overemphasized.

Wound Healing and Scar Remodeling

The first phase of wound healing, the acute inflammatory phase, is initiated within hours when the tissues are disrupted through injury or surgery, causing vasodilation and local edema as well as migration of white blood cells and phagocytic cells to the area. The phagocytes remove tissue fragments and foreign bodies and are critical to healing. The inflammatory process can subside or persist indefinitely depending on the degree of bacterial contamination.[66]

Fibroblasts in combination with associated capillaries begin to invade the wound within the first 72 hours and gradually replace the phagocytes, leading to the second phase: the collagen or granulation phase, between the fifth and fourteenth days. Collagen fiber formation follows the invasion by fibroblasts, so that by the end of the second week the wound is rich with fibroblasts, a capillary network, and early collagen fibers. This increased vascularization results in the erythema of the new scar.

During the third to sixth weeks fibroblasts are slowly replaced with scar collagen fibers and the wound becomes stronger and more able to withstand progressive stresses leading to the last phase of scar maturation. Strength continues to increase for 3 months or longer. The collagen metabolizes and synthesizes during this period of time, so that new collagen replaces old while the wound remains relatively stable. Covalent bonding between collagen molecules leads to dense scar adhesions and the formation of whorl-like patterns of collagen deposits which may be altered as the scar architecture and collagen fiber organization within the wound changes over time.[36] Myofibroblasts, which are fibroblasts with properties similar to smooth muscle cells, are contractile and cause a shortening of the wound.

Tissues that have restored gliding have different scar architecture from those which do not develop the ability to glide. With gliding the scar resembles the state of the tissues prior to injury, while the nongliding scar remains fixed on surrounding structures. Controlled tension on scar has been shown to facilitate remodeling. Scar formation is also influenced by age and the quantity of scar deposited.[53]

WOUND CARE AND DRESSINGS. There are many dressings that can be placed on a wound, including gauze that has been impregnated with petroleum, such as xeroform gauze or adaptic. Ointments such as Polysporin are also commonly applied. N-Terface[84] is a dry mesh fabric that looks and feels like interfacing that is used in sewing. Because it is nonadherent, it can be used directly over wounds and will not stick to them. Sterile dressings can be applied directly over the N-Terface without ointments or gels. Spenco Second Skin[93] is an inert gel sheeting made from 96% water and 4% polyethylene oxide. It removes friction between two moving surfaces and is said to clean wounds by absorbing secretions. It comes in sterile and nonsterile packs and is encased in a light plastic covering. It is especially effective with abrasions or areas of skin loss because it is cool and reduces itching. It can be used after burns. Spenco Dermal Pads[93] are artificial, fat pads that can be used to prevent pressure sores or can be cut to size to use around an existing pressure sore or wound to allow it to heal. Dermal pads are ⅛-inch thick (0.32-cm) and will adhere to the skin when the protective film is removed. The pad can be held in place with a dressing or with a pressure garment. It also can be washed without reducing its adherence. Dermal pads can be cut and placed around a healing wound to protect it under a splint or dressing. They are generally not needed after the wound is healed.

The wound can be cleaned with a solution of hydrogen peroxide and sterile saline, with dead tissue then being gently removed with sterile swabs. Sterile saline solution can be used to soak off adherent bandages rather than pulling them off the patient. The therapist should pour a very small amount of saline on the area that is sticking, wait a few moments, and gently pry the dressing off. Dead skin can be debrided using iris scissors and pickups. Betadine-impregnated scrub sponges may be used for cleaning and desensitization of the wound once it is healed and the stitches have been removed. The patient also can do this at home. Sterile whirlpool may also be used for debridement especially if the wound is infected.

PRESSURE. A hypertrophic scar or a scar that is randomly laid down and thickened is reduced by the application of pressure. Jobst garments are effective in providing pressure. Use of an insert of neoprene[85] fabric, or molds made from silastic Elastomer,[91] or Otoform[86] under the pressure garment will increase the conformity of the garment. Pressure should be applied for most of the 24-hour period, and with a hypertrophic burn scar this treatment should continue for a period of 6 months to 1 year following the injury. Other forms of pressure outlined in the section on edema control may also be used.

MASSAGE. Gentle to firm massage of the scarred area using a thick ointment, such as lanolin or Corrective Concepts Cream[25] will rapidly soften scar tissue and should be followed immediately with active hand use so that tendons will glide against the softened scar.[29] Vibration to the area with a small, low-intensity vibrator will have a similar effect.[51] Active exercise using facilitation techniques and against resistance or functional activity should follow vibration. Massage and vibration may be started at 4 weeks postinjury.

Thermal heat in the form of paraffin dips, hot packs, or Fluidotherapy immediately followed by stretching while the tissue cools will provide stretch to the scar tissue. Wrapping the scarred or stiff digit into flexion with Coban during the application of heat will often increase mobility in the area. Heat should not be used with insensate areas or if swelling persists.

ACTIVE ROM AND ELECTRICAL STIMULATION. Active ROM provides an internal stretch against resistant scar, and its use cannot be overemphasized. If the patient is unable to achieve active motion because of scar adhesions or weakness, use of a battery-operated neuromuscular electrical stimulator (NMES) may augment the motion. It may be done by the patient for several hours at home and has been shown to increase ROM and tendon excursion.[19]

High-voltage, direct current is used by many hand therapists as a treatment to increase motor activity and may be used for scar remodeling. Ultrasound phonophoresis treatments are often prescribed but may be more effective if done within the first few months following trauma. A continuous passive motion (CPM) device may be used at home to maintain passive ROM and promote tendon gliding. It should be used for several hours a day for maximum benefit.

Pain Syndromes

Pain is the subjective manifestation of trauma transmitted by the sympathetic nervous system, which may interfere with normal functioning. Because pain leads to overprotection of the affected part and disuse of the extremity, it should be treated early.

DESENSITIZATION. Stimulation of the large afferent A nerve fibers will lead to a reduction of pain by decreasing summation in the slowly-adapting, small, unmyelineated C fibers, which carry pain sensation. The A axons can be stimulated mechanically with pressure, rubbing, vibration, TENS, percussion, and active motion. Desensitization techniques are based on the amplification of inhibitory mechanisms.

Yerxa has described a desensitization program that "employs short periods of contact with three sensory modalities: dowel textures, immersion or contact particles, and vibration.[113] This program allows the patient to rank 10 dowel textures and 10 immersion textures on the degree of irritation produced by the stimulus. Treatment begins with a stimulus that is irritating but tolerable. The stimulus is applied for 10 minutes 3 or 4 times a day. The vibration hierarchy is predetermined and is based on cps of vibration, the placement of the vibrator, and the duration of the treatment. Complete instructions for assembling the Downey Hand Center desensitization kit can be found in the literature in the references. Downey Hand Center Hand Sensitivity Test can be used to establish a desensitization treatment program and to measure progress in decreasing hypersensitivity.[113]

NEUROMAS. Neuromas are a complication of nerve suture or amputation. A traumatic neuroma is an unorganized mass of nerve fibers which results from accidental or surgical cutting of the nerve. A neuroma in continuity occurs on a nerve that is intact.[97] They may be clinically identified by a specific, sharp pain. Stimulation of a neuroma will usually cause the patient to quickly pull the hand away; many patients report a burning pain that radiates up the forearm. Neuromas are disabling because any stimulation will cause intense pain and the patient avoids the sensitive area.

A generalized desensitization program may not work because the patient never develops a tolerance for stimulation of the neuroma. Injection of cortisone acetate may help break up the neuroma, making desensitization techniques more effective. Surgical excision of the neuroma or burying the nerve endings deeper may be necessary.

REFLEX SYMPATHETIC DYSTROPHY. Reflex sympathetic dystrophy (RSD) is a term used to describe a disabling reaction to pain that appears to be triggered by a cycle of vasospasm and vasodilation following an injury. The sympathetic nervous system plays a major role in the process.[82] The hallmarks of RSD are pain; edema; blotchy-looking, shiny skin; and coolness of the hand. There may be excessive sweating or dryness. The degree of trauma does not correlate with the severity of the pain and may occur following any injury. Abnormal edema and constrictive dressings or casts may be a factor in initiating the vasospasm. A vasospasm "causes tissue anoxia and edema and therefore more pain, which continues the abnormal cycle.[11,82] Circulation is decreased, which causes the extremity to become cool and pale. Fibrosis following tissue anoxia and protein-rich exudates results in joint stiffness. The patient may cradle the hand and prefers to keep it wrapped. There may be an exaggerated reaction to touch, especially light touch. Osteoporosis may be apparent on x-ray films by 8 weeks after trauma following active use of the

hand. Burning pain, associated with causalgia, is a symptom of RSD which can be alleviated by interruption of the sympathetic nerve pathways.

The first goal of treatment is reduction of the pain and hypersensitivity to light touch. This may be accomplished with application of warm (not hot) moist heat, Fluidotherapy, gentle handling of the hand, acupressure, and TENS. Narcotics may become addictive and should be avoided in favor of physical techniques that inhibit the perception of pain. Pain that cannot be controlled may be treated with the injection of stellate ganglion blocks by the surgeon. Stellate ganglion blocks may be beneficial in treating sympathetic symptoms but are usually a late treatment if other conservative measures fail to help.

Edema control techniques should be started immediately. Elevation, the Jobst intermittent compression pump, contrast baths, and high-voltage direct current in water have been found to be effective.

Biofeedback training for relaxation may help muscle spasming and ischemia as well as reduce anxiety.[35]

RSD will frequently trigger shoulder pain and stiffness, resulting in shoulder-hand syndrome or a "frozen" shoulder. Therefore as soon as pain is controlled active motion of the entire extremity and functional activities should be begun. Patients may benefit from several treatment sessions per week. Therapy should be coordinated with stellate ganglion blocks to take advantage of the pain-free period. Splints that reduce joint stiffness should be used as tolerated. A tendency to develop RSD should be suspected in any patient who seems to complain excessively about pain, appears anxious, and complains of profuse sweating and temperature changes in the hand. Patients will tend to overprotect the hand. Early intervention with a structured therapy program of functioinal activities, group interaction, and exercises that include the hand and shoulder may prevent the occurrence of a fully developed RSD. This is a problem that is best recognized early and treated with tempered aggressiveness and empathy.

TRANSCUTANEOUS ELECTRICAL NERVE STIMULATION. TENS is a treatment technique that is thought to stimulate the afferent A nerve fibers in the high-frequency mode and stimulate the release of morphinelike neural hormones, the enkephalins, in the low-frequency mode. Its efficacy as a treatment for pain control is well documented in medical literature. As with other electrical modalities that may be used by hand therapists, TENS should be correlated with functional use of the hand.

TENS should be used for treatment periods not to exceed 60 minutes at a time to achieve pain control.[53] A TENS diary should be used to record level of pain on a scale of 1 to 10 before and after treatment, as well as activities that exacerbate the pain. Use of TENS may be tapered down as the pain-free periods increase to avoid overuse. Treatment can be continued as long as necessary to provide pain control.

Joint Stiffness

Joint stiffness has been discussed in other sections of this chapter because it is seen following almost any hand trauma or disease. In the acute phase it may also result from "internal splinting" done unconsciously by the patient to avoid pain. It may be prevented by early mobilization, pain control, reduction of edema, active and passive ROM, and appropriate splinting techniques. Grade I and II joint mobilization is especially helpful in preparing for passive and active motion and for pain relief.

Treatment of established joint stiffness is more difficult. Thermal modalities, joint mobilization, ultrasound and electrical stimulation, dynamic splinting, serial casting, and active and passive motion in preparation for functional use should all be included in the treatment regimen.

Inflammatory Problems

Tendinitis may be the result of overuse of a muscle group, incorrect positioning for use, or trauma. It may be insidious or related to a specific injury. It is often the result of repetitive motions. Examples of soft tissue inflammatory problems are carpal tunnel syndrome, lateral epicondylitis (tennis elbow), de Quervain's disease, and trigger fingers. Treatment varies by the specific disorder, but general guidelines may be followed.[104]

Acute phase treatment is geared toward decreasing the inflammation through "dynamic rest." Splints are used for immobilization.

Splinting alone may relieve symptoms; splinting is often combined with cortisone injections to reduce inflammation. Icing, contrast baths, ultrasound phonophoresis, interferential and high-voltage electrical stimulation have all been found to be effective in reducing pain and decreasing inflammation. Nonsteroidal antiinflammatory drugs are also frequently used. When splints are used, they should be removed 3 times a day for stretching of the affected musculature (e.g., the extensor group with lateral epicondylitis) to maintain or increase muscle length and to avoid joint stiffness. Painful activities should be avoided during the dynamic rest phase. Vibration is contraindicated, since vibration may contribute to inflammatory problems.

When the inflammation has been controlled, the patient begins the exercise phase of treatment. After warming up the muscles by slow stretching, controlled progressive exercise is begun. Resistance should be given at the end of range when doing progressive resistive exercise. A tennis elbow armband can be worn over the extensor muscle bellies and will limit full excursion of the muscle during active use of the arm. Resistance should be increased slowly and should not cause an increase in pain.

Patients are instructed to continue stretching 3 times a day, especially before activity, for an indefinite time period. Proper body mechanics are critical in the long term control of inflammatory problems, so patients must become aware of what triggers their symptoms and learn early intervention if symptoms reappear. Icing, splints, stretching, and modified activities combined with correct body mechanics are usually effective. The key is that the patients learn self-management techniques and take an active role in their treatment.

An evaluation of the job site, tools used, and hand position during work activities may be indicated with the patient whose symptoms are related to job demands. Modification of the equipment used and strengthening of the dominant muscle groups and their antagonist muscles may permit continued employment while controlling the inflammatory problem.

Carpal tunnel syndrome is an example of a frequently seen inflammatory problem. Symptoms of this syndrome are caused by pressure on the median nerve as it travels beneath the transverse carpal ligament at the volar surface of the wrist.[46] It is associated with increased pressure in the carpal canal due to trauma, edema, retention of fluids as a result of pregnancy, flexor tenosynovitis, repetitive wrist motions, or static loading of the wrist.

Symptoms are night pain that is severe enough to waken the patient; tingling in the thumb and index and long fingers; and, if advanced, wasting of the thenar musculature caused by pressure on the motor branch of the nerve. Early carpal tunnel syndrome may be recognized by a thorough nerve evaluation.

Conservative treatment is usually attempted first and includes splinting the wrist in no more than 20° extension, contrast baths to reduce edema, wearing Isotoner gloves, and activity analysis. A custom fabricated semiflexible splint (Fig. 28-19), rather than a completely rigid splint, may be used to provide support while allowing a small amount of flexion and extension for greater functional use in carpal tunnel syndrome.

Ultrasound phonophonesis may be used to reduce inflammation, and icing techniques are beneficial. Specific strengthening exercises of the wrist, fingers,

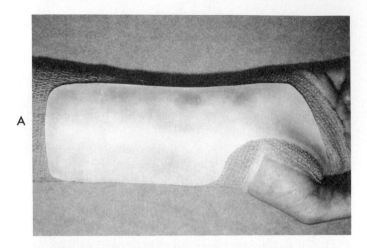

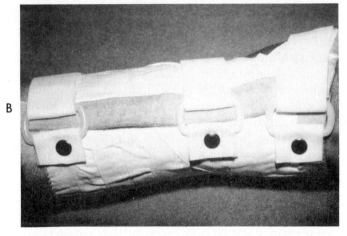

Fig. 28-19. A semiflexible splint may be constructed using Coban wrap, a thermoplastic insert (**A**) and finished with coach tape and straps (**B**). Detailed instructions for this splint are available from the RL Petzoldt Memorial Center for Hand Rehabilitation, 4155 Moorpark Ave., #21, San José, CA 95117.

and thumb should be given when the pain and inflammation have been controlled.

Diagnosis of carpal tunnel syndrome has increased,[62] and it is thought to occur more frequently in industrial settings with highly repetitive technical jobs that require the wrist to be held in dorsiflexion or palmar flexion while manipulating small objects. Occupational therapists may be asked to visit the job site and make recommendations for ergonomic adaptation of the workplace including tool modification and wrist position to reduce the incidence of this syndrome.

Surgical correction of carpal tunnel syndrome is done by releasing the transverse carpal ligament.

Myofascial pain and fibrositis are also conditions of pain elicited by activation of trigger points within the muscles and resulting in pain referred to a distal area; they are frequently encountered conditions. Travell[99] has studied myofascial pain and mapped out the traditional trigger points and their referral patterns. Poor posture and positioning of the body out of normal alignment are often the mechanism of injury in myofascial pain, so careful examination of the patient and his or her normal daily activities is indicated. The therapist should observe the patient performing the activity rather than rely on a verbal description. Myofascial pain should be considered in cases where direct treatment of the painful area does not relieve the pain. Evaluation for trigger points must be done meticulously, and mapping of the trigger points and the referral areas must be documented. Since the pain is referred, the trigger point must be treated, not the referral area. The treatments used for other inflammatory problems, such as ice and ultrasound phonophoresis, can be used. In addition, there are specific treatments for the trigger points, such as friction massage and TENS, which may relieve the pain. Activity analysis is an essential part of treatment to relieve the stresses on the affected tissues.

Strengthening Activities

Acute care is followed by a gradual return of motion, sensibility, and preparation to return to normal ADL. Strengthening the injured and neglected extremity is usually not accomplished by the patient at home, since he or she is often fearful of further injury and pain. Every hand clinic has its own armamentarium of strengthening exercises and media, and a few suggestions are provided here.

BTE WORK SIMULATOR. Baltimore Therapeutic Equipment (BTE) have made available the BTE work simulator[28] (Fig. 28-20), an electromechanical device that has more than 20 interchangeable tool handles and can be used for both work evaluation and upper extremity strengthening. Resistance can vary from no resistance to complete static resistance, with tool height and angle also adjustable. When used for strengthening, the resistance is usually set low and gradually increased, with concurrent increases in length of exercise. The BTE work simulator allows for close simulation of "real world" tasks that are easily translatable into physical demands common to manual work.

WEIGHT WELL. The weight well[3] was developed at the Downey Community Hospital Hand Center in Downey, California, and is available commercially.[60] Rods with a variety of handle shapes are placed through holes in the box and have weights suspended. The rods are turned against resistance throughout the ROM to encourage full grasp and release of the injured hand, wrist flexion and extension, pinch, and pronation and supination patterns. The weight well

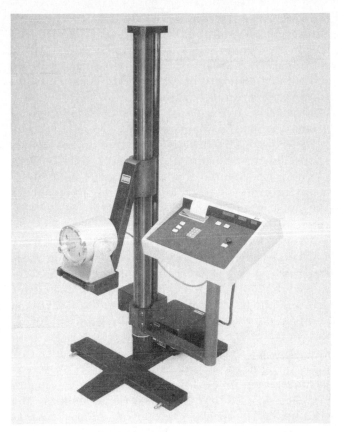

Fig.28-20. The BTE Work Simulator is an electromechanical device used to simulate "real life" tasks for upper extremity evaluation and strengthening. The patient's progress is monitored through a computerized print-out, and the program can be modified to increase resistance and endurance.

can be graded for resistance and repetitions and is an excellent tool for progressive resistive exercise.

THERABAND. Theraband is a 6-inch (15.2-cm) wide rubber sheet that is available by the yard and is color coded by degrees of resistance. It can be cut into any length required and used for resistive exercise for the upper extremity. Use of Theraband is limited only by the therapist's imagination; and it can be adapted to diagonal patterns of motion, wrist exercises, follow-up treatment of tennis elbow, and other uses. The Theraband can be combined with dowel rods and other equipment to provide resistance throughout the ROM. It is inexpensive and easy to incorporate into a home treatment program.

HAND STRENGTHENING EQUIPMENT. Hand grips of graded resistance are available from rehabilitation supply companies and sporting goods stores. Big Grips can be purchased in 10-, 15-, 30-, and 60-pound sizes and are recommended because they easily conform to the shape of the hand. They can be used for progressive resistive hand exercises. The Hand

Helper is also used, and resistance is varied by the addition of rubber bands. Small, hand-shaped rubber grippers are available and may be used for blocking exercises.

The therapist is cautioned against using overly resistive spring-loaded grippers often sold in sporting goods stores. These devices may be beneficial to the seasoned athlete but are usually too resistive for the recently injured.

Therapy putty can be purchased in bulk, and the amount given to the patient is geared to hand size and strength. Putty is also available in grades of resistance. It can be adapted to most finger motions and is easily incorporated into a home program.

Household items, such as spring-type clothespins and a toy called the "Obie Doll," have been used to increase strength of grasp and pinch. Imaginative use of common objects should present a challenge to the hand therapist.

Functional Activities

Functional activities are an integral part of rehabilitation of the hand. Functional activities may include crafts, games, dexterity activities, ADL, and work samples. Many of the treatment techniques described to this point are employed to condition the hand for normal use.

Activities should be started as soon as possible at whatever level the patient can perform them with adaptations to compensate for limited ROM and strength. They should be used as an adjunct to other treatments. The occupational therapist must continually assess the patient's functional capacities and initiate changes in the treatment program to incorporate activities as soon as possible in the restorative phase.

Vocational and avocational goals should be established at the time of initial evaluation and taken into account when planning treatment. The needs of a brick mason may be quite different from those of a mother with small children, and the environmental needs of the patient must not be neglected.

Crafts should be graded from light resistance to heavy resistance and from gross dexterity to fine dexterity. Crafts that have been found to work extremely well with hand injuries include macrame, turkish knot weaving, clay, leather, and woodworking.

All of these crafts can be adapted and graded to the patient's capabilities and have been found to have a high level of patient acceptance. When integrated into a program of total hand rehabilitation, they are viewed as another milestone of achievement and not as a diversion to fill up empty hours. For example, the pride of accomplishment for a patient who sustained a Volkmann's contracture caused by ischemia and who completed her first project in nearly four years is evidence that crafts belong in hand rehabilitation.

Activities that do not have an end product but provide practice in dexterity and ADL skills also fit into the category of functional activities. Developmental games and activities that require pinch or grasp and release may be graded and timed to increase difficulty. ADL boards that have a variety of opening and closing devices provide practice for use of the hand at home and increase self-confidence. String and finger games are challenging coordination activities that can be done in pairs and are fun to do.

Many times a hobby can be adapted for use in the clinic. Fly-tying is a difficult dexterity activity but one that will be enjoyed by an avid fisherman. Golf clubs and fishing poles can be adapted in the clinic to allow early return to a favorite form of relaxation.

Humor and patient interaction with the therapists and the other patients are factors that are vital but intangible benefits of treatment. Treatment should be planned to promote both.

Physical Capacity Evaluation

EVALUATION PHASE. The ultimate goal of therapy for an injured worker is to return to full employment. Many weeks or months may have elapsed between the time of the injury and the point at which the physician feels a return to work is appropriate from a medical standpoint. Despite the fact that x-ray examinations may show full healing and restored ROM, many patients do not feel they have the strength, dexterity, or endurance to return to their former jobs. Pain may continue to be a limiting factor, especially with heavy activities. Light duty or part-time positions may not be available; and the physician, therapist, industrial insurance carrier, and most of all, the patient are frustrated by the lack of an objective method of evaluating an individual's physical capacity for work. Occupational therapists with training in evaluation, kinesiology, and adaptation of environmental factors coupled with a functional approach to the patient may play a key role in physical capacity evaluation.

A renewed interest in evaluation of prevocational factors has brought the profession of occupational therapy full circle. Although one of the cornerstones of the profession in its early years, "prevocational evaluation" has been neglected in many centers during the last two decades. However, occupational therapists in the 1980s have rediscovered a need that the profession is in a unique position to provide. The term "prevocational evaluation" ambiguously implied that occupational therapists were involved in assessing the vocational needs of patients they treated. However, the development of the terms "physical capacity evaluation" (PCE) and "work tolerance screening" (WTS) more clearly describe the process of measuring an individual's ability to perform the physical demands of work. The results of this evaluation allow the therapist, worker, physician, and vocational counselor to establish a specific attainable employment goal using reliable data. This relieves the physician of the responsibility of returning the patient to work without objective information about the patient's ability to do a job. It also allows the patient to test his or her abilities for him- or herself and may result in increased self-confidence about returning to work.

Many techniques for performing a physical capacity evaluation have been proposed.[7,47,71,72] Some basic steps may be followed regardless of the specific technique adopted. The patient should be evaluated for grip and pinch strength, sensation, and ROM. Edema and pain must also be assessed and reassessed during the course of the evaluation. The GULHEMP (general physique, upper extremity, lower extremity, hearing, eye sight, mentality, and personality) Work Capacity Evaluation Worksheet[71] may be used as a general method of determining functional abilities. The GULHEMP Physical Development Analysis Worksheet[71] may be used to evaluate the job.

Job analysis may also be provided by a rehabilitation counselor and through information provided by the patient. The therapist should consult the *Dictionary of Occupational Titles* (DOT)[101] to obtain information about the worker traits required for the expected job. This dictionary contains 12,900 job descriptions and 20,000 job titles. If sufficient information about the job is not available through these methods, an on-site job analysis by the therapist may be necessary.

Once the physical demand characteristics of work have been documented, it is possible to evaluate the patient's ability to perform them.

Baxter[7] has described a physical capacity evaluation adapted for upper extremity injuries based on the physical capacity requirements found in the *Dictionary of Occupational Titles*. Following evaluation the therapist may recommend a work therapy program.[6] Work therapy can include simulated job tasks to increase job performance.

Matheson[71,72] has written several manuals and articles that describe Work Capacity Evaluation (WCE). This 8- to 10-day work assessment includes evaluation of the patient's feasibility for employment (worker characteristics, such as safety and dependability), employability, work tolerances (such as strength, endurance, and the effect of pain on work performance), the physical demand characteristics of the job, and the worker's ability to "dependably sustain performance in response to broadly defined work demands."[71]

Tests with well-accepted reliability, such as the Purdue Pegboard Test,[98] the Crawford Small Parts Dexterity Test,[26] the Minnesota Manual Dexterity Test,[79] and the Jebsen Hand Dexterity Test,[49] may be administered as a screening process. These tests will give the therapist valuable information through observation whether or not the normal tables are used or the test is adapted to an individual worker.

Many evaluation tests and job simulation devices are available and should be reviewed before establishing a physical capacity evaluation program. To choose appropriate work samples the job market in a specific area should be determined. This can be done by consulting with vocational schools, rehabilitation counselors, and employment agencies in the area.

Work samples, available through Jewish Employment and Vocational Service,[103] Singer,[42] Valpar,[102] and Work Evaluation Systems Technology (WEST)[112] may be used to test specific skills. Job samples may also be developed by the therapist using information on jobs in the local area. Discarded electronic assembly boards, a lawn mower motor, automobile engine, or other items from the local hardware store may provide valuable information about the worker's ability.

Work simulation using job samples or the BTE work simulator will assess the worker's specific physical capacities as well as his endurance and symptoms that become cumulative with prolonged use of the injured part—also called symptom response to activity (SRA). Monitoring the client's SRA may prevent loss of time and money expended in training for an inappropriate vocational goal.

A combination of "normed" tests, job samples, job simulation, and work capacity evaluation devices may provide the therapist with the best information about a worker's physical capacity. For more information about vocational evaluation and rehabilitation, the therapist should write to the Materials Development Center at the University of Wisconsin-Stout in Menomonie, Wisconsin.[70]

WORK HARDENING. Work hardening is the progressive use of simulated work samples to increase endurance, strength, productivity, and often feasibility. Work hardening may be performed for a period of weeks, and the progressive ongoing nature of the work usually results in improvements in physical capacity. It is an important contribution to vocational rehabilitation.

Since PCE is also performed over time, it may be difficult to identify the difference between PCE and work hardening. A PCE is generally done when the patient has stopped improving with traditional therapy methods and may have been released from acute medical care. The patient may be unable to return to his or her former employment or it may be questionable if the patient would be able to do his or her former work. A PCE may be initiated by a physician, rehabilitation counselor, insurance adjustor, or attorney.

Work hardening may be initiated earlier in the rehabilitation process, perhaps by the treating physician or therapist who recognizes that an individual may have difficulty returning to his or her former employment. It is performed before the end of medical care and may serve as a final "checkout" before discontinuing treatment.

Standards for work hardening services have been developed by the Commission on Accreditation of Rehabilitation Facilities (CARF)[24] to ensure that injured workers are being offered quality programs that are maximally effective in successfully returning them to gainful employment.

The Employment and Rehabilitation Institute of California (ERIC)[38] has many publications and resources available to therapists interested in establishing work capacity evaluation, work tolerance screening, or work hardening services. A publications and equipment listing is available on request.

It is important to stress that PCE and work hardening are adjuncts to the vocational rehabilitation process. Occupational therapists are trained to observe behavior and have the skills necessary to translate that observation into useful data. PCE and work hardening should not be a process that is in competition with the work of rehabilitation or vocational counselors but rather one that provides critical information about a worker's physical functioning and may serve as a program to foster reentry into the job market.

REVIEW QUESTIONS

1. Discuss three approaches to postoperative care of flexor tendon injuries. What would be the significance of each method in initiating occupational therapy?
2. To what does "joint dysfunction" refer? What are its causes?
3. List three treatment techniques that might be used in treatment of a pain syndrome.
4. Explain the three classifications of nerve injury.
5. Define the area referred to as "no-man's land." What is the significance of injury to this area?
6. What techniques would be employed to evaluate the physical demand characteristics of work?
7. List three methods of applying pressure to a hypertrophic scar.
8. What functional activities could be used for restoration of hand function following laceration and repair of the extrinsic finger flexors?
9. How does physical capacity evaluation differ from prevocational evaluation and vocational assessment?
10. List five components of hand evaluation.
11. List three objectives of splinting as they relate to injury of the radial, median, and ulnar nerves.
12. Describe the test for intrinsic and extrinsic muscle tightness.
13. What are the characteristics of a reflex sympathetic dystrophy? What are the treatment goals?
14. List four commonly used dexterity tests.
15. Define "work hardening." How can work hardening be incorporated into occupational therapy?
16. How is the presence of edema evaluated? List three methods used to reduce edema.
17. Explain the difference between acute phase and restorative phase treatment for an inflammatory problem. How would these factors influence occupational therapy?
18. What is the goal of sensory reeducation following nerve repair? List the hierarchy of nerve function return as it relates to sensory reeducation.

REFERENCES

1. Alon G: High voltage stimulation, Chattanooga, TN, 1984, Chattanooga Corp.
2. American Society for Surgery of the Hand: The hand examination and diagnosis, ed 2, New York, 1983, Churchill Livingstone, Inc.
3. Barber LM: Occupational therapy for the treatment of reflex sympathetic dystrophy and posttraumatic hypersensitivity of the injured hand. In Fredericks S and Brody GS, editors: Symposium on the neurologic aspects of plastic surgery, St Louis, 1978, The CV Mosby Co.
4. Barber LM: Desensitization of the traumatized hand. In Hunter JM et al: editors: Rehabilitation of the hand, ed 2, St Louis, 1984, The CV Mosby Co.
5. Basmajian JV: Practical functional anatomy. In Hunter JM et al, editors: Rehabilitation of the hand, ed 2, St Louis, 1984, The CV Mosby Co.
6. Baxter PL and Fried SL: The work tolerance program of the Hand Rehabilitation Center in Philadelphia. In Hunter JM et al, editors: Rehabilitation of the Hand, St Louis, 1984, The CV Mosby Co.
7. Baxter PL and McEntee PM: Physical capacity evaluation. In Hunter JM et al, editors: Rehabilitation of the hand, ed 2, St Louis, 1984, The CV Mosby Co.
8. Bell JA: Plaster cylinder casting for contractures of the interphalangeal joints. In Hunter JM et al, editors: Rehabilitation of the hand, ed 2, St Louis, 1984, The CV Mosby Co.
9. Bell JA: Sensibility testing: state of the art. In Hunter JM et al, editors: Rehabilitation of the hand, ed 2, St Louis, 1984, The CV Mosby Co.
10. Bell JA: Light touch-deep pressure testing using Semmes-Weinstein monofilaments. In Hunter JM et al, editors: Rehabilitation of the hand, ed 2, St Louis, 1984, The CV Mosby Co.
11. Benton LA, et al: Functional electrical stimulation: a practical clinical guide, ed 2, Downey, CA, 1981, Rancho Los Amigos Hospital.
12. Bennett GK: Hand-tool dexterity test, New York, 1981, Harcourt Brace, Jovanovich, Inc.
13. Bio-Concepts, 1016 S 23rd Street, Phoenix, AZ 85034.
14. Bora FW: Nerve response to injury and repair. In Hunter JM et al, editors: Rehabilitation of the hand, ed 1, St Louis, 1978, The CV Mosby Co.
15. Boyes JH: Bunnell's surgery of the hand, ed 5, Philadelphia, 1970, JB Lippincott Co.
16. Boyes JH and Stark HH: Flexor-tendon grafts in the fingers and thumb, J Bone Joint Surg 53A:1332, 1971.
17. Callahan AD: Methods of compensation and reeducation for sensory dysfunction. In Hunter JM et al, editors: Rehabilitation of the hand, ed 2, St Louis, 1984, The CV Mosby Co.
18. Cannon NM, et al: Control of immediate postoperative pain following tenolysis and capsulectomies of the hand with TENS, J Hand Surg 8:625, 1983.
19. Cannon NM and Mullins PT: Modalities in upper extremity rehabilitation. In Malick MH and Kasch MC: Manual on management of specific hand problems, Pittsburgh, 1984, AREN Publications.
20. Carroll D: A quantitative test of upper extremity function, J Chronic Dis 18:479, 1965.
21. Central Tool Company of Germany. (Available from Anthony Products, 7311 E 43rd St, Indianapolis, IN 46226.)
22. Chai SH, Dimick MP, and Kasch MC: A role delineation study of hand therapy, J Hand Ther 1:7, 1987.
23. Chusid JG: Correlative neuroanatomy and functional neurology, ed 15, Los Altos, CA, 1973, Lange Medical Publications.
24. Commission on Accreditation of Rehabilitation Facilities (CARF), 2500 N Pantano Rd., Tucson, AZ 85715.

25. Corrective Concepts, 3045 Park Lane, Suite 1084, Dallas, TX 75220.

26. Crawford JE and Crawford DM: Crawford small parts dexterity test manual, New York, 1981, Harcourt, Brace, Jovanovich, Inc.

27. Creelman G: Volumeters unlimited, Idyllwild, CA.

28. Curtis RM and Engalitcheff J: A work simulator for rehabilitating the upper extremity: preliminary report, J Hand Surg 6:499, 1981.

29. Cyriax JH: Clinical applications of massage. In Basmajian JV: Manipulation, traction and massage, ed 3, Baltimore, 1985, Williams & Wilkins.

30. Dellon AL: Evaluation of sensibility and reeducation of sensation in the hand, Baltimore, 1981, Williams & Wilkins.

31. Dellon AL, Curtis RM, and Edgerton MT: Reeducation of sensation in the hand after nerve injury and repair, Plast Reconstr Surg 53:297, 1974.

32. Dellon AL: Clinical use of vibratory stimuli to evaluate peripheral nerve injury and compression neuropathy, Plast Reconstr Surg 65:466, 1980.

33. Dellon AL: The vibrometer, Plast Reconstr Surg 71:427, 1983.

34. Digi-Sleeve. (Available from North Coast Medical, 450 Salmar Ave, Campbell, CA, 95008.)

35. Disk-Criminator. (Available from PO Box 16392, Baltimore 21210.)

36. Donatelli R and Owens-Burkhart H: Effects of immobilization on the extensibility of periarticular connective tissue, J Orth & Sports Phys Ther 3:67, 1981.

37. Duran RJ et al: Management of flexor tendon lacerations in zone 2 using controlled passive motion postoperatively. In Hunter JM et al, editors: Rehabilitation of the hand, ed 2, St Louis, 1984, The CV Mosby Co.

38. Employment and Rehabilitation Institute of California (ERIC), 1160 N Gilbert St, Anaheim, CA, 92801.

39. English CB, Rehm RA, and Petzoldt RL: Blocking splints to assist finger exercise, Am J Occup Ther 36:259, 1983.

40. Evans RB and Burkhalter WE: A study of the dynamic anatomy of extensor tendons and implications for treatment, J Hand Surg 11A:774, 1986.

41. Evans RB: Therapeutic management of extensor tendon injuries. In Hand Clinics, vol 1(2), Philadelphia, 1986, WB Saunders Co.

42. Ferraro MC, et al: Closed functional bracing of metacarpal fractures, Orth Rev 12:49, 1983.

43. Fess EE and Moran CA: Clinical assessment recommendations, Indianapolis, 1981, American Society of Hand Therapists.

44. Fields J: Anatomy and kinesiology of the upper extremity, lecture presented at San Jose State University, San Jose, CA, 1976.

45. Gelberman RH et al: Sensibility testing in peripheral-nerve compression syndromes, J Bone Joint Surg 65A:632, 1983.

46. Gelberman RH et al: The carpal tunnel syndrome, J Bone Joint Surg 63A:380, 1981.

47. Harrand G: The Harrand guide for developing physical capacity evaluations, Menomonie, WI, 1982, Stout Vocational Rehabilitation Institute.

48. Isotoner gloves by Aris, (Available from North Coast Medical, 450 Salmar Ave, Campbell, CA, 95008.)

49. Jebsen RH et al: An objective and standardized test of hand function, Arch Phys Med Rehabil 50:311, 1969.

50. Jobst Institute, Inc, PO Box 653, Toledo, OH 43694.

51. Kamenetz HL: Mechanical devices of massage. In Basmajian JV: Manipulation, traction and massage, ed 3, Baltimore, 1985, Williams & Wilkins.

52. Kasch MC: Clinical management of scar tissue, O.T. in Health Care 4(3/4):37, 1987.

53. Kasch MC and Hester LA: Low-frequency TENS and the release of endorphins, J Hand Surg 8:626, 1983.

54. Kessler RM and Hertling D: Joint mobilization techniques. In Kessler RM and Hertling D: Managment of common musculoskeletal disorders, New York, 1983, Harper & Row, Publishers, Inc.

55. Kellor M et al: Technical manual of hand strength and dexterity test, Minneapolis, 1971, Sister Kenney Rehabilitation Institute.

56. Kelsey JL et al: Upper extremity disorders: a survey of their frequency and cost in the United States, St Louis, 1980, The CV Mosby Co.

57. Kutz JE: Controlled mobilization of acute flexor tendon injuries: Louisville technique. In Hunter JM, Schneider LH, and Mackin EJ: Tendon surgery in the hand, St Louis, 1987, Times Mirror/Mosby College Publishing.

58. LaSalle WB and Strickland JW: An evaluation of the two-stage flexor tendon reconstruction technique, J Hand Surg 8:263, 1983.

59. Lister GL: The hand: diagnosis and indications, London, 1977, Churchill Livingstone, Inc.

60. LMB Hand Rehabilitation Products, Inc, San Luis Ohispo, CA.

61. Louis DS et al: Evaluation of normal values for stationary and moving two-point discrimination in the hand, J Hand Surg 99:552, 1984.

62. Lublin JS: Unions and firms focus on hand disorder that can be caused by repetitive tasks, The Wall Street Journal, January 14, 1983.

63. Lundborg G et al: Digital vibrogram: a new diagnostic tool for sensory testing in compression neuropathy, J Hand Surg 11A:693, 1986.

64. Mackin EJ and Maiorano L: Postoperative therapy following staged flexor tendon reconstruction. In Hunter JM et al editors: Rehabilitation of the

hand, ed 1, St Louis, 1978, The CV Mosby Co.

65. Mackinnon SE and Dellon AL: Two-point discrimination tester, J Hand Surg 10A:906, 1985.

66. Madden JW: Wound healing: the biological basis of hand surgery. In Hunter JM et al, editors: Rehabilitation of the hand, ed 2, St Louis, 1984, The CV Mosby Co.

67. Maitland GD: Peripheral Manipulation, Boston, 1977, Butterworth & Co, Ltd.

68. Malick MH and Carr JA: Flexible elastomer molds in burn scar control, Am J Occup Ther 34:603, 1980.

69. Mark One Health Care Products, Inc, Philadelphia.

70. Materials Development Center, Stout Vocational Rehabilitation Institute, University of Wisconsin-Stout, Menomonie, WI.

71. Matheson LN: Work capacity evaluation: a training manual for occupational therapists, Trabuco Canyon, CA, 1982, Rehabilitation Institute of Southern California.

72. Matheson LN and Ogden LD: Work tolerance screening, Trabuco Canyon, CA, 1983, Rehabilitation Institute of Southern California.

73. Mathiowetz V et al: Reliability and validity of grip and pinch strength evaluations, J Hand Surg 9A:222, 1984.

74. Mathiowetz V et al: Grip and pinch strength: normative data for adults, Arch Phys Med Rehabil 66:69, 1985.

75. Mathiowetz V, Rennells C, and Donahoe L: Effect of elbow position on grip and key pinch strength, J Hand Surg 10A:694, 1985.

76. Melvin JL: Rheumatic disease occupational therapy and rehabilitation, ed 2, Philadelphia, 1982, FA Davis Co.

77. Mennell JM: Joint pain, Boston,1964, Little, Brown & Co.

78. Mennell JM and Zohn DA: Musculoskeletal pain diagnosis and physical treatment, Boston, 1976, Little, Brown & Co.

79. Minnesota Manual Dexterity Test. (Available from Lafayette Instrument Co, PO Box 5729, Lafayette, IN, 47903.)

80. Moberg E: Objective methods of determining functional value of sensibility in the hand, J Bone Joint Surg 40A:454, 1958.

81. Moberg E: Aspects of the sensation in reconstructive surgery of the upper extremity, J Bone Joint Surg 46A:817, 1964.

82. Omer G: Management of pain syndromes in the upper extremity. In Hunter JM et al, editors: Rehabilitation of the hand, ed 2, St Louis, 1984, The CV Mosby Co.

83. O'Rain S: New and simple test of nerve function in the hand, Br Med J 3:615, 1973.

84. N-Terface made by Winfield Laboratories. (Available from North Coast Medical, 450 Salmar Ave, Campbell, CA, 95008.)

85. Neoprene. (Available from Orthopaedic Tech, Inc, 14670 Wicks Blvd, San Leandro, CA.)

86. Otoform K. (Available from WFR/Aquaplast Corp, PO Box 215, Ramsey, NJ, 07446.)

87. Parry CBW: Rehabilitation of the hand, ed 4, London, 1984, Butterworth & Co, Ltd.

88. Peacock, EE, Madden JW, and Trier WC: Postoperative recovery of flexor tendon function, Am J Surg 122:686, 1971.

89. Sarmiento A and Latta LL: Closed functional treatment of fractures, New York, 1981, Springer-Verlag, Inc.

90. Schneider LH and Hunter JM: Flexor tenolysis. In AAOS: Symposium on tendon surgery in the hand, St. Louis, 1975, The CV Mosby Co.

91. Silicone Elastomer. (Available from Smith-Nephew Medical Products, PO Box 555, Menomonie Falls, WI, 53051.)

92. Singer Education Division, Career Systems, Rochester, NY.

93. Spenco Medical Corp, Box 8113, Waco, TX, 76710.

94. Spinner M: Injuries to the major branches of peripheral nerves of the forearm, ed 2, Philadelphia, 1978, WB Saunders Co.

95. Strickland JW and Glogovac SV: Digital function following flexor tendon repair in zone II: a comparison of immobilization and controlled passive motion techniques, J Hand Surg 5:537, 1980.

96. Szabo RM et al: Vibratory sensory testing in acute peripheral nerve compression, J Hand Surg 9A:104, 1984.

97. Thomas CL, editor: Taber's cyclopedic medical dictionary, ed 14, Philadelphia, 1981, FA Davis Co.

98. Tiffin J: Purdue pegboard examiner manual, Chicago, 1968, Science Research Associates, Inc.

99. Travell JG and Simons DG: Myofascial pain and dysfunction; The tigger point manual, Baltimore, 1983, Williams & Wilkins.

100. Trombly CA, editor: Occupational therapy for physical dysfunction, ed 2, Baltimore, 1983, Williams & Wilkins.

101. US Department of Labor, Employment, and Training Administration: Dictionary of occupational titles, ed 4, Washington, DC, 1977, US Government Printing Office.

102. Valpar Corp, Tucson.

103. Vocational Research Institute, Jewish Employment and Vocational Service (JEVS), Philadelphia.

104. Walker SW: Treatment of soft tissue inflammatory problems of the forearm and hand, San Jose, 1983. Unpublished.

105. Waylett, J and Seibly D: A study to determine the average deviation accuracy of a commercially available volumeter, J Hand Surg 6:300, 1981.

106. Waylett-Rendall J: Sensibility evaluation and rehabilitation. In Orthopedic Clinics of North America, vol 19(1), Philadelphia, 1988, WB Saunders Co.

107. Wehbé MA and Hunter JM: Flexor tendon gliding in the hand, Pt II: Differential gliding, J Hand Surg 10A:575, 1985.

108. Wehbé MA: Tendon gliding exercises, Am J Occup Ther 41:164, 1987.

109. WFR Corp, Ramsey, NJ.
110. Wilson RE and Carter MS: Management of hand fractures. In Hunter JM et al, editors: Rehabilitation of the hand,

ed 2, St Louis, 1984, The CV Mosby Co.
111. Wolf SL: Electrotherapy, New York, 1981, Churchill Livingstone, Inc.
112. Work Evaluation Systems Tech-

nology (WEST), Huntington Beach, CA.
113. Yerxa EJ et al: Development of a hand sensitivity test for the hypersensitive hand, Am J Occup Ther 37:176, 1983.

Sample treatment plan

This sample treatment plan is not comprehensive. It deals with three of four identified problems. The reader is encouraged to add objectives and methods to complete the treatment plan.

CASE STUDY

Mr. D is a 69-year-old right-handed retired sales manager with an 8- to 10-year history of Dupuytren's contracture of both hands, the right being more involved than the left. He stated that the long, ring, and small fingers on his right hand became contracted 4 to 5 years ago and the contractures gradually progressed until the fingers were nearly in the palm. The ring and small fingers on the left hand have recently begun contracting. [Study hints: What are the characteristics of Dupuytren's contracture? Is there a known cause? Would it have been possible to prevent the progression of contractures in the right hand? Would treatment to the left hand help now?]

Six weeks prior to referral to occupational therapy, Mr. D had release and reconstruction of the contractures in the right palm including a Z-plasty that was left partially open at the time of surgery for drainage. [Study hints: What is a Z-plasty and how does it differ from a linear incision? What would be the benefits of this procedure for allowing skin closure versus a skin graft?] At the time of referral the surgeon noted that Mr. D also has underlying osteoarthritis of the small joints of his hands.

Mr. D has been retired for six years. He lives with his wife in their own home. They have three grown children and seven grandchildren whom they see frequently. Mr. D is independent in all his self-care activities. He enjoys fishing, golf, and cooking and likes to "putter" around the house. He does not smoke and drinks moderately. [Study hint: Does alcohol consumption have any correlation in Dupuytren's disease?] He is alert, pleasant, and cooperative.

TREATMENT PLAN

Personal data
Name: JD
Age: 69
Diagnosis: Dupuytren's contracture, both hands, with underlying osteoarthritis; status—postrelease and reconstruction of contractures with Z-plasty.

Disability: Unable to fully extend or flex fingers following surgery performed 6 weeks prior to referral.
Treatment aims stated in referral: Increase active and passive ROM; scar remodeling, static night splint and dynamic daytime splint; evaluate for compression garment. Frequency of 2 to 3 times per week for 4 weeks. [Note: This patient is insured by Medicare and has a $500 limit for outpatient occupational therapy as well as a secondary insurance that may or may not pay for additional therapy if needed. Some secondary or supplemental insurances pay only the 20% not paid by Medicare, and others will pay for services not covered by Medicare. How will that affect the services provided to him in your outpatient clinic?]

OTHER SERVICES
Physician: Performed surgery; prescribes medication and treatment; supervises rehabilitation.

FRAME OF REFERENCE:
Occupational performance.

TREATMENT APPROACHES:
Biomechanical and rehabilitative.

OT EVALUATION
Performance components
Motor functioning
Muscle strength: Test
Passive and active ROM: Test
Joint mobility: Test
Scar adhesions: Observe and palpate
Edema: Test
Sensory functioning
Sensation: Test
Cognitive functioning
Ability to follow directions: Observe
Psychological functioning
Chemical dependency: Observe behavior
Coping skills: Observe
Social functioning
Interpersonal skills: Observe
Performance skills
Self-care:
Interview
Home management:
Interview

Continued.

Sample treatment plan—cont'd

EVALUATION SUMMARY

Motor function (ROM)

Mr D had normal strength within a limited ROM at the time of his initial evaluation. Passive and active motion of the thumb, index, and long fingers was within normal limits. ROM of the ring and small fingers was as follows:

Digit	Passive	Active
Ring finger		
MP joint	22/75	30/75
PIP joint	30/80	33/85
DIP joint	0/45	0/34
Small finger		
MP joint	0/72	0/70
PIP joint	32/75	35/74
DIP joint	0/45	5/40

Joint Mobility: Joint accessory motion was limited [Study hint: How would the treatment plan be influenced by the presence of active joint inflammation caused by osteoarthritis in this patient?]

Scar adhesions: The surgical scar was dense and contractile in the palm and the volar surface of the ring and small fingers

Edema: Finger circumference was measured as well as hand volume to test for edema; circumferential measurements:

Ring finger

Proximal phalanx	7.0 cm
PIP joint	7.4 cm
Middle phalanx	6.5 cm

Small finger

Proximal phalanx	6.7 cm
PIP joint	6.7 cm
Middle phalanx	5.8 cm

Volume:

Right	595 ml
Left	530 ml

Sensory: Sensation tested in the diminished light-touch range on the ring and small fingers using the Semmes-Weinstein monofilaments

SUMMARY

Mr. D was highly motivated to have full use of his hand and was able to explain his home program to the therapist. His daughter is an RN and had helped him to understand the disease process and what to expect from therapy. He has coped well with the disease in the past and has adapted as needed to remain independent in all his activities, except for golf which is difficult because it has been hard to hold the club correctly. His use of alcohol is a general life-style coping mechanism that has not been exacerbated by his surgery. It did not interfere with his performance in OT.

ASSETS

Highly motivated and cooperative
Early postoperative referral allows scar remodeling
Scar and joints responded well to initial treatment
Good adherence to home treatment program

PROBLEM LIST

1. Limited active and passive ROM
2. Dense scar tissue
3. Edema
4. Decreased functional use of right hand

PROBLEM 1, 2

Limited ROM and dense scar tissue

Objective

Increase passive extension of ring and small PIP joints to 0° extension

Method

A removable static night extension splint was fabricated out of low-temperature thermoplastic material in maximum extension and lined with a silastic elastomer mold; the patient was instructed to wear this while sleeping and to bring it to therapy with him

Gradation

The splint was adjusted in greater extension as often as possible

As the scar softened, new molds were made

PROBLEM 1

Limited ROM

Objective

Increase passive extension of ring and small PIP joints to 0° extension

Method

The patient was fitted with two LMB finger extension splints and instructed to wear them each 3 times a day for 30 minutes; because of pain and edema tension on the spring wire was decreased

Gradation

Tension was increased on the splints as patient was able to tolerate it; if these splints had caused an increase in joint inflammation, a different splint would have been substituted

PROBLEM 3

Edema

Objective

Decrease edema by 5 to 10 ml per week

Method

Mr. D was instructed in retrograde massage and given an Isotoner glove to wear when not exercising or wearing a splint [Patients often wear gloves under their silastic molds if they have both. Be sure they understand that the mold must come in direct contact with the skin to be effective.]

Gradation

If the Isotoner were not effective, a custom garment could be ordered; the Jobst intermittent compression device might also be used at home several times a day or in the clinic; the patient must also continue to elevate the hand

Edema responds best to a variety of methods employed either at the same time or interchangeably, rather than to reliance on one method alone

29 Cardiac dysfunction

DENISE FODERARO
STEPHANIE O'LEARY

Coronary heart disease is the leading cause of death in the United States.[6] In 1984 over 1 million American deaths were attributed to cardiovascular disease. According to the National Center for Health Statistics that is more deaths than were recorded as a result of cancer, accidents, pneumonia, and influenza combined.[6]

Death rates related to coronary heart disease have been decreasing. As a result of improvement in modification of risk factors and in the treatment of patients with heart disease, survival rates are increasing. Rehabilitation of the coronary patient continues to be a problem of national concern.[39] Whereas accident victims need not fear recurrence of injury, patients with cardiac disease must attend to the continuing process of arteriosclerosis, which in many cases caused their injury.

Arteriosclerosis does not only affect the coronary circulation but often is manifest in the cerebral and peripheral circulation as well. It is not uncommon that a 65-year-old victim of a stroke also has a significant cardiac disease or that following a coronary episode a patient cannot engage in an aggressive conditioning program because of extensive peripheral vascular disease. These are the types of patients in general rehabilitation clinics who require special program modifications to accommodate their cardiovascular conditions and complications.

All occupational therapists working in the field of physical dysfunction must have a working knowledge of the cardiovascular system to provide safe, effective rehabilitation programs to all patients.

The principles of exercise physiology and work simplification used in treating the patient with a cardiac condition apply to the occupational performance of self-care, work, and play/leisure abilities for all patients.

This chapter provides a basic review of cardiovascular anatomy, physiology, and pathophysiology. Its purpose is (1) to enable the therapist to obtain the necessary medical information through chart review and patient interview and (2) to identify and understand the appropriate precautions when treating both the less serious or "uncomplicated" cardiac problems and the more involved or "complicated" cardiac conditions. The area of cardiac care has special terminology. Terms and definitions are included in the body of the text.

With background knowledge in cardiovascular anatomy, physiology, and pathophysiology, the therapist can plan an appropriate activity progression guided by accurate and continuous vital sign monitoring. In this way the patient may attain a maximal yet safe level of independent function.

The occupational performance frame of reference is used in evaluation and treatment of the patient with a cardiac condition. Evaluation focuses on the performance components of motor, sensory integrative, cognitive, psychological, and social functioning of the patient with cardiac dysfunction.[8] The patient's performance skills in the areas of self-care, work, and play/leisure are considered. During occupational therapy the patient will have the opportunity to learn and practice the tasks required for performance of role and developmental activities.

THE CARDIOVASCULAR SYSTEM
Normal Cardiovascular Function[9,29,34,50]

The cardiac cycle is an intricate interplay of events within the heart responsible for coordinating the direction and volume of blood flow. By this process the heart (1) delivers oxygen to vital organs and tissues of the body, (2) removes carbon dioxide and other byproducts, and (3) regulates body core temperature to maintain hemostasis.

ANATOMY AND CIRCULATION. The heart functions as a four-chambered pump.[41] The right side of the heart (right atrium and right ventricle) collects blood (venous return) and delivers it to the lungs where it can be reoxygenated. The left side of the heart (left atrium and left ventricle) collects blood

Judy Padé, OTR; Barbara Zoltan, MA, OTR; and Alison Fulmer, MD, are gratefully acknowledged for their support and assistance.

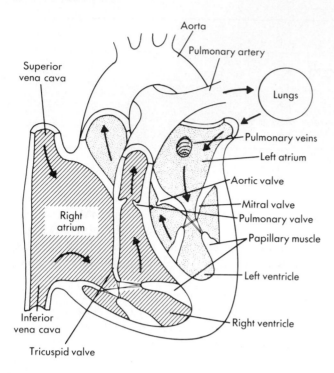

Fig. 29-1. Anatomy of the heart. From Andreoli KG et al: Comprehensive cardiac care: a text for nurses, physicians and other health practitioners, St Louis, 1983, The CV Mosby Co.

from the lungs and delivers it to the systemic circulation. Four heart valves assist in the passage and direction of blood flow within the heart (Fig. 29-1). The opening and closing of the valves depends on volume and pressure changes within the heart and on the papillary muscles. These muscles are connected to the inner myocardium and innervated by the conduction system. Although the heart muscle is always filled with blood, it receives its blood supply from the coronary circulation (Fig. 29-2).

The left main coronary artery and the right coronary artery are the major arteries that supply the outer layer of the heart muscle called the epicardium. These arteries divide further and extend into the myocardial wall called the endocardium. The small structure of these arteries predisposes them to arteriosclerotic disease, often referred to as coronary artery disease or CAD.

Cardiologists universally refer to these coronary arteries by abbreviations, such as LAD or left anterior descending coronary artery. The name of the artery describes the portion of the heart it supplies. A blockage in the LAD vessel interferes with blood supply to the left anterior aspect of the heart or the left ventricle. Since the left ventricle is responsible for pumping blood into the systemic circulation and to the brain, the consequences of LAD disease are often serious.

INNERVATION. Heart muscle, like skeletal muscle, requires nervous innervation to contract. A specialized nervous conduction network (Fig. 29-3) is responsible for causing myocardial contraction. This co-

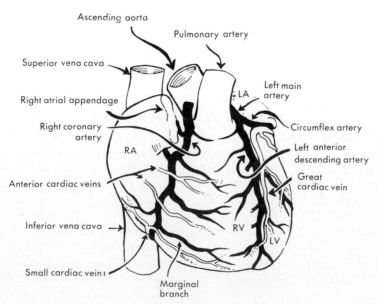

Fig. 29-2. Coronary circulation. From Underhill SL et al, editors: Cardiac nursing, Philadelphia, 1982, JB Lippincott Co.

ordinated sequence of depolarization and contraction is initiated by the sinoatrial (SA) node or pacemaker of the heart. From the SA node the impulse makes its way to the ventricles through the atrioventricular (AV) node, bundle branches, and Purkinje fibers.

Because depolarization is the result of electrical cellular changes, this process can be studied and recorded graphically by the electrocardiogram (ECG, EKG).[25] Surface electrodes are placed on the limbs and chest to monitor the sequence, timing, and magnitude of the impulse as it travels through the conduction system (Fig. 29-4). Each graphic segment, called P, ORS, and T waves, corresponds to the wave of depolarization as it travels through the various chambers of the heart. For instance, the P wave represents electrical stimulation arising from depolarization in the atria. The QRS complex corresponds to the wave of depolarization as it travels through the bundle of His to the ventricles. The timing of depolarization can be studied by counting the blocks on EKG paper. If the PR interval or QRS complex is longer than normal, a conduction abnormality or "block" in the system can be suspected.

The SA node adjusts its rate to meet the demands of the body and working muscle. It is sensitive to vagal and sympathetic nervous input.[9] This explains why heart rate increases during anxiety and with exercise. This mechanism also explains why heart rate decreases with deep breathing, meditation, or other relaxation techniques. Thus the ability to monitor, influence, and modify heart rate are important skills that can be learned by the patient with cardiovascular disease.

THE CARDIAC CYCLE.[17,23,29] The cardiac cycle maintains and adjusts cardiac output. The cardiac cycle occurs in two phases, input (diastole) and output (systole). The following discussion is a review of the cardiac cycle.

Input (diastole). During diastole the input valves (mitral and tricuspid) are open, and the output valves (aortic and pulmonary) are closed. This allows blood from the systemic pulmonary and coronary circulation to passively fill the ventricles. As ventricular volume increases, the pressure within the ventricles increases.

At this time the SA node initiates a wave of depolarization (P wave) which stimulates the atrial muscles to contract and "kick" their contents into the ventricle. The input valves close, and the first heart sound is heard.

The wave of depolarization (QRS wave) then stimulates the ventricles to contract. The output valves open, allowing blood flow into the systemic and pulmonary circulation. The numerical value assigned to the pressure required to open the output valves is the diastolic pressure or lower number of a blood pressure reading.

Output (systole). Once the aortic and pulmonary valves are open, the ventricles continue to contract. The pressure generated by the ventricles to eject blood is called the systolic blood pressure and is the upper number of the blood pressure reading. Once the ventricles empty, their volume and pressures decrease. When ventricular pressure falls, the output valves close and create the second heart sound. The total amount of blood ejected during one contraction is called stroke volume. The amount of blood ejected

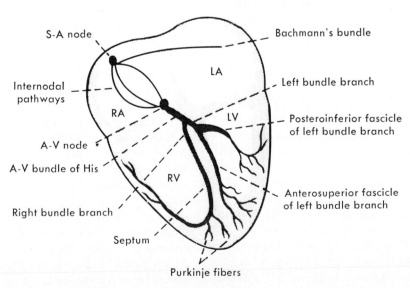

Fig. 29-3. Cardiac conduction. From Andreoli KG et al: Comprehensive cardiac care: a text for nurses, physicians, and other health practitioners, St Louis, 1983, The CV Mosby Co.

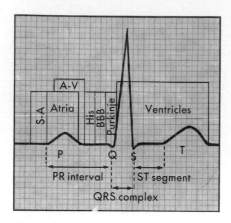

Fig. 29-4. Electrocardiography. Modified from Andreoli KG et al: Comprehensive cardiac care: a text for nurses, physicians, and other health practitioners, St Louis, 1983, The CV Mosby Co.

per minute is called cardiac output. The reader is referred to the references for a more detailed understanding of the factors influencing the cardiac cycle and ultimate cardiac output.

Pathophysiology

ISCHEMIC HEART DISEASE. The coronary circulation supplies oxygen to the heart muscle. An imbalance of oxygen supply and demand created by arteriosclerotic narrowing of the coronary arteries results in myocardial injury or myocardial infarction (death of tissue).

The consequences of ischemia include an excess accumulation in the myocardium of metabolic by-products. The presence of these metabolites may result in a decreased myocardial contractility, which can then decrease stroke volume.[35]

In addition, these circulating by-products predispose the myocardium to an increased occurrence of "ectopic" or irregular heart beats arising from irritable portions of the heart muscle. Depending on the origin and frequency of these ectopic beats, cardiac output may decrease and cardiac arrhythmias may develop.

Angina pectoris or chest pain is a clinical manifestation of ischemia and includes the characteristics described in Table 29-1.

Myocardial infarction (MI) occurs when severe ischemia lasts longer than 20 to 30 minutes. MIs can be either "transmural," in which the whole thickness of the myocardium is involved, or "nontransmural," in which a lesion is usually confined to the subendocardial layer of the myocardium. MIs are described by their location and size. An anterolateral MI affects both the anterior and lateral walls. Other types include septal, inferior, posterior, or any combination of these.

Nausea and vomiting are often associated with an acute MI. Other symptoms depend on the severity of MI (site and size) and the development of complications (congestive heart failure, arrhythmias, or cardiogenic shock). Additional characteristics of MI are compared with those of angina in Table 29-1. Those patients who develop complications are placed in a high-risk category, need close medical surveillance, and require slower progression in rehabilitation.

Congestive heart failure (CHF) can also be a manifestation of ischemia. When the heart tissue is damaged, the pumping function is impaired. The left ventricle is not able to move blood out of the lungs, causing pulmonary venous congestion.[44] If left heart failure continues, the system backs up further, causing the right ventricle to fail. The signs and symptoms of congestive heart failure are presented in Table 29-2.

VALVULAR DISEASE.[56,58] With age or in response to recurrent bacterial endocarditis the valve leaflets may become fibrous and prevent the valves from closing. A backward flow or "regurgitation" occurs, creating a valve "insufficiency." Clinically, this regurgitation can be heard as a murmur. Mitral insufficiency causes a congestion in the pulmonary circulation with resultant shortness of breath and susceptibility to erratic heart rates, such as atrial fibrillation. Such heart rates interfere with ventricular filling and complete emptying. Blood tends to stagnate, and emboli are common complications. Valvular disease with resultant emboli is a common cause of cerebral vascular accident (CVA).

Aortic insufficiency and regurgitation may result in CHF or ischemia. Aortic stenosis, if severe, will affect cardiac output. Symptoms caused by a decreased cardiac output include arrhythmias as a result of decreased coronary circulation perfusion; cerebral insufficiency or confusion; syncope, or "blacking out" when exerting effort; and dizziness related to a drop in blood pressure. Aortic stenosis warrants close medical management. Depending on severity exercise may be contraindicated and patients may require surgery, since these patients are at high risk for sudden death.

CARDIOMYOPATHY.[50,57] Cardiomyopathy means disease of the heart muscle. Although coronary arteries and valves may be intact, the cellular mechanics (actin and myosin) responsible for muscle contraction have been altered. This is usually the result of a virus or toxic substances, like alcohol, in the blood stream. There is a high incidence of cardiomyopathy among chronic alcoholics. Severe cases of cardiomyopathy, which cannot be medically controlled, produce a severely limited individual who is a prime candidate for occupational therapy intervention with energy conservation and equipment.

RISK FACTORS. The Framingham study[23] has cor-

Table 29-1 Characteristics of Angina Pectoris and Myocardial Infarction[21]*

	Characteristics of angina pectoris	Characteristics of myocardial infarction
Severity	Mild to moderate discomfort. The perception of the pain depends on the individual's age, culture, socialization, and previous experience. It is usually described as mild to moderate severity	Severe pain. A total loss of blood supply to a portion of the muscle results in severe pain and eventually necrotic tissue
Type and description	Squeezing, tightness, aching, burning, choking. This sensation is often described not as pain but discomfort. A classic description is for patient to clench their fist over their sternum in an attempt to describe the pain	Oppressive pressure, choking, strangling, feeling of impending doom. The greater intensity of the pain is evidence of a more complete and prolonged loss of blood supply and oxygen to heart muscle
Location	Substernal: the heart occupies a central location in the chest	Substernal: pain can be misinterpreted because many people think that heart pain has to be in the left chest
Radiation	Radiation **may** occur to the neck, arms, jaw, and epigastric area. If radiation occurs, it is due to the shared nerve innervation in the thoracic area. Occasionally the pain does not radiate in the chest	Radiation to the neck, arms, jaw, and epigastric area. The extensive damage with infarction increases the number of pain nerve receptors stimulated; MI pain may be misinterpreted as indigestion
Duration	Brief, usually less than 20 minutes. The ischemia is transient, causing pain of brief duration	Prolonged, usually greater than 20 minutes. The extent of ischemia is great, causing the duration of pain to be lengthened
Precipitating events	Emotions, exercise, extreme temperatures, heavy meals—these conditions increase the work of the heart, requiring an increased supply of blood and oxygen	Usually there may be precipitating factors; pain may occur at rest or during sleep. MI is the end result of the atherosclerotic process and is not affected by physical or emotional activity
Relief	Rest and/or nitroglycerin. Rest decreases the heart's work load and therefore the need for increased blood and oxygen supply. Nitroglycerin decreases the work of the heart by decreasing the resistance against which the heart has to pump	Pain is unrelieved by rest and nitroglycerin. Rest and nitroglycerin may decrease the intensity of the pain, but narcotics are usually required to eliminate it

*Adapted and reproduced with permission from Cornett S. and Watson J: Cardiac rehabilitation: an interdisciplinary team approach, New York, 1984, John Wiley & Sons, Inc.

related the presence of several risk factors to the progression of the arteriosclerotic process. The American Heart Association[3] divides them into two categories. Controllable risk factors of hypertension; smoking; obesity; sedentary or stressful life-style; diabetes; and other metabolic conditions (gout, hyperthyroidism, and lipidemia) can be controlled through medication, diet, and life-style modification. The second category includes uncontrollable factors: age, male sex, and heredity.

The Framingham study, a landmark study, inspired much research in an effort to understand the mechanisms responsible for arteriosclerosis. Medical science is now beginning to understand which factors control the development of arteriosclerosis. Much emphasis has been on prevention through exercise and diet. Consequently, much research has been performed on the cardiovascular benefits of aerobic conditioning at a target heart rate for a sustained 30- to 45-minute period.[10,24,27] Research shows that such conditioning alters metabolism and affects muscle mechanisms of oxygen transport and use, thus making the entire cardiovascular system a more efficient one.

Heart disease however is not solely the effect of arteriosclerosis. There are medical conditions and disabilities that have associated and secondary cardiac involvement. Some of these are as follows:[43]

Alcoholism
Anemia
Ankylosing spondylitis
Anorexia
Arteriosclerosis
Cerebrovascular disease
Cocaine use
Diabetes
Friedreich's ataxia

Table 29-2 Signs and Symptoms of Left and Right Heart Failure[21]*

Signs and symptoms of left heart failure	Signs and symptoms of right heart failure

1. Dyspnea (shortness of breath)
  a. Exertional (with exercise)
  b. Orthopnea (in supine)
  c. Paroxysmal nocturnal dyspnea (sudden shortness of breath at night)
2. Rales, wheezes
3. Dry hacking cough
4. Weakness, fatigue
5. Poor exercise tolerance
6. Daytime oliguria, nocturia
7. Tachycardia, weak pulses,
8. Behavioral changes
9. Chest pain
10. Pale or dusky, cool, moist skin
11. Changes in heart sounds (gallop rhythms)
	1. Weight gain
	2. Daytime oliguria (decreased urine output), nocturia (excessive urination at night)
	3. Dependent edema
	4. Jugular venous distention
	5. Hepatomegaly, right upper quadrant pain
	6. Anorexia, nausea
	7. Ascites (fluid in the peritonium)
	8. Changes in heart sounds (gallop rhythms)

*Adapted and reproduced with permission from Cornett S and Watson J: Cardiac rehabilitation: an interdisciplinary team approach, New York, 1984, John Wiley & Sons, Inc.

Gout
Hypertension
Marfan's syndrome
Obesity
Peripheral vascular disease
Progressive muscular dystrophy
Progressive systemic sclerosis (scleroderma)
Rheumatoid arthritis
Systemic lupus erythematosus
Patients in general rehabilitation clinics may require program modification and surveillance of vital signs because of these secondary diagnoses.

PATIENT MANAGEMENT
Medical and Surgical Management

The cardiologist's immediate concern is to preserve healthy heart tissue by controlling complications that may jeopardize healing and overall cardiac function. This is accomplished by a necessary period of bed rest during which the cardiac cycle is stabilized by medications.

Once the patient is stabilized at rest, medical surveillance continues through the cardiac program to assure medical stability during activity. If patients demonstrate significant CAD and are appropriate surgical candidates, coronary bypass surgery is performed. In this procedure a vein from another location (usually a leg) is placed in the heart to reroute blood around the occluded area to the myocardium (Fig. 29-5).

Other surgeries include valve replacement, aneurysm repairs, pacemaker inserts, and complete transplants. New techniques, like the pericutaneous transluminal arterioplasty (PTCA), float a balloon-tipped catheter to the point of occlusion. The balloon is inflated, and the occlusion is compressed against the arterial wall.[62] This noninvasive technique avoids costly open-heart surgery. Its long-term effectiveness is currently being examined.

Psychosocial Aspects

As with any physical disability, patients who experience a cardiac event progress through various stages of psychosocial reaction and adjustment. Anxiety produced by discomfort and imminent fear of death is often overwhelming. Patients may demonstrate their anxiety by asking many questions, acting out sexually, or pacing.

Anxiety places an increased physiological demand on the heart muscle at a time when it needs rest. It is most often noted during the first 48 hours of a pa-

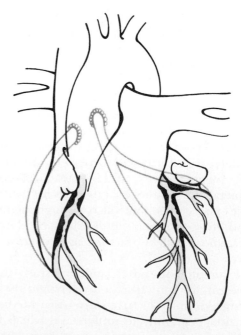

Fig. 29-5. Coronary artery bypass. From Heart Facts, 1986. ©Reproduced with permission. American Heart Association.

tient's admission and at times of changing environments, such as transfers to step-down units and at discharge. Sedation may be used to alleviate anxiety; however, excessive sedation may produce medical problems and interfere with integrating the realities of the event, which is a necessary step toward successful rehabilitation.[15]

Anxiety is best alleviated through supportive and educational communication.[8] Once a patient verbalizes his or her feelings and learns of the nature of the condition and ways to control it, anxiety usually diminishes.

Early ambulation and resumption of self-care activities can also help alleviate the feelings of helplessness which are common with patients experiencing a recent cardiac event. In the event of dysfunction, the patient draws on coping and defense mechanisms in order to respond to major life events. Some previously used coping behaviors may not be available to the patient in the hospital (i.e., smoking, drinking, taking a walk). The occupational therapist must therefore assist the patient in establishing new, healthy coping patterns.

Denial is a mechanism used when an individual cannot cope with the surrounding events. Denial is common in coronary disease because of the vague characteristics of symptoms and the hidden nature of the disability. At times denial is considered a healthy response,[51] and health professionals must be careful not to strip the patient of this coping mechanism by forcing the patient to face reality too quickly.[15] Careful monitoring of a patient's activities is important at this time to protect the patient from performing at unsafe, higher activity levels.

Depression is most commonly seen from the third to sixth day after MI[15] and may extend into the convalescent phase. A study of patients 6 months to 1 year following discharge found 88% of the patients reporting either anxiety or depression or both. The patients also reported that inactivity was the most frustrating experience following cardiac event.[18]

Family education is important. A patient's fears and feelings of inadequacy may be based on a misconception that may be reinforced from equally fearful and often noninformed family members.[13]

Although initial efforts are made to alleviate stress, patients must eventually be educated to handle it, not circumvent it.[15] Relaxation programs,[1] assisted therapeutic introspection and examination of coping patterns, changes in life expectations and beliefs, and self-help groups[42] are methods to effectively deal with stress. "It is only when the patient has confronted stress successfully that he can resume a fully functioning way of life."[15]

The entire health team has the responsibility to prepare the cardiac patient to deal with a new life. The medical and psychological training of occupational therapists enables them to be an integral part of the rehabilitation team.

CARDIAC REHABILITATION

Early mobilization of patients after coronary incidence is now standard cardiological practice. This differs from management of the patient with cardiac disease in the 1950s and 1960s. At that time strict bed rest was prescribed for 6 to 8 weeks. Pathologic studies quoted "6 weeks" as required for the transformation of necrotic myocardium to form scar tissue.[59]

The 1960s marked the advent of coronary care units with better monitoring techniques for the patient with acute coronary distress. At this time Wenger implemented her hallmark 14-step, early mobilization, activity program at Grady Memorial Hospital.[16] Programs across the country demonstrated that progressive activity under supervised conditions prevented the negative effects of bed rest, shortened hospital stays, facilitated earlier return to work, and reduced the anxiety and depression that often led to the "cardiac cripple" mind set.[59]

Following a "cardiac event" current medical management of patients includes an acute recovery phase (1 to 3 days) to stabilize cardiac conditions. This is followed by a subacute recovery phase called phase 1 of cardiac rehabilitation during which a course of progressive, low-energy expenditure hospital activity is prescribed.[51]

Following the subacute recovery phase patients usually undergo a predischarge graded exercise or treadmill test (GXT). By administering a symptom-limited GXT a safe target heart rate (THR) and functional capacity are identified and can be used as guidelines during home, vocational, and exercise activity programs. Patients continue this exercise program in phase 2, the outpatient phase of their convalescence. After a six-week program, the true benefits of cardiovascular conditioning occur.[24] The majority of patient education, risk factor modification, and life-style changes takes place during this phase of rehabilitation.[52]

Individuals continue to advance to greater exercise intensities in phase 3 and 4 programs. They further develop their own knowledge and self-monitoring techniques so that medical surveillance needs to occur only on an intermittent basis.

Optimally, as the rehabilitative process of recovery is completed, the once anxious and functionally limited patient becomes an educated individual who continues risk factor modification and exercise as a way of life. The patient consequently attains maximal functional capacity and can resume an active role in society.

Program Objectives[51]

PHASE 1—INPATIENT REHABILITATION

1. To provide a program of monitored low-level physical activity including exercise and activities of daily living
2. To decrease the effects of prolonged inactivity: such as thromboembolism, atelectasis, orthostatic hypotension, hypovolemia, muscle atrophy, osteoporosis, and negative nitrogen and protein balance
3. To identify medical problems and to monitor the patients during the various therapeutic regimes
4. To manage patient anxiety and depression related to heart disease and return the patient to previous life-style
5. To provide an educational program for patients and families to include cardiovascular anatomy, pathophysiology, and coronary risk factors
6. To provide appropriate dietary modifications and education to patient and family
7. To provide coordinated discharge that identifies home health, outpatient, and equipment needs
8. To administer GXT in order to establish appropriate exercise, prescription, and referral to outpatient rehabilitation program

PHASE 2—OUTPATIENT REHABILITATION

1. To provide an individualized exercise prescription based on patient's past medical history and results of GXT, as well as to facilitate an independent home exercise program
2. To provide continued follow-up for the patient after hospital discharge
3. To initiate and/or continue modification of risk factors
4. To initiate and/or continue patient surveillance concerning the effectiveness of therapeutic regimes for the referring physician
5. To initiate and/or continue training in energy-conservation techniques and use of self-care equipment to Class III and IV (New York Heart Association classification—see box, p. 524) cardiac patients
6. To initiate and/or continue diet education by means of regularly scheduled follow-up appointments with Outpatient Department
7. To provide simulated work evaluations and guidelines for return to work or avocational interests
8. To provide appropriate referrals to community based exercise program

Team Approach

Achieving such program objectives is a team endeavor and is not the sole responsibility of a single health profession.[21] In small community hospitals the cardiac rehabilitation team may include a physician and a nurse. In larger and more formalized rehabilitation programs other health professionals may be involved, including dietitians, exercise physiologists, occupational therapists, pharmacists, physical educators, physical therapists, psychologists, respiratory therapists, social workers, and vocational counselors.

The degree of the health professionals' involvement is largely dependent on (1) their availability, (2) their role as defined within the rehabilitation facility, (3) their specialty skills and experience in treating patients with cardiac disease, and (4) the financial resources available for the delivery of professional services.

Whichever health professionals are involved, the most important members of the cardiac team are the patient and family.

Patient Population

Following is a list of patients most often referred to medically supervised and "monitored" rehabilitation programs[51]:

I. Patient population for cardiac rehabilitation
    A. Myocardial infarction
    B. Angina pectoris
    C. Cardiac surgery
    D. Controlled congestive heart failure
    E. Cardiomyopathy
    F. Patients at high risk for development of coronary heart disease.
    G. Valve disorders
    H. Cardiac arrhythmias
    I. Hypertension
II. Patient population for general rehabilitation
    A. The 65-year-old paraplegic, amputee, and/or CVA patient with significant CAD and/or previous MI
    B. The 70-year-old patient with a fractured hip and a history of CHF and chronic atrial fibrillation
    C. The patient with muscular dystrophy or alcoholism and documented cardiac involvement
    D. General rehabilitation patients at high risk for coronary incidence

A monitored, graded activity progression is prescribed for all these patients: however, each condition varies, and activity progressions and modalities must reflect this. Therapists must be able to support their proposed rehabilitation programs and goals with sound physiological principles as documented in the literature discussing cardiac rehabilitation.

Program Guidelines

Graded activity is beneficial in minimizing the ill effects of bed rest and maximizing functional capacity. There are several conditions, however, for which exercise is absolutely contraindicated.[31,34] These conditions are:

1. Unstable angina
2. Resting diastolic blood pressure (DBP) 120 mm Hg or resting systolic blood pressure (SBP) 200 mm Hg
3. Uncontrolled atrial or ventricular arrhythmias
4. Second- or third-degree heart block
5. Orthostatic SBP drop of 20 mm Hg or more
6. Recent embolism, either systemic or pulmonary
7. Thrombophlebitis
8. Dissecting aneurysm
9. Fever greater than 100° Fa (37.7° or 38° C)
10. Uncompensated heart failure
11. Primary, active pericarditis
12. Severe aortic stenosis
13. Acute systemic illness
14. Resting heart rate greater than 120 beats per minute in the patient with a recent MI.
15. Resting heart rate greater than 130 beats per minute for patients with recent bypass surgery, cardiomyopathy, CHF, or valve surgery

Patients must be medically stable before initiating or continuing with any progressive activity program. Special considerations, however, do exist when a patient may be "relatively" stable on an optimal medical regime. These specific conditions require a modified rehabilitation program with close medical supervision:[28,51]

1. Resting diastolic blood pressure over 100 mm Hg or resting systolic blood pressure over 180 mm Hg
2. Hypotension
3. Fixed rate pacemaker
4. Intermittent claudication (cramps in legs)
5. Any neuromuscular, musculoskeletal, or arthritic disorders that could prevent activity

THE ROLE OF OCCUPATIONAL THERAPY

During phase 1 of a cardiac rehabilitation program, the occupational therapist is primarily responsible for encouraging the patient's self-care activity to achieve a safe yet maximal level of independent self-care. The process involves patient and family education and instruction in energy-conservation techniques to avoid stress to a healing myocardium. The occupational therapist's role is to evaluate the patient's technique of ADL performance and to identify ways to decrease

the energy used so the patient can begin to perform the task without symptoms. Adaptive aids and durable medical equipment are often necessary for these patients. Patient success with these simple activities, although using a varied technique, is of tremendous psychological benefit. Continued participation in their ADL gives them a sense of control and independence and thus alleviates the patient's and family member's fear and anxiety.

As with any other patient evaluation and treatment there are special evaluation tools and techniques pertinent to patients with cardiac disease.

Evaluation Procedures

CHART REVIEW. A thorough chart review is advised before meeting the patient. This implies that the therapist must be familiar with cardiac terminology and have a basic understanding of how a patient's clinical course and various test results affect program progression and treatment goals. Consultation with team members is important. The status of the phase 1 cardiac patient often changes rapidly. Current information may not yet be documented in the chart.

PATIENT INTERVIEW. Once a thorough chart review is completed, the therapist conducts an initial patient interview to obtain an activity history. Social, financial, architectural, psychological, cognitive-behavioral, vocational and/or avocational factors, and how they influence treatment planning may be further assessed. A sample evaluation as used at Santa Clara Valley Medical Center is included in Fig. 29-6.

The initial patient interview is frequently the patient's first contact with a member of the cardiac rehabilitation team. Moreover, it often occurs at a significantly anxious time; for instance, the patient has just been informed of the MI, has just been weaned from the ventilator, or has just been moved to the transitional care unit. The patient-therapist relationship is established. The therapist must outline the terms and expectations of the relationship so that the patient (1) understands the importance of gradually increasing activity; (2) understands the logistics of the cardiac rehabilitation program (scheduling and activity modalities); (3) begins to feel comfortable asking personal or repeated questions; and (4) begins to take an active part in the rehabilitation process, including reporting signs and symptoms experienced during activity.

MONITORED SELF-CARE EVALUATIONS. Self-care evaluations are most often performed in phase 1 of cardiac rehabilitation. They consist of ADL that require low energy expenditure and may include hy-

Santa Clara Valley Medical Center
Occupational Therapy

CARDIAC MONITORED EVALUATION

General Information *55 y/o male admitted 4/30 with shortness of breath, nausea, pedal edema*   Referral Date: *5/1/87*

Diagnosis *congestive heart failure, rule out myocardial infarction*

Precautions: *Call H.O. HR>100   SBP >140 <100*

Medical History: *CABG x2 1974. Follow up catheterization 1975 showed total occlusion LAD*

Pre-Admission Social Situation/Home Environment: *Lives locally with wife; 3 children, 6 grandchildren in area*   Language Spoken: *Spanish and English*

Activity History and Current Level of Function:

Activity	Pre-Admission Status	Current Status
Bed Mobility	*1 pillow orthopnea independent*	*2+ pillow orthopnea minimum assistance*
Transfers	*Independent (I)*	*Standby assist*
Functional Ambulation	*(I), two blocks s̄ rest*	*(I), < 20 feet*
Self-Care Hygiene Dressing Bathing Toileting	*Independent with standing shower until day of admission*	*Independent at 2.0 MET level bedside bathing*
Homemaking/Grocery Shopping	*Wife does homemaking. Independent carrying groceries with rest breaks.*	*not tested*
Vocational & Avocational	*Wire braider 30 hours per week; gardens, watches T.V.*	*not tested*
Endurance (typical day)	*Good; no rest breaks required (by report)*	*20 minutes unsupported sitting*

Risk Factors:

✓ obesity	✓ smoking *54* pkg yr	___ diabetes
✓ sedentary	___ caffeine	___ Fam Hx
___ HTN	___ Alcohol/drugs	___ COPD
___ cholesterol	✓ stress	___ gout
___ triglycerides	✓ Age/sex	

Instruction Needed:

① *Energy conservation*
② *Specific work simplification techniques to use at work.*
③ *Risk factor education*

Fig. 29-6. Santa Clara Valley Medical Center Occupational Therapy Cardiac Evaluation Form. Reproduced with permission, Santa Clara Valley Medical Center, OT Dept, San José, CA, 1987.

Continued.

Santa Clara Valley Medical Center
Occupational Therapy

Cardiac Monitored Self-Care Evaluation

ORTHOSTATS:

	Supine	Sit	Stand	Sit	Supine
HR	76	80	84	82	78
BP	116/76	102/76	118/76	110/76	104/74

ACTIVITY EVALUATION: Bedside basin bath   2.0 METS   RPE   12

Rest:

HR 77

Bp 118/76

Peak:

HR 86

Bp 120/74

Recovery

HR 83

Bp 112/76

Assessment

HR Appropriate increase with activity

Bp Appropriate increase with activity

EKG Normal sinus rhythm, no ectopic beats

Signs/Symptoms Pt c/o mild shortness of breath

PLANS/GOALS: ① Progress patient to 3.5 intermittent MET standing shower
② Provide instruction as needed

FREQUENCY & DURATION 1-2 daily, 30-60 minutes, 3-5 days

_____ , OTR _____   _____ , M.D. _____
        Ext.   Date   Date

Fig. 29-6 cont'd. Santa Clara Valley Medical Center Occupational Therapy Cardiac Evaluation
Form.

giene, grooming, simple bathing, dressing, and functional mobility tasks.[48]

The therapist chooses a combination of low-level self-care activities to both mobilize and evaluate the patient. The therapist's choice of activities is based on the patient's past medical and functional history, the patient's current clinical status and course of recovery, the therapist's knowledge of cardiovascular dynamics, and the metabolic energy costs of increasing activity.

For instance, a 74-year-old man is admitted to the hospital with a current bout of CHF. Before his admission to the hospital his activities were limited to independent seated bathing and dressing and walking for two blocks before experiencing shortness of breath. His hospital course is complicated by kidney problems. He has been resting in bed for 1 week, and his current hospital activity includes out-of-bed activity with assistance for short periods to use the commode.

The initial self-care evaluation for this patient may consist of a 30- to 60-minute treatment session. The activity history and patient interview will continue while the therapist monitors the patient's orthostats. Orthostats are the measurement of baseline vital signs (heart rate, EKG, and BP) and symptoms as the patient moves from supine to sitting to standing. Once it is established that the patient can tolerate positional changes with appropriate responses, the therapist can evaluate the patient during activity.

The patient may be asked to tolerate sitting on the edge of the bed unsupported for a sustained 15- to 20-minute period while performing intermittent upper and lower extremity tasks so the therapist can assess basic range, strength, coordination, and balance. The therapist encourages the patient to perform rhythmic ankle pumping to avoid venous pooling in the lower extremities and resultant dizziness. A significant drop in blood pressure related to sitting or standing up is called orthostatic hypotension. Slow transitional movements, support stockings, and rhythmical extremity movements help to prevent it. This patient may then be asked to stand for a 1- to 2-minute period and perform bed-to-chair or bed-to-commode transfers. The patient would have vital sign and symptoms recorded during the highest or peak level of activity and again 4 to 5 minutes after the activity was stopped. This is called the recovery phase. Patients will sometimes experience inappropriate responses in recovery despite good performance of self-care activity. The patient will be asked to report his or her perceived rate of exertion (RPE), which is discussed later in this chapter. Evaluation results are discussed with the patient, and activity guidelines are established to provide structure and reassurance. Mutually agreed upon discharge goals may be established at this time.

SIMULATED TASKS EVALUATION. Monitored task evaluations measure the cardiovascular response to a combination of lower and upper extremity work and variations in body position.[48] The tasks that are monitored simulate what the patient will actually be doing at home or at work to determine if this level of activity is safe to resume under nonmonitored circumstances. These tasks typically require more energy than that required during self-care and are therefore performed when the patient progresses to phase 2 or 3 of the cardiac rehabilitation program. Treadmill exercise tests are routinely used to evaluate a patient's functional capacity; however, the information obtained is based solely on lower extremity performance. Since upper extremity work elicits a different and more pronounced cardiovascular response,[10] simulated task evaluations can better evaluate a patient's response to specific vocational and leisure tasks.

A numerical scoring system of task analysis has been developed by Ogden.[46] She analyzes tasks by six variables: rate, resistance, muscle groups used, involvement of trunk muscles, arm position, and isometric work (straining). This system of analysis assists the therapist in evaluating which tasks demand the highest energy demand from the heart. Perhaps the application of this system is more useful to cardiac teaching and work simplification. Here the therapist reduces the energy demands of a task by altering the aforementioned variables. Other factors, such as environmental temperature, emotional stress related to the task, and length of time (sustained versus intermittent) the patient performs the task, must be considered.

The need for a simulated task evaluation most often arises when the patient is ready to return to work. For instance, Mr. J, a 53-year-old cafeteria dishwasher, had a coronary artery bypass following his MI 2 months ago. He has been involved in an aggressive cardiac rehabilitation program consisting of walking, bicycling, and arm ergometry (arm crank) at a target heart rate of 120 beats per minute. He can now tolerate sustained, 30-minute activities that are 4½ times the amount of energy he requires at rest. His treadmill test produced fatigue and a suboptimal blood pressure response. The question arises whether Mr. J's current activity tolerance is sufficient for a safe return to work as a dishwasher. The therapist performs a chart review, patient interview, and job analysis that may include an interview with the patient's employer and an on-site observation to determine the energy demands of the job. The therapist finds that the job is full-time employment performed in three parts daily:

1. Dish tray assembly for 2 hours (sustained standing and light upper extremity activity)
2. General cleaning of work stations for 2 hours (intermittent activity with frequent bending and reaching)
3. Dishwashing for 3 hours (sustained standing with frequent stacking and lifting 5 to 10 pounds at once on an assembly line)

These tasks take place in a warm environment; the patient has no control over pace or rest period because of the fixed-rate assembly line and union regulations concerning breaks. The therapist designs a simulated task evaluation that takes place over 3 hours. The therapist evaluates cardiovascular responses to (1) sustained standing and light upper extremity activity, (2) intermittent activity with frequent bending and reaching, and (3) sustained standing with moderate upper extremity work at a fixed, moderate pace. The therapist finds that the patient has significant difficulty and demonstrates abnormal cardiovascular responses. The therapist discusses this with the cardiologist who implements a medication change and suggests a change in the patient's physical conditioning program so it is geared toward those tasks the patient must perform at work. In this case the simulated task evaluation gave the cardiologist crucial information of functional performance which could not be obtained from a routine treadmill test. Occupational therapists are becoming more involved with simulated work evaluations for patients with cardiac disease.[12] Further methods, studies, and applications of such evaluations should be developed.

Evaluation Tools

Therapists assess a patient's cardiovascular response to activity by monitoring five parameters: heart rate, blood pressure, EKG readings, signs and symptoms of cardiac dysfunction, and heart sounds. In some facilities therapists are not required to monitor EKG and heart sounds. These authors believe that, if therapists are treating a cardiac population, they would benefit from workshops to develop skills in basic EKG interpretation and in recognition of abnormal heart sounds. Monitoring skills and techniques should be objective, expedient, and accurate.

HEART RATE. "Normal" heart rates vary with age, sex, activity, attitude, temperature, health status, emotion, amount of coffee or tobacco intake, and electrolyte and fluid imbalances.[24] Basically, normal adult heart rate is 60 to 100 beats per minute. Abnormal

heart rates are either too slow (called bradycardia: less than 60 beats per minute), too fast (called tachycardia: greater than 100 beats per minute), or irregular (called arrhythmias).

If the heart rate is bradycardic, the cardiac output may not be sufficient to meet the energy demands of the brain, systemic circulation, and working muscles. This results in fatigue; and if bradycardia is severe, dizziness, confusion, and syncope (loss of consciousness) can result. In highly trained athletes bradycardia is normal and reflects a highly efficient cardiovascular system. In other cases bradycardia that is symptom free at 50 to 60 beats per minute may be desired to decrease the work of the myocardium. This is often the result of medications, like propranolol (Inderal), in the beta blocker category. A sudden development of bradycardia, however, especially if associated with symptoms, warrants further medical workup and could be indicative of severe cardiac conduction dysfunction; that is, heart blocks that may necessitate inserting a cardiac pacemaker.

Tachycardic heart rates (HR) may be caused by general deconditioning or conditions that alter stroke volume (SV), the amount of blood ejected with each heart beat. Tachycardia may be the heart's attempt to maintain cardiac output (CO) since CO = SV × HR. Heart rates greater than 110 do not allow adequate filling time in diastole, which further impinges on stroke volume. Furthermore, tachycardic heart rates increase myocardial oxygen demand. The increase may exceed available supply and cause myocardial ischemia.

Heart rate can be monitored by several methods: palpation (feeling), auscultation (listening), and EKG monitoring (skin electrodes). Pulses can be palpated and counted at the radial, brachial, carotid, and temporal sites. Therapists must exercise caution if monitoring carotid pulse, since this site is close to the carotid sinus that if overstimulated, can cause bradycardia. If the pulse is regular, it is counted for 10 seconds and multiplied by 6, giving total beats per minute. Patients are routinely instructed in these techniques and precautions in order to begin self-monitoring.

Auscultation, or listening to the heart with a stethoscope to monitor heart rate, is recommended for patients with poor peripheral pulses or irregular heart beats. The stethoscope is placed over the apex of the heart (the fifth intercostal space at or just medial to the left midclavicular line).[11] This is the point of maximal impulse referred to as PMI. Apical pulses, if irregular, should be counted for a full 60-second period for accuracy. The EKG method of monitoring heart rate is a simple technique of reading heart rate from an accurate digital display. Heart rate can also be measured from EKG strips by counting blocks on the paper as they correlate to assigned heart rates[25] or by using a special rate ruler. Appropriate documentation of heart rate includes the number of beats per minute and a comment on regularity, such as "72 beats per minute and irregular."

BLOOD PRESSURE.[17,44,56] Blood pressure is simply the pressure of blood against the arteries created by the pumping of the heart and the peripheral resistance of flow. This pressure is responsible for driving the blood through the circulatory system to perfuse vital organs, tissues, and working muscle. The reader is referred to the discussion of the cardiac cycle. The diastolic blood pressure (lower number) is the amount of pressure generated by ventricular contraction which is responsible for opening the aortic and pulmonary valves. Systolic blood pressure (upper number) is the peak pressure that the ventricles continue to generate over and above the point at which the valves open. The amount of pressure generated from the time the valves open to peak pressure is the pressure available to move blood along the systemic circulation. This is called pulse pressure. If this pulse pressure becomes less than 20 mm Hg (90/80), perfusion to the distal tissues may not be sufficient. In severe cases circulatory shock or collapse may occur with permanent damage related to the amount of time the vital organs and tissues do not receive oxygen.

Normal blood pressures increase with age.[24] Since arteriosclerosis and a decrease in the distensibility of the arteries is often associated with age, more pressure is required to propel blood through the system. Pressures become hypertensive if they are between 160/90 to 200/110 mm Hg or greater. A particularly high systolic blood pressure may generate too much pressure in the arteries and could result in an aneurysm or CVA. In addition, diastolic hypertensive states require that the ventricles perform increased and often sustained contractions that may result in myocardial hypertrophy (enlargement). In this case the heart needs even more oxygen as a result of the increase in muscle fibers. If the oxygen cannot be supplied to meet this demand, ischemia may result.

If systolic blood pressure is less than 90 mm Hg, hypotension or low blood pressure exists. Similarly, low blood pressure affects perfusion and the delivery of blood to vital organs and peripheral tissues. Hypotension may be associated with dizziness and lightheadedness. In severe cases of hypotension caused by circulatory inadequacy hands and feet may become cold, the patient's color may be dusky or pale, lips may be cyanotic or bluish, and the patient may become confused, indicating degrees of cerebral anoxia.

When patients are admitted to a medical service, physicians will usually indicate vital sign precautions in the nursing orders. They are usually written as "Call H.O. (house officer or on-call physician) if SBP > 150 < 90; DBP > 90 < 50; HR > 120 < 50" (Systolic blood pressure greater than 150 or less than 90; diastolic blood pressure greater than 90 or less than 50; heart rate greater than 120 or less than 50).

Blood pressure is monitored by two methods: invasive and noninvasive. Invasive techniques require that an arterial line be placed into the artery for direct blood pressure monitoring. This is the most accurate method and is the most often used in acute care for the hemodynamically unstable patient. It is not feasible in a rehabilitation setting. Most often therapists will record blood pressure by the use of a sphygmomanometer or blood pressure cuff. Because this method is indirect, it is subject to sources of error which the therapist must attempt to minimize.

An indirect measurement is one that uses and examines associated factors (cuff pressure) to derive and define the desired measurement (blood pressure).[56] More simply, if a given blood pressure is 120/80 mm Hg and the therapist pumps the cuff to 200 mm Hg, the brachial artery will be completely occluded, since cuff pressure (200) exceeds peak arterial pressure (120). If a stethoscope is placed over the artery at this time, no sounds will be heard, since there is no blood flow. Once the therapist gradually releases the cuff pressure to 120 mm Hg, the artery's peak pressure may be able to move some blood through a now partially occluded artery and pulse sounds will be heard under the stethoscope. The point at which the first two sounds are heard corresponds to the point where the arterial pressure now exceeds the cuff pressure.[56] The therapist then reads the number on the dial as the systolic blood pressure. The systolic blood pressure is *not* the point where the needle or column of mercury visually bounces. Systolic blood pressure measurements are associated with auscultation or listening, not vision. As the therapist continues to release pressure, the artery becomes less occluded, enabling greater blood flow and louder sounds under the stethoscope. Once the artery is not occluded and full blood flow is established, the sounds will disappear (for example, 80 mm Hg). This point corresponds to diastolic blood pressure.

Sources of error can arise from faulty tools and techniques and errors in measurement.[37] The most common problems are noncalibrated meters and cracked or kinked tubing because of placement. All systems require calibration if the dial does not return to zero.

The relationship between the size of the cuff and circumference of the arm must be considered when choosing which cuff to use.[37] If a standard cuff is used on a very thin arm, the therapist will obtain a false, low pressure reading, whereas a standard cuff applied to an obese arm will result in a false, high reading. Alternate cuffs, for instance, pediatric or "large" adult cuffs, should be available in the clinic.

Additional sources of error may include placing the stethoscope underneath the cuff to hold it in place; varying the position of the arm during serial blood pressure monitoring; repeating inflation of the cuff to make sure measurement is correct; and deflating cuff too rapidly or slowly.[37]

Interpretation of blood pressure responses is based on accurate and expedient measurement. To ensure accuracy therapists are urged to use the same arm, position, evaluator, and equipment when measuring responses. In addition, therapists must be able to obtain a blood pressure response in 30 to 40 seconds. Once activity is stopped, blood pressure begins to recover and peak response will be missed.

EKG. Patients with cardiovascular disease are prone to arrhythmias, which, if frequent, can decrease cardiac output, cause symptoms, and affect overall cardiac function. If severe, they could be life threatening. All therapists must be trained in cardiopulmonary resuscitation as a basic life-support measure. Therapists working with patients who have known or suspected heart disease must be able to recognize signs and symptoms related to cardiac dysfunction. For therapists not trained in EKG interpretation this includes noting how irregular a pulse becomes (10 irregular beats per minute) during or after activity. Therapists using EKG during therapy should be familiar with monitoring equipment, including problems and artifacts (monitor interference). "They also should be capable of recognizing, at a minimum, the following EKG dysrhythmias:

1. Sinus tachycardia
2. Sinus bradycardia
3. Premature atrial complexes
4. Atrial tachycardia
5. Atrial flutter
6. Atrial fibrillation
7. Junctional rhythms
8. Atrioventricular blocks of all degrees
9. Premature ventricular complexes
10. Ventricular tachycardia
11. Ventricular fibrillation
12. Cardiac standstill or asystole."[4]

Changes in ST segments on the EKG should also be recognized, since these changes parallel cardiac ischemia and cardiac dysfunction. Because EKG interpretation is beyond the scope of this text, the reader is referred to Dubin's *Rapid Interpretation of EKG.*[25] Sample strips are shown in Fig. 29-7 so that the reader may gain an understanding that any arrhythmia either too fast, too slow, or too irregular interferes with cardiac output and function.

SIGNS AND SYMPTOMS OF CARDIAC DYSFUNCTION. The most important of all evaluation tools is the ability to observe and detect symptoms of cardiac dysfunction.

Whenever patients become symptomatic or display signs of intolerance to an activity, the therapist should evaluate and record the event by noting the following:[54]
1. Exact complaint
2. Body location
3. Quality
4. Quantity
5. Chronology
6. Setting
7. Aggravating or alleviating factors
8. Associated symptoms

Angina. Many chest pains are not associated with ischemia. Angina pectoris induced by ischemia has specific hallmark characteristics (see Table 29-1).[21] Patients should be asked to quantify the severity of the pain on an angina rating scale[11] with 10 being the worst pain felt. The surrounding activities that induce angina should be examined. Angina typically occurs during ambulation, shaving, bowel movement, stair climbing, observation of athletic events, arguing, or after a meal. Once these exacerbating factors are stopped, angina dissipates; prompt relief (3 minutes) may occur with sublingual nitroglycerin tablets, a quick-acting vasodilator. Associated symptoms may include nausea, palpitations, and dizziness. Angina is not the only indication of ischemia. Some patients never experience angina with MI. Instead, weakness or dyspnea (shortness of breath) may be a symptom.

Dyspnea.[11,54] Dyspnea, difficulty in breathing, is a common symptom in heart disease and may be indicative of left ventricular failure (see Table 29-2). When dyspnea is noted on exertion, the therapist must note the quantity of activity produces this. This functional method of recording dyspnea is preferred over the "numerical values" often used to describe dyspnea (for instance, +2 dyspnea). Orthopnea is shortness of breath created by resting in the supine position. Since this position creates a greater venous return, stroke volume increases, demanding more work from the myocardium. Often a diseased myocardium is not capable of handling the demand, and shortness of breath or orthopnea will result. "Two

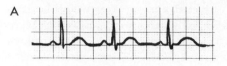

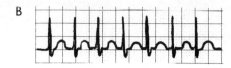

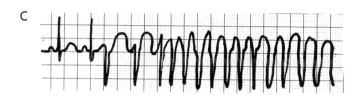

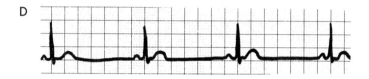

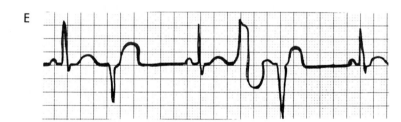

Fig. 29-7. Sample EKG readings of cardiac arrythmias. **A,** Regular sinus rhythm. **B,** Sinus tachycardia (too fast). **C,** Ventricular tachycardia (too fast). **D,** Sinus bradycardia (too slow). **E,** Multifocal premature ventricular contractions (too irregular).

pillow orthopnea" describes the propped-up position necessary to relieve this symptom.

Fatigue. Fatigue is often an initial sign of heart disease. When patients report fatigue, therapists must determine whether it is localized or generalized. Asking which muscles are fatigued will assist the patient in localizing it. If the patient has difficulty localizing the symptom and uses words like exhausted and drained and appears fatigued, the cause may be centralized, as in heart disease. One objective method of rating fatigue is Borg's rate of perceived exertion (RPE) scale[14] (see boxed material). Patients experiencing centralized fatigue are asked to assign a number to their fatigue based on their perception of the difficulty of activity. Myocardial oxygen consumption studies have correlated RPE scores of greater than 15 RPE to 75% of maximal myocardial oxygen con-

sumption.[14] RPE scores have been used during graded exercise tests and exercise training sessions to guide the clinician in grading or stopping the activity.[51] RPE has been successfully used during monitored self-care and simulated task evaluations. Such an objective rating scale warrants further examination and application to other physical disabilities, such as arthritis and multiple sclerosis.

In summary, whenever any sign or symptom is noted with activity, the therapist must accurately note its characteristics and associated factors for proper interpretation.

Assessment

If a patient has tolerated rehabilitation activities well, it implies that no adverse signs or symptoms were noted and that heart rate, blood pressure, and ECG

Rate of perceived exertion

6
7 Very, very light
8
9 Very light
10
11 Fairly light
12
13 Somewhat hard
14
15 Hard
16
17 Very hard
18
19 Very, very hard
20

From Borg G et al: Med Sci Sports Exerc 14:376, 1982.

responses were appropriate. Monitoring and assessing a *response* implies measuring and quantifying a change. Therefore therapists record each of these parameters before activity (resting phase), during activity (peak phase), and 4 to 5 minutes after the activity has stopped (recovery phase). To isolate the response to activity the therapist must monitor and record vital signs in the position of peak activity. For instance, if peak activity is performed while standing at the sink, baseline and recovery vital signs should be noted in the standing position.

Postural responses should also be noted, particularly since orthostatic hypotension is a common occurrence after immobility and is often a side effect of diuretic and antianginal medication regimes. Thera-

pists must be able to assess patient responses so they may establish appropriate treatment progressions for patients. The boxed material below lists appropriate (desired) and inappropriate cardiovascular responses to activity.[51]

In instances where significant maladaptive responses are noted, communication lines to the referring physician must be expedient. Emergency precautions and procedures[25] must be established in any program before placing any demand on patients with documented heart disease.

Treatment Progressions

GRADED ACTIVITIES. Program progressions are guided by the patient's current clinical status, prognosis, and tolerance of current activities with appropriate cardiovascular responses. The rate of progression is further guided by the patient's past functional history and severity of coronary event. The physician synthesizes this information and ultimately categorizes the patient into one of four functional categories (see boxed material p. 524).[43] Patients in Class I will obviously progress the most rapidly, depending on their continued demonstration to tolerate activities appropriately. Patients in Classes III and IV will progress slowly and may never achieve total independence in self-care.

Progressions are further guided by the energy costs of activities and the factors that influence them. Energy expenditure is measured by the amount of oxygen that is consumed. Years ago this was expressed in calories but has been refined recently to METs. One MET (basal metabolic equivalent) is equal to the

---

Cardiovascular responses to activity

APPROPRIATE

Heart rate: Increases with activity to a maximum of approximately 20 beats above resting rate

Blood pressure: Peak systolic blood pressure increases as work load increases

EKG readings: Absence of arrhythmias and segment changes

Symptoms: Absence of adverse symptoms

INAPPROPRIATE

Heart rate: Excessive heart rate response to activity (>20 beats above resting rate); resting tachycardia (>120); bradycardic response to activity (pulse drops or fails to rise with increased work loads)

Blood pressure: Hypertensive responses (220/110 mm Hg maximum); postural hypotensive responses (>10 to 20 mm Hg systolic blood pressure decrease); any drop in systolic blood pressure with activity; failure of systolic blood pressure to rise with activity

EKG readings: Any rapid arrhythmias or increase in ectopic activity; development of 2 or 3 degree heart blocks; ST segment depression (>3 to 4 mm); any ST segment elevation

Symptoms: Excessive shortness of breath; angina and/or associated symptoms of nausea, sweating, and extreme fatigue (RPE > 15); cerebral symptoms (confusion or ataxia)

From Santa Clara Valley Center: Cardiac rehabilitation program protocol, San Jose, CA, 1987. (Unpublished.)

Functional classification of cardiac disease

Class I: Patients with cardiac disease but without resulting limitations of physical activity. Ordinary physical activity does not cause undue fatigue, palpitation, dyspnea, or anginal pain

Class II: Patients with cardiac disease resulting in slight limitation of physical activity. They are comfortable at rest. Ordinary physical activity results in fatigue, palpitation, dyspnea, or anginal pain

Class III: Patients with the cardiac disease resulting in marked limitation of physical activity. They are comfortable at rest. Less than ordinary physical activity causes fatigue, palpitation, dyspnea, or anginal pain

Class IV: Patients with cardiac disease resulting in inability to carry on any physical activity without discomfort. Symptoms of cardiac insufficiency or of the anginal syndrome may be present even at rest. If any physical activity is undertaken, discomfort is increased

From New York Heart Association, Inc: Nomenclature and criteria for diagnosis of diseases of the heart and great vessels, ed 8, Boston, 1979, Little, Brown & Co.

energy consumed when a patient is at rest in a semi-Fowler position (semi-reclined with extremities supported). This is equal to 3.5 ml O_2 per minute per kilogram of body weight. As soon as one sits up, walks, or performs activities, this metabolic demand and oxygen consumption increases. For instance, dressing requires 2 METs or twice the amount of energy required at rest. Several MET lists establish a comprehensive catalog of a variety of activities that require 1 to 9 METs. Table 29-3 is an energy-cost list for activities at the 3.0 MET level.

This method of grading activity, however, is a general guideline. Caution must be exercised when ex-

trapolating the results of a treadmill test to apply to vocational and leisure tasks. For instance, if a patient achieves 5 METs on the treadmill, this does not necessarily mean that the patient can resume all activities listed at 5 METs on the energy-cost list. Hellerstein[32] found that the linear relationship between heart rate and oxygen use on a treadmill test may not remain linear during daily activity. Work-related factors such as emotion and use of small muscle groups produce a nonlinear relationship during vocational, leisure, and self-care activities. Astrand and Rodahl[10] reported consistently higher heart rates for all activities with the following conditions: hot environment, emotional stress, use of upper versus lower extremities, and use of isometric muscular efforts, especially during low to moderate levels of work (2-3 METS). Various factors, such as pace, position, muscles used, isometrics, techniques, and environmental factors, influence the energy cost of an activity.

Choosing "very light-light"[42] activities for a patient just recovering from an acute MI or cardiac surgery is essential. During a patient's acute recovery (phase 1) physicians wish to promote healing of the myocardium but also wish to avoid the deconditioning effects of inactivity. Physicians do not wish any activity to produce tachycardia or a heart rate response greater than 20 beats per minute above rest, since such myocardial work would interfere with healing. Patients in phase 1 rehabilitation should not be permitted to perform tasks greater than 3.5 METs. Most self-care can be achieved within this very light-light work category.

Note that sexual activity is listed at 5 METs. Patients just recovering from heart attacks often have questions concerning safe sexual activity. Since sexual activity is "intermittent" and does not require prolonged, sustained high levels of rhythmical physical

Table 29-3 Santa Clara Valley Medical Center's MET Levels of ADL and Vocational and Recreational Activities at the 3.0-MET Level

Daily activities	METs	Ref	Vocational tasks	METs	Ref
Walking 2 mph	3.0	—	Light janitorial	3.0	(26)
Walking 2.5 mph	3.0	—	Bartending	3.0	(26)
Bowel movement	3.6	(20)	Pressing	3.6	(22)
Warm shower	3.5	(26)	Auto repair	3.5	(26)
Stairs (24 ft/min)	3.5	(20)	Truck driving	3-4	(55)
Homemaking	**METs**	**Ref**	**Recreation**	**METs**	**Ref**
Preparing meals	3.0	(36)	Playing musical instrument	3.0	(26)
Hand laundry	3.5	(20)	Playing with children	3.5	(22, 38)
Mopping	3.5	(20)	Golfing	3.0	(26)
Ironing (standing)	3.5	(20)	Cycling at 5 mph level	3.0	(26)
Bed making	3.9	(36)			
Window washing	3-4	(26)			

activity, physicians advise return to sexual activity if patients can tolerate walking up and down two flights of stairs without symptoms.[52] Therefore patients may be able to perform 5-MET–level activity as long as performance is intermittent and can perform a lower level or 3.5-MET-level activity if performance is continuous or sustained. To ensure that patients gradually resume daily activities a step-by-step program similar to the one used at Santa Clara Valley Medical Center is advised (Table 29-4).

In phase 1 the therapist gradually progresses the patient from simple bed mobility and commode transfers to independent dressing and showering, listed at 3.5 METs, under controlled environmental conditions.

Myocardial healing and musculoskeletal and cardiac conditioning have occurred by 6 to 8 weeks after coronary event. At this time most patients can tolerate increased MET-level activities greater than 3.5 METs and are ready for simulated task evaluations.

Table 29-4 Santa Clara Valley Medical Center's Post MI and Post Open-heart Surgery Phase 1 Rehabilitation Program*

Stage	Physical therapy	Occupational therapy
Phase 1—inpatient program		
1 in ICU or on ward 1.5 METs	Check and record heart rate, blood pressure, and EKG readings in supine, sitting, and standing positions (orthostats) In semi-Fowler position: 5-10 times active assistive exercise Teach breathing patterns with exercises Postoperative: deep breathing exercises Chest: physical therapy as indicated	General mobility (bed mobility transfers to commode and position changes) with energy-conservation techniques (environmental setups, equipment, and pacing) Sedentary leisure tasks with arms supported (reading, writing, and cards) OT may not treat in the ICU. OT usually starts in stage 3
2 in ICU or on ward 1.5 METs	Same as stage 1 except exercises are active Orthostats Ambulate: 50-100 ft, with assistance, as tolerated	Stage 1 continued with focus on: Unsupported sitting (5-30 min) Standing tasks (seconds to 2 min) Simple hygiene, semi-Fowler sitting position
3 On ward 1.5-2 METs	Orthostats In sitting position: 5-10 times active upper extremity (UE) and lower extremity (LE) exercise with coordinated breathing Ambulate: 100-200 ft, with monitoring (2-3 min)	Unsupported sitting ½-1 hr Standing tasks (3-5 min) Bedside bathing (assist with feet and back) Bathroom privileges Light leisure tasks
4 2 METs	Orthostats In seated position: 5-10 times active UE and LE exercise with coordinated breathing Ambulate: 200-350 ft with monitoring (3-5 min)	Standing tasks (5-8 min) UE sustained activity (2-5 min) Total body bathing at sink
5 2 METs	Orthostats Same as stage 4 except ambulate 350-700 ft with monitoring (5-10 min)	Standing tasks (8-12 min) UE sustained activity (5-30 min) Total hygiene, bathing, and dressing at sink
6 2 METs	Orthostats Standing active UE and LE exercise (10-30 min) Ambulate: 700-1050 ft with monitoring (5-10 min) Stair climbing 1 flight monitored A predischarge GXT is recommended at this time	Standing tasks (10-30 min) with intermittent UE activity UE sustained activity (5-30 min) Total body mobility: bending for small object retrieval teaching Moderate leisure tasks
7 3-3.5 METs	Orthostats Same as stage 6, except ambulate 1050 feet for 10-20 minutes	Shower transfers Total showering task (hair washing, total body washing, drying, and dressing) Simple homemaking tasks Energy-conservation techniques with activity 3.5 METs (or greater as indicated by GXT) Home program with ADL guidelines and recommendations for equipment, as appropriate

From Santa Clara Valley Medical Center: Cardiac rehabilitation program protocol, San Jose, CA, 1987. (Unpublished.)
*Education program to be performed by all team members as per SCVMC *Cardiac Rehabilitation Education Manual.*

Energy Conservation

A balance of low-level activity and rest is essential to the healing myocardium, especially during phase 1 rehabilitation. Knowledge of how various activities evoke differing cardiovascular responses is the basis of energy conservation and work simplification principles.[7] Exercise physiology principles are included in many physiology texts,[10,24] but little is written concerning how these are applied to ADL, especially for the individual with severe cardiac disease.[49] For instance, UE work elicits a greater cardiovascular response than LE activity. Standing requires a greater cardiovascular positional adjustment and more energy than sitting. Any isometric muscular activity interferes with easy blood flow through the muscle and impinges a demand on the cardiovascular system, and Valsalva maneuvers (straining and breath holding) interfere with blood return to the heart and elicit large increases in blood pressure. In warm environments (for example, a hot shower or kitchen) the body has the added task of maintaining its core temperature and must direct blood to the periphery for cooling. This demands cardiovascular work and increased heart rate. Similarly, blood is shunted away from the muscles and to the stomach immediately after meals. Any activity immediately after a meal will elicit a higher heart rate and a higher myocardial oxygen demand. For a summary of additional cardiac research related to ADL the reader is referred to Table 29-5.

Energy conservation addresses patterns of activities. For instance, Mrs. R can perform a standing shower (3.5 METs) with good cardiovascular responses and no symptoms. However, as she dries herself and then attempts to redress, she experiences increased heart rates and fatigue. Therefore a shower chair may be necessary, and a system of work and rest (such as work 5 minutes and rest 2 minutes) can be introduced.

Patients need much guidance and education in this area. Once a patient understands the principles of work efficiency, anxiety is reduced and the patient feels in control of the events. For instance, Mr. J was extremely depressed because last evening he had chest pain during his shower; he now feels his cardiac condition is worse because this never happened before. On further examination the therapist discovers that Mr. J had to run up and down the steps twice to get the phone before taking a shower. It is under-standable that if he starts at a high heart rate, activity will certainly increase the rate further; in this case it was increased beyond Mr. J's angina threshold. Therapeutic intervention is to educate Mr. J in environmental and activity factors that increase heart rate and to instruct him in pulse monitoring. If Mr. J's pulse is greater than 90, he should wait to take a shower. Meditation or progressive relaxation 10 minutes before showering may be necessary so that showering begins at a heart rate of 70 beats per minute.

Patient education sheets can be used to instruct the patient in such principles. Furthermore a method of work simplification can be used to instruct patients in analyzing new tasks to be simplified at home or in their work environments.

PATIENT AND FAMILY EDUCATION. Patient and family education is of prime importance in cardiac rehabilitation. Topics covered include basic cardiac anatomy, basic exercise physiology, medications, pulse monitoring, diet and risk factor modification, energy conservation, and energy cost of activities.[42] The occupational therapist may be involved with instruction in several of these topics. Some occupational therapists coordinate cooking classes with the dietitian to address diet education and assess a patient's performance and use of energy conservation with kitchen tasks.

Patient and family education can be performed creatively in a variety of ways, such as direct instruction, experiential performance, demonstration, reinforcement, problem solving, and repeated practice. The reader is referred to the references that have evaluated the effectiveness of various presentation techniques geared toward patient education.[19,40]

SUMMARY

This chapter is designed to enable the therapist to establish a background and theoretical foundation in cardiac rehabilitation. The therapist is then able to provide safe activities for the patient with a primary or secondary cardiac diagnosis.

To assist the therapist in synthesizing and applying the foregoing information a sample treatment plan is provided. The sample treatment plan is not comprehensive, and the reader therefore may wish to apply information from this chapter to develop a more complete plan.

Table 29.5 Summary of Cardiac Research Related to ADL[49]

Authors	Study	(S/P)**	Methods	Results	Interpretation
Alteri 1984[2]	Comparison of recovery times to determine adequate rest periods following ADLs	10 men s/p** MI	Measured HR, BP responses @ 2-min intervals following activity, EKG monitor before and after activity	Time to return to baseline: after Shower 30.5 min Stairs 7.0 min Walking 10 min	Due to use of UEs and heat, shower demands more recovery time after activity
Harrington et al 1981[30]	Compared effectiveness of evaluation techniques	29 s/p** MI pts	Compared responses to monitored self-care, modified treadmill, Holter monitoring,* and exercise program	Highest HR produced during self-care BP responses during monitored self-care matched responses during GXT	Monitored self-care evaluation is effective method for screening for early mobilization
Johnston et al 1981[33]	Compared responses to basin, tub, and shower bathing	12 s/p** MI pts	Measured oxygen consumption, HR, BP, and EKG responses during activity	Showers require significantly more oxygen consumption & higher incidence of EKG ST segment depression (ischemia) esp for pts with inferior MI	Pts with EKG ST displacement during bathing may have diffuse disease and may benefit from GXT or Holter monitor to set guidelines for activity.
Sheldal et al 1984[53]	Heart rates during home activity	62 s/p** MI pts	Measured HR, symptoms on GXT and compared with postdischarge Holter monitor record	HR during self-care exceeded rate recommended at discharge without adverse symptoms of EKG abnormalities	HR and MET guidelines set at d/c by GXT may be too conservative
Winslow et al 1984[60]	Responses to in-bed and out of bed toileting	Normal, cardiac, medical, and outpatient men (53) & women (42)	Measured and compared oxygen uptake, HR, RPE, BP, and preference for use of urinal or bedpan vs bedside commode for urination	All methods of toileting were between 1.2 and 1.4 METs; all subjects preferred out of bed method	Out of bed toileting is safe low-level activity and can prevent orthostatic hypotension
Winslow et al 1985[61]	Responses to tub, basin, and shower bathing	22 normal and 18 s/p** MI pts	Monitored HR, BP, & oxygen consumption during 3 types of bathing	Energy costs of 3 methods are similar; Cardiac pts moved more slowly & had lower oxygen use	Stable MI pts who can tolerate upright and get in & out of tub can take a tub or shower bath if water temperature is controlled

* Holter monitor is a portable EKG worn for 24 hours.
** Status post

Sample treatment plan

CASE STUDY

DD is a 64-year-old man admitted 4 days ago with a 5-hour history of bilateral arm pain and tightness in his throat associated with fatigue and shortness of breath.

Diagnostic work-up disclosed an acute anterolateral MI with subsequent complications of CHF and arrhythmias.

This patient is divorced and lives alone. He is a retired plumber and enjoys doing maintenance jobs around the house.

He was referred to occupational therapy for ADL evaluation and activity progression per cardiac protocol.

He was transferred out of the ICU and onto a general medicine floor today.

TREATMENT PLAN

Personal data

Name: DD

Age: 64

Diagnosis: Acute anterolateral MI (post day 4) with complications

Disability: Altered functional capacity

Treatment aims as stated in referral: achieve maximal, functional level of ADL without adverse cardiovascular symptoms

OTHER SERVICES

Physician: Supervision of patient's progress and effectiveness of current medical regime with increasing activity and program adjustments as indicated

Nursing: Provision of nursing and supportive care: reinforcement of ADL and ambulation programs in accordance with rehabilitation progress; provision of educational program with nursing emphasis on anatomy and physiology, medications, tests, and wound care

Social service: Assistance in family and social adjustment; exploration of financial resources for follow-up services and arrangement for equipment; outpatient and home health and/or homemaker services as needed

Physical therapy: Graded exercise program with focus on musculoskeletal conditioning progressing to cardiovascular conditioning program with various use of modalities (such as ambulation, arm ergometer, and calisthenics); formulation of home program; ordering of exercise equipment for program as necessary

Dietary service: Diet evaluation and modification with follow-up patient and family education as needed

Respiratory therapy

Community support groups (for example, Mended Hearts)

FRAME OF REFERENCE

Occupational performance

TREATMENT APPROACH

Rehabilitative

OT EVALUATION

Performance components

Medical history and risk factors

Interview and chart review

Motor functioning

Blood pressure, heart rate, EKG, and symptomatic responses to activity: Observe, test, chart review

Functional capacity: Observe, interview, chart review, test

Muscle test: Observe functional task performance

ROM: Observe

Balance: Observe, test

Sensory integrative functioning

Sensation (touch, proprioception, thermal): Observe

Cognitive functioning

Safety awareness: Interview, observe

Memory: Test, observe

Insight into disability: Interview, observe

Psychological functioning

Self-identity: Interview

Coping skills: Interview, observe

Adjustment to disability: Observe, interview

Social functioning

Interpersonal skills: Observe and interview

Performance skills

Self-care

Dressing, bathing, transfers: Observe, test

Work-related skills

Work habits and attitudes: Interview, observe

Work tolerance: Interview, observe

Home management: Interview

Play/leisure

Past and present leisure interests/activities: Interview

Modes of relaxation and handling stress: Interview, observe

Continued.

Sample treatment plan—cont'd

EVALUATION SUMMARY

A chart review and interview reveal that Mr. D has positive risk factors for age, sex, borderline diabetes, smoking, and sedentary life-style. He has recurrent bouts of CHF due to poor compliance with medications. A chart review of recent tests shows normal heart rhythm, enlarged lungs, a small infarct, and diffuse coronary heart disease.

Cardiac monitoring during self-care activities show normal sinus heart rhythm with appropriate vital sign responses during seated basin bath at bedside. His functional capacity is at the 2.0-MET level.

By observation Mr. D has normal functional ROM, muscle strength, and balance. His endurance is limited to 15 minutes of unsupported sitting for eating. He transfers independently to the bedside commode.

Mr. D has strong denial of his disability resulting in poor safety judgment concerning his functional capacity and prognosis. He is sure he'll feel fine once he gets home where he can get a good night's rest. He would like to leave the transitional care unit for a cigarette, his usual method for handling stress.

Mr. D takes long, hot tub baths. He enjoys light housekeeping in his first floor apartment, and likes to work straight through until he gets his chores done. He eats most of his meals out and uses the bus for transportation. He sends his laundry out and hires someone to help with the heavy cleaning once a month. He tends to "keep to himself."

ASSETS

Potential for improved endurance
Good living situation
Presence of adults to assist with homemaking
Financial security

PROBLEM LIST

1. Decreased functional capacity for self-care
2. Little knowledge of current condition and associated signs and symptoms
3. Positive risk factors of smoking and sedentary life-style
4. Limited knowledge/practice of energy-conservation techniques
5. History of poor compliance with medications
6. Diet consists of food with high fat, high sodium content.
7. Lives alone; socially isolated

PROBLEM 1

Decreased functional capacity for self-care
Objective
Patient will be independent with seated shower at 3.0-MET level
Method
The patient will have daily practice in hygiene, dressing, and grooming with slow progression and close monitoring of blood pressure, heart rate, symptoms, and EKG; the patient will be instructed in energy-conservation techniques and provided with prescription for shower chair
Gradation
The patient will be progressed gradually according to

MET-level program, beginning with bathing UEs and dressing independently in a bedside chair

He will progress to full body bathing at bedside, seated shaving, and independent dressing in a chair; if he has appropriate cardiovascular responses to activity, he will progress to seated bathing in the bathroom with standing for oral hygiene; if he continues to have appropriate responses, he will increase his activity level to standing bathing and hygiene (shaving and dental care) in the bathroom

Finally he will progress to a seated shower, shampoo, drying, and dressing

PROBLEM 3

Positive history of smoking
Objective
The patient will be able to describe on interview the physical effects of nicotine on the cardiovascular system plus the risks of smoking and identify and demonstrate three alternative behaviors to use instead of smoking
Method
The therapist and patient will view and discuss The American Heart Association slide show on smoking, then review and discuss the patient's patterns of smoking behavior; the patient will identify alternative behaviors learned from the slide show and discussion

An activity analysis on prior coping patterns that were successful for the patient when smoking was not acceptable may be completed
Gradation
The patient will demonstrate alternative behaviors (deep breathing, gum chewing); the slide show may be repeated, with pauses to discuss different points in the program in order to individualize the material

Begin with neutral questions, then move slowly to more personal questions as a trusting relationship is developed

PROBLEM 4

Limited knowledge and/or practice of energy-conservation technique
Objective
The patient will be independent in energy-conservation and pacing techniques and will demonstrate this during performance of the shower
Method
Demonstration of energy-efficient ADL techniques with daily practice; the patient will be trained in body mechanics, work simplification, and relaxation techniques through the use of a tape and slide show

A written script that follows the slide show will be reviewed and discussed with patient; the patient will be reminded of environmental factors prior to each ADL treatment
Gradation
Initially the patient will have the entire treatment structured by the therapist (i.e., position, water temperature, duration of activity); as the patient begins to integrate information (as demonstrated during interview), allow the patient to set his own work pace and/or to set water temperature independently in order to assess his ability to put concepts into practice

REVIEW QUESTIONS

1. Describe the sequence of events (cardiac cycle) responsible for the heart's function as a systematic pump.
2. Name the symptoms and consequences encountered with prolonged cardiac ischemia.
3. Name the cardiac risk factors that can be controlled by medical and therapeutic intervention.
4. Which patients in general rehabilitation clinics may require special program modification as a result of secondary cardiac involvement?
5. Under what circumstances is exercise and activity absolutely contraindicated?
6. List the signs and symptoms of cardiac intolerance to activity.
7. Demonstrate and describe the method of taking an accurate blood pressure.
8. What are "METs," and how are they used in cardiac rehabilitation?
9. Design a cardiac rehabilitation activity program to be performed over 1 week for a 53-year-old man with cardiomyopathy. He has been described as a Class III cardiac case.
10. Name five factors that may alter the MET level and cardiovascular demand of an activity.
11. A patient with recent bypass surgery performs at a 3.5-MET level on a GXT the day before he goes home. Would you recommend that he take seated or standing showers? Why?

REFERENCES

1. Aiken LH and Henrichs TF: Systematic relaxation as a nursing intervention technique with open heart surgery patients, Nurs Res 20:212, 1971.
2. Alteri CA: The patient with myocardial infarction: rest prescriptions for activities of daily living, Heart Lung 13:355, 1984.
3. American Heart Association: Coronary risk handbook, Dallas, 1973, American Heart Association.
4. American Heart Association: Cardio-pulmonary resuscitation: advanced life support, JAMA Suppl Aug 1980.
5. American Heart Association: Recommendations for human blood pressure determination by sphygmomanometers, Dallas, 1980, American Heart Association Communications Division.
6. American Heart Association: Heart facts: 1986, Dallas, 1986, American Heart Association.
7. American Heart Association: The heart of the home, 1965, Dallas, American Heart Association.
8. American Occupational Therapy Association: A curriculum guide for occupational therapy educators, Rockville, MD, 1974, American Occupational Therapy Association.
9. Andreoli KG et al: Comprehensive cardiac care: a text for nurses, physicians, and other health practitioners, St Louis, 1983, The CV Mosby Co.
10. Astrand PO and Rodahl K: Textbook of work physiology, New York, 1970, McGraw-Hill, Inc.
11. Bates B: A guide to physical examination, ed 2, Philadelphia, 1979, JB Lippincott Co.
12. Beauchamp N, Creighton C, and Summers L: Cardiac work tolerance screening: a case study, Occup Ther in Health Care 1(2):99, 1984.
13. Bedsworth JA and Molen MT: Psychological stress in spouses of patients with myocardial infarction, Heart Lung 11:450, 1982.
14. Borg G et al: RPE collection of papers presented at ACSM Annual Meeting, 1981; Med Sci Sports Exerc 14:376, 1982.
15. Bragg TL: Psychological response to myocardial infarction, Nurs Forum 14:383, 1975.
16. Brock LL et al: Cardiac rehabilitation unit program guide, Dallas, 1977, American Heart Association.
17. Burch GE and De Pasquale NP: Primer of clinical measurement of blood pressure, St Louis, 1962, The CV Mosby Co.
18. Cassem NH and Hackett TP: Psychological rehabilitation of myocardial infarction patients in the acute phase, Heart Lung 2:382, 1973.
19. Chatham M and Knapp B: Patient education handbook, Bowie, MD, 1982, Robert J Brady Co.
20. Colorado Heart Association: Exercise equivalents, Denver, 1970, Cardiac Reconditioning and Work Evaluation Unit, Spalding Rehabilitation Center. (Pamphlet.)
21. Cornett SJ and Watson JF: Cardiac rehabilitation; an interdisciplinary team approach, New York, 1984, John Wiley & Sons, Inc.
22. University of Colorado Medical Center, Department of Physical Medicine and Rehabilitation: Coronary Heart Disease Rehabilitation/Cardiac Rehabilitation Unit, Denver, 1971, (Pamphlet.)
23. Dawber TR: The Framingham study: the epidemiology of arteriosclerotic disease, Cambridge, MA, 1980, Harvard University Press.
24. de Vries HA: Physiology of exercise, Dubuque, IA, 1978, Wm C Brown Co, Publishers.
25. Dubin D: Rapid interpretation of EKGs, Tampa, FL, 1974, C.O.V.E.R, Inc.
26. Fox SM, Naughton JP, and Gorman PA: Physical activity and cardiovascular health: the exercise prescription, frequency and type of activity, Mod Concepts Cardiovasc Dis 41:6, 1972.
27. Froelicher VF: Exercise in the prevention of atherosclerotic heart disease. In Wenger N, editor: Exercise and the heart, Philadelphia, 1978, FA Davis Co.
28. Gentry WD and Haney T: Emotional and behavioral reaction to acute myocardial infarction, Heart Lung 4:738, 1975.
29. Halpenny CJ: The cardiac cycle. In Underhill SL et al, editors: Cardiac nursing, Philadelphia, 1982, JB Lippincott Co.
30. Harrington K et al: Cardiac rehabilitation: evaluation and intervention less than six weeks after myocardial infarction, Arch Phys Med Rehab 62:151, 1981.
31. Haskell WL: Design of a cardiac conditioning program. In Wenger N, editor: Exercise and the heart, Philadelphia, 1978, FA Davis Co.
32. Hellerstein HK: Rehabilitation of

the cardiac patient, JAMA 164:225, 1957.

33. Johnston BL, Watt EW, and Fletcher GF: Oxygen consumption and hemodynamic and electrocardiographic responses to bathing in recent post-myocardial infarction patients, Heart Lung 10:666, 1981.

34. Kattus AA et al: Exercise testing and training of individuals with heart disease or at high risk for its development: a handbook for physicians, Dallas, 1975, American Heart Association.

35. Katz A: Effects of ischemia and hypoxia upon the myocardium. In Russak H and Zohman B, editors: Coronary heart disease, Philadelphia, 1971, JB Lippincott Co.

36. Kottke FJ: Common cardiovascular problems in rehabilitation. In Krusen FH, Kottke FJ, and Ellwood PM, editors: Handbook of physical medicine and rehabilitation, Philadelphia, 1971, WB Saunders Co.

37. Lancour J: How to avoid pitfalls in measuring blood pressure, Am J Nurs 76:773, 1976.

38. Maloney FP and Moss K: Energy requirements for selected activities, Denver, 1974, Department of Physical Medicine, National Jewish Hospital. (Unpublished.)

39. May GS et al: Secondary prevention after myocardial infarction: a review of long term trials, Prog Card Dis 24:331, 1982.

40. Megenity J and Magenity J: Patient teaching: theories, techniques and strategies, Bowie, MD, 1982, Robert J Brady Co.

41. Milnor WR: The heart as a pump. In Mountcastle VB, editor: Medical physiology, Vol. II, ed 14, St Louis, 1979, The CV Mosby Co.

42. Newton K and Sivarajan E: Cardiac rehabilitation: life style adjustments. In Underhill SL et al, editors: Cardiac nursing, Philadelphia, 1982, JB Lippincott Co.

43. New York Heart Association, Inc.: Nomenclature and criteria for diagnosis of disease of the heart and great vessels, ed 8, Boston, 1979, Little Brown & Co.

44. Niles N and Wills R: Heart failure. In Underhill SL et al, editors: Cardiac nursing, Philadelphia, 1982, JB Lippincott Co.

45. Ogden LD: Cardiac rehabilitation program design: occupational therapy, Downey, CA, 1981, Cardiac Rehabilitation Resources.

46. Ogden LD: Guidelines for analysis and testing of activities of daily living with cardiac patients, Downey, CA, 1981, Cardiac Rehabilitation Resources.

47. Ogden LD: Initial evaluation of the cardiac patient: occupational therapy, Downey, 1981, Cardiac Rehabilitation Resources.

48. Ogden LD: Procedure guidelines for monitored self-care evaluation and monitored task evaluation, Downey, CA, 1981, Cardiac Rehabilitation Resources.

49. O'Leary SS: Monitored showers during inpatient rehabilitation following cardiac events, San Jose, CA, 1986. (Master's thesis.)

50. Rushmer RF: Cardiovascular dynamics, Philadelphia, 1976, WB Saunders Co.

51. Santa Clara Valley Medical Center: Cardiac rehabilitation program protocol, San Jose, CA, 1983. (Unpublished.)

52. Scalzi C and Burke L: Myocardial infarction: behavioral responses of patient and spouses. In Underhill SL et al, editors: Cardiac nursing, Philadelphia, 1982, JB Lippincott Co.

53. Sheldahl LM et al: Heart rate responses during home activities soon after myocardial infarction, J Card Rehab 4:326, 1984.

54. Silverman M: Examination of the heart: the clinical history, Dallas, 1978, American Heart Association.

55. Sivarajan SE: Cardiac rehabilitation: activity and exercise programs. In Underhill SL et al, editors: Cardiac Nursing, Philadelphia, 1982, JB Lippincott Co.

56. Sokolow M and McIlroy MB: Clinical cardiology, Los Altos, CA, 1977, Lange Medical Publications.

57. Trobaugh G: Cardiomyopathies. In Underhill SL et al, editors: Cardiac nursing, Philadelphia, 1982, JB Lippincott Co.

58. Underhill SL: Valvular disorders. In Underhill SL et al, editors: Cardiac nursing, Philadelphia, 1982, JB Lippincott Co.

59. Wenger N: The physiological basis of early ambulation after myocardial infarction. In Wenger N, editor: Exercise and the heart, Philadelphia, 1978, FA Davis Co.

60. Winslow EH, Lane LD, and Gaffney FA: Oxygen consumption and cardiovascular response in patients and normal adults during in-bed and out-of-bed toileting, J Card Rehab 4:348, 1984.

61. Winslow EH, Lane LD, and Gaffney FA: Oxygen uptake and cardiovascular responses in control adults and acute myocardial infarction patients during bathing, Nurs Res 34:164, 1985.

62. Wulff K and Hong P: Surgical intervention for coronary artery disease. In Underhill SL et al, editors: Cardiac nursing, Philadelphia, 1982, JB Lippincott Co.

30 Low back pain

SALLY A. ROOZEE

Low back pain has probably plagued human beings since they stood upright.[9] Today low back pain has become a national health problem. In 1980, statistics from *Time*[9] predicted that 8 out of every 10 Americans will have a back problem some time in their lives. Anderson states that more people miss work because of back pain than because of any other disease or injury. In a study done by Frymoyer it was estimated that 217 million workdays are lost annually because of back pain.[5] In dollars and cents, *Forbes* magazine in a 1986 issue reported that backache is "business' silent crippler," costing an estimated 56 billion dollars annually in insurance, treatment, lost production, and employee retraining.[7]

With statistics as staggering as these, it can be easily recognized that low back pain is a surmounting economic and health concern. Because of this fact occupational therapists have become increasingly involved in the treatment and prevention of low back pain. The skills and knowledge that an occupational therapist possesses lend themselves well to the treatment of low back pain, and as the occupational therapist's involvement increases, he or she will find it to be an exciting and challenging field in which to work.

Why do individuals have back aches? Health care professionals cite many reasons that may be responsible for the prevalence of low back pain in America. The evolutionary predicament of human beings going from a quadruped to a biped stance with the back taking the abuse may be one of the causes for the prevalence of low back pain. Other causes or risk factors may be attributed to an ever increasing sedentary life-style. Because of the conveniences of modern technology Americans are physically not as active as their grandparents. Americans tend to be overweight, which contributes to extra stress on the spine. The back is further abused by the practice of bad habits, such as poor posture and the use of poor body mechanics in activities of daily living (ADL). Prolonged postures and certain repetitive motions can also contribute stress to the spine. Last but not least is the unavoidable accident or the trauma-induced injury to the back. Any or all of these factors contribute to the wear and tear of the structures of the spine which may result in low back pain or an injury to the back.

Low back pain is a complex and multifaceted problem. The patient who experiences low back pain may be affected physically, psychologically, economically, socially, and recreationally. As a result this disability requires medical professionals who are knowledgeable, sensitive, and versatile, for successful treatment.

MEDICAL MANAGEMENT
Anatomy of the Spine

To understand the medical and therapeutic management of low back pain, a brief review of anatomy and anatomical terms is necessary.

The spine comprises 33 vertebrae: 7 cervical, 12 thoracic, 5 lumbar, 5 sacral, and 4 coccygeal stacked on top of each other. The cervical, thoracic, and lumbar vertebrae remain distinct and separate from one another throughout life. The adult sacral and coccygeal vertebrae are fused or united with each other to form two bones, the sacrum and the coccyx.[4] Intervertebral disks separate the vertebrae, and a system of muscles and ligaments helps to provide alignment and mobility to the spine. The function of the vertebral column is to support human beings in an upright position that is mechanically balanced to conform to the stress of gravity.[3]

The vertebrae in the cervical, thoracic, and lumbar areas are all slightly different in size and shape, but they each have the same basic components. The vertebral body is the large portion of the vertebra and the area that is the weight-bearing surface. The transverse processes are located on both sides of the vertebral body. These processes serve as points of attachments for muscles. Slightly above and below the transverse processes are the facets. These articulations determine the direction of movement between two adjacent vertebrae. By their directional planes the facets prevent or restrict movement in a direction contrary to the planes of articulations.[3]

Two other areas on the vertebrae are the pedicles and the laminae, which are bony arches that help form the protective spinal foramen. The spinous process is the posterior portion of the vertebrae, which one feels as the "bumps" along the spine. These processes also serve as attachment sites for muscles.

In between the vertebrae are the intervertebral disks. The disks separate the vertebrae, act as shock absorbers, and serve as cushions on which the vertebrae may move. The disk is much like a jelly doughnut with a fibrous outer ring, the anulus, and the center, a colloidal gelatin, known as the nucleus pulposus. The mechanism by which a disk functions is similar to a water balloon between two hands. As compressive forces push evenly down on the vertebral body, the distribution of the nucleus is equal in all directions. If the force is exerted more on one side than another, however, the nucleus is forced predominately in the opposite direction of the force. This mechanism exists with the various movements of the spine, such as forward flexion, extension, and lateral flexion.

As an individual ages the disk loses some of its water and elastic properties. This results in the intervertebral disk space becoming narrower. The facets are closer and in some instances may touch each other; the mechanism of the disk becomes more sluggish; and the anulus is more brittle. All of these changes, which occur as a part of the natural aging process, make human beings more susceptible to back problems as they become older.

The most important factor to remember about a disk is that it is constantly under pressure. The pressure is increased every time an individual bends forward slightly. The repetitiveness with which one flexes forward every day continues to exert pressure on one area of the disk. Little tears gradually begin to appear in the anulus, and then one day a movement as simple as bending over to pick up a newspaper may result in a herniated disk. This process is insidious, painless, and there are no warning signs. However, it is a situation that can be prevented.

The ligaments of the spine run longitudinally along the vertebral column. They restrict movement in some directions and prevent any significant shearing action by their points of attachment.[3] The intervertebral disks are surrounded by ligaments anteriorly and posteriorly. The anterior longitudinal ligament runs anterior to the vertebral bodies and is broad and strong with intimate attachment to each vertebral body. In contrast the posterior longitudinal ligament is situated along the posterior surface of the vertebral bodies, which also forms the anterior surface of the spinal canal.[6] This ligament is intact throughout the entire length of the vertebral column until it reaches the lumbar region, which is of functional and potential pathological significance. At the first lumbar level

it begins to progressively narrow so that on reaching the last lumbar, first sacral interspace, the ligament is half of its original width. This ultimate narrow posterior ligamentous reinforcement contributes to an inherent structural weakness at the level where there is the greatest static stress and the greatest spinal movement producing the greatest kinetic strain.[3]

The muscles of the low back are numerous and interrelate and function together in many instances. For the purpose of this chapter muscles will be grouped together according to their action on the spine. The muscles that extend the spine include the quadratus lumborum; the sacrospinalis, also known as the erector spinae; the multifidus; the intertransversarii; and the interspinales.[4] These muscles work together to maintain an individual in an upright posture and to actively extend the lumbar spine. The primary flexors of the lumbar spine are the abdominal muscles that include the obliquus externus abdominis, the obliquus internus abdominis, the transversalis abdominis, and the rectus abdominis. Along with the abdominal muscles, the psoas major and minor are also considered flexors of the lumbar spine.[4] To classify a muscle as either a flexor or extensor of the lumbar spine implies bilateral simultaneous muscle action. However, unilateral action of some muscles will result in lateral bending or lumbar abduction. Therefore the abductors of the lumbar spine are the quadratus lumborum, psoas major and minor, musculi abdominis, and the intertransversarii.[4] The muscles of the lumbar spine function to allow motion to occur and help to maintain the upright posture.

The spinal cord is encased by the vertebrae and supporting structures. As the nerve roots descend the spinal canal, they cross the disk immediately above the intervertebral foramen.[3] As they emerge from the foramen, the nerves divide into the anterior and posterior primary divisions, and one branch goes immediately to the facets.[3] Because of this close relationship of the nerves to the structures of the spine, the nerve roots are susceptible to impingement and entrapment.

In summary the spine is composed of a network of structures, the vertebrae, disks, ligaments, and muscles all working together to keep a person upright, to allow movement to occur, and to provide stability. The lumbar spine withstands the greatest kinetic strain and it is also the area that is most vulnerable to trauma and injury.

Diagnosis

Medical diagnosis of a low back problem involves a multifaceted evaluation. Initially the physician will obtain a thorough history from the patient, which includes the following questions. When did the symptoms occur? What brought on the symptoms? Describe the pain. How often does the pain occur? What relieves the symptoms? What aggravates the symptoms? How does this limit functioning?

The physical examination, according to Finneson,[4] should consist of 12 steps.

1. Inspection—that is, observing the patient as he or she moves, walks, and sits as well as observing the spine and buttocks—is the first part of the examination.
2. The patient's gait is observed for a short distance, and then the physician may ask the patient to walk on his or her heels and then on the toes to detect any muscle weakness.
3. Mobility of the spine is examined next by having the patient go through the motions of trunk flexion, extension, lateral flexion, and rotation. Range of motion (ROM) or mobility of the spine is generally not recorded in degrees, but rather as "normal," "slightly" limited (moves through three-fourths ROM), "moderately" limited (moves through one-half ROM), or "severely" limited (moves through one-fourth or less ROM).
4. The patient squats with complete flexion of the knees and hips. Any pain produced in the low back, knees, or hips is noted.
5. Reflex testing of the deep tendon reflexes of the ankle and patella is conducted on the patient to determine if there are any nerve root problems.
6. Leg length is measured to determine that the low back pain is not produced by a discrepancy in the length of the patient's two legs.
7. Sensation testing for light touch and pain is performed on the individual with back pain symptoms.
8. Motor strength is evaluated by testing the muscles in the lower extremities. Measurement of the circumference of the thigh and the calf of both legs may also be done to determine if there is any significant difference in the size of the two extremities.
9. Straight leg raising is done on both lower extremities to determine if there is sciatic nerve involvement. This test will also indicate the tightness of the hamstring muscles.
10. Internal and external rotation of the hip is performed as part of the evaluation process to eliminate any hip disease. Pain with internal rotation of the hip indicates a sacroiliac dysfunction.
11. Spinal pressure is examined, which involves applying pressure over the spinous processes of the lumbar spine to determine areas of local tenderness or reproduction of sciatic pain.
12. Arterial pulses of the inguinal, popliteal, and dorsalis pedis sites are carefully checked.[4]

As an adjunct to the physical examination a physician may order other diagnostic tests to assist in the determination of the cause of the low back symptoms. An x-ray examination may be ordered to detect fractures, dislocation, infections, tumors, and other metabolic diseases. Common abnormalities seen on an x-ray film may include transitional vertebrae (either a sacralized lumbar vertebra or a lumbarized sacral vertebra), spina bifida, increased lumbar lordosis, scoliosis, intervertebral disk narrowing, asymmetrical lumbosacral facets, osteoarthritis, and spondylolisthesis.[4] In the majority of low back pain patients, however, a specific cause of the symptomatology is not clearly demonstrated by x-ray examinations. Therefore further testing may be necessary. Contrast x-ray studies, such as myelograms and diskograms, may be done to determine the condition of the spinal canal and the disks.

In recent years a computerized tomography (CT) scan has been developed which has many advantages over conventional x-ray films. The CT scan is noninvasive and permits visualization of fine anatomical detail by providing displays of thin slices of various planes. Furthermore, it permits discrimination of more differing tissue densities than conventional x-ray film techniques. Soft tissue organs, muscle, bone, fat, blood, metal, and iodinated contrast material all can be clearly distinguished on a CT scan.[4] Traditionally the lumbar myelogram has served as the primary diagnostic imaging method of the lumbosacral spine in the low back pain syndrome. However, a CT body scan of the lumbar spine has significant advantages over the earlier procedure in terms of accuracy, risk, accessibility, availability, and an ease of performance and is fast becoming one of the primary diagnostic tools in low back pain.[4]

Other diagnostic tests may be done to determine motor or sensory disorders. Electromyography and nerve conduction velocity studies are among the additional tests that the physician may order. Lumbar epidural or facet blocks may be done as a diagnostic procedure or as a method of treatment. These procedures generally involve injecting a peripheral nerve or facet with an anesthetic agent and sometimes a corticosteroid.

Nonsurgical Management of Low Back Pain

In the management of low back pain the physician's objectives are alleviating pain, restoring motion and mobility, minimizing residual impairment, preventing recurrence, and preventing entry into a chronic pain cycle.[3] One of the most important treatments in low back pain is rest. Patients who have low back discomfort from any cause will generally instinctively attempt to avoid activity and will rest. The method and extent of rest largely depend on the severity and nature of the symptoms. For example, an individual suffering from mild low back discomfort may only be restricted from heavy lifting, prolonged standing and flexion postures, excessive stooping, and long automobile trips.[4] In other cases however, strict bed rest at home or in a hospital may be necessary. In strict bed rest all meals are to be taken in bed and the patient is not allowed to get up except for toilet activities. Generally the preferred position in bed is lying supine with the knees and hips slightly flexed or lying on one side with the knees flexed. However, this may vary according to the patient's condition and the physician's preference. It must be recognized that in prolonged bed rest a certain degree of muscle atrophy will occur as a result of lack of activity and muscle disuse. Additionally there may be loss of calcium from the bones and loss of protein, and certain circulatory changes may cause light-headedness in some cases.[4] Once bed rest is discontinued, a program of strengthening and improving endurance will be necessary.

Traction is a time-honored procedure used in the conservative treatment of low back dysfunction. It has gained the reputation of being "specific" treatment for the herniated lumbar disk. However, traction in the manner and force usually applied does not distract the vertebrae but decreases the lordosis, thus separating the facets and opening the foramina. It also gradually overcomes the spasm of the erector spinae.[3]

Recently medical literature has advocated total body weight traction applied in the hospital environment in a mechanical circular bed. This uses the concept that 30% of the total body weight is found below the third lumbar vertebra. If the patient is suspended at the thoracic cage, this amount of weight is applied as lumbar traction.[3]

Modalities used in the conservative treatment of low back pain may include therapeutic cold, superficial heat, ultrasound, or transcutaneous electrical nerve stimulation. According to Finneson,[4] therapeutic cold is the most effective modality in the treatment of acute low back pain. He stated that physiologic cooling is associated with a decrease in the tissue metabolic rate and a vasoconstriction of the arterial system. The vasoconstriction leads to an effect that penetrates tissues deeper than does heat. Superficial heat can be effective in low back pain problems. However, it produces a vasodilation that can promote swelling. Therefore an individual with low back pain following trauma who may have tissue disruption has a tendency to produce swelling, and this treatment would be contraindicated.[4] Ultrasound is another method of providing heat to deeper tissues. This modality is generally not indicated in the acute phase of low back pain as a result of the tendency of heat to produce swelling.

Transcutaneous electrical nerve stimulation (TENS) is a modality that uses a mild electrical current to modulate the sensation of pain. TENS does not cure any of the symptoms causing the pain, but it can help reduce the severity and duration of the pain and may be used instead of medication. The device consists of a small pocket-size, battery-operated pulse generator that can be worn clipped to the clothing. Electrodes are adhered to the skin at or near the site of pain or over a nerve trunk representative of the painful area. Cables or leads attached to the electrodes run to the pulse generator where they are connected. TENS can be used only with the prescription of a physician.

Medications may be prescribed for individuals suffering from acute low back pain and may include analgesics, muscle relaxants, antiinflammatory drugs, and antidepressant drugs. Medications for the alleviation of pain are best used on a specified basis of every 4 to 6 hours depending on the life of the drug, rather than as requested by the patient. For patients susceptible to addiction or dependency, drugs become a reward for pain and are difficult in later periods of illness to decrease or discontinue.[3]

Most muscle relaxants are sedatives and are capable also of being depressants. It is recommended that they be given in limited doses and eliminated before too much depression occurs. Oral antiinflammatory medication is valuable when administered for a limited time. It, as other drugs, has side effects that must be carefully explained to the patients. Antidepressant drugs may be prescribed and are valuable in patients who have been premorbidly depressed or who react to their acute impairment with depression.[3]

Once a person has recovered from the painful acute stages of low back pain, bed rest has been discontinued, and the patient is on limited activity, then exercise becomes an important treatment in low back pain. As cited previously bed rest is a common treatment for the patient with low back pain, but even with bed rest the side effects of decreased strength and endurance are encountered. An exercise program may include specific exercises for the low back, strengthening exercises for supporting structures, and endurance exercises. Education of the patient with low back pain is another important facet in the treatment phase. The educational phase should include principles of body mechanics, energy conservation, simple anatomy of the spine, and principles of injury prevention.

The combination of rest, modalities, exercise, and education should help most patients suffering from low back pain. However, there will be a small percentage of patients who will have to undergo surgical intervention to alleviate the problem. Today most physicians are trying the conservative methods of treatment before recommending surgery. If a patient does undergo surgery, a recovery stage similar to that previously stated will be instituted as well. Immediately after surgery the patient will be ordered to rest in bed, progressing to limited activity, and later to an exercise and maintenance program, which will include the same components described earlier.

Acute versus Chronic Pain

Acute, symptomatic pain serves the useful purpose of warning an individual that something is wrong and serves as a diagnostic aid to the physician. Yet when the sudden, jabbing sharpness of acute pain persists and results in a chronic condition, pain then becomes a complex malady and a menace to the individual, his or her family, and ultimately to society. The point at which acute low back pain becomes chronic is a debatable issue. Finneson[4] stated that chronic low back pain can be defined as that which is present for more than 3 days. Cailliet[3] stated that low back pain considered to have existed less than 2 months can be termed acute. Since there is disagreement as to the exact timing when acute pain becomes chronic, perhaps it is better to state that chronic intractable low back pain is more of an attitude on the part of the patient.[10] Acute pain demands a need for immediate relief. Medication, rest, modalities, and often surgery will accomplish this goal. Chronic pain may have mechanical irritating factors, such as structural defects, disk herniations, and congenital or disease problems. Contributing nonmechanical factors include anxiety, depression, frustration, and paranoia.[10] No matter when acute low back pain becomes chronic, the individual with chronic pain has a complex condition.

The patient with chronic low back pain may have some of the same symptoms and restrictions as the individual with acute pain. For example, the patient is suffering from pain, which restricts his or her ADL, such as tying shoes, driving a car, and performing yard activities and household tasks. The pain further restricts the patient's social and recreational events because he or she is unable to sit through a movie or church service, for example. The patient cannot play ball with his or her children and is unable to work because the pain restricts the activities required for the job. Once the pain persists for a length of time, however, unlike the patient with acute low back pain, the person suffering from chronic pain soon may undergo a change in income status because he or she can no longer work. The spouse may have to take a job or increase the number of hours working, and there may be a reversal of roles in the family. The patient continues to make trips to physicians only to have more of the same tests, more medication, and possibly to have initial or recurrent surgery only to end up feeling the same. The patient becomes frustrated, feels hopeless, and develops a mistrust of the medical profession. The constant pain makes him or her irritable. The inability to work and function as previously makes him or her depressed, despondent, and angry. The increasing isolation from activities, friends, and even family members makes the patient fearful. The pain is ever present, serving as a reminder of all of his or her inabilities and slowly eroding self-esteem, motivation, and courage. It is obvious then that the patient suffering from chronic low back pain presents a picture of physical, psychological, economic, and social limitations.

REHABILITATION

Since the patient with low back pain, and especially chronic low back pain, has a myriad of symptoms and disabilities and because the syndrome is such a complex one, it is best dealt with by a variety of professionals. A team approach to treating low back pain is the best and preferred method of handling this syndrome. The team might include a physician, physiatrist, neurologist, orthopedist, psychiatrist or psychologist, physical therapist, occupational therapist, recreational therapist, social worker, and vocational counselor.

Role of Occupational Therapy

The goal of an occupational therapist in the treatment of any patient is to help the patient achieve the maximal level of functional independence. In treating patients the occupational therapist makes an assessment of the person's limitations and problems, and a treatment program is designed around these facts to help alleviate or at least improve the existing conditions. No matter what problem or diagnosis exists or what methods of treatment are used, the occupational therapist's role is to provide the patient with the best opportunity to achieve maximal functional independence.

As noted previously, the patient with chronic low back pain has physical, psychological, social, and economic limitations. The occupational therapist has the skills to work with people who are depressed, angry, or have low self-esteem; the skills to assess joint restrictions, muscle weakness, and nerve involvement; and the skills to help people accomplish their daily activities with minimal effort and as independently as possible. With these skills the occupational therapist is a vital and important member of the health care team in the treatment of low back pain.

Assessment

The assessment of a patient with low back pain should include a four-part evaluation. If the occupational therapist is working as a member of a team, part of the assessment process may be done by another team member, such as the physical therapist. The entire assessment process is described here but it can be adapted according to the division of responsibilities and the facilities available in the treatment environment (Fig. 30-1).

SUBJECTIVE ASSESSMENT. The first part of the evaluation consists of the "subjective assessment." This involves obtaining information from the patient through an interview and reading the medical records. First the therapist should obtain a pain history from the patient. A blank chart showing the outline of a person with front and back views may be given to the patient with the instructions to draw in the areas of pain. Many times the manner in which the patient marks in his or her pain on the chart provides the evaluator with insight as to how the patient perceives the pain. For example, some patients merely mark the chart with a light line or "X" to represent where the pain is located. Other people will mark in the painful area heavily, practically coloring in the entire back or extremity. Although having the patient mark on the pain chart is not meant as an interpretative measure, the evaluator can surmise that when the patient colors in most of the chart as the area of pain-marking that the patient views the pain as all-encompassing.

After the patient has marked the pain on the chart, the evaluator should follow through by asking the patient some additional questions. When did the pain occur? What caused the pain? Next, a description of the pain is obtained to include the quality of the pain, such as sharp, burning, or jabbing; the frequency of the pain, such as constant or intermittent; and the intensity of the pain, such as excruciating, moderate, or mild. Next, a series of questions can be asked to determine when the pain is worse, what exacerbates the condition, and what alleviates the pain. The evaluator will also want to know how the patient perceives that his or her ADL are interrupted or limited because of the low back pain. Furthermore, the therapist will want to know if this condition has existed in the past, and if so, what treatments seemed to help and which aggravated the condition. Finally, the evaluator needs

to ascertain if the patient is taking any medication, what kind, and how often it is used. It is also important to ask the patient if he or she is using any orthotic or bracing devices.

Once the pain history has been obtained, it is important to ascertain what a typical day for the patient entails. This can be done by using the daily schedule described in Chapter 3. The patient is asked to describe in detail a typical day. Another method is to present the patient with a chart that breaks the day into small increments on which he or she can complete a daily schedule.

Finally, the evaluator should determine what the home and work situations entail. If the patient is still working or hopes to return to work, the evaluator should ask for a job description. Detail is necessary. Does the patient sit, stand, walk, or climb? Does the patient have to lift or carry objects, and if so, how much weight is he or she required to lift or carry, for how long, and for what distances? The evaluator should ask the patient to describe any problem tasks that he or she is involved with now or that her or she expects as problem tasks once the patient returns to work. It is also important to determine what the home atmosphere is like. Does the spouse work? Are there small children at home? What household or yard tasks does the patient typically engage in on a routine basis?

PHYSICAL ASSESSMENT. The second phase of the evaluation is the physical assessment. In this category if the therapist is working as a member of a team, it should be determined definitely which discipline will undertake which parts of the evaluation. It is not fair to the patient for two disciplines to perform the same tests or procedures, especially if both services charge for the evaluation. Furthermore, it is a waste of time to duplicate certain procedures. If two or more disciplines work closely together to determine what the evaluation should include and what procedures will be followed, cooperation can be achieved and redundancy can be avoided.

ROM is the first part of the physical assessment. Even though a patient is suffering from low back pain, a quick assessment of the upper extremities is indicated. Certain motions do put a strain on the lower back, and the evaluator will want to know this. For example, shoulder flexion exceeding 90° causes a shift in the center of gravity, resulting in increased lordosis, which may aggravate a patient's symptoms. The upper extremity ROM test can be done actively with the patient standing and mimicking the evaluator's motions. Any limitations in ROM are noted in degrees, and any exacerbation of pain is recorded. ROM testing of the lower extremities should be done with more exactness than ROM for the upper extremities. Hip

Name: _____

Room number: _____

Physician: _____

O.T. AND P.T. LOW BACK EVALUATION

Subjective assessment

Age: _____ _____.   Date of onset: _____

Mechanism of injury: _____

_____

Description of pain: _____

_____

What aggravates pain? _____

What eases pain? _____

What time of day is pain worse? _____

Is pain better or worse when:

    Lying _____   Position _____ Lying to sit _____

    Sitting _____   Sitting time _____ Sit to stand _____

    Standing _____   Standing time _____

Description of daily routine: _____

_____

Which tasks can or cannot be done?

    Sleeping _____   Household tasks _____

    Dressing _____   Yard tasks _____

    Sink activities _____   Driving _____

    Sitting _____   Working _____

    Lifting _____   Reaching _____

Previous history

    Back injuries or problems: _____

    Hospitalizations: _____

    Physical therapy: _____

    Chiropractor: _____

    Surgeries or procedures: _____

    What treatments increased pain? _____

    What treatments decreased pain? _____

    Present medications: _____ Frequency: _____

Fig. 30-1. Low back evaluation.

Physical assessment

Range of motion
  Upper extremities (gross): _____

    Lower extremities:

	Left	Pain	Right	Pain
Hip flexion				
Hip extension				
Straight leg raise test in lying position				
Straight leg raise test in sitting position				
Hip external rotation				
Hip internal rotation				

  Trunk:
    Trunk flexion (standing) _____
    Trunk flexion (supine) _____
    Trunk extension (standing) _____
    Trunk extension (supine) _____
    Trunk hyperextension _____
    Lateral flexion (right) _____ (left) _____
    Trunk rotation (to right) _____ (to left) _____

Sensation (sharp to dull): _____
_____

Strength:
  Upper extremity (gross) _____
_____

  Trunk (functional) _____

  Lower extremity:

	Left	Pain	Right	Pain
Hip flexion (L2)				
Knee extension (L3)				
Dorsiflexion (L4)				
Extensor hallucis longus (L5)				
Plantar flexion (S1)				
Quad set (functional)				

Fig. 30-1, cont'd. Low back evaluation.

Functional assessment

ADL assessment:

	Level	Body mechanics	Pain
Lying			
Sitting			
Standing			
Supine lying to sitting			
Sitting to standing			
Tying shoes			
Sink activities			
Sweeping and vacuuming			
Reaching overhead			

Level code: IE = Independent
IG = Independent but movements guarded
A = Assisted
U = Unable
ND = Not done

Lifting:

0-36 inches _____

36-72 inches _____

0-72 inches _____

Endurance walk:

Time _____

Distance _____

Treadmill incline:

Minutes _____

mph _____

Upper extremity weights:

Bench press _____

Elbow flexion _____

Shoulder flexion _____

right _____

left _____

Lower extremity weights:

Leg press _____

Static quad _____

Carrying:

Weight _____

Time _____

Distance _____

Treadmill level:

Minutes _____

mph _____

Bicycle:

Resistance _____

Time _____

Distance _____

Abduction:

right _____

left _____

_____

Posture (standing): _____

Sitting tolerance: _____ Standing tolerance: _____

Low back exercises: _____

Fig. 30-1, cont'd. Low back evaluation.

Psychological assessment

    Cooperative:_____   Motivated:_____

    Hostile:_____   Withdrawn:_____

    Outgoing:_____

    Remarks:_____

Treatment goals

    _____   _____

    _____   _____

    _____   _____

    _____   _____

    _____   _____

    _____

Plan _____

    _____

    _____

    _____

    _____

    _____

    _____

    _____ OTR

    _____ RPT

    _____ DATE

Fig. 30-1, cont'd. Low back evaluation.

flexion, hip extension, straight leg raise, and hip internal and external rotation, which are key motions, should be tested passively, noting any limitations in degrees and any pain on execution of the test. Hip flexion should be tested with the patient lying supine, knee flexed, and then the hip flexed through the available ROM. Hip internal and external rotation are also done with the patient lying supine. The straight-leg-raise test should be done with the patient lying supine and both legs extended. When the lower extremity is to be tested, the knee should remain fully extended with movement occurring at the hip through the patient's available ROM. A sitting straight-leg-raise test may be done to observe any inconsistencies in the patient's performance. For a sitting straight-leg-raise test the patient should be sitting on the edge of a firm surface. The evaluator asks the patient to sit up straight so 90° hip flexion is present, then asks the patient to straighten out the knee and lift the leg as high as he or she can without tilting backward. The evaluator will watch that the patient does not compensate by leaning backward, thus decreasing the angle at the hip joint. If the patient can achieve only 40° straight leg raise in a supine position and 90° in a sitting position, this indicates a discrepancy and should be noted and investigated. Active ROM should be evaluated for trunk flexion, trunk extension, trunk hyperextension, lateral bending, and trunk rotation. The results for trunk extension, rotation, and hyperextension should be recorded in degrees. Results from trunk flexion and lateral bending can be recorded either in degrees or in inches from a set landmark. For example, on trunk flexion the distance from the patient's fingertips to the floor can be measured and recorded. Lateral bending can be measured as inches above or below the knee joint. For all the previously mentioned motions any complaints of pain expressed during the testing should be recorded according to location and motion that evoked the pain.

Sensation testing is another part of the physical assessment. Generally sharp and dull sensation is tested. Using a pinwheel the examiner tests the patient's lower extremities in the dermatomal distributions. Any sensory abnormalities may help to indicate any possible nerve problems.

Evaluating the patient's strength is another important part of the assessment. Generally specific muscle testing of the trunk and lower extremities is performed, and a quick muscle test of the upper extremities should be done. Instead of testing the individual muscles in the entire trunk and lower extremities, the evaluator selects muscle groups that represent each nerve root in the lower extremity. Muscle testing is typically done on trunk flexion, hip flexion, knee extention, dorsiflexion and plantar flexion of the ankle, and extension of the great toe. Dorsiflexion and plantar flexion of the ankle may also be done by asking the patient to walk on the toes and the heels.

FUNCTIONAL ASSESSMENT. In the functional assessment as in the physical assessment, if the therapist is working with other team members, it must be determined who will be doing each part of the evaluation. The functional assessment can be thought of as the current status of the patient. What can the patient do now? What are the patient's capabilities and shortcomings?

To start, a functional assessment of the patient's ADL capabilities is necessary. Some of this can be done through observation, and part of the assessment data may be obtained by interviewing and performing simulated tasks. It is not uncommon for patients with low back pain to complain or demonstrate difficulty in tying shoes, putting on shoes and socks, standing at a sink to shave or apply makeup, standing to wash dishes, sweeping, vacuuming, washing windows, and mowing the lawn. It is best for the evaluator to ask the patient to actually try these tasks or to simulate them as closely as possible.

As the evaluator is having the patient try certain tasks, he or she must always be observant of the manner in which the patient attempts the tasks. Does the patient use proper body mechanics? Does the patient do the task with ease, guardedly, with much effort, or is he or she unable to attempt the task at all? Is there any facial grimacing visible or sound of effort audible? All these factors should be noted. Even during the initial interview and physical assessment the evaluator should observe the patient's movements. How does the patient get in and out of a chair? What sitting posture does the patient assume? How long can the patient sit before he or she must adjust his or her posture? In the physical assessment how does the patient get up from and down to the supine position?

In evaluating the use of body mechanics the evaluator should have the patient lift a box or object weighing no more than 5 pounds (2.3 kg) from the floor to a tabletop and then from a tabletop to a position 72 inches (182.9 cm) overhead. Again the way the task is accomplished should be observed and recorded. After instructing the patient in proper lifting techniques, the evaluator should gradually increase the amount of weight the patient is handling to obtain a maximal weight that the patient can lift to and from the three different heights (floor, tabletop, and overhead).

The patient's carrying capacity needs to be assessed. This can be done by asking the patient to carry the amount of weight he or she was able to lift to the tabletop. The evaluator asks the patient to walk a measured course until he or she becomes tired or starts to feel the pain becoming aggravated. This task is timed. The distance the patient was able to travel with the weight, the amount of weight carried, and the time are recorded.

The patient's posture should be evaluated. This can be accomplished by asking the patient to stand next to a plumb line. If a plumb line is not available, the evaluator asks the patient to stand erect and observes the patient's posture, noting any increases or decreases in the normal curves of the spine. The sitting posture can also be observed and noted. The patient's sitting and standing tolerances should be determined. If the evaluator has the opportunity to have the patient sit for a class, workshop, or interview, the therapist can document the amount of time the patient was able to sit. If the evaluator is unable to observe the patient in such a situation, then the evaluator asks the patient how long he or she thinks he or she can sit but compares it to something with a time frame, such as "Can you sit through a 30-minute television program?" The evaluator will want to determine the tolerance for standing as well, and the same techniques or questioning can be used.

PSYCHOLOGICAL ASSESSMENT. During the evaluation process the evaluator has an opportunity to talk with and become acquainted with the patient. From this contact with the patient, the evaluator will be able to obtain an idea of the patient's psychological state. The patient throughout the evaluation process may express anger, frustration, hostility, or depression, and these attitudes should be noted as part of the evaluation. If there is a psychiatrist or psychologist on the rehabilitation team, however, a specific psychological assessment should be carried out by that professional.

On completion of the assessment treatment goals and a treatment program need to be established. The overall goal in treating the individual with low back pain is to help the patient reach the maximal level of independence. Of course the goals established for each individual may differ according to the findings of the assessment. However, there are a few general goals that will apply to most patients suffering from low back pain. The goals are to improve and maintain ROM and flexibility; to improve endurance; to develop proper ways of using the body (body mechanics); to understand the structures of the spine, how they work, and what the adverse forces are that should be avoided; and to improve functional capabilities.

Treatment

EDUCATION. One of the most important phases of the treatment program for a patient with low back pain is education. The person who has injured his or her back is 10 times more likely to reinjure the back again within 1 year following the initial injury. Therefore teaching the patient how the back works, how to use proper body mechanics, and how to avoid unnecessary stresses are all important in preventing reinjury. The educational phase of a treatment program should include five areas of concentration. The first area is back anatomy, that is, teaching the patient the simple anatomy of the spine and the interrelationship of the structures and how they work together. Body mechanics, or how to use the body to obtain the most from it with the least amount of physical stress to the spine, is a vital part of the educational program. This includes discussion about the correct ways to stand, sit, sleep, lift, carry, stoop, climb, reach, sweep, vacuum, and rake.

Since psychological and emotional stresses can aggravate pain, sessions on stress management should be offered to the patient with low back pain. This can be done by using biofeedback, relaxation techniques, and classes on how to cope and reduce the everyday stresses of daily life.

Sessions about time management can be offered to the patient as a way of helping the patient learn how to pace his or her day and work tasks to avoid fatigue and overexertion. This is especially important for the patient who is just beginning to resume regular activities. This person may have the impulse or desire to immediately step back into a regular routine before he or she is physically ready to take on the stresses following surgery, a period of prolonged bed rest, or a period of limited activity. Besides helping the patient manage his or her time, discussion of realistic goal planning is imperative and complements the sessions of time management.

The last area of the educational phase should include a session on energy conservation. These sessions can help the person learn to reorganize home and office space to reduce the stresses placed on the back. For example, the individual should minimize the amount of reaching, bending, and twisting which is done in the daily activities while at work. Many times by simply reorganizing a cupboard or desk much of the reaching, bending, or twisting is eliminated.

The educational part of the patient's treatment program can be taught by any of several professionals. If the therapist is working in a team environment, the anatomy, time management, and stress management classes can be shared or presented by the individual most qualified and comfortable with the material, such as the occupational therapist or the physical therapist. The body mechanics and energy conservation sessions are generally instructed by the occupational therapist, but the physical therapist may also instruct patients in these areas. Again it is important to accomplish the goals set forth without conflict or duplication of services.

EXERCISE. In a setting in which a team approach to the treatment of low back pain is being used, the endurance training and lower extremity strengthening is customarily done by the physical therapist, whereas the upper extremity strengthening and functional training is done by the occupational therapist.

Treatment programs for patients with low back pain usually involve instructing patients in specific exercises. The primary physician usually prescribes the type and frequency of exercises to be given to the patient. Depending on the diagnosis and condition of the patient's back the physician may prescribe flexion or extension exercises or even a combination of the two. Flexion and extension exercises refer to the action of the trunk and back. Flexion exercises generally involve trunk flexion exercises, such as sit-ups and single and double knee-to-chest exercises. Extension exercises refer to extension of the spine and include trunk hyperextension and hip extension exercises (Fig. 30-2). If any of the exercises aggravates a patient's pain beyond normal stretching or pulling sensation, the patient should stop, and the physician should be consulted.

In addition to specific exercises for the low back, exercises to improve the patient's upper and lower extremity strength may be a part of the treatment plan. Strengthening both the upper and lower extremities helps the patient lift, carry, and manage weighted objects better, and because the stronger muscles are doing the work, it eliminates stress that otherwise might be exerted to the back. Strengthening of the upper extremities can be done by using weight equipment or by merely using barbells or cuff weights. Generally the areas to strengthen are the elbow flexors, shoulder depressors, scapular stabilizers, and pectoralis major and minor. Strengthening of the lower extremities should be done by using specific equip-

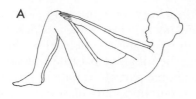

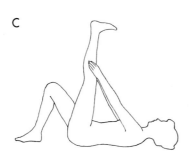

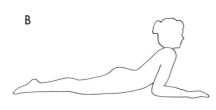

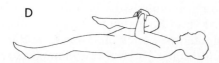

Fig. 30-2. Low back exercise. **A,** Partial sit-up. **B,** Back extension exercise. **C,** Straight leg raise exercise. **D,** Single knee-to-chest exercise.

ment, such as a leg press. Static setting of the quadriceps muscles (quad sets) can be used as part of the strengthening program for the lower extremities.

Since many patients with low back pain have been on limited activity during their convalescence, there is usually a need to improve endurance. Endurance training can be done with a variety of activities, such as walking, riding a stationary bicycle, walking on a treadmill, or climbing stairs. The important factor in endurance training is that the patient should be started slowly and progressed at a steady, slow rate to allow him or her to build up tolerance and to prevent the creation of more pain and discomfort.

FUNCTIONAL PRACTICE. Another important phase of any treatment program is to provide the patient with the opportunity to practice many of the body mechanics techniques he or she has been taught. Standing, sitting, and lying posture should be practiced. If there is a video camera and monitor available, videotaping the patient's posture in various positions can be a valuable adjunct to therapy. Even taking a picture with an instant print camera can be beneficial and provide immediate feedback to the patient.

Functional practice of lifting, reaching, and carrying techniques is necessary in the treatment of low back pain. Not only does this practice help teach the patient the correct way to handle objects safely, but the activity can be graded so the patient gradually increases the amount of weight lifted and learns what he or she can and cannot handle. In the functional practice different size objects should be used, such as a box, suitcase, laundry basket, and grocery bag. Differing amounts of weight can be added or subtracted according to the patient's tolerance for the particular activity. For any patients who were injured on the job the carrying and lifting practice results are important information for the employer or the insurance agency. The information in many cases may determine whether the patient may return to the former occupation or not.

Functional practice of body mechanics can also be carried out in a "par course." This is a set of activities put together in an orderly sequence that the therapist asks the patient to perform. Many times this activity lends itself to videotaping and can be used for comparative testing before and after treatment. Depending on the purpose of the par course activity, a sequence of tasks are combined which requires a variety of body mechanic techniques. For example, the par course may start with the patient going to a cupboard or shelf and reaching for a few items, putting them into a box or sack, carrying it to a table, and setting it down. Then the patient may be asked to sweep paper shreds and pick the debris up in a dustpan.

Any combination of activities can be put together. Generally patients like this type of activity because it is not repetitive, it simulates real situations, and it sparks some interest. Functional practice activities are usually designed and administered by the occupational therapist, especially since so many of the activities are actual or simulations of ADL.

To include job simulation as part of the treatment program, special equipment and space may be needed. If the occupational therapy department serves a large number of worker's compensation cases, the work simulation may be an integral part of the program. Providing accurate, relevant, and well-documented data to an employer or insurance carrier is important in helping to determine the feasibility of return to employment. Simple job simulations can be devised for some people. For example, for a secretary, it would be easy to set up a situation in which the patient can type, file, and answer phones. However, some of the manual, heavy labor occupations entail more sophisticated equipment and space than is available in many facilities. Since work simulation in some cases is vital, the patient may have to be referred to another agency for a thorough work evaluation assessment.

Work hardening and functional capacity evaluation are terms more commonly used today, especially in clinics or hospitals that service large numbers of worker-compensation or work-related back injuries. Work hardening, according to Blakenship, is a systematic program of gradually progressive work-related activities performed with proper body mechanics, which reconditions the person's musculoskeletal, cardiorespiratory, and psychomotor systems to prepare that person for return to work.[2] The work hardening program may take days or weeks to accomplish the end results.

The functional capacity evaluation is an intensive systematic evaluation process that determines a worker's physical ability to perform work.[2] There are standard tests that may be given and specialized equipment, such as West and Valpar, to augment the process. This evaluation is done in the course of 1 day, and results are sent to the physician and/or employer stating the return to work potential for the individual tested.

PSYCHOLOGICAL SUPPORT. The approach that a therapist takes with low back pain patients will set the atmosphere for the entire treatment environment. A direct, honest, and sincere approach is always best. A therapist should strive always to inform the patient about any procedure in which the patient is about to become involved. Sharing with the patient why a certain task or procedure is about to be undertaken and

relating it specifically to his or her condition will help alleviate the patient's apprehension, fear, or mistrust. This is especially true with those patients experiencing chronic low back pain. A therapist should not make promises of eliminating a patient's pain. A better approach to take is one that acknowledges the presence of the pain but focuses more on the functional goals and improvements. In dealing with patients with chronic pain a therapist may have to discourage the patient's "pain behavior," such as talking incessantly about the pain, holding back with every movement, or moaning and grimacing. Generally if the therapist is sincere and honest, the patients will respond with cooperation and trust.

In the treatment plan for a patient with low back pain psychological support is vital. Many times patients will exhibit anger, frustration, depression, and low self-esteem. Depending on the extent of these symptoms, a psychologist or psychiatrist may be dealing with the patient. Engaging the person in leisure time activities or crafts, however, can do much to improve the outlook and feelings about him or herself. The occupational therapist can structure activities for the patient which are at a level that he or she can handle and which will provide him or her with a challenge so the patient has a feeling of accomplishment and self-worth. If a department has a workshop or craft area available, this is an ideal setting to allow patients with low back pain to participate in crafts. It is especially beneficial if two or more patients can work together while making crafts, because interaction and socialization will occur.

Recreational therapy through the use of leisure activities can play an equally important part in the psychological support of individuals. Socialization, interaction, and accomplishment of a project all contribute to a patient's feelings of self-worth.

Group or individual counseling sessions may be conducted with patients who are experiencing chronic low back pain and who are exhibiting anger, frustration, and depression. However, trained personnel, such as a psychiatrist or psychologist, should be involved in these sessions. Family members may be encouraged to attend these or similar sessions to help them cope with the changes the patient and the family are experiencing.

Family members may also become involved in the educational process if time, circumstances, and situations allow this or if special sessions for family education can be established. Helping the family understand the anatomy and mechanisms of the spine will enhance their understanding of what a loved one might be encountering and may prevent another back problem in the family.

PAIN MODULATION. Pain modulation or pain reduction may be another part of the treatment program for the patient with low back pain. Any increase, decrease, or elimination of medications is handled by the physician, but it is important for other team members to be aware of this so they can be alerted to any changes in behavior which might indicate a drug reaction. With proper training and preparation therapists may become involved in pain reduction or modulation through the modalities of biofeedback, TENS, and relaxation. These can all be used in conjunction with other phases of the treatment program.

Progression of Treatment

When to start a patient on certain phases of the treatment program and when to progress the patient in his or her activities once he or she is on a full treatment program are decisions based on the physician's recommendations, the therapist's knowledge, and the individual's performance. When a patient is in the acute stages of low back disability, the activities are limited and often the patient is resting in bed and in so much pain that even the educational phase of treatment will be of no benefit. At this stage rest and control of the pain are the primary objectives of the treatment program. The patient with chronic pain has different treatment goals. This person generally is not resting in bed but has been on limited activities for an extended period of time, and to start the patient on a full treatment program may be detrimental. Once a physician has permitted the patient to participate in activities, the therapist must pay close attention and progress the patient at a slow, steady pace. Many of the therapist's clues to treatment progression will be given by the patient, and an alert, observant therapist will watch for the clues and grade the activities accordingly. For example, if a therapist is asking the patient to walk a certain distance and the first day the patient completes the task he or she is flushed, out of breath, and complaining of increased pain, the program should not be progressed and perhaps the activity level should be reduced. If on the third or fourth day, however, the patient completes the task with no increased symptoms and does not appear flushed or breathless, then perhaps the patient is ready to progress. When using weights in strengthening activities, progressive resistive exercise programs (PRE) are the safest for patients with low back pain. When a patient has successfully completed a maximal amount of weight on the PRE method, the therapist can ask the patient to try a few more repetitions at the maximal amount of weight. If the patient succeeds in completing 10 more repetitions at his or her maximal amount of weight, then it is time

for the patient to progress to a higher weight limit. This type of progression can apply to any activity, even if it does not involve weight lifting. For example, if the patient has been riding on a stationary bicycle at 1 speed for 5 minutes with no difficulty and has even been increasing the mileage, the therapist can grade the program by increasing one of the parameters. In this case the therapist would probably increase the time and later the amount of resistance.

In any activities that are done with the patient it will be helpful to record and obtain as much objective data as possible, because the data give an accurate picture of the patient's performance. For example, with an endurance walk activity the course should be measured for distance, and the patient and therapist should keep account of the number of laps the former does in a specified amount of time. On a stationary bicycle resistance, time, and mileage can all be recorded. On a treadmill incline, speed, and time are the available parameters.

By carefully progressing patients in their programs there should be no aggravation of pain and little muscle soreness. By meticulously progressing patients the therapist will instill confidence while allowing good habits and techniques to become ingrained.

Body Mechanic Techniques

Posture is the basic foundation of all good body mechanics. As stated earlier, the spine is composed of a column of vertebrae, which is a curved column rather than a straight one. The curves serve a purpose and provide strength to the column. Therefore for proper alignment of the spine and good posture, it is important that these curves be maintained. Since the purpose of this chapter is to discuss low back pain, the focus of attention will be on the lumbar spine.

The lumbar spine withstands the most stresses. It supports the weight of the body and allows several motions to occur. The lumbar spine is also the most vulnerable area because it does not have the same ligamentous support as the other areas of the spine. Therefore it is especially important to be aware of the curves in the lumbar area. Any exaggeration of the curve contributes additional stresses to the structures of the lumbar area.

For proper posture one must be aware of the curves in the spine and the factors that influence these curves. The position of the pelvis plays an important role in the curves of the low back. By rotating the pelvis forward and backward, the lumbar curve is increased and decreased. Flexibility of the muscles in the lumbar, pelvic, and lower extremities is another factor that influences the curve of the lumbar spine. For example, tight hamstring muscles exert a pull on the pelvis which results in a flattening of the lumbar curve. The amount of weight an individual carries and the condition of the abdominal muscles are still other factors that can influence the lumbar curve. Finally it is important to remember that the body is a system of interrelated and connecting parts and that movement or position of one structure is likely to influence the position of another structure. This holds true in the back and extremities. For example, by flexing the knees and hip joints, the pelvis is influenced, which affects the low back. Likewise raising the arms above shoulder level changes the center of gravity and changes the curve in the low back. Even the height of the heel on a shoe can affect the lumbar curve. Keeping these facts in mind, Figs. 30-3 to 30-8 and the boxed material on p. 548 demonstrate basic principles for posture and body mechanics.

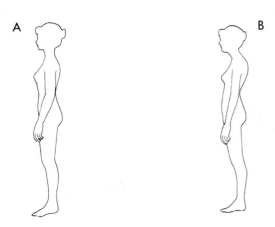

Fig. 30-3. Standing. **A,** Correct. **B,** Incorrect.

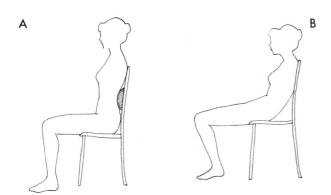

Fig. 30-4. Sitting. **A,** Correct. **B,** Incorrect.

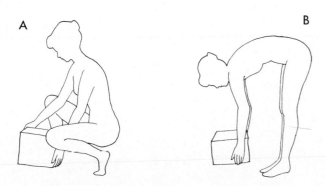

Fig. 30-5. Lifting. **A,** Correct. **B,** Incorrect.

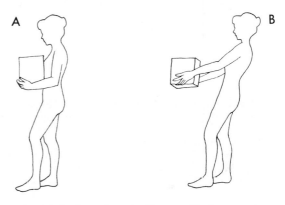

Fig. 30-6. Carrying. **A,** Correct. **B,** Incorrect.

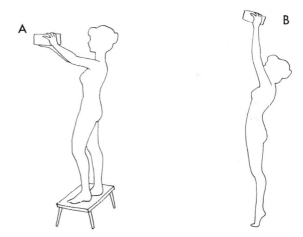

Fig. 30-7. Reaching. **A,** Correct. **B,** Incorrect.

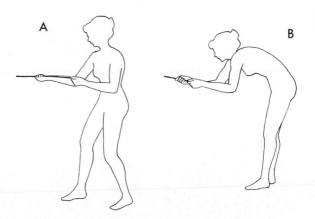

Fig. 30-8. Pulling. **A,** Correct. **B,** Incorrect.

Correct posture for body mechanic techniques

Standing posture (Fig. 30-3)	Stomach should be flat. With a plumb line dropped all curves must transect the line to be gravity balanced. Observe the spine and check that the curves are not exaggerated.
Prolonged standing posture	Avoid prolonged standing, especially in shoes with a high heel. Move about and stretch whenever possible. Use a footstool to prop one foot on from time to time.
Sitting posture (Fig. 30-4)	Avoid prolonged sitting. Get up every 45 minutes to stretch in the opposite direction. Use a lumbar support in the chair to maintain the lumbar curve. Use a footstool as an alternative to lumbar support.
Lying posture	Lie on one side. When lying on the back, put pillows under the knees.
Principles for lifting (Fig. 30-5)	Feet should have a wide base of support. Squat and bend the knees, not the back. Lift with the legs. Tighten the abdominal muscles. Avoid twisting. Keep object close. Be sure the lumbar curve is present.
Carrying (Fig. 30-6)	Carry the object close to you. Use the arms and carry at waist level. Avoid torquing or twisting movements. Check to be sure lumbar curve is present.
Reaching (Fig. 30-7)	Avoid reaching above the shoulders without taking precautions. Use a footstool or ladder when possible. Rearrange an area so you do not have to reach across a desk or cabinet for commonly used items.
Pushing	Push instead of pull when possible. Use mechanical devices to help push heavy or large items. Push with legs or entire body to break the inertia.
Pulling (Fig. 30-8)	Avoid pulling an object if possible. Keep the knees partially bent. Maintain a wide base of support. Shift the body weight to give extra pull. Do not pull with the back muscles. Try to keep the lumbar curve present.

Sample treatment plan

The following treatment plan is modeled after the program at Saint Francis Memorial Hospital in San Francisco, in which back rehabilitation is a team effort between occupational and physical therapies. This treatment plan is merely an example and would not be suitable for any and every patient with low back pain. Each patient needs to be evaluated and then be the recipient of a treatment plan designed specifically to meet his or her needs.

CASE STUDY

Mr. M is a 29-year-old single man who was injured on the job 2 years ago. When he was lifting a 50-pound box, he lost his balance and felt a pull in his low back. Subsequently he underwent two lumbar laminectomies, one 3 months following his injury and the other one 6 months ago. Currently he continues to complain of pain in his right lower back and complains that he is unable to function and be as active as he was before his injury. His diagnosis is low back strain.

Mr. M is a picture framer and would like to return to work. He enjoys fishing, skiing, and basketball and he wants to be able to engage in these sports again.

He was referred to an inpatient back rehabilitation program. The goals were to improve ROM, flexibility, strength, endurance, and body mechanics and to restore him to his maximal level of independence so that he can resume his former work and leisure roles.

TREATMENT PLAN

Personal data

Name: Mr. M
Age: 29
Diagnosis: Low back strain
Disability: Constant pain in lower right back; decreased functional capabilities
Treatment aims as stated in referral: Restoration to maximal functional independence through increased ROM and flexibility; improved strength and endurance; and participation in proper body mechanics in self-care, work, and leisure activities

OTHER SERVICES

Physician: Prescribe treatment, modalities, and any medication if necessary; supervise rehabilitation services
Nursing: Assist inpatient's orientation to nursing floor; administer medications; reinforce and follow through with body mechanic techniques in patient's ADL
Psychiatrist: Evaluate patient's psychological status; recommend any medication.
Physical therapy: Evaluate physical potential of patient; strengthen lower extremities; increase endurance in conjunction with occupational therapy
Social worker: Explore financial problems; help family and patient adjust to hospital setting; provide support, education, and encouragement to family members
Family: Provide support and encouragement to the patient
Recreational therapy: Provide leisure time activities to help improve patient's self-esteem and decrease depression

Vocational rehabilitation: Explore feasibility of return to present occupation or explore new job possibilities and retraining

FRAME OF REFERENCE

Occupational performance

TREATMENT APPROACHES

Biomechanical, Rehabilitative, Educational

OT EVALUATION

Performance components

Motor functioning
  Muscle strength: Test
  Passive and active ROM: Test
  Physical endurance: Test, observe UE and LE
  Standing tolerance: Observe, interview
  Walking tolerance: Observe, interview
  Sitting tolerance: Observe, interview
  Lifting tolerance: Test, observe, interview
  Carrying tolerance: Test, observe, interview
  Functional movement patterns: Observe body mechanics
Sensory integrative functioning
Sensation (touch): Test
Cognitive functioning
Judgment: Observe for correct use of body mechanics
Safety awareness: Observe
Psychological functioning
Adjustment to disability: Observe, interview
Coping skills: Observe
Self-identity: Observe, interview
Social functioning
Interpersonal skills: Observe with family and peers

Performance skills

Self-care
Observe, interview
Work/work-related skills
Work habits and attitudes: Interview
Potential work skills: Interview, possibly test; referral
Work tolerance: Test if ordered or indicated; refer to appropriate agency
Home management: Observe, interview
Play/leisure
Interview

EVALUATION SUMMARY

Muscle testing revealed that strength was normal throughout except for right ankle dorsiflexion and right extensor hallucis longus; both were graded as fair plus (F+)

Patient demonstrates limited ROM in trunk flexion, trunk extension, and lateral flexion; all are limited to within one-half normal range on the right and three-fourths normal range on the left. Trunk rotation is limited to one-half normal range on the right and three-fourths normal range on the left. He experiences an increase of pain with these motions. LE limitations include right straight leg raise of 0° to 45°, left straight leg raise of 0° to 90°, right hip flexion of 0° to 100°, and right hip abduction of 0° to 50°

Further physical endurance skills were evaluated as follows:

Continued.

Sample treatment plan—cont'd.

Lifting: Patient is able to lift 10 pounds (4.5 kg) from 0 to 36 inches (0 cm to 91.4 cm) and 36 inches to 72 inches (91.4 cm to 182.8 cm) with only a "pulling" sensation.

Carrying: Patient is able to carry 10 pounds (4.5 kg) for 5 minutes for 323 feet (98.4 meters) with no complaints of pain

LE weights: Patient is able to extend leg with 75-pound (34-kg) weights and hold a 90° static quadriceps set for 12 seconds.

UE weights: Patient is able to flex elbow with 15-pound (6.8-kg) weight, depress scapula with 20-pound (9.1-kg) weights, and flex shoulder with 45-pound (20.4-kg) weights

Treadmill: Patient able to walk 1.5 mph for 10 minutes with no aggravation of pain

Stationary bicycle: Patient is able to resist with 3.3 pounds (1.5 kg) for 2 miles in 15 minutes but experienced right leg pain

Endurance walk: Patient is able to walk 947 feet (328 meters) in 30 minutes with some stopping because of pain

Sensory testing reveals no deficits in LEs.

Patient is independent but guarded in dressing and sink activities. He complains of pain when donning shoes and socks and demonstrated poor body mechanics with these activities. He has difficulty with sweeping, vacuuming, and mopping and used poor body mechanics. Outdoor tasks and driving are not attempted, since in the past they have aggravated his pain. He further demonstrates improper body mechanics when sitting and when moving from a sitting to standing position. His standing posture demonstrates increased lordosis with head jutting forward.

The patient complains of constant burning pain in his right lower back. The pain is aggravated by prolonged standing and is relieved somewhat by lying down. The patient intermittently wears a back brace. He has attempted to return to work but has to take time off or quit because of pain. He lives by himself; when not working he does daily chores and watches television.

Patient expresses some anger at his insurance company. He is pleasant, but withdrawn, and has lost social contact with many of his friends.

ASSETS

Expresses desire to get better
Expresses desire to return to work
No exhibition of muscle atrophy or gross loss of strength
Limitation in ROM because of inactivity; no bony problems
Young
Cooperative; appears motivated to follow treatment program

PROBLEM LIST

1. Constant pain in right low back
2. Some limitation in ROM
3. Slight decrease in strength
4. Low lifting and carrying capabilities
5. Poor endurance

6. Improper body mechanics
7. Some display of anger, withdrawal, low self-esteem
8. Change or loss in vocational role

PROBLEM 1

Pain
Objective

Given appropriate modalities, pain will be modulated or reduced so that patient can increase functional activities and return to work

Method

Trial use of TENS for pain modulation

Biofeedback to aid the patient's ability to relax, thereby reducing pain

Teach patient several relaxation methods: may include progressive relaxation, visualization techniques, or a form of meditation. Stress-reduction techniques such as energy conservation and time management may also be instructed

Gradation

Start and use TENS as needed for pain relief; may be weaned from device as pain decreases

Daily biofeedback training until patient can maintain a relaxed state for 5 minutes; increase time to 20 minutes

Daily trials and practice of various relaxation techniques until find one that is effective and can maintain a state of relaxation for 5 minutes; increase time to 20 minutes

PROBLEM 1, 2

Pain, decreased ROM and flexibility
Objective

ROM will increase and pain will be reduced so that normal ROM is attained in the LEs
Method

Occupational or physical therapist to instruct patient in low back exercises for trunk mobility, hamstring stretching, and hip flexibility; exercises are as follows:

1. Lumbar rotation: Patient supine, both knees bent, head and shoulders on mat; bring both knees to the right by rotating the pelvis; repeat on left side
2. Double knee to chest: Patient supine with both knees bent; bring right knee to chest, hold with right hand; bring left knee to chest, hold with left hand; lift head up toward knees, hold for 5 seconds; lower head and legs one at a time to mat
3. Straight-leg stretch: Patient supine, one leg bent, one leg straight out on mat; bend straight leg toward chest, straighten and lift as high as possible without bending knee; tilt toes toward nose, hold for 5 seconds and return; repeat with other leg
4. Pelvic roll: Patient supine, one leg bent, one leg straight, head and shoulders on mat; bring bent knee toward straight leg by rotating pelvis (keep foot on mat); hold for 5 seconds, return to starting position; repeat with other leg
5. Back extension: Patient prone, elbows bent, hands by shoulders; slowly push up with arms to a position that can be tolerated; hold for 5 seconds

Gradation

Start with 5 repetitions for each exercise unless exercise aggravates pain; repetitions increased 1 per day until a total of 10 is reached; progression holds for all of the five exercises

Continued.

Sample treatment plan—cont'd.

If pain at certain level, decrease number of repetitions and maintain a lower level for several days

PROBLEM 3

Decreased strength

Objective

Abdominal strength will improve so patient will be able to complete 20 sit-ups with ease; LE strength will improve so patient can do 15 exercise repetitions with ease

Method

Occupational or physical therapist to instruct patient in exercises to strengthen abdominal and LE muscles; exercises that may be used:

1. Pelvic tilt with sliding legs: Patient supine, both knees bent; tilt pelvis backward; flatten back against mat; slowly straighten legs down to the mat to a count of 5; *must* be able to maintain pelvic tilt throughout the exercise; if unable, straighten legs only to the point that the pelvic tilt can be maintained
2. Partial sit-up: Patient supine, both knees bent, arms straight in front, tuck chin in, sit up toward knees only enough to clear head and upper back from mat; hold for 5 seconds
3. Diagonal sit-up: Patient supine, both knees bent, arms straight in front; sit up toward right side enough to clear head and upper back from mat; hold for 5 seconds
4. Quad sets/straight-leg raise: Patient supine, one knee bent, one leg straight; tighten thigh muscle on the straight leg to set the quadriceps muscle; while holding the set lift leg straight up about 6 inches (15.2 cm) from mat; hold for 5 seconds; return to start position; repeat with other leg
5. Hip abduction: Patient lying on one side, bottom leg slightly bent forward; lift top leg up toward ceiling; hold for 5 seconds; return; repeat with other leg

Gradation

Start at 5 repetitions and increase 1 each day until reach 20 sit-ups and 15 LE exercise repetitions

If pain at certain level, decrease number of repetitions, and maintain at lower level for several days

For quad sets/straight-leg raise and hip abduction, add cuff weight at ankle for more resistance when patient can do 15 repetitions with ease; start patient at 10 repetitions with new weight

PROBLEM 4

Low lifting and carrying capability

Objective

Ability to lift weight with arms will increase from 10 pounds (22 kg) to 20 pounds (44 kg) and individual weight exercises will increase by 20%

Method

Occupational or physical therapist to instruct patient in any or all of the following UE strengthening exercises:

1. Curls (elbow flexion): With long-weight bar patient to stand against a wall, pelvis tilted, back flat against wall, feet 12 inches (30.5 cm) to 15 inches (38.1 cm) away from wall, arms at sides with elbows bent; on receiving the bar patient to flex arms toward chest and then slowly return arms to sides

2. Bench press (shoulder flexion and pectoralis major and minor): If bench press equipment available use equipment, otherwise long-weight bar sufficient; patient supine on mat, arms at sides, elbows bent 90°; therapist to hand weight bar to patient, asks patient to push straight up into full elbow extension and 90° shoulder flexion; hold for 5 seconds, slowly return to starting position

Gradation

PRE method of exercise used for the following strengthening exercises; determine the patient's maximal weight at 10 repetitions

When patient can comfortably perform the progressive method for 1 maximum, ask patient to do several more repetitions at the same maximum; if can comfortably handle the increased repetitions, progress him to a new level; if cannot do 10 repetitions, have him continue at the current level

PROBLEM 5

Poor endurance

Objective

General endurance will improve and work tolerance will increase to 4 hours

Method

Use activities such as endurance walk, stationary bicycle, treadmill, and stair climbing

Patient to start any of these activities until notices an aggravation of pain or until reaches level of endurance exhibited by shortness of breath, perspiration, flushing, or fatigue

Gradation

Progress patient at own pace; use as many parameters, such as distance, time, and weight

When patient ready to progress, increase only one parameter at a time; for example, all activities can be timed, to progress patient increase amount of time spent on the activity

PROBLEM 4, 6

Low lifting and carrying capabilities; improper body mechanics

Objective

Body mechanic techniques will improve so that proper body mechanics are used consistently in ADL and simulated work tasks

Method

Occupational or physical therapist to instruct back anatomy class, providing a foundation for later body mechanics teaching

Occupational therapist to instruct principles of body mechanics

Occupational therapist to provide practical application of body mechanic principles by having patient try activities such as standing, sitting, lying, lifting, carrying, and reaching posture; and ADL such as dressing, hygiene, vacuuming, sweeping, and washing windows

Patient to run through a "par course" of activities, such as carrying a bag of groceries, unloading the groceries on varying shelf heights, sweeping a floor, and washing dishes

Continued.

Sample treatment plan—cont'd.

Gradation

Provide 30- to 45-minute sessions for classes; use variety of media if possible

In teaching posture techniques, start with standing posture; progress to sitting and lying; instruct in dynamic postures for lifting, carrying, and reaching

Start with demonstration, progress to patient participation; use as many real situations as possible

PROBLEM 7

Display of anger, withdrawal, low self-esteem

Objective

Anger, depression, and low self-esteem will decrease and interaction with others will increase so that patient expresses less anger and displays a more positive attitude half of the time

Method

Use a supportive, honest approach with patient; explain procedures carefully and thoroughly

Workshop activities of woodburning, leather crafts, and mosaics to improve self-esteem; socialization and expression encouraged in group situations

During workshop activities or recreational therapy, sitting and standing tolerances can be observed and recorded

Gradation

Simple, short-term crafts that the patient can accomplish easily and quickly; interact with patient

Progress to more difficult crafts, being sure to structure the activity of success

Patient to perform activities in a group situation

PROBLEM 8

Change or loss of vocational role

Objective

Given selected activities, physical tolerance and capabilities will be documented and aid determination of feasability of future employment

Method

Give patient task, such as woodburning during workshop time; patient to stand while working on project; observe patient and record amount of standing time tolerated

While patient engages in a craft activity and is sitting, observe and record the amount of time patient able to sit comfortably

Provide patient with variety of lifting and carrying situations: for example, carry a weighted box for a given distance and lift a weighted box to various heights

Patient to lift weighted tool box from floor to 36 inches (91.4 cm) and then to a shelf at 72 inches (183 cm)

Patient to carry a weighted toolbox for a given period of time and set distance

Patient to lift and carry different sizes and shapes of wood or other objects, such as long but light-weight objects and bulky objects

Gradation

Encourage patient to gradually increase standing time; patient to try using a footstool and varying work heights while standing

Encourage patient to gradually increase sitting tolerance; patient to try different types of chairs, lumbar supports, work heights, and angles

Patient to lift and carry to tolerance; amount of weight gradually increased as strength and endurance improve

Patient to start lifting and carrying objects that are easily manageable; progress to more awkward sizes and shapes

---

REVIEW QUESTIONS

1. List three risk factors that may contribute to the incidence of low back pain.
2. Name the major components of the spine.
3. Explain the mechanism of an intervertebral disk.
4. List the four areas of assessment which the therapist evaluates on an individual with low back pain.
5. What are some of the problems that a person with chronic low back pain encounters?
6. List five possible treatment phases for a patient suffering from low back pain.
7. How is an individual progressed when on a treatment program?
8. What is the foundation for good body mechanics?
9. List the principles of proper body mechanics for lifting, carrying, reaching, pushing, and pulling.
10. In a team environment what other disciplines might be seeing or treating the person with low back pain?

REFERENCES

1. Anderson GBJ, editor: Symposium: low back pain in industry, Spine 6:52, 1981.
2. Blankenship KL: Functional capacity evaluation, seminar presented San Francisco, May 14-16, 1987.
3. Cailliet R: Low back pain syndrome, Philadelphia, 1982, FA Davis Co.
4. Finneson B: Low back pain, ed 2, Philadelphia, 1980, JB Lippincott Co.
5. Frymoyer JW et al: Risk factors in low back pain J Bone Joint Surg 65A:213, 1983.
6. Keim HA: Low back pain, vol 2, Summit, NJ, 1973, CIBA Pharmaceutical Co.
7. Lappen AA: Oh, my aching back, Forbes 137:102, February 24, 1986.
8. Mines S: The conquest of pain, New York, 1974, Grosset & Dunlap, Inc.
9. Toufexis A: That aching back, New York, 1974, Grosset & Dunlap, Inc.
10. Trigiano LL: Treatment of chronic pain, paper presented at International Congress on Natural Medicine, Rome, March 25, 1983.

31 Hip fractures and total hip replacement

KAREN PITBLADDO
ELIZABETH MARIA BIANCHI
SHERI L. LIEBERMAN
JAN POLON NOVIC
HELEN BOBROVE

The occupational therapist plays a key role in defining and remediating the many functional problems imposed by both acute and chronic orthopedic conditions, thus sharing in the goal of returning the orthopedic patient to optimal performance of safe and independent daily living activities.

This chapter discusses hip fractures and total hip replacement, their medical and surgical management, the psychological implications of hospitalization and disability, and the health care team-approach in an acute hospital setting.

FRACTURES

It is important for the therapist working with orthopedic patients to have a good understanding of the site, type, and cause of the fracture before starting treatment. A basic understanding of fracture healing and medical management is also necessary to appreciate risks, precautions, and complications involved.

Fractures occur in bone when the bone's ability to absorb tension, compression, or shearing forces is exceeded. Fractures are classified according to the type of fracture sustained and the direction of the fracture line[4] (Fig. 31-1).

Fracture Healing

Grossly, bone tissue occurs as cancellous or cortical. Cancellous or spongy bone surrounds spaces filled with bone marrow in the metaphysis of long bones and in the bodies of short bones and the flat bones of the pelvis and ribs. Cortical or compact bone is on the outer surface of the bone, giving it strength. It is covered with periosteum, and the inner surface is lined with endosteum.[4]

The authors extend their appreciation to Karen Donaldson, OTR, for the illustrations and to Susan Sitko, RPT, and Annie Affleck, MA, OTR, for their consultations.

At the time of fracture blood vessels are torn across the fracture site, causing bleeding then clotting; this situation is called a fracture hematoma. The repair cells or osteogenic cells form an internal and external callus from the endosteum and periosteum respectively.[4] This callus begins to form from the time of injury, and its maturation rate is dependent upon the specific bone that is fractured. Primary woven bone is initially formed from osteoblasts and eventually matures through the action of osteoclasts and osteoblasts into compact or cortical bone. With maturation of the fracture comes bone stability, which is termed *union*.[4,8] Immobilization is required throughout this maturation period. In some cases additional protection may be necessary to confirm maturation of the callus.

The fracture matures many months later when excess callus is reabsorbed and the bone returns to almost its normal diameter. Remodeling of bone occurs in response to physical stress referred to as Wolff's law.[8] Bone is deposited in sites where there is stress, such as weight bearing, and reabsorbed where there is little stress.

Cancellous bone is structurally different from cortical bone, so the healing process differs. The internal callus plays a greater role in forming primary woven bone; because of greater blood supply and larger surface area, healing occurs more rapidly.

As a result of the lack of blood supply, articular cartilage cannot regenerate into hyaline cartilage but instead forms fibrous tissue and fibrocartilage. This form of scar tissue cannot withstand normal wear-and-tear stresses. If the structural change is significant, degenerative changes may develop.[4]

The time required for fracture healing varies with the age of the patient, site and configuration of the fracture, initial displacement of the bone, and the blood supply to the fragments. The fracture healing may be abnormal in one of three ways: a bony deformity develops (called a malunion), the healing pro-

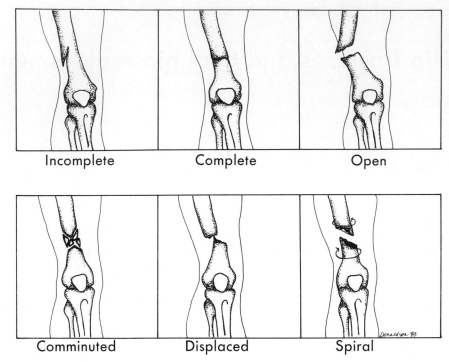

| Incomplete | Complete | Open |
| Comminuted | Displaced | Spiral |

Fig. 31-1. Types of fractures. Modified from Gartland JJ: Fundamentals of orthopaedics, Philadelphia, 1979, WB Saunders Co.

cess takes longer than normal (called a delayed union), or the fracture fails to heal (called a nonunion).

Etiology of Fractures

Trauma is the major cause of fractures. The force may be transmitted directly or through torsion. A forceful muscle contraction may also break a bone, as in certain patella fractures. Stress fractures occur when bone fatigues from repeated loading, as seen in some metatarsal fractures. Osteoporosis, a type of metabolic bony atrophy, is a common bone disease of people over 65 years of age. It involves mostly the vertebral bodies and cancellous metaphyses of the neck of the femur, humerus, and distal end of the radius. Because the bone becomes porous and thereby fragile, the affected bones are prone to fracture. A pathological fracture can occur because of a bone weakened by disease or tumor. This can occur in diseases, such as osteomyelitis and lytic tumors of bone caused by deposition of metastatic carcinoma.[4]

Medical Management

The aims of fracture treatment are to relieve pain, maintain good position of the fracture, allow for bony union for fracture healing, and restore optimal function to the patient.[8] Occupational therapy provides a significant role in the restoration of function of the

patient; that role will be discussed later in this chapter.

Reduction of a fracture refers to restoring the fragments to normal alignment.[4] This can be done by a closed procedure (manipulation) or by an open procedure (surgery). A closed reduction is performed by applying a force to the displaced bone opposite to the force that produced the fracture. Depending on the nature of the fracture, the reduction is maintained in a cast, cast brace, skin traction, skeletal traction, or skeletal fixation.

With open reduction the fracture site is exposed surgically so that the fragments can be aligned. The fragments are held in place with internal fixation by pins, screws, a plate, nails, or a rod. Further immobilization by a cast or a cast brace may be necessary. Usually an open reduction and internal fixation (ORIF) must be protected from excessive forces, so weight-bearing restrictions are indicated.[5] In the hip fracture the articular fragment of the hip may need to be removed and replaced by a prosthesis called an endoprosthesis. This is necessary when there are complications of avascular necrosis, nonunion, or degenerative joint disease.

Hip Fractures

A knowledge of hip anatomy is necessary to understand medical management of hip fractures. The

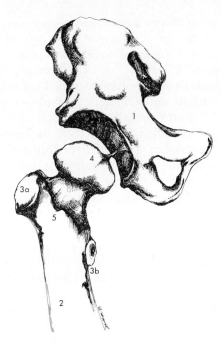

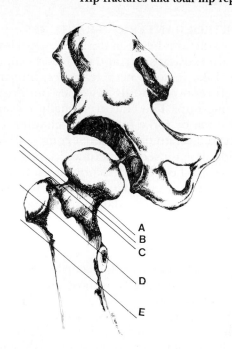

Fig. 31-2. Normal hip anatomy. *1*, Acetabulum; *2*, femur; *3a*, greater trochanter; *3b*, lesser trochanter; *4*, ligamentum teres; *5*, intertrochanteric crest. Modified from Crouch JE: Functional human anatomy, ed 3, Philadelphia, 1978, Lea & Febiger; and Grant LC: Grant's atlas of anatomy, ed 6, Baltimore, 1972, Williams & Wilkins.

Fig. 31-3. Levels of femoral fracture. *A*, Subcapital; *B*, transcervical: *C*, basilar; *D*, intertrochanteric; *E*, subtrochanteric. Modified from Crow I: Fracture of the hip: a self study, ONA J 5:12, 1978.

articular capsule of the hip joint refers to the dense connective tissue enclosing the joint. It provides stability and assists with hip motion. The capsule extends from the margins of the acetabulum downward anteriorly to the intertrochanteric ridge and posteriorly to the middle of the neck. The greater trochanter serves as the point of attachment for the hip abductors; gluteus minimus, gluteus medius, and external rotators; piriformis; gemellus; and obturators. The iliopsoas tendon, a hip flexor, attaches to the lesser trochanter. Blood supply to the femoral head is via the ligamentum teres, capsular vessels, and vessels from the femoral shaft (Fig. 31-2).

The levels of fracture lines are shown in Fig. 31-3. The names of the fractures generally reflect site and severity of injury. These terms are frequently indicators of which medical treatment will be used. For example, femoral neck fracture will be treated with femoral neck stabilization.

FEMORAL NECK FRACTURES. Femoral neck fractures are common in adults over 60 years old and occur more frequently in women. The bone is osteoporotic, and only slight trauma or rotational force causes the fracture.[2] Treatment of a displaced fracture in this area is complicated by poor blood supply, the osteoporotic bone that is not suited to hold metallic

fixation, and the thin periosteum limiting fracture healing. The type of surgical treatment used is based on the amount of displacement and the circulation in the femoral head.

The age and health of the patient are of course considered in deciding on the surgical procedure. Generally hip-pinning or use of a compression screw and plate is employed when displacement is minimal to moderate and blood supply is intact. With a physician's approval a patient is usually able to begin out-of-bed activities 2 to 4 days after surgery. Weight-bearing restrictions must be observed with the aid of crutches or a walker for at least 6 to 8 weeks while the fracture is healing. Limited weight bearing may be necessary beyond this time if precautions are not observed or delayed union occurs.[5]

With severe displacement or an avascular femoral head the femoral head is excised and replaced by an endoprosthesis. Several types of metal prostheses can be used; each has its own shape and advantages. Weight-bearing restrictions are sometimes indicated. Because of the surgical procedure used, precautions for positioning the hip must be observed to avoid dislocation. The precautions will vary according to the surgical approach used. Patients who have had a prosthesis implanted can usually begin out-of-bed activity with a physician's approval about 2 to 4 days after surgery.[5]

INTERTROCHANTERIC FRACTURES. Intertrochanteric fractures between the greater and lesser trochanter are extracapsular, and the blood supply is not affected. Like femoral neck fractures, intertrochanteric fractures occur mostly in women but in a slightly older age-group. The fracture usually is caused by direct trauma or force over the trochanter. ORIF is the preferred treatment. A nail or compression screw with a sideplate is used. Sometimes as long as 4- to 6-months weight-bearing restrictions must be observed when a patient is ambulating. Again the patient is allowed out of bed 2 to 4 days after surgery pending the physician's approval.[5]

SUBTROCHANTERIC FRACTURES. Subtrochanteric fractures 1 to 2 inches (2.5 cm to 5.0 cm) below the lesser trochanter usually occur because of direct trauma. These fractures are most often in younger people less than 60 years old. Skeletal traction followed by an ORIF is the usual treatment. A nail with a long sideplate or an intramedullary rod is used, and the condition may possibly require further immobilization after surgery.

Total Joint Replacement

Restoration of joint motion and treatment of pain by total hip replacement is sometimes indicated in osteoarthritis, rheumatoid arthritis, and ankylosing spondylitis. Osteoarthritis or degenerative joint disease may develop spontaneously in middle age and progress as the normal aging process of joints is exaggerated. It may also develop as the result of trauma, congenital deformity, or a disease that damages articular cartilage. Weight-bearing joints, such as the hip, knee, and lumbar spine, are usually affected. There is a loss of cartilage centrally on the joint surface and formation of osteophytes on the acetabulum, peripherally, producing joint incongruity. Pain arises from the bone, synovial membrane, fibrous capsule, and muscle spasm. When movement of the hip causes pain, the muscles are not normally used and shorten from disuse. The osteoarthritic hip may assume a flexed, adducted, and externally rotated position that also causes a painful limp.[9]

Ankylosing spondylitis, a chronic progressive polyarthritis, primarily involves the sacroiliac and spinal joints. The soft tissues eventually ossify, producing a bony ankylosis. The proximal joints of the extremities, particularly the hips, may be affected, which could also progress to bony ankylosis.[9]

Rheumatoid arthritis (covered in Chapter 27) is another type of arthritis which may involve the hip joint. Surgery is often performed early in the disease process to avoid fibrotic damage to joint and tendon structures.[9]

Total joint replacement or replacement arthroplasty may be necessary in various types of arthritis. This surgery is designed to alleviate pain and regain joint motion. There are two components to a "total hip." A high-density polyethylene socket is fitted into the acetabulum, and a metallic prosthesis replaces the femoral head and neck. Methylmethacrylate or bone-like cement fixes the components to the bone. Various surgical approaches are used according to the surgical skill or technique of the orthopedist, severity of the joint involvement and past surgery to the hip. With an anterolateral approach the patient will be unstable in external rotation, adduction, and extension of the operated hip and usually must observe precautions to prevent these movements for 6 to 12 weeks. If a posterolateral approach is used, the patient must be cautioned not to move the operated leg in specific ranges of flexion (usually 60° to 90°) and not to internally rotate or adduct the leg. Failure to maintain these precautions during muscle and soft tissue healing may result in hip dislocation. Most surgeons do not restrict weight bearing postoperatively when cement fixation is used. One of the major problems with total joint replacement is the loss of fixation at the prothesis interface. The most recent development is the use of biological fixation. This involves the use of bony ingrowth instead of cement, to secure the prosthesis. The precautions following the surgery are those of the anterior or posterior hip replacements with an additional restriction on weight bearing for 6 to 8 weeks. The restrictions on weight bearing will vary in terms of amount of pressure and length of time. A walking aid, usually a walker or crutches, is necessary for at least the first month while the hip is healing and muscles are becoming stronger.[9]

It is important to be aware of complications or special procedures that occurred during surgery. For example, a trochanteric osteotomy may have been necessary. In this case, if the greater trochanter was removed and rewired down, active abduction would be prohibited. Patients with total joint replacements usually begin out-of-bed activity 1 to 3 days after surgery.[6]

Total joint surface replacements, which are rarely used, are a variation of the total hip replacement.[4] The surface of the femur is capped by a metallic shell, and the acetabular cavity receives a plastic cup. Both are held in place by methylmethacrylate. This technique preserves the femoral head and neck. With this technique, no weight bearing restrictions apply.

PSYCHOLOGICAL FACTORS

Psychological issues are critical considerations in the overall treatment of the orthopedic patient. A large number of patients in this population are faced with either a chronic disability (such as rheumatoid arthritis), a life-threatening disease (such as cancer), or the aging process. Therefore loss or potential loss of physical ability is a predominant problem faced by most of these patients. This is a stressful process, requiring an enormous amount of physical and emotional energy.[7] Therefore an awareness of and a sensitivity toward the orthopedic patient is critical to the delivery of optimal patient care.

When dealing with this patient population the therapist must realize that each patient's experience of loss will depend on that patient's intrinsic makeup (personality, physical diseases, specific changes, or experience of body dissolution) and the environmental factors affecting the patient (personal losses or gains, family dynamics, or the home environment).[7] For example, the losses experienced by a young woman with rheumatoid arthritis would create an entirely different psychosocial picture than the losses experienced by an elderly man suffering from a fractured femur.

Those patients suffering from a chronic orthopedic disability often experience one or all of the following: body dissolution, deformity, disease of a body part, change in body image, decreased functional ability, and pain. The onset of these factors may occur at a relatively young age and often in rapid succession. Orthopedic patients often consider themselves prisoners of their own bodies, left with accumulated layers of unresolved grief, fatigue, and a sense of emptiness.[2] Thus when treating a patient with a chronic orthopedic disability, it is important to address these issues and provide the support needed for the mourning and grieving process to take place. Without an opportunity to resolve these conflicts, the patient becomes depressed, filled with guilt and anxiety, and paralyzed with fear. These emotions inhibit the patient's progress and enhance the development of poor self-image. Therapists can help reintegrate some of these conflicts, which will give the patient a feeling of accomplishment and pride, enhancing the treatment process.

The same holds true for the elderly patient dealing with disability. In addition to the issues just discussed, however, the elderly also face psychological issues specific to the aging process. The elderly patient often experiences the need to reflect on and review past life experiences.

This life review is conceived of as a naturally occurring universal mental process characterized by the progressive return to consciousness of past experiences, and particularly the resurgence of unresolved conflicts; simultaneously and normally, these revived experiences and conflicts are surveyed and reintegrated. It is assumed that this process is prompted by the realization of approaching dissolution and death.[1]

A second important issue experienced by the elderly, disabled individual is dependency. With the onset of a disability late in life the patient is forced to face the realities of the aging process and let go of years of independence and self-sufficiency.[7] For some this can be a devastating experience, but others use these negative changes to acquire benefits that are satisfying to them. Examples of this are patients who remain in the hospital because they enjoy the extra attention in contrast to those who use their illness to manipulate their support systems and avoid taking responsibility for themselves and others.

A third psychosocial phenomenon experienced by the aged when hospitalized is relocation trauma. This presents itself through confusion, emotional lability, and disorientatioin. Older people, when removed from their familiar environment, will often decompensate cognitively. Therefore it is important that their new environment be made as familiar as possible. Decorating it with familiar objects from the patient's home and providing the patient with a calendar and current newspapers and magazines are often helpful in reducing this traumatic effect.

Learning to cope and adjust to the changes resulting from chronic disability or the aging process is a critical part of patient treatment. Therapists must realize that a great deal of a patient's functional independence has been relinquished as a result of disease or disability. For this reason it is critical that the psychosocial issues resulting from these losses be addressed while focusing on increasing a patient's functional level of independence.

REHABILITATION MEASURES[6,9]

Good communication and clear role delineation among members of the health care team are essential for an efficient and smooth therapy program. The health care team usually consists of a primary physician, nursing staff, a physical therapist, an occupational therapist, a nutritionist, a pharmacist, a discharge planner, and possibly a social worker. Regular team meetings to discuss each patient's ongoing treatment, progress, and discharge plans are necessary to coordinate individual treatment programs. Members from each service usually attend to provide information and consultation.

The role of the physician is to inform the team of the patient's medical status. This includes information regarding a previous medical history, diagnosis of the present problem, complete account of the surgical procedure performed which would include the type of appliance inserted, the anatomical approach, and any movement or weight bearing precautions that could endanger the patient. The physician is also responsible for ordering specific medications and therapies. Any change or progression in therapy or changes in the patient's medication regime should be approved by the physician.

The nursing staff is responsible for the actual physical care of the patient during hospitalization. Responsibilities of the nurse include administering medications, assisting the patient with bathing and hygiene, and constant monitoring of vital signs and physical status. Each patient's blood pressure, pulse, and respiratory status are checked every 1 to 2 hours immediately after surgery.[6,9] During the rehabilitation phase, vital signs are usually checked once every 8 hours unless otherwise ordered by the physician.[6] Wound and skin care, such as the changing of dressings or the sterilization of wounds, are performed by the nurse. The orthopedic nurse must have a thorough understanding of the surgical procedures and movement precautions for each patient. Proper positioning using pillows, wedges, and ski boxes is carried out by the nurse, especially in the first few days following surgery. As the patient's therapy program progresses, the patient starts to take more responsibility for proper positioning and physical care. The nurse works closely with the physical and occupational therapists to help establish a self-care program that implements skills that the patient has already learned in therapy.[6,9]

The physical therapist is responsible for evaluation and treatment in the areas of musculoskeletal status, sensation, pain, skin integrity, and locomotion (especially gait). In many cases involving total hip replacements and surgical repair of hip fractures, physical therapy is initiated on the first day after surgery. The therapist obtains baseline information including range of motion (ROM), strength of all the extremities, muscle tone, mental status, and mobility, adhering to the prescribed precautions of protocol. A treatment program that includes therapeutic exercises, ROM activities, and progressive gait activities is established. The physical therapist is responsible for recommending the appropriate assistive device to be used during ambulation. As the patient's ambulation status advances, instructions in stair climbing, managing curbs, and outside ambulation are given.[6,9]

The nutritionist consults with each patient to assure that adequate and appropriate nutrition is received to aid the healing process, and the pharmacist monitors the patient's drug therapy and provides information and assistance with pain management.[6]

The role of the discharge planner is to assure that each patient is being discharged to the appropriate living situation or facility. Usually the discharge planner is a registered nurse with a thorough knowledge of community resources and nursing care facilities available. With input from the health care team the discharge planner makes the arrangements for ongoing therapy after hospitalization, for admission to a rehabilitation facility for further intensive therapy, or for nursing home care if necessary. The discharge planner works closely with the health care team and is instrumental in coordinating the program after the patient's discharge from the hospital.[6,9]

The Role of Occupational Therapy

Following a total hip replacement or surgical repair of a fractured hip, occupational therapy is usually initiated when the patient is ready to start learning the proper technique of getting out of bed. Occupational therapy is usually initiated 2 to 4 days after surgery. The average time varies depending on the age, general health, surgical events, and motivation of the individual patient. Before any physical evaluation, it is important for the therapist to introduce and explain the role of occupational therapy, establish a rapport, and then gather by interview any pertinent information regarding the patient's prior functional status, home environment, and living situation. The goal of occupational therapy is for the patient to return home independent in activities of daily living (ADL) with all movement precautions observed during activities. It is the role of the occupational therapist to teach the patient ways and means of performing ADL safely.[6,9]

A baseline physical evaluation is necessary to determine whether any physical limitations not related to surgery might prevent functional independence. Upper extremity (UE) ROM, muscle strength, sensation, coordination, and mental status are assessed before a functional evaluation is made. It is also important to consider the patient's pain and fear at rest and during movement. Occupational therapy is then a progression of functional activities that simulate a normal, daily regime of activity that is in accordance with all the movement precautions.[6,9] The reader should refer to the Medical Management section of this chapter for a review of the different prescribed precautions.

GUIDELINES FOR TRAINING[6,9]
Total hip replacement—anterolateral approach
POSITIONS OF HIP STABILITY: Flexion, abduction to neutral, and internal rotation
POSITIONS OF HIP INSTABILITY: abduction, external rotation, and excessive hyperextension
Bed mobility. It is recommended that the patient lie in bed in the supine position. The appropriate wedge and ski box

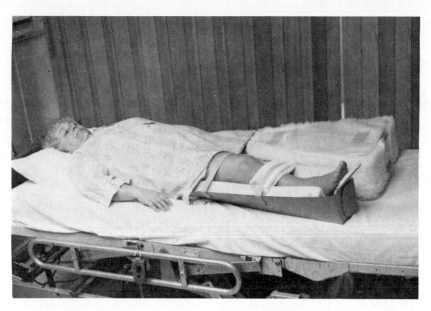

Fig. 31-4. Bed positioning with wedge and ski box.

should be in place (Fig. 31-4). It is not recommended that a patient sleep on the side, although it is possible for a patient to roll if the wedge is in place and the operated extremity is supported by someone to maintain hip abduction. The patient is instructed in getting out of bed on both sides, although initially it may be easier to observe precautions by moving toward the nonoperated leg. Careful instruction is given to avoid adduction past midline and to maintain the operated extremity in internal rotation.

Transfers. It is always helpful for the patient to first observe the proper technique for transfers.

CHAIR: A firmly based chair with armrests is preferred. Before sitting, the patient is to extend the operated leg, reach back for the armrests, and then sit down slowly (Fig. 31-5). To stand from sitting the patient is instructed to first slide forward to the edge of the chair, then extend the operated leg and push off from the armrests. Low-seated or sling-seated chairs should be avoided.

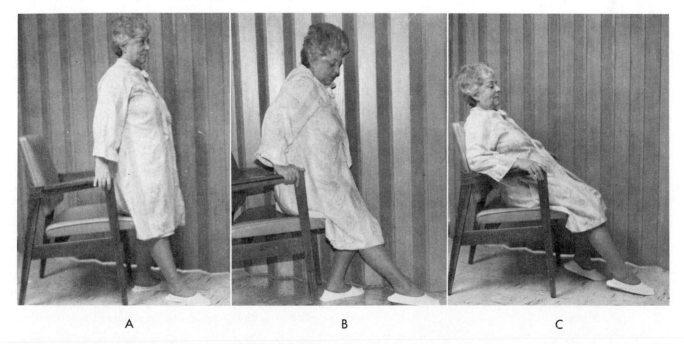

A   B   C

Fig. 31-5. Chair transfer technique. **A**, patient extends operated leg and reaches for arm rests. **B** and **C**, Bearing some weight on arms, patient sits down slowly, maintaining some extension of operated leg.

COMMODE CHAIR: An over-the-toilet commode chair is used initially while in the hospital. Usually by the time of discharge the patient will have enough hip mobility to safely use a standard toilet seat. It is recommended not to twist while wiping. To flush the toilet the patient should stand up and turn around to face the flusher.

SHOWER STALL: Nonskid stickers are recommended in all shower stalls and tubs. To transfer, walker or crutches go in first, then the nonoperated leg followed by the operated leg. For patients with weight-bearing precautions, the operated leg should lead.

SHOWER-OVER-TUB: The patient is instructed to stand parallel to the tub, facing the shower fixtures. Using a walker or crutches, the patient should transfer in sideways by bending one knee at a time over the tub. For patients with weight-bearing precautions or poor balance this transfer is not recommended. Such patients are advised to sponge bathe.[6]

CAR: A bench-type seat is recommended. The patient is instructed to back up to the passenger seat, sit down slowly with the operated leg extended, and then slide buttocks toward the driver's seat. The upper body and lower extremities move as one unit until the patient is squarely seated. Patients should avoid prolonged sitting in a car.

(LE) dressing. It is usually recommended to sit in a chair or on the side of the bed to dress. The patient is instructed to avoid externally rotating or crossing the legs to dress. Crossing the operated extremity over the nonoperated extremity at either the ankles or knees is to be avoided. Assistive devices may be necessary to observe precautions (see Fig. 31-6).

Homemaking. Heavy housework, such as vacuuming, lifting, and bed making, should be avoided. Kitchen activities are practiced with suggestions made to keep commonly used items at counter top level. Carrying items can be done by using aprons with large pockets, sliding items along the counter top, or attaching a small basket to a walker if necessary.

Family orientation. A family member or friend should be present for at least one occupational therapy treatment session so that any questions may be answered. Appropriate supervision recommendations and instruction regarding activity precautions are given at this time.

Total hip replacement—posterolateral approach

POSITIONS OF HIP STABILITY: Flexion (within limitations of precautions), abduction, and external rotation

POSITIONS OF HIP INSTABILITY: Adduction, internal rotation, and flexion greater than limitations of precautions

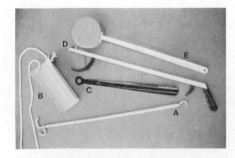

Fig. 31-6. Assistive devices useful for hip fracture. *A,* Dressing stick; *B,* sock aid; *C,* long-handled shoe horn; *D,* reacher; *E,* long-handled bath sponge.

Bed mobility. The supine position with the appropriate wedge and ski box in place is recommended (see Fig. 31-4). It is not recommended that a patient sleep on the side. If a skin rash is present, sidelying is possible by assisting the patient to roll toward the uninvolved extremity with the wedge or larger pillows between the legs and someone holding the operated extremity to maintain hip abduction.

Transfers

CHAIR: A firmly based chair with armrests is recommended. The patient is instructed to extend the operated leg forward, reach back for the armrests, and sit slowly, being careful not to lean forward (see Fig. 31-5). To stand, the patient extends the operated leg and pushes off from the armrests, being careful not to lean forward. Because of the hip flexion precaution, the patient should sit on the front part of the chair and lean back. Firm cushions or blankets can be used to increase the height of chairs, especially if the patient is tall. Low chairs, soft chairs, reclining chairs, and rocking chairs should be avoided.

COMMODE CHAIR: Over-the-toilet commode chairs with armrests are to be used in the hospital and at home. The height and angle are adjusted so that the front legs are one notch lower than the back legs; thus, with the patient seated, the precautionary hip angle of flexion is not exceeded. The patient should wipe between the legs in a sitting or standing position to avoid twisting. The patient is to stand up and turn to face the toilet to flush.

SHOWER STALL: To enter, the walker or crutches go first, then the operated leg followed by the nonoperated leg. The patient is provided with a long-handled sponge to reach the feet safely. Grab bars should be installed if balance is a problem.

SHOWER-OVER-TUB: The patient is instructed to stand parallel to the tub facing the shower fixtures. Using the walker or crutches, the patient is to transfer in sideways by bending at the knees, not at the hips. For patients with weight-bearing precautions or poor balance, this transfer is not recommended. They should take a sponge bath.

CAR: Bucket seats in small cars should be avoided. Bench-type seats are recommended. The patient is instructed to back up to the passenger seat, hold onto a stable part of the car, extend the operated leg, and slowly sit in the car. Remembering to lean back, the patient then slides the buttocks toward the driver's seat. The upper body and lower extremities then move as one unit to turn to face the forward direction. It is helpful to have the seat slid back and reclined to maintain the hip flexion precaution. Prolonged sitting in the car should be avoided.

LE dressing. To maintain hip precautions a dressing stick is used to aid in donning and removing pants and shoes. For pants, the operated leg is dressed first by using the dressing stick to bring the pants over the foot and up to the knee. A reacher, elastic laces, and a long-handled shoehorn are also provided. A sock aid is given if the patient lives alone. The patient is instructed to sit in a chair with arms or on the edge of the bed for dressing activities.

Homemaking. This is the same as for anterolateral approach. Reachers are provided to reach items in low cupboards or on the floor.

Family orientation. This is also the same as for anterolateral approach.

Special equipment

The occupational therapist should be familiar with the following equipment that is commonly used in the treatment of hip fracture and total hip replacement.

NELSON BED: An adjustable bed that allows for chair or 90° vertical tilt positions in comparison with regular hospital beds may be used in some programs in the initial postoperative days to facilitate a change in the patient's position and allow a progressive tilting program before ambulation. It continues to be used until the patient has been instructed in transfer skills on and off the side of the bed.

HEMOVAC: During surgery a plastic drainage tube is inserted at the surgical site to assist with drainage of blood postoperatively. It has an area for collection of drainage and may be connected to a portable suction machine. The unit should *not* be disconnected for any activity, since this may create a blockage in the system. The Hemovac is usually left in place for 2 days following surgery.

ABDUCTION WEDGE: Large and small triangular wedges are used when the patient is supine to maintain the LEs in the abducted position. The large wedge is also used postoperatively to assist with stretching of hips into increased abduction.

SKI BOX: The box is made of cardboard with foam padding inside and Velcro attachments to secure the leg in place. It is used to maintain the operated extremity in a position of neutral hip rotation.

BALANCED SUSPENSION: The balanced suspension device is an alternative to the use of the abduction wedge and ski box initially. It is fabricated and set up by the cast room technician and physician and is usually used for about 3 days following surgery. Its purpose is to support the affected LE in the first few postoperative days. The patient's leg should *not* be taken out of the device for exercise until the device's use has been discontinued by the physician.

RECLINING WHEELCHAIR: A wheelchair with an adjustable backrest that allows a reclining position while in the chair is used for patients who have hip flexion precautions while sitting.

COMMODE CHAIRS: The use of a commode chair instead of the regular toilet aids in safe transfers and allows the patient to observe necessary hip flexion precautions. The two front legs of the commode chair may be adjusted slightly lower than the back legs to increase the patient's ability to observe hip flexion limitations and decrease the risk of dislocation.

BOLSTERS: Large, firmly folded blankets are used to assist with positioning the patient for passive hip stretching exercises.

DRESSING AIDS: Dressing aids are used to encourage independence in performing ADL while maintaining precautions against specific hip motions. These include a dressing stick, reacher, long-handled sponge, long-handled shoehorn, and sock aid (Fig. 31-6).

SEQUENTIAL COMPRESSION DEVICES (SCDs). SCDs are used postoperatively to reduce the risk of deep vein thrombosis. They are inflatable, external leggings that provide intermittent pneumatic compression of the legs.[6]

ANTIEMBOLUS HOSE. This device is thigh-high hosiery that is worn 24 hours a day and removed only during bathing. Its purpose is to assist circulation, prevent edema, and thus reduce the risk of deep vein thrombosis.[6]

SUMMARY

Occupational therapy is determined by the surgical procedure performed and by the precautions prescribed by the physician. For patients who have an ORIF, weight-bearing precautions must be observed during all ADL. Particular attention should be paid to the patient's weight-bearing during bathing activities. It is often safest for the patient to bathe in the sitting position. A tub bench or shower seat may be necessary for safe and independent bathing. A simulation of the home environment is helpful to prepare the patient for potential problems that may arise when discharged. Recommendations to remove throw rugs and slippery floor coverings are made since the patient will most likely be going home using an ambulatory assistive device.

Sample treatment plan

This sample treatment plan is not comprehensive. It deals with four of eight problems identified. The reader is encouraged to add objectives and methods to the plan, dealing with these and the other problems.

CASE STUDY

Mr. B is an 82-year-old man who has noticed increased right hip pain over the past year. He had a hip x-ray examination 3 months ago, and a diagnosis of degenerative arthritis was confirmed. He has been admitted to the orthopedic unit of the hospital for elective right total joint replacement using the anterolateral approach.

Mr. B is a widower from Kentucky whose wife died shortly after they moved to California 6 months ago. Mr. B lives in his own cottage behind his son's home. Mr. B has been independent in meal preparation, self-care, and homemaking. He enjoys gardening, walking in the neighborhood, and visiting with his two grandchildren. His increased hip pain has limited his daily activity so that he must take frequent rests during the day and use a cane.

Mr. B has been admitted to the hospital 1 day before surgery for a preoperative assessment. OT staff will evaluate the patient's present function, describe the rehabilitation program as it will progress following surgery, and carry out functional training after surgery.

Personal data

Name: Mr. B

Age: 82

Diagnosis: Degenerative arthritis affecting right hip; elective right total hip replacement

Disability: Limited ROM and ambulation

Precautions: Avoidance of right hip external rotation and adduction for 6 weeks after surgery

Treatment aims as stated in referral

1. Orientation of patient to rehabilitation program preoperatively
2. Evaluation of patient's function preoperatively
3. Instruction of patient in maintaining hip precautions for ADL postoperatively

OTHER SERVICES

Medical: Perform total hip replacement surgery; prescribe rehabilitation therapies and medication

Nursing: Nursing care; positioning; supervise patient in activities and exercises following therapist's instruction of the patient

Physical therapy: ROM and strengthening exercises and gait training

Discharge planner: Arrange for home care follow-up

Family: Provide emotional support and physical assistance after discharge from hospital; encourage patient to observe precautions for hip movements at home

FRAME OF REFERENCE/TREATMENT APPROACH

Occupational performance/rehabilitative approach

OT EVALUATION

Before surgery

General appearance: Observe ease of movement, personal hygiene, hospital equipment in use, and patient's position and expression

Mental and behavioral state: Observe

Communication, vision, and hearing: Observe

Sensation and pain: Test, observe

Strength of extremities and trunk: Test

Muscle tone: Test

Posture: Observe

Bulbar function: Screen

Perceptual and cognitive function: Test, observe

Avocational and vocational activities and endurance: Interview

Home layout and accessibility: Interview

Rehabilitation program after surgery: Orient patient

Patient's goals from this surgery: Interview

Specific evaluation

Bed mobility: Demonstrate, interview

Transfers (bed, chair, toilet, shower, and car): Demonstrate or interview

Dressing: Interview

Self-care: Interview

After surgery

The presurgical evaluation and evaluation of the patient's ability to observe hip precautions during functional activities and simulated work or avocational activities are repeated. The need and use of assistive devices is also assessed

EVALUATION SUMMARY

Before surgery. UE active ROM was limited to 160° of shoulder flexion bilaterally. Active ROM of the right LE was limited to 5° to 85° of hip flexion, 5° of internal rotation, 10° of external rotation, and 15° of abduction. All other ranges were within normal limits (WNL). Strength in UEs and both LEs was 4 to 5 (G to N).

All sensory and perceptual functions were WNL. Mr. B reported forgetfulness (especially of dates, places, and phone numbers) at times in daily activities. He described the forgetfulness as more "bothersome" than a significant problem.

The patient was anxious about the hospital stay and surgery but appeared motivated to gain increased function and decreased pain. He showed an interest in the rehabilitation program by asking appropriate questions during the evaluation.

Mr. B was able to do most ADL independently, except for difficulty with tying shoes and donning socks. He required frequent rests during meal preparation and homemaking because of pain. For heavy household tasks he required assistance.

After surgery. UE ROM and strength remains at grades 4 to 5 (G to N). ROM of the right LE is the same as before surgery except that hip flexion is limited to 10° to 65°.

The patient is very cooperative during treatment. He is tearful at times when he discusses the loss of his wife.

Mr. B requires adaptive equipment for independence in dressing. Endurance is improved for homemaking, but assistance is still required for heavy household tasks because of hip precautions. After 6 weeks of recovery he is expected to be independent in most household tasks and in all ADL without equipment.

For the first 6 weeks of recovery, Mr. B will be cautioned against activities such as gardening and heavy lifting which may violate hip precautions. After 6 weeks he will be allowed to resume all of his leisure activities with less pain and increased endurance expected.

Continued.

Sample treatment plan—cont'd

ASSETS

Well-motivated for independence
Good understanding of rehabilitation program
Supportive family
Good safety awareness and judgment

PROBLEM LIST

Before surgery
1. Pain
2. Limited independence due to pain
3. Anxiety about surgery and dependence

After surgery
4. Limited motion of right hip
5. Unable to ambulate without aids
6. ADL dependence
7. Limited leisure activities
8. Mild memory deficit

PROBLEM 3

Anxiety about surgery and functional dependence

Objective

Patient will understand hip precautions as related to functional activity and progression of rehabilitation following surgery

Method

Surgery and hip precautions are described to the patient

The occupational therapy program and progression of functional activities both in the hospital and at home are explained; a sound-slide module is used to help clarify explanations

PROBLEMS 4, 6

Limited motions of right hip, ADL dependence

Objective

Patient will consistently demonstrate good safety skills in shower transfers

Method

Correct shower transfer is demonstrated to the patient; walker or crutches lead, then the nonoperated leg, followed by the operated leg

Patient practices the transfer

PROBLEMS 4, 7

Limited motion of right hip; limited leisure activities

Objective

The patient will understand and demonstrate how he may modify gardening, visiting with grandchildren, and walking in the neighborhood to ensure observance of hip precautions and safety

Method

Patient participates in simulated gardening by bending, reaching, and carrying items in clinic

Safety skills for ambulating with crutches around children are discussed and demonstrated; patient practices maneuvering in clinic obstacle course

Therapist discusses the methods for pacing and awareness of safe surfaces for ambulating in neighborhood with patient; patient practices pacing and maneuvering on various surfaces in hospital

Gradation

Patient solves problems through discussion, then in simulated situations

---

REVIEW QUESTIONS

1. Why is it critical for an occupational therapist to understand hip anatomy and treatment of hip fractures?
2. When reviewing the patient's medical history, what information should be obtained?
3. Define "clinical union." How does it relate to weight bearing and activity?
4. Identify four factors that will influence fracture healing.
5. What is a pathological fracture, and in which diseases can it occur?
6. Describe the differences in approach and maintenance of closed and open reductions.
7. Femoral neck fractures are common in women greater than 60 years old. The type of surgical treatment used is based on the amount of displacement and what other factor?
8. Why would a compression screw and plate not be a surgical choice when there is poor blood supply to the femoral head?
9. Why are weight-bearing precautions observed with ORIF hip pinnings?
10. Which surgical procedure is generally used with a severely displaced femoral neck fracture or with an avascular femoral head?
11. Why must hip position precautions be observed during activity in patients with total hip replacements?
12. In which diagnostic groups other than fractures will there be frequent indication for total joint replacement? What are the goals for this surgical approach in these diagnostic conditions?
13. Briefly describe the positions of instability in both the anterolateral and posterolateral approaches to hip replacement orthoplasty.
14. Briefly describe a total joint surface replacement and indications for its application.
15. Briefly describe a wedge and ski box and the indications for its use and application.
16. Following initial postoperative assessment, which functional activities are generally assessed in planning the initial treatment program?
17. Briefly describe the transfer method to a chair for a person after total hip replacement using posterolateral approach. What is the rationale applied here? What types of chairs should be avoided? Why?
18. Briefly describe a car transfer recommended for the patient with hip replacement orthoplasty using an anterolateral approach.

19. Which pieces of adaptive equipment might help a patient who has had a posterolateral total hip replacement achieve independence in LE dressing?
20. What suggestions could be made concerning carrying items when ambulation aids are necessary?

REFERENCES

1. Butler RN: The life review: an interpretation of reminiscence in the aged. In Kastenbaum R, editor: New thoughts on old age, New York, 1964, Springer Publishing Co, Inc.
2. Butler RN: Aging and mental health, ed 3 St Louis, 1982, The CV Mosby Co.
3. Crow I: Fractures of the hip: a self study, ONA J 5:12, 1978.
4. Garland JJ: Fundamentals of orthopedics, Philadelphia, 1979, WB Saunders Co.
5. Hogshead HP: Orthopaedics for the therapist, Gainesville, 1973, University of Florida. (Unpublished.)
6. Jones M and Lieberman S: The total hip replacement protocol, Stanford, CA, 1986, Stanford University Hospital, Department of Physical and Occupational Therapy. (Unpublished.)
7. Lewis SC: The mature years: a geriatric occupational therapy text, Thorofare, NJ, 1979, Charles B Slack, Inc.
8. Salter RB: Textbook of disorders and injuries of the musculoskeletal system, Baltimore, 1970, Williams & Wilkins.
9. Sitko S and Pitbladdo K: The total hip replacement protocol, Stanford, 1982, Stanford University Hospital, Department of Physical and Occupational Therapy. (Unpublished.)

Chapter

32 Lower motor neuron dysfunction

GUY L. McCORMACK

The lower motor neuron system[3] includes the anterior horn cells of the spinal cord; spinal nerves and their associated ganglia; and 10 pairs of cranial nerves and their nuclei, which are housed in the brainstem (cranial nerves 1 and 2 are fiber tracts in the brain).[12] The motor fibers of the lower motor neurons are divided into the somatic and autonomic components. The somatic motor components include the alpha motor neurons, which innervate skeletal (extrafusal fibers) muscles, and gamma motor neurons, which innervate muscle spindles (intrafusal fibers). The autonomic component innervates the glands, smooth muscles, and heart musculature.[13,16,41] A lesion to any of these neurological structures consitutes a lower motor neuron dysfunction.[13]

Lower motor neuron dysfunction can result from several different causes, including traumatic injury, such as bone fractures and dislocations, contusions, compression of nerve roots, lacerations, traction (stretching), penetrating wounds, and friction. Vascular deficiencies may also cause lower motor neuron dysfunction. Examples of these deficiencies include arteriosclerosis, diabetes mellitus (sensory loss), peripheral vascular anomalies, and polyarteritis nodosa. Furthermore, toxic agents, such as lead, phosphorus, alcohol, benzene, and sulfonamides, can cause lower motor neuron dysfunction. Other contributing factors may include neoplasms, such as neuromas and multiple neurofibromatosis, and inflammatory processes, such as polyneuritis or mononeuritis. Degenerative diseases of the central nervous system (CNS) and congenital anomalies can also produce lower motor neuron dysfunction.[23,53]

Since the occupational therapist traditionally treats a variety of lower motor neuron dysfunctions that affect the upper extremities, this chapter deals with the conditions commonly seen in clinical practice.

DISEASES OF THE LOWER MOTOR NEURON
Poliomyelitis

Poliomyelitis is a contagious viral disease that affects the anterior horn cells of the gray matter of the spinal cord and the motor nuclei of the brainstem. The cervical and lumbar enlargements of the cord are affected the most. Because of the active immunization program (Salk and Sabin vaccines) in the United States, new cases of poliomyelitis are rare. However, the recent complacency about immunization has created some new cases, and "old cases" are frequently referred to occupational therapy for rehabilitation or improvement of the quality of life.[19]

Clinically patients who have poliomyelitis initially have flaccid paralysis that may be local or widespread. The lower extremities, accessory muscles of respiration, and muscles that promote swallowing are primarily affected. Marked atrophy may be seen in the involved extremities, and deep tendon reflexes may be absent. Since poliomyelitis destroys the anterior horn cells, sensory roots are spared and sensation is intact. Contractures can occur very early in the course of the disease. In cases of local paralysis the asymmetry of muscles pulling on various joints may promote deformity complications, such as subluxation, scoliosis, and contractures. In severe cases osteoporosis (bone atrophy) may weaken the long weight-bearing bones and pathological fractures can occur.[32]

The medical treatment for poliomyelitis during the acute phase includes bed rest, positioning, and applications of warm packs to reduce pain and promote relaxation. Since there is no known cure for poliomyelitis, the disease must run its course. There is an incubation period of 1 to 3 weeks, and the recovery is dependent on the number of nerve cells destroyed. Paralysis may begin in 1 to 7 days after the initial symptoms. The medical aspects of rehabilitation may include reconstructive surgery, such as tendon transfer; arthrodesis; and surgical release of fascia, muscles, and tendons. Although the lower extremities are primarily affected, the hand splinting techniques were developed and codified at Rancho Los Amigos Hospital in the West and at Georgia Warm Springs Hospital in the East. Other medical procedures may include therapeutic stretching, casts, muscle reeducation, and bracing for standing or stability.[25]

OCCUPATIONAL THERAPY INTERVENTION.

During the acute phase the patient receives symptomatic treatment and is confined to bed. The therapist should assist the nurse in providing good bed positioning to prevent contractures and protect weakened joints. Because the poliomyelitis virus is infectious during this stage, isolation procedures should be carefully followed. The therapist should provide gentle passive range of motion (ROM) at the patient's physical tolerance level to prevent contractures, joint stiffness, and deformities. Care should be taken not to grasp the involved muscle bellies, because they will be extremely tender and painful. The muscles may also be prone to spasm when painfully stimulated.[19]

The primary emphasis should be placed on the avoidance of muscle fatigue. Fatigue at this point can result in further residual weaknesses. If the patient has bulbar poliomyelitis, which affects the muscles of respiration, a respirator may be used to facilitate ventilation of the lungs or a tracheostomy may be performed. If the muscles necessary for swallowing are impaired, tube feeding may also be prescribed. The therapist should collaborate treatment procedures with the nursing staff to ensure proper functioning of the equipment necessary for the life support systems.[12,19,25,28]

The treatment program should include psychological support. The patient's fears and anxieties about the crippling effects of the disease should not be underestimated. The patient may need encouragement and positive experiences to promote an optimistic outlook during the rehabilitation process. The family may also need assistance in adjusting to the patient's disability.

As the rehabilitation process progresses, the precautions against physical and body fatigue continue. Assistive devices, splints, and mobile arm supports may be used to gain independence in daily activities. The long-range rehabilitation program should follow a functional course of action. After the acute medical problems have subsided, the recovery stage may last as long as 2 years.[12] Since the damage to the anterior horn cells is permanent, the therapist should assist the patient in making the best possible use of whatever muscular function remains. Before treatment is started, an evaluation of the existing disability must be obtained. A thorough manual muscle test not only provides a baseline for muscle strength but moreover detects joint deformities caused by contracted muscles, ligaments, tendons, and joint capsules. Manual muscle tests should be repeated monthly for the first 4 months and bimonthly for the next 4 months. After 8 months of therapeutic exercises the average patient has probably responded to his or her maximal ability.[8,12,23] In short the therapeutic regime includes combinations of rest, movement, muscle reeducation, functional activities, and psychological support. Consequently the prognosis of poliomyelitis depends on the personality of the patient and the perseverance of the therapist.

Movement for the patient who is recovering from acute poliomyelitis proceeds from passive to active ROM, depending on the patient's level of voluntary control. Muscle reeducation should be preceeded by gentle stretching exercises. For the upper extremity emphasis should be placed on stretching the pectoralis major and minor and latissimus dorsi to ensure free motion of the shoulder region. All active motions should be performed under careful supervision of the therapist. Compensatory movement should be avoided. A limited but correct movement is preferred to an ampler but incorrect movement. Active movements should be done in front of a mirror, which enables the patient to observe and correct motions accordingly.[19,25,28]

Muscle reeducation is accomplished in a graded fashion. At first the patient should learn "muscle-setting" exercises, that is, alternating contraction and relaxation of muscles without moving the joints. Isometric exercises and electromyographic (EMG) biofeedback may be beneficial at this juncture. As the patient progresses, light resistance can be applied manually by the therapist before the use of pulleys and weights. This allows the therapist to develop an empirical understanding of the patient's physical strengths and weaknesses. Weakened muscles must be protected at all times. Muscles that cannot resist the forces of gravity are supported during exercise and rest periods. As a rule of thumb, resistive exercises are not attempted until the muscle is able to carry out a complete ROM against gravity. Weakened or flaccid muscles can be splinted at night to counteract the forces of gravity or the pull of the stronger antagonist muscles. During resistive exercises the therapist should stress correct body positioning, joint alignment, and energy conservation. Periods of rest should be included in the exercise program, as well as activities that incorporate the same movements and musculature.[18]

The rationales for resistive exercises in the rehabilitation of the patient who has poliomyelitis are to cause hypertrophy of the undamaged muscle fibers and give usefulness to the slightest contraction by integrating it into the global movement that permits the performance of a given activity. Emphasis is placed on strengthening individual weakened muscles. After the 8-month period if the muscle is unable to contract completely against gravity, it is doubtful that additional muscle strength will return. At this point the emphasis should be placed on maintenance of existing muscles and functional activities of daily living (ADL). Again a self-care evaluation should be administered to achieve a baseline of function. Dressing activities may include putting on braces, prostheses, or orthoses. Assistive and adaptive devices should be tailored to the needs of the patient. The adaptation of assistive devices should begin where the patient's functional abilities are limited. Assistive and adaptive devices should provide the patient with the most ability within the limits of the disability.[40] It may also be advantageous to begin activities for prevocational and vocational exploration. The patient's quality of life can be improved if he or she is employed and productive.

Today therapists are seeing more "post polio syndrome" patients in rehabilitation centers. Some of the patients are experiencing additional weakness and paralysis. The phenomenon is not fully understood, but it is believed to be the normal loss of neurons in later life. Since the poliomyelitis victim has a diminished number of neurons in the anterior horn cells, further loss can be debilitating. This problem may pose some new challenges to the therapist in the future.

Guillain-Barré Syndrome

Guillain-Barré syndrome, also known as either infectious polyneuritis or Landry's syndrome, is an acute inflammatory condition involving the spinal nerve roots; peripheral nerves; and, in some cases, selected cranial nerves. The Guillaine-Barré syndrome often follows an afebrile illness. It is probably caused by a virus that produces a hypersensitive response that results in patchy demyelination of lower motor neuron pathways. The axons are generally spared, so recovery often follows a predictable course. In severe cases, however, Wallerian degeneration of the axon results in a slow recovery process. This disease affects men and women equally from ages 30 to 50.[8,12,19,42,53]

Clinically Guillain-Barré syndrome is characterized by a rapid onset. Initially there is an absence of fever, pain and tenderness of muscles, and weakness and decrease in deep tendon reflexes. As the disease progresses, it produces motor weakness or paralysis of the limbs, sensory loss, and muscle atrophy. The prognosis is varied. In severe cases cranial nerves 7, 9, and 10 may be involved and the patient may have difficulty speaking, swallowing, and breathing. If vital centers in the medulla are affected, the patient may experience respiratory failure.

In the majority of the cases the patient completely recovers within 3 to 8 months. Some slight exacer-

bation can occur, producing residual weaknesses and muscular atrophy.[25]

OCCUPATIONAL THERAPY INTERVENTION. Once the patient is medically stabilized, treatment goals should be coordinated with the nurse, physical therapist, and other members of the team to implement a comprehensive rehabilitation program. The occupational therapist should grade the activity to the patient's physical tolerance level. Physical fatigue should be avoided at all costs. Gentle, nonresistive activities can be introduced to alleviate joint stiffness and muscle atrophy and prevent contractures.[19,50] Resistive activities should not be introduced until the manual muscle test reveals a fair plus grade or better.[7]

Treatment should always begin with a thorough evaluation of the patient's level of functioning. During the early stages of recovery the evaluation process itself may be fatiguing. It is often best to spread the evaluation process over the course of a few days. For example, testing may begin by gently squeezing the muscle bellies of the large muscle groups to determine the extent of muscle tenderness and atrophy. Since the muscles of the limbs are usually affected symmetrically, this test can be grossly administered. Manual muscle testing should not be done in one session. It is best to test a few muscles at a time and allow the patient periods of rest. Particular attention should be paid to the intrinsic muscles of the hands to determine residual weakness. If swallowing or speech is impaired, a tongue depressor may be used to apply light resistance against the tongue to estimate the motor involvement in the twelfth (hypoglossal) cranial nerve.

Manual muscle testing should follow the strict definitions for grading strength. The patient's previous physical condition and occupation should be taken into account when calibrating the muscle strength.[19] It is important to establish an objective baseline for all of the clinical findings and record the progression of the affected muscles on a standardized chart.

Sensory testing should also be conducted because the sensory pathways are often affected. Sensory tests should include light touch, stereognosis, pain and temperature, proprioception, and two-point discrimination. Test findings should be recorded and deficits should be noted.

Passive ROM should begin with gentle movement of the proximal joints and should proceed only to the point of pain. As the patient's tolerance level increases, active ROM and light exercises may be introduced. The program should stress joint protection, and the therapist should look for muscle imbalance and substitution patterns. Progressive resistive exercises should be used conservatively. Throughout the course of recovery the therapist should guard against fatigue and irritation of the inflamed nerves. As the patient's strength and tolerance level increase, more resistance can be employed, but to a moderate degree. The therapist may also introduce sedentary or table-top activities during the early stages of recovery. As the patient's strength increases, activities promoting more resistance, such as leather work, textiles, and ceramics, can be incorporated into the treatment regime. Grooming, self-care, and other ADL should be included as the need and desire arise. Slings and mobile arm supports may be employed to alleviate muscle fatigue and gain independence.

Van Dam,[51] an occupational therapist who experienced Guillain-Barré at the age of 14, underscores the importance of psychosocial support. According to Van Dam the therapist should try to facilitate the feeling of self-worth throughout the therapeutic process. Because the prognosis for recovery is good, the activities should be mentally stimulating and purposeful to the patient. The therapist should also respect the patient's level of pain tolerance during stretching and ROM exercises.

Bell's Palsy

Bell's palsy is an acute inflammatory disorder that affects the seventh (facial) cranial nerve. It is commonly attributed to exposure to cold, herpes zoster of the middle ear, traumatic conditions, and in some cases there is a familial tendency.[12,18] The course of the disease is usually short in duration, lasting 2 to 8 weeks. Approximately 70% of Bell's palsy patients experience spontaneous recovery whereas 30% do not. During the acute onset of the disorder one side of the patient's face is expressionless with an inability to close the eye. The patient may have difficulty eating and speaking, and the eye on the affected side may produce tears.[12,18]

OCCUPATIONAL THERAPY INTERVENTION. The occupational therapist may play an important role in the treatment of the patient with Bell's palsy. Beals[5] developed a treatment program based on phylogenetic facial expression. Since the facial musculature is controlled by both cortical and subcortical centers, facial expression represents a reflex action of high complexity. Therefore the treatment plan should first emphasize subcortical facial reactions of a spontaneous or reflexive nature. The treatment should promote gross patterns of expression facilitated by high-intensity stimuli. For example, a small slice of lemon is used to stimulate the buccal area. This stimulus affects the maxillary portion of the trigeminal nerve and is transmitted to the brainstem where synaptic connections are made with motor neurons of the facial nerve.[3,17] In addition, strong smells, such as ammonia,

cause the sensory endings of the trigeminal nerve to discharge into reflex arcs that stimulate the action of the nares and depressor septi. Thus the facial musculature can be stimulated reflexively through indirect synaptic connections via the trigeminal and olfactory cranial nerves.

The conscious component of facial expression can be activated in a graded fashion by reciting the alphabet, reading prose, or through activities that use pantomine.

Brown et al[10] described a successful program using EMG biofeedback for the reduction of facial paralysis. This program used visual and auditory feedback signals to allow the patient to gain functional control of facial musculature. The patients were trained to use EMG biofeedback and to practice facial expressions and verbalizations while viewing themselves in a mirror. This program reported successful results within a 3-month training period.

The occupational therapist may also work with the orthotist to fabricate a temporary facial splint to prevent stretching of the delicate muscle fibers. The affected facial muscles can also benefit from gentle, upward massage for 5 to 10 minutes 2 to 3 times a day to increase circulation and maintain muscle tone. Electrical stimulation and infrared treatments by the physical therapist may also be included in the patient's treatment regime. The therapist should assist the patient in carrying out his or her normal personal hygiene tasks. The lack of facial sensation on one side will require careful visual awareness while shaving. Brushing the teeth will require careful visual attention because food particles can collect on the affected side. Some patients may wear a patch over the affected eye, so visual awareness should be stressed to compensate for the temporary loss of sight and sensation.

Trigeminal Neuralgia (Tic Douloureux)

Trigeminal neuralgia is characterized by sudden attacks of excruciating pain in the sensory distribution of one or more branches of the trigeminal nerve. The cause of this disorder is multifaceted. There are reports of degenerative changes in the trigeminal ganglia, aberrant arteries impinging on the nerve roots, tumors, demyelinating conditions, and mechanical causes.[12,18,23] Statistically trigeminal neuralgia affects middle-aged and elderly people. It is more common in women and frequently affects the right side of the face. In 90% of the cases it affects the second and third divisions of the trigeminal nerve distribution.[18]

At the present time it is not understood why the neurons that subserve pain sensation for the trigeminal nerve suddenly discharge. In many cases there is a "trigger zone" in the facial or oral region which is extremely sensitive to temperature changes, light touch, or facial movement. Any irritation to the trigger zone can cause paroxysmal pain of brief durations.[13]

The medical management for trigeminal neuralgia includes alcohol injections, surgery, and drugs.

OCCUPATIONAL THERAPY INTERVENTION. Treatment should begin with a thorough interview and sensory evaluation to identify the location of the "trigger zones" and the stimuli that precipitate the pain attacks. In cooperation with the medical treatment prescribed by the physician, the therapist may implement one of several approaches. First the therapist may attempt to systematically desensitize the patient to the stimuli that trigger the pain attacks. This would require a carefully graded program using relaxation techniques and biofeedback. The EMG biofeedback machine can monitor muscle tightness in selected muscles, such as the temporalis or upper trapezius, to watch for muscle tension following pain.[20] Galvanic skin resistance biofeedback may also be used, since it measures the activity of the sympathetic nervous system. The combined effects of biofeedback and relaxation techniques enable the patient to obtain information about his or her body's physiologic responses and to establish some cortical control over the intensity of pain sensation. Recent studies on pain management suggest that when the patient feels he or she is able to do something to control the pain, the pain perception is decreased.[14,29,31,49] It has also been suggested that placebos may stimulate the release of endogenous opiates (enkephalins) and contribute to pain reduction.[54]

A second approach is to incorporate a consistent program of graded cutaneous stimulation. The therapist should avoid noxious stimuli, such as icing and electrical brushing, since they will activate the C and A delta-size pain fibers.[35] Instead, the therapist may try stretch pressure and low-frequency vibration (60 Hz) over the facial muscles to activate the large fibers of the proprioceptive system. According to the gate control theory of pain mechanisms, pain sensation may be suppressed in the neurons of the spinal cord and the brainstem.[29] Another benefit of graded sensory stimulation is that the cutaneous receptors will eventually adapt and perhaps raise their threshold to stimuli that trigger pain responses.[36]

A third and important treatment is the implementation of a daily program of purposeful activities. The therapist may want to administer an activity configuration to identify the periods in which the patient is most inactive. Most patients experience more pain sensation during the evenings or when they are inactive.[14] During these junctures the patient tends to

focus on the pain experience. This is the best time to engage the patient in routine activities to direct the conscious energies toward a purposeful task. Cortical distraction during painful episodes is a proven method of alleviating pain sensation.[14,54]

Transcutaneous electrical nerve stimulation (TENS) is an effective modality for reducing acute and chronic pain.[31,49] The role of the occupational therapist in the uses of TENS is controversial at this time. In many settings nurses and therapists use TENS under the prescription of a physician.

INJURIES TO PERIPHERAL NERVES
Clinical Signs of Peripheral Nerve Injuries

Regardless of the origin of the injury peripheral nerve lesions produce similar clinical manifestations. Seddon[43] describes three categories of peripheral nerve injury: 1) neuropraxia, 2) neurotmesis, and 3) axonotmesis. Neuropraxia is a nerve lesion that is usually caused by orthopedic injuries resulting in compression, concussion, and traction injuries. Neuropraxis results in a block of neuronal transmission, usually in the larger myelinated nerve fibers. Although it produces muscle paralysis, there is usually some sparing of sensory modalities and an absence of peripheral degeneration. Neuropraxia usually has a good prognosis for recovery if causal factors are removed.[7] Neurotmesis is a complete severance of the nerve root or division of all the essential neuronal structures. This injury usually results from traumatic mechanisms such as severe traction forces or open lacerations. Axonotmesis represents disruption of nerve fibers (axons) causing peripheral (Wallerian) degeneration. Because the epineurium and surrounding connective tissues are preserved, spontaneous regeneration is likely to occur. Axonotmesis usually follows traction injuries, closed fractures or dislocations, or results from ischemia.[35,43]

The most obvious manifestation is muscle weakness or flaccid paralysis, depending on the extent of the nerve damage. Because of the loss of muscle innervation, atrophy will follow and deep tendon reflexes will be absent or depressed. Sensation along the cutaneous distribution of the nerve will also be lost. Trophic changes, such as dry skin, hair loss, cyanosis, brittle fingernails, painless skin ulcerations, and slow wound healing in the area of involvement, may also be present as clinical signs. Occasionally minute muscle contractions called fasciculations may be seen on the surface of the skin overlying the denervated muscle belly. As a result of disturbances of sympathetic fibers of the autonomic nervous system, there will be a loss of the ability to sweat above the denervated skin surfaces.

The patient may experience paresthesias, that is, sensations such as tingling, numbness, and burning or pain (causalgia), particularly at night. In addition, if the nerve damage was caused by trauma, edema will be a prominent clinical manifestation. EMG examinations may reveal extremely small muscle contractions called fibrillations.*

Extensive peripheral nerve damage may produce deformity if contractures, joint stiffness, and poor positioning are allowed to occur. Disfigurement of the hands is particularly noticeable and may produce some psychological complications. Other complications may include osteoporosis of the bony structures and epidermal fibrosis of the joints.

All of the clinical manifestations just discussed may not be present. The clinical findings may vary with the underlying cause of the lesion.

Clinical Signs of Peripheral Nerve Regeneration

Peripheral nerve regeneration begins about 1 month after the injury occurred. The rate of regeneration depends on the nature of the nerve lesion.

If the nerve root has been cleanly severed and surgically repaired, the rate of regeneration will vary from ½ inch (1.3 cm) to 1 inch (2.6 cm) per month. Peripheral nerve injuries caused by burns, sepsis, or crushing will present other complications to the healing process. Age is another factor: Children usually have a faster rate of regeneration than adults.[38] In addition, proximal lesions regenerate faster than distal lesions and injuries to mixed nerves are slower to recover than single nerves.[7,33] Early medical treatment may require suturing the nerve and immobilizing the involved extremity to ensure good opposition of the severed nerves. The introduction of microsurgery has brought new advancements to the process of peripheral nerve regeneration. An experimental technique of nerve grafting called the mesothelial tube promotes nerve regeneration across an extended gap.[27] The mesothelial tube is a silicone chamber that protects the severed nerve endings so the newly formed nerve has a larger diameter. Another newly developed surgical technique called direct neurotization has shown that a denervated muscle will accept an implanted motor nerve and functional innervation can be attained.[11] This innovative surgical technique offers new hope for patients with significant muscle paralysis as a result of peripheral nerve lesions.

In most postsurgery cases the therapist may fabricate resting splints and assist in the proper positioning of the extremity to reduce edema. The therapist may also supervise the patient in active ROM to maintain the strength of the uninvolved muscles and joint mobility. Active rehabilitation begins about 7 weeks after the incision or graft has healed. In the past full recovery of muscles was not probable because regenerated fibers lose about 20% of their original diameter and conduct impulses at a slower rate.[13,35] Newer surgical techniques may improve the regenerative process.

Since peripheral nerves have the capacity to regenerate, the course of recovery can be somewhat predictable. The clinical signs of regeneration do not always abide by a specific sequence. Yet one might expect to see the following clinical signs:

Skin appearance: As the edema subsides and collateral blood vessels develop, the circulatory system should become more normalized. The skin should improve in its color and texture.

Primitive protection sensations: The first signs of cutaneous sensation will usually be the gross recognition of crude pain, temperature, pressure, and touch.

Paresthesias (Tinel's sign): Tapping or percussing from distal to proximal along the course of the damaged nerve route can be used to detect recovery. If the patient feels paresthesias (pins and needles) distal to the presumed site of lesion, regeneration is occurring—whereas a painful Tinel sign at the lesion may indicate neuroma formation.[7,12,23]

Scattered points of sweating: As the parasympathetic fibers of the autonomic nervous system regenerate, the sweat glands will recover their functions.

Discriminative sensations: The more refined sensations, such as the ability to identify and localize touch, joint movements (proprioception), recognition of objects in the three-dimensional form (stereognosis), speed of movement (kinesthesia), and two-point discrimination, should be returning at this juncture.

Muscle tone: As nerve fibers regenerate and tie into their respective musculature via their motor end plates, flaccidity will decrease and tone will increase. An important principle is that paralyzed muscles must first sense pressure before tone and movement can be realized.

Voluntary muscle function: The patient will be able to move the extremity first with gravity eliminated, and as strength increases, he or she may actively move the extremity through full ROM. At this point graded exercises can begin.

Full recovery of muscle power is not probable, because the possibility that thousands of regenerating

---

*References 3, 4, 12, 13, 17, 26

fibers will find their previous connections is unlikely.*

Phelps and Walker[38] reported that for complete laceration of peripheral nerves, the two-point discrimination test and the wrinkle test are viable methods of monitoring sensory return. The two-point discrimination test provides a quantitative measure of sensation. An earlier study by Moberg reveals the normal distance to discriminate one point from two points on the distal fingertip is 2 to 4 mm. A two-point discrimination of greater than 15 mm denotes tactile agnosia (absent sensation). This test can be achieved with the use of a high-quality caliper with blunted tips so that the pain sensation is not elicited. Light application of the calipers to the patient's skin in a random pattern can help the therapist map out the cutaneous, topographical areas that are innervated and denervated.

Another test that can be clinically significant is the wrinkle test. This test is performed by immersing the patient's hand in plain water at 108° F (42.2° C). The hand remains submerged for about 20 to 30 minutes until wrinkling occurs. At this point the patient's hand is dried, graded on a scale of 0 to 3, and photographed. The "0" on the scale represents an absence of wrinkling, whereas "3" represents normal wrinkling. The wrinkle test appears to provide an objective method of testing innervation of the hand with recent complete and partial peripheral nerve injuries. The actual physiologic mechanism that causes the wrinkling is not fully understood, and the test is not appropriate for patients with traumatic peripheral nerve compression injuries.[38] Nevertheless, the test can be significant in determining the rate of sensory regeneration and can provide a graphic record of denervated areas.

MEDICAL MANAGEMENT OF PERIPHERAL NERVE INJURIES. The medical-surgical management of peripheral nerve lesions depends on the type of injury that has occurred. Lacerations may be treated with microsurgery to suture the severed nerve. Exploratory surgery (neurolysis) may be conducted to remove unwanted scar tissue from the site of the lesion. Nerve grafts and transplants are performed for severe traumatic injuries. Alcohol injections, vitamin B_{12}, and phenol are used to alleviate the pain that might accompany peripheral neuropathy. For inflammatory processes high caloric diets with liberal use of vitamin B complex is the treatment of choice.[8,12,18]

Specific Peripheral Nerve Injuries

BRACHIAL PLEXUS INJURY. The nerve roots that innervate the upper extremity originate in the ante-rior rami between C4 and T1. This network of lower anterior cervical and upper dorsal spine nerves is collectively called the *brachial plexus*. This very important nerve complex can be palpated just behind the posterior border of the sternocleidomastoid as the head and neck are tilted to the opposite side.[8,12,25,46]

Lesions to the brachial plexus usually result from a variety of traumatic injuries. Most brachial plexus injuries in children are caused by birth trauma. The more classic of these brachial plexus injuries are called Erb's palsy and Klumpke's paralyses. Erb's palsy is indicative of lesions to the fifth and sixth plexus roots. Paralysis and atrophy occur in the deltoid, brachialis, biceps, and brachioradialis muscles. Clinically the arm hangs limp, the hand rotates inward, and functional movement is extremely limited.

Klumpke's paralysis affects the more distal aspect of the upper extremity. The disorder results from injury to the eighth cervical and first thoracic plexus roots. Consequently there will be paralysis to the distal musculature of the wrist flexors and the intrinsic muscles of the hand.[8,12]

LONG THORACIC NERVE INJURY. The long thoracic nerve (C5-7) innervates the serratus anterior (magnus) muscle, which anchors the apex of the scapula to the posterior of the rib cage. Although injury to this nerve is not common, it has been injured by carrying heavy weights on the shoulder, neck blows, and axillary wounds. The resulting clinical picture is threefold: First, winging of the scapula occurs when the arm is extended and pressed against a stabilized object in front of the patient. Second, the patient will have difficulty flexing the outstretched arm above the level of his or her shoulder. Third, the patient will have difficulty protracting the shoulder or performing scapula abduction and adduction.

Injuries involving the long thoracic nerve are usually treated by stabilizing the shoulder girdle to limit scapula motion. The therapist must avoid using activities that promote shoulder movements. If nerve regeneration is not complete, surgery may be indicated to relieve the excessive mobility of the scapula. After medical treatment the occupational therapist encourages maximal functional independence and teaches the patient to use long-handle devices to compensate for shoulder limitations.

AXILLARY NERVE INJURY. The axillary nerve is composed from the C5-6 spinal nerves and derived from the posterior region of the brachial plexus. The motor branches of the axillary nerve innervate the superior aspect of the deltoid muscle and the teres minor muscle. Although the axillary nerve is rarely damaged by itself, it is often damaged along with traumatic lesions to the brachial plexus. As a result, the

---

*References 3, 8, 12, 13, 26, 35

patient will experience weakness or paralysis of the deltoid muscle, which causes limitations in horizontal abduction and hyperesthesia on the lateral aspect of the shoulder. In addition to the loss of muscle power, atrophy of the deltoid muscle produces asymmetry of the shoulders. If the nerve damage is permanent, a muscle transplantation may be required to provide some abduction of the arm.[8,12,42]

The occupational therapist should maintain ROM to prevent deformity and improve circulation. Passive abduction of the shoulder should be done daily. The teres minor and deltoid muscles should be protected from stretch during the manual ROM activities. The patient may be taught to use long-handled assistive devices to compensate for the abduction deficit. If a surgical transplant is performed, the therapist should be familiar with the surgical procedure and assist in muscle reeducation. An EMG biofeedback machine can be beneficial in providing the patient with visual and auditory incentives during muscle reeducation sessions. The occupational therapist may also assist the patient in dressing activities. If the asymmetry of the shoulders presents a cosmetic problem when wearing shirts or jackets, a foam rubber or Orthoplast pad can be fabricated to fill in the space that was once filled by the deltoid muscle. The patient should be encouraged to learn self-ranging techniques and implement an exercise program to maintain the integrity of the unimpaired muscles of the involved extremity.

RADIAL NERVE INJURY. The radial nerve represents the largest branch of the brachial plexus and descends along the humerus in the musculospiral groove. Below the elbow it bifurcates into the superficial radial nerve and the deep radial nerve. The superficial radial nerve terminates in the first, second, and third phalanges, whereas the deep radial nerve descends along the posterior region of the forearm, branching out to supply the extensor-supinator group of muscles.

The sensory branches innervate cutaneous receptors along the dorsal aspect of the arm and forearm and the posterior surface of the thumb, index, and middle fingers, and half of the ring finger. The motor branches innervate the triceps, brachioradialis, anconeus, extensor digitorum communis, extensor carpi ulnaris, supinator, abductor pollicis longus, and extensor indicis proprius muscles.

The actions produced by the radial nerve are wrist extension, metacarpophalangeal (MP) extension, thumb abduction and extension, ulnar and radial deviation, and release of grasping actions.

The most common types of injury to the radial nerve are fractures of the humerus or lacerations across the dorsum of the forearm.

The most blatant clinical feature of radial nerve injury is extensor paralysis. The patient will exhibit "wrist drop" and an inability to extend the thumb, proximal phalanges, and elbow joint. In addition, the patient will have difficulty pronating the hand and grasping objects.[4,12,34,35,50]

MEDIAN NERVE INJURY. The median nerve originates in the lateral and medial cords of the brachial plexus. The two cords unite, forming one nerve trunk that descends along the medial part of the arm to the anterior region of the forearm, branching out until it terminates in the hand.

The sensory branches of the median nerve supply the volar surface of the thumb, the index and middle fingers, and half of the ring finger. The motor branches innervate the pronator teres, flexor carpi radialis, palmaris longus, flexor digitorum sublimis, flexor pollicis longus, half of the flexor digitorum profundus, lumbricales 1 and 2, and pronator quadratus.

The actions produced by the median nerve are thumb opposition and abduction, interphalangeal (IP) flexion of the index finger, distal interphalangeal (DIP) flexion of the thumb, wrist flexion, forearm pronation, MP flexion of the second and third fingers, and IP flexion of the third, fourth, and fifth fingers.

The most common types of injury for the median nerve are forearm lacerations, wrist trauma, and deep lacerations to the flexor pollicis brevis muscle.[4,12,35,50]

Clinically one would expect to see loss of thumb opposition, thenar atrophy, and ape hand deformity. Furthermore the patient would have difficulty making a fist because the second and third fingers would remain extended while the fourth and fifth would flex.

CARPAL TUNNEL SYNDROME. The carpal tunnel represents a small passage in the volar aspect of the wrist formed by the concavity of carpal bones and bridged by the transverse carpal ligament. The tunnel provides a restricted space for the tendons of the long flexors of the fingers, the flexor pollicis longus, and the median nerve.[12,18] Anytime the wrist is flexed or extended the transverse ligament tightens over the wrist.[18]

The so-called carpal tunnel syndrome can result from several factors. For instance, a dislocation of the lunate bone or a malunited Colles' fracture can cause narrowing of the passage. Arthritic complications, such as tenosynovitis, following rheumatoid arthritis can cause enlargement of the tendons. Other causes would include trauma, spur formation, lipomas and hypertrophy of the wrist because of occupational hazards.[18,23,25] These conditions result in compression or entrapment of the median nerve in the carpal tunnel. Carpal tunnel syndrome may also obstruct venous return causing edema, increased pressure, and ischemia. This may result in permanent damage to the median nerve.

Clinically the onset of carpal tunnel syndrome can be sudden or occur over a long time. The patient may feel numbness, paresthesias, or pain, especially at night. Physical examination of the hand would reveal diminished sensation on the radial half of the hand, atrophy of the thenar eminence, fasciculations in the area of wasting, and trophic changes on the first, second, and third fingertips.[12,18,23] Medical management would be contingent on the cause of the pressure or entrapment of the median nerve.

The occupational therapist can provide supportive devices, such as splinting if indicated, and can teach the patient the use of assistive devices for one-handed activities and adaptive devices for daily activities. It is also important to engage the patient in purposeful activities to maintain function, joint mobility, and muscular strength in the uninvolved extremities. The patient should be instructed to visually compensate for sensory loss so further damage does not occur in the denervated tissues. For some patients prevocational exploration may be appropriate to maintain gainful employment during the period of recovery.

ULNAR NERVE INJURY. The ulnar nerve is the largest branch of the medial cord of the brachial plexus. It travels down the medial side of the arm and passes posteriorly to the medial epicondyle of the humerus. From the elbow it descends along the ulnar side of the forearm to innervate the small muscles of the hand.

The sensory branches of the ulnar nerve innervate cutaneous receptors in the little finger, half of the ring finger, and the medial portion of the hand. The motor branches innervate the flexor carpi ulnaris half of the flexor digitorum profundus, adductor digiti minimi, opponens digiti minimi, flexor digiti minimi, lumbricales 3 and 4, interossei, adductor pollicis, flexor pollicis brevis, and palmaris brevis muscles.

The actions produced by the ulnar nerve are finger adduction and abduction, wrist flexion, and MP extension. Grasp and pinch are achieved by proximal interphalangeal (PIP) flexion of the fourth and fifth phalanges and thumb adduction and opposition.

The usual sites of injury of the ulnar nerve are the posterior elbow region and the palmar region of the hand from the MP joint of the fifth finger to the carpal joint.[4,12,50]

COMBINED ULNAR AND MEDIAN INJURY. Since the ulnar and median nerves are anatomically close to each other in the wrist region, they are often injured together. The clinical picture depends on the severity of the lesion and which nerve has undergone the most damage. If both nerves suffer a complete transection, ape hand deformity would be present, the wrist would be hyperextended, and flexor movements and abduction and adduction of the fingers would be greatly impaired.[4,12,35,50]

VOLKMANN'S CONTRACTURE. A fracture of the lower end of the humerus (supracondylar region) may result in a diminished supply of well-oxygenated blood to the muscles of the forearm. This phenomenon can occur when the fracture has been tightly cast and bandaged. Edema sets in near the site of the injury and shuts down the blood supply to the muscle bellies because the site of injury cannot swell outward. Ischemia will deprive tissues of oxygen and nourishment. The muscle can become necrotic, causing atrophy and contractures of the wrist, fingers, and forearm. The flexor digitorum profundus and flexor pollicis longus muscles are severely affected. The median nerve is often more impaired than the ulnar nerve.[12,25]

Shortly after a fracture of the humerus has been immobilized, the patient may have a cold, distal extremity with a smooth, glossy, or dusky appearance of the skin. If the therapist cannot detect a radial pulse, the physician should be informed immediately, and the cast should be removed. Early detection and prevention of this problem can eliminate a very severe deformity. If, for example, the ischemia lasts 6 hours, some contracture will follow. Ischemia lasting 48 hours or more will result in a permanent deformity of the forearm.

If mild ischemia has occurred, the physician may prescribe vigorous, active exercises to increase circulation, activate musculature, and prevent joint stiffness.

The occupational therapist may be involved in the treatment of acute peripheral nerve injury or may be involved later in the rehabilitation process. Treatment during the acute postoperative phase is aimed at preventing deformity. Initially static splints are used to immobilize the extremity and protect the site of injury.[19,50] During this phase the reduction of edema may be of primary importance. The first step in the reduction of edema is to elevate the extremity above the level of the heart. This will decrease the hydrostatic pressure in the blood vessels and promote venous and lymphatic drainage. Manual massage while the extremity is elevated may also reduce edema. The massage should entail centripetal strokes to gently force the excess fluids toward the proximal aspects of the body. Care must be taken not to disturb the healing process of the site of injury. External elastic support can also be used to alleviate the edema. Furthermore, passive ROM will assist in the prevention of edema by promoting venous return.[52]

Table 32-1 Clinical Manifestations of Peripheral Never Lesions

Spinal nerves	Nerve roots	Motor distribution	Clinical manifestations
Brachial plexus			
C5-7	Long thoracic	Shoulder girdle, serratus anterior	"Winged scapula"
C5-6	Dorsal scapular	Rhomboid major and minor, levator, scapulae	Loss of scapular adduction and elevation
C7-8	Thoracodorsal	Latissimus dorsi	Loss of arm adduction and extension
C5-6	Suprascapular	Supraspinatus, infraspinatus	Weakened lateral rotation of humerus
C5-6	Subscapular	Subscapularis, teres major	Weakened medial rotation of humerus
C6-8, T1	Radial	All extensors of forearm, triceps	"Wrist drop," extensor paralysis
C5-6	Axillary	Deltoid, teres minor	Loss of arm abduction, weakened lateral rotation of humerus
C5-6	Musculocutaneous	Biceps brachii, brachialis, coracobrachialis	Loss of forearm flexion and supination
C6-8, T1	Median	Flexors of hand and digits, opponens pollicis	Ape hand deformity, weakened grip, thenar atrophy, unopposed thumb
C8, T1	Ulnar	Flexor of hand and digits, oppenens pollicis	Claw hand deformity, interosseus atrophy, loss of thumb adduction
Lumbosacral plexus			
L2-4	Femoral	Iliopsoas, quadriceps femoris	Loss of thigh flexion, leg extension
L2-4	Obturator	Adductors of thigh	Weakened or loss thigh adduction
L4-5, S1-3	Sciatic	Hamstrings, all musculature below the knee	Loss of leg flexion, paralysis of all muscles of leg and foot
L4-5, S1-2	Common peroneal	Dorsiflexors of foot	Foot-drop, steppage gait, loss of eversion
L4-5, S1-3	Tibial	Gastrocnemius, soleus, deep plantar flexors of foot	Loss of plantar flexion and inversion of foot

Occupational Therapy Intervention for Peripheral Nerve Injuries

The treatment goals for peripheral nerve injuries are generally similar. The aim is to assist the patient in regaining the maximal level of function. The rate of return and the residual impairments depend largely on the severity of the lesion and the quality of care during the rehabilitation process. Table 32-1 is a useful summary of the major nerve roots and clinical manifestation of their lesions.

As the patient's muscle tone returns, a mild progressive resistive exercise program can be established. Resistive activities, such as woodworking, ceramics, leatherwork, and copper tooling, may be used in conjunction with isometric and isotonic exercises. The therapist should not overtax the returning musculature and should protect the weaker muscle groups from stretch and fatigue.

The peripheral nerve injury may create some challenging problems in ADL that the therapist and patient must overcome. If one upper extremity is impaired (flaccid paralysis), the therapist may design a temporary "static sling" to be worn during shower activities or anytime the extremity needs to be securely positioned so that the person can move about. Static slings have some disadvantages. They should not be worn for long periods because they hold the arm in a flexed position, interfere with the postural support of the arm during some activities, limit proprioceptive feedback, and change the body image. Some therapists are fabricating "dynamic slings," designed by Farber[15] for hemiplegic patients, which can also help the patient with peripheral nerve injury. Elastic straps are used instead of webbing straps, and a cone is secured in the patient's hand to maintain a functional position. Tourniquet hosing has also been used in place of a rigid shoulder strap to allow some mobility of the joints, yet allow enough support to keep the arm flexed and close to the trunk. This elasticity allows better circulation to the extremity and better tactile, proprioceptive, and kinesthetic stimulation.

Assistive devices, such as long-handled reaching

aids and one-handed kitchen tools used in the treatment of hemiplegia, have also been found to be beneficial.

Sensory Reeducation

The occupational therapist can use sensory reeducation to assist the patient in establishing appropriate responses to sensory stimuli. In many cases surgical intervention such as skin island transfers results in crossed reinnervation. Thus the patient may have difficulty identifying touch localization. This phenomenon may also affect fine motor skills if the proper sensory feedback is not accurate. The therapist may start by applying more primitive sharp-dull stimuli and progress to moving touch stimuli. Lastly, as touch acuity improves, the therapist uses touch localization. The patient closes his eyes; the therapist applies a touch stimulus. The patient identifies where he has been touched by pointing to the spot. If the patient makes an incorrect touch response, the therapist allows him to look at where he pointed so he can use visual input to learn or "reeducate" the somatosensory pathways.[55] (Also see Chapter 11.)

PERIPHERAL NERVE PAIN SYNDROMES

Pain is a common complication in peripheral nerve injuries.[9,56] For some patients the pain itself becomes an overwhelming disability. Two types of pain have been associated with peripheral nerve injuries: causalgia and neuroma pain.[43,47,56] Causalgia is pain of great intensity originating from peripheral lesions affecting the fibers of the autonomic nervous system.[17] The most common sites for peripheral nerve injuries producing causalgia are the brachial plexus, sciatic, tibial, median, and ulnar nerves.[7] Because the sympathetic and parasympathetic fibers travel in the walls of blood vessels until they reach their respective organs, the pain can radiate to quadrants of the body served by these major blood vessels. In the upper extremity, causalgia is described as an intense burning sensation so excruciating that the patient holds the affected limb immobile for fear of stimulating the pain. The affected limb becomes extremely sensitive to temperature change, wind, and even noise.[16,33] Causalgia is also exacerbated by emotional stress. Because of its origin in the sympathetic division of the autonomic nervous system, even mood changes alter the pain sensitivity levels.[16]

Neuromas are incompletely regenerated nerve endings and fibers at the site where the peripheral nerve was damaged. Neuromas are particularly problematic in nerve endings serving the fingers and in amputated limbs. Phantom limb pain is often the result of neuroma formation. Neuromas are exquisitely painful and tender when they develop in the extremities that bear weight or are easily traumatized. In some cases, surgical resection is necessary to remove neurons that adhere to fascia and subcutaneous tissue.

Occupational Therapy Intervention

Recent research on pain management has revealed that certain activities and noninvasive techniques can modulate pain perception.[47,48] Today a better understanding of pain control mechanisms and the discovery of endogenous opiate-like substances (endorphins, enkephalins, and substance P) in the body, have provided therapists with new techniques for patients suffering from peripheral nerve pain.[1,9,37,45]

The occupational therapist can modulate pain perception in several ways. Pain perception travels from pain receptors (nociceptors) along ascending pathways to the thalamus to the cerebral cortex where the messages reach the conscious mind. Several intervention techniques can alter pain messages or neuronal transmission within these pathways. Peripheral pain emitting from neuromas can be alleviated by increased input to mechanoreceptors in the skin. This works because the sensory neurons transmitting pain messages must synapse in the dorsal horn of the spinal cord. The synapse to the secondary neurons in the dorsal gray matter is conducted through the release of substance P, one of the opiate-like neurotransmitters. Increased input to the mechanoreceptors in the skin inhibits the release of substance P.[37,47] The therapist can utilize several techniques to increase mechanoreceptor input. Graded light local percussion and therapeutic vibration over neuromas have been used to expedite this process.[1,29,30] TENS has been found to provide relief from pain related to neuromas, peripheral nerve injuries, stump pain, and phantom limb syndromes.[24,44] The occupational therapist can use TENS when it is prescribed by a physician.

Research evidence also supports the use of localized stimulation to acupoints and trigger points to modify neuroma pain.[45,47] Melzak has studied these pain relief mechanisms in support of the gate control theory. Many patients also obtain pain relief by protecting the tender regions of the body. The therapist can fabricate protective devices from splinting materials. Some patients find relief when the extremity is wrapped with a cloth material that has been soaked in water.[7]

Pain management for causalgia uses a different rationale and different neurophysiologic systems. As previously mentioned, causalgia arises from the autonomic nervous system. Increased activity in the sympathetic division of the autonomic nervous system exacerbates causalgia. In addition, the neuronal connections to the limbic system suggest that emotions play an important role in causalgia.[7,16,33,37]

The neurophysiologic rationale for alleviating causalgia is very complex because it involves at least two distinct systems. Both systems originate in areas of the cortex. One system is more direct in that it projects to neurons in the reticular formation and to motor pathways terminating on excitatory and inhibitory neurons in the dorsal gray matter of the spinal cord. The other system includes neurons in the cortex projecting to cell bodies in the limbic system which go on to transmit to the midbrain. The first cortical modulating system is very responsive to physical and emotional stress. Consequently, stress increases blood concentrations of catecholamines (dopamine, epinephrine, and norepinephrine) via the autonomic nervous system. As a result, this triggers the release of enkephalins that inhibit transmission of afferent interneurons in the dorsal gray matter. The second cortical modulating system involving the limbic system and midbrain responds by releasing endorphins to inhibit pain transmission.[1,9,45,47] The release of these endogenous opiates (enkephalin and endorphins) gives credence to the utilization of purposeful activities to modulate the perception of pain.

By involving the patient in successful and purposeful activities the occupational therapist provides cognitive diversion from the pain exerience. Engagement in purposeful activities can afffect moods and emotions, an effect that in turn will alter the perception of pain intensity and ultimately modify the pain threshold.[33,47] The therapist can also use background music as a therapeutic modality. Concentration on music affects the cortical modulating system through connections with the limbic system. In addition, music can be used with earphones. While the patient is engaged in activities, it provides a control factor over the pain stimulus because the volume can be increased or decreased to accommodate the pain intensity.

Since causalgia is related to tension and stress, the therapist can also employ relaxation techniques.[9,16] Deep breathing and progressive relaxation can promote a dominance of the parasympathetic system.[33,47] By eliciting the relaxation response, the patient's muscles relax, heart rate and respiration rate slows, and the patient experiences a sense of well-being. By learning relaxation techniques the patient can control emotional tension and depression: Both are contributors to causalgia and the perception of pain.

MYASTHENIA GRAVIS

Although myasthenia gravis is not a true lower motor neuron disease, it warrants some discussion in this chapter.

Myasthenia gravis is a chronic neuromuscular condition characterized by abnormal voluntary muscle fatigue. The cause of this disease is unknown at the present time. However, the defect occurs at the myoneurojunction where the presence of IgG autoantibodies seems to block acetylcholine receptors on the postsynaptic membrane.[18] Another theory suggests that there is a defect in the resynthesis of acetylcholine in the presynaptic membrane of the myoneurojunction.[41] In addition, many patients develop concurrent complications of the thyroid and thymus glands. It is not understood how the thymus gland affects the disease, but surgical removal causes significant improvement in 70% to 80% of the patients.[12]

Statistically this disease affects women between age 20 and 40 and men between age 50 and 70. It affects all races. The prevalence in the United States is estimated to be about 20,000 persons.[23]

Clinically myasthenia gravis produces a variety of symptoms. The disease can affect any of the striated skeletal muscles of the body. Yet it seems to have an affinity for the muscles innervated by the brainstem nuclei. Therefore the muscles most often affected are those that move the eyes, eyelids, tongue, jaw, and throat. The muscles that are used most often fatigue the earliest.[18] Therefore the patient may have double vision, drooping of the eyelids, and difficulty with speech or swallowing as the day goes on.

Medical management includes a long list of drugs, such as anticholinesterase, prednisone, and possibly corticosteroid therapy. A thymectomy is performed on patients not responding to anticholinesterase therapy. A new therapy called plasmapheresis entails filtering the blood to remove the IgG autoantibodies. This treatment may be accompanied by cytotoxic immunosuppressive therapy.[21,22]

Occupational Therapy Intervention

The prognosis for myasthenia gravis varies with each individual. Spontaneous remissions have been reported with thymectomy, but for most it is a progressively disabling disease.[12] It is important for the therapist to monitor the patient's muscle strength on a regular basis. The therapist need not evaluate all of the muscles because the evaluation will contribute to fatigue. Instead, the therapist can test the strength of a few muscles during each visit and keep a running chart to note any significant changes. If the patient is taking oral cholinergic drugs, optimal strength is expected about 1 or 2 hours after the medication has been ingested.[2] Therefore the therapist should coordinate muscle testing with the drug treatment regime so the test results are not confounded by the medication. The therapist should also record any changes in the patient's physical appearance, such as ptosis of the eyelids, drooping facial muscles, or alterations of breathing or swallowing. The therapist should provide gentle nonresistive activities that are intellectually and psychologically stimulating. The activities should be graded so they do not fatigue the patient. The treatment plan should include energy conservation, work simplification, and an array of adaptive and assistive devices to reduce effort during daily activities. If appropriate, electronic communication devices can be installed in the patient's home so he or she can maintain contact with community agencies. In addition, the therapist may assist with home planning to determine architectural barriers, bathroom adaptations, and furniture rearrangements. Supportive devices can also be fabricated to prevent overstretching the weakened musculature.

The therapist should assist in educating the patient about the disease. The patient should avoid emotional stress, fatigue, and excessive heat or cold because they may exacerbate the symptoms of the disease. Women may experience an increase in symptoms during menstruation because of hormonal changes taking place. The patient may need additional rest during this time. The therapist should also follow infection control procedures, since minor infections can also exacerbate the symptoms.

REVIEW QUESTIONS

1. Describe the components of the lower motor neuron system.
2. Describe the pathology and major clinical findings of poliomyelitis.
3. Compare and contrast poliomyelitis with Guillain-Barré syndrome.
4. List some treatment strategies for Guillain-Barré syndrome.
5. List at least six clinical manifestations of peripheral nerve injury.
6. Describe the sequential signs of recovery following peripheral nerve injury.
7. Describe some evaluations to determine sensory loss.
8. Identify the classic deformities associated with the radial, ulnar, and median nerves.
9. Describe some treatment strategies for peripheral nerve injuries.
10. List some contraindications when treating peripheral nerve injuries.
11. Describe the clinical signs of Bell's palsy.
12. Discuss some treatment strategies used to rehabilitate the facial muscles.
13. Describe the clinical signs of trigeminal neuralgia.
14. List three treatment techniques that can be used for trigeminal neuralgia.
15. Describe two new surgical techniques that may improve peripheral nerve regeneration.
16. Describe the pathophysiology of carpal tunnel syndrome.
17. Discuss some treatment intervention techniques for occupational therapists.
18. Describe the pathophysiology of myasthenia gravis.
19. Discuss the clinical signs of myasthenia gravis.
20. Describe the role of occupational therapy for patients who have myasthenia gravis.
21. Differentiate between causalgia and neuroma.
22. Describe four noninvasive methods of modulating pain perception.

REFERENCES

1. Adler M: Endorphins, enkephalins and neurotransmitters, Med Times 110:32, June 1982.
2. Barone D: Steroid treatment for experimental autoimmune myasthenia gravis, Arch Neurol 37:663, 1980.
3. Barr ML: The human nervous system, ed 2, New York, 1974, Harper & Row, Publishers, Inc.
4. Bateman J: Trauma to nerves in limbs, Philadelphia, 1962, WB Saunders Co.
5. Beals R: A study of occupational therapy in Bell's palsy, Am J Occup Ther 5:185, 1951.
6. Bickerstaff E: Neurology, ed 3, London, 1978, Hodder & Stoughton, Ltd.
7. Birch R and Grant C: Peripheral nerve injuries—clinical. In Downie P, editor: Cash's textbook of neurophysiology for physiotherapists, ed 4, Philadelphia, 1986, JB Lippincott Co.
8. Brashear RH and Raney RB: Shands' handbook of orthopaedic surgery, ed 9, St Louis, 1978, The CV Mosby Co.
9. Brena SF, editor: Chronic pain: America's hidden epidemic, New York, 1978, Atheneum Publishers.
10. Brown MD, et al: Electromyographic biofeedback in the reeducation of facial palsy, J Am Phys Ther Assoc 57:183, 1978.
11. Brunelli G: Direct neurotization of severely damaged muscles, J Hand Surg 7:572, 1982.
12. Chusid JG: Correlative neuroanatomy and functional neurology, ed 18, Los Altos, CA, 1982, Lange Medical Publications.
13. Clark RG: Clinical neuroanatomy and neurophysiology, ed 5, Philadelphia, 1975, FA Davis Co.
14. Evans FJ: Placebo response in pain reduction, Adv Neurol 4:289, 1974.
15. Farber S: Neurorehabilitation: a multisensory approach, Philadelphia, 1982, WB Saunders Co.
16. Gandhavadi B: Autonomic pain: features and methods of assessments, Postgrad Med 71:85, Jan 1982.
17. Gardner E: Fundamentals of neurology, ed 6, Philadelphia, 1975, WB Saunders Co.
18. Gilroy J and Meyer J: Medical neurology, ed 3, New York, 1979, Macmillan Publishing Co, Inc.
19. Hopkins HL and Smith HD:

Willard and Spackman's occupational therapy, ed 5, Philadelphia, 1978, JB Lippincott Co.

20. Jacobs A and Felton GS: Visual feedback of myoelectric output to facilitate muscle relaxation in normal patients and patients with neck injuries, Arch Phys Med Rehabil 50:34, 1969.

21. Khana E et al: Creutzfeldt-Jakob disease: focus among Libyan Jews in Israel, Sci 183:90, 1974.

22. Kornfeld P: Plasmapheresis in refractory generalized myasthenia gravis, Arch Neurol 38:478, 1981.

23. Krupp MA and Chatton MJ: Current medical diagnosis and treatment, ed 16, Los Altos, CA, 1977, Lange Medical Publications.

24. Lampe G: Introduction to the use of transcutaneous electrical nerve stimulation devices, Phys Ther 1:357, 1975.

25. Larson CB and Gould M: Orthopedic nursing, ed 9, St Louis, 1978, The CV Mosby Co.

26. Laurence TN and Pugel AV: Peripheral nerve involvement in spinal cord injury: an electromyographic study, Arch Phys Med Rehabil 59:209, 1978.

27. Lundborg G et al: Nerve regeneration across an extended gap: a neurobiological view of nerve repair and the possible involvement of neuronotrophic factors, J Hand Surg 7:500, 1982.

28. Melville ID: Clinical problems in motor neurone disease. In Obeham, P and Rose FC, editors: Progress in neurological research, London, 1979, Pitman Publishing, Ltd.

29. Melzack R and Wall PD: Psychophysiology of pain, Int Anesthesiol Clin 8:3, 1970.

30. Melzak R: Prolonged relief from pain by brief, intense transcutaneous somatic stimulation, Pain 1:357, 1975.

31. Moore DE and Backer MM: How effective is TENS for chronic pain, Am J Nurs 83:1175, 1983.

32. Morrison D, Pathier P, and Horr K: Sensory motor dysfunction and therapy in infancy and early childhood, Springfield, IL, 1955, Charles C Thomas, Publishers.

33. Newberger P and Sallan S: Chronic pain: Principles of management, J Pediatr 98:180, 1981.

34. Nichols HF: Manual of hand injuries, Chicago, 1955, Year Book Medical Publishers, Inc.

35. Noback CR and Demares RJ: The nervous system: introduction and review, ed 2, New York, 1977, McGraw-Hill, Inc.

36. Pertovaara A: Modification of human pain threshold by specific tactile receptors, Acta Physiol Scand 107:339, 1979.

37. Piercey MF and Folkers K: Sensory and motor functions of spinal cord substance P, Sci 214:1361, Dec 1981.

38. Phelps PE and Walker C: Comparison of the finger wrinkling test results to establish sensory tests in peripheral nerve injury, Am J Occup Ther 31:465, 1977.

39. Rathenberg E: Dynamic living for the long term patient, Dubuque, IA, 1962, Wm C Brown Co, Publishers.

40. Robinault I: Functional aids for the multiply handicapped, New York, 1973, Harper & Row, Publishers, Inc.

41. Schmidt RF: Fundamentals of neurophysiology, ed 2, New York, 1978, Springer-Verlag, Inc.

42. Schumacher B and Allen HA: Medical aspects of disabilities, Chicago, 1976, Rehabilitation Institute.

43. Seddon HJ: Surgical disorders of the peripheral nerves, ed 2, Edinburgh, 1975, Churchill Livingstone, Inc.

44. Shealy C: Transcutaneous electrical nerve stimulation for control of pain, Surg Neurol 2:45, 1974.

45. Sjolund B and Erikson M: Electroacupuncture and endogenous morphines, Lancet 2:1985, 1976.

46. Smith B: Differential diagnosis in neurology, New York, 1979, Arco Publishing, Inc.

47. Swerdlow M: The therapy of pain, Philadelphia, 1981, JB Lippincott Co.

48. Tappan FM: Healing massage techniques: a study of eastern and western methods, Reston, VA, 1978, Reston Pub Co, Inc.

49. Taylor AG, et al: How effective in TENS for acute pain, Am J Nurs 83:1171, 1983.

50. Trombly CA and Scott AD: Occupational therapy for physical dysfunction, Baltimore, 1977, Williams & Wilkins.

51. Van Dam A: Guillain-Barré syndrome: a unique perspective, Occup Ther Forum 2:6, Feb 1987.

52. Vasudevan S and Melvin JL: Upper extremity edema control: rationale of the techniques, Am J Occup Ther 33:520, 1979.

53. Walter JB: An introduction to the principles of disease, Philadelphia, 1977, WB Saunders Co.

54. West A: Understanding endorphins: our natural pain relief system, Nurs 12:50, 1981.

55. Wynn-Parry CB and Salter M: Sensory reeducation after median nerve lesions, Hand 8:250, 1976.

56. Wynn-Parry CB and Withrington R: Painful disorders of peripheral nerves, Postgrad Med J 60:869, 1984.

Sample treatment plan

CASE STUDY

John is a 23-year-old man employed as a construction worker. He is a high school graduate, is married, and has two children. Recently while working he sustained a deep laceration of the right anterior forearm. This injury resulted in a severed ulnar nerve and partial damage to the median nerve. The patient has undergone microsugery, and the severed nerves have been repaired with moderate success.

John is energetic and has difficulty adjusting to the hospital environment and to a sedentary existence.

He was referred to occupational therapy for services during the acute and rehabilitation phases of his treatment program. The goals are to prevent deformity, restore joint and muscle function to the maximal level possible, facilitate adjustment to hospital and disability, and evaluate potential for return to former employment.

Personal data
Name: John
Age: 23
Diagnosis: Laceration to right forearm, peripheral nerve injury
Disability: Unlar and median nerve dysfunction; moderate to severe motor paralysis
Treatment aims as stated in referral
To pevent deformity
To restore joint and muscle function to maximal level possible
To facilitate adjustment to hospital and disability
To evaluate potential for return to employment

OTHER SERVICES

Medical-surgical: Surgery, medication, supervision of rehabilitation program
Nursing: Nursing care during acute phase of treatment, psychological support
Physical therapy: ROM, muscle reeducation, edema control
Social service: Financial arrangements, counseling to patient and family
Vocational rehabilitation counselor: Explore vocational potential, vocational counseling

FRAME OF REFERENCE

Occupational performance

TREATMENT APPROACHES

Biomechanical and rehabilitative

OT EVALUATION

Sensation: Test (light touch, stereognosis, proprioception, two-point discrimination, pain)
Nerve regeneration: Wrinkle test
Muscle strength: Manual muscle test
ROM: Measure
Grip and pinch strength: Test with instruments
Hand evaluation: Observation, Jebsen-Taylor Test of Hand Function; tests of speed and dexterity
ADL: Observe performance
Psychosocial adjustment: Observe
Muscle function: EMG biofeedback evaluation to obtain quantitative information for baseline function

EVALUATION SUMMARY

Muscle testing revealed that the right upper extremity has considerable weakness in the distal musculature. Wrist flexors, finger adductors, finger abductors, and opposition of thumb are P(2). Muscles innervated by the radial nerve such as the wrist extensors are G(4) to N(5).

The joint motions are within normal limits, but some tightness is noted in the thumb and long finger flexors. Visual inspection shows some edema and marked muscle atrophy of the interossei (web space) and moderate atrophy of the thenar muscles. The pattern of denervation has produced a muscle imbalance and the ape hand deformity.

Grip strength registers at 10 pounds (4.2 Kg) in the right hand and 120 pounds (54 Kg) in the left. Palmar pinch strength using lateral pinch is 4 pounds (1.8 Kg) on the right and 24 pounds (10.8 Kg) on the left.

The Jebsen Hand Function Test reveals below standard norms for age in gross grasp, fine prehension, and manual dexterity.

Sensory testing shows that light touch, proprioception, and two-point discrimination are absent in the ulnar aspect of the right hand. The medial aspect is impaired, especially in the thenar region. Stereognosis sensibility is impaired when comparing nickels with quarters and pennies with dimes. Superficial pain sensitivity (pinprick) is intact on medial anterior surface of the right hand and absent along ulnar nerve root distribution.

Tinel's sign is present distal to the laceration on the right forearm. The wrinkle test shows absence of wrinkling along the cutaneous sensory distribution of the ulnar nerve; some wrinkling is noted in the medial nerve root distribution. Photos of wrinkle distributions are included in record for visual inspection and documentation.

The accident does not appear to have had any effect on the patient's cognitive functions. He has performed within normal limits for a 23-year-old male of average intelligence. He exhibits normal long term and short term memory, good judgment, and problem-solving skills. He attended to cognitive perceptual tasks, followed directions effectively, and demonstrated the ability to concentrate for extended periods of time.

Psychosocial adjustment appears to be normal. John is married and has two children. His marriage appears to be stable, and his wife has been supportive. John has had difficulty adjusting to his hospitalization. He has a high level of energy and is accustomed to being active. At times, he seems to be agitated, impatient, and mildly depressed because of his inactivity. The patient's leisure interests consisted of automechanics and playing handball and baseball. He also enjoyed home improvement projects such as painting, decorating, and light construction. John and his wife have many friends and engage in social activities on weekends.

The patient appears to have good vocational potential. He is very motivated for recovery and to return to his former occupation in the field of construction. Because he was injured while on the job, he is presently receiving workmen's compensation and disability insurance for financial support. If residual weakness prevents his return to employment, further prevocational testing will be conducted to determine an alternative occupation.

In functional skills John is somewhat independent in most self-care actitivies. He has attempted to use one hand for personal hygiene skills. Assistive devices have been recommended to ease difficulty in cutting food, attaching buttons, and managing soap in the shower.

Continued.

Sample treatment plan—cont'd

ASSETS

Very motivated
Good manual dexterity in uninvolved hand
Good strength in uninvolved hand
Good attention span and working tolerance
Independent in self-care
Family support
Good potential for reemployment
Age
Intelligence
Financial Support

PROBLEM LIST

1. Muscle weakness and atrophy in right hand
2. Slight muscle imbalance
3. Sensory loss
4. Edema
5. Loss of ROM
6. Difficulty adjusting to inactivity
7. Decreased independence in personal hygiene activity
8. Decreased work capacity

PROBLEM 1

Muscle weakness

Objective

Strength of affected wrist flexors and hand muscles will increase from P to G

Method

Active exercise to wrist flexors, thumb flexors, finger abductors, and adductors; thumb abduction; opposition

Construction of small jewelry box with mosaic tile top; ceramics—pinch pot or coil project; therapeutic putty exercises

Gradation

Increase resistance as F + muscle grades are attained; commence PRE program; increase time of activity; increase variety of activities

PROBLEM 2

Muscle imbalance

Objective

Muscle imbalance at the wrist will be prevented and muscles will be maintained at normal length

Method

Static resting splint to maintain functional position of wrist and hand: to be worn at night and during periods of inactivity

Teach gentle passive ROM 4 times a day for 15 minutes each session to stretch tight soft tissues

Gradation

Decrease use of static splint and manual stretching as hand function increases; integrate functional hand activities

PROBLEM 3

Loss of sensation

Objective

Sensation in hand will increase to normal limits

Method

Massage intrinsic muscles to maintain good circulation and elasticity of soft tissues; sensory stimulation and sensory reeducation to skin areas supplied by median and ulnar nerves

Gradation

Touch and tactile sensation are graded, beginning with crude touch and pinprick; increase discriminative touch stimuli to two-point discrimination less than 10 mm, stereognosis, and touch localization

PROBLEM 4

Slight hand edema

Objective

Edema in the right hand will be reduced or remain minimal

Methods

Retrograde massage of hand from distal to proximal; application of vibratory stimuli to promote venous drainage; overhead sling attached to headboard of bed, which supports forearm and hand in elevated position; allow some movement to increase blood circulation

Gentle passive ROM exercises to thumb, fingers, and wrist after sufficient healing of nerve has occurred to allow some traction on the nerve; teach client ROM exercises and proper positioning of hand

Gradation

Decrease massage and manual stimulation of hand as it recovers normal circulation and skin color

Decrease then eliminate use of overhead sling when active rehabilitation program commences

PROBLEM 5

Loss of active ROM

Objective

Increase joint mobility and ROM of hand and wrist

Method

Gentle passive ROM to all affected joints; 5 to 10 repetitions 3 times daily; immediately follow with active ROM of each joint or isolated active motion of affected joints and muscles to within practical limits

Gradation

Decrease passive exercise; increase active exercise as strength improves

Promote functional hand activities

PROBLEM 6

Difficulty adjusting to hospitalization and inactivity

Objective

Patient will be more relaxed and less depressed, resulting in tolerance for hospital routines and social interactions

Method

Isometric exercises for shoulder and elbow muscle groups; isometric resistive exercises for unaffected extremities; supportive approach to patient, positive reinforcement for participation in activities: puzzles, games (cards, checkers, chess, dominoes, Atari television sports games), reading (sports magazines)

Gradation

Decrease extrinsic motivation and initiation of activities; increase number of persons participating with patient

Elicit ideas on improving physical arrangement of clinic; draw up plans and material list

PROBLEM 7

Decreased independence in personal hygiene activities.

Sample treatment plan—cont'd

Objective

Given assistive device patient will perform personal hygiene and eating activities independently

Method

One-handed rocker knife, rubber placemat for stability of plate, plate guard, suction soap holder to fix soap to wall, wash mitt, built-up handle on razor for shaving

Gradation

Decrease use of assistive devices as right hand function increases

PROBLEM 8

Decreased work capacity

Objective

Feasibility for return to employment or related job will be explored

Method

Construction of a large wood chest or bookshelf; patient is to plan and perform all operations; activities should be performed standing; purpose is to evaluate handling and use of hand tools, safety awareness, standing tolerance, and physical endurance

Engage patient in construction of closet or shelves for health care facility under direction of maintenance supervisor, as a job trial; aspects of the actual construction duties can be simulated in the clinic; weighted objects similar to construction materials will be lifted, carried, and manipulated and will be graded according to gained strength and endurance

Gradation

Increase weight of loads and requirements for bending, lifting and carrying large objects

33 Spinal cord injury

CAROLE ADLER
LORRAINE WILLIAMS PEDRETTI

Rehabilitation of the spinal-cord-injured (SCI) individual is a lifelong process that requires readjustment to nearly every aspect of life. Occupational therapists play an integral role in maximizing physical and psychosocial restoration as well as in enhancing functional performance to an optimal level of independence. Through analyzing, retraining, and adaptive techniques, occupational therapists provide patients with the tools and resources to pursue their optimal physical and functional potentials.

Spinal cord injuries are caused by a multitude of factors. The most common are trauma from automobile accidents, gunshot and stab wounds, falls, sports, and diving accidents. Spinal cord functions may also be disturbed by diseases, such as tumors, myelomeningocele, syringomyelia, multiple sclerosis, and amyotrophic lateral sclerosis.[16] Some of the treatment principles outlined in this chapter may have application to these conditions. The emphasis, however, will be on rehabilitation of the individual with traumatic injury.

RESULTS OF SPINAL CORD INJURY

Spinal cord injury results in quadriplegia or paraplegia. Quadriplegia is any degree of paralysis of the four limbs and trunk musculature. There may be partial upper extremity (UE) function, depending on the level of the cervical lesion. Paraplegia is paralysis of the lower extremities (LEs) and possibly of some trunk musculature, depending on the level of the lesion.[16]

Spinal cord injuries are referred to in terms of the regions (cervical, thoracic, and lumbar) of the spinal cord in which they occur and the numerical order of the neurological segments. The level of spinal cord injury designates the last fully functioning neurological segment of the cord: for example, C6 refers to the sixth neurological segment of the cervical region of the spinal cord as the last fully intact neurological segment. Thus in this instance all muscles innervated by segments below the C6 neurological level will be paralyzed.[15]

Complete lesions result in total dysfunction of the spinal cord below the level of the injury. Incomplete lesions may involve several neurological segments and some spinal cord function may be partially or completely intact, which allows for some function below the level of the injury.[2,15]

Complete versus Incomplete Classifications

The extent of neurological damage depends on the location and severity of the injury (Fig. 33-1). In a *complete* injury, total paralysis and loss of sensation result from a complete interruption of the ascending and descending nerve tracts below the level of the lesion. In an *incomplete* injury there is some degree of preservation of the sensory and/or motor nerves below the lesion. Frankle Classification refers to the degree of incompleteness and is usually stated after the neurological level: that is, C6 Frankle Class B.[5]

The Frankle classes are defined as follows:
Frankle Class A: Motor and sensory complete
Frankle Class B: Motor complete, sensory incomplete
Frankle Class C: Motor and sensory incomplete—nonfunctional motor control
Frankle Class D: Motor and sensory incomplete—functional voluntary motor control
Frankle Class E: No remaining neurological deficit—complete recovery

Incomplete injuries are categorized according to the area of damage: central, lateral, anterior, or peripheral.

CENTRAL CORD SYNDROME. Central cord syndrome results when there is more cellular destruction in the center of the cord than in the periphery. There is greater paralysis and sensory loss in the UEs because these nerve tracts are more centrally located than nerve tracts for the LEs. This syndrome is often seen in older people in whom arthritic changes have caused a narrowing of the spinal canal; in such cases cervical hyperextension without vertebral fracture may precipitate central cord damage.

BROWN-SEQUARD SYNDROME. Brown-Sequard syndrome results when only one side of the cord is

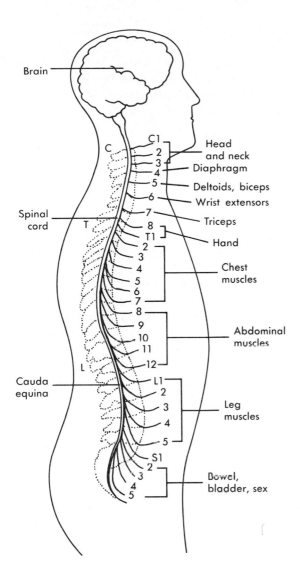

Brain

C1
C 2
3
4
5
6
7
8
T1
2
3
4
5
6
7
8
9
10
11
12

Head
and neck
Diaphragm

Deltoids, biceps

Wrist extensors

Triceps

Hand

Chest
muscles

Abdominal
muscles

Spinal
cord

T

Cauda
equina

L

L1
2
3
4
5
S1
2
3
4
5

Leg
muscles

Bowel,
bladder, sex

Fig. 33-1. Spinal nerves and the major areas of the body they supply. From Phillips R, editor: Spinal cord injury home care manual, ed 2, San José, CA, 1986, Santa Clara Valley Medical Center.

damaged, as in a stabbing or gunshot injury. Below the level of injury there is motor paralysis and loss of proprioception on the ipsilateral side and loss of pain, temperature, and touch sensation on the contralateral side.

ANTERIOR SPINAL CORD SYNDROME. Anterior spinal cord syndrome results from injury that damages the anterior spinal artery or the anterior aspect of the cord. There is paralysis and loss of pain, temperature, and touch sensation. Proprioception is preserved.

CAUDA EQUINA. Cauda equina injuries involve peripheral nerves rather than the spinal cord directly. Since peripheral nerves possess a regenerating capacity that the cord does not, there is better prognosis

for recovery. Patterns of sensory and motor deficits are highly variable and asymmetrical.*.[8]

After spinal cord injury the victim enters a stage of spinal shock that may last from 24 hours to 8 weeks. This spinal shock phase is a period of areflexia, the cessation of all reflex activity below the level of the injury.[15] During this phase there is loss of sensation and voluntary motor function below the level of the injury, which results in complete flaccid paralysis. The bladder and bowel are atonic or flaccid. Deep tendon reflexes are decreased, and sympathetic functions are disturbed. This disturbance results in decreased constriction of blood vessels, low blood pressure, slower heart rate, and absence of perspiration below the level of the injury.[18] Since the spinal cord is usually not damaged below the level of the lesion, there is continued loss of motor function after spinal shock; but muscles that are innervated by the neurological segments below the level of injury usually develop spasticity because the monosynaptic reflex arc is intact but separated from higher inhibitory influences.[18] Deep tendon reflexes become hyperactive, and clonus may be evident. Sensory loss continues, and the bladder and bowel usually become spastic in patients whose injuries are above T12. The bladder and bowel usually remain flaccid or atonic in lesions at L1 and below.[18] Sympathetic functions become hyperactive. Spinal reflex activity (mass muscle spasms) becomes evident in the limbs. Reflex erections may develop in patients with thoracic and cervical injuries but usually do not occur in patients with lumbar and sacral injuries, since the essential reflex arc is usually interrupted in these individuals.[2,15]

Prognosis for Recovery

Prognosis for significant recovery of neuromuscular function after spinal cord injury depends on whether the lesion is complete or incomplete. In complete lesions if there is no sensation or return of motor function below the level of lesion 24 to 48 hours after the injury occurs, then no motor function return is expected. Partial to full return of function to one spinal nerve root level below the fracture is the usual gain and may occur in the first 6 months after injury. In incomplete lesions progressive return of motor function is possible, however uncertain.[18] When improvement begins immediately and return of muscle function appears consistently, prognosis for recovery

*Reprinted in part with permission from Hanak M and Scott A: Spinal cord injury, an illustrated guide for health care professionals, New York, 1983, Springer Verlag, Inc.

is better than if return of motor function occurs sporadically and inconsistently several months after the injury occurred.[15,18]

MEDICAL AND SURGICAL MANAGEMENT OF THE PERSON WITH SPINAL CORD INJURY

After a traumatic event in which spinal cord injury is a possibility, the conscious victim should be carefully questioned about cutaneous numbness and skeletal muscle paralysis before being moved. Emergency medical technicians and paramedics are trained in spinal cord injury precautions and extrication techniques when moving a possible SCI victim from an accident site. Flexion of the spine must be prevented during the transfer procedures. A firm stretcher or board to which the victim's head and back can be strapped should be procured before moving the victim. After transferring the victim to the stretcher or board, while maintaining axial traction on the neck and preventing any flexion of the spine and neck, the victim is strapped to the board or stretcher and transferred carefully to the hospital emergency room.

Careful examination, stabilization, and transportation of the person with spinal injury may prevent a temporary or slight spinal cord injury from becoming permanent or more severe.

Initial care in the hospital is directed toward preventing further damage to the spinal cord and reversing neurological damage if possible by stabilization or decompression of the injured neurological structures.[11,15] A careful neurological examination is carried out by the examining physician to aid in determining the site and type of injury. This is done with the patient in a supine position with the neck and spine immobilized. A catheter is placed in the patient's bladder for drainage of urine. Anteroposterior and lateral x-ray films may be taken, with the patient's head, neck, or spine immobilized, to obtain a rough idea of the type of injury. A CAT scan or Magnetic Resonance Imaging (MRI) may be required for further evaluation.

In early medical treatment the goals are to restore normal alignment of the spine, maintain stabilization of the injured area, and decompress neurological structures that are under pressure.

Bony realignment and stabilization usually occur by placing the patient on a kinetic bed (Roto Rest) that allows for skeletal traction and immobilization. The bed's design allows for continuous pressure relief and easy access to the patient's entire body for bowel, bladder, and hygiene care.

Open surgical reduction with wiring and spinal fusion is sometimes indicated. The goals of surgery are to decompress the spinal cord and achieve spinal sta-

bility and normal bony alignment.[15] Surgery, however, is not indicated in many cases, and the patient will heal with proper immobilization. As soon as possible a means of portable immobilization (halo vest or cast for cervical injuries and a thoracic brace or body jacket for thoracic injuries) is provided. This enables the patient to be transferred to a standard hospital bed and subsequently to be up in a wheelchair and involved in an active therapy program in as little as 1 to 2 weeks after injury. Being up in a wheelchair shortly after injury can significantly reduce the incidence and severity of further medical complications such as deep vein thrombosis, joint contractures, and the general deconditioning that can result from prolonged bed rest.

Complications of Spinal Cord Injury

PRESSURE SORES OR DECUBITUS ULCERS. Sensory loss enhances the development of pressure sores. The patient cannot feel the pressure of prolonged sitting or lying in one position or pressure from splints or braces. Pressure causes loss of blood supply to the area, which can ultimately result in necrosis. The areas most likely to develop pressure sores are bony prominences over the sacrum, ischium, trochanters, elbows, and heels. It is important for rehabilitation personnel to be aware of the signs of developing pressure sores. At first the area reddens yet blanches when pressed. Later the reddened area becomes blue or black and does not blanch. This indicates that necrosis has begun. Finally a blister or ulceration appears in the area and it may become infected. If allowed to progress, these sores may become very severe.

Pressure sores can be prevented by relieving and eliminating pressure points and protecting vulnerable area from excessive shearing. Turning in bed, special mattresses, foam "booties" to protect the heels, and shifting weight when sitting are some of the methods used to prevent pressure sores.

The use of hand splints and other appliances can also cause pressure sores. The therapist must inspect the skin, and the patient must be taught to inspect the skin, using a mirror, to watch for signs of developing pressure sores. Reddened areas can develop within 30 minutes, so frequent shifting, repositioning, and vigilance are essential if pressure sores are to be prevented.[15,18]

DECREASED VITAL CAPACITY. Decreased vital capacity will be a problem in people who have sustained cervical and high thoracic lesions. Such individuals will have markedly limited chest expansion and decreased ability to cough because of weakness or paralysis of the diaphragm and the intercostal and latissimus dorsi muscles. This can result in proneness to respiratory tract infections. The reduced vital capacity will affect overall tolerance level for activity. This problem may be alleviated by methods of assisted breathing and by teaching the patient glossopharyngeal or "frog" breathing. Strengthening of the sternocleidomastoids and the diaphragm and deep breathing exercises are helpful. Manually assisted coughing and mechanical suctioning of chest secretions may be required if there are excess secretions or a respiratory tract infection.[15,18]

OSTEOPOROSIS OF DISUSE. Because of disuse of long bones, particularly of the lower extremities, osteoporosis is likely to develop in patients with spinal cord injuries. A year after the injury the osteoporosis may be sufficiently advanced for pathological fractures to occur. Pathological fractures usually occur in the supracondylar area of the femur, proximal tibia, distal tibia, intertrochanteric area of the femur, and neck of the femur. Pathological fractures are usually not seen in UEs. Daily standing helps to prevent or delay the osteoporosis by placing the weight load on the long bones of the LEs.[15,18]

ORTHOSTATIC HYPOTENSION Lack of muscle tone in the abdomen and LEs leads to pooling of blood in these areas with resultant decrease in blood pressure. This occurs when the patient is sat up too quickly. Symptoms are dizziness, nausea, and loss of consciousness. The patient must be reclined quickly and if sitting in a wheelchair, must be tipped back with legs elevated until symptoms subside. With time this problem will diminish as sitting tolerance and level of activity increases. Abdominal binders, leg wraps, antiembolism stockings, and/or medications can aid in reducing symptoms.

AUTONOMIC DYSREFLEXIA. Autonomic dysreflexia is a phenomenon seen in persons whose injuries are above the T4 to T6 level. It is caused by reflex action of the autonomic nervous system in response to some stimulus, such as a distended bladder, fecal mass, bladder irrigation or rectal manipulation, thermal and pain stimuli, and visceral distention. The symptoms are perspiration, flushing, chills, nasal congestion, paroxysmal hypertension, pounding headache, and bradycardia. Autonomic dysreflexia is a *medical emergency.* If any of these symptoms appear, the patient should be attended to at once with administration of the appropriate prophylactic measures. The patient should not be left alone.[15,18]

Autonomic dysreflexia is treated by placing the patient in an upright position to reduce blood pressure. The bladder should be drained or legbag tubing checked for obstruction. Blood pressure and other symptoms should be monitored until back to normal. The occupational therapist must be aware of symp-

toms and treatment because dysreflexia can occur at any time after the injury.

SPASTICITY. Spasticity is involuntary muscle contraction below the level of injury which results from lack of inhibition from higher centers. Patterns of spasticity change over the first year, gradually increasing in the first 6 months and reaching a plateau about 1 year after the injury. A moderate amount of spasticity can be helpful in the overall rehabilitation of the patient with a spinal cord injury. It helps to maintain muscle bulk, assists in joint ROM, and can be used to assist during wheelchair and bed transfers and mobility. A sudden increase in spasticity can alert the patient to other medical problems, such as bladder infections.

Severe spasticity can be very frustrating to both the patient and the therapist in that it can interfere with function. It may be treated more aggressively with medication. Surgical procedures that involve cutting or lengthening spastic muscles and peripheral and spinal nerve blocks designed to paralyze the spastic muscle also may be used to eliminate problems of severe and disabling spasticity.[15,18]

HETEROTOPIC OSSIFICATION. Heterotopic ossification, also called "ectopic bone," is the abnormal deposition of osseous material. Usually it occurs in the muscles around the hip and knee but occasionally it can be noted also at the elbow and shoulder. The first symptoms are heat, pain, swelling, and decreased joint ROM. The ossification may progress to ankylosis of the affected joint. Treatment is the maintenance of joint ROM during the early stage of active bone formation to maintain the functional ROM necessary for good wheelchair positioning, symmetrical position of pelvis, and maximization of functional mobility.

If the ossification progresses to ankylosis and severely limits function because of joint immobility, surgical intervention may be pursued at a later date if necessary criteria and conditions are met.[15]

SEXUAL FUNCTION

The sexual drive and need for physical and emotional intimacy are not changed by spinal cord injury; but problems of mobility, dependency, and body image, plus complicating medical problems and the attitudes of partners and society affect social and sexual roles, access, and interest. Sexuality is an important part of life, and rehabilitation is not complete until a person is comfortable with his or her sexual and social role.

Lack of sensation over one part of the body is accompanied by increased or altered sensation over other parts of the body. The sexual response of the body after spinal cord injury needs to be explored the same way a person learns what muscles are working and where he or she can feel.

In males erections and ejaculations are often affected by the spinal cord injury. This is variable, however, and needs to be evaluated individually. Independent of these individual differences are changes in function, and for reasons that are not well understood, the viability of sperm in SCI males is frequently decreased even when other function is near normal.

In females there is usually an interval of weeks to months after injury during which menstruation ceases. It will usually start again and return to normal in time. There may also be changes in lubrication of the vagina during sexual activity. In contrast to males, however, there is no change in female fertility. SCI females can conceive and give birth. Special attention must be given to the interaction of pregnancy and childbirth with spinal cord injury, especially in regard to blood clots, respiratory function, bladder infections, dysreflexia, and use of medications during pregnancy and breast-feeding. To avoid pregnancy SCI women must take precautions, and the type of birth control used must be considered very carefully. Birth control pills are associated with blood clots, especially when combined with smoking, and probably should not be used. The intrauterine device (IUD) is not recommended even for able-bodied females. Diaphragms may be difficult to position properly when there is loss of sensation in the vagina or decreased hand function. Foams and suppositories are not very effective. The use of condoms by the male partner is probably the safest method.*[14]

Physically disabled individuals quickly sense the attitudes of professional helpers toward their sexuality. Traditionally professionals have viewed disabled persons as asexual and often communicated a sense that it was not all right to discuss sexual functioning. Professionals tended to put the topic off, whereas their patients waited for them to bring it up, thus granting permission for this important concern to be aired.[13] Fortunately these tendencies and attitudes are changing, and sexual counseling and education are a regular part of many rehabilitation programs for all types of physical disabilities.

Some patients lack basic sex education. Others feel asexual because of their disabilities and are isolated from peers; thus they may fear any type of sexual interaction. For these reasons sexual counseling must be geared to the needs of the individual patient. In some instances social interaction skills will need improvement before sexual activity can be considered. Occupational therapy can play an important part in improving social skills.

Since occupational therapists are concerned with the functional aspects of their patients' lives, they are in an excellent role to provide information and counseling on sexual functioning. Specific education and personal-attitude assessment of the counseling therapist are critical preliminaries to initiating sexual counseling and education.[13]

OCCUPATIONAL THERAPY INTERVENTION
Evaluation

Assessment of the patient is an ongoing process that begins the day of admission and continues until discharge. The occupational therapist is informally assessing the patient's functional progress and appropriateness of treatment and equipment on a day-to-day basis. An accurate formal initial evaluation is essential to determine baseline neurological, clinical, and functional status from which to formulate a treatment program and substantiate progress. Initial data gathering from the medical chart will provide personal information, a medical diagnosis, and a history of other pertinent medical information. Discharge planning begins during the initial evaluation; therefore the patient's social and vocational history as well as past and anticipated living situation is vital information necessary to plan a treatment program that meets the patient's individual needs.

PHYSICAL STATUS. Prior to evaluating the patient's physical status, very specific medical precautions should be obtained from the primary physician. Skeletal instability and related injuries of medical complications will affect the way in which the patient is moved and the active or resistive movements allowed.

Passive range of motion (PROM) should be measured prior to manual muscle testing to determine available pain-free movement. This evaluation also identifies the presence of or potential for joint contractures which could suggest the need for preventive or corrective splinting and positioning.

Shoulder pain, which will ultimately cause decreased shoulder and scapular ROM, is extremely common in C4-7 quadriplegia. It can be caused by several factors such as scapular immobilization resulting from prolonged bed rest or nerve root compression subsequent to the injury. Shoulder pain should be thoroughly assessed and diagnosed so that proper treatment can occur prior to the onset of chronic discomfort and functional loss.

An accurate assessment of the patient's muscle strength is critical in determining a precise diagnosis

---

*Reprinted in part with permission from Philips R: The spinal cord injury home care manual, Santa Clara Valley Medical Center, CA, 1983.

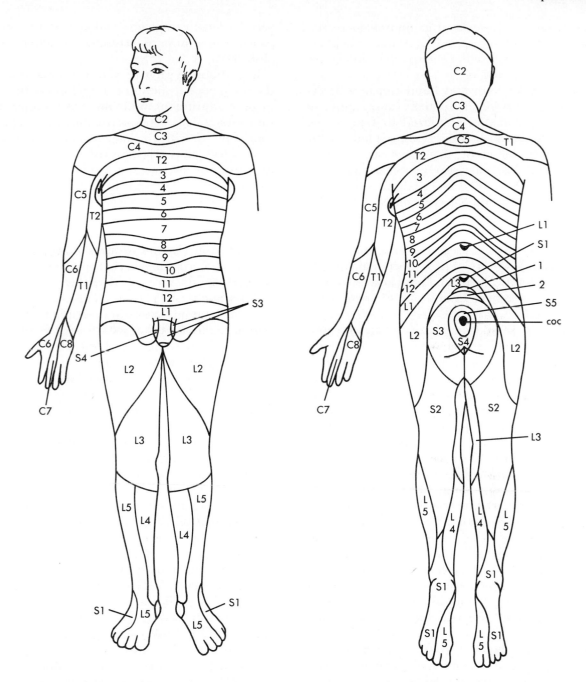

Fig. 33-2. Dermatomes of man. From Yashon D: Spinal injury, Norwalk, Conn, 1978, Appleton-Lange.

of neurological level and to establish a baseline for physical recovery and functional progress. Since the occupational therapist's skills with activity analysis will greatly enhance his or her effectiveness in treating the SCI individual, a precise working knowledge of musculoskeletal anatomy and specific manual muscle-testing techniques are essential. Utilizing accepted muscle-testing resources during testing is encouraged to ensure accurate technique while performing this complex evaluation. The muscle test should be re-

peated as often as necessary to provide an ongoing picture of the patient's strength and progress.

Sensation is evaluated for light touch, superficial pain (pinprick), and kinesthesia. This will determine areas of absent, impaired, and intact sensation. These findings will be useful in establishing the level of injury and in determining functional limitations (Fig. 33-2).

Immediately after injury, spasticity is rarely noted since the patient is still in spinal shock. When that subsides (from 6 to 8 weeks after injury), increased tone may be present in response to stimuli. The therapist should evaluate whether the spasticity interferes with or enhances function.

An evaluation of wrist and hand function determines the degree to which a patient can manipulate objects. This information is utilized to suggest the need for equipment such as positioning splints, cuffs, or, later, consideration of the tenodesis orthoses. Gross grasp and pinch measurements indicate functional abilities and are used as an adjunct to manual muscle testing to provide objective measurements of baseline status and progress if necessary muscles are innervated.[9]

Clinical observation is used to assess endurance, head and trunk control, LE functional muscle strength, oral motor control, and total body function. More specific assessment in any one of these areas may be required.

As a result of recent documentation of an increased number of combined spinal cord injury/head injury diagnoses, a specific cognitive and perceptual evaluation may be necessary.[10] Assessing a patient's ability to initiate tasks, follow directions, carry over learning day to day and problem solve contributes to the information base required for realistic goal setting.

FUNCTIONAL STATUS. Performing activities of daily living (ADL) is an important part of the occupational therapy evaluation. The purpose is to determine present and potential levels of functional ability. The evaluation should begin as soon as possible after injury, with light activities such as feeding and object manipulation. In later stages, activities may progress to hygiene at the sink, bed and wheelchair mobility, transfers, toileting, bathing, dressing, cooking, homemaking, child care, community reintegration, prevocational assessment, and driving.

Durable medical equipment such as wheelchairs, beds, and bathing equipment can be anticipated at this time. Such equipment should be specifically evaluated, however, and ordered only at the time when specific goals and expectations are known. Frequently equipment is not used or will hinder function because a therapist has not thoroughly taken into account all functional, environmental, psychological, and financial considerations when evaluating the patient's equipment needs.

Direct interaction with the patient's family and friends will provide valuable information regarding the patient's support systems while in the hospital and more importantly after discharge. This will have im-

pact on later caregiver-training in areas where the patient will require the assistance of others to accomplish ADL.

In addition to physical and functional assessments, the occupational therapist should assess the patient's stage of adjustment to the disability and psychosocial functioning skills.[15] The occupational therapist should communicate with the patient initially and continuously during the early phase of the evaluation process regarding needs, interest, aspirations, and feelings about the disability and the hospital and its personnel.[16] This is an important time to establish rapport and mutual trust, which will facilitate participation and progress in later and more difficult phases of rehabilitation. An individual's motivation, determination, socioeconomic background, education, family support, acceptance of disability, problem-solving abilities, and financial resources prove to be invaluable assets or limiting factors in determining the outcome of rehabilitation. A therapist must carefully assess the patient's status in each of these areas before determining the course of treatment.[9]

Establishing Treatment Objectives

It is important to establish treatment objectives in concert with the patient and with the rehabilitation team. The primary objectives of the rehabilitation team are often not those of the patient. Psychosocial factors, cultural factors, cognitive deficits, environmental limitations, and individual financial considerations must be identified and integrated into the development of a treatment program that will meet the unique needs of each individual. Every patient is different; therefore remedial or compensatory treatment methods should be planned to address each factor that may interfere with or affect goal achievement.[9] More participation can be expected if the patient's priorities are respected to the extent that they are achieveable and realistic.

The general objectives of treatment for the person with spinal cord injury are (1) to maintain or increase joint ROM and prevent deformity; (2) to increase strength of all innervated and partially innervated muscles through the use of prefunctional and functional activities; (3) to increase physical endurance; (4) to train the patient in the use of necessary adaptive equipment; (5) to develop the patient's maximal independence in all aspects of self-care and mobility skills; (6) to explore leisure interests and vocational potential; (7) to aid in the psychosocial adjustment to physical disability; (8) to evaluate and recommend necessary equipment; (9) to ensure for safe and independent home accessibility through home modification recommendations; (10) to instruct the patient in communication skills necessary for training caregivers to provide safe assistance.

Treatment Methods

ACUTE PHASE. During the acute or immobilized phase of the rehabilitation program the patient may be in traction or wearing a stabilization device such as a halo brace or body jacket. Medical precautions must be in force during this period. Flexion, extension, and rotary movements of the spine and neck are contraindicated.

Evaluation of total body positioning and hand splinting needs should be initiated at this time. In quadriplegics scapular elevation and elbow flexion as well as limited shoulder flexion and abduction while on bed rest will cause potentially painful shoulders and ROM limitations. Upper extremities should be intermittently positioned in 80° of shoulder abduction, external rotation with scapular depression, and full elbow extension to assist in alleviating this common problem. At Santa Clara Valley Medical Center, a device was designed and fabricated by the Occupational Therapy Department which will maintain the arm in an appropriate position while the patient is immobilized on a kinetic or Roto Rest bed (Fig. 33-3).

Selection of appropriate splint style and its accurate fabrication and fit by the occupational therapist will enhance patient acceptance and optimal functional gain. If musculature is not adequate to support wrist and hands properly for function and/or cosmesis, then splints should be fabricated to properly support the wrist in extension, thumb in opposition, and maintain the thumb web space while allowing the fingers to flex naturally at the metacarpophalangeal (MP) and proximal interphalangeal (PIP) joints. Splints should be dorsal rather than ventral in design to allow maximal sensory feedback while the patient's hand is resting on any surface. If at least F+ (3+) strength of wrist extension is present, then short opponens splints should be fabricated to maintain the web space and support the thumb in opposition. This same splint can be used functionally while training the patient to utilize a tenodesis grasp.

Active and active-assisted ROM of all joints within strength, ability, and tolerance levels should be performed. Muscle reeducation techniques to wrists and elbows should be employed. Progressive resistive exercises to wrists may be carried out. The patient should be encouraged to engage in self-care activities such as feeding, writing, and hygiene if possible, using simple devices such as a universal cuff or a custom

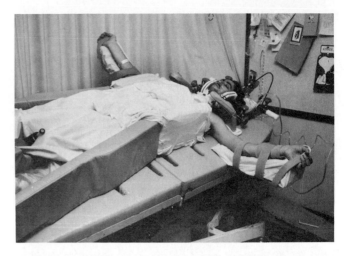

Fig. 33-3. ROTO Rest bed with arm positioner. Designed and fabricated by Occupational Therapy Department, Santa Clara Valley Medical Center, San José, CA.

writing splint. The occupational therapist may introduce leisure activities such as reading and provide prism glasses so that this and other activities may be pursued while in a supine position.[16]

ACTIVE PHASE. During the active or mobilization phase of the rehabilitation program, the patient can sit in a wheelchair and should begin developing upright tolerance. It is at this time that a method of relieving sitting pressure for the purpose of preventing decubitis ulcers on the ischial, trochanteric, and sacral bony prominences should be initiated. If the patient is quadriplegic yet has at least F+ (3+) shoulder strength bilaterally, pressure can be relieved on the buttocks by leaning forward over the feet. Simple cotton webbing loops are attached to the back frame of the wheelchair (Fig. 33-4). A paraplegic with intact UE musculature can perform a full depression weight shift off of the arms or wheels of the wheelchair. Weight shifts should be performed at least every 30 minutes until skin tolerance is determined.

Active and passive ROM exercises should be continued regularly to prevent undesirable contractures. Stretching may be indicated to correct contractures that are becoming established. In patients who have wrist extension, which will be used to substitute for absent grasp through tenodesis action of the long finger flexors, it is desirable to develop some tightness in these tendons in order to give some additional tension to the tenodesis grasp. The desirable contracture is developed by ranging finger flexion with the wrist fully extended and finger extension with the wrist

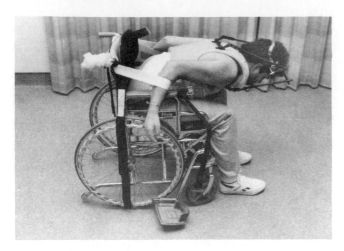

Fig. 33-4. Forward weight shift using loops attached to wheelchair frame.

flexed, thus never allowing the flexors or extensors to be in full stretch over all of the joints that they cross[17,18] (Fig. 33-5).

Elbow contractures should never be allowed to develop. Full elbow extension is essential to allow "propping" to maintain balance during static sitting and to assist in transfers. With zero triceps strength a C6 quadriplegic can maintain forward sitting balance by shoulder depression and protraction, external rotation, and full wrist extension (Fig. 33-6).

Progressive resistive exercise and resistive activities can be applied to innervated and partially innervated muscles. Shoulder musculature may be exercised with emphasis on the shoulder depressors, rotators, and abductors needed to perform sliding board and depression-type transfers.[1,16] The triceps, pectoralis, and latissimus dorsi muscles are needed for transfers and for shifting weight when in the wheelchair. Wrist extensors should be strengthened to maximize natural tenodesis function, thereby maximizing hand function.

The treatment program should be graded to increase the amount of resistance that can be tolerated during activity. As muscle power improves, increasing the amount of time in wheelchair activities will help the patient gain upright tolerance and endurance.

There are many assistive devices and equipment items that can be useful to the person with a spinal cord injury. However, it is important to note that every attempt should be made to have the patient perform the task with as little or no equipment as possible. Modified techniques are available which enable an individual to perform efficiently without the need for costly or bulky equipment. When appropriate the universal cuff for holding eating utensils, toothbrushes, pencils, and paintbrushes is a simple and versatile device that offers increased independence (see Fig. 15-38). A wrist cock-up splint to stabilize the wrist with attachment of the universal cuff can be useful for persons with little or no wrist extension. A plate guard, cup holder, extended straw with strawclip, and nonskid table mat can facilitate independent feeding (see Fig. 15-34). The wash mitt and soap holder or soap-on-a-rope can make bathing easier; however, the added difficulty of donning and doffing such equipment must be considered (see Fig. 15-12). Many people with quadriplegia can use a button hook to fasten clothing (see Fig. 15-6). A transfer board is an option for safe transfers. Through treatment, optimal muscle strength and coordination can occur, enabling the patient to potentially "grow out of" equipment that was initially provided.

The ADL program may be expanded to include independent feeding with devices; oral hygiene and upper body bathing; bowel and bladder care, such as suppository insertion and application of the urinary collection device; UE dressing; and transfers using the sliding board. Communication skills in writing and using the telephone, tape recorder, electric typewriters, and personal computer should be an important

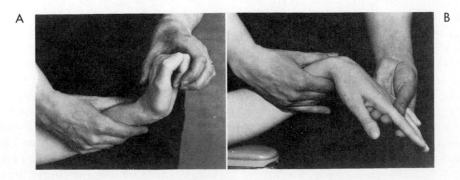

Fig. 33-5, A, Wrist is extended when fingers are passively flexed. **B,** Wrist is flexed when fingers are passively extended.

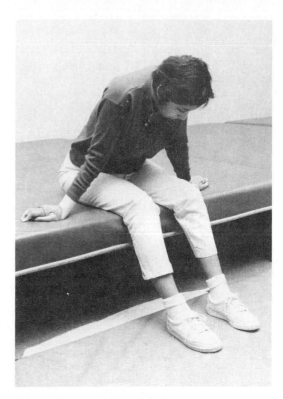

Fig. 33-6. Forward sitting balance is maintained by locking elbows. A valuable skill for bed mobility and transfers.

part of the treatment program.[16] Training in the use of the mobile arm support (MAS), flexor hinge splint (tenodesis), and assistive devices is also part of the occupational therapy program.

The occupational therapist should continue to provide psychological support by allowing and encouraging the patient to express frustration, anger, fears, and concerns. The occupational therapy clinic could provide an atmosphere where patients can establish support groups with other patients and rehabilitated individuals who can offer their experiences and problem-solving advice to those in earlier phases of their rehabilitation.

SCI individuals spend most of their time sitting in wheelchairs; it is imperative that the therapist involved in the evaluation and ordering of this costly and highly individualized equipment be familiar with what is currently on the market and be creative in ordering a wheelchair that will provide optimal function and body positioning to the patient. Advancements in technology and design have provided a wide variety of wheelchairs from which to choose. The desired wheelchair and positioning modifications should be available for demonstration by the patient prior to final ordering.

In addition to enhancing respiratory function by supporting the patient in an erect, well-aligned po-

sition and maximizing sitting tolerance and optimizing function, wheelchair seating must also assist in the prevention of deformity and pressure sores. An appropriate and adequate wheelchair cushion will help to distribute sitting pressure, stabilize the pelvis as necessary for proper trunk alignment, and provide comfort. Whether it is the occupational therapist's or the physical therapist's role to evaluate and order the wheelchair and cushion, both should work closely together to ensure consistent training and use for the individual needs of each patient.

An increasing number of high-level SCI individuals, C4 and above, are surviving and participating in active rehabilitation programs. Their equipment needs are unique and extremely specialized, ranging from mouthsticks and environmental control systems to ventilators and sophisticated electric wheelchairs and drive systems. (See Table 33-1, levels C1-3 and C3-4.) The utilization of experienced resources in determining appropriate short and long term equipment needs will enhance the quality and functional ability of an otherwise totally dependent individual. Rehabilitation centers specializing in the care of the ventilator-dependent quadriplegics should be sought for their expertise in addressing all aspects of care for this unique patient population.

EXTENDED REHABILITATION PHASE. During the extended phase of the rehabilitation program driving evaluation and training and home management activities may be introduced. Leisure activities should be further explored.[16] Activities such as cards, table games, or workshop activities using hand or power-based tools are feasible and very appropriate treatment modalities employed to evaluate and increase UE strength, coordination, and trunk balance. Such activities can improve socialization skills and assess problem-solving skills and potential work habits.

The patient should be introduced to home and community by the occupational therapist before discharge from the treatment facility. The therapist can offer recommendations for major and minor modifications in the home, such as installation of ramps, grab bars, bathtub seats, and guardrails around the toilet. The therapist can assist in family education and adjustment by training family members or attendants in proper techniques of skin care and inspection, use of special equipment, bed mobility, positioning, transfers, dressing, and toileting activities that require supervision or assistance.

Occupational therapy services can offer valuable evaluation and exploration of the vocational potential of SCI individuals. By the sheer magnitude of the physical disability vocational possibilities for these persons are limited.

Table 33-1 Functional Potential in Spinal Cord Injury[3, 4, 6, 7, 11, 12, 15, 16]

Level*	Muscles innervated	Movements possible	Pattern of weakness	Functional capabilities and limitations
C1-3	Sternocleido-mastoids Trapezius (upper) Levator scapulae	Neck control	Total paralysis of arms, trunk, and LEs Dependence on respirator	Total ADL dependence—can instruct in care Can drive electric wheelchair equipped with portable respirator and chin or breath controls Communication devices & environmental control systems with mouthstick or pneumatic control Require full-time attendant care
C3-4	‡Trapezius (superior, middle and inferior) ‡Diaphragm (C3-5) Cervical and para-spinal muscles	Neck movements, scapula elevation Inspiration	Paralysis of trunk, UEs, and LEs Difficulty in breathing and coughing	Confined to wheelchair—can talk through all set-ups and train caregivers in care Only head-neck and some scapula movement Respiratory assistance may be required—at least part-time Maximal assistance for skin inspection (patient cannot position mirrors but should inspect himself) Activities can be accomplished through use of mouth-stick (e.g., typing, page turning, and manipulation of checkers, chess & cards) Can operate electric wheelchair with chin controls Require full-time attendant care
C5	All muscles of shoulder at least partially innervated except latissimus dorsi and cora-cobrachialis ‡Partial deltoids ‡Biceps brachii Brachialis Brachioradialis Levator scapula, diaphragm, and scaleni now fully innervated Rhomboid (major and minor) Serratus anterior (C5-7)	Shoulder extension and horizontal abduction (weak) Shoulder flexion Shoulder abduction to 90° Elbow flexion and supination Scapular adduction and downward rotation (weak) Scapular abduction and upward rotation (weak)	Absence of elbow extension, pronation, and all wrist and hand movements Total paralysis of trunk and LEs Endurance low because of paralysis of intercostals and low respiratory reserve	Confined to wheelchair Unable to roll over or to come to sitting position independently and has no independent hand functions Need assistance in transfers If good muscle power, may be able to perform UE dressing with some success Dependent for skin inspection Manual wheelchair with handrim projections or electric wheelchair with joystick or adapted arm controls Cannot apply own hand splints, but with standard mobile arm support or elevating proximal arm functional activities are possible: feeding, light hygiene, applying makeup, and shaving; handwriting (sufficient for legal signature); telephoning (touch tone telephone); and typing if set up by an attendant

Continued.

*Each level includes the muscles and functions of the preceding levels.
‡ Key muscles.

Table 33-1 Functional Potential in Spinal Cord Injury—cont'd

Level*	Muscles innervated	Movements possible	Pattern of weakness	Functional capabilities and limitations
C5— cont'd	Teres major (C5,6) Subscapularis (C5,6)	Shoulder internal rotation (weak)		Require at least part-time attendant care; can instruct caregivers in all self-care, mobility, and functional set-ups
	Pectoralis major (C5-8, T1)	Shoulder horizontal adduction (weak)		
	Infraspinatus Supraspinatus Teres minor (C5,6)	Shoulder external rotation		
C6	All partially innervated C5 muscles now fully innervated except serratus and pectoralis major	Full strength to shoulder flexion and extension, abduction and adduction, internal and external rotation, and elbow flexion	Absence of elbow extension and ulnar wrist extension	Still confined to wheelchair—will be able to perform many activities on own with equipment Flexor hinge splint or universal cuff aid in self-feeding with regular utensils; personal hygiene & grooming (oral & upper body); UE dressing; handwriting; typing; telephoning; light kitchen activities; driving, with equipment Roll from side to side in bed with aid of bed rails and assist in rolling over Can perform supine to sidelying to sit with minimal assistance
	Partial but significant innervation to serratus anterior (C5-7)	Scapular abduction and upward rotation		Independent in wheeling wheelchair on level terrain and minimum-grade inclines
	Latissimus dorsi (C6-8)	Shoulder extension and internal rotation	Endurance may be low because of reduced vital capacity	Propel standard wheelchair with adapted rims Relieve pressure independently when sitting, using loops & forward weight shift (see Fig. 33-4)
	‡Pectoralis major (C5-8, T1)	Shoulder horizontal adduction and internal rotation		Independent in managing communication device with adapted equipment Assist in transfers by substituting shoulder adduction and rotation for elbow extension and may be independent with aid of transfer board Drive with adaptations Independet skin inspection— mirrors May manage bladder care Employment possible Some assistance required for bathing & bowel care May require attendant care mornings & evenings only
	Coracobrachialis (C6,7)	Shoulder flexion		
	Pronator teres (C6,7)	Forearm pronation		
	Supinator	Complete innervation for forearm supination		

Continued.

Table 33-1 Functional Potential in Spinal Cord Injury—cont'd

Level*	Muscles innervated	Movements possible	Pattern of weakness	Functional capabilities and limitations
C6—cont'd	‡Extensor carpi radialis longus and brevis (C6,7)	Radial wrist extension	Absence of wrist flexion usually Total paralysis of trunk and LEs	
C7-8	Shoulder prime movers now fully innervated, as well as the rest of the partially innervated C6 muscles	Full strength of all shoulder movements, radial wrist flexors and extensors, and strong pronation	Full strength of shoulder muscles but lack of trunk fixation for the origins of the shoulder prime movers	Essentially confined to wheelchair, but many attain complete wheelchair independence Can come to sitting position in bed Can perform transfers to & from bed and wheelchair independently
	‡Triceps brachii Extensor carpi ulnaris (C6-8)	Elbow extension Ulnar wrist extension		
	‡Flexor carpi radialis	Radial wrist flexion		Can roll over, sit up, and move about in sitting position
	‡Flexor digitorum superficialis and profundus (C7-8, T1)	PIP & DIP flexion	Limited grasp, release, and dexterity because of incomplete innervation of hand intrinsics	Can dress independently & perform personal hygiene activities Self-feeding (usually with no assistive devices) Wrist-driven flexor hinge splint may still be helpful for some patients because of weakness of grasp
	‡Extensor digitorum communis (C6-8)	Metacarpophalangeal (MP) extension		Can propel standard wheelchair (may need friction tape on handrims for long distances; may need assistance on rough ground)
	Extensor pollicis longus and brevis	Thumb extension (MP & IP)	Total paralysis of LEs Weakness of trunk control	Drive with adaptations Independent bladder & bowel care and skin inspection
	Abductor pollicis longus	Thumb abduction	Limited endurance because of reduced respiratory reserve	Employment outside home possible Light housework possible
C8-T1	All muscles of UEs now fully innervated			
	Pronator quadratus	Forearm pronation	Paralysis of LEs	Independent in bed activities, wheelchair transfers, self-care and personal hygiene
	Flexor carpi ulnaris	Ulnar wrist flexion	Weakness of trunk control	Can manage standard wheelchair up & down ramps
	‡Lumbricales and ‡interossei dorsales and palmares	MP flexion	Endurance reduced because of low respiratory reserve	Can move from wheelchair to floor and return with standby assistance Nonfunctional ambulation for standing or exercise may be possible but still not a practicable mode of mobility
	‡Interossei dorsales and abductor digiti minimi	Finger abduction		Can get up & down from standing in standing frame independently Independent bladder & bowel care and skin inspection Work in a wheelchair-accessible environment possible
	‡Interossei palmares	Finger adduction		Light housekeeping can be done independently Drive with adaptations

Continued.

Table 33-1 Functional Potential in Spinal Cord Injury—cont'd

Level*	Muscles innervated	Movements possible	Pattern of weakness	Functional capabilities and limitations
C8-T1—cont'd	Flexor pollicis longus and brevis Adductor pollicis ‡Opponens digiti minimi ‡Opponens pollicis	Thumb flexion (MP and IP) Thumb adduction Opposition of fifth finger Thumb opposition		Independent in management of communication devices
T4-T6	All muscles of upper extremities plus partial innervation of intercostal muscles and long muscles of the back (sacrospinalis and semispinalis)	All arm functions Partial trunk stability Endurance increased because of better respiration	Partial trunk paralysis and total paralysis of LEs	Self-care independence Independence in standard wheelchair and transfers May stand with braces & crutches and ambulate for short distances but not practical for mobility Can work and do some heavy lifting from sitting position Drive car with adaptations Independent in light housekeeping
T7-L2	Intercostal muscles fully innervated Abdominal muscles partially to fully innervated (rectus abdominis, internal and external obliques)	Partial to good trunk stability Increased physical endurance	Paralysis of LEs	Independence in self-care, personal hygiene, sports, work & housekeeping activities possible Ambulates with difficulty using braces and crutches, but wheelchair is ambulation of choice for speed & energy conservtion
L3-L4	Low back muscles Hip flexors, adductors, quadriceps	Trunk control and stability Hip flexion Hip adduction Knee extension	Partial paralysis of lower extremities; hip extension, knee flexion, and ankle and foot movements	Independent in all activities outlined above Can ambulate with short leg braces, using crutches or canes May still use a wheelchair for convenience, energy conservation & sports
L5-S3	Hip extensors—gluteus maximus and hamstrings Hip abductors—gluteus medius and gluteus minimus Knee flexors—hamstrings, sartorius, and gracilis Ankle muscles—tibialis anterior, gastrocnemius, soleus, and peroneus longus Foot muscles	Partial to full control of LEs	Partial paralysis of LEs, most notable in distal segment	Independent in all activities No equipment needed if plantar flexion is sufficiently strong for push-off in ambulation

Many patients with spinal cord injuries must change their vocation or alter former vocational goals. Lack of intelligence, poor motivation, and lack of interest and perseverance on the part of many patients make vocational rehabilitation challenging.

The occupational therapist, during the process of the treatment program and through the use of ADL, craft, and work sample activities, can help to assess the patient's level of motivation, functional intelligence, aptitudes, attitudes, interests, and personal vocational aspirations. The occupational therapist can observe the patient's attention span, concentration, manual ability with splints and devices, accuracy, speed, perseverance, work habits, and work tolerance level. This information can be provided to the vocational counselor, who can counsel the patient regarding vocational potential and future possibilities, perform specialized vocational testing, and suggest feasible educational and vocational training possibilities.[15]

The occupational therapy service can offer a work adjustment program in which work tolerance level and work habits can be developed while specific job testing and trials are under the direction of the vocational counselor.

For the person with quadriplegia who is of adequate intelligence and motivation, further education is often the solution to the vocational future. Such individuals may perform successfully in occupations such as teaching, engineering, business management, research, psychology, counseling, and sales. Adaptive equipment and a barrier-free environment may be essential to the performance of these jobs.[15]

When suitable vocational objectives have been selected, they may be pursued in an educational setting, at the treatment facility if it is equipped for vocational training, or in a work setting. This phase of rehabilitation is beyond the scope of occupational therapy.

Maximal self-care independence, personal satisfaction through leisure activities, and socialization should be the end goals of the rehabilitation program for those persons who lack the intelligence for further education or vocational training and essential personal skills and habits for good work adjustment.[15]

REVIEW QUESTIONS

1. List three causes of spinal cord injury. Which is most common?
2. Describe the patterns of weakness in quadriplegia and paraplegia.
3. Describe the functional and prognostic differences between complete and incomplete lesions.
4. When reference is made to "C5" in quadriplegia, what is meant in terms of level of injury and functioning muscle groups?
5. What are the characteristics of spinal shock?
6. What physical changes occur following the spinal shock phase?
7. What is the prognosis for recovery of motor function in complete lesions and incomplete lesions?
8. What are the purposes of surgery in management of spinal injury?
9. What are some medical complications, common to patients with spinal cord injuries, which can limit achievement of functional potential?
10. How should postural hypotension be treated?
11. How should autonomic dysreflexia be treated?
12. What is the role of the occupational therapist in the prevention of pressure sores?
13. Why is vital capacity affected in patients with spinal cord injuries?
14. What effect will reduced vital capacity have on the rehabilitation program?
15. Which level of injury has full innervation of rotator cuff musculature, biceps, and extensor carpi radialis and partial innervation of serratus anterior, latissimus dorsi, and pectoralis major?
16. What additional muscle power does the patient with C6 quadriplegia have over the patient with C5 quadriplegia? What is the major functional advantage of this additional muscle power?
17. What are the additional critical muscles that the patient with C7 quadriplegia has, as compared with the patient with C6 quadriplegia?
18. What additional functional independence can be achieved because of this additional muscle power?
19. What is the first spinal cord lesion level that has full innervation of UE musculature?
20. Which evaluation tools does the occupational therapist use to assess the patient with a spinal cord injury? What is the purpose of each?
21. List five goals of occupational therapy for the patient with a spinal cord injury.
22. How is wrist extension used to effect grasp by the patient with quadriplegia?
23. How does the patient with C6 quadriplegia substitute for the absence of elbow extensors?
24. What is the "contracture" that is encouraged in patients with spinal cord injuries? Why? How is it developed?
25. What is the splint that allows the C6 quadriplegic to achieve functional grasp?
26. What are some of the first self-care activities that the patient with a C6 spinal cord injury should be expected to accomplish?
27. List four assistive devices commonly used by persons with quadriplegia, and tell the purpose of each.
28. Describe the role of occupational therapy in the vocational evalua-

tion of a patient with a spinal cord injury.

REFERENCES

1. Bedgrook GM, editor: Lifetime care of the paraplegic patient, New York, 1985, Churchill Livingstone, Inc.
2. Bromley I: Tetraplegia and paraplegia: a guide for physiotherapists, ed 3, New York, 1985, Churchill Livingstone, Inc.
3. Chusid JG: Correlative neuroanatomy and functional neurology, ed 19, Los Altos, CA, 1985, Lange Medical Publications.
4. Daniels L and Worthingham C: Muscle testing, ed 5, Philadelphia, 1986, WB Saunders Co.
5. Frankle H et al: The value of postural reduction in the initial management of closed injuries to the spine with paraplegia and tetraplegia, Paraplegia 7:179, 1969.
6. Functional goals in spinal cord lesions, Downey, CA, Physical Therapy Department, Rancho Los Amigos Hospital. (Unpublished.)
7. Greb M and Mueller JM: Functional goals at specific levels of spinal cord injury, Denver, Craig Hospital.
8. Hanak M and Scott A: An illustrated guide for health care professionals, New York, 1983, Springer Verlag, Inc.
9. Hill JP, editor: Spinal cord injury, a guide to functional outcomes in occupational therapy, Rockville, MD, 1986, Aspen Publishers, Inc.
10. Institute for Medical Research, Santa Clara Valley Medical Center: Severe head trauma, a comprehensive medical approach, Project 13-9-59156/9, report to National Institute for Handicapped Research, Nov 1982.
11. Malick MH and Meyer CMH: Manual on management of the quadriplegic upper extremity, Pittsburgh, 1978, Harmarville Rehabilitation Center.
12. McKenzie MW: The role of occupational therapy in rehabilitating spinal cord injured patients, Am J Occup Ther 24:257, 1970.
13. Neistadt M and Baker MF: A program for sex counseling the physically disabled, Am J Occup Ther 32:646, 1978.
14. Phillips R, editor: Santa Clara Valley Medical Center spinal cord injury home care manual, ed 2, San Jose, CA, 1986, Santa Clara Valley Medical Center.
15. Pierce DS and Nickel VH: The total care of spinal cord injuries, Boston, 1977, Little, Brown & Co.
16. Spencer EA: Functional restoration. In Hopkins HL and Smith HD, editors: Willard and Spackman's occupational therapy, ed 7, Philadelphia, 1988, JB Lippincott Co.
17. Venegas N and Del Pilar-Christian M, editors: Proceedings of the workshop "Occupational therapy for patients with physical dysfunction," PR, 1967, Occupational Therapy Department, University of Puerto Rico.
18. Wilson DJ, McKenzie MW, and Barber LM: Spinal cord injury: a treatment guide for occupational therapists, rev ed, Thorofare, NJ, 1984, Slack, Inc.
19. Yashon D: Spinal injury, New York, 1978, Appleton-Century-Crofts.

Sample treatment plan

The treatment plan deals with four of ten identified problems. The reader is encouraged to add objectives and methods for the remaining problems to make a more comprehensive treatment plan.

CASE STUDY

Mr. H is a 37-year-old male who sustained a cervical fracture in a diving accident. He suffered a C5-6 fracture dislocation, Frankle class A, with resultant paralysis of hands, trunk, and LEs.

Prior to his injury he worked full-time as a policeman in a small town. He has been married for 13 years and has no children. His wife is an RN. Mr. H has led a very active lifestyle. His hobbies include raising horses, weight lifting, racquetball, and cycling. He has always been an extremely independent gentleman with a good sense of humor and with a large circle of friends, mostly fellow police officers. His parents and two sisters live in a nearby town and visit frequently.

Immediately after his injury Mr. H was flown to a nearby community hospital, where after diagnosis his neck was surgically stabilized. A posterior fusion of C5 on C6 with laminar wiring was performed. A halo vest traction device was applied postsurgically, and he was subsequently transferred to a regional spinal cord injury center for further medical management and total spinal cord injury care. A referral for occupational therapy was received the day of admission, and a full evaluation was initiated.

Personal data

Name: Mr. H

Age: 37

Diagosis: C5-6 Fracture dislocation resulting in C6 complete quadriplegia, Frankle class A

Disability: Paralysis and sensory loss of hands, trunk, and LEs

Treatment aims stated in referral: Occupational therapy evaluation and treatment

OTHER SERVICES

Physician: Maintenance of general health, prescription of medication, coordination of rehabilitation team

Nurse: Administer medication, manage bowel and bladder program, attend to skin and self-care needs as necessary, follow through on ADL program as instructed by OT

Physical Therapy: UE and LE ROM, strengthening of available musculature, standing program, increase vital capacity through breathing exercise program

Social service: Discharge and community resource planning, individual and family counseling

Psychology: Individual and family counseling

Recreation Therapy: Develop leisure skills

FRAME OF REFERENCE

Occupational performance

TREATMENT APPROACH

Biomechanical and rehabilitative

OT EVALUATION

Performance components

Motor functioning

Muscle strength: Test

Passive ROM: Test

Physical endurance: Observe, interview

Movement speed: Observe

Coordination: Test, observe

Functional movement: Test, observe

Sensory integrative functioning

Sensation (touch, pain, thermal, proprioception): Test

Cognitive functioning

Judgment: Observe

Safety awareness: Observe

Motivation: Observe, interview

Psychological functioning

Coping skills: Observe

Adjustment to disability: Observe, interview

Social skills

Interpersonal relationships: Observe

Performance skills

Self-care

Observe, interview

Home management

Observe, interview

EVALUATION SUMMARY

Patient's PROM is within normal limits (WNL) in all joints of the UEs. Slight tightness at the MP and PIP joints will be encouraged to facilitate finger stability for natural tenodesis action. Specific manual testing revealed symmetry in all innervated UE muscle groups with the exception of elbow extension and wrist flexion. (See Table 33-2.)

Sensory tests performed were pain, light-touch, and kinesthesia, with the following findings:

Pain (pinprick)

L	R
C6 and above—intact	C5 and above—intact
C7 and below—absent	C6—impaired
	C7 and below—absent

Continued.

Table 33-2 Occupational Therapy Manual Muscle Evaluation

	RIGHT	CA					CA	LEFT	
		CA		EXAMINERS INITIALS			CA		
				DATE					
			N E C K	FLEXION					
				FLEXION/ROTATION: Sternocleidomastoid	C2-3,CRXI	Spinal Accessory			
				EXTENSION	C1-8	Dorsal Rami			
		4	S C A P U L A	ELEVATION: Upper Trapezius	C3-4	Spinal Accessory	4		
		3+		DEPRESSION: Lower Trapezius	C3-4	Spinal Accessory	3+		
				ADDUCTION:					
		3		Rhomboids	C5	Dorsal Scapular	3		
		3+		Middle Trapezius	C3-4	Spinal Accessory	3+		
		4		ABDUCTION: Serratus Anterior	C5-7	Long Thoracic	4		
		3+	S H O U L D E R	FLEXION: Anterior Deltoid	C5-6	Axillary	3+		
				EXTENSION: Latiss/Teres Major	C5-7	Lower Subscapular/ Thoracodorsal	3+		
		4		ABDUCTION: Middle Deltoid	C5-6	Axillary	3+		
		3+		HORIZONTAL ABDUCTION: Posterior or post. Deltoid	C5-6	Axillary	4		
				HORIZONTAL ADDUCTION					
		0		Pectoralis Major-Clavicular	C5-T1	Med. Lat. Ant. Thoracic	0		
		0		Pectoralis Major-Sternal	C5-T1	Med. Lat. Ant. Thoracic	0		
		4		EXTERNAL ROTATION: Inf. Sp/T Min	C5-6	Axillary/Subscap.	3+		
		3+		INTERNAL ROTATION: Subscap.	C5-T1	Subscap./Thoracic	3+		
			E L B O W	FLEXION:					
		4		Biceps/Brachialis	C5-6	Musculocutaneous	4		
		4		Brachioradialis	C5-6	Radial	4		
		2−		EXTENSION: Triceps	C6-8	Radial	0		
		4		SUPINATION	C5-7	Radial	4		
		3		PRONATION: Pro. Teres/Pro Quad.	C6-T1	Median	3		
			W R I S T	FLEXION					
		0		Flexor Carpi Radialis	C6-8	Median			
		0		Flexor Carpi Ulnaris	C8-T1	Ulnar	0		
				EXTENSION					
		4 > ®		Extensor Carpi Radial Longus/Brevis	C6-8	Radial	4		
		1		Extensor Carpi Ulnaris	C7-8	Radial	0		

Continued.

Table 33-2 Occupational Therapy Manual Muscle Evaluation—cont'd

	RIGHT									LEFT	
					FLEXION:						
			0		Flexor Digitorum Superficialis	C7-T1	Median		0		
			0		Index				0		
			0		Long				0		
			0	F	Ring				0		
			0	I	Little				0		
			0	N	Flexor Digitorum Profundus				0		
			0	G	Index	C8-T1	Median		0		
			0	E	Long	C8-T1	Ulnar		0		
			0	R	Ring	C8-T1	Ulnar		0		
			0	S	Little	C8-T1	Ulnar		0		
			0		Lumbricales				0		
			0		Index	C6-7	Median		0		
			0		Long	C6-7	Median		0		
			0		Ring	C8	Ulnar		0		
			0		Little	C8	Ulnar				

Sample treatment plan—cont'd

Light Touch

L	R
C6 and above—intact	C6 and above—intact
C7—impaired	C7 and below—absent
C8 and below—absent	

Kinesthesia

L	R
Wrist, elbow, shoulder—intact	same
radial fingers—impaired	radial and ulnar fingers—absent
ulnar fingers—absent	

Although physical endurance is low as observed in frequent rest periods during a 60-minute treatment session, the patient's wheelchair tolerance is 8 hours per day.

Sitting balance is fair on the mat or edge of bed. However, Mr. H requires a chest strap while pushing his wheelchair to maintain good sitting balance.

Coordination and muscle control are good in available musculature as evidenced by performance in tabletop and sink activities.

LE spasticity is severe, requiring medication to regulate since it interferes with bed mobility and transfer progress.

Although finger function is absent bilaterally, Mr H is able to pick up light objects of varied sizes and textures, utilizing natural tenodesis grasp in both his dominant right and nondominant left hands.

Mr. H's judgment, safety awareness, and problem-solving abilities are good. However, he occasionally has difficulty in sequencing frustrating activities such as transferring from wheelchair to bed. His motivation varies daily in conjunction with the degree of despair he feels over his injury. His coping skills are generally very good in that his sense of humor and high level of intelligence help him through the "bad days." He is having difficulty adjusting to his disability and accepting himself in a less physically capable and traditionally masculine role than prior to his injury. Ironically, he becomes very passive around his wife who assumes her nursing role when with him. On occasion Mr. H is easily angered and makes critical comments about himself and his body. In contrast, he is a great motivator with other patients, assuming more of a leadership role. Using appropriate humor, he takes charge of most group interactions. He has a large circle of close friends, several of whom drive 2 or more hours to visit.

Mr. H is independent in feeding with the exception of cutting meat. The only adaptive equipment he uses is a universal cuff. He requires minimal assistance for his hygiene setup at the sink. He requires moderate assistance with UE dressing secondary to the interference of the halo vest. He is dependent for LE dressing.

He currently requires moderate assistance of one person to perform sliding board transfers and wheelchair mobility to and from level surfaces; he requires maximal assistance on uneven surfaces.

He requires moderate to maximal assistance for bed mobility because of the halo vest which is in place for approximately 3 months from the day of surgery.

Prior to his accident Mr. H had an excellent work record and habits. He continues to demonstrate this by his consistent timeless and attendance to therapy sessions. His work potential is good as demonstrated by the clerical tabletop tasks he performs diligently although slowly. He would of course not be able to return to his prior job duties.

Mr. H has been unwilling to participate in community reintegration activities subsequent to feeling self-conscious in public; therefore his community mobility skills have not been assessed.

Assessment of light meal planning and preparation as well as some housekeeping skills will occur when the halo vest is removed.

Mr. H lives in a single story house that will require only bathroom modifications for safe accessibility.

The majority of Mr. H's leisure activities were very active, and appropriate leisure interests after discharge will be assessed by recreation therapy.

ASSETS

Symmetrical UE strength
Strength of 3+ to 4 in innervated musculature
Relatively good coordination and dexterity in hand skills
Good living situation
Strong family and community support
Good coping skills
Good problem-solving skills
Marketable job skills
High level of education
Good potential for independent driving

PROBLEM LIST

1. Poor prognosis for recovery
2. Paralysis of fingers, trunk, and LE
3. Sensation absent below C7 dermatome
4. Requires the assistance of one person for mobility when out of the wheelchair (bed mobility and transfers)
5. Requires the assistance of one person for dressing, bathing, bowel and bladder program; dependent on wheelchair for all mobility
6. Potential for skin breakdown
7. Lack of assertiveness in directing wife in his care; lack of knowledge regarding durable medical equipment
8. Requires the assistance of one person for kitchen and homemaking skills
9. Requires assistance for community mobility
10. Inability to return to former vocational and avocational activities

PROBLEM 4

Dependent on moderate physical assistance for transfers

Continued.

Sample treatment plan—cont'd

Objective

Patient will require standby assistance only for all level surface transfers, including pretransfer and posttransfer setup

Method

Pretransfer and posttransfer setup: Patient backs wheelchair to bed and applies brakes and loosens chest and hip strap; he hooks arm behind push handle for balance and leans forward hooking hand and wrist under ipsilateral leg

Using wrist extension and elbow flexion to "kick" foot off footplate and onto opposite foot, patient then removes whole footrest using power from wrist extension; with one footplate off of chair, he then removes brake and positions wheelchair appropriately next to bed and relocks brake

Patient then repeats same sequence of movement, putting foot on floor; patient hooks other arm behind push handle and repeats sequence until both feet are on the floor

With modified depression, patient scoots buttocks forward in seat so as to clear wheel during transfer; he then places slideboard under leg midway between knee and hip, angled toward opposite hip; patient then finds stable handholds, one on wheelchair and one on slideboard, leans forward while maintaining balance and locked elbows (Fig. 33-6)

By using momentum of swinging head and shoulders away from slideboard, patient slides across board, periodically adjusting feet with arms and repositioning UEs

Caregiver is in front of the patient within arms length to provide assistance if necessary

Gradation

Therapist initially provides more assistance while patient moves through each step; gradually reduce amount of assistance and amount of time and energy required by patient

PROBLEM 6

Potential for skin breakdown

Objective

Patient will be independent in forward weight shifts using loops attached to back frame of wheelchair

Method

Using method just described for removing feet from footplates and putting flat on floor, patient then places both arms in loops (approximately 24-inch × 1-inch (60-cm × 2.5-cm) cotton webbing sewn into loops and screwed into top upholstery screws of back frame of wheelchair)

Patient pulls self forward using arms against armrests and slowly lowers self toward knees, using loops to control the speed in which he drops forward; patient lays completely across knees and remains down for 1 to 2 minutes to allow capillary blood flow to return over bone prominences of ishial tuberosities and sacrum

When ready to sit up, patient pulls symmetrically against loops first using elbow flexion and then shoulder abduction and flexion to pull upper body upright, returning to a sitting position

Arms must then be removed from loops; patient must then place feet back on footplates by reversing procedure

described previously; seatbelts must then be secured tightly and brakes removed

Gradation

Initially therapist sits in front of patient to provide assistance and security while patient is lowering self and pulling back to sitting

Gradually withdraw assistance as patient gains strength and confidence; time spent performing activity should decrease to no more than 5 minutes

PROBLEM 2

Paralysis of fingers

Objective

Patient will increase wrist extension strength to at least a grade 4, sufficient for successful natural tenodesis for grasping light objects and donning and doffing adaptive equipment and splints

Method

Patient is seated in wheelchair with arm supported on armrest; hand is hanging over end of armrest; patient self-ranges wrist by actively extending wrist through full ROM against gravity; this is done prior to resistive exercise to ensure full active ROM; a wrist cuff and small weights are placed on the hand

Patient actively extends wrist through full available ROM 10 times; repeat repetitions 3 times

Weight is then decreased, and repetitions are repeated; therapist ensures that full ROM occurs upon each repetition; if not, then weight should be decreased

Weights are then removed and functional activities are then performed such as board games and object manipulation tasks using same motion

Gradation

Increase resistance; goal is reached at approximately 5 lbs

Increase repetitions; increase complexity and duration of subsequent functional activity

PROBLEM 7

Lack of assertiveness in directing wife in care

Objective

Patient will be independent in talking through, instructing, and critiquing wife in all aspects of his care when indicated

Method

Therapist instructs patient in the specific sequence of a dependent activity such as LE dressing; this includes predressing setup, such as bathing and legbag application

Patient then talks therapist through entire activity; therapist role-plays predictable responses of wife relating to body mechanics and other aspects of the procedure which may prove difficult; therapist then arranges for wife to be present when patient can be successful

Patient then instructs wife in all aspects of the procedure and critiques the process; therapist observes entire process and intervenes when necessary

Gradation

Decrease therapist's physical and verbal cues and decrease amount of time taken to perform task

Decrease amount of stress on patient and wife so that process and interaction is positive and successful

34 Cerebral vascular accident

LORRAINE WILLIAMS PEDRETTI

Cerebral vascular accident (CVA) or stroke is the most common disabling neurologic disease of adulthood.[32,55] It accounts for at least half the patients hospitalized with neurologic disease. An estimated 400,000 to 500,000 new strokes occur every year in the United States. The fatality rate of acute stroke victims is about 15%, and at least 50% of the survivors suffer permanent neurologic disability. Because of the very limited success in the reversal of the effects of brain damage, prevention is the key to reducing mortality and morbidity resulting from CVA.[32]

Factors associated with a high risk for CVA are hypertension, coronary artery disease, carotid bruits, transient ischemic attacks (TIAs), congenital artery wall weakness, diabetes mellitus, hyperlipidemia, cigarette smoking, age and gender, race, heredity, alcohol consumption, polycythemia, obesity, and use of oral contraceptives.[26,32,50]

Definition of CVA

Cerebral vascular accident (CVA) is a complex dysfunction caused by a lesion in the brain. It results in an upper motor neuron dysfunction that produces hemiplegia or paralysis of one side of the body, limbs, and sometimes the face and oral structures that are contralateral to the hemisphere of the brain that has the lesion. Thus a lesion in the left cerebral hemisphere, or left CVA, produces right hemiplegia, and vice versa. When referring to the patient's disability as *right* hemiplegia, the reference is to the paralyzed body side and *not* to the locus of the lesion.[50]

Accompanying the motor paralysis may be a variety of other dysfunctions. Some of these are sensory disturbances, perceptual dysfunctions, visual disturbances, personality and intellectual changes, and a complex range of speech and associated language disorders.[51,53]

EFFECTS OF CVA

The outcome of the CVA depends on which artery supplying the brain was involved in the vascular disease.

Internal Carotid Artery

Occlusion of the internal carotid artery, in the absence of adequate collateral circulation, results in contralateral hemiplegia, hemianesthesia, and homonymous hemianopsia.[17] Additionally, involvement of the dominant hemisphere is associated with aphasia, agraphia or dysgraphia, acalculia or dyscalculia, right-left confusion, and finger agnosia. Involvement of the nondominant hemisphere is associated with visual perceptual dysfunction, unilateral neglect, anosognosia, constructional or dressing apraxia, attention deficits, and loss of topographic memory. A tendency to tilt space in a counterclockwise direction is seen in some left hemiplegics, making ambulation and two-dimensional constructional tasks difficult.[51]

Middle Cerebral Artery

Involvement of the *middle cerebral artery* (MCA) is the most common cause of CVA.[11,31] Ischemia in the area supplied by the MCA results in contralateral hemiplegia with greater involvement of the arm, face, and tongue, sensory deficits, contralateral homonymous hemianopsia; and aphasia, if the lesion is in the dominant hemisphere.[11,18,50,51] Perceptual deficits such as anosognosia, unilateral neglect, impaired vertical perception, visual spatial deficits, and perseveration are seen if the lesion is in the nondominant hemisphere.[17]

Anterior Cerebral Artery

Occlusion of the *anterior cerebral artery* (ACA) produces contralateral lower extremity weakness that is more severe than that of the arm. Apraxia, mental changes, primitive reflexes, and bowel and bladder incontinence may be seen. Total occlusion of the ACA results in contralateral hemiplegia with severe weakness of the face, tongue, and proximal arm muscles and marked spastic paralysis of the distal lower extremity. Cortical sensory loss is present in the lower extremity. Intellectual changes such as confusion, disorientation, abulia, whispering, slowness, distractibility, limited verbal output, perseveration, and amnesia may be seen.[17,51]

Posterior Cerebral Artery

The potential scope of posterior cerebral artery (PCA) symptoms is broad and varied because this artery supplies the upper brain stem region, as well as the temporal and occipital lobes. Possible results of posterior cerebral artery involvement depend on the arterial branches involved and the extent and area of cerebral compromise. Some possible outcomes are sensory and motor deficits, involuntary movement disorders (hemiballism, postural tremor, hemichorea, hemiataxia, intention tremor), memory loss, alexia, astereognosis, dysesthesia, akinesthesia, contralateral homonymous hemianopsia or quadrantopsia, anomia, topographic disorientation, and visual agnosia.[17,18,51]

Cerebellar Artery

Cerebellar artery occlusion results in ipsilateral ataxia, contralateral loss of pain and temperature sensitivity, ipsilateral facial analgesia, dysphagia and dysarthria due to weakness of the ipsilateral muscles of the palate, nystagmus, and contralateral hemiparesis.[11,17,18]

Vertebrobasilar Artery System

A CVA in the vertebrobasilar artery system affects brain stem functions. The outcome of the stroke is some combination of bilateral or crossed sensory and motor abnormalities, such as cerebellar dysfunction, loss of proprioception, hemiplegia, quadriplegia, and sensory disturbances, with unilateral or bilateral cranial nerve involvement of nerves III to XII.[51]

ETIOLOGY

CVA, sometimes called shock, stroke, or apoplexy, is caused by some pathology in the cerebral vasculature. A compromise in the blood supply to the brain caused by thrombus, embolus, or hemorrhage results in cerebral ischemia and ultimately, in secondary brain abnormality. The onset of CVA is often unanticipated and sudden.[51]

Cerebral anoxia and aneurysm also can result in hemiplegia.[10,13,50] Some of the treatment approaches outlined in this chapter may be applicable to hemiplegia that results from causes other than CVA or stroke, such as head injuries, neoplasms, and infectious diseases of the brain.[10]

Vascular disease of the brain can result in a completed CVA or cause transient ischemic attacks (TIAs).

A TIA occurs as mild isolated or repetitive neurologic symptoms that disappear within 24 hours. The TIA is seen as a sign of impending CVA. Most TIAs occur in those with atherosclerotic disease. An estimated 25% to 40% of patients who experience TIAs go on to a completed stroke within 5 years.[51]

If the TIA is caused by extracranial vascular disease, surgical intervention to reestablish patency of arteries may be effective in preventing the CVA and the resultant disability.[51]

MEDICAL MANAGEMENT

Specific treatment of CVA depends on the type and location of the vascular lesion, the severity of the clinical deficit, concomitant medical and neurologic problems, availability of technology and personnel to administer special types of treatment, and the cooperation and reliability of the patient.[16]

General treatment includes bladder care, prevention of pressure ulcers, prevention of contractures, possible use of elastic hose to prevent venous thrombosis, measures to prevent pain and dislocation of the shoulder on the hemiplegic side, emotional support, and medication or psychotherapy for depression.[16]

The physician's responsibility is to make the diagnosis and apply the early life-saving measures. These may include ordering appropriate nourishment and hydration and establishing an airway. The physician also prescribes medication to treat or prevent infection or concomitant medical problems.[10]

During the acute illness the need for urinary drainage should be determined and catheterization carried out, if necessary. The physician also should order early mobility, adequate diet and fluids, and use of suppositories and medication to prevent or treat fecal impaction.[10]

The physician should see that appropriate measures are instituted to prevent contractures. This means writing orders for appropriate positioning, splints, and passive exercise in the early phases of rehabilitation. Pressure sores should be vigilantly guarded against by early mobilization, use of an air or water flotation mattress, frequent repositioning in bed or chair, excellent hygiene, and skin inspection. The physician is responsible for ordering these measures, seeing that they are carried out, and inspecting the patient's skin on a regular basis.[10,16]

It is important for the physician not to overlook the possibility of disability of unaffected parts because of disuse and immobility. The physician should see to it that the patient is involved in physical activities and exercises that are commensurate with his or her medical status and abilities as early as possible in the rehabilitation program.[10]

Evaluating the residuals of the CVA, writing orders for the rehabilitation therapies, and reevaluating the patient's progress are the responsibilities of the physician, who supervises the rehabilitation program.[10]

MOTOR DYSFUNCTION AFTER CVA

Bobath outlined four major factors that interfere with normal motor performance in an adult hemiplegia: sensory disturbances, spasticity, disorder of the normal postural reflex mechanism, and loss of selective movement patterns.[9]

The degree of sensory involvement has a profound influence on the degree of spontaneous motor recovery and the results of treatment. All movement is in response to sensory stimuli acting on the central nervous system (CNS) from the external and internal environments.[9,14] These sensory stimuli progress through the CNS and are integrated at the cortical level, where they produce an effective, coordinated motor response to meet the demands of the environment. Sensations arising from the movement response serve to guide it through its course, determine its effectiveness, and give cues for the need for any revision of the movement response.[9]

Because of this critical sensory-motor relationship and interdependence, it is important to think of the sensorimotor cortex as one functional unit of the brain.[9] The sensory disturbance in patients with hemiplegia aggravates the motor dysfunction even in the absence of severe spasticity. The patients lack the urge to move; probably in part because they cannot sense and interpret the environmental stimuli that normally evoke movement.[9]

Characteristics of the Motor Disturbance after CVA

After CVA upper motor neuron paralysis follows a one-sided distribution and includes musculature of the trunk and limbs on the affected side. The muscles of the face and mouth also may be involved. The paralysis is usually characterized by increased muscle tone or spasticity. In some cases, hypotonicity of flaccidity may be apparent. Even in these instances some spasticity may be evoked in the finger and wrist flexors and the ankle extensors, if prolonged and strong stretch stimuli are applied. In cases in which apparent flaccidity persists indefinitely, it usually combined with severe sensory loss, making active motion impossible.[9]

Coordination or control of smooth, rhythmic movement is lost. Rather, the spasticity occurs in gross patterns of flexion and extension called *synergies* (Chapter 19). Synergies are released when cortical control of motion is interrupted. All muscles in the synergy are neurophysiologically linked, and when one of the movements is performed, some or all of the movement components are likely to occur simultaneously.[13,29]

Normal postural reflex mechanisms are disturbed after CVA. Normal righting, equilibrium, and protective reactions (Chapter 9) are lost on the hemiplegic side. This affects the patient's ability to maintain and recover balance and make the normal postural adjustments that accompany movement and activity. Primitive reflexes (Chapter 9) may be released so that changes of the position of the head and body in space have an abnormal influence on muscle tone.

Bobath described the loss of "adaptive changes of muscle tone as a proteciton against the forces of gravity."[9] This is the ability to control slow, unresisted movements in the direction of gravity. For example, in lowering the upraised arm the antigravity muscles contract and hold while their antagonist muscles relax. The person with hemiplegia has lost this mechanism of automatic control on the affected side. He or she tends to compensate for the loss with the automatic reactions of the unaffected side. The patient does not initiate movement with the affected side, does not support him or herself on the affected arm and hand, and bears little weight on the affected leg.

Because of the spasticity and release of abnormal synergistic movement patterns, loss of selective, discriminative, and isolated movement occurs after CVA. This loss is most apparent in the arm and hand, probably because of the nature of the normal function of this part.[9] However, selective movement is also lost in the leg and foot and is evident in the inability to dorsiflex the ankle and toes regardless of the position of the hip and knee or in the inability to flex the knee while the hip is extended.[9] In function this is evidenced by the gait pattern, which is usually performed with the leg held in stiff extension or in the extensor synergy pattern. The person with hemiplegia lacks ability to perform a wide variety of movement combinations to effect normal motor performance.[9]

Recovery Period

Spontaneous recovery of voluntary motor function occurs primarily in the first 3 months after the onset of the CVA.[33] Recovery may continue up to 1 year and in rare instances is seen somewhat longer. This does not imply that motor behavior cannot be influenced by appropriate therapy after a year, however.

Prognosis for Functional Recovery

The physician and therapist may wish to estimate the potential for recovery of function for purposes of planning rehabilitation goals. Factors associated with poor prognosis at onset are unconsciousness, severe weakness of affected side, inability to perform conjugate gaze to the affected body side, and advancing age. Following the initial period of acute illness, factors that adversely affect prognosis for functional recovery are prolonged hypotonia and severe spasticity, apraxia, sensory disturbances,[33] receptive aphasia, dementia, homonymous hemianopsia, unilateral neglect, body scheme disturbance, disturbance of spatial perception, and lack of use of the hand after 3 weeks.[53]

Conversely, prognosis for functional recovery is good when the patient has early return of muscle tone and motor function (within 2 weeks), intact sensation and perception, good cognitive functioning, intact body scheme, minimal spasticity, no contractures, some spontaneous use of the arm in bilateral activities, and development of some selective motion.[33]

CONCOMITANT DYSFUNCTIONS

In the rehabilitation program of patients with stroke, much emphasis is placed on treating the motor dysfunction, which is the part of the disability that can easily be seen and assessed. However, the disability is complicated by many invisible problems, which have a significant impact on the patient's performance and prognosis for rehabilitation. If the therapist fails to recognize the problems concomitant to the motor disability, rehabilitation efforts result in frustration and failure for the patient and the therapist.[20] On the basis of a comprehensive evaluation, realistic rehabilitation goals and methods can be planned with the patient.

Sensory Disturbances

Disturbances in the senses of touch, pain, temperature, pressure, and vibration and proprioception may occur as a result of CVA.[33] Such disturbances prohibit the sensory feedback that is so important to the perceptual-motor functioning of the person and thus may be one cause of disuse of the affected extremities, even when motor recovery is apparently good.

Information about sensation and sensory reeducation methods is included in Chapter 11.

Perceptual Dysfunction

The ability to learn and make continuous adaptation to the ever-changing environment is dependent on intact perceptual processes. Perception is complex and involves processes of transforming, organizing, and structuring sensory information from the environment. Adaptation is dependent on intact perceptual processing. A hemiplegic patient who lacks adequate perceptual processing skills fails to adapt adequately to the tasks of daily living.[20]

Evaluation of visual perception and perceptual motor skills is discussed in Chapter 12. Some of the perceptual dysfunctions that commonly affect patients with hemiplegia are outlined below.

TACTILE PERCEPTION. Tactile perception is the ability to recognize, localize, and make discriminations about touch stimuli to the skin surface. It includes the ability to recognize and localize light touch stimuli, ability to recognize symbols "written" on the skin (graphesthesia), ability to recognize two stimuli in close proximity (two-point discrimination), ability to recognize two simultaneous stimuli, and ability to identify common objects and geometric forms through manipulation without the aid of vision (stereognosis).[18] The inability to perceive the tangible properties of an object tactually (astereognosis) interferes with perceptual-motor functioning of the patient in that he or she receives no sensory feedback about the objects he or she is manipulating unless vision is used to compensate for the sensory loss. This compensation is often ineffective, because it is difficult to visually supervise the hand performing an activity while trying to watch the activity and focus on its goal.

BODY SCHEME DISORDERS. Body scheme disorders are disturbances in the neurologic function that include knowledge of body construction, its anatomic elements, and spatial relationships; ability to visualize the body in movement and its parts in different positional relationships; ability to differentiate right from left; and ability to know body health and disease.[3] Body scheme disorders are found frequently enough in patients with hemiplegia to make routine evaluation for the presence of this dysfunction advisable.[35] Because knowledge of the body scheme is basic to all motor function, a disturbance in body scheme has a profound effect on the success of the patient's rehabilitation. Patients with body scheme disturbances have difficulty with ADL, especially self-care and dressing activities that require a good knowledge of the body.[35] They may have difficulty following directions related to their own bodies.[5] They may be unable to correctly localize body parts, recognize right and left, and visualize and plan how to move their bodies to accomplish a given activity.

APRAXIA. The disturbance in praxis, or the ability to plan motor acts, is often intimately associated with the body scheme disorder.[3,58] Three types of apraxia have been identified. In *ideomotor apraxia*, the patient is unable to carry out a purposeful movement on command even though the concept of the task is understood and even though it may be possible to carry out the act automatically.[29,58] If *ideational apraxia* is present as well, the patient is not able to carry out routine activities, such as combing hair automatically, or on command because the concept of the task is not understood.[58]

Constructional apraxia is difficulty or inability to produce two- or three-dimensional designs in copying, constructing, or drawing. Constructional apraxia is often related to body scheme problems and is associated with difficulties in ADL, particularly dressing.[56,58]

When apraxia is present, often the person cannot formulate a plan of movement to accomplish an act. He or she may be unable to imitate movements of the therapist in demonstrated instructions.

VISUAL FIELD DEFECT—HOMONYMOUS HEMIANOPSIA. Homonymous hemianopsia is blindness of the nasal half of one eye and the temporal half of the other eye.[18] The affected side of the vision corresponds to the paralyzed side of the body. A patient with left hemiplegia with left homonymous hemianopsia cannot see things in the left visual field unless the patient turns the head toward the affected side to compensate for the deficit. In practical activity things placed on the left side may not be seen. Objects moving toward the patient from the left may be startling. The patient may bump into things on the left when walking. Some patients with hemiplegia compensate for this deficit automatically by turning their heads. Others need to be trained to turn the head, using the intact visual field to compensate for the visual loss.[53]

VISUAL ATTENTION. The ability to attend visually to elements in the environment depends on visual fixation, a voluntary act for the normal adult. The normal adult is able to select objects in the environment that demand attention and to focus on them appropriately.[6,58] The process of selecting objects on which to focus attention involves visual search and scanning. Visual search is the process of scanning the environment to gather information for identification or to select elements that demand attention or response. Deficits in visual search and the oculomotor skills necessary for its performance are seen frequently in patients with CVA.[8] The patient with a visual attention deficit has difficulty shifting the gaze or attention and has slowed eye movements and loss of the visual fixation point.[46]

UNILATERAL NEGLECT. Unilateral neglect, also called unilateral inattention, is the inability to integrate and utilize perceptions from the hemiplegic side of the body or of space and is most frequently seen in persons with left hemiplegia. Homonymous hemianopsia can be a complicating factor but unilateral neglect occurs in the absence of hemianopsia.[54,58]

The cause of unilateral neglect is not exactly known. It has been attributed to body scheme disorder and to visual scanning disorders.[43,53,58]

Unilateral neglect poses serious problems in rehabilitation. It is associated with deficits in reading, writing, arithmetic, and self-care skills. Some studies have shown that the presence of unilateral neglect in patients with right hemisphere lesions is a predictor of poor outcome in recovery of performance skills in ADL.[54]

The patient with unilateral neglect ignores the affected limbs and the affected side of space. The patient may fail to shave the affected side of the face or to dress that side of the body. Food on the affected side of the tray may be ignored and the patient may read only one side of a page of printed material. Communication from the hemiplegic side may be ignored or poorly integrated.[58]

SPATIAL RELATIONSHIPS. The ability to recognize the relationship between one form and another and between form and self in spatial areas may be lost as a result of CVA.[25,58] Disturbances in the perception of visual-spatial relationships are particularly common among patients with left hemiplegia.[51] The result is difficulty with tasks such as drawing or constructing three-dimensional objects and designs. The patient with this deficit has difficulty or failure with tasks involving spatial analysis. The ability to follow a familiar route may be lost because of a lack of spatial orientation.[51] Dressing failures are common because understanding of space words such as over, under, through and behind, may be lost.[53]

The problem may be compounded by the patient's inability to perceive the shape and relationship of the clothing to his or her body. Tasks such as matching parts in a sewing or woodworking project are impossible, as is matching puzzle parts or block designs.

VISUAL PERCEPTION OF VERTICAL. The perception of vertical lines and elements in the environment is essential to visual orientation in space. Patients with hemiplegia often have difficulty making visual judgments of what is vertical or horizontal. Patients with left hemiplegia tend to misjudge the vertical in a counterclockwise direction.[7,51] Because visual orientation to vertical is important to the optical righting reactions that help in the maintenance of upright posture, directional disturbances in perception of vertical and horizontal may interfere with balance and ambulation.[7]

FIGURE-BACKGROUND PERCEPTION. Figure-background perception is the recognition of forms hidden within a gestalt[25] and the ability to attend to a relevant visual stimulus while separating it from and ignoring background stimuli.[58] Some patients with hemiplegia have difficulty distinguishing a figure from its background. The result is that they cannot always select the most relevant visual cue to which to respond.[5] The patient may appear distractible but, in truth, he or she is responding to many irrelevant visual stimuli.[22,58] The patient may have difficulty selecting items from a cabinet or refrigerator because he or she cannot perceive the desired object as separate from the surrounding objects that constitute its background.[53,58]

VISUAL SEQUENCING. Visual sequencing is the ordering of visual patterns in time and space and involves temporal concepts, such as first, second, and third, and spatial ordering, such as top to bottom, left to right, and around.[4] A disturbance in sequencing skills may affect the patient's ability to plan steps and anticipate consequences of tasks and activities that require ordering of objects and steps in a procedure.

Cognitive Dysfunctions

Because CVA may interfere with integrative processes of the brain, and intelligence and cognitive abilities depend on the integrative functions of the brain, some patients with hemiplegia show impairment of specific intellectual functions. These may be demonstrated by a drop in intelligence test scores and an overall change in organization, mental abilities, and ability to do abstract reasoning.[29]

Evaluation of cognitive dysfunction is discussed in Chapter 13.

MEMORY. The reception, registration, integration, and retrieval of information is disrupted in stroke patients, at least in part, by factors such as language disorders, visual perceptual problems, alertness, motivation, and mental stamina, to name a few. Psychological reactions to stroke such as anxiety and depression can also affect memory adversely.[8]

Memory disturbance retards rehabilitation efforts. The patient may have difficulty recalling persons, objects, and procedures learned from day to day. Retrieval of information may be reduced, and learning ability may be impaired.

Patients with deficits in memory require much repetition of activity before training can be retained.[5] The therapist needs to discover each patient's best mode of sensory learning and provide the necessary sensory and perceptual cues and methods of instruction to suit the individual patient.

JUDGMENT. Poor judgment may be easily detected or may be masked by good social or verbal skills.[5] The patient may be unable to abstract the future and make judgments about the consequences of certain behaviors. The patient may not be able to judge, for example, that not locking his or her wheelchair may have grave consequences.

ABSTRACT THINKING. Abstract thinking and reasoning also may be impaired. Stroke patients are very concrete, dealing best with the realities of concrete objects and situations than with ideas and speculations about them. They may not be able to generalize learning from one situation or another and may be unable to comprehend the abstract ideas.[27]

Personality and Emotional Changes

REGRESSION. The patient who regresses does not appear to use his or her full adult capacities to deal with personal difficulties. The patient seems to regress to a lower level of emotional maturity. This is not an uncommon reaction to illness and may be due in part to sensory loss.[5,8]

RIGIDITY. Rigidity is an inability to be flexible or adapt to change. The patient feels most secure in a familiar and unchanging environment. This phenomenon manifests itself in inability to function with a changed time schedule, in disturbance at lack of symmetry or change in personnel, and in a tenacity to old and familiar methods of performing familiar activities.[21]

DENIAL. Denial is an unawareness of the hemiplegia and a denial of the defective performance of the paralyzed side. It manifests itself when the patient neglects the affected side. The patient may move the normal side and claim he or she is moving the affected arm or leg. The patient may declare that his or her arm belongs to someone else or may regard it as an object.[46] This phenomenon may be a psychological reaction to an unbearable truth or may be due to sensory and perceptual dysfunctions.[5]

PERSEVERATION. Perseveration is the meaningless, nonpurposeful repetition of an act.[18,42] The patient does not stop unless someone or something intervenes. It becomes particularly apparent during activities that are repetitive by nature, such as sanding wood, but can manifest itself in ADL such as buttoning and sponge bathing.

DEPRESSION. Depression is usually a reaction to a catastrophic illness. The patient may feel inadequate in dealing with his or her problems and may be overwhelmed by them. The patient feels a loss of control over life and a sense of helplessness. He or she has experienced not only a loss of control, but a significant loss of function and must mourn for the loss. The depression usually lifts and rehabilitation progresses as the patient rediscovers his or her assets and gains confidence and self-esteem.[5,8]

EMOTIONAL LABILITY. The patient with CVA may lose the cortical control of emotional responses and thus may manifest loss of emotional control more easily than he or she did formerly. Emotional lability may exhibit itself in automatic laughing or crying that seems inappropriate. Situations of stress often provoke crying. The patient is embarrassed by these outbursts and requires the reassurance and understanding of family and rehabilitation workers.[5,8]

REDUCTION IN BEHAVIORAL AND EVALUATIVE STANDARDS. The patient demonstrating a reduction in behavioral and evaluative standards may exhibit a reduced level of goal aspiration. He or she may seem satisfied with shoddy performance. His or her pride and perseverance in working toward goals may be poor. Inadequate performance and poor products may be acceptable to the patient in contrast to standards held before the illness occurred. This problem may be organic in origin but is enhanced by inactivity and the psychological trauma of the illness.[22]

MOTIVATION. Many patients with hemiplegia manifest an apparent defect in *intrinsic* motivation, or the inner drive to act spontaneously. This may be organic in origin or related to depression and should not be regarded as something that the patient can modify at will. This lack of motivation may cause rehabilitation workers to overestimate the disability. It may cause them to regard the patient as "stubborn" or "unwilling to try" and may reduce their motivation to help the patient. The problem may be related to the patient's readiness to deal with the overwhelming problems of the disability and to the tremendous amount of energy it takes every day for these patients to put their all into everything they attempt to do.

Motivation can be enhanced by establishing treatment goals that are realistic and meaningful. The patient and therapist should plan treatment goals together. The experience of success in the treatment program facilitates motivation. The therapist should explain the purposes of treatment so that the patient can understand the relevance of the treatment methods to goal attainment and should remind the patient frequently to practice newly learned motor skills and functional activities.[23]

Therapists must approach motivation problems with patience and perseverance. Patients need encouragement, reassurance, praise for success, and a lot of *extrinsic* motivation in prodding, cuing, and the planning of activities by therapists and caretakers.

FRUSTRATION TOLERANCE. Because of the numerous difficulties in performance posed by motor, sensory, perceptual, and cognitive impairments, the patient with hemiplegia understandably experiences much stress and frustration. Excessive stress and frustration are experienced when the patient is confronted with tasks that are above the capacity for performance and success. It is important for the therapist to select relevant activities difficult enough to challenge the patient to improve function, yet not so difficult as to evoke undue stress or frustration. Also, the therapist should monitor the effect that any given treatment method has on the patient. It is important for the patient to experience success in the treatment program.

Speech and Language Disorders

CVA may result in a wide variety of speech disorders and disturbances in the ability to deal with symbols and may vary from mild to severe. These dysfunctions occur most frequently in right hemiplegia, or damage to the left hemisphere of the brain, but also may occur in left hemiplegia. All persons with CVA should be evaluated by the speech pathologist for the presence of speech and language disorders. The speech pathologist can provide valuable information to other members of the rehabilitation team regarding the best ways to communicate with a particular patient. The occupational therapist should carry over the work of the speech therapist in the treatment sessions, as it is appropriate. This may occur in reinforcing communication techniques that the patient is learning, presenting instruction in ways that the patient is able to integrate, and instructing and practicing writing, which often is the responsibility of the occupational therapist.

When reading the descriptions of the specific speech and language dysfunctions that follow, it is important to remember that these dysfunctions can exist in mild to severe form and in combination with one another.

APHASIA. Aphasia is a language disorder that results from neurologic impairment. It can affect auditory comprehension, reading comprehension (alexia), oral expression, written expression (agraphia) and ability to interpret gestures. Mathematical deficits (acalculia) can also be present in aphasia. There are several different types of aphasia.

Global aphasia is characterized by a loss of all language skills. Oral expression is lost except for some persistent or recurrent utterance. Global aphasia is usually the result of involvement of the middle cerebral artery of the dominant cerebral hemisphere. The patient with global aphasia may be sensitive to gestures, vocal inflections, and facial expression. As a result the patient may appear to understand more than he or she actually does.[28]

Broca's aphasia is characterized by speech apraxia and agrammatism. The apraxia is manifested by slow, labored speech with frequent misarticulations. Syntactical structure is simplified because of the agrammatism, sometimes referred to as *telegraphic speech*. There is good auditory comprehension except when speech is rapid, grammatically complex, or lengthy. Reading comprehension and writing may be severely involved, and deficits in monetary concepts and ability to do calculations are usually present.[28]

Wernicke's aphasia is characterized by impaired auditory comprehension and feedback and fluent, well-articulated paraphasic speech. Paraphasic speech consists of word substitution errors. Speech may occur at an excessive rate and may be hyperfluent. The patient uses few substantive words and many function words. The speech is a running speech composed of

English words in a meaningless sequence. Some patients produce neologisms (non-English nonsense words) interspersed with real words. Reading and writing comprehension is often limited and impairment of mathematical skills may occur.[28]

Anomic aphasia is characterized by difficulties with word retrieval. Anomia or word finding difficulty occurs in all types of aphasia. However, patients in whom word finding difficulty is the primary or only symptom may be said to have anomic aphasia. The speech of these patients is fluent, grammatically correct, and well articulated, but there is significant difficulty with word finding. This can result in hesitant or slow speech and the substitution of descriptive phrases for actual names of things. Mild to severe deficits in reading comprehension and written expression occur and mild deficits in mathematical skills may be present.[28]

DYSARTHRIA. Patients with dysarthria have an articulation disorder because of a dysfunction of the CNS mechanisms that control speech musculature in the absence of aphasia.[53] This results in paralysis and incoordination of the organs of speech that make it sound thick, sluggish, and slurred.[10]

COMMUNICATION WITH APHASIC PATIENTS. Although the speech pathologist is responsible for the treatment of speech and language disorders, the occupational therapist can facilitate communication and meaningful interaction with aphasic patients.

Patients respond best to intelligent and sympathetic understanding from professional staff and family members. Those communicating with the patient should adopt an attitude of patience, relaxation, and acceptance. When talking to the patient, simple, short, concrete sentences should be used. Instructions and explanations should be kept simple. The patient can be encouraged, but not pressured, to respond in any way possible. The use of gestures for communication should be encouraged. Having the patient demonstrate through performance is the best way to ensure that instructions are understood. The patient should never be ridiculed nor forced to make correct responses. Bizarre, inaccurate language and the use of profanity should be accepted without amusement or anger. It is not necessary to raise the voice when speaking to aphasic patients. Hearing is usually not defective. Professional staff and family members should not talk about the patient in his or her presence. The patient can probably understand all or part of what is being said and should be included in conversations. Rapid, complicated speech with abstract and esoteric words should be avoided. Direct questions requiring one word answers are useful.[30].

The occupational therapist can use routine ADL as opportunities to encourage speech. The patient needs to be reassured that the language disorder is part of the disability and is not a manifestation of mental illness.[30]

Contrast Between Right and Left Hemiplegia

There is an apparent difference between the performance and learning styles of persons with right hemiplegia and those with left hemiplegia. This contrast is related to the difference in hemispheric function.

The right cerebral hemisphere is concerned with the perception of the whole or Gestalt processing.[17] It is associated with perceptual skills such as the body scheme and visual spatial analysis. Therefore, right hemisphere lesions involving the parietal lobe result in body scheme disturbance, spatial perceptual disorders, and inattention to the left side.[1,53] Lesions of the right cerebral hemisphere result in difficulties with tasks of spatial analysis and spatial orientation and in dressing apraxia.[53,58]

There is a significant correlation between extremely poor performance on perceptual organization tasks and failures in dressing and grooming.[34] The patient with left hemiplegia may retain good verbal skills, which may tend to mask the perceptual dysfunction and give the impression of good performance. The therapist needs to require performance evaluation of self-care skills and not rely on the interview as a means of determining the patient's ability to function.

The left cerebral hemisphere of most right-handed persons is primarily responsible for analytical processing of individual elements rather than perception of the whole. It is also responsible for temporal sequencing.[17] The control of language and complex voluntary movement resides primarily in the left hemisphere. Left hemisphere lesions result in varying degrees of aphasia.[1,53] The ability to deal with visual spatial tasks may be undisturbed, and the patient may benefit from demonstrated or pantomimed instructions rather than verbal ones. He or she is usually more successful in achieving self-care independence earlier than the patient with left hemiplegia.

Conclusion

When the patient has some or all of the perceptual and psychological problems discussed, the traditional rehabilitation goals for motor and functional retraining may be more than can be mastered. Rehabilitation goals cannot be based on the motor evaluation alone. Rather, the total scope of the disability must be considered, including sensory, perceptual, psychological, emotional, and intellectual impairments and the patient's social and family situation. If evaluation of the patient is inadequate and inappropriate goals are set, the result is frustration for the therapist, patient, and family.

Therapists must evaluate and observe the effect of all of the concomitant dysfunctions, as well as the motor dysfunction. If the limitations of the patient are clearly recognized and identified, realistic rehabilitation goals may be set. Retraining to the degree possible can be achieved, and the therapist, patient, and family will feel a sense of achievement rather than failure in the rehabilitation program.

OCCUPATIONAL THERAPY INTERVENTION

The role of the occupational therapist in the treatment of CVA that results in hemiplegia revolves around facilitating symmetric motor function, use of the affected side, and restoring the patient to his or her maximal level of independence.

Each patient must be evaluated for his or her residual abilities and disabilities. A treatment program must be especially tailored to the patient's particular needs, because the range of possible motor, sensory, perceptual, and cognitive dysfunctions after CVA is wide. The selection of treatment objectives and treatment methods depends on factors, such as stage of motor recovery, sensory perceptual status, cognitive functions, age, date of onset, concomitant illness, social and economic factors, and potential for further recovery.

The occupational therapist may be involved in the acute care of the patient and the early mobilization aspects of treatment. Later occupational therapy may be a primary service in extended rehabilitation when the emphasis is on achieving self-care independence and performance skills for work or leisure activities.

Goals of Occupational Therapy

The overall goals of occupational therapy for the hemiplegic patient are to prevent complications and deformities, to remediate psychosocial dysfunction, to achieve maximal physical function, and to facilitate maximal independence in self-maintenance.[43] More specific goals are

1. to prevent deformity caused by spasticity and poor positioning
2. to inhibit abnormal patterns of posture and movement
3. to achieve maximal active ROM, strength, and coordination of the affected extremities and body side.
4. to achieve maximal voluntary bilateral and unilateral use of affected extremities in correct functional patterns
5. to correct or compensate for perceptual and cognitive dysfunction

6. to achieve maximal functional independence in self-care
7. to facilitate realistic acceptance of and adjustment to disability
8. to improve functional communication skills and social interaction
9. to facilitate reentry to meaningful roles in family and community
10. to facilitate a balance between work, rest, and play.[43,50,53]

Occupational Therapy Evaluation

The occupational therapist begins the program with a thorough evaluation of the patient's deficits and assets to establish a baseline for progress. The evaluation process is continuous, beginning with the evaluation of motor and sensory status and simple self-care skills and progresses to perceptual, cognitive, and more complex performance evaluations.[10]

MOTOR FUNCTIONS. The degree of spasticity in a patient with CVA should be evaluated (Chapter 8). Brunnstrom's test (Chapter 19) can be used to determine the stage of motor recovery, the presence of synergistic movement, and associated reactions. Abnormal movement patterns, the presence of primitive reflexes, abnormal motor patterns, abnormal coordination, righting reactions, equilibrium and protective reactions, and in general, the postural reflex mechanism should be evaluated according to methods outlined by Bobath.[9,52] Joint ROM may be measured or estimated, but the therapist should be aware that ROM often is limited by transient and variable degrees of spasticity at any given time. In recording joint ROM, the therapist must differentiate between apparent limitations due to temporary spasticity and actual limitations due to structural changes.[20] When the patient has achieved some voluntary control of movement, the therapist should evaluate the ability to perform selective movement. Spontaneous use of the affected extremities should be observed during testing and functional activities, because this is a good sign of improving sensorimotor status.

SENSATION. Senses of touch, superficial pain, temperature, pressure, stereognosis, and proprioception should be tested.[53] Olfactory and gustatory sensation may be tested, because these senses are disturbed in some patients and often overlooked. Methods for evaluating sensation can be found in Chapter 11.

PERCEPTION. Body scheme, and motor planning should be routinely evaluated. Tests for visual perception problems, such as hemianopsia and visual-spatial relationships, figure-ground perception, visual attention, and unilateral neglect, should be included in the battery of evaluation procedures.

Methods for evaluating perception are described in Chapter 12.

COGNITION. Cognitive skills such as memory, attention, initiation, planning and organization, mental flexibility and abstraction, insight and impulsivity, problem-solving skills, and ability to do calculations should be evaluated.[43] Methods for evaluating cognition are described in Chapter 13.

PSYCHOSOCIAL FACTORS. Through observation and interview of the patient, family members, friends, and other rehabilitation team members, the occupational therapist should ascertain the patient's vocational and recreational histories, role in the family and community, amount of family support, adjustment to disability, and frustration tolerance and coping skills.

Regressive behavior and functioning should be assessed because CVA can cause regression to childlike physical and mental levels. The patient may deny the necessity to engage in apparently simplistic activities to regain motor, sensory, perceptual, cognitive, performance, and communication skills. Coping with the multitude of personal and social changes brought about this catastrophic illness may be more than the patient can do. It is also possible that the brain damage has affected areas that subserve motivation and adjustment.[50]

COMMUNICATION AND ORAL MOTOR FUNCTION. An oral motor evaluation, carried out according to methods described in Chapter 10 may be necessary for many CVA patients. Such an evaluation helps to determine the need for facilitation and inhibition of oral structures in a prefeeding program and the need for feeding training. If speech is affected, information about specific speech impairments should be gleaned from the evaluation of the speech pathologist. This specialist can recommend appropriate methods of adapting and modifying instruction to best suit the patient's deficits. The patient's attempts at nonverbal communication may be hampered by altered muscle tone and sensation, lack of movement, and facial paralysis.[52]

The occupational therapist should make an assessment of functional communication skills in the course of the evaluation process and treatment. The therapist can observe the patient's ability to interpret spoken and written language, ability to speak and write, difficulty with motor control of oral structures due to paralysis or mouth apraxia, difficulty with auditory perception and determining direction of auditory stimuli, and loss of hearing.[50]

PERFORMANCE SKILLS. Performance skills should be evaluated by interview and, more importantly, by actual performance of test items. Self-care and home management skills, mobility and transfer techniques, physical endurance, and work-related activities, when appropriate, should be included in the performance evaluation. It may take several weeks to complete the performance evaluation, which is an ongoing part of the treament program.

Methods of evaluating performance skills are described in Chapter 15.

Treatment

THE MOTOR DYSFUNCTION

Motor retraining. The occupational therapy program may include one or a combination of the sensorimotor approaches to treatment such as the Brunnstrom (Chapter 19), Bobath (Chapter 20), and PNF (Chapter 21) approaches. The purposes of the motor retraining program are to facilitate movement and use of the affected side, develop more normal postural reflex mechanisms, and inhibit abnormal reflexes and movement patterns.

Range of motion. The maintenance of joint ROM and prevention of deformity is an important early goal in the treatment program and should be continued indefinitely if a substantial amount of spontaneous voluntary movement is not regained. This is achieved through positioning techniques, such as those recommended by Bobath and passive, assistive, and self-administered ROM procedures.[9]

ROM exercises usually are carried out using principles of the selected treatment approach. In the Brunnstrom approach, positioning, passive movement through the synergy patterns, trunk and bilateral shoulder movements described in Chapter 19, and the facilitating patterns of movement used in treatment all serve to maintain ROM.[12]

The Bobath approach utilizes bilateral movement with clasped hands to release spasticity and maintain full passive shoulder flexion and scapula movement. In this method, the patient clasps the hands together with fingers interlaced and the hemiplegic thumb on top in some abduction. Abduction of the affected fingers and thumb may help to reduce flexor spasticity of the entire limb. The patient is taught to begin by pushing the clasped hands forward and protracting the scapula before lifting the arms. With elbows extended, the arms are then raised to the level of comfort. These maneuvers can be practiced many times during the day to maintain full pain-free shoulder ROM.

The advantages of the Bobath exercise are improved sensation and awareness of the affected arm as it is brought to midline and into the field of vision, and prevention of scapula and trunk retraction.[20] Proper positioning, and the patterns of movement used during treatment prevent loss of ROM. All the patterns of normal movement are incorporated into the motor retraining program. Thus, upper extremity

ROM is an integral part of the total treatment program.[19]

In the PNF approach, performance of antagonistic pairs of diagonal upper extremity patterns activates all muscle groups in the upper extremities. Ten repetitions of antagonistic diagonals maintain ROM of all joints of the arm. To perform ROM of the wrist and hand, the therapist grasps the side of the patients thumb with the thumb and one finger of one hand. The patient's thumb is pulled into palmar abduction. The therapist places his or her fingers across the palmar surface of the patient's fingers in a diagonal direction. The patient's hand is then moved in partial diagonal patterns so that the forearm is supinated with wrist and finger flexion and pronated with wrist and finger extension.[38]

Shoulder pain and subluxation. The Bobath, Brunnstrom, and PNF approaches caution against the traditional passive ROM exercises to the shoulder. Passive flexion, abduction, and rotation of the glenohumeral joint to extreme ranges in the absence of good scapula mobility can be more harmful than helpful.[52]

Normal abduction and upward rotation of the scapula are prevented by spacticity of scapula musculature when the glenohumeral joint is flexed or abducted. Shoulder joint motion without the normally associated scapula movement results in faulty mechanics and can cause joint trauma. Bicipital tendinitis, coracoiditis, brachial plexus traction, or supraspinatus tendinitis caused by compression of the tendon between the humeral tuberosities and the acromion can result from joint trauma.[15,52]

Reciprocal pully exercises are contraindicated, because they are forced passive exercise and can cause joint pain and possibly damage if there is inadequate scapular mobility.[13,20,47] Inappropriate exercise and incorrect handling of the upper extremity by professional staff during transfers, ambulation, and bed mobility activities are some causes of trauma to the shoulder joint.[20,43]

Subluxation of the humerus from the glenoid fossa is a common problem in hemiplegia. The rotator cuff muscles are probably of primary importance in the maintenance of joint stability. The function of the supraspinatus muscle is especially important in the prevention of subluxation. Brunnstrom recommended procedures to activate the muscles surrounding the shoulder joint as a means of preventing subluxation.[13]

In the past occupational therapists prescribed and applied arm slings to the patient for wear when the arm is in a dependent position for the purpose of preventing or reducing subluxation. Smith and Okamoto reported that there are more than 22 hemiplegic sling designs.[48] The benefits of such a sling are doubtful.[2,43] Bobath maintains that subluxation cannot be prevented if the muscles are weak and that slings contribute to poor positioning, pain, and swelling.[9] Todd and Davies stated that a sling should never be worn because it reinforces flexor spasticity and immobilizes the upper limb, both of which are factors contributing to shoulder pain.[52] The sling is not effective for reducing pain or preventing subluxation.

Hand edema. Hand edema, resulting from fluid accumulation in the hand of the hemiplegic patient, should be prevented. Lymphatic pumps located proximally and distally in the upper extremity are dependent on muscle tone and contraction for their function. The hypotonicity and inactivity of the hemiplegic upper extremity can result in faulty pumping action of the lymphatic system and subsequent hand edema. Edema can be prevented by elevation of the hand above the heart level to facilitate venous return. The hand can be propped on pillows at night and supported on a wheelchair arm or a distally elevated lapboard during the day when the patient is not involved in activity or treatment. Passive and active assisted ROM exercises also help to prevent edema. Because immobilization contributes to the development of edema, splints and positioning devices should be closely monitored. More aggressive techniques for edema reduction which may be used by both physical and occupational therapists are air splints, the Jobst pump, distal to proximal massage, elastic gloves,[13] centripetal wrapping of the fingers and hand with string, and immersion in a bucket of ice and water. Davies recommended the use of a small cock-up splint to prevent wrist flexion, which is thought to contribute to edema.[20] The splint is held in place with an elastic bandage.

Flexor spasticity of the hand. Flexor spasticity in the hand musculature can result in wrist flexion and a fisted position, which can progress to contracture and deformity if not prevented. Orthotic devices may be used to protect joints and prevent deformity, particularly if there is no active motion. Orthotic devices also have been used for the purpose of reducing flexor spasticity. The use of orthotic devices for this purpose has been controversial.[36,43]

Todd and Davies stated that splints can reduce sensory stimulation and decrease the need for activity.[52] This in turn can inhibit the return of voluntary control and prevent normal movement. In their review of the literature, Mathiowetz and colleagues pointed out that others have claimed that several types of splints are useful for inhibition of spasticity.[36]

Some of the devices used to reduce flexor spasticity are the volar resting splint, the dorsal resting splint, a firm cone held in the hand, a finger spreader, and the Snook spasticity reduction splint.[36,49] The effects of the volar versus the dorsal resting splint on spasticity have been contradictory.[36] Snook modified the dorsal platform splint to make her spasticity reduction splint.[49] Preliminary findings indicated the splint was effective in reducing spasticity.[37,49] The use of a firm cone in the hand was first advocated by Rood. It provides constant pressure to the flexor surface of the hand and on the insertions of the spastic wrist and finger flexors. This is thought to have an inhibitory effect on the muscles[36] (see Chapter 18). The foam rubber finger spreader was first advocated by Bobath because it maintained the fingers and thumb in abduction and extension. Finger abduction is thought to facilitate finger extension and reduce flexor spasticity throughout the upper extremity.[36]

No definitive study compares the long-term effects of various positioning devices on the spastic hands of hemiplegic patients.[36,40] Clinical research is greatly needed to test the effectiveness of various positioning devices for their effectiveness in reducing flexor spasticity in the hemiplegic hand.[40]

Techniques to facilitate relaxation of spastic wrist and finger musculature followed by gentle, passive ROM, which is done to avoid stretch of the relaxed musculature, may be adequate to prevent the flexion deformity of the hand if done regularly.

A broad wheelchair armrest or lapboard may be used to support the arm and hand when the patient is inactive and is sitting or moving about in the wheelchair. These armrests are commercially available or may be custom made at the treatment facility.

Armrests and lapboards made of clear plastic are recommended because they allow the patient to see their legs, their feet, and the floor.

Therapeutic activities. The use of therapeutic activities to enhance motor retraining is advocated in the Bobath, Brunnstrom, and PNF approaches to treatment. Bobath advocated the close cooperation of the physical and occupational therapists in coordination of an integrated treatment program.[9] She recommended that occupational therapy could use bilateral activities with hands clasped such as pushing a roll or a ball to inhibit flexor spasticity. Activities which involve trunk rotation weight-bearing on the affected arm, such as moving objects from one side of a bench to the other, are also useful to decrease tone and prevent associated reactions. Positioning of the sound arm well forward and in the field of vision is recommended during one-handed activities such as eating or sponge bathing at the wash basin.[9] Eggers described many very creative activities appropriate for the hemiplegic at each stage in the recovery process.[24] Positioning, transfers, bilateral activities, unilateral ac-

tivities, and activities for hand retraining are included in Eggers' work. All of the activities are directed to the inhibition of abnormal tone and reflexes, and the facilitation of normal movement patterns.

Brunnstrom advocated the use of the limb synergies and other available movement patterns in ADL.[12] Activities such as sanding, sawing, using a carpet sweeper, and dusting furniture make use of movement patterns similar to the limb synergies. Symmetric bilateral activities facilitate the hemiplegic upper extremity and can elicit and reinforce extension. For the patient in the earlier stages of recovery, the hand can stabilize or hold objects while the unaffected hand does the skilled work. Activities for patients in more advanced stages of recovery should be designed to include combined movements of increasing complexity.[12]

In the PNF approach, activities are analyzed for the diagonal patterns. Activities of daily living and therapeutic activities that elicit desired diagonal patterns of movement can be used to reinforce motor learning taking place in physical therapy.[38] When planning therapeutic activities, the therapist needs to take into account the patient's motor, sensory, perceptual, and cognitive dysfunctions. It is important for the patient to be successful at accomplishing the tasks. This can be achieved if the tasks are within his or her capabilities.

Early use of therapeutic activities enhances development of alertness, interest, and motivation and provides opportunities for socialization and communication.

SENSORY RETRAINING. The occupational therapy program for the hemiplegic patient may include sensory reeducation and compensation techniques to remediate sensory dysfunction. Methods for sensory reeducation and compensation techniques are described in Chapter 11. Techniques of sensory retraining have met with limited success.

PERCEPTUAL RETRAINING. Occupational therapists have used perceptual retraining since the 1950s. They have focused on retraining specific perceptual skills and incorporating perceptual retraining into functional tasks such as ADL skills. Occupational therapists use perceptual training because performance of functional activites is assumed to be dependent upon perceptual skills and, conversely, that perceptual deficits affect functional performance. Also, remediation of or compensation for perceptual deficits is assumed to improve functional performance, and improvement of perception is assumed to be effected through occupational therapy. The relationship between perceptual deficits and functional performance has been demonstrated in several studies. However, the effectiveness of the various approaches to the re- mediation of perceptual deficits has not been well doc- umented and requires scientific investigation.[39]

Treatment of perceptual problems can be difficult and complex. The best results are obtained when the treatment is done on a daily basis. Zoltan, Siev, and Frieshtat described four approaches that are used for perceptual training of the hemiplegic patient.[58] These are the sensory integrative approach, the neurode- velopmental (Bobath) approach, the transfer of train- ing approach, and the functional approach.

The sensory-integrative approach is based on neu- rophysiologic and developmental principles and was described by A. Jean Ayres as a treatment approach for children with sensory-integrative dysfunction.[3] It assumes that controlled sensory input can be used to elicit specific motor responses. Thus the sensory- integrative functions of the brain can be influenced by selected activities that provide the necessary input and evoke the desired motor responses. This ap- proach may be impractical for adults because it takes much treatment time to be effective. It is also likely that the adult's CNS does not have the same capacity for learning as a child's CNS, because it is thought that it does not have the same degree of plasticity. Some therapists use modifications and selected tech- niques from this approach with adults with some re- ported success.[58]

In the neurodevelopmental (Bobath) approach, perceptual retraining is integral to the handling tech- niques and feedback about correct movement during the motor retraining program.[58] The experience of the sensation of normal movement and the feedback about correct performance enhances the retraining of perceptual functions. Bilateral activities used in the motor retraining program stimulate total body aware- ness and help to remediate problems of unilateral neglect and homonymous hemianopsia. Weight-bear- ing activities, an important part of the motor retrain- ing program, enhance proprioception.

The transfer of training approach assumes that practice in a particular perceptual task carries over to performance of similar tasks or practical activities re- quiring the same perceptual skill. For example, prac- tice in reproducing pegboard designs for spatial re- lations training could carry over to dressing skills that require spatial judgment (for example, matching blouse to body and discriminating right from left shoe). This is a common approach to the treatment of perceptual problems in occupational therapy clin- ics. Conflicting reports of its effectiveness exist, and further research is needed to determine its benefits.[58]

The repetitive practice of particular tasks that help the patient become more independent in the perfor-

mance of ADL characterizes the functional approach. This is probably the most common approach in deal- ing with perceptual problems. The therapist does not do specific perceptual training. Rather, the therapist helps the patient to adapt to or compensate for his or her perceptual deficits. The patient is made aware of the problem and taught to compensate for it. For example, if the patient has an homonymous hemi- anopsia, the therapist may cue him or her to turn the head to see the blind visual field. Adaptation of en- vironment or methods is another way to compensate for a perceptual deficit. If the patient is distractable because of visual or auditory figure-ground deficits, the therapist may arrange for treatment or training to take place in a quiet and uncluttered room to min- imize distractions and create the best environment for learning.[58]

Principles of treatment for perceptual deficits are outlined in Chapter 12. Zoltan, Siev and Frieshtat described several methods for the remediation of perceptual deficits.[58] A few of these are outlined here.

Body scheme disorder. Using the transfer of train- ing approach, the therapist may touch the patient's body parts and have him or her identify them as they are touched. Practice in assembling human figure puzzles and quizzing the patient on body parts are other methods in this approach.

Unilateral neglect. In a unilateral deficit, the ther- apist engages the patient in activities that focus his or her attention on the neglected left side. Examples are giving tactile stimulation to the affected extremities, using precautions for not increasing spasticity, placing work materials to the left side, and approaching the patient from the left side for conversation and during treatment. To use adaptation or compensation the therapist may place food, utensils, and work materials on the unaffected side and give all instructions from that side.

Spatial relations. Using a transfer of training ap- proach, the therapist might have the patient copy par- quetry block design, matchstick designs, or pegboard patterns that the therapist arranges; connect dots to make a design using a stimulus design to follow; or construct puzzles.[58] To compensate for a spatial def- icit, the therapist might use colored dots to mark the route to a specific location.

Dressing apraxia. To overcome dressing apraxia, the therapist teaches a set pattern for dressing and gives cues that help the patient to distinguish right from left or front from back. A helpful method is to have the patient position the garment the same way each time, such as a shirt with the buttons face up and pants with the zipper face up. Labels can be used as cues to differentiate the front from the back of the garment. The garment may be color coded with small buttons or ribbons for front and back or right and left side.

Ideational and ideomotor apraxia. Treatment of ideational and ideomotor apraxia disorders is difficult. Use of short, clear, concise, and concrete instructions is necessary, because this apraxia is usually the result of a dominant hemisphere lesion, and often aphasia is present as well. The task should be broken down into its component steps, and each stop should be taught separately. Verbal and demonstrated instructions may be ineffective, and it can be helpful to guide the patient through the correct movements, giving tactile and proprioceptive input to the instruction. This can be done while also giving brief verbal instruction. After the patient has performed each step of the task separately, the therapist can begin to combine the steps, grading to the complete task.[58]

An example of a complete task is hair combing. The therapist can break the task into steps: lift comb; bring comb to hair; move comb across top of head, down left side, down right side, down back; and replace comb on table. Much repetition is necessary to be effective.

COGNITIVE RETRAINING. Cognitive rehabilitation is an emerging field in which the neuropsychologist, speech pathologist, and occupational therapist have parts to play. Much of the effort in cognitive rehabilitation has been concerned with head injury patients. Cognitive rehabilitation is a complex, multidimensional process, which involves the patient and his or her human and nonhuman environment.[41,45] Methods of evaluation and treatment of selected cognitive dysfunctions are described in Chapter 13. For a detailed discussion of cognitive rehabilitation, see the references.[8,57,58]

PERFORMANCE SKILLS. Training in ADL is a primary function of the occupational therapy service. Specific procedures are described in Chapters 15 and 20. Early in the rehabilitation process this may include wheelchair mobility and transfer skills (Chapter 22) and simple self-care activities, such as feeding and oral hygiene. Training in more complex bathing and dressing skills might be added later. As the patient progresses in independent performance of the skills of self-maintenance, evaluation and training in appropriate home management activities should be included in the ADL program.

Affected limbs and the affected side of the body should be employed in ADL training as much as possible. However, motor, sensory, perceptual, and cognitive deficits may influence the feasibility of use of the affected limbs. The effect of the activity on frustration and muscle tone should be assessed.

Coordination and skill training in one-handed performance may be necessary when the dominant upper extremity is affected and a change of dominance is necessary or when motor recovery is so limited as to preclude any functional use of the affected arm. Such patients may have to rely on one-handed performance indefinitely.[9]

The patient must learn methods of stabilizing objects and equipment for one-handed performance. He or she must learn to use assistive devices and equipment adapted to ease functioning with one hand. It is the role of the occupational therapist to acquire the necessary assistive devices and train the patient in their use.

Home evaluation. As the patient nears discharge to home and community, the occupational therapist should be involved in a home evaluation (Chapter 15), and vocational or leisure skills potential should be explored. A living situation is recommended that accomodates the patient's needs. The occupational therapist, having evaluated self-care and home management skills performance, is the most qualified to estimate the patient's potential for independent living. Patients with hemiplegia range from those who can resume living independently to those who require continuous supervision and assistance. The outcome depends on the severity of the CVA, success in rehabilitation, mental status, and social factors.

PSYCHOSOCIAL ADJUSTMENT. An important role of the occupational therapist is to aid in the patient's adjustment to hospitalization and, more important, to disability. A patient and supportive approach by the therapist is essential. The therapist must be empathetic to the fact that the patient has experienced a devastating and life-threatening illness. Sudden and dramatic changes in life roles and performance have resulted. The therapist must be cognizant of the normal adjustment process (Chapter 2) and gear approach and performance expectations to the patient's stage of adjustment. Frequently the patient is not ready to engage in rehabilitation measures with whole-hearted effort until several months after onset of the disability.

Many patients dwell on the possibility of full recovery of function and need to be made aware gradually that some residual dysfunction is very likely. The therapist may approach this by discussing what is known about prognosis for functional recovery from CVA in objective terms. This may have to be reviewed many times with the patient before the patient begins to apply the information to his or her own recovery and should be done in a way that is honest, yet does not destroy all hope.

The occupational therapy program should focus on the skills and abilities of the patient. The patient's attention should be focused, through the performance of activity, on his or her remaining and newly learned skills. Therapeutic group activities for socialization and sharing common problems and their solutions can be included.

The discovery that there are residual abilities and perhaps new abilities and success at performing many daily living skills and activities that were initially thought to be impossible can have a beneficial effect on the patient's mental health and outlook. The occupational therapy program can be thought of as a laboratory for real living in which skills are learned and practiced and abilities are recovered or discovered.

TREATMENT GRADATION. Treatment of the motor dysfunction is directed toward the reintegration of the postural reflex mechanism and the recovery of controlled, coordinated movement. The manner and speed with which treatment is graded depends on the patient and the treatment approach. In general, inhibition and facilitation techniques should be decreased as voluntary control of motion is improved. The amount of assistance in exercise and activity should be decreased as control and coordination are gained. The difficulty of performance skills demanded can be increased as synergistic movement subsides, and isolated voluntary motion is possible.[44]

Treatment time and time spent in standing and ambulation activities can be gradually increased to improve endurance. The complexity and number of ADL can be increased as physical, perceptual, and cognitive functioning improves. The amount of assistance given during transfers and for all activities should be decreased as independence is increased.

Conclusion

CVA is a complex disability, which challenges the skills of professional health care workers. Although a significant increase in the number and effectiveness of approaches for the remediation of affected motor, sensory, perceptual, cognitive, and performance dysfunctions has occurred, many limitations in treatment remain. The occupational therapist must bear in mind that the degree to which the patient achieves treatment goals depends on the CNS damage and recovery, psychoneurologic residuals, psychosocial adjustment, and the skilled application of appropriate treatment by all concerned health professionals.

Some patients remain severely disabled in spite of the noblest efforts of rehabilitation workers, and others recover quite spontaneously with minimal help in a short period of time. Most benefit from the professional skills of occupational therapists and other rehabilitation specialists to achieve improvement of performance skills and resumption of meaningful occupational roles.

REVIEW QUESTIONS

1. Define CVA.
2. List three other dysfunctions that could accompany the motor dysfunction in hemiplegia.
3. List the disturbances that are likely to result from occlusion to the anterior cerebral artery, middle cerebral artery, posterior cerebral artery, and cerebellar arteries.
4. Which artery is most frequently affected in CVA?
5. Define "transient ischemic attack."
6. Describe the dependence of motion on sensation in the normal sensorimotor process.
7. Besides the upper motor neuron paralysis of limbs and trunk after CVA, what other important motor disturbances can result?
8. List three poor prognostic signs for functional recovery.
9. List three good prognostic signs for functional recovery.
10. What differences in performance can be expected between persons with right and left hemiplegia? What accounts for these differences?
11. How does body scheme disorder interfere with rehabilitation?
12. How would training be approached if there is a memory loss?
13. Describe apraxia. Give examples of apraxic behavior. How would it interfere with rehabilitation.
14. What is the difference between unilateral neglect and visual inattention?
15. Describe what is meant by "lability." How can it be dealt with during a treatment session?
16. How does aphasia differ from dysarthria?
17. Describe four suggestions for more effective communication with an aphasic patient.
18. What is the importance of comprehensive occupational therapy evaluation of patients with hemiplegia?
19. Describe two methods that are used to maintain ROM.
20. List four major elements of the occupational therapy program for hemiplegia. Describe the purposes of each.
21. How can occupational therapy assist with the psychosocial adjustment of the hemiplegic patient?

REFERENCES

1. Almli CR: Normal sequential behavioral and physiological changes throughout the developmental arc. In Umphred DA editor: Neurological rehabilitation, St Louis, 1985, The CV Mosby Co.
2. Andersen LT: Shoulder pain in hemiplegia, Am J Occup Ther 39:11, 1985.
3. Ayres AJ: Perceptual motor training for children. In Approaches to the treatment of patients with neuromuscular dysfunction, Proceedings of study course IV, Third International Congress, World Federation of Occupational Therapists, Du-

buque, Iowa, 1962, Wm C Brown Co, Publishers.

4. Banus BS, editor: The developmental therapist, Thorofare, NJ, 1971, Charles B Slack, Inc.

5. Bardach JL: Psychological factors in hemiplegia, J Am Phys Ther Assoc 43:792, 1963.

6. Baum B et al: Perceptual motor evaluation for head injured and neurologically impaired adults, San José, 1983, Santa Clara County, Santa Clara Valley Medical Center.

7. Birch HG et al: Perception in hemiplegia. I. Judgment of the vertical and horizontal by hemiplegic patients, Arch Phys Med Rehabil 41:19, 1960.

8. Bleiberg J: Psychological and neuropsychological factors in stroke management. In Kaplan PE and Cerullo LJ: Stroke rehabilitation, Boston, 1986, Butterworth & Co.

9. Bobath B: Adult hemiplegia: evaluation and treatment, ed 2, London, 1978, William Heinemann Medical Books, Ltd.

10. Bonner C: The team approach to hemiplegia, Springfield, Ill, 1969, Charles C Thomas, Publisher.

11. Branch EF: The neuropathology of stroke. In Duncan, PW and Badke MB: Stroke rehabilitation: the recovery of motor control, Chicago, 1987, Year Book Medical Publishers, Inc.

12. Brunnstrom S: Motor behavior in adult hemiplegic patients, Am J Occup Ther 15:6, 1961.

13. Brunnstrom S: Movement therapy in hemiplegia, New York, 1970, Harper & Row Publishers, Inc.

14. Buchwald J: General features of nervous system organization, Am J Phys Med 46:89, 1967.

15. Cailliet R: The shoulder in hemiplegia, Philadelphia, 1982, FA Davis Co.

16. Caplan LR: Care of the patient with acute stroke. In Kaplan PE and Cerullo LJ: Stroke rehabilitation, Boston, 1986, Butterworth & Co.

17. Charness A: Stroke/head injury. Rehabilitation Institute of Chicago Procedure Manual, Rockville, MD, 1986, Aspen Publishers, Inc.

18. Chusid J: Correlative neuroanatomy and functional neurology, ed. 19, Los Altos, Calif., 1985, Lange Medical Publications.

19. Davis JZ: Personal communication, November 21, 28, 1988.

20. Davies PM: Steps to follow: a guide to the treatment of adult hemiplegia, New York, 1985, Springer-Verlag.

21. Delacato CH: Hemiplegia and concomitant psychological phenomena, Part I, Am J Occup Ther 10:157, 1956.

22. Delacato C and Doman G: Hemiplegia and concomitant psychological phenomena, Am J Occup Ther 11:186, 196, 1957.

23. Duncan PW and Badke MB: Therapeutic strategies for rehabilitation of motor deficits. In Duncan PW and Badke MB: Stroke rehabilitation: the recovery of motor control, Chicago, 1987, Year Book Medical Publishers, Inc.

24. Eggers O: Occupational therapy in the treatment of adult hemiplegia, Rockville, MD, 1984, Aspen Systems Corporation.

25. Gilfoyle E and Grady A: Cognitive-perceptual-motor behavior. In Willard H and Spackman C, editors: Occupational therapy, ed. 4, Philadelphia, 1971, JB Lippincott Co.

26. Haberman S, Capildeo R, and Rose FC: Risk factors for cerebrovascular disease. In Rose FC: Advances in stroke therapy, New York, 1982, Raven Press.

27. Hague HR: An investigation of abstract behavior in patients with cerebral vascular accident. Part II, Am J Occup Ther 13:83, 1959.

28. Halper AS and Mogil SI: Communication disorders: diagnosis and treatment. In Kaplan PE and Cerullo LJ: Stroke rehabilitation, Boston, 1986, Butterworth & Co.

29. Hopkins HL: Occupational therapy management of cerebral vascular accident and hemiplegia. In Willard HS and Spackman CS, editors: Occupational therapy, ed 4, Philadelphia, 1971, JB Lippincott Co.

30. Horwitz B: An open letter to the family of an adult patient with aphasia, Rehabil Lit, 23:141, 1962.

31. Larson CB and Gould M: Orthopedic nursing, ed 9, St Louis, 1978, The CV Mosby Co.

32. Levine RL: Diagnostic, medical and surgical aspects of stroke management. In Duncan PW and Badke MB: Stroke rehabilitation: the recovery of motor control, Chicago, 1987, Year Book Medical Publishers, Inc.

33. Lieberman JS: Hemiplegia: rehabilitation of the upper extremity. In Kaplan PE and Cerullo LG: Stroke rehabilitation, Boston, 1986, Butterworth & Co.

34. Lorenze E and Cancro R: Dysfunction in visual perception with hemiplegia: relation to activities of daily living, Arch Phys Med Rehab 43:514, 1962.

35. MacDonald JC: An investigation of body scheme in adults with cerebral vascular accidents, Am J Occup Ther 15:75, 1960.

36. Mathiowetz V, Bolding DJ, and Trombly C: Immediate effects of positioning devices on the normal and spastic hand measured by elecromyography, Am J Occup Ther 37:247, 1983.

37. McPherson JJ: Objective evaluation of a splint designed to reduce hypertonicity, Am J Occup Ther 35:189, 1981.

38. Myers B: Proprioceptive neuromuscular facilitation, Unit III: Patterns and their application to occupational therapy (videotape), Chicago, 1982, Rehabilitation Institute of Chicago.

39. Neistadt ME: Occupational therapy for adults with perceptual deficits, Am J Occup Ther 42:434, 1988.

40. Neuhaus BE et al: A survey of rationales for and against hand splinting in hemiplegia, Am J Occup Ther 35:83, 1981.

41. Novack TA et al: Cognitive stimulation in the home environment. In Williams JM and Long CJ, editors: The rehabilitation of

cognitive disabilities, New York, 1987, Plenum Press.

42. Olson DA: Management of non-language behavior in the stroke patient. In Kaplan PE and Cerullo LJ, editors: Stroke rehabilitation, Boston, 1986, Butterworth & Co.

43. Pelland MJ: Occupational therapy and stroke rehabilitation. In Kaplan PE and Cerullo LJ, editors: Stroke rehabilitation, Boston, 1986, Butterworth & Co.

44. Perry C: Principles and techniques of the Brunnstrom approach to the treatment of hemiplegia, Am J Phys Med 46:789, 1967.

45. Sbordone RJ: A conceptual model of neuropsychologically-based cognitive rehabilitation. In Williams JM and Long CJ, editors: The rehabilitation of cognitive disabilities, New York, 1987, Plenum Press.

46. Schlesinger B: Higher cerebral functions and their clinical disor-ders, New York, 1962, Grune & Stratton.

47. Sharpless JW: Mossman's a problem-oriented approach to stroke rehabilitation, ed 2, Stringfield, Ill, 1982, Charles C Thomas, Publisher.

48. Smith RO and Okamoto GA: Checklist for the prescription of slings for the hemiplegic patient, Am J Occup Ther 35:91, 1981.

49. Snook JH: Spasticity reduction splint, Am J Occup Ther 33:648, 1979.

50. Spencer EA: Functional restoration. In Hopkins HL and Smith HD, editors: Willard and Spackman's occupational therapy, ed 7, Philadelphia, 1988, JB Lippincott Co.

51. Sutin JA: Clinical presentation of stroke syndromes. In Kaplan PE and Cerullo LJ: Stroke rehabilitation, Boston, 1986, Butterworth & Co.

52. Todd JM and Davies PM: Hemiplegia—assessment and approach. In Downie PA editor: Cash's textbook of neurology for physiotherapists, Philadelphia, 1986, JB Lippincott Co.

53. Turner A: The practice of occupational therapy, ed 2, New York, 1987, Churchill Livingstone.

54. Van Deusen J: Unilateral neglect: suggestions for research by occupational therapists, Am J Occup Ther 42:441, 1988.

55. Wade JPH: Clinical aspects of stroke. In Downie PA, editor: Cash's textbook of neurology for physiotherapists, ed 4, Philadelphia, 1986, JB Lippincott Co.

56. Warren M: Relationship of constructional apraxia and body scheme disorders to dressing performance in adult CVA, Am J Occup Ther 35:431 and 35:671, 1981.

57. Williams JM and Long CJ, editors: The rehabilitation of cognitive disabilities, New York, 1987, Plenum Press.

58. Zoltan B, Siev E, and Freishtat B: Perceptual and cognitive dysfunction in the adult stroke patient (rev. ed.) Thorofare, NJ, 1986, Charles B Slack, Inc.

Sample treatment plan

This treatment plan is not a comprehensive one for the hypothetical patient. It deals with six of the identified problems. The reader is encouraged to add objectives and methods to make a more comprehensive plan.

CASE STUDY

Mr. S is a 59-year-old man who worked as a trucker until he suffered a CVA 6 weeks ago. He lives with his wife and teenage daughter in a modest, three-bedroom suburban home. He is their sole support.

Before the onset of CVA Mr. S was a very hard worker and enjoyed working around the house doing repairs and gardenting. Cooking and furniture refinishing were his hobbies.

His wife and teenage daughter are very loving but are exhibiting signs of oversolicitiousness and denial of Mr. S's limitations and the potential residual disability. Mr. S is depressed and is expressing feelings of worthlessness because of the loss of his role as worker and breadwinner. He is beginning to sense his family's unrealistic attitude and feels he has to "play along" with them. He resents this and would prefer to be open and get on with the business of dealing with life adjustments.

The CVA resulted in right hemiplegia and mild expressive aphasia. Mr. S is now able to ambulate with a quadruped cane under supervision. He walks slowly and occasionally loses his balance. He tolerates standing and walking activities up to 10 minutes. His right upper extremity exhibits beginning spasticity and some evidence of the flexor and extensor synergies, which can be elicited reflexly.

Mr. S has been in the occupational therapy program since the first week of hospitalization for maintenance of ROM, development of sitting balance, and training in simple self-care skills. He is now referred for improvement of the function of the right upper extremity, improvement of standing balance and tolerance, increased performance of self-care skills, and aid with adjustment to the disability.

Personal Data

Name: Mr. S
Age: 59
Diagnosis: CVA, 6 weeks after onset
Disability: Right hemiplegia, expressive aphasia
Treatment aims as stated in referral:
Improve function of right limbs and body
Improve standing balance and tolerance
Improve performance of ADL

OTHER SERVICES

Physician: Supervision of rehabilitation team and provision of care
Nursing: Provision of nursing and supportive care; follow through in self-care skills
Social service: Assistance in family and social adjustment
Speech therapy: Treatment of expressive aphasia
Physical therapy: Gait training and improvement in LE function

FRAME OF REFERENCE

Occupational performance

TREATMENT APPROACHES

Bobath neurodevelopmental and rehabilitative

OT EVALUATION

Performance components

Motor functioning
  Stage of motor recovery: Test
  Muscle tone: Test and observe
  Attempts at spontaneous use of involved upper extremity: Observe
  Reflexes/reactions: Test
  Standing tolerance: Observe
  Standing balance: Observe
  Walking tolerance: Observe
Sensory integrative functioning
  Touch: Test
  Pain: Test
  Temperature: Test
  Stereognosis: Test
  Proprioception: Test
  Body scheme: Test
  Visual fields: Test
  Visual-spatial relationships: Test
  Memory: Test and observe
  Motivation: Observe
Cognitive functioning
  Judgment and reasoning: Observe
  Problem solving: Test and observe
  Expression: Observe
Psychological functioning
  Adjustment to disability: Observe

Performance skills

Self-care: Test
Homemaking: Test

Continued.

Sample treatment plan—cont'd

EVALUATION SUMMARY

Physical evaluation revealed ROM of upper extremity within normal limits except for shoulder flexion and abduction, which are limited by spasticity to 90°. Mr. S is unable to stand or walk without his cane and fatigues after 10 minutes of walking. He can sit in an armless chair without losing his balance. The right upper extremity shows beginning spasticity in flexor and extensor synergy patterns with greater tone in the flexor synergy. In the lower extremity, moderate spasticity in the extensor synergy pattern is present. Muscle tone is influenced by the assymetric tonic neck and tonic labyrinthine reflexes.

Primary sensory modalities are intact but mild impairment of stereognosis and proprioception is present. Body scheme and motor planning are intact. All visual perceptual skills are within functional limits except that there is a right homonymous hemianopsia at 60°, which Mr. S compensates for without cuing.

Visual memory for demonstrated instructions is intact. There is some difficulty with memory for auditory instructions. Mr. S needs to have these instructions repeated and accompanied by demonstrated instructions. Judgment, reasoning, and problem-solving skills are adequate for daily living skills. Reading skills for everyday needs are accurate but slow. Mr. S has difficulty writing because he cannot use the right dominant upper extremity. Mr. S's speech is limited but comprehensible for communication of basic needs. He has difficulty with word finding. With cues, questioning, and some use of pictures, it is possible to elicit Mr. S's ideas.

Mr. S is discouraged and shows some lack of motivation. He responds well to praise and encouragement. He has expressed feelings of worthlessness related to the loss of his role as worker. His family denies the extent of his limitations and is overanxious to help. Before his stroke, Mr. S was a kindly man who enjoyed working around the house, cooking, and refinishing antique furniture. Because of his age and disability, Mr. S has realized that he probably will not return to work and is considering retirement. He has expressed some interest in expanding his home and leisure activities to use his retirement purposefully.

In self-care, Mr. S is partially independent. He needs help with some dressing activities and transfers. In the OT clinic, Mr. S demonstrated ability to prepare a sandwich and pour juice while sitting, if all of the materials were brought to the table for him. Use of the stove has not been evaluated because of limited standing and walking tolerance. He shows ability to use assistive devices to enhance one-handed performance.

Mr. S attempts to use the right upper extremity when confronted with bilateral tasks about 50% of the time. However, limited voluntary movement makes success impossible at this time.

ASSETS

Intact sensation
Intact perception
Good cognitive functions
Positive attitude
Supportive family
Ability to learn new methods
Realistic outlook about limitations
Leisure interests

PROBLEM LIST

1. Limited standing and walking tolerance
2. ADL dependence
3. Lack of selective movement in the right upper extremity
4. Limited scapula mobility and shoulder ROM
5. Right-sided spasticity and decreased postural reflex mechanism
6. Right visual field defect
7. Lack of coordination in nondominant (unaffected) upper extremity
8. Loss of worker role
9. Low sense of self-worth

PROBLEM 4

Limited scapula mobility and shoulder ROM
Objective
Decrease spasticity and increase scapula mobility so that 120° shoulder flexion and abduction is possible

Continued.

Sample treatment plan—cont'd

Methods

Bobath positioning techniques during sitting; clasps hands together with affected thumb on top and unaffected arm guides affected right arm into a position of full elbow extension with shoulder flexion and scapula protraction,[9] arms on wheelchair lapboard or on table in this position when patient not engaged in activity

Following scapula mobilization by the therapist, patient's arm gradually brought into the reflex inhibiting pattern of scapula protraction, shoulder abduction, flexion, and external rotation, elbow extension, forearm supination, wrist and finger extension, and thumb abduction[9,24] (Chapter 20)

Method

Self-administered ROM; with hands positioned as described previously, patient to bring both arms down between knees; then move arms from side to side, rotating trunk, and gradually elevating arms to 90° shoulder flexion with elbows extended

Methods

Participation in activity group; using pegboard checkers and oversized checkerboard, play with another patient using the bilateral arm positioning pattern described previously; move the checkers by grasping them between the palms of his hands[24]; also facilitates trunk rotation and looking over the entire visual field

Gradation

Decrease facilitation and assistance as spasticity declines and active motion improves

PROBLEM 7

Lack of left-handed coordination

Objective

Improve left hand coordination so that Mr. S can write his name and address legibly and with ease.

Method

Left-hand writing practice beginning with large round forms such as circles, ovals, and figure 8s performed in horizontal, vertical, and diagonal directions; may begin on chalkboard or large paper on tabletop[24]

Gradation

Introduce straight lines and rectangular shapes. Progress to smaller-sized paper with lines and to letters and then words[24]; begin writing practice with right hand if recovery of function permits

PROBLEM 6

Right visual field defect

Objective

Patient to spontaneously compensate for visual field defect 80% of the treatment time

Methods

Patient to cover small (2 feet × 2 feet, or 6.096 mm × 6.096 mm) tabletop with mosaic tiles (1 inch or 2.5 cm); tiles placed directly to right side of the body; table placed in front and slightly to left of the body; glue placed on left side of body; patient to reach across body to obtain tiles for placement on tabletop; affected arm positioned forward, used for weight-bearing on edge of wide chair; as right arm function improves, patient to reach for tiles with right hand; facilitates trunk rotation and visual attention to affected side

Room arranged so patient must look to affected side to get belongings, look to doorway for staff and visitors

Therapist to stand on affected side when talking to patient or giving instructions

PROBLEM 2

ADL dependence

Objective

The patient to dress himself independently within 30 minutes

Method

Teach dressing techniques for pants, T-shirt, shirt, shoes, socks, and shorts, using Bobath methods for dressing (Chapter 20)

Gradation

Begin with one garment, T-shirt; progress to shirt, then shorts, socks, pants, and shoes; progress to normal bilateral techniques as function improves.

PROBLEM 1

Limited standing and walking tolerance

Objective

With a quadruped cane for support, the patient's balance to improve and standing tolerance to increase to 30 minutes

Methods

Light home-making activities that require walking for short distances: meal preparation, table setting, and dusting, with supervision; grooming activities in a standing position under supervision

Gradation

Decrease supervision as balance and stability are gained

PROBLEM 9

Low sense of self-worth

Objective

The patient to achieve an increased sense of self-worth, expressing two positive things about self during group activities

Method

A group of 5 to 8 patients to meet biweekly for 1½ hours; the therapist to act as group facilitator; the group initially to be task-oriented; activities such as exercises to music, simple crafts, and cooperative meal preparation to be used

Gradation

Increase responsibility for planning the activities

Method

The group to move from the activity into discussion of the problems encountered during the activity, feelings about these, and solutions; the therapist to facilitate expansion of the discussion to include problems encountered beyond the activity and the treatment facility

Gradation

As group support and cohesiveness grows, discussion can include deeper feelings, and group members can act as facilitators

Chapter

35 Head injury in adults

BARBARA ZOLTAN
DIANE MEEDER RYCKMAN

During the evolution of rehabilitation medicine, various metabolic, systemic, and traumatic injuries have come into focus. Sociologic occurrences or changes in life styles can have a major effect on the types of disabilities that prevail. For example, with the advent of war an increased number of gunshot wounds or amputations could occur. In recent years changes in diet and exercise regimen altered the attention of medical and allied health professions to cardiac and stroke management. As society became more mobile, and the automobile developed into a necessity of life, again the focus of medical care was altered. Recent statistics on the occurrence of spinal cord injury and head trauma have forced those involved in acute and rehabilitation medicine to deal with a whole new set of concerns. The material presented in this chapter deals with the concerns of head trauma.

The mechanism and occurrence of head injury, surgical management, and a description of the levels of recovery are briefly outlined. The patient's clinical picture, including physical, cognitive, perceptual, functional, and psychosocial aspects, is described. The occupational therapy evaluation and treatment of these problems are also provided.

In 1975, 10 million people, or 3.68% of the U.S. population, sustained a head injury significant enough to require medical attention.[11] In 1976 7.56 million Americans sustained a head injury.[14] A breakdown of the place and occurrence and severity of these injuries is presented in Tables 35-1 and 35-2. The occurrence and severity of head injury are sufficient to warrant the attention of medical and allied health personnel working in acute and rehabilitation medicine.

MECHANISM OF HEAD INJURY

Most head injuries are "blunt injuries caused either by the moving head striking a static surface . . . or by the head being struck by a moving object."[26,27] The degree of deformation and damage sustained by the brain after the injury depends on the amount of acceleration or deceleration of the skull and its contents.[33,35] *Deceleration* refers to the sudden, rapid slowing of the moving head when it strikes a solid surface. *Acceleration* refers to the movement of the brain inside the skull when the stationary head is struck. An additional type of head injury is a penetrating injury, which may be a result of "low-velocity agents" or sharp objects or high-velocity ballistic missiles. Low-velocity penetrating injuries generally result in local damage, whereas high-velocity and acceleration-deceleration injuries usually result in diffuse damage.

Forces can injure the brain by (1) compression (pushing the tissues together), (2) tension (tearing the tissues apart), or (3) shearing (sliding of portions of tissues over other portions). These three types of injuries can occur simultaneously or in succession.[35] Damage can occur where the blow was sustained (coup lesion) or to the intact skull opposite to where the blow was applied (contrecoup lesion).[27]

In addition to the primary damage sustained on impact, secondary events often follow that may develop a few hours or days after onset, for example, hemorrhage, infection, and brain swelling.

For a detailed analysis and description of the mechanism and pathology of head injury, including primary and secondary damage, anoxia, and infectious encephalitis, see the references.* Although it is not vital for the reader to have a detailed knowledge of the mechanisms of head injury, the concepts and terms used should be understood.

MEDICAL AND SURGICAL MANAGEMENT

The medical and surgical management of a person who sustains a severe head injury begins when the victim is rescued and brought into the emergency room. The patient with a severe head injury may experience many complications. Some major compli-

The valuable contributions of Karen Nelson and Rosemary Shaw for their editorial assistance in the preparation of this chapter are greatly appreciated.

---

*References 8, 13, 21, 26, 35, 37, 41.

Table 35-1 Head Injuries, 1976 (Total 7,560,000)

Place of occurrence	No. of injuries
Motor vehicle accident	1,202,000
At home	3,828,000
At play, in school, or in public domain	2,472,000
At work	196,000

Based on data from Caveness W: Incidence of craniocerebral trauma in the United States with trends from 1900 to 1975, Adv Neurol 22:1, 1979.

Table 35-2 Types of Injury Sustained, 1976 (Total 7,560,000)

Types of injuries		No. of injuries
Superficial or minor		6,305,000
Lacerations of head	4,686,000	
Contusions of scalp, face, and neck, except eye	1,619,000	
Major		1,255,000
With concussion	644,000	
With skull fractures, extradural, subdural, or subarachnoid hematomas	611,000	

Based on data from Caveness W: Incidence of craniocerebral trauma in the United States with trends from 1970 to 1975, Adv Neurol 22:1, 1979.

cations are increased intracranial pressure, wound infection or osteomyelitis, pulmonary infections, hyperthermia, shock, and associated injuries or fractures.[15]

When the patient arrives at the hospital, the first concern is to establish an unobstructed airway, which may require suctioning, intubation, or tracheostomy. The patient may be in shock and may require intravenous fluids, plasma, blood transfusions, or vasopressor agents. The neurosurgeon then performs a neurologic examination to determine the extent and severity of the head injury. The neurosurgeon may have to perform an emergency craniotomy after arteriography to reduce increased intracranial pressure and any demonstrated hematoma.[21]

Because of the patient's decreased level of awareness and decreased oral-bulbar status, nasogastric tube feedings or a gastrostomy procedure may be required to ensure that the patient receives adequate nutrition.

Posttraumatic seizures are also complications of head injury. These may begin as early as 1 week after sustaining a head injury in some patients and as late as 1 week to 10 years or more after injury in others.[21] In some cases seizures following head injury may

never occur at all or may be controlled by medication prescribed by the physician. The patient often is incontinent and may require catheterization; later in the rehabilitation phase, as these functions start to return, a bowel and bladder program is initiated.

After the patient has been medically stabilized and cleared by the physician, the occupational therapist begins the evaluation and treatment program. It is important for the therapist to be aware of the medical and surgical management problems and precautions before establishing a treatment plan. Usually a patient with an open head injury requires a helmet before getting up for the first time to protect the open skull from further brain injury as soon as the patient is medically stable. Treatment should start while the patient is in the intensive care unit but should be closely coordinated with the physician and nursing staff.

DESCRIPTION OF THE DYSFUNCTION
Recovery Stages

Recovery following severe brain injury can be extensive and involve the physical, cognitive, visual-perceptual, psychosocial, and behavioral functions. The adult with head injury can regain lost functions rapidly, over a period of many years, or not at all. Moving out of coma through the rehabilitation stages to reenter the community is often a complicated and difficult process. No two patients have the same clinical picture, problems, needs, and family support systems. There are many different methods for analyzing the stages of recovery or the changes in level or awareness that lead to a higher level of functioning. The following is an overview of some of the different methods of rating recovery in patients with head injury.

NEUROLOGIC EXAMINATION. In general the neurologic examination performed by the physician describes the states of awareness as follows[21]:

Head injury with loss of consciousness
Coma: No response to painful stimuli
Semicoma: Withdrawal of a body part from a painful stimulus
Stupor: Spontaneous movement and groaning in response to various stimuli
Obtundity: Arousal by stimuli and response to a question or command; confusion and disorientation with poor judgment
Full consciousness: Recovery of orientation and memory; full recovery

Glasgow coma scale.[49] The Glasgow Coma Scale is the method most frequently used by physicians to categorize the levels of consciousness following a traumatic injury to the brain. This test is an attempt to quantify the severity of the brain injury and establish a baseline from which to predict the outcome of the patient. The physician using this scale assesses consciousness by three major areas: (1) motor responses, (2) verbal responses, and (3) eye opening. The patient is then rated and assigned the corresponding number of points for the best response elicited.

Levels of awareness. Still another system used for evaluating a patient's level of awareness is one that was developed at Rancho Los Amigos Hospital in Downey, California. The Rancho Los Amigos scale uses the following eight levels: (1) no response, (2) generalized response, (3) localized response, (4) confused-agitated, (5) confused, inappropriate, nonagitated, (6) confused-appropriate, (7) automatic-inappropriate, and (8) purposeful-appropriate.[39] (See box.)

The mechanism of a traumatic head injury and the resulting neurologic impairment vary so much that it is extremely difficult to label or categorize the person with brain damage. Whereas general trends for recovery can be seen in patients with head injuries, no two persons have the same set of problems, rate of recovery, environment, disposition, and neurologic deficits.

THE PATIENT EMERGING FROM COMA

The coma-emergent patient is functioning at a very low level, displaying one or a combination of the following deficit areas:

1. *Severe motor impairment.* The patient may have severe spasticity, abnormal reflexes, and loss of motor control in any or all four limbs. Head and

---

Levels of cognitive functioning*

I **No Response** Patient appears to be in a deep sleep and is completely unresponsive to any stimuli presented to him.

II **Generalized Response** Patient reacts inconsistently and nonpurposefully to stimuli in a nonspecific manner. Responses are limited in nature and are often the same regardless of stimulus presented. Responses may be physiologic changes, gross body movements and/or vocalization. Often the earliest response is to deep pain. Responses are likely to be delayed.

III **Localized Response** Patient reacts specifically but inconsistently to stimuli. Responses are directly related to the type of stimulus presented as in turning head toward a sound, focusing on an object presented. The patient may withdraw an extremity and/or vocalize when presented with a painful stimulus. He may follow simple commands in an inconsistent, delayed manner, such as closing his eyes, squeezing or extending an extremity. After external stimulus is removed, he may lie quietly. He may also show a vague awareness of self and body by responding to discomfort by pulling at nasogastric tube or catheter or resisting restraints. He may show bias by responding to some persons (especially family; friends) but not to others.

IV **Confused-Agitated** Patient is in a heightened state of activity with severely decreased ability to process information. He is detached from the present and responds primarily to his own internal confusion. Behavior is frequently bizarre and nonpurposeful relative to his immediate environment. He may cry out or scream out of proportion to stimuli even after removal, may show aggressive behavior, attempt to remove restraints or tubes or crawl out of bed in a purposeful manner. He does not, however, discriminate among persons or objects and is

unable to cooperate directly with treatment effort. Verbalization is frequently incoherent and/or inappropriate to the environment. Confabulation may be present; he may be euphoric or hostile. Thus gross attention is very short and selective attention is often nonexistent. Being unaware of present events, patient lacks short-term recall and may be reacting to past events. He is unable to perform self-care (feeding, dressing) without maximum assistance. If not disabled physically, he may perform motor activities as in sitting, reaching, and ambulating, but as part of his agitated state and not as a purposeful act or on request necessarily.

V **Confused, Inappropriate, Nonagitated** Patient appears alert and is able to respond to simple commands fairly consistently. However, with increased complexity of commands or lack of any external structure, responses are nonpurposeful, random, or at best fragmented toward any desired goal. He may show agitated behavior, not on an internal basis (as in Level IV), but rather as a result of external stimuli, and usually out of proportion to the stimulus. He has gross attention to the environment, but is highly distractible and lacks ability to focus attention to a specific task without frequent redirection back to it. With structure, he may be able to converse on a social, automatic level for short periods of time. Verbalization is often inappropriate; confabulation may be triggered by present events. His memory is severely impaired, with confusion of past and present in his reaction to ongoing activity. Patient lacks initiation of functional tasks and often shows inappropriate use of objects without external direction. He may be able to perform previously learned tasks when structured for him, but is unable to learn new information. He responds best to self, body, comfort-

---

*Reproduced with permission from Rancho Los Amigos Hospital, Downey, California.

Continued.

Levels of cognitive functioning—cont'd

and often family members. The patient can usually perform self-care activities with assistance and may accomplish feeding with maximum supervision. Management on the ward is often a problem if the patient is physically mobile, as he may wander off either randomly or with vague intention of "going home."

VI **Confused-Appropriate** Patient shows goal-directed behavior, but is dependent on external input for direction. Response to discomfort is appropriate and he is able to tolerate unpleasant stimuli (as NG tube) when need is explained. He follows simple directions consistently and shows carryover for tasks he has relearned (as self-care). He is at least supervised with old learning; unable to maximally assist for new learning with little or no carryover. Responses may be incorrect due to memory problems, but they are appropriate to the situation. They may be delayed and patient shows decreased ability to process information with little or no anticipation or prediction of events. Past memories show more depth and detail than recent memory. The patient may show beginning awareness of his situation by realizing he doesn't know an answer. He no longer wanders and is inconsistently oriented to time and place. Selective attention to tasks may be impaired especially with difficult tasks and in unstructured settings, but is now functional for common daily activities (30 min with structure). He shows at least vague recognition of some staff, has increased awareness of self, family, and basic needs (as food), again in an appropriate manner as in contrast to Level V.

VII **Automatic-Appropriate** Patient appears appropriate and oriented within hospital and home settings, goes through daily routine automatically, but frequently robotlike; with minimal to absent confusion, but has shallow recall of what he has been doing. He shows increased awareness of self, body, family, foods, people, and interaction in the environment. He has superficial awareness of, but lacks insight into his condition, demonstrates decreased judgment and problem-solving, and lacks realistic planning for his future. He shows carryover for new learning, but at a decreased rate. He requires at least minimal supervision for learning and for safety purposes. He is independent in self-care activities and supervised in home and community skills for safety. With structure he is able to initiate tasks in social and recreational activities in which he now has interest. His judgment remains impaired; such that he is unable to drive a car. Prevocational or avocational evaluation and counseling may be indicated.

VIII **Purposeful and Appropriate** Patient is alert and oriented, is able to recall and integrate past and recent events and is aware of and responsive to his culture. He shows carry-over for new learning if acceptable to him and his life role, and needs no supervision after activities are learned. Within his physical capabilities, he is independent in home and community skills, including driving. Vocational rehabilitation, to determine ability to return as a contributor to society (perhaps in a new capacity), is indicated. He may continue to show a decreased ability, relative to premorbid abilities, reasoning, tolerance for stress, judgment in emergencies or unusual circumstances. His social, emotional, and intellectual capacities may continue to be at a decreased level for him, but are functional for society.

---

trunk control are severely impaired, contributing to total dependence in self-care activities.

2. *Severe impairment of perceptual-motor skills.* The patient may have poor gross visual skills and perceptual-motor skills that prevent involvement in any self-care or higher level functional activities. For example, severe motor planning problems prevent the patient from self-feeding or dressing.

3. *Decreased functional cognition and inappropriate behavior.* The patient may exhibit cognitive and behavioral deficits such as poor judgment, safety awareness, and impaired problem-solving resulting in dependence in most functional tasks despite good physical abilities.

The coma-emergent, low level patient is totally dependent or requires maximum assistance because of physical, visual, preceptual, and cognitive deficits.

THE HIGHER LEVEL PATIENT

The higher level patient has cognitive, perceptual, motor, and behavioral deficits; however, they are not significant enough to cause total dependence in activities of daily living (ADL). The occupational therapist working with the higher level patient must be able to correlate the underlying neurologic problems with the patient's functional status. The higher level patient, unlike the coma-emergent patient, has the potential to make an adaptive motor response and carry over learning in therapy toward achieving a functional goal. For example, the patient now may have sufficient equilibrium reactions and upper extremity (UE) function to work on UE dressing while sitting with legs over the edge of the bed.

The overall level of awareness of the patient at an advanced level is higher, allowing the ability to control more aspects of the environment and participate in the treatment program. The patient still has significant cognitive, perceptual, and motor deficits, but therapy can now be structured toward working on a functional goal, such as feeding or dressing.

Clinical Picture

PHYSICAL ASPECTS. The physical deficits encountered in patients with head injury can be severe and complex. The patient has motor involvement in one to four extremities; decreased total body function, impaired oral-bulbar status, impaired sensation, coordination, balance, endurance, and range of motion (ROM); abnormal reflexes, motor patterns, and muscle tone; muscle weakness; and poor isolated muscle control. The occupational therapist must have a good theoretical knowledge of these physical deficits in order to design an effective treatment program.

Limitation of joint motion. Loss of ROM that results in contractures is a common problem. During the coma or acute rehabilitation phase, patients can develop decorticate or decerebrate rigidity or posturing.[9] The failure of the brain to control or inhibit abnormal postural reflexes and hypertonicity may cause joint deformities and contractures. The prolonged immobilization of the comatose patient with severe spasticity can lead to the development of possible joint ossification and calcification. It is extremely important in the early period after onset to become aware of and start to control potential loss of ROM.

Muscle weakness. Most adults with head injury do not have muscle weakness. Rather, there is severe spasticity or excessive abnormal muscle tone. A specific manual muscle test is therefore inappropriate for most head-injured patients.

Abnormal reflexes and tone. Abnormal postural reflexes are a common problem after head injury. Postural reflexes regulate the degree and distribution of muscle tone. The brain, depending on the site of the lesion, can no longer inhibit certain reflexes that were integrated at an earlier developmental stage.[7] The most common abnormal reflexes and reactions found are asymmetric tonic neck reflex (ATNR), symmetric tonic neck reflex (STNR), and tonic labyrinthine reflex (TLR); associated reactions; positive support reaction; extensor thrust; and decreased equilibrium, righting, and protective reactions. These abnormal reflexes and reactions affect ROM, muscle tone, and selective movements. Unless prevented or controlled, they may prevent the patient from making even basic physical and functional gains. Detailed description of these reflexes, their effect on function, and their evaluation are covered in Chapter 9.

Patterns and isolated muscle control. Patients with head injury usually have severe flexor patterning of the upper extremities and extensor patterning of the lower extremities. Often a patient has a combined flexor-extensor pattern in the upper or lower extremities. The patient, for instance, may have spasticity in both the triceps and the biceps. The muscle group with a greater degree of hypertonicity has the stronger action. Until gross motor skills develop, the patient does not perform well in fine motor activities. Controlled movement usually develops from proximal to distal, although at times it can occur distal to proximal or concurrently. For example, without good, selective shoulder control, hand function and coordination is limited. Gross grasp and release usually return before prehension in the adult with head injury.[7]

Many patients have deficits in coordination at the trunk, head, and hips in addition to that typically seen in the upper and lower extremities. The origin of the incoordination must be analyzed to establish an effective treatment plan.

Ataxia. Ataxia is an abnormality of movement and disordered muscle tone seen in patients with damage to the cerebellum or the sensory pathways and results in a cerebellar or sensory ataxia. A patient may have ataxia of the total body, trunk, or upper or lower extremities or may have gait ataxia. The normal flow of a smooth voluntary movement is destroyed by errors in the direction and speed of movement.[31] Ataxia ranges from mild to severe and can be a significant impediment to achieving a functional goal. A detailed description of the evaluation and treatment of ataxia is covered in Chapter 8.

Spasticity. Spasticity is one of the most common and damaging physical problems encountered in head injuries. Spasticity is the activation of a hyperactive stretch reflex with resultant hypertonicity.[50] It ranges from minimal to severe in any particular muscle or muscle group. Spasticity may occur in combined flexor and extensor patterns, thus making its inhibition more complicated.

See Chapter 8 for detailed information on spasticity, its evaluation, and treatment.

Loss of sensation. The most common sensory losses seen are decreased proprioception, response to deep pain, superficial pain, touch, and stereognosis; and diminished temperature sense, two-point discrimination, and kinesthesia. The patient also may have impaired senses of taste and smell, depending on cranial nerve involvment. The low level patient's response to pinprick or deep pain can help to establish a level of awareness. Evaluation of the low level patient is discussed later in this chapter.

Abnormal posturing. Along with the abnormal reflexes and hypertonicity, postural problems can develop. The nature of the abnormal patterns can be much more severe than those seen in the patient with CVA. Abnormal postures frequently exhibited in adults with head injury are as follows:

Head: Forward flexion or hyperextension may rotate to preferred side because of the influence of the ATNR. Lateral flexion of the neck often accompanies lateral flexion of the trunk.

Trunk: Lateral flexion and retraction of one side, kyphotic posture, scoliosis, and extension are exhibited.

Scapula: Humeral depression is common with either protraction and elevation or retraction patterns.

Upper extremities: Bilateral involvement with asymmetry between sides or unilateral involvement may be seen, depending on the areas of brain damage. A strong flexor pattern usually predominates; however, patients may exhibit an UE extensor pattern or a combination flexor-extensor pattern.

Pelvis and hip: Usually a posterior pelvic tilt exists, causing too much sacral sitting. Some patients tend to slide forward in the wheelchair when sitting and have the appearance of extending over the backrest. Pelvic obliquity is often a problem because of asymmetry of muscle tone. Aside from these problems, hip flexors or adductors are often contracted.

Lower extremities: Knee flexor contractures are frequently present. On the other hand, there also can be an extensor pattern in the lower extremity. The pattern usually is affected by a change in position, for example, supine versus sitting.

Feet: Inversion, plantar flexion, with a downward clawing of the toes may be seen. A positive supporting reaction is present in some cases.

It is important to know the biomechanics of the body and prevent deformities rather than try to deal with them after poor posture has developed.

Decreased physical capacity. Decreased vital capacity, endurance, and general tolerance for an exercise or activity are common problems of head injury. Having gone through medical complications, such as pneumonia, prolonged bed rest, and immobilization, the patient with head injury who suddenly starts getting up in a wheelchair is easily fatigued or overloaded. The comatose patient or the low level patient must be closely monitored for changes in blood pressure and vital signs the first few times he or she sits up.

Loss of total body function control. Total body function skills are head and trunk control, sitting and standing balance, reaching, bending, stooping, and functional ambulation. During the acute phase of the patient's recovery, decreased head and neck, trunk, and hip control are encountered along with the upper and lower extremity losses. Sitting balance and the

ability to support oneself with the legs over the edge of the mat or bed are poor. The low level patient has a tendency for excessive foward flexion of the neck or too much hyperextension. The patient at a more advanced level exhibits problems such as poor sitting or standing balance and difficulty bending, stooping, and reaching to high or low areas. Total body function skills are necessary for performing higher level functional skills, such as functional ambulation during a kitchen activity.

COGNITIVE-BEHAVIORAL ASPECTS. As previously described, there are several levels of awareness that the patient with head trauma may exhibit. As the patient begins to progress from a semicomatose state, more formal cognitive testing can be administered. At this state the therapist may begin to observe severe cognitive and behavioral problems.

The occupational therapist should direct intervention to areas that may affect the patient's functional status. Some problems that are frequently seen are disorientation; decreased level of attention, safety awareness, and insight into disability; impaired memory, sequencing, judgment, and problem-solving skills; and decreased ability to process information accurately and think abstractly. These and other cognitive deficits are evaluated by the occupational therapist through structured clinical evaluation, activity analysis, and, when appropriate, standardized testing.

Reduced attention level and concentration ability. Persons may have problems with attention to task, attention to control of their behavior, and the attentional aspects of memory. Reduced level of attention and the ability to concentrate may seriously affect functional independence. Most normal persons find it difficult to concentrate on reading while the radio or television is on or while people are talking nearby. A person must be able to tune out nonessential stimuli in the environment and attend to stimuli that are important to the task at hand. Patients with head trauma may be unable to distinguish those stimuli that are pertinent to successful performance. The patient with head injury often loses not only the ability to filter out distraction but also the ability to concentrate for any length of time.

Impaired sequencing. Sequencing is the ability to accurately process information in steps or sequentially. One does this automatically, primarily through the visual and auditory modes. Because of the extensive disruption of central nervous system (CNS) functions, these skills may be severely disturbed in the patient with a head injury. The patient may be able to process information presented visually but not information presented auditorily. The patient may be able to process the information through both systems, but with extreme delay. For example, the patient may understand a request even though a significant time lag may occur before the message has been processed and a response made. At times the patient may be able to process information only when it is presented in the simplest manner. Instructions involving long explanations, specific sequence of direction, or complex, unfamiliar vocabulary may hinder performance. It is vital for the occupational therapist to know exactly what the patient's processing abilities are to establish an appropriate treatment approach.

Decreased safety awareness. The patient with head injury often displays unsafe behavior. This may be a result of impulsiveness, decreased insight into the disability, impaired judgment, or a combination of all of these. Decreased insight, disorientation, and impaired memory can contribute to the patient's inability to recognize limitations for specific situations or analyze the consequences of his or her actions. It is therefore imperative that all members of the treatment team assist the patient in structuring the environment and understanding limitations to maximize relearning of appropriate, safe behavior.

Impaired memory. Impaired memory is probably one of the most devastating problems that the patient with head injury must face. There are several types of memory impairments, ranging from the inability to recall a few words just heard to remembering events that occurred a few months or years before the injury. Although the degree of severity differs with each patient, most patients have some level of impaired memory. This manifests in the inability to learn and carry over new tasks and contributes to confusion and inability to interact effectively with the environment.

Impaired intellectual functions and abstract thinking. An additional aspect of impaired cognition is that of reduced intellectual functioning. The patient has lost the ability to solve problems, analyze information presented, and come up with appropriate solutions. The patient is unable to structure thoughts or formulate a good cognitive strategy. Relearning these skills may require external structure from staff and family. The patient may be able with some assistance, to recognize errors, but unable to resolve the errors without external cuing. Patients with head injury tend to analyze problems in concrete terms, interpreting all information at the most literal level. The ability to think abstractly and generalize knowledge and experience is usually significantly impaired. Functional independence demands the mastering and manipulation of basic cognitive and academic skills, such as categorizing, calculating, and generalizing experiences. The occupational therapist must consider and incorporate these critical cognitive skills into the treatment plan. Detailed information on the evaluation and treatment of these and other cognitive deficits are covered in Chapter 13.

Behavior disorders. Common aberrant behavior which the patient with head injury displays includes distractibility, agitation, combativeness, emotional lability, inappropriate affect, and socially unacceptable behavior. The patient who is unable to filter distractions becomes agitated in a noisy environment. The patient with limited insight becomes frustrated and at times combative when unable to perform simple tasks. Most patients with head injury are unable to process and respond to excessive stimulation, and as a result, a turning off, or shutdown of systems, occurs. When this happens, the patient is no longer able to participate effectively with the task at hand.

Depending on the area of the brain affected, the patient may show an inability to control emotions. The patient may show inappropriate outbursts of anger, tears, and laughter and may show socially inappropriate behavior, shouting obscenities or making indiscriminate sexual advances. At the other extreme the patient may display flat affect or passivity or may lack initiative, interest, or participation in the environment. This lack of participation may be interpreted as poor motivation on the patient's part when in fact this apparent lack of responsiveness is the result of organic damage. It is important to recognize that the behavior exhibited by the patient with head injury correlates significantly with the level of cognitive function.

Cognitive and behavioral aspects of head injury are vast and complicated. This chapter constitutes an overview of areas that pertain to occupational therapy. For a detailed analysis of cognitive functions as they relate to head injury, see references.[23,30] Practical remediation techniques are discussed in the treatment section of this chapter and in Chapter 13.

PERCEPTUAL-MOTOR ASPECTS. The ability to accurately perceive and respond to people and objects within the environment is necessary for successful, independent function. Disruption of various pathways within the CNS can cause the head injury patient to have difficulty with a multitude of perceptual-motor skills that previously were taken for granted. Depending on the nature and extent of damage, the impairment may involve visual, perceptual and/or perceptual-motor skills.

IMPAIRED VISUAL SKILLS

The head injury patient is likely to exhibit problems in one or more of the following areas: acuity, binocularity, convergence, saccades, attention, nystagmus, and field of vision. The occupational therapist specifically evaluates visual attention, pursuits and saccades, visual fields, visual neglect or imperception, and depth of vision. Acuity, double vision, and nystagmus also are evaluated during functional tasks. A detailed description of the evaluation and treatment of pertinent visual deficits is covered in Chapter 12.

PERCEPTUAL MOTOR SKILLS
Apraxia

The ability to determine the appropriate type and sequence of movement to perform a task is praxis or motor planning. Despite intact sensation, motor power, or coordination, the patient with head injury may exhibit impaired motor planning skills, or apraxia. One or more types of apraxia may be apparent. The patient may be able to carry out tasks that involve one limb and at the same time may be unable to perform tasks that involve total body movement. The patient may be unable to blow out a match but can cut paper with scissors. If asked to pantomime, some patients are unable to demonstrate how a task is performed unless allowed to use the necessary objects. For example, at the most concrete level a patient may be unable to demonstrate taking a drink of water from a glass unless provided with a full glass of water when he or she happens to be thirsty.

Categories of motor planning skills generally include four areas of possible body involvement. These are buccofacial, unilateral limb, bilateral limb, and total body movements. Each of these four areas of the body may be tested with five classes of actions. These actions can be defined as follows[48].

Transitive: Gestures and actions demonstrating the use of a missing object

Conventional: Gestures that are representative or symbolic of culturally specific concepts, for instance, a salute

Natural: Gestures that are nonculturally specific, for instance, a stomachache

Real object: Actions demonstrating the use of a real object (same as transitive only with object)

Nonrepresentative: Actions that convey no message, for example, puffing cheeks

The presence of any of these motor planning impairments, combined with additional cognitive problems, can be a source of extreme frustration for the patient. Apraxia often is unjustly interpreted by members of the team as uncooperative behavior. It is vital, therefore, for the occupational therapist to accurately assess the patient's motor planning abilities to avoid unrealistic expectations and mislabeling of behavior.

Constructional apraxia is "the inability to produce designs in two or three dimensions by copying, drawing or constructing, upon command, or spontaneously."[58] The patient with a head injury with dam-

age to the right side of the brain may show a lack of perspective and poor spatial relations. Patients with damage to the left side of the brain may show a tendency toward simplicity of design and difficulty in the execution of the requested tasks. There has been considerable documentation on the relationship between constructional praxis abilities and the ability to dress.[29,55] Because of this high correlation between abilities, the occupational therapist must include a constructional praxis evaluation in the perceptual-motor testing.

Impaired Body Scheme

Impaired body image and impaired body scheme are related but are not identical perceptual disorders. Body image is the "visual and mental memory image of one's body."[58] A patient's body image, often tested by the Draw a Man test, reveals that person's feelings and perceptions about himself or herself. Body scheme relates to the ability to perceive one's body position and the relationship of body parts. To deal effectively with objects within the environment, the patient must develop an internal awareness of the body and its parts.[41] The patient with impaired body scheme does not know how to move around in the environment effectively.[1]

Impaired Figure-Ground Perception

The ability to visually distinguish an object from its background is figure-ground perception. The patient with figure-ground deficit may have difficulty locating an item on a supermarket shelf or finding an item in a cluttered drawer.

Impaired Position-In-Space Perception

Position-in-space perception is the "ability to understand and deal with concepts of spatial position such as up-down, in-out, right-left, before-behind."[58] The therapist who is treating the patient with impaired position-in-space perception must carefully analyze how to instruct the patient to follow commands. For example, the patient may not be able to conceptualize a command, such as "Get your toothbrush, which is behind your comb." Taken at its extreme the patient with severely impaired perception of position in space may be unable to make a sandwich, because he cannot place the lunchmeat "in between" two slices of bread.

Additional areas of impaired perception that may appear in the patient with head injury are form and size discrimination, part-whole visualization, and depth perception. A classic example of impaired form perception is the patient who mistakes a water pitcher for a urinal.[58] The patient with impaired part-whole perception, when presented visually with only part of an object, may not be able to synthesize the parts to identify the object correctly. A hair dryer may be mistaken for a telephone. Impaired depth perception affects the patient's ability to ambulate on stairs or on uneven surfaces, such as the ground.

From this summary of perceptual problems found in patients with head injury, it may appear that impairments occur in an isolated manner. This is rarely the case. Rather, the therapist usually is presented with a patient who has a constellation of problems. The therapist's job is to carefully observe the patient's behavior and interpret the reasons or impairments underlying abnormal responses.

It is also important to formulate an awareness of the cognitive functions and their relationship to perceptual-motor abilities. Essentially it is impossible to separate cognition from language, perception, or behavior, because all these areas are instrumental in the learning process. The significance of the interaction between cognition and perception is that "the object of perception does not come to us as a given, but rather, that it must actively be sought after and constructed through cognitive processes."[10] For example, the therapist who is evaluating praxis with a block design test can at the same time be assessing the cognitive strategy that the patient uses to duplicate the design. Aside from analyzing only the perceptual skills, the cognitive functions of sequencing and problem solving also should be assessed.

Many clinicians have found that visual cognitive and perceptual-motor skills involve the integration of sensory, motor, perceptual, and cognitive modalities into a meaningful mode to create successful interactions with the environment. Perceptual motor skills should be considered as building blocks or significant components of cognition.[33] On the other hand, it can also be stated that cognitive skills are significant components of perception. For example, during a task the patient might be able to visually discriminate the correct object (perceptual skill) from a set of pictures but have no memory (cognitive skill) for what that object or person was in the past or is in the present. Cognition, language, vision, and perception are integrated for function. Without the integration of visual, perceptual, and cognitive skills the person will fail to function optimally in any environment.

PSYCHOSOCIAL FACTORS

The psychosocial aspects of head injury are frequently overlooked but can be key components to the success of the patient's recovery process. It is important to know the family and social histories along with personality characteristics before head injury.

Family support is an important factor in dealing with the head-injured patient. It can determine the patient's level of motivation to achieve functional independence. Family and friends are an integral part of the rehabilitation process, especially in the beginning stages, because they may be able to elicit a response from the patient when no one else can.

Family role alterations and the patient's coping mechanisms for dealing with these role changes must be considered. The patient may go from being an extremely independent person to being totally dependent, which is frustrating and degrading. It is difficult for the patient and the family members or significant others to cope. No matter how cognizant the family and the patient are of the disability, it disrupts the family structure. It is often difficult for family members to understand the uncontrolled behavior that they observe in their loved one.

The patient may be unable to control variations in emotion. The patient may be inappropriately friendly and indiscriminate in showing affection. As the patient becomes more aware of self and the environment again, depression sets in and the patient may suddenly perceive the confinements of the current world.

The alteration of sexual function and the ability to deal with sexual needs and feelings can occur. The patient may lack the impulse control to keep from making sexual advances toward others. These impulsive advances may be combined with verbal abuse, and often the patient is not cognitively aware of this behavior. Memory deficits further complicate this problem. The male patient may not remember that the woman he is making advances toward is his therapist or nurse.

Previous educational status and values play an important part in the patient's progress toward independence. These factors must be incorporated into the long-term treatment plan. Eventual discharge plans must be set up to meet the needs of the patient. For example, a patient who had a learning disability before the head injury and always had difficulty in school may not benefit from a traditional college program but rather from a disabled students' program, directed toward the specific problem areas, at a community college.

Lack of insight into the disability can be a serious problem affecting adults with head injury. The patient may not even be aware of the deficits or the necessity of working on a certain functional activity or exercise. The patient may be embarrassed by performing a certain task or may simply refuse to do it. In general the psychosocial aspects of the patient with head injury go hand in hand with the cognitive and behavioral aspects and contribute to or retard recovery throughout the overall rehabilitation process.

FUNCTIONAL LIMITATIONS

A patient with head injury may have problems in all peformance skills. Possible areas of deficit are listed as follows:

Self-care
    Feeding
    Dressing
    Hygiene
    Grooming
    Bathing
    Toileting
Mobility
    Bed
    Wheelchair
    Transfer skills
    Functional ambulation
Home management
    Kitchen tasks
    Housekeeping
    Child care
Communication
    Speech
    Symbolic language
Transportation
    Public modes
    Driving ability
Community function
    Shopping
    Street safety
    Community facilities
Work skills
    Prevocational activities
    Work activities
Leisure activities
    Social activities
    Sports and games
    Hobbies

Functional disabilities cannot be separated from cognitive, perceptual, sensory, motor, and behavioral problems. A problem in one of these areas can cause or contribute to the functional deficit. For instance, a kitchen activity requires a combination of skills, such as UE function, wheelchair mobility, figure-ground and form perception, scanning, sequencing, direction following, memory, safety awareness, and judgment. The person with head injury struggles to put even the most basic components of the process together in some meaningful and orderly fashion.

Another example of a functional task that can be analyzed for areas of function that interact for effective performance is feeding ability. If decreased feeding ability is present, improvement in some or all of the following areas is necessary to independent functioning: oral reflexes, level of awareness, oral sensation such as hypersensitivity, head and trunk control in sitting, UE function, and cranial nerve functions.

It becomes extremely important, then, for the therapist to identify the underlying components that relate to the functional deficit so that the best treatment approach can be established. The therapist must have good observational skills and the ability to do formal testing to help pinpoint how the functional task should be broken down into steps and structured to gain optimal results in performance.

EVALUATION

Joint measurement, muscle testing, evaluation of reflexes and equilibrium reactions, sensory testing, ADL, home management, and home evaluations are described in Chapters 9, 11, and 15. Evaluation for degree of spasticity is described in Chapter 8. All these assessments are applicable to the patient with head injury.

GUIDELINES FOR EVALUATION OF THE LOW LEVEL PATIENT
Position and posture

Test position:
Note whether the patient is supine, sitting, or upright in a wheelchair. The response may vary with proprioceptive, kinesthetic, labyrinthine, and visual input. The best response usually occurs when the patient is optimally positioned and sensory input is more normalized. Note symmetry between the two sides of the body and check for any abnormal postural reflexes. Note tonus changes and differences from one position to another, and estimate ROM and spasticity. Note if there is decorticate or decerebrate posturing or rigidity. A detailed description of the evaluation of postural reflexes is contained in Chapter 9.

Balance and control:
Check for sitting balance, trunk control, head control, and any balance reactions. After looking at all these areas together, evaluate head and trunk control separately in the wheelchair after hips and lower extremities are properly positioned. Head and neck control develop along with visual skills. Measure head control by the amount of support required. This helps determine the type of device needed to support the head. The length of time that the head can be held erect by itself or during an activity, the number of times per day without head device, and the length of time without head device are also important to note for assessing improvement. Set up a flow sheet to keep a record of progress.

Motor picture

Observe ROM, spasticity, rigidity, and contractures. Note the presence of movement response and the presence of any spontaneous movements. If a response is present, is it (1) to a stimulus, (2) with sensory input and imitation, (3) to imitation only, or (4) on command? Note also whether the movement is (1) reflexive, (2) generalized, or (3) localized and voluntary.

Sensory picture

Pain:
Evaluate for response to pinprick on upper and lower extremities and face. Is the response generalized or localized?

Assess whether the response is away from or toward the body, delayed or absent.

Deep pain:
Either pinch the patient on the leg, arm, or neck and note response (same as for pain), or put pressure on fingernail with a hard object like a pen.

Oral area:
See Chapter 10 for a detailed description of oral bulbar evaluation.

Olfactory:
See whether the patient can be aroused with noxious odors. Watch out for rebound phenomenon. Noxious stimuli have an arousing effect, whereas pleasant odors have a calming effect. Various smells may be used to arouse the patient before a treatment session.

Gustatory:
Check out response to taste. This can be used as a stimulation technique or for working on the oral feeding mechanisms, for example, sour tastes help with lip pursing, which in turn helps with sucking. This area is mentioned because the patient may need to be aroused to truly assess level of awareness.

Auditory:
Use a bell, jingle keys, clap hands, or simply talk to see whether the patient responds to sound. Note whether the patient turns the head or eyes toward the sound or whether there is merely a startle response. Note whether a generalized, localized, delayed, or absent response is present. Abnormal postural reflex mechanisms may prevent the patient from responding. Positioning should be optimal.

Tactile:
Note the presence of any response to touching, rubbing, vibration, or different textures. Response could be the same as for auditory. Fine tactile discrimination cannot be assessed with the patient with head injury at the primary level, but responses can be observed to combine with observations of other responses to come up with a clinical picture.

Refer to Chapter 11 for a detailed description of sensory testing and evaluation.

Visual skills

Test position:
Patient should be sitting with the head upright for testing visual skills.

Attentiveness:
See whether the patient can attend to a bright object or to the therapist. Be sure to measure attentiveness according to the amount of time it takes for response to appear so that future tests can be measured against this baseline to show progress. Keep a flow sheet, noting the time that it takes to respond.

Tracking:
See whether the patient can track a large, bright object of side-to-side or up-down. Note the specific quality of the movement, that is, jerkiness, nystagmus, convergence, completeness, or delay. Also note and be aware of any other clues the therapist is giving to the patient to encourage tracking of the object, such as giving verbal clues or standing on one side of the patient. Keep a flow sheet of the kind of cuing used and the length of the delay from introduction of stimulus to the response. Tracking requires attentiveness.

Visual fields:
It is difficult to test specifically for field deficits or visual-spatial neglect in the low level patient, but generally it can be noted whether the patient tends to neglect one side or responds better on the other side. The therapist may want

to work initially on the more responsive side progressing towards the neglected side to facilitate head turning and body awareness.

Form and color perception:
The therapist may want to evaluate basic perceptual skills, such as color discrimination and form perception. Color perception may be assessed by asking the patient to select a color from two colored objects, such as blocks or pegs. A higher level of color discrimination can be demanded by asking the patient to match colored cubes to design cards. Form perception can be evaluated with a form board that uses basic shapes, such as the circle, square, triangle, and diamond.

Communication:
Before commencing any evaluation, establish a system of responses with the patient. For tasks that require simple "yes" or "no" responses or the choice of one object over another, signals such as eye blinks, gazing toward the correct answer, hand signals, and shaking of the head in different directions may be used. The therapist must establish beforehand which is the easiest for the nonverbal patient to give an optimal response.

Summary

In general it is important to provide consistent sensory input to evaluate the quality of the motor output. It is best to structure the environment or task to demand a motor response after sensory stimulation. Keep track on a flow sheet of which sensory stimulation is being used, its frequency, duration, sequence, and combinations. Then on the flowsheet, note the response after specific stimulation techniques. Keep track of progress by consistency (how often) and by timing (how long) the various responses. Most of all, record observations to note the quality of the response. Is the response to a specific stimulus, with sensory input and imitation, to imitation only, or to command? Note whether a delay in processing occurs, and be sure to allow time for the delay. The patient needs time to make the adaptive response and therefore to increase the level of awareness.

Oral Reflexes/Dysphagia

Oral functions of the adult with head injury may be affected and have an influence on the ability to eat, drink, swallow, and speak. The evaluation and treatment of dysphagia deficits are described in Chapter 10.

Perceptual Motor Evaluation

The perceptual motor evaluation should be administered when the therapist has a clear understanding of the patient's sensory, motor, language, and visual status. The evaluation should follow an established progression with motor planning evaluated before body scheme, which is evaluated before higher level discrimination skills. A detailed description of perceptual motor evaluation is contained in Chapter 12.

Cognition

The occupational therapist administers a cognitive evaluation that relates to function. As with perceptual evaluation, cognitive evaluation follows a hierarchy of testing. The recommended testing progression is attention, memory, initiation, planning and organization, mental flexibility and abstraction, insight and impulsivity, problem solving, and acalculia. Specific techniques for cognitive evaluation are covered in Chapter 13.

Hand Function

After muscle tone, ROM, muscle strength, and selective movements have been assessed, hand function can be examined. The therapist must analyze first whether the hand has isolated control for (1) gross grasp and release, (2) lateral pinch, (3) palmar prehension, and (4) fingertip prehension. A good test used for this purpose is the Quantitative Test of Upper Extremity Function by Carroll.[12] When evaluating hand function, assess the effects of proximal stabilization versus no stabilization.

Higher level skills are assessed only when full isolated muscle control is possible. Manipulation of objects and fine finger dexterity are examples of these skills.

It is also important to assess speed of movement and any other complicating clinical signs, such as ataxia and shoulder weakness, because these will affect hand function. A test frequently used is the Jebsen-Taylor Test of Hand Function.[26] This test assesses speed and coordination by timing the patient's performance of a variety of simulated functional tasks, such as writing, feeding, and fine prehension activities. The specific evaluation of coordination and ataxia is covered in Chapter 8.

Total Body Function

It is important for the occupational therapist to assess total body function to relate it to ADL. Depending on the patients level of function, one of the first things that the therapist should evaluate is head and trunk control while sitting over the edge of the bed, along with total body patterning to see what kind of wheelchair is appropriate. Next, the therapist should assess sitting balance when unsupported, noting equilibrium and protective reactions. As the patient progresses, the therapist needs to assess standing balance when unassisted and standing balance while performing a UE activity, such as bending or reaching for an item in a kitchen cupboard. It is one thing to ambulate forward and backward between the parallel bars, but it is much more complex to maneuver in tight spaces when performing an activity. Functional ambulation should be assessed in various settings, such as the kitchen and bathroom and the community. It is essential for the therapist to know which perceptual-motor skills are significant to total body function to be able to break them down and work on the deficit

areas. A patient may be able to climb stairs, but the coordination, speed, and perception needed to step on a city bus or to get on an escalator in a shopping center are considerably more complex.

Kitchen Evaluation

The patient's ability to be safe and independent in the kitchen may determine a future living place. In evaluating the head-injured patient in the kitchen, that person's cognitive status is of the utmost importance. Adapting utensils and equipment and adapting and structuring the environment may be necessary to compensate for the patient's safety, judgment, and problem-solving impairments. The components of the kitchen evaluation used for the patient with head injury are not very different from those used with other patient populations. The major difference is the need for the occupational therapist to closely evaluate the amount and type of supervision and structuring and the degree of physical assistance required in these tasks.

Prevocational Evaluation

Before a formal prevocational evaluation is administered, it is important to assess the patient's overall physical capacity. This evaluation reveals areas that may pose problems in future job training and placement. The wheelchair-bound patient should be assessed for indoor and outdoor mobility, reaching height, ability to retrieve items from the floor, and sitting tolerance. The ambulatory patient must be evaluated for the ability to alternately stand and sit, stoop, crouch, carry objects, and maintain standing balance. Patients should be evaluated in communication skills, unilateral and bilateral strength and coordination, and overall endurance. Some tests that can be used for measuring hand function and coordination and speed in performance are the Purdue Pegboard, the Bennett Hand Tool Test, and the Minnesota Rate of Manipulation Test.[5,36,40]

After the occupational therapist has completed a comprehensive disability evaluation, including overall physical capacity, structured prevocational evaluations can be administered when appropriate. A useful tool for the evaluation is the Micro-TOWER system.[2] The evaluating therapist often has to modify and structure the test for optimal success. By doing so the therapist is unable to use the standardized methods of scoring but can describe the patient's performance and how the testing was altered to get a general picture of the patient's skills. It is also advisable for the patient with head injury to be evaluated separately from other patient populations. In this way the therapist can provide special guidance, structure, and support that the patient may require without causing the patient embarrassment and frustration.

Driving Evaluation

The first step in the driving evaluation of the patient with head injury is a complete disability evaluation. The patient's visual, cognitive, and perceptual status are extremely important, because the task of driving requires complex visual functions and because vision influences more than 90% of the decisions of the person who is driving.[3]

In addition to the previously mentioned perceptual tests, it is helpful to use specific visual-perceptual exercises that depict various street scenes and driving situations. These can be indicative of a previous driving style and can demonstrate some problem-solving abilities. Specific techniques for driver's evaluation are covered in Chapter 15.

GENERAL PRINCIPLES OF OCCUPATIONAL THERAPY INTERVENTION

Although there is no set of magic answers concerning the treatment of head-injured patients, certain principles and guidelines for occupational therapy intervention can be generalized for most patients. All patients require structured, normalized sensory input from their environment. For example, the semicomatose patient must not remain in bed indefinitely but must be placed upright and positioned to inhibit abnormal muscle tone. As a result, the patient can begin to perceive the environment from the proper perspective and consequently may display an increased level of awareness. During treatment of the low level patient the therapist should assume that at least some information is getting through. In approaching all patients with head injury, the therapist should not relate to them in a condescending manner. They are adults and as such deserve respect. They do not respond any better if they are yelled at or patronized.

The occupational therapist treating the head-injured patient must constantly observe, reevaluate, interpret behavior and response, and alter treatment accordingly. This patient population demands a great deal of flexibility and astute observation skills from the treating therapist.

When establishing a treatment plan, the therapist is faced with a long list of problems regarding the patient's physical, cognitive, perceptual, psychosocial, and ADL functioning. The therapist must place these problems in order of priority and set up realistic goals for the patient. The therapist must analyze the treatment tasks and activities that were chosen and structure the treatment sessions to facilitate maximal function.

Treatment strategies for each problem can vary, and a strategy must be chosen that is best for the therapist and the patient. Common impairments already discussed can be treated functionally with table-top activities and/or with sensorimotor approaches. However, most therapists who treat this population feel that any combination of methods may be the most beneficial. To minimize patient confusion and agitation and facilitate carry-over of learned tasks, constant communication must occur among team members. If the nursing staff is instructing a patient in one type of transfer and the occupational therapist is instructing in another type, the patient can become confused and show limited progress. A consistent, repetitive, and appropriately structured approach to the patient by all members of the treatment team yields optimal results.

General Aims and Methods of Treatment

LOW LEVEL PATIENTS. The aims of treatment for the low level patient are to increase the patient's level of response and overall awareness. Input must be well structured, timed, and broken down into simple steps, and enough time must be allowed for a response, which often is delayed during this phase of treatment.

Sensory stimulation program. After the patient has been evaluated, a baseline for treatment is established. Treatment of the low level patient should start as soon as the patient is medically stable. Often the patient is still comatose or semicomatose. The goal of treatment is to increase the patient's level of awareness by trying to arouse the patient with controlled sensory input. Sensory stimulation increases input into the reticular activating system, which increases arousal to the threshold necessary for responsiveness.[53] The occupational therapist needs to provide visual, auditory, tactile, olfactory, and gustatory stimulation. In addition to these, it is important to start getting the patient into a wheelchair to normalize sensory input through the kinesthetic and labyrinthine systems.

Many patients who appear semicomatose when lying supine in bed suddenly respond when sitting erect in a wheelchair. The therapist is changing the position of the body in space and placing the patient in a position to start to visually perceive the environment. After the patient is up, the therapist starts to work on gross visual skills, starting first with visual attentiveness. The goal is that the patient attend to an object and to people in the environment. Next it is important to elicit visual tracking by using a bright object and sometimes the additional input of an auditory stimulus. The different levels or ways and analysis of the patient's response should be noted according to guidelines given in the preceding section on evaluation.

AUDITORY AND TACTILE STIMULATION. Auditory and tactile stimulation are used to see whether the patient can localize the specific stimulus given. Even when working with a comatose patient with a head injury, the therapist should talk as if the patient can understand. Even if the patient is not responsive, verbal commands that are clear and simple should be given. Examples of auditory stimuli are ringing a bell, clapping hands, cassette tape recordings of familiar sounds, and therapist's voice.

The goal is to get the patient to localize the sound or respond to it voluntarily. Usually the automatic responses, such as turning the head toward a loud noise, occurs before the voluntary responses. Tactile stimulation includes superficial pain (pinprick), deep pain (pressure on the fingernails), rubbing an affected limb with cloths of various textures, and stroking body parts while giving verbal cues to increase overall body awareness.

OLFACTORY STIMULATION. Olfactory stimulation may be done with relatively "pure" olfactory stimulants, such as musk ketone, exaltolide (musk perfume), linalyl acetate, and coumarin (floral). Common odors that are trigeminal nerve stimulants should not be used when evaluating olfactory nerve impairment; these include ammonia, camphor, anisole, menthol, cloves, and peppermint.[22,37] The therapist generally starts with vanilla and banana odors.[18] Olfactory as well as gustatory stimuli are generally more effective before the patient has been fed.[47] A 30-second delay is recommended between each stimulus. A positive neutral, or negative response to stimuli and specific observations of behavioral response are noted.

GUSTATORY STIMULATION. Taste stimuli can include sodium chloride solution (salt), sucrose solution (sweet), quinine (bitter), and vinegar or lemon juice (sour).[51] Containers should be coded, and stimuli should be given in a water solution. Salty and sweet stimuli usually are recognized within 2 or 3 seconds. Sour takes a little longer, and recognition of bitter could take as long as 5 seconds.[52] A dental tweezer or cotton swab to appropriate oral structures can be used for gustatory input[18] As with olfactory evaluation, the therapist should note positive, negative, or no response and observe specific behaviors.

VESTIBULAR STIMULATION. The use of vestibular stimulation and sensory-integrative therapy for the adult with head injury is essential for progress. The vestibular system, that is, the vestibular pathways running throughout the brain stem and cerebellum, has a major influence on posture and equilibrium responses.[4] Vestibular stimulation also facilitates eye movement tone and arousal.[47]

By providing vestibular stimulation via slow spin-ning, rocking, or inversion activities, tone in the antigravity muscles can be reduced, followed by muscle cocontraction.

The vestibular reflexes have three major roles: (1) the body acts to oppose or compensate for changes in the direction of the force of gravity (negative geotrophic movement); (2) through kinetic action the muscles cocontract to maintain equilibrium and ocular stability during movement; and (3) the vestibular reflex activity helps maintain posture and regulate muscle tone.[4] Therefore the vestibular system can be used to reduce or inhibit abnormal muscle tone or spasticity, facilitate equilibrium and righting reactions, and enhance gross visual skills. "The maintenance of body equilibrium and posture and appreciation of spatial orientation in everyday life are complex functions involving multiple receptor organs and neural centers in addition to the labyrinths. Visual and proprioceptive reflexes in particular must be integrated with vestibular reflexes to ensure postural stability."[4]

It is important that the occupational therapist use a neurophysiologic basis for the treatment of head injury. The goal is not to develop specific or splinter skills or simply learn to compensate for a visual or motor problem but to try to reintegrate or redevelop the impaired function. For example, asking a patient to lift the foot may be ineffective, because it is a cortical level approach to treatment. The problem must be approached from a lower level of the brain for its integration there, if the skill is to be mastered. Rood stated that the cortex is not the highest control center of motor activity. Rather, she believed that treatment should be aimed at the cerebellum and basal ganglia to gain effective and long-lasting results.[41]

It is important to monitor the patient's vital signs closely during activities that provide vestibular stimulation, such as when the patient is inverted over a bolster while bearing weight on the upper extremities or is rocking on an equilibrium board.

In some cases continued vestibular stimulation can cause seizures, nausea, fatigue, dizziness, blood pressure changes, and associated reactions. The patient's level of awareness is an important factor. The low level patient may not be able to voluntarily give cues to the therapist as to when enough stimulation has been given. The therapist should communicate closely with the physician, nursing staff, and other members of the rehabilitation team before, during, and after vestibular stimulation has been initiated in the treatment program to determine and monitor its effects on the patient.

Rood stated that after cocontraction has been established through the use of the inverted position, stability in space is gained, and this is the basis for kinesthetic figure-ground perception. Kinesthetic figure-ground perception serves as a foundation for orientation of the body in the dimensions of space and time. After a person separates figure from ground internally, he or she can begin to deal with the external environment and to gain bilateral integration and proper body image.[41]

The use of vestibular stimulation in conjunction with NDT is an important tool for changing and maximizing the patient's response. Ayres stated that the primary cerebellar function is that of an integrating and regulating servomechanism whose action frequently has been linked to motor output.[41] As in any type of sensorimotor stimulation, it is important to demand a motor response, after giving the stimulation, to help facilitate CNS integration. It is important in the treatment of the patient with head injury to provide stimulation in a structured and goal-oriented way and to help regulate the response toward the desired outcome. At all times during treatment application, precautions and contraindications to specific treatment modalities should be kept in mind.

The use of vestibular stimulation in the treatment of adults with head injury is important to the patient's recovery. However, this area of treatment is complex and requires specific study and training before it is used. The beginning therapist *should not* attempt to incorporate vestibular stimulation into the treatment program unless supervised by an experienced therapist.

DYSPHAGIA TREATMENT. The therapist should have special training in appropriate facilitation-inhibition techniques for improving oral-bulbar status before attempting to treat a patient. The therapist should evaluate the patient's outer oral status, oral sensation, facial musculature, oral reflexes, inner oral structures, tongue musculature, palatal function, swallowing, and food management. A detailed description of the evaluation and treatment of all these areas is covered in Chapter 10.

Positioning

With the release of abnormal postural reflexes, abnormal muscle tone, and decreased isolated muscle control, it becomes very difficult for the adult with head injury to control the body or maintain good posture (Fig. 35-1). The parts of the body that are usually affected were previously described in the section on abnormal posturing. The occupational therapist must help inhibit this abnormal muscle tone and facilitate voluntary movement through proper wheelchair positioning.

PELVIS. Wheelchair positioning should begin at the pelvis, because poor hip placement alters head and

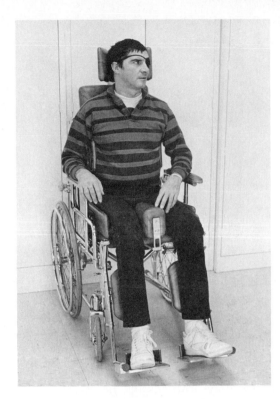

Fig. 35-1. Improved posture and trunk alignment is achieved with positioning devices.

trunk alignment and influences tone in the extremities. A seat insert that is slightly wedged (the downward slope pointing toward the back of the wheelchair) can be used to flex the hips, to help inhibit extensor tone in the hip and lower extremities. A solid seat wedge placed underneath a standard wheelchair cushion can be used to facilitate anterior pelvic tilt. A lumbar roll or a solid back insert can also be used, if needed, in conjunction with a solid seat insert. A knee abductor, side wedges, or a seat cushion with the sides slightly sloped toward or away from center, depending on the pattern of abnormal tone, can be beneficial in controlling lateral hip placement.

TRUNK. After the pelvis is properly positioned, trunk positioning can follow. Lateral trunk supports or a chest strap can be employed to decrease kyphosis or scoliosis. Generally a three-point pressure system is used for a scoliosis in which the pressure is applied to the apex of the curve on the one side and then distributed to two points above and below the curve on the opposite side. A solid seat (homemade or commercially made) or a firm wheelchair cushion (for example, dense cell foam) may be all that is needed to facilitate a more erect posture of the spine. If a great deal of difficulty in positioning the trunk remains, it may prove helpful to recheck hip placement.

LOWER EXTREMITIES. Lower extremity (LE) po-

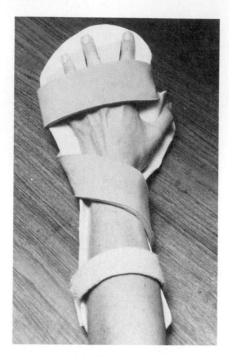

Fig. 35-2. Stretch splint.

sitioning is done to break up the abnormal postural patterns or reflexes that affect the lower extremities and trunk, such as excessive plantar flexion and inversion of the ankle. To inhibit this pattern, a foot cast with an inhibitive toe plate is used. For an abnormal positive supporting reaction, a foot wedge is attached to the wheelchair footrest to equally distribute the weight throughout the foot, taking the pressure off the ball of the foot.

UPPER EXTREMITIES. After good trunk and LE alignment are accomplished, an effort to gain UE control can be made. The application of a lap tray may support the upper extremities for those patients with only a slight problem. The upper extremities should be placed in positions opposite to reflex or spastic patterns. Using cones or straps as needed, the positioning can be done on a lap tray, on a one-half lap tray, or with an arm trough made out of a rain gutter pipe or Kydex (Fig. 35-2).

To position the arms out of a flexor pattern the shoulders must be protracted and slightly flexed with some external rotation, elbows extended, forearms in neutral, and wrists and fingers extended to submaximal stretch with thumb abducted.[28] A stretch splint or a bivalved elbow cast can be used in conjunction with the positioning device, such as the arm trough on the wheelchair, to break up the total pattern (Figs. 35-2 and 35-3). It is important to maintain both upper extremities on the same height surface so as not to disturb trunk alignment.

HEAD. Head positioning is often done before po-

sitioning of the upper and lower extremities because of the influence of tonic reflexes. Head positioning is one of the most difficult tasks for the therapist. The patient with poor head control usually needs to be in a recliner wheelchair that is in the upright or slightly reclined position. The standard head extension found on the recliner wheelchair is a good base from which to work when making the head device. If possible, without causing resistance, the head should be kept in midline, and the force used to keep the head erect is best applied around the occipital region of the skull and at the forehead. A circumferential (bicycle-helmet shape without the outer helmet) or a U-shaped device that extends around the occipital areas and has a forehead strap can be fabricated out of Kydex and fastened to the headrest bars. The traditional neck collars do not work for head positioning. In head positioning caution must always be taken to avoid overstressing the cervical area or causing excessive resistance to spastic neck musculature. It is essential to look at the placement of the shoulders and upper trunk when working on correct positioning, because they can influence neck muscle tone.

Positioning the patient is a key factor to normalizing sensory input from the evnironment. Positioning is in concert with neurodevelopmental techniques done on the mat and with other sensorimotor integration techniques. The devices should be removed gradually as the patient starts to actively control the body and to manipulate more aspects of the environment. A patient may not require the devices while engaged in therapy, such as during wheelchair mobility or when increasing head control. It is critical to make a schedule for the use of the head device. The patient can then learn to control the head and not merely rely on the static device for support. Positioning is done in a graduated sequence; the devices are slowly phased out or made less complicated, offering less support. Positioning needs change rapidly, for example, and a patient discharged from the hospital may no longer require positioning devices a month later. This constant change in status requires close monitoring, especially after discharge from the hospital.

BED POSITIONING. Bed positioning is a crucial component of the total positioning program. The head-injured patient has bilateral involvement requiring a program for side-lying on both sides. A proning schedule is also indicated to maintain normal hip and knee extension range. See Chapter 20 for specific bed positioning techniques.

Splinting and Casting

Splinting and casting for the spastic upper or lower extremities are effective means of reducing muscle tone, preventing contractures, increasing ROM and coordination, and complementing mat activities. The most frequently used splints and casts for the upper extremity are the elbow cast (see Fig. 35-3), stretch splint, and stretch splint-cast. For the lower extremities the posterior knee shell, dropout cast, foot cast, and inhibitive foot-toe plate are used. The elbow cast is usually fabricated to break up an upper extremity flexor pattern and increase ROM. Serial casting of the elbow should be done every 24 to 48 hours to progressively stretch out the flexor muscles.

The stretch splint is used to break up the UE flexor pattern by placing wrist and fingers in maximal extension with the thumb radially abducted (see Fig. 35-2). A stretch splint also can be used during weight-bearing activities, such as mat work or bed mobility. Maintained stretch accomplished through splinting or casting changes the muscle bias and therefore facilitates muscle relaxation.[50]

After selective hand movements have started to develop, a cock-up splint or cast can be used to promote hand skills, such a prehension. A cock-up splint is also useful in cases in which ataxia or intention tremors are present at the wrist.

LE splinting or casting is usually done to break up an extensor pattern or a positive support reaction. The goal is to extend the knee and place the ankle in midline with the foot dorsiflexed to neutral. In cases in which severe plantar flexion is present, serial casting should be used in conjunction with foot wedges to distribute the weight equally from the ball of the foot to the heel. LE casts also may be bivalved.

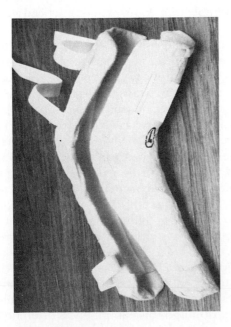

Fig. 35-3. Bivalved cast.

It is important to establish a splint schedule for the nursing staff to follow, with regular splint checks for potential pressure areas. In cases of severe spasticity the initial splint schedule may be only 2 hours on and 2 hours off until the patient can tolerate it for longer periods. The patient should never be locked up in the splints, casts, or positioning devices all the time, because they are only static tools to help the patient become more mobile. Splinting and casting for patients with head injury and severe spasticity must always be done in a progression, from initially breaking up the abnormal pattern to eventually aiding the person to improve UE function and coordination.

Functional Cognition

One fundamental aspect of functional cognition retraining is to reacquaint the disoriented patient to the environment. With the disorientation, confusion, and decreased memory that the patient may experience, the therapist must consistently provide structure and familiarize the patient with the environment, self, and current events. Many clinicians also use computer programs for functional cognitive retraining of the head-injured patient. See Chapter 13 for detailed information on computer cognitive retraining.

Communication Systems

As a result of head trauma, language impairment and inability to communicate may be severe.[21,24] Communication involves many different modalities, such as speech, writing, and sign language. Several communication systems are available to the adult with head injury to compensate for nonfunctional speech.

Communication systems range from simple to complex. There are three major approaches to consider when developing a nonoral communication system: direct selection, scanning, and encoding.[45] By direct selection a patient directly selects the desired choice. For example, the patient might directly select pictures or letters to spell a word on a communication board. The occupational therapist must work closely with the speech pathologist in adapting the communication system to allow for a maximal response based on perceptual and motor abilities.

When a scanning system is used, the patient signals when a desired choice is present or directs an indicator toward the choice.[45] Various control systems, such as the puff and sip mechanism, may be adapted to be a scanner system so that a light scans across a row of letters or symbols until the desired choice is reached. At that time the patient signals the light to stop.

The third kind of system is the encoding system in which the patient indicates a choice by a code of input symbols.[45]

The inability to communicate needs to others is one of the most frustrating problems that the adult with head injury faces. It is extremely important for the therapist to assess the patient's level of awareness, gross visual skills, visual perception, and motor status before working on adapting a communication system. The communication system allows the patient to interact again with the environment and should be geared to the patient's level of function. For example, a patient who could respond "yes" and "no" to questions by nodding may not be able to do so until good head control is developed or proper head positioning is provided.

HIGHER LEVEL PATIENTS. The higher level patient has progressed to a point to tolerate formal evaluations and full treatment sessions. Obviously the evaluation results, specific to each patient, outline which areas are priorities for treatment. Usually the patient will have some degree of deficit in all major categories. The following is a description of the areas that may require treatment and the general principles of occupational therapy interventions for these.

Self-care. When the patient begins to enter a more advanced stage, the therapist can begin to analyze the patient's ability to manipulate and effectively use familiar objects. With this in mind, light hygiene and early dressing activities can be initiated. Not only is this an effective means of identifying possible difficulty in motor planning, but it is also an avenue to increase the patient's functional independence and improve body image.

Because of the patient's cognitive status, hygiene or dressing activities must be broken down into segments and done repetitively in the same way. Depending on the patient's balance and total body function, training in dressing should progress from in bed to the wheelchair to the bed edge to standing. During training it is necessary to decide which techniques to use.

The therapist must be aware of techniques that increase functional independence but cause the reinforcement of abnormal motor patterns. The therapist must constantly assess the techniques at each stage in recovery with other team members and decide whether the goal is normalization or compensation. For example, teaching the patient to place the unaffected leg under the affected leg to enable removing the legs from the bed improves functional independence but reinforces an abnormal pattern of movement. Incorporation of normal movement patterns in ADL is important to the patient's recovery.

Feeding. To reinforce the neuromuscular facilitation techniques used in oral-bulbar training and increase the patient's functional independence, training in feeding is initiated when appropriate. Numerous factors should be considered when feeding the patient who has CNS dysfunction. See Chapter 10 for a detailed description of feeding training.

Mobility. Mobility training can be subdivided into bed mobility, transfer training, wheelchair mobility, and functional ambulation.

When working on *bed mobility*, the occupational therapist must aim for improving independence while using the sensorimotor approaches to improve sensory and motor function previously described. It is of little benefit to simply teach the patient to compensate for a loss of function or to develop splinter skills. The bed mobility skills that the patient with head injury may need to work on are scooting in supine position, rolling, bridging, moving from supine to sitting position and back, sitting over the bed edge, and sitting balance.

Transfer training. Transfer training has been described in Chapter 22. Cognitive, perceptual, and physical status affects the type of transfer used in training. Memory and limited carry-over require training to be consistent in type and sequence among all staff members treating the patient. When the patient has begun to master the mechanics and sequence of the bed-to-chair transfer, toilet, bathtub, and car transfers can be initiated. At this stage the therapist becomes involved with evaluating the need for equipment. Bathroom dimensions and layouts are discussed with the family, and a home visit is planned. Architectural barriers, which are a constant issue for the wheelchair-bound person, are considered at this time. It is preferable that transfers be practiced moving in either direction, if possible. Often a patient becomes proficient in a transfer with an approach to one side and is dismayed in a public bathroom to discover that the particular approach is not possible. An additional reason for practicing transfers to both sides is that by doing so, more normal sensory input is provided by encouraging the patient to bear weight on the affected leg and use the trunk muscles of the affected side. Thus the therapist is encouraging normalization of tone and movement, rather than compensation.

Bathtub transfers are practiced with both a dry surface and the more realistic wet surface. Generally it is safer to have the patient in the bathtub before filling it with water. Also, the water should be emptied and the patient should be dry before attempting to get out of the bathtub. Bathtub mats can aid in safety by making the bathtub surface less slick. A variety of bathtub, shower, and toilet equipment is commercially available. Although this equipment is often necessary, the therapist should remember that the ultimate goal is to eliminate the need for as much equipment as possible without creating a safety hazard for the patient or family.

The car transfer is one of the most important transfers to the patient. Patient motivation for this area is rarely a problem, because this is the patient's ticket out for a day or a weekend. The patient and an appropriate family member should be cleared by the occupational therapist in car transfers before the patient is allowed out on a weekend pass. This depends on the patient's *functional* level and may take more than one session for the necessary arrangements, which should be made in advance. Teaching the family member car transfers is only one of the many areas in which the therapist and the family are involved. This ongoing communication alleviates many of the family's and patient's fears and decreases the chances of failure during the initial visits home.

Though not a common occurrence, the patient may at some time fall to the floor. It is therefore necessary that the occupational therapist instruct the patient and his family in wheelchair mobility techniques, for example, getting from the floor back to the wheelchair. The patient needs sufficient gross motor skills and balance to be able to accomplish this task. Generally, if lying on the side, the patient has to get in the all fours or kneeling position. The patient can use the wheelchair, if stabilized, or a sturdy piece of furniture to assist. Next the patient must prop both elbows on the seat of the wheelchair and bring one or both legs into position as if to stand. Pushing up into a bent stand–pivot position, the patient can reach for an armrest, pivot, and then sit. Floor-to-wheelchair transfers can be done only with a patient who is advanced in motor skills. Any abnormal patterns that the patient might have should be kept in mind. The method described is only one general technique, and each transfer should be worked out for the person's unique set of problems and assets.

UE function. The types of motor impairment present in the patient with head injury are numerous. Weakness, synergistic movement, spasticity, rigidity, ataxia, primitive reflexes, and impaired sensation affect the patient's ability to perform UE activities. Treatment techniques for the patient with synergistic movements, spasticity, or the presence of primitive reflexes are described. The general aims of treatment for the upper extremity of the primary-level patient and the CVA patient were presented earlier.

The key to designing a treatment program that increases UE function is the analysis of normal movement. The amount of UE selective control that a patient displays usually relates closely to the degree of tone and postural reflexes present, which affect the head, trunk, and lower extremities. For example, normalization of tone in the trunk before working with the upper extremity often yields optimal results. Although the UE program for each patient with head injury is individualized, the common principles of treatment are to analyze the degree of selective control that is present and to inhibit and/or facilitate specific movements or combinations of movements as appropriate (for example, to decrease abnormal movement patterns and subsequently facilitate normal movement). To initiate beginning hand function, the patient must have the ability for controlled alternating flexion and extension of the fingers. These controlled alternating movements facilitate a light, controlled grasp and release rather than the uncontrolled primitive grasp usually seen.

During the treatment session, the therapist is continually evaluating the patient's response and altering techniques, depending on the patient's response. The therapist must observe and feel for the patient's reaction to the treatment. Specific modalities and techniques used to obtain normal upper extremity movement are limited only by the therapist's creativity.

Ataxia is a common and frustrating problem that often develops early, persists into the late rehabilitation phase, and may remain permanently. Although various treatment methods have been tried, it is difficult to assess their ultimate long-term value. Weighting of body parts and use of resistive activities appear to improve control during performance of tasks but show inconsistent carry-over of control when the weights are removed. When applying weights to the patient, the therapist must carefully evaluate at which joint or joints the tremor originates. Applying weights to a patient's wrists when the tremor originates in the trunk or shoulder is ineffective. The amount of weight applied also affects results. Generally 2 to 2.5 pounds (0.91 to 1.14 kg) is the optimal weight that can be applied without causing additional tremor. Resistive bracing, in which resistance is applied at each joint throughout the ROM, has been tried with some success. By adding continued resistance throughout the ROM, muscle groups are forced into cocontraction, and tremor decreases. Unfortunately, bracing is expensive and often is not cosmetically acceptable to the patient.

A detailed description of the evaluation and treatment of movement, tone, and coordination impairments is contained in Chapters 8 and 9.

Perceptual training. Most occupational therapy literature on the treatment of perceptual-motor dysfunction pertains to remediation of these deficits in adults with CVA and children. The following four treatment approaches, however, can be applied to the treatment of perceptual-motor deficits in adult patients with head injury:

1. Neurodevelopmental or sensorimotor[1,58]
2. Transfer of training[58]
3. Behavioral or social
4. Functional[58]

The sensorimotor approach is based on neurophysiologic and developmental principles. A major assumption of this approach is that controlled sensory input followed by facilitation and demand of a specific motor response increases integration of the sensorimotor functions of the brain.[1] The premise of the NDT approach is the facilitation of more normal movement patterns on a subcortical-automatic level to gain the desired motor response or integration. Neurodevelopmental principles can be applied to both the performance of functional activities and the development of perceptual skills, because most of the patient's performance requires movement as part of the response. The assistance given by the therapist in the NDT approach is primarily manual rather than verbal, thus putting less stress on the patient and encouraging a more automatic response.

The transfer of training approach assumes that repeated practice of a perceptual training task affects the patient's performance on similar tasks.[58] For example, practice in doing simple shape matching during a tabletop or computer activity may carry over to performance skills requiring similar perceptual skills, such as matching clothing shape to body parts. However, if the patient is not closely monitored and structured, splinter skills may develop, which are isolated and have no functional carryover.

Behavioral techniques are an integral part of the perceptual training program. Some factors that lead to behavioral problems in patients with head injury are fatigue, low frustration tolerance, sensory overloading, lack of control of the environment, defective cognitive processing, perseveration, lack of insight, and poor memory. A classic conditioning approach can be used in which the therapist pairs a neutral stimulus with the stimulus that elicits the desired response. For example, a patient became extremely agitated and refused to get out of bed when someone tried to get him up to go to the clinic for therapy. As a solution, the rehabilitation team started to provide meals for the patient only in the therapy clinic. The original problem of the refusal to get out of bed was resolved in 5 days. A system of token economy or positive reinforcement also can be incorporated into the perceptual training program.

The last major approach to the treatment of perceptual deficits is the functional approach. In this approach there is repetitive practice of specific functional skills, such as transferring from a wheelchair, cooking a meal, or making change. The functional approach can include compensatory training that involves making the patient aware of the problem and teaching the patient to work with the deficit. It can also involve adaptation of the environment to compensate for the patient's symptoms, or it can involve adaptation of the patient's behavior. In other words, the patient can formulate a new scheme or strategy for performing the task.

Probably the best way to handle functional treatment is to incorporate NDT, transfer of training, and behavioral approaches into the process. For example, when working on dressing or transfer skills, the patient can also be prompted to improve sequencing, following directions, and memory for steps of the task and to decrease visual spatial neglect. The incorporation of kinesthetic, proprioceptive, visual, and tactile information through total body movement and weight-bearing can facilitate improved body scheme and the development of visual discrimination skills.

The use of computers in cognitive perceptual training programs has become popular in recent years. The computer primarily uses visual and auditory stimulation and feedback. It does not provide adequate tactile and proprioceptive stimulation, which are vital sensory stimuli for training. Computers have an integral place in cognitive-perceptual training but should be used in conjunction with the approaches described previously.

There are no prescribed formulas for the treatment of perceptual deficits associated with head injury. Rather, the therapist must work to improve specific skills on an individual basis and subsequently combine these skills for application in functional situations. In this way learning is carried over from treatment to the real environment.

A detailed description of the evaluation and treatment of specific visual perceptual, and perceptual motor deficits is contained in Chapter 12.

Home management. As the patient gains increased skills and independence in dressing, feeding, and functional mobility, treatment is expanded to include kitchen and home-making tasks. As in other areas of treatment, kitchen training is graded to suit the patient's progress. Beginning tasks might include simple sandwich preparation. Depending on the patient's cognitive status, the therapist may place all food items on the table and have the patient verbally review the task before doing it for the first time. At the end of the session the following day's activities can be discussed. A session such as this requires simple sequencing, organizing, and memory for the task. As the patient improves, more demands are made until the patient reaches the final stages in the progression. Then the patient should be able to plan and cook a complete meal with no verbal cuing or structure given by the therapist.

Total body function and endurance also are important aspects of kitchen activities. Standing endurance and ability for bending to low shelves or reaching for high shelves are measured. Safety becomes a key issue in this setting. The patient's judgment in handling sharp utensils and using the stove can become key issues in selecting a living place after discharge.

Homemaking activities can include light housekeeping, such as dusting, vacuuming, and making the bed. As in other functional training, energy conservation and work simplification are stressed.

Child care is an area of treatment that is often overlooked. Family involvement is vital if a woman is to return effectively to her role as wife and mother. Sensory overload is a common problem that must be handled. Most people agree that sensory overload is a problem even for the mother who has not sustained a head injury. One-handed diapering techniques or commercially available strollers, cribs, and child care equipment that can be handled more easily by the handicapped woman are examples of the areas that might be covered by occupational therapy services.

Community reintegration. In the rehabilitation process, the patient with the head injury often reaches a maximal level of independence in the protected and structured atmosphere of the hospital and, when discharged into the community, is faced with people, situations, and problems that have not yet been encountered and resolved. It is therefore vital that the occupational therapist initiate a community reintegration program before discharge. The training can begin with the basic skills involved in a simple purchase, that is, handling money or communicating needs. As the patient's cognitive, perceptual, and physical status changes, the therapist can help the patient to progress to a more demanding activity or setting. The transition of treatment from an initial setting, such as a hospital gift shop to a community store, not only demands skills in the areas listed but also presents new psychosocial issues with which the patient must deal. It is often of benefit for an appropriate family member to accompany the therapist and the patient on a community trip. The family member can gain increased insight into the patient's level of functioning and into the way in which the outside world views the disability. The therapist must be aware of the patient's and family's attitudes toward a community reintegration program. The therapist may become frustrated when a cooperative patient suddenly refuses to participate in the program. The patient may not feel ready for the outside world to view the handicap, and the therapist's responsibility is to give the patient the support and guidance needed for the easiest transition possible.

Many occupational therapists are now working in new transitional living programs for head-injured persons. As a final phase in the health care continuum, these programs are designed to develop daily life skills within the community. The patient lives initially within a supervised group home setting and progresses, if possible, to independence within an apartment set-up.

Prevocational training and placement. Vocational training and placement of the patient with head injury are extended processes that require the involvement of an occupational therapist, vocational evaluator, and other allied health professionals usually under the coordination of a vocational counselor. Each professional brings to the case a different expertise that is essential to successful job placement. Many patients with head injury are not immediately ready for sheltered workshop or competitive employment, therefore it may be more appropriate for them to be involved in an adapted learning program at a local university or community college. Job placement, as well as work-site evaluation and training, are generally handled by the occupational therapist with the transitional living programs.

Family training and follow-up. The participation of the family members in the recuperation of the patient with head injury is extremely important. Frequently, the familiar faces of the patient's relatives are among the first that the patient is able to remember when coming out of coma. Education of family members starts from the first time the professional meets them; however, the information provided should be given in gradual steps.

Family involvement in treatment should occur throughout the patient's rehabilitation. Constant communication between the therapist and the patient's family aids in appropriate follow-through of newly acquired skills that the patient has learned. Constant communication also provides feedback to the therapist and enables the family to show the unique ways they solve a given problem. This often happens after a patient has been home and returns for an assessment or for outpatient therapy. The family often discovers methods that the therapist has never considered.

Sample treatment plan

CASE STUDY

KB is a 24-year old male who sustained a gunshot wound to the head during an altercation 4 months ago. The bullet entered the left occipital area and traversed to the right temporal-parietal area. An emergency craniotomy and decompression were performed 1 week later. Craniotomy and debridement with removal of devitalized brain tissue, foreign bodies, and bone chips were performed 3 weeks after the injury.

KB was living in a city about 30 miles from the rehabilitation facility and had been married for 4 years. Presently he is divorced. He has a high school education and has worked as a bricklayer for 6 years. When initially interviewed by the occupational therapist, he stated that he would be returning to work "in a couple of weeks."

KB was referred to occupational therapy for evaluation and appropriate treatment to facilitate maximal function and independence.

TREATMENT PLAN

Personal data

Name: KB

Age: 24

Diagnosis: Traumatic injury to the head

Disability: Motor, sensory-perceptual-cognitive dysfunction

Treatment aims as stated in the referral:

Evaluation

Facilitate maximal function and independence

OTHER SERVICES

Physical therapy: Ambulation, mat mobility, strengthening exercises

Nursing: Nursing care, reality orientation

Speech: Cognitive skills, language retraining

Psychology: Intelligence, memory testing

Social service: Counseling, community placement, financial arrangements

Educational program: Academic skills retraining

FRAME OF REFERENCE

Occupational performance

TREATMENT APPROACHES

Rehabilitative, biomechanical, sensory-integrative

OT EVALUATION

Performance components

Motor functioning

ROM: Measure

Abnormal muscle tone: Test and observe

Selective functioning

Hand function: Test

Sensory integrative functioning

Sensation: Test (pain, temperature, stereognosis, proprioception)

Visual perceptual functioning

Visual attention, oculomotor (pursuits, saccades), visual fields, visual imperception, depth of vision, acuity: Test and observe

Praxis: Test and observe

Body scheme: Test and observe

Visual discrimination (form, size, depth, figure-ground, position-in-space): Test and observe

Cognitive functioning

Attention, memory, initiation, problem solving, planning and organization, mental flexibility/abstract thinking, acalculia: Test and observe

Judgment: Observe

Safety awareness: Observe

Motivation: Observe and interview

Psychological functioning

Coping skills: Observe

Adjustment to disability: Observe and interview

Social functioning

Interpersonal relationships: Observe

Performance skills

Self-care: Observe

Home management: Test and observe

Community skills: Test and observe

Driving evaluation: Test and observe

Prevocational: Test and observe

Physical capacities: Test and observe

Sample treatment plan—cont'd

EVALUATION SUMMARY

KB has full isolated motion and normal strength in the right UE. He displays in the left UE a moderate flexor pattern with mild to moderate spasticity at the shoulder and elbow joints and wrist and finger flexors. With the left upper extremity he is able to perform the following selective movements with difficulty: shoulder flexion to 90°, hand behind back, and hand to opposite shoulder. Incomplete motion is possible when performing hand behind head and wrist flexion and extension with the elbow relaxed. KB's passive ROM for both upper extremities is within normal limits. His right hand functions normally. With the left hand, KB can perform gross grasp and lateral prehension, but these are weak. He is unable to put the prehension patterns to functional use. He is also unable to perform fine manipulative skills with the left hand.

All sensory modalities are intact in the right upper extremity. In the left upper extremity, impairment of superficial pain (pinprick) sensation is present. Proprioception and stereognosis in the left upper extremity are absent. Visual scanning is slow and jerky and reduced to the left. KB has extreme difficulty with motor planning, as well as with figure-ground perception and perception of position in space. Body scheme deficits of poor right-left discrimination and unilateral left neglect also are present.

KB is generally cooperative, in spite of his difficulty in following simple commands. Impaired safety awareness, judgment, and limited insight into his disability are apparent. He becomes extremely frustrated when unable to perform simple tasks.

KB requires minimal physical assistance for all dressing, hygiene, and grooming activities. He has a severe dressing apraxia, that is, he puts on his shirt upside down or backwards or puts his shoes on the wrong foot, unless given cues by the therapist. He requires assistance with all fastenings. For feeding he requires assistance for opening containers and cutting meat. Bed, chair, tub, and toilet transfers, as well as bed mobility, require moderate physical assistance and verbal cues to compensate for apraxia, difficulty with sequencing, and decreased perception of position in space and figure-ground perception.

KB requires minimal physical assistance and moderate verbal cues for kitchen and community tasks.

ASSETS

Good function of right upper extremity
Good motivation
Intact memory
Supportive family
Supportive employer and possibility for reemployment
Intact functional communication skills

PROBLEM LIST

1. Self-care dependence
2. Dependence for functional mobility transfers, that is, bed mobility and wheelchair management

3. Sensory impairments
4. Lack of selective control of the left upper extremity
5. Decreased left hand function
6. Deficit in postural mechanism and equilibrium
7. Visual perceptual dysfunction
8. Apraxia
9. Body scheme disorder
10. Cognitive deficits

PROBLEM 1

Self-care dependence

Objective

Minimum verbal cues and no physical assistance with upper extremity dressing

Method

Daily ADL training in the patient's room with the door or curtain closed to reduce distraction; sensory stimulation to left arm through rubbing with a washcloth or cream prior to dressing; use of solid color shirts only (for figure-ground deficit) with clearly marked labels or adaptations as necessary for dressing apraxia

Gradation

Decrease verbal cues and have patient provide his own sensory stimulation of left arm progressing to no longer needing stimulation; expand to use of print shirts and decrease need for adaptations as patient improves

PROBLEM 4

Decreased left hand function

Objective

Increase left hand function sufficient for a good functional assist to dominant right hand

Method

Weight-bearing and joint compression activites as needed to reduce spasticity in left UE and hand prior to active movement activities; patient sitting at table with arm extended and placed on a pillow for proximal stabilization; repetitive activities (lifting objects such as paper cup or ping-pong ball) for increased isolated wrist control. After wrist control is accomplished, begin activities for three-point and lateral pinch with proximal stabilization remaining.

Gradation

Reduced need for weight-bearing and joint compression activities as well as for proximal stabilization

PROBLEM 7

Visual perceptual dysfunction (poor visual scanning)

Objective

Increase visual scanning sufficient for reading, driving, and community activities

Method

Visual scanning exercises with worksheets, magazines, or newspaper using anchoring[58] (cuing the patient where to begin the visual search) or red tape or marker; slowing the patient down through pacing to prevent jerky scanning by having the patient call out and/or place a sticker over a number or letter as he sees it,[58] then changing the distance between each adjacent letter or number

Gradation

Reduce the amount of anchoring, pacing, and overall cuing required for effective scanning

REVIEW QUESTIONS

1. Describe what is meant by acceleration and deceleration injuries.
2. When is a gastrostomy performed?
3. What are the three major assessment areas of the Glasgow Coma Scale?
4. Name five major physical impairments that may be present in the patient with head injury.
5. Define "spasticity" and "ataxia."
6. How does the patient's cognitive status affect the patient's function?
7. Define the following: visual neglect, hemianopsia, praxis, constructional praxis, body scheme, figure-ground, and position in space.
8. List four psychosocial variables that influence the patient's behavior.
9. What are the major clinical areas that affect function?
10. How are gross visual skills evaluated?
11. What is included in a physical capacity evaluation?
12. What type of approach do all patients with head injury require?
13. Give examples of auditory, visual, and olfactory stimulation.
14. Where should the therapist start with wheelchair positioning? Why?
15. What are some examples of methods of reality orientation?
16. What would be the splinting-casting plan for the patient with decorticate posturing?
17. When in the treatment progression are kitchen activities appropriate?
18. How can the Bobath theory of treatment be incorporated in bed mobility tasks?
19. What are the three treatment approaches to perceptual impairment?

REFERENCES

1. Ayres AJ: Sensory integration and learning disorders, Los Angeles, 1972, Western Psychological Services.
2. Backman ME: The development of the Micro-TOWER, New York, 1977, ICD, Rehabilitation and Research Center.
3. Ballard SS and Knoll HA, editors: The visual factors in automobile driving, National Research Council, Publication no 574, Washington, DC, 1958, National Academy of Sciences.
4. Baloh RW and Honrubia V: Clinical neurophysiology of the vestibular system, Philadelphia, 1979, FA Davis Co.
5. Bennett GK: Hand tool dexterity test, manual of directions, New York, 1965, Psychological Corp.
6. Bliss CK: Semantography (Blissymbolics), ed 2, Sydney, Australia, 1965, Semantography (Blissymbolics) Publications.
7. Bobath B: Adult hemiplegia: evaluation and treatment, London, 1978, William Heinemann Medical Books, Ltd.
8. Brain L and Walton JN: Brain's diseases of the nervous system, ed 7, New York, 1969, Oxford University Press, Inc.
9. Bricolo A et al: Decerebrate rigidity in acute head injury, J Neurosurg 47:680, 1977.
10. Brown J: Aphasia, apraxia and agnosia: clinical and theoretical aspects, Springfield, Ill, 1972, Charles C Thomas, Publisher.
11. Bruce D, Gennarelli T, and Langfitt T: Resuscitation from coma due to head injury, Crit Care Med 6:254, 1978.
12. Carroll D: A quantitative test of upper extremity function, J Chron Dis 18:479, 1965.
13. Cave E, Burke JF, and Boyd RJ: Trauma management, Chicago, 1974, Year Book Medical Publishers, Inc.
14. Caveness W: Incidence of craniocerebral trauma in the United States with trends from 1970 to 1975, Adv Neurol 22:1, 1979.
15. Chusid JG: Correlative neuroanatomy and functional neurology, ed 15, Los Altos, Calif, 1973, Lange Medical Publications.
16. Denny-Brown D: The nature of apraxia, J Nerv Ment Dis 126:9, 1958.
17. Farber S: Neurorehabilitation: a multisensory approach, Philadelphia, 1982, WB Saunders Co.
18. Farber S: Sensorimotor evaluation and treatment procedures for allied health personnel, 1986, Indiana University Foundation.
19. Gatz AJ: Manter's essentials of clinical neuroanatomy and neurophysiology, ed 4, Philadelphia, 1970, FA Davis Co.
20. Geschwind N: Disconnexion syndromes in animals and man, Brain 88:237, 1965.
21. Gilroy J and Meyer JS: Medical neurology, New York, 1969, Macmillan, Inc.
22. Gordan C: Practical approach to the loss of smell, Am Fam Physician 26:192, 1982.
23. Groher M: Language and memory disorders following closed head trauma, J Speech Hear Res 20:212, 1977.
24. Halpern H, Darley FL, and Brown JR: Differential language and neurological characteristics in cerebral involvement, J Speech Hear Disord 38:162, 1973.
25. Harrington DO: The visual fields, ed 4, St Louis, 1976, The CV Mosby Co.
26. Jebsen RH et al: An objective and standardized test of hand function, Arch Phys Med Rehabil 50:311, 1969.
27. Jennett B: An introduction to neurosurgery, ed 3, London, 1977, William Heinemann Medical Books, Ltd.
28. Johnstone M: Restoration of motor function in the stroke patient, New York, 1978, Churchhill Livingstone, Inc.
29. Lorenze E and Cancro R: Dysfunction in visual perception with hemiplegia: its relation to activities of daily living, Arch Phys Med Rehabil 43:514, 1962.
30. Luria AR: Higher cortical functions in man, New York, 1966, Basic Books, Inc.
31. Marsden CD: The physiological basis of ataxia, Physiotherapy J 61:326, 1965.
32. McLaurin R: Head injuries, proceedings of the second Chicago Symposium on neural trauma, New York, 1975, Grune & Stratton, Inc.
33. Meeder D: Cognitive perceptual motor evaluation research findings for adult head injuries. In

Trexler, LE, editor: Cognitive rehabilitation, conceptualization and intervention, New York, 1982, Plenum Publishing Corp.

34. Meyer JS: An orientation to chronic disease and disability, New York, 1965, Macmillan, Inc.

35. Meyer JS: Medical neurology, New York, 1969, Macmillan, Inc.

36. Minnesota Rate of Manipulation Tests: examiner's manual, Circle Pines, Minn, 1969, American Guidance Service, Inc.

37. Pinching AJ: Clinical testing of olfaction reassessed, 1977.

38. Plum F and Posner J: Diagnosis of stupor and coma, Philadelphia, 1966, FA Davis Co.

39. Professional Staff Association of Rancho Los Amigos Hospital: Rancho Los Amigos Hospital Head Trauma Rehabilitation Seminar, Downey, Calif, 1977.

40. Purdue Pegboard: examiner's manual, Chicago, 1968, Science Research Associates, Inc.

41. Randolph S and Heineger M: A psychoneurologically integrated model for learning capacity, lectures on the Rood Treatment Approach, White Plains, NY, May 1975, Burke Rehabilitation Foundation.

42. Ryckman DM: Various approaches to cognitive re-training, Paper presented at the Sixth and Seventh Annual Post Graduate Head Trauma Rehabilitation Courses, Williamsburg, Va., June, 1982 and 1983, Medical College of Virginia.

43. Shaw R: Persistent vegetative state: principles and techniques for seating and positioning, Head Trauma Rehabil 1:1, 31, 1986.

44. Shires TG: Care of the trauma patient, ed 2, New York, 1979, McGraw-Hill, Inc.

45. Sinatra K: Nonoral communication systems, lecture given at Santa Clara Valley Medical Center, San Jose, Calif, Feb 8, 1980.

46. Smith SS: Traumatic head injuries. In Umphred DA, editor: Neurological rehabilitation, St Louis, 1985, The CV Mosby Co.

47. Solet J: The Solet test for apraxia, Boston, 1975, Copyright by author.

48. Sterno-occipital mandibular immobilizer: United States Manufacturing Co., Glendale, Calif, Commercially available head device.

49. Teasdale G and Jennett B: Assessment of coma and impaired consciousness, Lancet 2:81, 1974.

50. Trombly CA, and Scott AD: Occupational therapy for physical dysfunction, Baltimore, 1977, Williams & Wilkins.

51. Wall N et al: Hemiplegia evaluation, Boston, 1979, Massachusetts Rehabilitation Hospital.

52. Weiffenbach JM: Variation in taste thresholds with human aging, JAMA 247:775, 1982.

53. Westerman T: How I do it—head and neck: an objective approach to subjective testing for sensation of taste and smell, Laryngoscope 91:301, 1981.

54. Whyte J, Glenn MB: The care and rehabilitation of the patient in a persistent vegetative state, Head Trauma Rehabil 1:1; 39, 1986.

55. Williams N: Correlation between copying ability and dressing activities in hemiplegia, Am J Phys Med 46:1332, 1967.

56. Zoltan B et al: Perceptual motor evaluation for the neurologically impaired adult 1983, Copyright by Santa Clara Valley Medical Center, may be purchased through Santa Clara Valley Medical Center, 751 South Bascom Avenue, San Jose Calif.

57. Zoltan B: The establishment of reliability and validity of a perceptual motor evaluation on a sample of adult head injured patients, 1985. (Unpublished paper).

58. Zoltan B, Siev E and Freishtat B: Perceptual and cognitive dysfunction in the adult stroke patient, revised edition, Thorofare NJ, 1986, Charles B Slack, Inc.

36 Degenerative diseases of the central nervous system

LORRAINE WILLIAMS PEDRETTI
GUY L. McCORMACK

Degenerative diseases are characterized by chemical changes and deterioration of neurons and supporting tissues.[28] This chapter discusses five of the most common degenerative diseases seen in occupational therapy: multiple sclerosis, amyotrophic lateral sclerosis, Parkinson's disease, Alzheimer's disease, and Pick's disease. Although these diseases are unrelenting and incapacitating, the occupational therapist can offer much in the form of supportive care, maintenance of physical resources, compensatory measures, preventive measures against further complications, and retention of the quality of life.

MULTIPLE SCLEROSIS

Multiple sclerosis (MS) is a diffuse, chronic, slowly progressive disease of the central nervous system characterized by the development of disseminated, demyelinated glial patches resulting in disruption of neurotransmission. The development of multiple plaques or scar tissue on the myelin sheath leads to diversified symptoms, which are frequently transient in nature. For this reason, multiple sclerosis is often classified as a demyelinating disease.[2,27,57]

Incidence

Multiple sclerosis is one of the most common neurologic diseases of young adults.[3] The figures vary, but in the United States about 500,000 persons are affected with multiple sclerosis and about 2 million world-wide. Some sources estimate 50 to 60 cases per 100,000 of the population in areas of high incidence.[23,43] Reliable statistics are difficult to attain because it is not easy to diagnose multiple sclerosis.[27]

Multiple sclerosis usually affects persons between the ages of 20 and 50. Females are affected more than males at a ratio of 3:2. The geographic distribution of the disease appears to be related to latitude.[4] According to Kurland, MS is most prevalent in North America, Europe, and southern Canada between latitudes 65° and 45°.[43] Whites are at higher risk for multiple sclerosis, and the incidence among blacks and Asians is lower. Some evidence suggests that incidence of MS is related to socioeconomic conditions.[4,69]

At the present time, there is no known cause of multiple sclerosis but three main theories are under investigation. The most prominent theory postulates that MS is caused by a slow-acting virus infection suppressing the body's immune system. Another theory suggests that an autoimmune response occurs because a virus passes through the blood-brain barrier and produces a localized destruction of myelin. The breakdown products of myelin act as antigens stimulating systemic immunologic mechanisms targeted at the myelin sheath of the central nervous system. A genetic predisposition also has been suggested. Current research is focusing on a multifactorial approach with the possibility of a triggering event such as allergy, emotional stress, infection, and trauma.[3,5,16,24,46]

In acute cases of MS, demyelination occurs in a scattered fashion throughout the white matter located near the ventricles. The myelin sheath is broken down and chemically degraded, thus causing inflammation. After the initial onset, the demyelination may subside at some sites leaving sclerotic plaque formation.[27] In chronic cases, the increased demyelination causes shrinkage of the hemispheres with widening of sulci and dilatation of the ventricles. The plaques of demyelination disrupt nerve transmission. In addition, unmyelinated axons conduct impulses more slowly because the electrical current is insufficient for depolarization. Eventually, formation of sclerotic plaques and enzymatic activity disrupt neurotransmission in extensive locations.[44,57]

The signs and symptoms of MS depend on the variability and anatomic sites of the lesions. Onset may be sudden and symptoms may develop over a period of weeks. The manifestations are variable degrees of motor disturbances such as weakness, spasticity, intention tremors, and ataxia. Some patients also experience swallowing problems due to brain stem involvement. Sensory symptoms vary from numbness and tingling to dysesthesia of specific sensory modalities such as temperature perception, touch, and position sense. Visual symptoms result from optic neuritis. Patients may experience blurring of vision, double vision, delayed blink reflex, nystagmus, and ocular pain. Urinary bladder and bowel symptoms include urinary incontinence, urinary retention, bowel incontinence, urinary urgency, and recurrent urinary infection. Speech problems resulting from bulbar involvement may precipitate dysarthria and scanning speech. Sexual symptoms constitute varying degrees of impotence and decreased sensation in the genital area. Emotional and mental symptoms vary considerably. An estimated 31% of persons with MS experience euphoria, 26% intellectual deterioration, 16% lability, and 7% depression.[3,24,57,69]

Medical management of multiple sclerosis remains empiric or symptomatic. Because of the frequency of remissions and exacerbations, the course of treatment must respond to the needs of the patient. During exacerbations, patients are treated with bed rest and limited activity until symptoms subside. Steroid and hormone therapy is recommended during acute exacerbations. However, there is no evidence that long-term steroid therapy reduces the risk of relapse, and a risk of respiratory infections exists during the use of corticosteroids. Immunosuppressive and diet therapy have been employed with some success. Antiinflammatory drugs are administered to reduce inflammation of the myelin sheath. Muscle relaxants are used to reduce spasticity. Anticholinergic drugs and intermittent catheterization are used for bladder management. Bowel complications are managed by adequate fluid intake, diet, and occasional enemas.[2,5,10,66]

OT Intervention

The severity and progression of multiple sclerosis varies from one person to the next. The disease is characterized by exacerbations and remissions of numerous central nervous system symptoms, resulting in temporary, transient, or permanent loss of function. Because of its variability, the occupational therapy program must be individualized and based on the assessment of each patient. The physiologic changes and symptoms and psychological effects of the uncertainty of the disease course affect all areas of the patient's life.[22]

Occupational therapy for MS patients is concerned primarily with functional disabilities. Improving the quality of life and productivity of the patient and minimizing complications are the goals of occupational therapy.[72] The focus of treatment is directed toward minimizing disability and facilitating maximal independence of function within the patient's limited physical capacities.[22] Occupational therapy focuses on

five areas: (1) energy conservation and work simplification methods, (2) coordination and strength, (3) ADL and assistive devices, (4) home management and work evaluation and training, and (5) wheelchair evaluation and training.[72]

OT Evaluation

Because the course and symptoms of MS vary from time to time, evaluation must be done at intervals in the course of the disease. Factors such as fatigue, temperature, mood, and time of day also must be taken into consideration when evaluating the patient.[24]

The occupational therapy assessment for the MS patients should include evaluation of strength, physical endurance, range of motion, muscle tone, hand function, coordination, reflexes, and balance. The presence of tremor, ataxia, sensory loss, paresthesias, perceptual problems, and visual dysfunctions also should be assessed. In some instances a feeding and oral motor evaluation is indicated. The evaluation of ADL, work, and leisure skills is necessary to assess the patient's level of function in performance skills. Cognitive and intellectual functions, mental status, behavior, emotional stability, and adjustment to disability are included in the psychosocial evaluation.[24,62,72]

OT Goals

The overall goal of occupational therapy for the MS patient is to maintain the maximal level of function throughout the disease process. Specific objectives are (1) to increase or maintain ROM, (2) to increase or maintain strength, (3) to diminish abnormal spastic patterns, (4) to prevent contractures, deformity, and decubiti, (5) to facilitate maximal coordination and function of extremities, (6) to maintain maximal level of ADL, (7) to maintain ability to work, (8) to aid with psychosocial adjustment, and (9) to provide patient and family education and support.[22,56,62,67]

Treatment Methods

The selection of treatment methods for the MS patient depends on the symptoms and the level of function. The variability of the disease necessitates continual reestablishment of treatment goals and methods in response to therapy and changes in the patient's condition, home environment, and family situation.[24] The patient's problems must be solved as they arise, and life changes necessitated by the disease should be made gradually.[67]

SENSORIMOTOR DYSFUNCTION. Passive and active stretching and active range-of-motion exercises should be performed several times a day to decrease spasticity and maintain joint mobility of the MS patient. Engagement in daily living and leisure activities also should be encouraged to help maintain joint mobility. Prolonged icing and inhibition techniques, and the use of positioning to influence tone, can be used to reduce spasticity. The Bobath neurodevelopmental handling techniques using key points of control also are used to reduce spasticity.[24,56]

Strengthening exercises and activities are used to increase or maintain strength and flexibility. Exercises and activities done in the proprioceptive neuromuscular facilitation (PNF) diagonal patterns are helpful. Strengthening exercises are useful to increase strength of nonaffected muscle groups, to overcome spastic antagonists, and to prevent weakness secondary to disuse. Energy conservation techniques are taught to prolong strength and avoid fatigue.[24]

The occupational therapist should encourage the MS patient to engage in activities that involve all extremities. Poor sensation, tremor, and incoordination can be discouraging and cause frustration in the performance of hand activities.[62] Coordination and stability may be improved by strengthening fixation musculature, adapting techniques for proximal stabilization, and facilitating proximal cocontraction.[24] Distal mobility can be superimposed on proximal stability as improvement occurs. The application of wrist weights often is used to increase proprioceptive feedback, and decrease forearm tremor during upper extremity activity.[56,72] A specially designed hand cuff has been used to reduce hand tremors and is useful for tremor control during feeding.[72] General coordination activities graded from gross to fine may be helpful.[24] As in any treatment program, the effectiveness of treatment must be monitored and evaluated by its effect on the patient. Increased fatigue, spasticity, and frustration are undesirable and are indicators for analysis of their causes and possible changes in treatment media and methods.

Orthotic devices may be helpful for some MS patients. A resting splint may be used in the presence of finger extensor weakness to allow the flexor tendons to remain at a functional length and prevent overstretching of the extensors. The wrist cock-up splint may be used for weak wrist extensors to place the hand in a functional position for activities and prevent overstretching of weak extensors. (These splints are shown in Chapter 24.) A mobile arm support, described in Chapter 23, is useful to compensate for significant weakness of the upper extremities.[72]

Sensory problems are treated with a compensatory approach. Safety measures using visual feedback and increasing the patient's awareness of areas of sensory impairment must be taught. The patient and the family need to be educated about the sensory deficits and

how to employ safety techniques during routine ADL such as bathing, preparing meals, and nail care. Skin breakdown must be prevented by regular pressure relief, use of appropriate cushions and air or water mattresses, and daily skin inspection.[24,56]

SELF-CARE. Specific training in dressing, bathing, toileting, personal hygiene, and feeding can improve or maintain independence in ADL for the MS patient.[24] The patient should be trained in suitable methods and advised about the need for special equipment and assistive devices. Such devices should be introduced only when absolutely necessary.[67] Weighted silverware, a large-handled cup, a plate guard, and a nonskid mat may be helpful for feeding. Button hooks, reachers, stocking aids, and Velcro closures may be useful for increasing dressing independence.[24,67,72] The selection and use of assistive devices require a cooperative problem-solving approach by both patient and therapist. Problems must be identified and alternative solutions explored. This may require a trial-and-error approach, resulting in the adoption and discarding of various assistive devices.[72] Specific suggestions for assistive devices and ADL methods, according to the predominant symptom, can be found in Chapter 15.

HOME EVALUATION. A home evaluation is necessary to assess the MS patient's ability to function maximally in the home environment. Occupational and physical therapists can make recommendations for equipment that improves safety and independence. Furniture may have to be rearranged or eliminated to allow easy mobility and access within the home. Grab rails and banisters may have to be installed to ensure the patient's safety on stairs and during toilet and tub transfers.[67]

MOBILITY. The ambulation ability of the patient with MS is likely to decline as the disease progresses. Ambulation aids may progress from the use of a cane to crutches and then a walker. Ultimately, acquisition of a wheelchair may be a necessary part of the rehabilitation program for many patients. The patient's current status and potential progression of the disease, as well as life style and living environment, are important considerations in wheelchair selection. Obtaining a wheelchair necessitates training in wheelchair mobility and transfers that can be coordinated by occupational and physical therapists.[24]

COMMUNICATION. As tremor and incoordination increase, adaptations for communication become necessary for the MS patient. Built-up pencils, an electronic typewriter or personal computer with keyboard shield, universal cuff, clipboard and nonslip mat are devices that may be helpful for written communication. If severe dysarthria is present along with the motor dysfunction, communication boards with scanners, page turners, speaker phones, and other telephone adaptations may be necessary.[24,67]

LEISURE SKILLS. The use of previous leisure interests or the development of new ones can be helpful for satisfying instrinsic gratification needs and socialization for the MS patient. It is important to select leisure activities within the capabilities of the patient. Activities with the family or in a group can afford opportunities for socialization and support. The patient's activity configuration and interest history are important tools for discovering appropriate leisure activities.

WORK SKILLS. A vocational evaluation may be necessary for MS patients whose capacities do not preclude employment. Whether the same employment can be continued or whether a change is necessary, the need for modification of the workplace or work schedule can be determined by vocational evaluation. Psychological adjustment, perceptual, and cognitive problems influence the feasibility for continued employment or reemployment.

The ability to work not only contributes to the family economy, but also enhances self-esteem, maintains contact with work peers, and provides daily social interaction. The possibility of alternative jobs with the same employer can be explored as work tolerance and motor abilities decrease.[24,67]

PSYCHOSOCIAL ADJUSTMENT. To be informed of the diagnosis of MS is a significant and perhaps shocking event. It is well known that MS is likely to lead to progressive disability, and it is generally regarded with dread and apprehension.[49] Some patients regard the news of the diagnosis with relief following a long period of diagnostic evaluation and unexpressed fears of mental dysfunction, brain tumor, and accusations of fabricating the symptoms.[49,67]

Initially, the MS patient may feel that the future is hopeless and intolerable and may become depressed and despondent. Many patients rally and resolve to combat the disease, which now has a name and some known approaches to its management. The occupational therapist can be a valuable resource for helping the patient to make the most of remaining capabilities and for giving appropriate advice, support, and treatment.[49,67] The occupational therapist must assist the patient in adjusting to the progression of the disability.[62] Stress management techniques can be taught by the occupational therapist. These have both physical and psychological benefits.[72]

The therapist, patient and family must bear in mind that a diagnosis of MS does not mean that there is going to be a steady, rapid decline. Often there are long periods of remission, and the patient may remain stable for many years.[67] The disease has a benign course in some patients, making it possible to retain complete or partial working capacity for many years after the initial diagnosis is made.[8,49]

Euphoria is the mental change often associated with MS, though it is not common.[67] The patient who is euphoric may overestimate abilities and underestimate the seriousness of problems and potential hazards, making safety awareness poor.[62]

Patients can benefit from the opportunity to talk about their concerns and fears to someone who is knowledgeable about MS. Group counseling techniques are suitable for some MS patients. Support of rehabilitation team members and psychological or psychiatric intervention can be helpful.[49]

TREATMENT PRECAUTIONS. Patients with MS should avoid fatigue, stress, heat, and chill.[62] Heavy resistance exercise and activity are contraindicated. Exercises should be planned in conjunction with physical therapy to avoid fatigue from the cumulative efforts of the patient.[72] Rest periods should be provided during evaluation and treatment. A daily schedule of rest and activity designed within the endurance level and capabilities helps to keep the patient at an optimal level of function. The therapist should be aware that euphoria, or a denial of the severity of the symptoms, and decline in function may result in a lack of acceptance of assistive devices, safety measures, and mobility aids.[62]

PARKINSON'S DISEASE

The condition called Parkinson's disease was originally described by James Parkinson in 1817.[30] Parkinson's disease, also called parkinsonism, paralysis agitans, and shaking palsy, refers to a variety of conditions of different causes that show a similar clinical appearance. For this reason, some physicians have suggested that it be more accurately termed parkinsonian syndrome.[28]

Parkinson's disease is a slowly progressive degenerative disorder affecting the pigmented cells in the cerebral gray masses, basal ganglia, and selected midbrain nuclei. In essence, it results from a deficiency of the chemical dopamine and produces three main clinical features: (1) rigidity, (2) tremor, and (3) bradykinesia.[28,48]

In the United States, the incidence of the Parkinsonian syndrome is about 1% of the population over the age of 50 years. The incidence is approximately 187 cases per 100,000 of the population. Presently, an estimated 36,000 new cases of parkinsonism occur annually. Because it affects older persons, its incidence will most likely increase as the overall population lives longer. Parkinson's disease does not appear to be restricted to a particular sex, race, or geographic region(s) of the world.[18,48]

Many etiologic factors are associated with the parkinsonian syndrome. Primary Parkinson's disease is idiopathic. Another category called secondary or acquired parkinsonism includes postencephalitis, arteriosclerosis, infectious diseases, toxic agent exposure, and hypoparathyroidism.[48] Another group of parkinsonian syndromes are drug-induced and related to phenothiazines, reserpine, butyrophenones and α-methyldopa.[28] Some evidence of familial tendency also exists. Moreover, parkinsonism has been associated with a host of neurologic disorders such as Alzheimer's disease, Huntington's disease, Wilson's disease, olivopontocerebellar syndrome, and Shy-Drager syndrome.[74]

The pathophysiology of Parkinson's disease is well documented.[30,50] Dopamine is normally produced in the neurons of the substantia nigra located in the midbrain. A pathway called the *nigrostriatum*, transmits the dopamine to the corpus striatum (putamen, globus pallidus, caudate nucleus), where excitatory and inhibitory synapses occur. The corpus striatum is an important relay station for the extrapyramidal system, which normally modulates posture, righting reactions, and associated movements. Dopamine acts as a precursor to the inhibitory transmitter norepinephrine and is responsible for balancing the excitatory action of acetylcholine. Normally, dopamine and acelytcholine work antagonistically, inhibiting and exciting neurons to regulate normal movements. Depletion of dopamine in the extrapyramidal system results in the transmission of uncontrolled excitatory impulses. This causes an imbalance in the activity of the alpha and gamma motor systems.[28] In addition to the chemical imbalance, degenerative changes occur in the globus pallidus, the substantia nigra, and the locus ceruleus.[50] As previously mentioned, the most common clinical manifestations of the parkinsonian syndrome are tremor, rigidity, and bradykinesia.

Tremor is the most common symptom seen in Parkinson's disease.[30] Resting tremors usually begin in the upper extremities. The so-called pill-rolling tremor is the constant rubbing together of the thumb and index fingers at a rate of 4 to 10 times per second. Tremors are also seen in the lower extremities and are rhythmic or slow and often suppressed by voluntary effort.

Rigidity causes increased tone in both agonist and antagonist muscles. Muscle rigidity impedes voluntary actions and results in slow, deliberate movement. Lead-pipe rigidity is seen as a plasticlike resiliency when the extremity is moved passively. Cogwheel rigidity is less common and provides intermittent resistance to passive movement.[28]

Rigidity of the trunk is seen in Parkinson's disease, and trunk rotation is severely diminished. The patient experiences decreased chest expansion. This factor, together with inactivity, often results in bronchopneumonia, a serious and somewhat common complication of Parkinson's disease.[51]

Bradykinesia is slowness of movements and difficulty in initiating voluntary actions. In Parkinson's disease, bradykinesia is the result of increased inhibitory influences projecting from the ventrolateral nucleus of the thalamus onto gamma motor neurons.[48]

Parkinson's patients may also exhibit diminished righting and balance reactions, causing them to fall frequently. The festinating gait is another characteristic problem associated with mobility. The patient may have difficulty starting the first few steps, but after that the gait pattern speeds up considerably—a phenomenon called *propulsion*. *Retropulsion* is less common and is a shuffling gait occurring in a backward direction.

Some patients with Parkinson's disease appear to have a masked facial appearance because of cranial nerve involvement. These patients do not blink normally, and the eyes may be fixed in a downward or lateral gaze. Autonomic nervous system involvement may produce drooling, dysphagia, oily skin, excessive sweating, and bladder dysfunction.[28,48]

Dementia occurs in about one third of patients with Parkinson's disease.[50] Most patients remain mentally alert and have little, if any, loss of sensation. Medical management for Parkinson's disease involves the use of drug therapy, surgery, and symptomatic intervention. One of the most important treatments for the condition has been the use of levodopa, which passes through the blood-brain barrier and is converted to dopamine in the brain.[70] Combined drug therapy using Sinemet, which is carbidopa and levodopa, reduces the amount to be administered daily. This approach has reduced the side-effects (insomnia, mental confusion, depression, nausea, cardiac arrythmia, and hypotension) associated with levodopa replacement therapy.[50,70]

Early surgical procedures such as thalamotomy (stereotaxis) are seldom used today.[28] New surgical procedures currently being investigated offer more hope for Parkinson's victims. One very controversial approach involves fetal tissue implants.[15] Researchers hope that by implanting the brain tissues of dead fetuses to the basal ganglia, new dopamine will be produced.[39] This approach has created many heated ethical debates among medical researchers.

A more promising neurosurgical procedure involves tissue autotransplantation. This procedure was originally tried in Sweden, and more recently performed in Mexico with moderate success. The surgery requires the transplantation of tissue from the adrenal glands to the caudate nucleus of the basal ganglia. Surgeons in Mexico used surgical staples to anchor the adrenal tissue to a site within the ventricular cavity where the cells are continually bathed in cerebrospinal fluid. This nourishing bath of cerebrospinal fluid may have contributed to the success of the tissue graft.[52,53,68]

The preliminary results of tissue autograft have been viewed with optimism. The small number of patients who have undergone this procedure have shown remarkable functional recovery. A group of American surgeons, with Mexican surgeons in attendance, will begin testing the procedure in patients young enough to withstand neurosurgery.[68]

OT Intervention

The role of occupational therapy in the patient who has Parkinson's disease is to increase and maintain the patient's highest level of function throughout the disease process. Because the disease progresses over a long period of time, the occupational therapist and other rehabilitation specialists may be in contact with the patient over a period of months or years.[67] The illness is now expected to last an average of 10 years or more.[25] During this time, the patient can be maintained at home with a regimen of exercises and activities, which can be carried out independently or with the aid of the care giver. Patients may be seen for intermittent short periods of intensive therapy when necessary. This approach facilitates maintenance of the highest level of function possible at each stage in the disease process.[21,67]

OT Evaluation

The evaluation of the patient with Parkinson's disease should focus on the degree of rigidity and its distribution, tremors, and bradykinesia, and the extent to which these interfere with performance of occupational roles in self-care, leisure, and work activities.[51,56] The occupational therapy evaluation should include an assessment of (1) rigidity (muscle tone), (2) passive and active joint range of motion, (3) movement speed, (4) posture, (5) equilibrium and protective reactions, (6) mobility (ambulation), (7) tremor, (8) sitting and standing tolerance, (9) pain or other discomfort, (10) gait pattern and speed, (11) activities of daily living, (12) home and community living situation, (13) psychosocial adjustment, (14) leisure skills, and (15) work skills, if applicable.[26,51,56,62] The occupational therapist may be asked to assess the patient's function before and after drug or surgical treatment.[67] Such an evaluation can aid in determining the effect of the medical treatment on function.

OT Goals

The goals of occupational therapy are related to the data gathered in the patient assessment. To achieve the ultimate goal of maintaining the highest level of functional performance, the objectives of occupational therapy are (1) to increase movement rhythm, coordination, and speed, (2) to increase joint ROM and prevent contractures, (3) to increase trunk rotation, (4) to improve equilibrium reactions, (5) to encourage therapeutic breathing patterns and integrate these with daily living activities, (6) to maintain maximal independence in ADL, (7) to aid with sexual adjustment, (8) to increase endurance, (9) to aid in psychosocial adjustment, and (10) to involve and educate the patient's family in the treatment program.[51,62,67]

Treatment Methods

IMPROVING MOVEMENT. The occupational therapy program may use relaxation techniques such as gentle, slow rocking, and rotation of the trunk and extremities before the therapist has the patient engage in activities.[51,56] Relaxation techniques are best done in a sitting position because the supine position may increase rigidity.[51]

When relaxation has been achieved, active motion through the wide range should be carried out. These motions may begin distally and progress to gradually include proximal joints and trunk motion. Bilateral symmetric patterns of motion should be used first, and later reciprocal movement patterns should be included.[67] Proprioceptive neuromuscular facilitation (PNF) patterns, (shown in Chapter 21) are effective with Parkinson's patients. These patterns also introduce trunk rotation, which decreases proximal rigidity. The facilitation of righting and protective reactions in developmental patterns of movement is emphasized.[56] The use of rhythm and auditory cues is helpful to facilitate movement in alternating patterns without the patient becoming rigid. Rhythmic exercises, ball playing, and calisthenics to recorded music can be beneficial.[51,56] Music can be used to encourage mobility through marching, dancing, clapping, and singing. Singing with forced lip movements can help to mobilize facial musculature. Such activities are appropriate for group treatment.[56,62]

Walking with wide steps and arm swing should be

encouraged in activities that require ambulation.[51] The size and rhythm of the gait pattern can be improved by practicing a slightly broader-based gait and large, rhythmic, nonresistive movements. There should be conscious dorsiflexion of the toes and encouragement of associated arm swing.[26,56,67] Activities such as cycling and treadle devices and walking practice over foot outlines at paced intervals on the floor are possibilities. Other activities that encourage walking should be included in the treatment program to give the patient the opportunity for gait practice.[67]

Sports and games can be used for socialization and motivation and for improving movement. Activites such as ball or dart throwing, ping-pong, and shuffleboard have therapeutic value because they incorporate some of the upper and lower extremity PNF patterns and encourage trunk rotation.[62] Activities such as printing or collating can be used to encourage trunk rotation and lateral flexion.[67] In all gross motor activities, balance, coordination, and breathing patterns are emphasized.[62]

Daily physical exercise and activity aid in maintaining joint ROM, cardiovascular fitness, breathing, and bladder and bowel function. Parkinson's patients tend to withdraw from activity, gradually participating in less and less. This tendency to inertia can result in a sedentary life with increased rigidity and decreased function and may be attributed to rigidity and bradykinesia, which make activity so difficult. To combat this tendency, the therapist must provide an appropriate home program of exercise and activity and enlist the patient's cooperation and the assistance of care-givers in carrying it out. An advantage in keeping active can be cultivation of previously held or new leisure interests. Such activities engage the patient's interest and motivation and make an exercise program more acceptable.[21]

Exercise and activity programs should be coordinated between the physical and occupational therapist.[67] Physical exercise and activity do not alter or reverse the course of the disease but can aid in keeping the patient more physically fit, can forestall potential deformity, loss of function, and mental deterioration, and can enhance the quality of life.[21,51]

IMPROVING ADL PERFORMANCE. Bradykinesia, tremors, and rigidity make it tiring and time-consuming to perform ADL. Because of the difficulties, it is often easier for the patient to get assistance with many ADL. Care-givers may find it easier to do for the patient rather than watch the struggle and take the time to have the patient do the tasks independently. This arrangement needs to be examined with the patient and the care givers. Complete dependence on

others results in increased inactivity and decreased self-esteem.

On the other hand, excessive struggling with ADL for independence can leave the patient exhausted, frustrated, and unable to participate in leisure and social activities, which may be therapeutic and bring needed gratification. Therefore, it is necessary to thoroughly evaluate ADL and determine problems and their causes. After this assessment is made, the occupational therapist and the patient can determine which activities can be performed independently with relative ease, which require some assistance, and which activities should be done for the patient. Here, the occupational therapist can introduce assistive devices that may ease or bypass performance. Elastic shoelaces to eliminate the need for shoe tying is an example. The goal is to achieve a balance between rest and activity, which satisfies needs for independence, self-respect, and personal reward or pleasure.[67]

Dressing should be done in the sitting position with feet on the floor and back supported. The room should be warm and well lit. The patient should be given plenty of time to complete dressing but should not continue to the point of exhaustion. Clothing should be made of lightweight and stretchy fabrics and should be large enough to be put on easily. Styles with wide openings and a minimum of fasteners are recommended. Fasteners should be front opening and easy to see.[67] Velcro may be used to replace small snaps or buttons.

Eating may be slow and dribbling of food and slowness in chewing may occur. This can lead to embarrassment and reduced food intake. A well-balanced diet of easily managed foods is recommended. A dietitian should be consulted after eating difficulties with particular types of foods have been identified. Food can be kept warm while the patient is served small amounts at one time. Built-up utensils and a mat to stabilize the dish can be used. If tremors are a problem, wrist weights, weighted utensils or cups, and cups with bilateral handles may help to increase control. Raising the eating surface or plate and positioning the patient to use one elbow as a pivot can enhance control of the upper limbs during feeding.[67]

The home environment should be evaluated for safety and convenience features. On a home visit the occupational therapist can make recommendations for increased safety and function in the home. Floor coverings should be even, smooth and nonskid materials. Small carpets should be removed. Grab rails should be installed for toilet and tub or shower safety. Banisters should be installed for any steps or stairs in or outside the home. Home management must be simplified to reduce stress and fatigue. Assistance from other family members or outside agencies may be required.[67] The patient should be instructed in energy conservation and work simplification methods. Assistive devices such as a utility cart, electric appliances, and stabilizing devices may be helpful.

As the patient's condition deteriorates, the occupational therapist's role shifts to giving instruction to care givers. Proper bed positioning and ROM exercises should be demonstrated. Equipment such as a hospital bed, mechanical patient lifter, and wheelchair may be necessary. The therapist may make recommendations for needed equipment, assist the family in securing it, and instruct them in its use.[21]

PSYCHOSOCIAL ADJUSTMENT. Depression is common in Parkinson's disease, especially as communication skills and mobility decline. When dealing with the depressed patient, the occupational therapist must have a positive and supportive approach. Treatment sessions must be purposeful, and the patient needs to see the relevance of the activities. Familiar activities that are interesting to the patient should be used. A variety of stimuli such as color, touch, and sound are helpful. The therapist should consider the patient's activity tolerance and attention span when planning the treatment session. The patient should be introduced gradually to small group treatment for maintenance of social contact. At home and in the community, hobbies, visitors, outings, and attendance at community activity programs, senior centers, or day treatment programs may be ways to meet social needs. The occupational therapist can be instrumental in surveying available programs and making the appropriate referral.[67]

Sexual dysfunction may occur in patients with Parkinson's disease as a result of disruption of nervous system control or as a side-effect of various medications. Psychological factors such as the depression, anxiety, and frustration of the disease affect the libido. Treatment with Levodopa may provide partial or satisfactory improvement of libido in some patients, or possibly excessive libido. Limitations of movement because of rigidity and bradykinesia may cause problems in the mechanical aspects of sexual functioning.[21]

The patient should be given the opportunity to express sexual concerns. Whether the sexual problems are caused by nervous system dysfunction, medication, or mechanical difficulties can be determined by the physician and the appropriate rehabilitation professionals. Possible solutions can be offered, such as suggestions for positioning or exploring changes in medication.[21] The occupational therapist, trained in sexual counseling, may encourage the patient to

share concerns as a part of the ADL evaluation and may offer information about and solutions for mechanical difficulties.

COMMUNICATION. Group treatment provides support and offers opportunities to practice communication. An apparent lack of verbal responsiveness can be caused by slow thought processes, depression, and weak facial movement. Family members and friends need to be informed of the problem and its causes, and the patient needs to be given time to formulate and make a reply. Questions should be direct and be phrased so that a long and complex response is not required. For those whose speech is very slow and weak, a word chart or other communication device can be used to avoid undue frustration of the patient and the listener. Singing, board games, quizzes, and discussion groups are activities that can encourage speech. During such activities, deep breathing, articulation, speech volume, swallowing, and breaking up sentences into short segments should be emphasized.[26,27]

Writing skills may decline as tremors and rigidity increase. Writing practice can be introduced by using the chalkboard or large sheets of paper. Rhythmic writing in wide-spaced lines are practiced progressing to letters and words. A built-up pencil and paper stabilizer may be helpful.[67]

GROUP TREATMENT. Because of the tendency to social isolation and a sedentary life in Parkinson's patients, a group approach to treatment can be more beneficial than individual treatment. Gauthier, Dalziel, and Gauthier studied the effects of a group treatment program on patients with idiopathic Parkinson's disease.[25] They compared a rehabilitation group that received group treatment with a control group that did not. Both groups were receiving pharmacologic management. Group treatment sessions of 2 hours twice a week over a 5-week period were carried out. Each treatment session consisted of a period of welcome and socialization, general mobilization activities, rest and socialization, dexterity activities, functional activities, and departure. During most activities, visual and auditory cues were used such as watching and following the therapist's movements, music, a metronome, and verbal cues. Rhythm, music, singing, and dancing were used to initiate movement and increase postural stability. Dexterity tasks included games, writing exercises, and crafts. Activities of daily living were discussed, demonstrated, and practiced. Educational information about the disease was presented by the occupational therapists or other invited health professionals.

The results of group treatment on maintenance of

functional status, perception of psychological well-being, and maintenance or regression of physical symptoms were significant compared with results of the control group. Follow-up evaluations were done at 6 months and again at 1 year. Changes that were observed, but not assessable, were improved appearance, better understanding of the disease process with decreased fear and increased self-confidence, and decreased egocentricity. Long-term benefits were attributed to patient education and participation in the prescribed home program. The group treatment setting provided a supportive environment and afforded opportunities for communication and socialization.[25]

FAMILY EDUCATION. Family members or other care givers need information on the symptoms and course of Parkinson's disease and how these affect the patient's ability to function. The occupational therapist should instruct the family about the prescribed home exercise and activity programs, about how and when to give assistance in ADL, about making adjustments in the home environment, and about how to obtain and use assistive devices. Family education is critical to carry-over of the treatment program outside the rehabilitation setting. Without the interest, support, supervision, and encouragement of a concerned family member or care-giver, the patient is not likely to perform prescribed exercise and activity at home.[56] The occupational therapist should offer the patient and the family support and encouragement, as well as instruction. The therapist can act as a resource and can be instrumental in finding community activity programs for the patient. The therapist can assist the patient and the family in coping with the limitations imposed by Parkiinson's disease.[51]

TREATMENT PRECAUTIONS. The therapist should observe for drug side-effects of Levodopa such as gastrointestinal disturbances, dystonic movements, mental disturbances, orthostatic hypotension, and cardiac arrhythmias.[51,56] The therapist should also monitor any increase in rigidity as a result of exercise or activity and make appropriate changes in the program to prevent this. Fatigue and frustration should be avoided.[51]

Conclusions

The patient with Parkinson's disease is a challenge for the rehabilitation team. The progression of the disease over a period of several years necessitates intervention that is directed toward maintaining the highest possible level of function at every stage of the disease. The maintenance or improvement of the physical, functional, and psychosocial status of the patient is the overall goal of rehabilitation. Such a therapeutic program can improve the quality of life

for the patient and the family. A variety of exercises and activities is used in individual and group treatment and at home to achieve these ends.

AMYOTROPHIC LATERAL SCLEROSIS

Amyotrophic lateral sclerosis (ALS) has been referred to as Lou Gehrig's disease, progressive muscular atrophy, and motor neuron disease.[34] In the United States, amyotrophic lateral sclerosis is one of the most common neuromuscular disorders affecting adults.[45] Three clinical variants of this disease are (1) primary lateral sclerosis, (2) progressive muscular atrophy, and (3) progressive bulbar palsy.[64] In short, ALS is a progressive neurologic disease affecting both upper motor and lower motor neurons.[42]

The incidence of ALS is about 5 to 7 per 100,000.[71] Epidemiologic data reveal that ALS occurs more frequently in males than in females at a ratio of 2:1. Most victims are between the ages of 40 and 70, with an average age of onset of 57.[54] Although ALS is well distributed throughout the world, it is reportedly most prevalent among the people of Guam and the Mariana Islands in the western Pacific.[28]

The etiology of ALS is unknown, but several possible causes have been proposed. Some theories of its cause presently under investigation include a slow-acting virus infection, a toxic degeneration, an autoimmune reaction, hormonal abnormalities, circulating lead toxicity, and deficiency of a repair enzyme in the blood.[35,42]

The pathophysiology shows that ALS is a bilateral, degenerative disease restricted to motor neurons primarily in the corticobulbar, corticospinal tracts and anterior horn cells of the spinal cord. The motor nuclei of the cranial nerves also are involved. Marked atrophy of distal muscles is characteristic, with loss of muscle fibers and fascicles in the distribution of motor units.[45,71]

The clinical manifestations conform to the three variations of the disease. The progressive muscular atrophy patients exhibit progressive weakening and wasting of distal musculature. Atrophy can begin in either upper or lower extremities. A combination of spasticity and wasting results from the effects of upper and lower motor neuron involvement. Although sensory pathways are preserved, painful muscle spasms and paresthesias are common complaints. Bladder dysfunction is usually absent.

ALS patients with progressive bulbar palsy exhibit difficulty in swallowing, coughing, speaking, and breathing. There is marked wasting of the musculature innervated by the cranial nerves, particularly the tongue.[35]

In some ALS patients, progressive involvement of

the laryngeal and pharyngeal muscles produces dysphagia, aspiration problems, and respiratory insufficiency. This variation of ALS runs a rapid course, and the patient rarely survives more than 18 months from the onset of the symptoms.[37]

Primary lateral sclerosis is rare and may be a familial predisposition. In this type of ALS spasticity in all four extremities with little wasting in the early stages of the disease may be present. Usually little loss of intellectual capacity occurs except in cases in which degeneration of the corticobulbar pathways, which lends to emotional lability, is present.[35]

There is no specific medical treatment for amyotrophic lateral sclerosis.[37] Treatment is symptomatic, with medications to decrease the discomfort of muscle spasms. Gastrostomy or tracheostomy or both is used for patients with malnutrition resulting from swallowing difficulties. Tranquilizers and antidepressant drugs are used to alleviate anxiety and depression.[55,64]

OT Intervention

As with the four other degenerative CNS diseases, the role of occupational therapy in ALS patients is to maintain an optimal level of function during the relentless progression of motor impairment. The occupational therapy program addresses symptomatic care and includes graded exercise and activity, energy conservation and work simplification techniques, selection and management of appropriate ambulation aids and orthotics, and provision of assistive devices necessary for communication and self-care independence. In addition, psychological support for the patient and the family and family education are important elements of the occupational therapy program. The occupational therapist should work within a multidisciplinary team for a comprehensive approach to disease management.[37]

The complexity and progressive nature of ALS make each patient unique in terms of degree of weakness, rate of progression, and order and severity of clinical manifestations. Therefore each patient needs an individualized treatment program.[37] Janiszewski and colleagues found it useful to classify ALS progression into four clinical stages according to symptoms and level function.[37]

Neuro Scale 1—Free ambulatory. The patient is able to perform normal life activities, although mild discomfort or limitations of performance and endurance may be apparent.
Neuro Scale 2—Ambulatory with mild-to-moderate limitation of function. The patient demonstrates muscle imbalance, increased muscle fatigue caused by excessive energy expenditure, decreased mobility and function.
Neuro Scale 3—Wheelchair-bound and ADL-dependent.

This stage is characterized by progressive weakness of axial muscles, and deterioration of mobility and endurance. The patient requires a wheelchair to go long distances, and later in this stage, becomes wheelchair bound.
Neuro Scale 4—Bedridden. The patient is totally ADL-dependent. Gastrostomy, tracheostomy, and some form of respiratory assistance may be needed.

OT Evaluation

The occupational therapy evaluation should include the assessment of muscle strength, muscle tone, active and passive ROM, ADL performance, and a home evaluation.[37] Activity tolerance and possible cranial nerve involvement also should be evaluated. The latter includes a dysphagia evaluation. Motor assessment for the use of nonvocal communication devices should be carried out when communication skills weaken.[65] Information from the evaluation of pulmonary function and gait should be obtained from physical and respiratory therapists. The evaluation results are used as a baseline for functional endurance and performance. From this, progression of limitations can be measured and the treatment program modified.[37]

OT Goals

The goals of the occupational therapy program are to (1) maintain strength, (2) prevent contractures, (3) reduce spasticity, (4) maintain independence in ADL, (5) facilitate psychosocial adjustment, and (6) provide family education and support.[62]

Treatment Methods

Janiszewski and colleagues outlined a multidisciplinary treatment program for each stage of ALS previously outlined.

In the first stage of the disease (Neuro Scale 1), the patient should be taught work simplification and energy conservation methods. Mild aerobic exercise for uninvolved muscles to maintain ROM and compensate for weakness in other muscles may be helpful. Swimming and bicycling are recommended for general conditioning.[37] Progressive resistive exercises are not recommended because these usually cause cramping and fatigue. Fatigue should be avoided in any exercise or activity program because it seems to increase the rate of motor unit degeneration.[37,75] Simple assistive devices and orthotics may be provided.[37]

In the second stage (Neuro Scale 2) of ALS, progressive muscle atrophy of particular muscles is noted. Pain and discomfort from spasticity or pressure neuropathies may be present. Adaptive equipment and bracing are needed to support weak muscles and conserve energy. Such devices also can help to improve the patient's performance at home and at work. A cane, tripod, or quad cane, a rolling walker, and short-leg braces are necesary for ambulation.[37]

The treatment program for ALS patients may include active range-of-motion (ROM) exercise to prevent contractures, active exercise and moderate activity to maintain strength, and teaching of positioning for comfort and function.[62,65] Exercise is monitored and patients are advised to have several brief exercise periods each day rather than a single strenuous exercise session. Swimming and limited bicycling are continued.[37]

In the third stage (Neuro Scale 3), the patient is confined to a wheelchair for all or part of the time. A wheelchair with a reclining back, headrest, elevating padded legrests, padded armrests, safety belt, and lapboard may be necessary to accommodate the patient's increasing functional limitations and need for rest and special positioning. Active and passive range-of-motion exercises and breathing exercises are included in the treatment program. Considerable psychological support is necessary for both patient and family.[37]

In the fourth stage (Neuro Scale 4) of ALS, breathing and swallowing difficulties are common. Assistive techniques for breathing, coughing, and swallowing are employed. Breathing assistance by respirator or tracheostomy is used for some patients. Special feeding techniques and devices, as well as special diet, are introduced. Communication devices become necessary.[37]

ORTHOTICS AND ASSISTIVE DEVICES. Splints commonly used to prevent deformity and support weak musculature in the ALS patient are the wrist cock-up splint, opponens splint, soft cervical collar, and ankle-foot orthosis.[37,75]

Some assistive devices that may be helpful are the long-handled comb, brush, and bath sponge, bath and shower chairs, grab bars in tub and around toilet, flexible shower hose, and raised toilet seat. Takai recommended that padded drop-arm commode for use over the toilet while the patient is still ambulatory but has difficulty rising from a standard toilet seat.[65] For dressing, the long-handled shoe horn, sock aid, zipper pull, and button hook can be helpful. Clothing should be chosen for comfort as well as ease of putting on and removing.[13] Devices to ease home management tasks may be appropriate in the early stages of the illness.

Feeding can be managed with the assistance of a nonskid mat, plate guard, universal cuff, and cups with one or two handles. Food consistency must be modified to accomodate progressive difficulty with swallowing. In the intermediate stages of ALS, puréed foods are easier to manage than liquids. The patient must be allowed adequate time for eating because rushing increases the chances of choking. If eating is tiring, six small meals may be taken.[11]

When evaluating the ALS patient for the use of assistive devices, the occupational therapist must consider the fatigue and frustration that the patient experiences in using the device, its cost, appearance, acceptability to patient and family, and convenience of use. The stage of the disease, rate of progression, current motor status, endurance, and positioning are other important considerations in the selection and use of assistive devices. Whether the device is going to be helpful should be determined before it is ordered or fabricated, if possible.[65]

COMMUNICATION. All ALS patients ultimately become limited in communication. Problems with writing, using the telephone, speaking, or signaling for attention eventually arise. The occupational therapist should examine the problems and their causes and advise the patient about available alternatives. The patient needs reassurance that no matter how severe the communication difficulty, it is possible to convey needs and ideas to others. Different types of telephones are available such as the speaker phone, the automatic dialer, and the receiver holder. Communication boards, eye-gaze charts, electronic scanners, and personal computers are aids that can be used to augment communication.[65] As the patient loses more and more mobility, environmental control systems and attendant care may be necessary.[62]

PSYCHOSOCIAL ADJUSTMENT. Progressive muscular weakness creates feelings of hopelessness, discouragement, and despair in the ALS patient.[75] Adjustment to the disease is especially difficult because of its progressive nature. Because no disability is static, adjustments must be made over and over again.[11] Reactive depression is common, but suicide is rare among ALS patients.[37]

To facilitate psychosocial adjustment, the therapist must promote continued appropriate activity and exercise, and provide support and encouragement.[75] Keeping the ALS patient as active as possible and reducing dependency lessens depression and hopelessness and enhances self-image.[37] The provision of a concrete assistive device, for example, which makes an immediate change in performance has a positive psychological effect on the patient.[65] The maintenance or recovery of function has a good effect on self-esteem and improves the sense of independence. The occupational therapist can support the development of coping mechanisms and help both patient and family to confront a terminal illness.[62]

The pursuit of recreational and leisure skills should

be encouraged for diversion, fitness, and a sense of personal gratification. Johnson described an aquatic therapy program for an ALS patient.[38] The aquatics program was used to improve strength, ROM, and endurance. Functional ambulation and balance activities were facilitated by the buoyancy of the water. The program also allowed opportunity for recreation and socialization. The warm water was soothing and promoted muscle relaxation. The patient's feelings of self-esteem and well-being were improved by the program. Swimming is a very good multisystem conditioning activity for the ALS patient.[38]

Conclusions

ALS is a progressively disabling disease for which there is no known cause or cure. Rehabilitation efforts for these patients are directed toward maintaining performance at a level submaximal to the patient's endurance to save energy and avoid fatigue. Toward these ends, the patient is taught energy conservation and work simplification methods, is provided with orthotics and assistive devices, and is involved in an individualized graded exercise and activity program.[37]

Involvement of patient and family in the rehabilitation process is an essential part of the treatment program. Emotional support and encouragement of rehabilitation team members are necessary to help both patient and family deal with the progressive severity of the disability and terminal illness.

ALZHEIMER'S DISEASE

In 1907, a German physician named Alvis Alzheimer described a condition resulting in an early onset of senility in a 51-year-old woman.[47] Today Alzheimer's disease is one of the most common forms of the dementias.[12] Alzheimer's disease is a progressive, degenerative disease that ravages the brain. It is characterized by progressive loss of memory, cognitive impairment, and changes in personality.[14,41]

In the United States, Alzheimer's disease affects one person in every six over the age of 65. It is estimated that the disease affects 880,000 to 1,200,000 persons, and at least 100,000 succumb each year.[41,58] Females are affected twice as often as males. It occurs with equal frequency in all racial, ethnic, and socioeconomic groups.[17]

The etiology of Alzheimer's disease is unknown, but there are several theories about causal factors. One theory suggests a deficiency of the neurotransmitter acetylcholine. Autopsies have shown that an enzyme catalyst needed for the production of acetylcholine is 70% to 90% below normal levels. Another theory suggests that a slow-acting virus may be the cause. Toxic substances such as aluminum also have been found in high concentrations in some of the brain tissue of diseased Alzheimer's patients.[41] Head trauma may be another predisposing factor to Alzheimer's disease in later life.[14,33,40]

The pathophysiology studies show that the brain undergoes atrophy, especially in the frontal and temporal lobes. Widening of sulci and narrowing of gyri result in a brain that is underweight. The cerebral ventricles are dilated, which causes pressure on the hippocampal formation. Histologic studies show loss of neurons in the cortex, nucleus basalis, and locus ceruleus. Other microscopic signs are senile plaques, which are ringlike structures resulting from gliosis; neurofibrillary tangles, which are coiled filaments twisted in helical configurations; and intraneuronal granulovacular degeneration, which signifies the formation of cavities within the cytoplasms of neurons.[12,36,63]

The clinical features of Alzheimer's disease may vary and the course of the disorder may range from 5 to 25 years. The course of the disease is usually categorized into three stages.[1,17,20] Stage 1 is the forgetfulness phase. The patient may be absent-minded, lack concentration, and experience mood changes and functional loss of orientation. Stage 2, the confusional phase, shows marked loss of memory, episodic bouts of irritability, aphasia, apraxia, neurologic movement disorders, inability to communicate effectively, sleep disturbances, and night wandering. Stage 3 represents the dementia phase. The patient becomes apathetic, unresponsive to stimuli, incontinent, prone to seizures, agitated, and severely disoriented. Eventually, the patient may succumb to an infectious disorder.[7]

The medical management tends to be experimental and symptomatic.[47] Phenothiazines (tranquilizers) are the mainstay of treatment. Medical management also is aimed at helping the patient to function at an optimal level throughout the course of the disease. Therefore, treatment includes maintaining the patient's general health, independence, basic orientation, personal safety, and dignity.[1,7]

OT Intervention

Alzheimer's disease affects not only the person who has it but the primary care-giver and all family members. The professional helper must consider the needs of all those involved, if treatment is to be effective.[29] The role of occupational therapy with the dementias focuses on self-care, independent living skills, and assessment of potential for continued employment if the patient is still in the early stages of the disease.[6] Family education and support are also essential parts of the occupational therapy program.

Occupational therapy provides a graded program

of environmental modification and task simplification, which keeps pace with the patient's declining capacities. Such an approach allows the patient to maintain as much control over life as possible at each stage of the disease and to retain a sense of personal dignity. An important component of the occupational therapy program is teaching care-givers how to manage the progressive incapacities of the patient.[6]

OT Evaluation

The purposes of the occupational therapy evaluation of an Alzheimer's patient are to assess the level of cognitive and motor functioning and to assess performance skills of self-care, home management, and leisure activities.[6] The occupational therapist administers tests of perceptual and cognitive abilities and observes for deficits of these functions during activity performance. Evaluation of ROM, coordination, equilibrium, muscle tone, gait, posture, and movement speed and rhythm are used to assess motor functioning.[76]

A comprehensive evaluation of performance skills includes assessment of self-care including feeding, swallowing, dressing, toileting, hair and nail care, bathing, shaving or make-up application, and mobility. Home management evaluation may include telephoning, meal preparation, doing laundry, housecleaning, gardening, and money management.[6,76] Performance of leisure skills is assessed through expressed interests, interest history, and observation of performance to determine the potential for participation. If intervention is early, when cognitive impairment is minimal, evaluation of work skills is indicated. An assessment of environmental factors such as space, equipment, and objects should be a part of the occupational therapy evaluation to determine how the environment helps or hinders the patient's performance.[6,76] Recommendations for changes in space, equipment, and furniture arrangement to enhance the function of the patient may be made by the occupational therapist.

Data for the occupational therapy evaluation is obtained by interviewing the Alzheimer's patient, family members, or care-givers. Performance skills are evaluated by observing the patient during task performance. The performance observation yields information about tasks that the patient performs easily, tasks performed with moderate difficulty, and tasks that are not possible. The occupational therapist should determine factors that underlie dysfunctional performance. The balance of activity in the patient's day needs careful consideration. Too much activity may precipitate confusion or a catastrophic reaction, and too little activity may induce lethargy.[6]

The occupational therapy evaluation serves as a guide for selecting objectives and intervention strategies that are within the realm of the Alzheimer's patient's capabilities. In addition, the evaluation may be used to determine the level of supervision or care that the patient needs. The occupational therapy evaluation also can contribute valuable information for decision making about the feasibility of independent living and the need for attendant care or guardianship. Work evaluation can determine the feasibility of continued employment or the need for work adaptations. The effect of medical treatment on behavior can be assessed by controlled observation of patient performance in the occupational therapy clinic.[6]

OT Goals

The goals of occupational therapy for the patient with Alzheimer's disease are (1) to improve or maintain functional capacities for as long as possible, (2) to maintain level of attention and memory, (3) to promote participation in activities that enhance physical and mental health, (4) to aid in socialization, (5) to increase patient comfort, and (6) to increase ease of activities for care-givers.[6,20]

Treatment Methods

ACTIVITY PROGRAMS. Activities selected should be voluntary and relevant to the patient and should offer a reasonable chance for success. To be successful, an activity must be within the patient's physical and mental capacities. The activity should never be childish or demeaning. Its purpose should be obvious to the patient. One way of grading activities for this population is by the degree of task involvement of the patient. Involvement can range from merely attending to a task that is presented, to initiating, planning, and executing an entire task independently. Activities most suitable for grading in this way are those involving several steps. To determine their suitability, activities must be analyzed for their physical, sensory, perceptual, and cognitive demands.[76]

Patients with Alzheimer's disease should be encouraged but not coerced to participate in an activity program. The therapist should use a structured approach with clear, concise instructions. The patient's habitual skills can be used advantageously. Although some habitual skills may be lost, the loss tends to be patchy and significant abilities may be intact.[76] Active exercise, supervised activities of daily living, simple leisure activities related to past hobbies and interests, and structured social activities are useful for maintenance of physical and mental capacities.[6,20,76] Performance is sometimes better when rhythmic activities such as dancing, sawing wood, and threading beads are used. Rhythmic walking may be done with more ease and instructions followed more accurately if given simply and in a rhythmic tone.[76]

As deterioration progresses, tasks must be analyzed to their component parts. It is then determined whether the patient with Alzheimer's disease is capable of any part of the given task. In an activity group, each member may be assigned one part of a process so that the entire group completes a given activity. Care-givers must avoid the tendency to take over all the patient's activities, because this leads to inactivity and depression and hastens deterioration. Continued engagement in activity has a reality-orienting influence on the patient's behavior. Exercise, games, crafts, sensory stimulation, and rhythm activities may be used to maintain joint mobility, strength, mental alertness, and self-esteem. The debilitating effects of contractures, decubiti, fatigue, and depression can be forestalled by engaging the patient in activities at an appropriate level.[6] Zgola offers several specific guidelines for activities, the activity program, and suitable environment and routine.[76]

ENVIRONMENTAL MODIFICATION. The occupational therapist can not only simplify tasks but also structure the environment to maximize the Alzheimer's patient's performance. The environment should be kept predictable and familiar, consistent, and free of ambiguities. Furniture should have clear limits, and traffic areas should be free of obstacles. Contrasting colors can be used effectively to help the patients distinguish figure from background.[6,20,76]

ACTIVITIES OF DAILY LIVING. As Alzheimer's disease progresses, the patient may require some assistance with ADL. Simple assistive devices may make independent performance of some activities possible. Frequent orientation to time and place and frequent changes of activity may be helpful. Patterning of social interactions and structuring is important for maintaining daily living skills. Activities should be broken down into very short steps. Instructions must be clear, concise, and brief. Verbal, visual, or physical prompting may help the patient to initiate and perform activities. Care-givers can be taught these methods for helping the patient initiate and sustain activity.[6,20]

BEHAVIORAL CONTROL. It is important to eliminate sources of agitation and thus to avoid or reduce catastrophic reactions characteristic of this disease. These reactions consist in a refusal to cooperate, often accompanied by outbursts of crying, stubbornness, and combative behavior.[19,20] Catastrophic reactions are caused by sensory or cognitive overload, misinterpretation of sensory information or of a request, fatigue, and frustration over the inability to perform. The therapist must try to reduce the reaction, because

the patient cannot change. This is done by getting the patient's attention and verbalizing what is happening with assurance. Information must be given step by step, slowly and clearly. The patient must be able to see the therapist clearly. Activity and noise should be reduced, and choice making must be limited. Arguing should be avoided, and the therapist or care-giver should respond sympathetically to the patient's stress. If the patient is about to throw an object, Davis recommends that the therapist should clap loudly and say "Look! Behind you!"[19] This diverts attention and often patients forget what they were about to do.[19] The occupational therapist, the occupational therapy assistant, and the care-givers should take note of the kinds of stimuli or activity that provoke such reactions. Human contact, social interaction, and frequent changes of activity may be helpful. Those responsible for treatment and care should use a calm, slow, and soft voice and allow adequate response time.[20]

FAMILY EDUCATION. The family should be made aware of the causes and handling of catastrophic reactions. It should be reinforced that their loved one is not in control of this behavior and it should not be personalized.[19] In the final stages of the disease, the occupational therapist can make a contribution to patient safety and comfort by assisting care-givers with life maintenance functions. The therapist can instruct the care-giver in bed positioning, ROM exercises, dysphagia management, lifting and moving skills, and assistance with ADL. The use of touch, gentle speech, and tender loving care gives comfort to the patient.[6,20]

The rehabilitation team members must offer as much support as possible to the patient and the family. Recommendations for home modifications, safety factors, and handling catastrophic reactions need to be made at the appropriate time and with respect by members of the rehabilitation team. Determination of the care-giver's willingness and ability to care for the patient, the need for respite care, and potential plans for institutional placement must be handled by members of the rehabilitation team.[6,36]

RECOMMENDATIONS FOR THE THERAPIST. Glickstein offers several tips to professional helpers working with patients who have Alzheimer's disease.[29] She recommends that therapists should be realistic and develop plans of action based on the patient's current level of function. Expectations that treatment can alter the course or outcome of the disease leads to frustration. It is important for professional helpers to work with others and to have ongoing reinforcement. The therapist should identify the patient's needs and all the barriers to fulfilling those needs. Communication can be enhanced if the therapist addresses the patient directly by name and identifies self by name as well. Eye contact should be established with the patient before communication is attempted. The patient needs time to respond. Repetition is helpful and directions should be short and simple. The patient should not be offered choices unless he or she is capable of making a choice. Consistency of approach and of activities is very helpful in handling the patient with dementia.[29]

DAY CARE. Day care programs for patients with Alzheimer's disease and related disorders are increasing in number. Occupational therapists and occupational therapy assistants may be part of the staff of such programs. The purposes of day care programs are to increase socialization, maintain physical and mental well-being, and promote reality orientation and task participation for the clients. In addition, the programs offer respite care to the primary care-giver and family members.[60] Rudolph describes such a program.[60] It is open 3 days a week and accepts clients at all functional levels except those who are hazardous to themselves or others or are in need of constant attention and maximal physical assistance. The program includes a morning coffee time, which incorporates reality orientation activites such as reading and discussing the newspaper. Following this, the clients are engaged in gross motor activity such as walking or simple chair exercises. The rest of the day includes relaxation and quiet time, music, entertainment, table games, and crafts. Clients also assist in preparing lunch and snacks. Participation in various activities is encouraged. Parallel programming allows clients at different functional levels to participate. The center provides nurturing and improved quality of life for the clients and their families.

Respite care has resulted in decreased depression in clients and families. The center serves as an interim step between home care and institutional placement.[60] Rabinowitz described a day care program on Saturdays only in New York City.[59] This program uses activities such as reality orientation, reminiscence, exercises that use concrete objects such as an elastic jump rope for stretching, activities such as balloon toss, meal preparation, crafts, and structured games. Outdoor activities are sometimes used, and a special event such as pet therapy or live concert is planned once a month.[59]

Conclusions

In the treatment of patients with Alzheimer's disease and related disorders, the role of occupational therapy is for support, maintenance, and improve-

ment of the quality of life. The therapist must accept the progressive deterioration of the patient while providing intervention that stimulates maximal function in all phases of the disease process. The therapist must be one who cares about the patient and strives to make life as comfortable and fulfilling as possible in spite of the fact that the disease is incurable and decline is inevitable.

PICK'S DISEASE

Pick's disease is a type of dementia that is less common than Alzheimer's disease. Pick's disease is an organic brain disorder of rapid progression that may be inherited as an autosomal dominant trait.[28] It affects people in the 40 to 60 age group and runs an unrelenting course of about 7 to 10 years from onset to death. The exact cause of the neuronal degeneration is unknown, but increased concentrations of zinc in brain tissues are presently being investigated.[12] The brain shows marked atrophy in the temporal and frontal lobes. The neurofibrillary tangles and senile plaques seen in Alzheimer's disease are infrequent or absent in Pick's disease. Clinically, patients with Pick's disease have the same symptomatology as those with Alzheimer's disease.[7,14,58]

OT Intervention

Occupational therapy intervention for patients with Pick's disease is essentially the same as that outlined for Alzheimer's disease.

FUTURE DIRECTIONS

Although the prognosis for patients with degenerative diseases has been dim, discoveries in the neurosciences are producing a more positive outlook. Research is now suggesting that thinking processes and attitudes affect health and the ability to combat diseases.[9,31,32,61] The occupational therapist is in a position to promote positive thinking and attitudes, and even to use humor, in spite of adversity. Through the use of guided imagery, relaxation techniques, and breathing practices, the therapist can help the patient to achieve a physiologic state called the *relaxation response*.[32] By reducing stressful thoughts and behaviors, the body produces lower levels of the hormone norepinephrine and a higher ratio of helper T cells, an important balance in the immune system.[9] By developing hopeful patterns of thinking, the patient may activate protective healing from within.[31] These new approaches may make a significant contribution to change in the course of catastrophic illness in the future.[61]

Sample treatment plan

The following treatment plan is not a comprehensive one for the hypothetical patient. It deals with five problems on the Problem List. The reader is encouraged to add objectives and methods to deal with the additional problems to make a more comprehensive plan.

CASE STUDY

Mr. D is a 30-year-old man who has multiple sclerosis, onset 3 years ago. Since then, there have been some short periods of remission, but generally a steady decline in function. Present symptoms are blurred vision, ataxia, upper extremity tremors, low physical endurance, limited standing tolerance, and occasional urinary incontinence.

Present functional limitations include difficulty with ambulation and transfers, meal preparation, and feeding. He moves about the house with an ataxic gait while holding on to furniture, appliances, and door frames.

Prior to onset of the disease, Mr. D worked as an inspector in a high-technology electronics factory. The job required long periods of sitting, walking about, excellent visual acuity, and fine hand coordination. Mr. D has left the job and is being compensated by disability insurance.

Mr. D is not married and lives at home with his parents. His leisure activities were dating, dancing, sports, rock music, and CB radio operation. After the onset of the disease, he has tried to continue with the CB radio but is having difficulty operating dials and switches. He enjoys collecting and listening to rock music tapes and listening to sporting events on the radio.

Following the diagnosis of MS, Mr. D was in a reactive depression for several weeks. This lifted as he became involved in early rehabilitation efforts. At this time Mr. D demonstrates cheerfulness, a good sense of humor, and garrulousness.

He was referred to occupational therapy for evaluation and training in ADL, physical conditioning, and exploration of possible leisure activities. Treatment precautions include avoidance of fatigue, stress, heat, and cold.

Personal Data

Name: Mr. D
Age: 30
Diagnosis: Multiple sclerosis
Disability: Ataxia, tremors, poor vision
Treatment aims as stated in referral: Evaluation and training in ADL, physical conditioning, and exploration of leisure activities

OTHER SERVICES

Physician: Prescription of medication; oversee rehabilitation program; maintenance of general health
Physical therapy: Exercise, gait training with aids, transfer training.
Social service: Family and patient counseling; assistance with financial arrangements for treatment. Contacts with community support groups.
Community social group: MS Society support group and education program

FRAME OF REFERENCE

Occupational performance

TREATMENT APPROACH

Rehabilitative

OT EVALUATION

Performance components

Motor functioning
  Functional strength: Observe and test
  ROM: Test
  Physical endurance: Observe and interview
  Muscle tone: Test and observe
  Hand function: Test
  Coordination: Test and observe
  Involuntary movement: Observe
Sensory integrative functioning
  Sensation: Test and interview
  Visual perception: Test
  Functional visual acuity: Test and observe
Cognitive functioning
  Judgment: Observe
  Safety awareness: Interview and observe
  Motivation: Interview and observe
  Intellectual functions: Observe

Continued.

Sample treatment plan—cont'd

Psychological functioning
Adjustment to disability: Observe
Emotional stability, affect: Observe
Coping skills: Observe
Social functioning
Interpersonal relationships: Observe and interview
Performance skills
Self-care: Observe and interview
Mobility: Test and observe
Home management: Observe and interview
Leisure skills: Observe and interview

EVALUATION SUMMARY

Evaluation of motor function revealed ataxia of the lower extremities with mild spasticity in hip flexor and adductor groups. Gait is unsteady due to ataxia. Upper extremity strength is good (4), and movement is affected by mild tremors especially when patient attempts to perform fine movements. Scores on the Jebsen Test of Hand Coordination were 3 standard deviations below the norm, showing a mild coordination disturbance.[72] Passive range of motion is within normal limits for all upper extremity joint motions. Physical endurance is limited to one half hour of moderate activity (eg, standing, or light bicycling) before the patient experiences fatigue and needs a rest.

Tests of sensation revealed that touch, pain, pressure, and thermal and proprioceptive senses are intact. Stereognosis is intact. Accurate testing of visual perception was not possible because of blurred vision. Functional visual acuity is adequate for moving about in the environment, recognizing faces and large objects, and performing gross motor activities. Reading, identifying paper money, and working with small objects are not possible because of visual limitation.

According to the report of patient and parents, intellectual functioning is the same as before onset of illness. Mr. D is not always aware of potential hazards at home. He gets about by holding onto furniture, walls, and door frames and believes that this is safe. He tends to overestimate his capabilities and resists the use of aids or assistance. He is well motivated for rehabilitation and seems to enjoy getting out and having contact with the staff and other patients.

Mr. D is independent in dressing activities. He has some difficulty raising a full glass to his mouth and managing some types of food from hand to mouth. His responsibilities for meal preparation are minimal. His mother leaves a sandwich for him, and he prepares coffee at lunch time. He has some difficulty managing the kettle from sink to stove to table while maintaining his balance.

He spends his time listening to tapes, attempting to operate the CB radio, and listening to the television. He has difficulty with the CB radio because of poor vision and incoordination for fine tuning it. Because of easy fatigability, he takes two or three naps each day.

ASSETS

Good intelligence
Family support
Good family relationships
Comfortable living situation
Good sensation
Motivation
Good range of motion
Positive affect

PROBLEM LIST

1. Ataxia
2. Tremors
3. Incoordination
4. LE spasticity
5. Low physical endurance and standing tolerance
6. Difficulty with mobility and transfers
7. Poor safety awareness
8. Partial dependence in ADL
9. Not realistic about potential hazards and own abilities
10. Loss of social activities
11. Loss of work role
12. Loss of leisure skills

PROBLEM 5

Low physical endurance
Objective
Physical endurance for moderate activity will be maintained or increased from 30 to 40 minutes.
Method
Stationary bicycle with no resistance for two 10-minute periods followed by 10 minutes of rest during the treatment hour. Patient listens to music on personal radio while cycling. Standing table with back and knee support, for 20 minutes with 10-minute rest. Patient explores CB radio while standing.
Gradation
Maintain same time schedule or increase time spent in activities if endurance allows

Continued.

Sample treatment plan—cont'd

PROBLEMS 1, 6
Ataxia, difficulty with mobility and transfers
Objective
Patient will use a walker safely with minimal to moderate supervision.
Method
Following gait training with walker by a physical therapist, patient does clinic activities using the walker in performance of ADL. This includes using the walker while making coffee and to reach the table, bed, standing table, and stationary bicycle. Cues for safety and correct use of walker are given repeatedly by therapist.

Educate parents about correct use of walker and necessary supervision. Walker is to be taken home for moving about in the house during ADL following a home visit to assess patient's use of the walker there.
Gradation
Decrease verbal cues and supervision as safety awareness and correct procedure increase; introduce a wheelchair for mobility as function declines

PROBLEM 8
Partial dependence in ADL
Objective
Increase safety and independence in lunch preparation and clean-up, and feeding
Method
To prepare lunch, patient uses walker and pushes a utility cart ahead of it to gather premade sandwich, dishes, and silverware and bring them to the table. Soiled dishes and silverware are placed on the utility cart and returned to the sink after he has eaten. Dishes are left for Mrs. D to wash later. Prepare hot water for coffee with electric tea kettle. Kettle should be slid along the counter, to the sink, filled, and plugged in. Patient leans on counter, stabilizes his arm by leaning on elbow and tilts tea kettle on its edge to pour water. Drinking liquid is accomplished by using a broad-based, weighted cup

and a long plastic straw, eliminating the necessity to pick up the cup.

For independent feeding of the evening meal, use a nonskid mat, plate guard, and weighted swivel spoon-fork combination.
Gradation
When function declines, Mrs. D will leave a thermos of coffee to be used with the long straw. If independent feeding becomes more difficult because of increasing upper extremity weakness, a suspension sling or mobile arm support and wrist splint may be tried.

PROBLEM 12
Loss of leisure skills
Objective
Patient will engage in meaningful leisure activity and initiate participation without prodding.
Method
Explore possibility of CB radio use. Teach patient to memorize switch settings and dial positioning, using tactile cues. Explore adaptation of radio receiver with stops or raised dots to indicate dial and switch positions. Use weighted wrist and hand cuff to decrease tremors in hands.

Listen to sporting events on radio and discuss them with other patients and therapist during socialization group.

Organize tape collection by artist or type of music. Tape cases can be color-coded with large stickers in geometric shapes.

Explore possibility of talking book services at local library.
Gradation
Increase passive activities such as listening to music, sports programs, and talking book; decrease use of CB radio to listening only, as tremors and vision problems become worse.

REVIEW QUESTIONS
Multiple Sclerosis (MS)
1. Briefly describe the pathology of MS.
2. List three theories of the possible causes of MS.
3. Which psychological problem is sometimes associated with MS?
4. What is the overall goal of occupational therapy?
5. List the elements of the occupational therapy assessment.
6. Describe appropriate treatment procedures for maintenance or improvement of motor functioning?
7. List the treatment precautions.

Parkinson's disease
8. List and describe the three main clinical features of Parkinson's disease that interfere with function.
9. A depletion of which neurotransmitter in the brain is thought to be responsible for Parkinson's symptoms?
10. Describe "pill-rolling tremor."
11. How does muscle rigidity impede voluntary movement?
12. List five symptoms of autonomic nervous system involvement.
13. How can the occupational therapy evaluation be used to assess

the effects of medical treatment?
14. Describe some methods for improving movement in patients with Parkinson's disease.
15. Is complete independence in ADL possible and realistic? What are the alternatives?
16. What is the role of the occupational therapist when the patient becomes completely dependent?
17. How can the occupational therapist facilitate psychosocial adjustment?
18. List the treatment precautions.

Amyotrophic Lateral Sclerosis (ALS)

19. What is the pathology of ALS?
20. Describe the outstanding clinical manifestations.
21. How are speech and respiration affected in ALS?
22. Define the Neuro Scale.
23. Describe the OT evaluation of a patient with ALS.
24. List six goals of OT for ALS.
25. How is treatment graded for ALS?
26. What are some alternatives for loss of verbal communication?

Alzheimer's disease

27. What is the pathophysiology of Alzheimer's disease?
28. List the clinical features of the disease.
29. What is the characteristic progression?
30. What are the purposes of occupational therapy?
31. Describe what is meant by "environmental modification"?
32. List the elements of the occupational therapy evaluation.
33. What are the goals of occupational therapy?
34. Describe the principles of an activity program for Alzheimer's.
35. Define catastrophic reaction.
36. How can such reactions be managed?

REFERENCES

1. Aaron MM: Alzheimer's disease: care of the patient and her family, The Female Patient, 8(11)36, 1983.
2. Abissi C and Scheinberg L: Multiple sclerosis: diagnosis and treatment, Medical Times 7:109, 1981.
3. Allen I: The pathology of multiple sclerosis—fact, fiction and hypothesis, Neuropathol Appl Neurobiol, 7:169, 1982.
4. Alter M: Migration and risk of multiple sclerosis, Neurology 28:1089, 1978.
5. Alter M, Yamoor M, and Harshe M.: Multiple sclerosis and nutrition. Arch Neurol 31:267, 1974.
6. American Occupational Therapy Association: Occupational therapy services for Alzheimer's disease and related disorders, Am J Occup Ther 40:822, 1986.
7. Beam IM: Helping families survive. Am J Nurs 84:229, 1984.
8. Beisel K: Multiple sclerosis—factors that affect activity performance: a patient survey. Physical Disabilities Special Interest Section Newsletter, 6:1, 1983, Rockville, MD, The American Occupational Therapy Association.
9. Blair J: Who gets sick: thinking and health, Houston, 1987, Peak Press.
10. Blaivas JG: Management of bladder dysfunction in multiple sclerosis, Neurology 30:12, 1980.
11. Blount MN, Bratton C, and Luttrell N: Management of the patient with amyotrophic lateral sclerosis, Nurs Clin North Am 14:157, 1979.
12. Bowen DM: Accelerated aging or selective neuronal loss as an important cause of dementia? Lancet 8106(1):11, 1979.
13. Brammell CA: Assistive devices for patients with neuromuscular diseases: the role of occupational therapy. In Maloney FP, Burks JS, and Ringel SP, editors: Interdisciplinary rehabilitation of multiple sclerosis and neuromuscular diseases, Philadelphia, 1985, JB Lippincott Co.
14. Charles R, Truesdell ML and Wood EL: Alzheimer's disease: pathology, progression and nursing process. Gerontol Nurs 8:69, 1982.
15. Clark M: Should medicine use the unborn? Newsweek 110:63, 1987.
16. Cole M and Ross RJ: Plaque of multiple sclerosis seen in computerized transaxial tomography, Neurology 27:360, 1977.
17. Cybyk ME: Alzheimer's disease, Nurs Times 76:280, 1980.
18. Davis JC: Team management of Parkinson's disease. Am J Occup Ther 32(10):300, 1977.
19. Davis CM: The role of the physical and occupational therapist in caring for the victim of Alzheimer's disease. In Taira ED, editor: Therapeutic interventions for the person with dementia, Phys Occup Ther Geriatr 4:3, 15, 1986.
20. Dorey MM: Alzheimer's disease the "new" old approach, Phys Ther Forum 4:32, 1985.
21. Duvoisin RC: Parkinson's Disease, A guide for patient and family, ed. 2, New York, 1984, Raven Press.
22. Ekberg PS: Neurologist's perceptions of and referrals to occupational therapy for persons with multiple sclerosis. Unpublished thesis, Department of Occupational Therapy, San José State University, December 1985.
23. Fischman HR: Multiple sclerosis: a new perspective on epidemiologic patterns, Neurology (NY) 32:864, 1982.
24. Frankel D: Multiple sclerosis. In Umphred DA, editor: Neurological rehabilitation, St Louis, 1985, The CV Mosby Co.
25. Gauthier L, Dalziel S, and Gauthier S: The benefits of group occupational therapy for patients with Parkinson's disease, Am J Occup Ther 41:360, 1987.
26. Gersten JA: Rehabilitation for degenerative diseases of the central nervous system. In Kottke FJ, Stillwell GK, and Lehmann JF, editors: Krusen's handbook of physical medicine and rehabilitation, Philadelphia, 1982, WB Saunders Co.
27. Gilman S: The diagnosis of multiple sclerosis, JAMA 246(10): 1122, 1981.
28. Gilroy I and Meyer JS: Medical neurology, ed 3, New York, 1979, Macmillan Publishing Co, Inc.
29. Glickstein JK: Therapeutic interventions in Alzheimer's disease, Rockville, MD, 1988, Aspen Publishers, Inc.
30. Gresh C: Parkinson's disease, Nursing 10(1):26, 1980.
31. Hall N and Goldstein: Thinking well: chemical links between emotions and health, The Sciences 26:34, 1986.
32. Hammer S: The mind as healer, Science Digest 24:44, 1984.
33. Harris R: Genetics of Alzheimer's disease, Brit Med J 284:1065, 1982.
34. Hopkins H: ALS: "Lou Gehrig's disease" still needs a cure, FDA

Consumer 17(12):23, 1984.

35. Hudson AJ: Amyotrophic lateral sclerosis and its association with dementia, parkinsonism and other neurological disorders: a review, Brain 194:36, 1981.

36. Jackson-Klykken O: Brain function, aging and dementia. In Umphred, DA, editor: Neurological rehabilitation, St Louis, 1985, The CV Mosby Co.

37. Janiszewski DW, Carosico JT, and Wisham LH: Amyotrophic lateral sclerosis: a comprehensive rehabilitation approach, Arch Phys Med Rehabil 64:304, 1983.

38. Johnson CR: Case report—aquatic therapy for an ALS patient, Am J Occup Ther 42:115, 1988.

39. Josephs PJ: Brain transplants, Neurology 32(10)1205, 1982.

40. Katzman R: Banbury report 15: biological aspects of Alzheimer's disease, New York, 1983, Cold Spring Harbor Laboratory, Inc.

41. Kent S: What causes Alzheimer's? Geriatrics 38:33, 1983.

42. Kraft G: Diseases of the motor unit. In Rosse C and Clawson DK: The musculoskeletal system in health and disease, New York, 1980, Harper & Row.

43. Kurland LT: The frequency and geographic distribution of multiple sclerosis as indicated by mortality statistics and morbidity surveys in the US and Canada, Am J Hygiene 55:457, 1952.

44. Leibowitz U, Kahana E, and Altes M: Changing frequency of multiple sclerosis in Israel, Arch Neurol 29:197, 1973.

45. Lenox AC: When motor nerves die, Am J Nurs 4:540, 1983.

46. Lisak RP: Multiple sclerosis: evidence for immunopathogenesis, Neurology 30(2):99, 1980.

47. Mallison MB: Alzheimer's disease: theories and therapies. Am J Nurs 84:223, 1984.

48. Marttila RJ and Rinne UK: Epidemiology of Parkinson's disease: an overview, J Neurotrans 51(1):135, 1981.

49. Matthews WB, Acheson ED, Batchelor JR, and Weller RO: McAlpine's multiple sclerosis, New York, 1985, Churchill Livingstone.

50. Mayeax R, Stern Y, Rosen J, and Lenenthal J: Depression, intellectual impairment and Parkinson's disease, Neurology 31(5):645, 1981.

51. Melnick MA: Basal ganglia disorders: metabolic, hereditary, and genetic disorders in adults. In Umphred DA: Neurological rehabilitation, St Louis, 1985, The CV Mosby Co.

52. Merz B: Adrenal-to-brain transplants improve prognosis for Parkinson's disease, JAMA 257:2691, 1987.

53. Moore RY: Parkinson's disease—a new treatment? N Engl J Med 316(2):872, 1987.

54. Mulder DW: Clinical limits of amyotrophic lateral sclerosis, Adv Neurol 36:151, 1982.

55. Mulder DW: Treatment of anterior horn cell disease, Modern Treatment 3:243, 1966.

56. O'Sullivan SB, Cullen KE, and Schmitz TJ: Physical rehabilitation: evaluation and treatment procedures, Philadelphia, 1981, FA Davis Co.

57. Patzold V and Pocklington PR: Course of multiple sclerosis, Acta Neurol Scand 65(4):248, 1982.

58. Penel C: Alzheimer's disease, Nursing Times 71(3):667, 1975.

59. Rabinowitz E: Day care and Alzheimer's disease: a weekend program in New York City. In Taira ED, editor: Therapeutic interventions for the person with dementia, Phys Occup Ther Geriatr 4(3)95, 1986.

60. Rudolph M: Alzheimer center replaces depression with dignity for clients and their families, OT Week 2(23):16, 1988.

61. Siegel B: Love, medicine and miracles, New York, 1986, Harper & Row.

62. Spencer EA: Functional restoration—specific diagnosis. In Hopkins HL and Smith HD: Willard and Spackman's occupational therapy, ed 7, Philadelphia, 1988, JB Lippincott Co.

63. Sulkova R, Haltia M, Paetau A, Wistrom J, and Palo J: Clinical and neuropathological features in Alzheimer's disease, Acta Neurol Scand(suppl 90)65:294, 1982.

64. Svien HJ and Cody DT: Treatment of spasmatic torticollis by suppression of labyrinthine activity: report of a case, Mayo Clin Proc 44:825, 1969.

65. Takai V: ADL and adaptive equipment for the ALS patient. Physical Disabilities Special Interest Section Newsletter, 6:2, 1983, Rockville, MD American Occupational Therapy Association.

66. Tourtenotte WW: Therapeutics of multiple sclerosis, South Deerfield, Mass, 1981, Channing L Bete Co, Inc.

67. Turner A, editor: The practice of occupational therapy, ed 2, New York, 1987, Churchill Livingstone.

68. Wallis C: Therapy by transplant, Scientific American 256(2):29, 1987.

69. Weeks C: Multiple sclerosis: the malignant uncertainty, Am J Nurs 80(2):298, 1980.

70. Weiner M: Update on antiparkinsonism agents, Geriatrics 37:81, 1982.

71. Wikstrom N, Paetau A, Palo J, Sulkava R, and Haltia M: Classic amyotrophic lateral sclerosis with dementia, Arch Neurol 39:681, 1982.

72. Wolf B: Occupational therapy for patients with multiple sclerosis. In Malony FP, Burks JS, and Ringel SP: Interdisciplinary rehabilitation of multiple sclerosis and neuromuscular disorders, Philadelphia, 1985, JB Lippincott Co.

73. Wurtman RJ: Alzheimer's disease, Scientific American 252(11)62, 1985.

74. Yahr JO: Early recognition of Parkinson's disease, Hosp Pract 16(7):65, 1981.

75. Zawodniak J: Recommended exercises and ambulation aids for people with ALS, Physical Disabilities Special Interest Section Newsletter, 6:2, 1983, American Occupational Therapy Association.

76. Zgola JM: Doing things, Baltimore, 1987, The Johns Hopkins University Press.

Index

Page numbers in *italics* indicate illustrations and boxed material.
Page numbers followed by *t* indicate tables.

Synesthesia, 304
Synkinesis
  homolateral limb, 337
  imitation, 337
Synovial membrane, proliferation of, in wrist in rheumatoid
      arthritis, 464
Synovitis
  elbow, in rheumatoid arthritis, 464-465
  shoulder, in rheumatoid arthritis, 465
  wrist, 463-464
Systole of cardiac cycle, 509-510

T

Tactile perception
  disorders of, from cerebral vascular accident, 606
  test for, 187-189
Tactile stimulation for head injured patient, 636
Tactile system in motor learning, 366
Tapping in proprioceptive facilitation, 321
Taste, mechanisms of, 303-304
Taste reflexes, 304
Taste sensation, test for, 186
Team management in dysphagia treatment, 162
Temperature
  and pain, proprioception compared to, 283*t*
  in sensorimotor techniques, interoceptors and, 292
Tendinitis in acute hand injury, 497
Tendinous pressure as inhibition technique, 325
Tendon(s)
  action of, position of hand and, 407
  injuries of, in acute hand injury, 489-492
  transfers of, in acute hand injury, 489
Tensor fascia latae, manual muscle testing of, 120-121,
      123
Teres major
  functional muscle testing of, 127, 128
  manual muscle testing for, 102, *103*, 104
Teres minor
  functional muscle testing of, 128
  manual muscle testing of, 103-104
Terminal devices (TDs) of UE prosthesis, 422-423
  checkout of, 426-428
Thalamus, 287
Theraband in acute hand injury, 499
Therapeutic activity(ies), 210-228
  after cerebral vascular accident, 614
  for perceptual skills, 222-223
Therapeutic exercise
  active stretch in, 216
  classification of, 213-215
  coordination, 216-218
  isometric, 216
  muscle contraction used in, types of, 212-213
  prerequisites for use of, 212
  principles of, 211-212
  purposes of, 212
  requirements for, 217
  stretching or forced, 215
Therapeutic touch, 306, 330

Therapeutic vibration in proprioceptive facilitation, 320-
      321
Thermal sensation, test for, 183-184
Thermoplastic, cutting hand splint out of, 412, *413*, 415-
      416
Thinking, abstract
  disorders of, from cerebral vascular accident, 608
  impaired, in head injury, 629
Thoracic spine, range of motion of
  average normal, 65*t*
  measurements for, 68, *69-70*
Thumb
  adduction of, 118, *119*, 128
  deformity of, in rheumatoid arthritis, 463
  interphalangeal extension of, 115-116, 128
  interphalangeal flexion of, 116-117, 128
  metacarpophalangeal extension of, 114-115, 128
  metacarpophalangeal flexion of, 116, 128
  movement of, in hemiplegic, evaluation of, 342
  opposition of, 118-120, 128
  palmar abduction of, 117, 128
  radial abduction of, 117-118
  range of motion of
    average normal, 65*t*
    measurements for, 80, *81-83*
Tibialis anterior
  functional muscle testing of, 129
  manual muscle testing of, 125-126
Tibialis posterior
  functional muscle testing of, 129
  manual muscle testing of, 126
Tic douloureux, 568-569
Tinel's sign, 570
  in acute hand injury evaluation, 480
Tolerance, therapeutic activities for, grading and adaptation
      of, 222
Tone
  muscle; *see* Muscle tone
  postural, in neurodevelopmental treatment of adult
      hemiplegia, 352
Tongue, movement of, in oral evaluation of dysphagia, 153-
      154
Tonic labyrinthine reflex (TLR), evaluation of, 142
Tonic neck reflex(es)
  asymmetrical, evaluation of, 141-142
  effects of sensory stimulation and, 312-313
  symmetrical, evaluation of, 142
Tonic reflexes, 301
Total active motion (TAM) in acute hand injury evaluation,
      492
Total hip replacement, 556
Total passive motion (TPM) in acute hand injury evaluation,
      492
Touch
  light, test for, 181, 183
  light moving, in cutaneous faiclitation, 316
  therapeutic, 306, 330
  types of, 328
Touch communication, 306